**ELSEVIER**

# evolve

*To access your Student Resources, visit:*

## http://evolve.elsevier.com/Potter/basic/

Evolve® Student Resources for *Potter, Perry: Basic Nursing,* 6th Edition offers the following features:

## Student Resources

- **NCLEX® Review**
  includes questions and answers to help prepare for the NCLEX examination.

- **Audio Glossary**
  provides definitions of key terms.

- **English/Spanish Audio Glossary**
  provides audio pronunciations of important nursing terms as well as their definitions in both English and Spanish.

- **Video Clips**
  demonstrate important steps in various nursing skills throughout the textbook.

- **WebLinks**
  are an exciting resource that lets you link to hundreds of websites carefully chosen to supplement the content of the textbook.

- **Content Updates**
  include the latest content updates from the authors of the textbook to keep you current with recent developments in this area of study.

# Get more out of your textbook with these **innovative resources!**

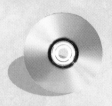

### Companion CD
**FREE** *inside this textbook!*

The interactive **Companion CD** offers you instant access to practical resources including video clips, a searchable audio glossary, a Spanish/English audio glossary, *Butterfield's Fluids & Electrolytes Tutorial*, and NCLEX® examination-style review questions.

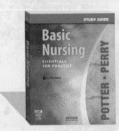

### Study Guide
*Patricia Castaldi, RN, BSN, MSN; Patricia A. Potter, RN, MSN, PhD, CMAC, FAAN; and Anne Griffin Perry, RN, MSN, EdD, FAAN*

Corresponding chapter-by-chapter to the text, this **Study Guide** helps you master the content presented in this textbook. It includes case studies, chapter reviews with assorted matching, short answer, multiple-choice, and true/false questions, study group discussion questions, a study chart, and performance checklists for each skill and procedural guideline in the text.

May 2006 • Approx. 400 pp. • ISBN: 0-323-04121-3 • ISBN-13: 978-0-323-04121-8

*Sold separately.*

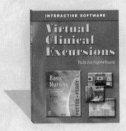

### Virtual Clinical Excursions 3.0 for *Basic Nursing: Essentials for Practice, 6th Edition*
*Patricia A. Potter, RN, MSN, PhD, CMAC, FAAN; and Jay Tashiro, PhD, RN*

This interactive workbook and CD-ROM package complements the textbook and guides you through a multi-floor virtual hospital for a true-to-life, hands-on clinical learning experience. You can assess and analyze information, diagnose, set priorities, and implement and evaluate care. NCLEX® examination-style review questions provide immediate testing of clinical knowledge.

June 2006 • Approx. 168 pp. • ISBN: 0-323-04616-9 • ISBN-13: 978-0-323-04616-9

*Sold separately.*

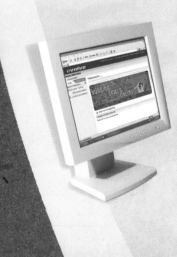

### Nursing Skills Online for *Basic Nursing: Essentials for Practice, 6th Edition*
*Patricia A. Potter, RN, MSN, PhD, CMAC, FAAN; and Anne Griffin Perry, RN, MSN, EdD, FAAN*

This one-of-a-kind interactive learning tool offers 17 distinct media-rich modules that correspond to the textbook and cover key nursing skills. Each user-friendly module challenges you with a series of realistic, case-based lessons that consist of objectives, a content overview, reading assignments, numerous interactive exercises, and a post-test. It's a great way to review and evaluate your competency before performing skills in the clinical setting.

May 2006 • ISBN: 0-323-04242-2 • ISBN-13: 978-0-323-04242-0

*Sold separately.*

**MOSBY**
**ELSEVIER**

# Basic Nursing

## ESSENTIALS FOR PRACTICE

**Patricia A. Potter PhD, RN, CMAC, FAAN**
Siteman Cancer Center Research Scientist
Barnes-Jewish Hospital
St. Louis, Missouri

**Anne Griffin Perry, EdD, RN, FAAN**
Professor and Chair
Department of Primary Care and Health Systems Nursing
Southern Illinois University
Edwardsville, Illinois

## **6**TH EDITION

With *over 700* illustrations

## MOSBY
ELSEVIER

11830 Westline Industrial Drive
St. Louis, Missouri 63146

*Basic Nursing: Essentials for Practice*

ISBN-13: 978-0-323-03937-6
ISBN-10: 0-323-03937-5

---

**Notice**

Knowledge and best practice in this field are constantly changing. As new research and experience broaden our knowledge, changes in practice, treatment and drug therapy may become necessary or appropriate. Readers are advised to check the most current information provided (i) on procedures featured or (ii) by the manufacturer of each product to be administered, to verify the recommended dose or formula, the method and duration of administration, and contraindications. It is the responsibility of the practitioner, relying on experience and knowledge of the patient, to make diagnoses, to determine dosages and the best treatment for each individual patient, and to take all appropriate safety precautions. To the fullest extent of the law, neither the Publisher nor the Authors assume any liability for any injury and/or damage to persons or property arising out or related to any use of the material contained in this book.

---

Previous editions copyrighted 1987, 1991, 1995, 1999, 2003

NCLEX®, NCLEX-RN®, and NCLEX-PN® are registered trademarks of the National Council of State Boards of Nursing, Inc.

ISBN-13: 978-0-323-03937-6
ISBN-10: 0-323-03937-5

*Executive Editor:* Susan Epstein
*Senior Developmental Editor:* Robyn L. Brinks
*Publishing Services Manager:* John Rogers
*Senior Project Manager:* Beth Hayes
*Design Direction:* Andrea Lutes
*Text Designer:* Kathi Gosche

Printed in Canada

Last digit is the print number:  9  8  7  6  5  4  3  2

# Section Editors

**Amy Hall, RN, BSN, MS, PhD**
Associate Professor
Saint Francis Medical Center College of Nursing
Peoria, Illinois

**Patricia A. Stockert, RN, BSN, MS, PhD**
Professor, Associate Dean BSN Program
Saint Francis Medical Center College of Nursing
Peoria, Illinois

# Contributors

**Jeanette Spain Adams, RN, PhD, CRNI, APRN**
Faculty
University of Miami School of Nursing and Health Sciences
Coral Gables, Florida

**Marjorie Baier, PhD, RN**
Associate Professor
Southern Illinois University–Edwardsville
Edwardsville, Illinois

**Sylvia Baird, RN, BSN, MM**
Manager Patient Safety
Spectrum Health
Grand Rapids, Michigan

**Julia Balzer Riley, RN, MN, AHN-C, CET**
Adjunct Faculty
University of Tampa
Tampa, Florida
President, Constant Source Seminars
Ellenton, Florida

**Janice Colwell, RN, MS, CWOCN**
Clinical Nurse Specialist
University of Chicago Hospital
Chicago, Illinois

**Kelly Jo Cone, RN, BSN, MS, PhD**
Associate Professor
Graduate Program
Saint Francis Medical Center College of Nursing
Peoria, Illinois

**Eileen Constantinou, MSN, RN**
Consultant
Barnes-Jewish Hospital
St. Louis, Missouri

**Roslyn Corcoran, RN, BSN**
Registered Nurse
Barnes-Jewish Hospital
St. Louis, Missouri

**Christine Durbin, RN, MSN, JD**
Faculty
School of Nursing
Southern Illinois University–Edwardsville
Edwardsville, Illinois

**Margaret Ecker, RN, BA, MS, PNP**
Director of Education
Saint John's Health Center
Santa Monica, California

**Sharon J. Edwards, RN, BSN, MSN, PhD**
Assistant Professor
University of South Florida
Tampa, Florida

**Susan Fetzer, BA, BSN, MSN, MBA, PhD**
Associate Professor
University of New Hampshire
Durham, New Hampshire

**Victoria N. Folse, PhD, APRN, BC, LCPC**
Assistant Professor
School of Nursing
Illinois Wesleyan University
Bloomington, Illinois

**Leah Frederick, MS, RN, CIC**
Consultant
Infection Control Consultants
Scottsdale, Arizona

**Amy Hall, RN, BSN, MS, PhD**
Associate Professor
Saint Francis Medical Center College of Nursing
Peoria, Illinois

**Maureen Huhmann, MS, RD**
Clinical Nutrition Instructor
University of Medicine and Dentistry of New Jersey
Newark, New Jersey

**Judith Ann Kilpatrick, RN, MSN, DNSc**
Assistant Professor
Widener University
Chester, Pennsylvania

**Kristine L'Ecuyer, RN, MSN, CCNS**
Assistant Professor
Saint Louis University
St. Louis, Missouri

**Elaine Neel, BSN, MSN**
Nursing Instructor
School of Nursing
Graham Hospital
Canton, Illinois

**Dula F. Pacquiao, EdD, RN, CTN**
Professor and Director
Transcultural Nursing Institute and MSN Program
Kean University
Union, New Jersey

**Nancy Panthofer, RN, BSN, MSN**
Lecturer
Kent State University
Kent, Ohio

**Patricia A. Stockert, RN, BSN, MS, PhD**
Professor/Associate Dean BSN Program
Saint Francis Medical Center College of Nursing
Peoria, Illinois

**Riva Touger-Decker, PhD, RD, FADA**
Associate Professor and Program Director
Graduate Programs in Clinical Nutrition
Dept of Primary Care, SHRP
Division of Nutrition, Department of Diagnostic Sciences
New Jersey Dental School
Newark, New Jersey

**Pamela Becker Weilitz, RN, MSN(r), BC, ANP, M-SCNS**
Private Practice
Adult Nurse Practitioner
St. Louis, Missouri

**Joan Domigan Wentz, MSN, RN**
Assistant Professor
Barnes-Jewish College
St. Louis, Missouri

**Rita Wunderlich, MSN(r), PhD, RN**
Assistant Professor
Saint Louis University
St. Louis, Missouri

**Barbara Yoost, RN, BSN, MSN, CNS**
Lecturer, Fundamentals Course Coordinator
Kent State University College of Nursing
Kent, Ohio

# Reviewers

**Marianne Adam, MSN, RN, CRNP**
Assistant Professor
Moravian College
Bethlehem, Pennsylvania

**Pamela Adamshick, MSN, APRN, BC**
Assistant Professor of Nursing
St. Luke's School of Nursing at Moravian College
Bethlehem, Pennsylvania

**Kate Allen, RN, BSc, MSc, PGCE**
Lecturer in Critical Care
University of East Anglia
Norwich, England

**Doris Bartlett, BSN, MS**
Adjunct Faculty
Bethel College
Mishawaka, Indiana

**Julie Baylor, PhD, RN**
Assistant Professor
Bradley University
Peoria, Illinois

**Anna Brock, BSN, MSN, PhD**
Professor
University of Southern Mississippi
School of Nursing
Hattiesburg, Mississippi

**Vickie Carrington, BSN, MSN**
Clinical Instructor
Southern State Community College
Hillsboro, Ohio

**Elizabeth Weaver Casazza, AS, BS, MS, CAS**
Nursing Instructor
Crouse Hospital School of Nursing
Syracuse, New York

**Brigitte Casteel, RN, BSN**
Associate Professor
Program Director
Mountain Empire Community College
Big Stone Gap, Virginia

**Barbara Daniel, BSN, MED, MS, CRNP**
Professor of Nursing
Cecil Community College
North East, Maryland

**Mary Ann Deb, MSN, MBA**
Professor of Nursing
Trocaire College
Buffalo, New York

**Debra DeMaria, RN MSN, APN-C**
Assistant Clinical Professor
College of Nursing and Health Professions
Drexel University
Philadelphia, Pennsylvania

**Catherine Eddy, MSN, RN**
Assistant Professor
University of South Dakota
Rapid City, South Dakota

**Barbara Elkins, MS, RN, APRN**
Instructor
State University of New York–Ulster
Stone Ridge, New York

**Susan Erue, RN, BSN, MS, PhD**
Professor
Department of Health and Natural Sciences
Iowa Wesleyan College
Mt. Pleasant, Iowa

**Susan Fairchild-Charalambous, EdD, MSN-Ed, APRN, CNOR, CS**
Professor
Lester L. Cox College of Nursing and Health Sciences
Springfield, Missouri

**Marianne Fasano, RN, BSN, MEd, MSN, CRNI, CWOCN, PCCN**
Assistant Director of Nursing
Pasco Hernando Community College
New Port Richey, Florida

**Mary B. Gallagher, RN, MSN, CCRN**
Critical Care/Trauma Clinical Educator
Abington Memorial Hospital
Abington, Pennsylvania

**Cathy Garcia, BSN, RN, BC, CAN, BC**
Director of Neuroscience and Orthopedic Services
East Texas Medical Center–Tyler
Tyler, Texas

**Shirley Lyon Garcia, RN, BSN**
Nursing Program Director
McDowell Technical Community College
Marion, North Carolina

**Marcia Gardner, MA, RN, CPN, CPNP**
Assistant Professor
Drexel University College of Nursing and Health Professions
Philadelphia, Pennsylvania

**Yvette Glenn, MSN, FNP, CWS, APRN, BC**
Wound Care Specialist
VA Illiana Medical Center
Danville, Illinois

**Carol Greenway, MA, BSc**
Senior Lecturer
School of Nursing and Midwifery
De Montfort University
Leicester, United Kingdom

**Stephanie Greer, RN, MSN**
ADN Instructor
Southwest Mississippi Community College
Summit, Mississippi

**Suzy Harrington, RN, MS, CHES**
Director of Education
Central Colorado Area Health Education Center
Denver, Colorado

**Adrienne Hentemann, BSN, MS**
Administrative Associate
Spectrum Health
Grand Rapids, Michigan

**Monica M. Hentemann, RN, BSN**
Registered Nurse
Spectrum Health Downtown
Grand Rapids, Michigan

**Dorothy Herron, PhD, RN, APRN**
Assistant Professor
University of Maryland School of Nursing
Baltimore, Maryland

**Crystal Higgins, MSN, BSN, RN**
Program Chair, Practical Nursing
Southeast Community College
Beatrice, Nebraska

**Linda Kerby, BSN, MA, BA, RNC**
Educational Consultant
Mastery Educational Consultants
Leawood, Kansas

**Priscilla Killian, RN, MSN, APNP**
Assistant Professor
Drexel University College of Nursing and Health Professions
Philadelphia, Pennsylvania

**Joyce Kunzelman, BScN, GNC(C), RN**
Clinical Nurse Educator
Interior Health Authority
Vernon, British Columbia, Canada

**Ronnette Langhorne, RN, MS**
Instructor
Norfolk State University
Norfolk, Virginia

**Virginia Lester, BSN, MSN, CNS**
Assistant Professor
Angelo State University
San Angelo, Texas

**Rosemary Macy, RN, PhDc**
Associate Professor
Boise State University
Boise, Idaho

**Rosanna L. Marker-Faour, MSN, BSN, CSN**
Adjunct Faculty
Duquesne University
Pittsburgh, Pennsylvania

**Barbara Maxwell, RN, BSN, MS, MSN, CNS**
Associate Professor of Nursing
State University of New York–Ulster
Stone Ridge, New York

**Lesia D. McBride, BSN, RN**
Clinical Research Coordinator and Clinical Educator
Community Hospital–Anderson
Anderson, Indiana

**Nancy McCartney, AS, RN**
Registered Nurse
Hillsboro, Oregon

**Teri Murray, BSN, Med, MSN, PhD**
Clinical Professor and Director
Undergraduate Nursing Program
University of Missouri
St. Louis, Missouri

**Kristen Newman, BSN, RN**
Director of Recruitment and Retention
Southern Maryland Hospital Center
Clinton, Maryland

**Sue Owensby, RN, PhD**
Professor of Nursing
University of North Carolina Wilmington
Wilmington, North Carolina

**Lynn Painter, DNSc, RN**
Assistant Professor
Bloomsburg University
Bloomsburg, Pennsylvania

**Elaine Princevalli, RN, BSN, MS**
Instructor
Eli Whitney Practical Nurse Education Program
State of Connecticut Department of Education
Hamden, Connecticut

**Beth Hogan Quigley, RN, MSN, CRNP**
Associate Course Director
University of Pennsylvania School of Nursing
Philadelphia, Pennsylvania

**Anita K. Reed, MSN, RN**
Clinical Instructor
St. Elizabeth School of Nursing
Lafayette, Indiana

**Mary Tedesco-Schneck, MSN, CPNP**
Assistant Professor
Husson College
Bangor, Maine

**Ruth Novitt-Schumacher, BSN, MSN**
Instructor
University of Illinois–Chicago
Chicago, Illinois

**Scott Thigpen, RN, MSN, CCRN, CEN**
Assistant Professor of Nursing
South Georgia College
Douglas, Georgia

**Susan Scholtz, BSN, MN, DNSc**
Associate Professor of Nursing
St. Luke's School of Nursing at Moravian College
Bethlehem, Pennsylvania

**Michelle Schutt, MSN, RN**
Instructor
Auburn University Montgomery
Montgomery, Alabama

**Tamara Shields, RN, MSN, CFNP**
Instructor of Nursing
St. Elizabeth School of Nursing
Lafayette, Indiana

**Patti Simmons, RN, MN, CHPN**
Assistant Professor of Nursing
North Georgia College and State University
Dahlonega, Georgia

**Mimi Snyder, RN, MSN, FNP**
Assistant Professor of Nursing
St. Joseph College
West Hartford, Connecticut

**Donna B. Titus, RN, MSN**
Clinical Instructor
Valdosta State University
Valdosta, Georgia

**Mary Grace Umlauf, RN, PhD, NP-C, APRN, BC, FAAN**
Professor, Graduate Program
University of Alabama School of Nursing
Birmingham, Alabama

**Kathleen Upham, BSN, MSN, ONC**
Associate Professor
Coastal Georgia Community College
Brunswick, Georgia

**Anne Vaughan, MSN, RN**
Clinical Instructor
Bellarmine University
Louisville, Kentucky

**Shellye Vardaman, BSN, MSN**
Instructor and Laboratory Coordinator
Troy University
Troy, Alabama

**Roberta Waite, RN, MSN, EdD**
Assistant Professor
Drexel University
Philadelphia, Pennsylvania

**Diane Welch, RN, BSN, MS**
Associate Professor of Nursing
Linfield Good Samaritan School of Nursing
Portland, Oregon

**Katherine West, BSN, MS, Ed, CIC**
Infection Control Consultant
Infection Control/Emerging Concepts Inc.
Manassas, Virginia

**Margaret Wilson, RN, MSN, EdD**
Professor of Nursing
Cypress College
Cypress, California

**Gail L. Withers, RN, MSN, ARNP-CNS**
Dean of Nursing and Allied Health
Pratt Community College
Pratt, Kansas

**Janice Womack, AS, RN**
Nurse Executive Associate
Northwest Georgia Regional Hospital
Rome, Georgia

# Contributors to Previous Editions

**Elizabeth A. Ayello, RN, BSN, MS, PhD, CS, CETN**
Clinical Assistant Professor of Nursing
New York University School of Education, Nursing
Clinical Associate, Enterostomal Therapy Service
New York University Medical Center
New York, New York

**Judith C. Brostron, RN, BA, JD, LLM**
Attorney
Lashly & Baer, P.C.
St. Louis, Missouri

**Peggy Breckenridge, MSN, FNP**
Associate Professor of Nursing
College of Health Sciences
Roanoke, Virginia

**Victoria M. Brown, RN, BSN, MSN, PhD, HNC**
Professor of Nursing
Georgia College and State University
Milledgeville, Georgia

**Gale Carli, MSN, MSHed, BSN, RN**
Assistant Professor
Ohlone College
Fremont, California

**Rick Daniels, RN, BSN, MSN, PhD**
Professor of Nursing
Oregon Health Sciences University at Southern Oregon University
Ashland, Oregon

**Carolyn Ruppel D'Avis, RN, BSN, MSN**
Director, Baccalaureate Program, Adjunct Assistant Professor
The Catholic University of America, School of Nursing
Washington, DC

**Martha Keene Elkin, RN, MSN, IBCLC**
Lactation Counselor
Stephens Memorial Hospital
Norway, Maine

**Linda Fasciani, RN, BSN, MSN**
Assistant Professor of Nursing
County College of Morris
Randolph, New Jersey

**Cynthia S. Goodwin, RN, BSN, MSN**
Instructor, School of Nursing at Health Professions
University of Southern Indiana
Evansville, Indiana

**Lois C. Hamel, BS, MS**
Assistant Professor of Nursing
Westbrook College
University of New England
Portland, Maine

**Carl A. Kirton, RN-C, BSN, MA, ACRN, ANP**
Clinical Assistant Professor, Adult Nurse Practitioner
New York University
New York, New York

**Ruth Ludwick, RN, BSN, MSN, PhD, RN-C**
Associate Professor
Kent State University School of Nursing
Kent, Ohio

**Mary Kay Knight Macheca, RN, BSN, MSN(R), CS, CDE**
Certified Adult Nurse Practitioner
The Health Care Group of St. Louis/Unity Medical Group
St. Louis, Missouri

**Rita G. Mertig, RNC, MS, CNS**
Professor of Nursing
John Tyler Community College
Chester, Virginia

**Mary Dee Miller, RN, BSN, MS, CIC**
Regional Director, Epidemiology Services
Mercy Regional Health System
Cincinnati, Ohio

**Geralyn A. Ochs, RN, AND, BSN, MSN**
Assistant Professor of Nursing
Saint Louis University School of Nursing
St. Louis, Missouri

**Marsha Evans Orr, RN, MS, CS, CNSN**
Zone Clinical Manager
Apria Healthcare
Phoenix, Arizona

**Janice J. Rumfelt, BSN, MSN, EdD, RNC**
Assistant Professor of Nursing
Southern Illinois University–Edwardsville
Edwardsville, Illinois

**Sharon Souter, RN, BSN, MSN**
Nursing Program Director
New Mexico State University–Carlsbad
Carlsbad, New Mexico

**Elizabeth Speakman, RN, EdD**
Associate Professor of Nursing
Community College of Philadelphia
Philadelphia, Pennsylvania

**Rachel E. Spector, BS, MS, PhD, CTN, FAAN**
Associate Professor
Boston College School of Nursing
Chestnut Hill, Massachusetts

**Susan Speraw, RN, PHD, CNP**
Associate Professor of Pediatrics
University of Tennessee College of Medicine–Chattanooga Unit
Chattanooga, Tennessee

*To the professional nursing staff of Barnes-Jewish Hospital. They inspire me and challenge me to search for ways to improve the lives of our patients.*

**Patricia A. Potter**


*To the nursing faculty at Southern Illinois University, Edwardsville, and Saint Louis University. Your commitment to nursing and nursing education inspire us all to be the guardians of the discipline.*

*To my grandaughter, Cora Elizabeth Bryan, March 1, 2006.*

**Anne Griffin Perry**

# Student Preface

*Basic Nursing* was developed to provide you with all of the fundamental nursing concepts and skills in a visually appealing, easy-to-use format. We know how busy you are and how precious your time is. As you begin your nursing education, it is very important that you have a resource that includes all the information you need to prepare for lectures, classroom activities, clinical rotations, and exams—and nothing more. We've designed this text to meet all of those needs. This book has been designed to help you succeed in this course and prepare you for more advanced study. In addition to the readable writing style and abundance of full-color photographs and drawings, we've incorporated numerous features to help you study and learn. We've made it easy for you to pull out important content. **Check out the following special learning aids:**

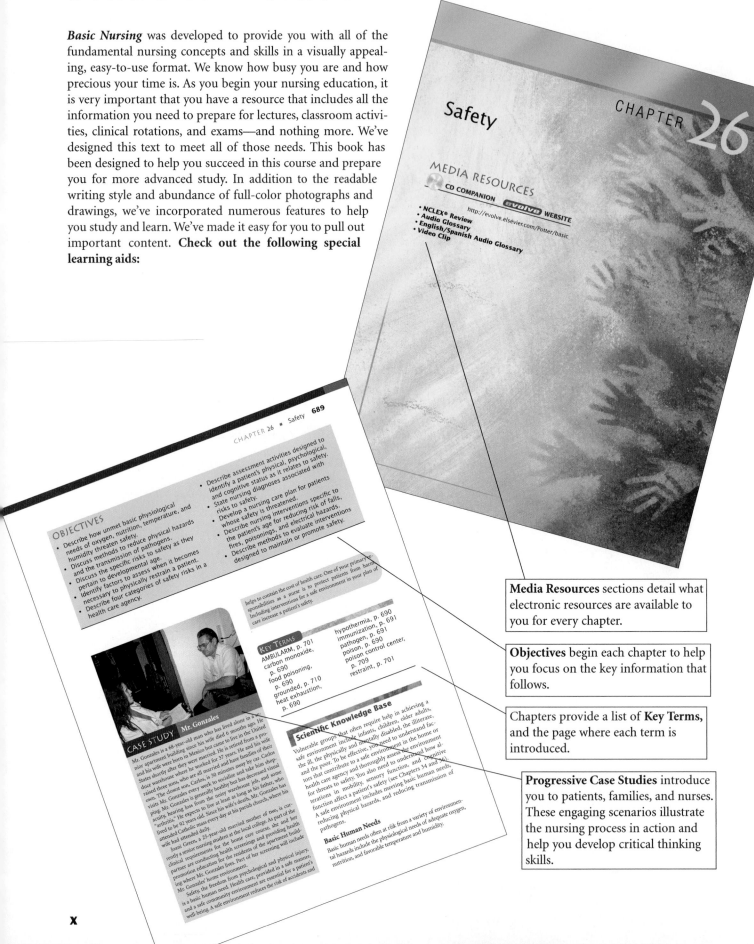

Safety
CHAPTER 26

MEDIA RESOURCES
CD COMPANION    evolve WEBSITE
http://evolve.elsevier.com/Potter/basic
• NCLEX® Review
• Audio Glossary
• English/Spanish Audio Glossary
• Video Clip

CHAPTER 26 ■ Safety **689**

## OBJECTIVES
- Describe how unmet basic physiological needs of oxygen, nutrition, temperature, and humidity threaten safety.
- Discuss methods to reduce physical hazards and the transmission of pathogens.
- Discuss the specific risks to safety as they pertain to developmental age.
- Identify factors to physically restrain a patient.
- Describe four categories of safety risks in a health care agency.
- Describe assessment activities designed to identify a patient's physical, psychological, and cognitive status as it relates to safety.
- State nursing diagnoses associated with risks to safety.
- Develop a nursing care plan for patients whose safety is threatened.
- Describe nursing interventions specific to the patient's age for reducing risk of falls, fires, poisonings, and electrical hazards.
- Describe methods to evaluate interventions designed to maintain or promote safety.

helps to contain the cost of health care. One of your primary responsibilities as a nurse is to protect patients from harm. Including interventions for a safe environment in your plan of care increase a patient's safety.

KEY TERMS
AMBULARM, p. 701
carbon monoxide, p. 690
food poisoning, p. 690
grounded, p. 710
heat exhaustion, p. 690
hypothermia, p. 690
immunization, p. 691
pathogen, p. 690
poison, p. 690
poison control center, p. 709
restraint, p. 701

CASE STUDY    Mr. Gonzales

Mr. Gonzales is a 68-year-old man who has lived alone in a senior apartment building since his wife died 6 months ago. He and his wife were born in Mexico but came to live in the United States shortly after they were married. He is retired from a produce warehouse where he worked for 37 years. He and his wife raised three sons, who are all married and have families of their own. The closest son, Carlos, is 30 minutes away by car. Carlos visits Mr. Gonzales every week to socialize and take him shopping. Mr. Gonzales is generally healthy but has decreased visual acuity, hearing loss from the noisy warehouse job, and some "arthritis." He expects to live at least as long as his father, who lived to be 92 years old. Since his wife's death, Mr. Gonzales has attended Catholic mass every day at his parish church, where his wife had attended daily.

Joani Green, a 25-year-old married mother of two, is currently a senior nursing student at the local college. As part of the clinical requirements for the home care course, she and her partner are conducting health screenings and providing health promotion education for the residents of the apartment building where Mr. Gonzales lives. Part of her screening will include Mr. Gonzales' home environment.

## Scientific Knowledge Base

Vulnerable groups that often require help in achieving a safe environment include infants, children, older adults, the ill, the physically and mentally disabled, the illiterate, and the poor. To be effective, you need to understand factors that contribute to a safe environment in the home or health care agency. You also need to understand how alterations in mobility, sensory function, and cognitive function affect a patient's safety (see Chapters 34 and 36).

A safe environment includes meeting basic human needs, reducing physical hazards, and reducing transmission of pathogens.

### Basic Human Needs

Basic human needs often at risk from a variety of environmental hazards include the physiological needs of adequate oxygen, nutrition, and favorable temperature and humidity.

Safety, the freedom from psychological and physical injury, is a basic human need. Health care, provided in a safe manner, and a safe community environment are essential for a patient's well-being. A safe environment reduces the risk of accidents and

**Media Resources** sections detail what electronic resources are available to you for every chapter.

**Objectives** begin each chapter to help you focus on the key information that follows.

Chapters provide a list of **Key Terms**, and the page where each term is introduced.

**Progressive Case Studies** introduce you to patients, families, and nurses. These engaging scenarios illustrate the nursing process in action and help you develop critical thinking skills.

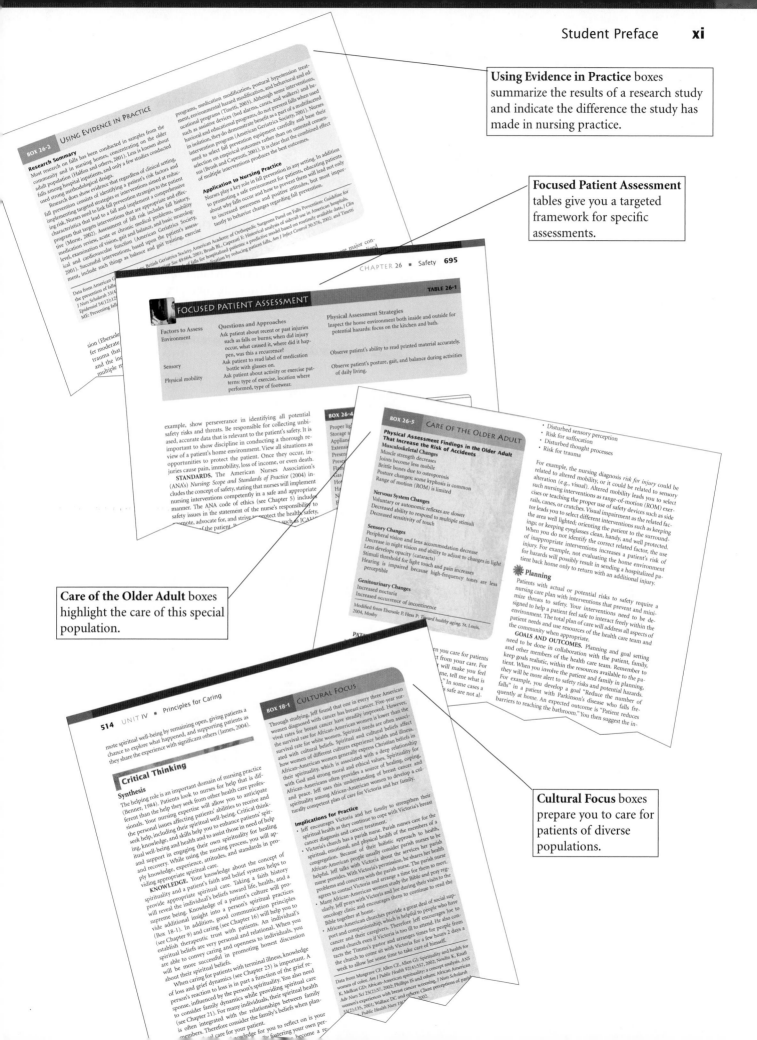

**Using Evidence in Practice** boxes summarize the results of a research study and indicate the difference the study has made in nursing practice.

**Focused Patient Assessment** tables give you a targeted framework for specific assessments.

**Care of the Older Adult** boxes highlight the care of this special population.

**Cultural Focus** boxes prepare you to care for patients of diverse populations.

---

BOX 26-2
USING EVIDENCE IN PRACTICE

**Research Summary**
Most research on falls has been conducted in samples from the community and in nursing homes, concentrating on the older adult population (Halfon and others, 2001). Less is known about falls among hospital inpatients, and only a few studies conducted used strong methodological design.
Research does show evidence that regardless of clinical setting, fall prevention consists of identifying strategies or interventions aimed at reducing risk. Nurses need to link fall risk factors and implementing targeted strategies that are appropriate and effective (Morse, 2002). Assessment of fall risk includes fall history, characteristics that lead to a fall and implement a comprehensive program that targets interventions that are appropriate and effective (Morse, 2002). Assessment of fall risk includes fall history, medication review, acute or chronic medical problems, mobility level, examination of vision, gait and balance, and basic neurologic and cardiovascular function (American Geriatrics Society, 2001). Successful interventions, based upon the patient's assessment, include such things as balance and gait training, exercise

**Application to Nursing Practice**
Nurses play a key role in fall prevention in any setting. In addition to promoting a safe environment for patients, educating patients about why falls occur and how to prevent them will lead not only to increased awareness and positive attitudes, but most importantly to behavior changes regarding fall prevention.

---

CHAPTER 26 • Safety **695**

TABLE 26-1
FOCUSED PATIENT ASSESSMENT

| Factors to Assess | Questions and Approaches | Physical Assessment Strategies |
|---|---|---|
| Environment | Ask patient about recent or past injuries such as falls or burns; when did injury occur, what caused it, where did it happen, was this a recurrence? | Inspect the home environment both inside and outside for potential hazards: focus on the kitchen and bath. |
| Sensory | Ask patient to read label of medication bottle with glasses on. | Observe patient's ability to read printed material accurately. |
| Physical mobility | Ask patient about activity or exercise patterns: type of exercise, location where performed, type of footwear. | Observe patient's posture, gait, and balance during activities of daily living. |

---

example, show perseverance in identifying all potential safety risks and threats. Be responsible for collecting unbiased, accurate data that is relevant to the patient's safety. It is important to show discipline in conducting a thorough review of a patient's home environment. View all situations as opportunities to protect the patient. Once they occur, injuries cause pain, immobility, loss of income, or even death.

**STANDARDS.** The American Nurses Association's (ANA's) *Nursing: Scope and Standards of Practice* (2004) includes the concept of safety, stating that nurses will implement nursing interventions competently in a safe and appropriate manner. The ANA code of ethics (see Chapter 5) includes safety issues in the statement of the nurse's responsibility to promote, advocate for, and strive to protect the health, safety,

---

BOX 26-5
CARE OF THE OLDER ADULT

**Physical Assessment Findings in the Older Adult That Increase the Risk of Accidents**

**Musculoskeletal Changes**
Muscle strength decreases
Joints become less mobile
Brittle bones due to osteoporosis
Posture changes; some kyphosis is common
Range of motion (ROM) is limited

**Nervous System Changes**
Voluntary or autonomic reflexes are slower
Decreased ability to respond to multiple stimuli
Decreased sensitivity of touch

**Sensory Changes**
Peripheral vision and lens accommodation decrease
Decrease in night vision and ability to adjust to changes in light
Lens develops opacity (cataracts)
Stimuli threshold for light touch and pain increases
Hearing is impaired because high-frequency tones are less perceptible

**Genitourinary Changes**
Increased nocturia
Increased occurrence of incontinence

Modified from Ebersole P, Hess P: *Toward healthy aging*, St. Louis, 2004, Mosby.

---

• Disturbed sensory perception
• Risk for suffocation
• Disturbed thought processes
• Risk for trauma

For example, the nursing diagnosis *risk for injury* could be related to altered mobility, or it could be related to sensory alteration (e.g., visual). Altered mobility leads you to select such nursing interventions as range-of-motion (ROM) exercises or teaching the proper use of safety devices such as side rails, canes, or crutches. Visual impairment as the related factor leads you to select different interventions such as keeping the area well lighted; orienting the patient to the surroundings; or keeping eyeglasses clean, handy, and well protected. When you do not identify the correct related factor, the use of inappropriate interventions increases a patient's risk of injury. For example, not evaluating the home environment for hazards will possibly result in sending a hospitalized patient back home only to return with an additional injury.

**Planning**
Patients with actual or potential risks to safety require a nursing care plan with interventions that prevent and minimize threats to safety. Your interventions need to be designed to help a patient feel safe to interact freely within the environment. The total plan of care will address all aspects of patient needs and use resources of the health care team and the community when appropriate.

**GOALS AND OUTCOMES.** Planning and goal setting need to be done in collaboration with the patient, family, and other members of the health care team. Remember to keep goals realistic, within the resources available to the patient. When you involve the patient and family in planning, they will be more alert to safety risks and potential hazards. For example, you develop a goal "Reduce the number of falls" in a patient with Parkinson's disease who falls frequently at home. An expected outcome is "Patient reduces barriers to reaching the bathroom." You then suggest the in-

---

**514** UNIT IV • Principles for Caring

mote spiritual well-being by remaining open, giving patients a chance to explore what happened, and supporting patients as they share the experience with significant others (James, 2004).

**Critical Thinking**

**Synthesis**
The helping role is an important domain of nursing practice (Benner, 1984). Patients look to nurses for help that is different than the help they seek from other health care professionals. Your nursing expertise will allow you to anticipate the personal issues affecting patients' spiritual well-being. Critical thinking, knowledge, and skills help you to assist those in need of help and support in engaging them using the nursing process, you will apply knowledge, experience, attitudes, and standards in providing appropriate spiritual care.

**KNOWLEDGE.** Your knowledge about the concept of spirituality and a patient's faith and belief systems helps to provide appropriate spiritual care. Taking a faith history will reveal the individual's beliefs toward life, health, and a supreme being. Knowledge of a patient's culture will provide additional insight into a person's spiritual practices (see Chapter 9) and caring (see Chapter 16). An individual's spiritual beliefs are very personal and relational. When you establish therapeutic trust with patients, you are able to convey caring and promoting honest discussion about their spiritual beliefs.

When caring for patients with terminal illness, knowledge of loss and grief dynamics (see Chapter 23) is important. A person's reaction to loss is in part a function of the grief response, influenced by the person's spirituality. You also need to consider family dynamics while providing spiritual care (see Chapter 21). For many individuals, their spiritual health is often integrated with the relationships between family members. Therefore consider the family's beliefs when planning care for your patient.

---

BOX 18-1
CULTURAL FOCUS

Through studying, Jeff found that one in every three American women diagnosed with cancer has breast cancer. Five-year survival rates for breast cancer have steadily improved. However, the survival rate for African-American women is lower than the survival rate for white women. Spiritual needs are often associated with cultural beliefs. Spiritual and cultural beliefs affect how women of different cultures experience health and illness. African-American women generally express Christian beliefs in their spirituality, which is associated with a deep relationship with God and strong moral and ethical values. Spirituality for African-Americans often provides a source of healing, coping, and peace. Jeff uses this understanding of breast cancer and spirituality among African-American women to develop a culturally competent plan of care for Victoria and her family.

**Implications for Practice**
• Jeff encourages Victoria and her family to strengthen their spiritual health as they continue to cope with Victoria's breast cancer diagnosis and cancer treatment.
• Victoria's church has a parish nurse. Parish nurses care for the spiritual, emotional, and physical health of the members of a congregation. Because of their holistic approach to health, African-American people usually consider parish nurses to be helpful. Jeff talks with Victoria about the services her parish nurse provides. With Victoria's permission, he shares her health problems and concerns with the parish nurse. The parish nurse agrees to contact Victoria and arrange a time for them to meet.
• Many African-American women study the Bible and pray regularly. Jeff prays with Victoria and Joe during their visits to the oncology clinic and encourages them to continue to read the Bible together at home.
• African-American churches provide a great deal of social support and companionship, which is helpful to people who have cancer and their caregivers. Therefore Jeff encourages Joe to attend church even if Victoria is too ill to attend. He also contacts the Timms's pastor and arranges times for people from the church to come sit with Victoria for a few hours 2 days a week to allow Joe some time to take care of himself.

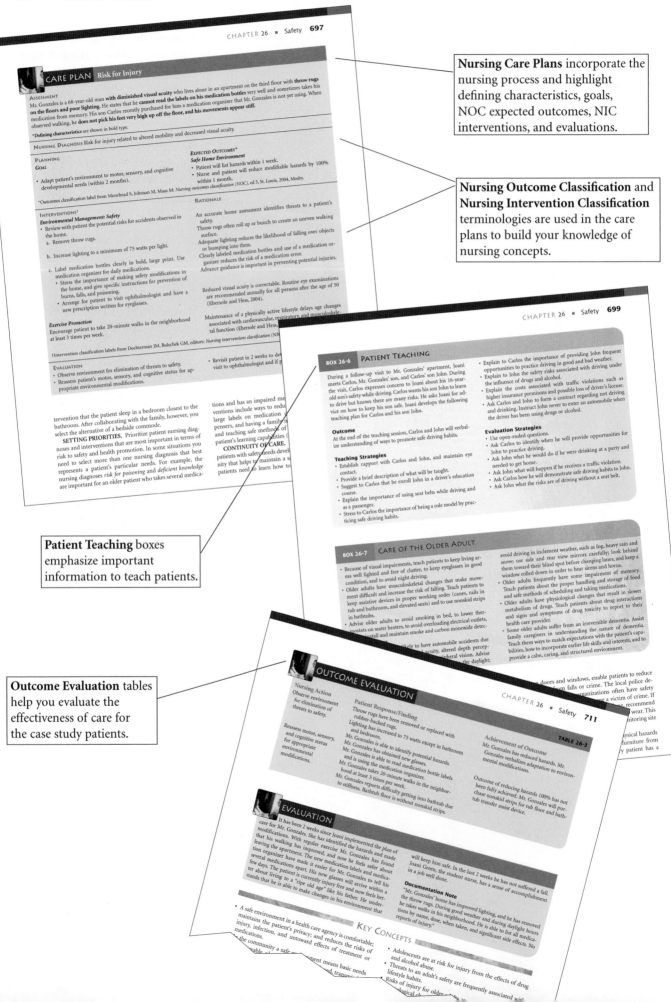

**Nursing Care Plans** incorporate the nursing process and highlight defining characteristics, goals, NOC expected outcomes, NIC interventions, and evaluations.

**Nursing Outcome Classification** and **Nursing Intervention Classification** terminologies are used in the care plans to build your knowledge of nursing concepts.

**Patient Teaching** boxes emphasize important information to teach patients.

**Outcome Evaluation** tables help you evaluate the effectiveness of care for the case study patients.

**Nursing Skills** are presented in a clear, two-column format with steps and rationales so you learn why as well as how.

**Delegation Considerations** guide you in delegating tasks to assistive personnel.

**Equipment** lists show specific items needed for each skill.

**Video Icons** indicate video clips associated with specific skills that are available on the free Companion CD and Evolve Student Learning Resources website.

**Critical Decision Points** alert you to important information to consider as you perform a skill.

Clear, close-up **photos** help you learn to perform important techniques.

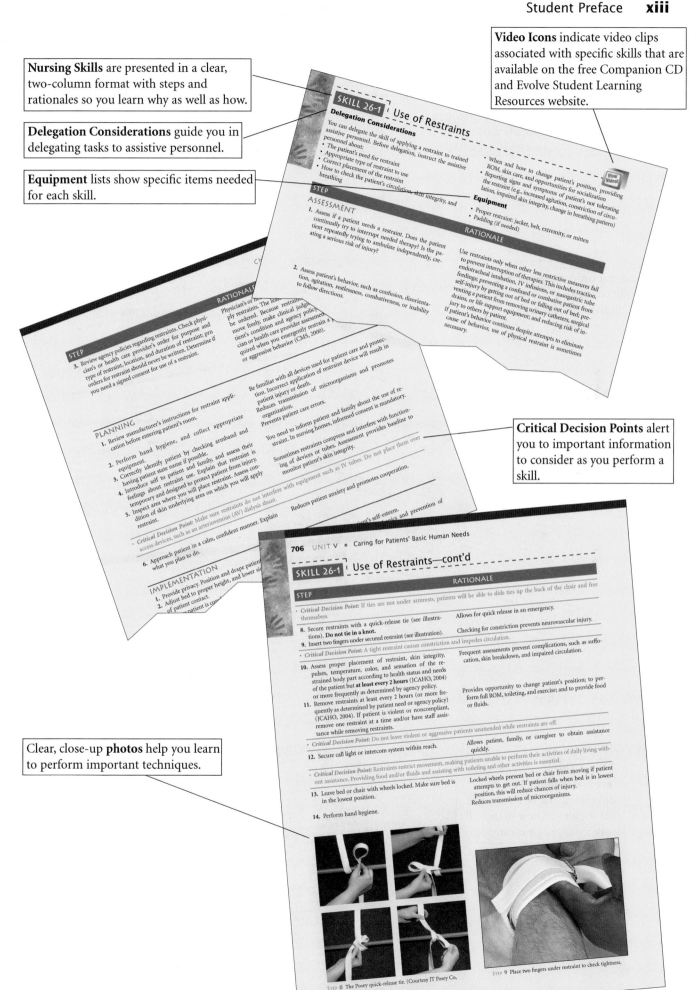

**SKILL 26-1  Use of Restraints**

**Delegation Considerations**

You can delegate the skill of applying a restraint to trained assistive personnel. Before delegation, instruct the assistive personnel about:
- The patient's need for restraint
- Appropriate type of restraint to use
- Correct placement of the restraint
- How to check the patient's circulation, skin integrity, and breathing

- When and how to change patient's position, providing ROM, skin care, and opportunities for socialization
- Reporting signs and symptoms of patient's not tolerating the restraint (e.g., increased agitation, constriction of circulation, impaired skin integrity, change in breathing pattern)

**Equipment**
- Proper restraint: jacket, belt, extremity, or mitten
- Padding (if needed)

| STEP | RATIONALE |
|---|---|
| **ASSESSMENT** | |
| 1. Assess if a patient needs a restraint. Does the patient continually try to interrupt needed therapy? Is the patient repeatedly trying to ambulate independently, creating a serious risk of injury? | Use restraints only when other less restrictive measures fail to prevent interruption of therapies. This includes traction, endotracheal intubation, IV infusions, or nasogastric tube feedings; preventing a confused or combative patient from self-injury by getting out of bed or combative patient from venting a patient from removing urinary catheters, surgical drains, or life support equipment; and reducing risk of injury to others by patient. |
| 2. Assess patient's behavior, such as confusion, disorientation, agitation, restlessness, combativeness, or inability to follow directions. | If patient's behavior continues despite attempts to eliminate cause of behavior, use of physical restraint is sometimes necessary. |
| 3. Review agency policies regarding restraints. Check physician's or health care provider's order for purpose and type of restraint, location, and duration of restraint; prn orders for restraint should never be written. Determine if you need a signed consent for use of a restraint. | Physician's or ... ply restraints. The lea... be ordered. Because restrain... move freely, make clinical judg... tient's condition and agency poli... cian or health care provider assessm... quired when you emergently restrain a ... or aggressive behavior (CMS, 2000). |
| **PLANNING** | |
| 1. Review manufacturer's instructions for restraint application before entering patient's room. | Be familiar with all devices used for patient care and protection. Incorrect application of restraint device will result in patient injury or death. |
| 2. Perform hand hygiene, and collect appropriate equipment. | Reduces transmission of microorganisms and promotes organization. |
| 3. Correctly identify patient by checking armband and having patient state name if possible. | Prevents patient care errors. |
| 4. Introduce self to patient and family, and assess their feelings about restraint use. Explain that restraint is temporary and designed to protect patient from injury. | You need to inform patient and family about the use of restraint. In nursing homes, informed consent is mandatory. |
| 5. Inspect area where you will place restraint. Assess condition of skin underlying area on which you will apply restraint. | Sometimes restraints compress and interfere with functioning of devices or tubes. Assessment provides baseline to monitor patient's skin integrity. |
| *Critical Decision Point:* Make sure restraints do not interfere with equipment such as IV tubes. Do not place them over access devices, such as an arteriovenous (AV) dialysis shunt. | |
| 6. Approach patient in a calm, confident manner. Explain what you plan to do. | Reduces patient anxiety and promotes cooperation. |
| **IMPLEMENTATION** | |
| 1. Provide privacy. Position and drape patien... | ...nt's self-esteem. ...ics and prevention of ... |
| 2. Adjust bed to proper height, and lower si... of patient contact. ...patient is co... | |

---

**SKILL 26-1  Use of Restraints—cont'd**

| STEP | RATIONALE |
|---|---|
| *Critical Decision Point:* If ties are not under armrests, patients will be able to slide ties up the back of the chair and free themselves. | |
| 8. Secure restraints with a quick-release tie (see illustrations). **Do not tie in a knot.** | Allows for quick release in an emergency. |
| 9. Insert two fingers under secured restraint (see illustration). | Checking for constriction prevents neurovascular injury. |
| *Critical Decision Point:* A tight restraint causes constriction and impedes circulation. | |
| 10. Assess proper placement of restraint, skin integrity, pulses, temperature, color, and sensation of the restrained body part **at least every 2 hours** (JCAHO, 2004) of the patient but at least every 2 hours (JCAHO, 2004) or more frequently as determined by agency policy. | Frequent assessments prevent complications, such as suffocation, skin breakdown, and impaired circulation. |
| 11. Remove restraints at least every 2 hours (or more frequently as determined by patient need or agency policy) (JCAHO, 2004). If patient is violent or noncompliant, remove one restraint at a time and/or have staff assistance while removing restraints. | Provides opportunity to change patient's position; to perform full ROM, toileting, and exercise; and to provide food or fluids. |
| *Critical Decision Point:* Do not leave violent or aggressive patients unattended while restraints are off. | |
| 12. Secure call light or intercom system within reach. | Allows patient, family, or caregiver to obtain assistance quickly. |
| *Critical Decision Point:* Restraints restrict movement, making patients unable to perform their activities of daily living without assistance. Providing food and/or fluids and assisting with toileting and other activities is essential. | |
| 13. Leave bed or chair with wheels locked. Make sure bed is in the lowest position. | Locked wheels prevent bed or chair from moving if patient attempts to get out. If patient falls when bed is in lowest position, this will reduce chances of injury. |
| 14. Perform hand hygiene. | Reduces transmission of microorganisms. |

STEP 8 The Posey quick-release tie. (Courtesy JT Posey Co, Arcadia, Calif.)

STEP 9 Place two fingers under restraint to check tightness.

# xiv   Student Preface

**Recording and Reporting** provides guidelines for what to chart and report.

**Unexpected Outcomes and Related Interventions** identify possible undesired results and provide appropriate nursing actions.

**Procedural Guidelines** provide streamlined, step-by-step instructions for performing the most basic skills.

**Critical Thinking in Patient Care** and **Nursing Process** provide a dynamic framework that shows you how to logically work through client care.

---

CHAPTER 26 • Safety **707**

## EVALUATION

1. Inspect patient for any injury, including all hazards of immobility, while restraints are in use.
2. Observe IV catheters, urinary catheters, and drainage tubes to determine that you positioned them correctly.
3. Reassess patient's need for continued use of restraint at least every 24 hours with the intent of discontinuing restraint at the earliest possible time (see agency policy) (CMS, 2000; JCAHO, 2004).
4. Provide appropriate sensory stimulation, and reorient patient as needed.

Ensures patient is free of injury and does not exhibit any signs of immobility complications.

Reinsertion is uncomfortable and increases risk of infection or interruption of therapy.

Face-to-face reassessment by physician or health care provider is required and new order obtained if continuing restraint.

Use of restraints further increases disorientation.

## RECORDING AND REPORTING

■ Record patient behaviors before you applied restraints.
■ Record restraint alternatives you attempted and the patient's response.
■ Record patient's and/or family's understanding of and consent to restraint application.
■ Record type and location of the restraint and time applied.
■ Record times that you performed assessments and releases while patient in restraints.
■ Record findings from your assessments related to orientation, oxygenation, skin integrity, circulation, and positioning.
■ Record patient's behavior and expected or unexpected outcomes after you applied the restraint.
■ Record patient's response when you removed restraints.
■ Also see behavioral restraint flow sheet (Figure 26-1).

## UNEXPECTED OUTCOMES AND RELATED INTERVENTIONS

■ Skin integrity becomes impaired.
 • Reassess the continued need for the restraint; use a different...
 • ...sary, make sure you apply restraint ...adequate padding

• Assess skin, provide appropriate therapy, or remove restraints more frequently.
 • Change wet or soiled restraints.
■ Patient becomes more confused and agitated after you apply restraints.
 • Determine the cause of the behavior and eliminate the cause, if possible.
 • Determine the need for more or less sensory stimulation.
 • Reorient as needed and/or attempt other restraint alternatives.
■ Neurovascular status of an extremity is altered, manifested by cyanosis, pallor, edema, or coldness of skin, or patient complains of tingling, pain, numbness, or loss of ROM.
 • Remove the restraint immediately, stay with the patient, and notify the physician or health care provider.
■ Patient releases the restraint and suffers a fall or other injury.
 • Protect extremity from further injury.
 • Attend to patient's immediate physical needs.
 • Notify the physician or health care provider.
 • Assess the type of restraint, correct application, and whether alternatives will be useful.

*Side Rails.* When used properly, side rails increase a patient's mobility and stability in bed when moving from a bed to a chair. Raising only the top two side rails gives the patient room to exit a bed safely and maneuver within the bed. Side rails also help to prevent the unconscious or sedated patient from rolling out of bed. Always check agency policy about the use of side rails; they are a restraint when used to prevent the patient's desired movement or activity, such as getting out of bed. Side rails also have the potential to trap the head and body in gaps and openings between the bed frame and body (Brush and Capezuti, 2001). Use side rail netting or protective padding to prevent the mattress from sliding to one side. The use of side rails alone for a disoriented patient often causes only more confusion and further injury. Frequently a

---

**710** UNIT V • Caring for Patients' Basic Human Needs

BOX 26-9 **PROCEDURAL GUIDELINES FOR**
### Intervening in Accidental Poisoning

1. Assess for signs or symptoms of accidental ingestion of harmful substances, such as nausea, vomiting, drooling, difficulty breathing, sweating, lethargy.
2. Terminate the exposure by emptying the mouth of pills, plant parts, or other material.
3. If poisoning is due to skin contact or eye contact, irrigate the skin or eye with copious amounts of tap water for 15 to 20 minutes. In the case of an inhalation exposure, safely remove the victim from the potentially dangerous environment.
4. Identify the type and amount of substance ingested to help determine the correct type and amount of antidote needed.
5. **If the victim is conscious and alert, call the local poison control center or the national toll-free poison control center number (1-800-222-1222) before attempting any intervention.** Poison control centers have information needed to treat poisoned patients or to offer referral to treatment centers. The administration of ipecac syrup is no longer recommended for routine home treatment of poisoning (American Academy of Pediatrics, 2003).
6. If the victim has collapsed or stopped breathing, call 911 for emergency transportation to the hospital. Initiate CPR, if indicated, until emergency personnel arrive. Ambulance personnel will be able to provide emergency measures if needed. In addition, parent or guardian is sometimes too upset to drive safely.
7. Position victim with head turned to side to reduce risk of aspiration.
8. Never induce vomiting if the victim has ingested the following poisonous substances: lye, household cleaners, hair care products, grease or petroleum products, and furniture polish, paint thinner, or kerosene.
9. Never induce vomiting in an unconscious or convulsing victim because vomiting increases risk of aspiration.

Modified from Hockenberry MJ: *Wong's Essentials of Pediatric Nursing,* St. Louis, 2005, Mosby and; American Academy of Pediatrics, Committee on Injury, Violence and Poison Prevention: Poison Treatment in the home, *Pediatrics* 112(5): 1182, 2003.

BOX 26-10 **Mercury Spill Cleanup Procedure**

In the event of a mercury spill, follow these steps:
1. Evacuate the room except for a housekeeping crew (if available).
2. Cleanup personnel need to wear rubber (latex or vinyl) gloves while handling the mercury.
3. Spray the spill area with a mist of water. This diminishes vaporization of mercury.
4. Ventilate the area. Close interior doors, and open any outside windows.
5. Use a suction device, such as a syringe without a needle, to extract mercury in a leakproof glass or plastic container with a nonmetallic cap or lid. **DO NOT VACUUM THE SPILL.**
6. Mop the floor with a mercury cleaner (see agency policy).
7. Dispose of collected mercury according to local environmental safety regulations.

ground. Teach patients and family how to reduce their risk of electrical injury in the home. For example, discuss prevention of electrical shock by...ting use of grounded appliances, near a water source, the...grounding appliances, and avoiding operati...

**Evaluation**
PATIENT CARE. ...reducing threats...sponse to the...When the expe...interventions...have develop...patient's pro...of a goal, o...Patient's...cognitive...goal is...100%...

restraint when they are not a ...ment plan. You must have...restraint, and it must be a...l treatment and plan of...der's order is required...ment of the patient....e duration and cir-...e restraints. Your...complications of...reased sense of...te with other...ntion pro-...atient. The...possible.

---

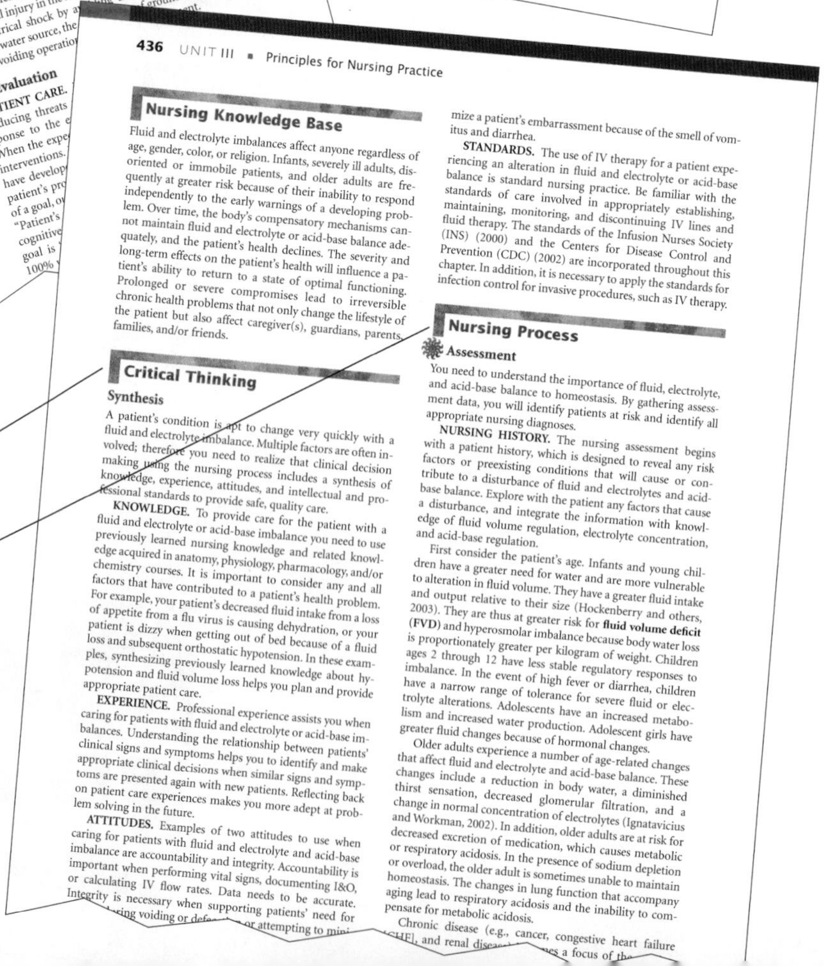

**436** UNIT III • Principles for Nursing Practice

## Nursing Knowledge Base

Fluid and electrolyte imbalances affect anyone regardless of age, gender, color, or religion. Infants, severely ill adults, disoriented or immobile patients, and older adults are frequently at greater risk because of their inability to respond independently to the early warnings of a developing problem. Over time, the body's compensatory mechanisms cannot maintain fluid and electrolyte or acid-base balance adequately, and the patient's health declines. The severity and long-term effects on the patient's health will influence a patient's ability to return to a state of optimal functioning. Prolonged or severe compromises lead to irreversible chronic health problems that not only change the lifestyle of the patient but also affect caregiver(s), guardians, parents, families, and/or friends.

### Critical Thinking

**Synthesis**

A patient's condition is apt to change very quickly with a fluid and electrolyte imbalance. Multiple factors are often involved; therefore you need to realize that clinical decision making using the nursing process includes a synthesis of knowledge, experience, attitudes, and intellectual and professional standards to provide safe, quality care.
KNOWLEDGE. To provide care for the patient with a fluid and electrolyte or acid-base imbalance you need to use previously learned nursing knowledge and related knowledge acquired in anatomy, physiology, pharmacology, and/or chemistry courses. It is important to consider any and all factors that have contributed to a patient's health problem. For example, your patient's decreased fluid intake from a loss of appetite from a flu virus is causing dehydration, or your patient is dizzy when getting out of bed because of a fluid loss and subsequent orthostatic hypotension. In these examples, synthesizing previously learned knowledge about hypotension and fluid volume loss helps you plan and provide appropriate patient care.
EXPERIENCE. Professional experience assists you when caring for patients with fluid and electrolyte or acid-base imbalances. Understanding the relationship between patients' clinical signs and symptoms helps you to identify and make appropriate clinical decisions when similar signs and symptoms are presented again with new patients. Reflecting back on patient care experiences makes you more adept at problem solving in the future.
ATTITUDES. Examples of two attitudes to use when caring for patients with fluid and electrolyte and acid-base imbalance are accountability and integrity. Accountability is important when performing vital signs, documenting I&O, or calculating IV flow rates. Data needs to be accurate. Integrity is necessary when...sing voiding or def...or attempting to mini-

...mize a patient's embarrassment because of the smell of vomitus and diarrhea.
STANDARDS. The use of IV therapy for a patient experiencing an alteration in fluid and electrolyte or acid-base balance is standard nursing practice. Be familiar with the standards of care involved in appropriately establishing, maintaining, monitoring, and discontinuing IV lines and fluid therapy. The standards of the Infusion Nurses Society (INS) (2000) and the Centers for Disease Control and Prevention (CDC) (2002) are incorporated throughout this chapter. In addition, it is necessary to apply the standards for infection control for invasive procedures, such as IV therapy.

### Nursing Process

**Assessment**

You need to understand the importance of fluid, electrolyte, and acid-base balance to homeostasis. By gathering assessment data, you will identify patients at risk and identify all appropriate nursing diagnoses.
NURSING HISTORY. The nursing assessment begins with a patient history, which is designed to reveal any risk factors or preexisting conditions that will cause or contribute to a disturbance of fluid and electrolytes and acid-base balance. Explore with the patient any factors that cause a disturbance, and integrate the information with knowledge of fluid volume regulation, electrolyte concentration, and acid-base regulation.
First consider the patient's age. Infants and young children have a greater need for water and are more vulnerable to alteration in fluid volume. They have a greater fluid intake and output relative to their size (Hockenberry and others, 2003). They are thus at greater risk for **fluid volume deficit (FVD)** and hyperosmolar imbalance because body water loss is proportionately greater per kilogram of weight. Children ages 2 through 12 have less stable regulatory responses to imbalance. In the event of high fever or diarrhea, children have a narrow range of tolerance for severe fluid or electrolyte alterations. Adolescents have an increased metabolism and increased water production. Adolescent girls have greater fluid changes because of hormonal changes.
Older adults experience a number of age-related changes that affect fluid and electrolyte and acid-base balance. These changes include a reduction in body water, a diminished thirst sensation, decreased glomerular filtration, and a change in normal concentration of electrolytes (Ignatavicius and Workman, 2002). In addition, older adults are at risk for decreased excretion of medication, which causes metabolic or respiratory acidosis. In the presence of sodium depletion or overload, the older adult is sometimes unable to maintain homeostasis. The changes in lung function that accompany aging lead to respiratory acidosis and the inability to compensate for metabolic acidosis.
Chronic disease (e.g., cancer, congestive heart failure [CHF], and renal disea...

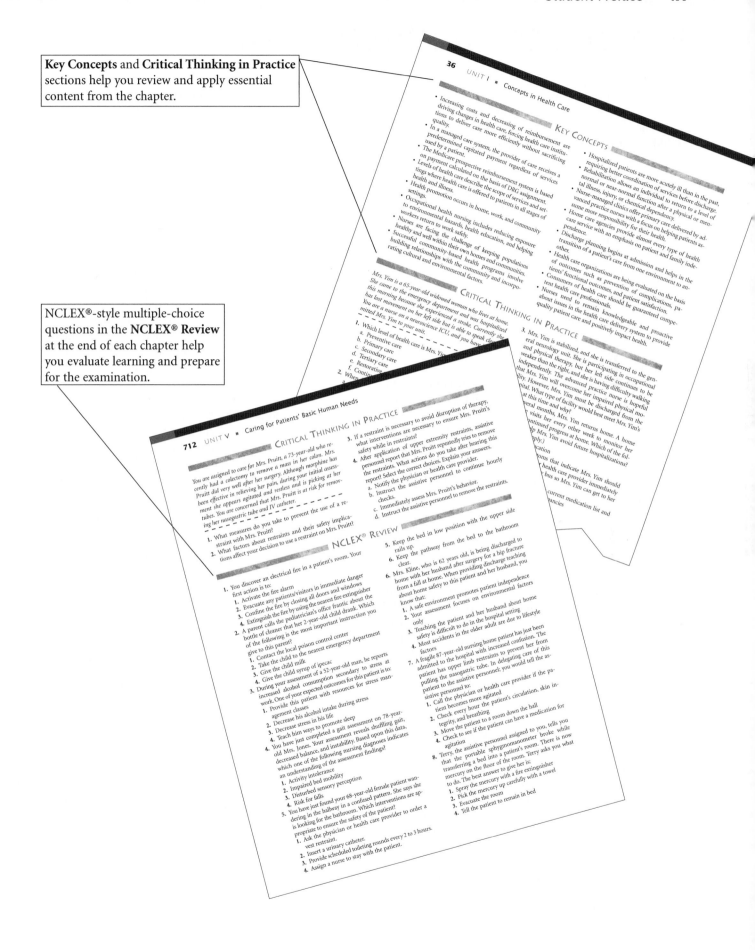

**Key Concepts** and **Critical Thinking in Practice** sections help you review and apply essential content from the chapter.

NCLEX®-style multiple-choice questions in the **NCLEX® Review** at the end of each chapter help you evaluate learning and prepare for the examination.

# Preface to the Instructor

"Traditional nursing" is a thing of the past. Today's nurses must be prepared to adapt to the continual changes occurring in health care. They play a vital role in the delivery of multidisciplinary health care services. The practice arena is changing—moving more and more to the community setting. The focus of care is changing as well—more emphasis is being placed on health promotion and restorative care. Even the patients are changing—more cultural diversity exists, and the percentage of older adult patients continues to increase. Patients are far more involved in and informed about health care.

Despite these changes—perhaps because of these changes—it is essential that the basics of nursing must remain the foundation of practice. Nurses must be knowledgeable and professional. They must be both technically proficient and personally caring. And they must be able to synthesize a broad array of knowledge and experiences when providing care for their patients.

We continue to cover all of the fundamental nursing concepts, skills, and techniques that students must master before moving on to other areas of study. We address changes in practice that affect how and where nurses use the skills and knowledge they acquire.

## FEATURES

We have designed this text to welcome the new student to nursing, communicate our own love for the profession, and promote learning and understanding. We know that today's students are busy and, too often, overwhelmed by all that they must learn and do. They want their texts to focus on the most current, factual, and essential content and skills. We want to ensure that these students are ready to continue with their education and will, ultimately, be prepared for all of the challenges of practice. To this end, we have included the following key features:

- Students will appreciate the **clear, engaging writing style.** We have totally revamped the narrative so that it speaks to the reader, making this edition more of an active instructional tool than a passive reference. Students will find that even complex technical and theoretical concepts are presented in language that is easy to understand.
- The **attractive, functional design** will appeal to today's visual learner. The clear, readable type and bold headings make the content easy to read and follow. Each special element is consistently color-keyed so students can readily identify important information.
- Hundreds of **large, clear, full-color photographs and drawings** reinforce and clarify key concepts and techniques.

- The **five-step nursing process** serves as the organizing framework for all clinical chapters. This logical, consistent framework for narrative discussions is further enhanced by special boxes that highlight assessment, care plans, and evaluation of outcome achievement.
- **Critical thinking** is presented in a separate chapter, then incorporated as a consistent partner to the nursing process in each clinical chapter. This application of critical thinking provides a practical, clinical decision-making guide that is easy for even the beginning student to understand.
- **Ongoing case studies** in each clinical chapter introduce "real-world" patients, families, and nurses. The chapter follows the case study through the steps of the nursing process, helping students see how to apply the process, along with critical thinking, to the care of patients. Cases take place in both acute and community settings, and include patients and nurses from a variety of cultural backgrounds.
- **Expected outcomes** are addressed in care plans, special boxes, and narrative to help students understand and apply these key clinical measures.
- Implementation narrative consistently addresses health promotion, acute care, and restorative and continuing care to reflect the current focus on **community-based nursing** and **health promotion.**
- **More than 45 nursing skills** are presented in a clear, two-column format with steps and rationales. Skills include delegation guidelines and critical decision points that alert students to steps requiring special assessment or specific technique for safe and effective administration.
- **Procedural guidelines** provide streamlined step-by-step instructions for performing very basic skills.
- Care of the **older adult** and **patient teaching** are stressed throughout the narrative, as well as highlighted in special boxes.
- **Learning aids** to help students identify, review, and apply important content in each chapter include Objectives, Key Terms, Key Concepts, Critical Thinking in Practice questions, and an NCLEX® review.

### New to This Edition

- **Active, engaging writing style** speaks to the student, enhancing learning and understanding.
- Each student text is packaged with a free **Companion CD** that contains additional NCLEX®-style review questions, an audio glossary, an English/Spanish audio glossary, video clips, and Butterfield's Fluids and Electrolytes tutorial.
- **Using Evidence in Practice** boxes summarize the results of a research study and indicate the difference the study has made in nursing practice.

- **NCLEX®-style multiple-choice review questions** at the end of each chapter help students evaluate learning and incorporate the new NCLEX®-style questions.
- **New chapter on "Community-Based Nursing"** and the increased emphasis on caring throughout the text highlight this fundamental principle of nursing.
- **Briefer coverage of higher-level concepts** provides just the right amount of detail on research, theory, professional roles, and management to maintain a strong "essentials" focus.

## TEACHING AND LEARNING PACKAGE

In recognition of the incredible challenges faced by both students and educators, we have developed an unsurpassed array of teaching and learning materials.

- The **Instructor's Electronic Resource** on CD-ROM by Gale Carli includes a comprehensive Instructor's Manual, a Test Bank, and an impressive collection of PowerPoint lecture slides and images from the text to enhance classroom lectures. These **Course Resources** are also available online for faculty only.
- **Mosby's Nursing Skills Video Series** provides engaging, action-packed demonstrations of how to perform key nursing procedures in real-life clinical situations. Actual nurses perform each skill as they work through contemporary concepts such as delegation, critical thinking, patient rights, and communication techniques.
- **Evolve Website** provides content updates and a reliable source of annotated current nursing weblinks for class assignments and independent study.

- **Study Guide** by Patricia A. Castaldi provides students with a wide variety of exercises and activities to enhance learning and comprehension. This study guide features learning activities; chapter review sections with matching, fill-in-the-blank and NCLEX®-style multiple-choice questions; study group questions; Skills Performance Checklists; instructions for creating and using study charts; and Case Studies with related questions.
- **TEACH Lesson Plan Manual** link all parts of the educational package by providing you with customizable lesson plans and lecture outlines based on learning objectives.
- **Virtual Clinical Excursions** is a groundbreaking new workbook and CD-ROM experience that brings learning to life in a virtual hospital setting. The workbook guides students as they care for clients, providing ongoing challenges and learning opportunities. Each lesson in *Virtual Clinical Excursions* complements the textbook content and provides the perfect environment for students to practice what they are learning in the text for a true-to-life, hands-on learning experience. This CD/workbook is available separately or packaged at a special price with the textbook.
- **Nursing Skills Online** offers 17 distinct media-rich modules that cover key nursing skills. Throughout the lessons, students encounter over 700 interactive self-assessment exercises that provide immediate feedback. Modules end with a comprehensive examination that evaluates student comprehension, with results automatically entered into your online gradebook.

# Acknowledgments

This edition of *Basic Nursing* is the result of collaboration among authors, section editors, nursing editorial, design, production editing, electronic media, and marketing. Each of these divisions and individuals within these groups contributed their commitment, talent, and time to create a unique text. As always the advanced planning and design has ensured our readers a quality textbook.

- We wish to acknowledge Suzi Epstein, Executive Editor, for her vision, organization, creativity, and support to develop a text that offers a state-of-the-art approach to the design, organization, and presentation of *Basic Nursing*. Her skill as an editor enables us to be innovative; her skillful and thoughtful editing provided needed attention to detail in designing such a comprehensive text.
- Robyn Brinks, Senior Developmental Editor, whose organization skills and attention to detail are the best in the business. Her patience and gracious manner skillfully tracked manuscript, authors, and deadlines, all the while maintaining her cool and a wonderful sense of humor. We acknowledge and appreciate her professionalism; she kept us on time and on target.
- Kathi Gosche, our book designer, contributed to a clear, crisp, colorful, and visually distinctive design. Involved from the beginning, her work helped us avoid numerous pitfalls and achieve a finished produce that is visually appealing and easy to use.
- Andrea Lutes, for her creativity and vision for the design of the cover art and her direction in implementing the overall design of the text.
- Many thanks and gratitude to the Production Team.
  - John Rogers, Publishing Services Manager, for support throughout the editing and final pages.
  - Beth Hayes, Senior Project Manager, who is an accomplished production editor. Beth juggles multiple aspects of the book while keeping the book and the authors on deadline. She is talented and calm under pressure and through her sense of humor and commitment to excellence guided this text to completion.

- To Mike DeFilippo, for his photographic excellence, and to the Saint Francis Medical Center, Peoria, Illinois for the generous use of their facility for our photo shoot.
- To the sales and marketing team and Kathy Mantz, Nursing Product Manager, who continually offer market insight into the design elements to enhance the quality of the text.
- Tricia Kinman, readability specialist, whose editing and knowledge helped us to create a text that is informative and maintains a consistent reading level for our students.
- To our contributors, excellent clinicians and educators, who share their valuable experiences and knowledge in the chapters they create. Their attention to detail within their areas of specialization help us achieve a state-of-the art textbook. We are fortunate to be associated with excellent nurse authors who are able to convey standards of nursing excellence through the printed word.
- Amy Hall and Patricia Stockert, section editors, whose talents help to take this text to the next level. Their attention to detail, knowledge of the nursing literature, and commitment to excellence were integral components of this text from planning to publication. Amy and Patti, thank you for a wonderful partnership.
- To our nursing colleagues, who educate the next generation of nurses and who care for our patients, help them through their fears, assist in their recovery, and practice excellence every day. You influence us greatly.
- To our reviewers, for their expertise, candor, and astute comments that assist us in developing a text with high standards that reflect professional nursing practice today.

As always, we would like to acknowledge a friendship that enables us to collaborate as coauthors. Together our friendship encourages us to seek new challenges and to extend our boundaries. A friendship built on caring, consideration, respect, and compassion is unbeatable, and for that we are truly blessed.

**Patricia A. Potter**
**Anne Griffin Perry**

# Contents

# CHAPTER 1

# Health and Wellness

## MEDIA RESOURCES

**CD COMPANION** *evolve* **WEBSITE**

http://evolve.elsevier.com/Potter/basic

- **NCLEX® Review**
- **Audio Glossary**
- **English/Spanish Audio Glossary**

## OBJECTIVES

- Discuss the health belief, health promotion, and holistic health models of health and illness to understand the relationship between patients' attitudes toward health and health practices.
- Discuss the meaning of determinants of health status.
- Describe the variables influencing health beliefs and health practices.
- Describe health promotion and illness prevention activities.
- Discuss the three levels of prevention.
- Discuss four types of risk factors and the process of risk factor modification.
- Describe the variables influencing illness behavior.
- Describe the impact of illness on the patient and family.
- Discuss the nurse's role in health and illness.

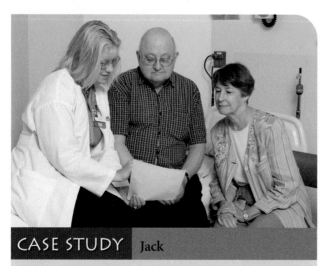

## CASE STUDY   Jack

Jack is a 62-year-old obese man with diabetes. He is married, and he and his wife baby-sit for their 3-year-old grandson 3 days a week while their daughter works. He also has known cardiovascular disease and peripheral vascular disease. He was admitted to the hospital with a foot wound. Kathy, the wound care specialist nurse, is completing her evaluation, which includes a history and physical. Jack describes walking barefoot in his basement about 2 weeks ago. He stepped on a nail. He did not notice the severity of the injury for almost a week. He knew he had an appointment with his physician in a few days, so he thought it could wait until his appointment. By the time he went to the physician, he had a fever, loss of appetite, and his blood glucose levels had been running high. In addition, the foot injury had progressed into a large foot ulcer. Kathy reviews the chart and learns that further tests have found positive blood cultures and altered laboratory work, including increased erythrocyte sedimentation rate (ESR) and blood count. An x-ray film of the foot reveals bone destruction beneath the wound, and a bone scan confirms osteomyelitis. His physician has prescribed broad-spectrum antibiotics and has planned a surgical debridement.

Postoperatively Kathy continues to follow Jack's course of treatment. Because of lengthy wound healing time, Kathy suggests using an amorphous hydrogel dressing instead of the traditional wet-to-dry normal saline gauze dressing. Kathy reviewed the wound care literature and learned that the hydrogel dressings are significantly more cost-effective and are equally effective at promoting wound healing (Box 1-1). Jack remains on a 4- to 6-week course of intravenous (IV) antibiotics and is discharged home with daily visits from a home care nurse.

## KEY TERMS

active strategies of health promotion, p. 8
acute illness, p. 13
chronic illness, p. 13
determinants of health, p. 7
health, p. 4
health belief model, p. 4
health beliefs, p. 4
health promotion, p. 9
health promotion model, p. 4
health status, p. 7
holistic health, p. 5
illness, p. 12
illness behavior, p. 13
illness prevention, p. 9

Maslow's hierarchy of needs, p. 3
negative health behaviors, p. 4
passive strategies of health promotion, p. 8
positive health behaviors, p. 4
primary prevention, p. 9
risk factor, p. 10
secondary prevention, p. 10
tertiary prevention, p. 10
wellness, p. 2
wellness education, p. 9

In the past most individuals and societies viewed good health or **wellness** as the opposite or absence of disease. We now understand that some conditions of health lie between disease and good health. Therefore we view health from a broader perspective. As a nurse you will use concepts of health, health promotion, wellness, and illness to assist your patients in achieving and maintaining an optimal level of health. You will use models of health and illness to understand and explain these concepts. In addition, you will assist patients in making changes to their current health state to bring about improved health and wellness.

One way to understand an individual's motivation to achieve optimal health is to review Abraham Maslow's hierarchy of needs (1954). This model is a means to understand human behavior. Businesses use it to understand the motiva-

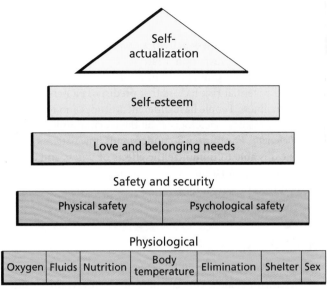

| BOX 1-1 | USING EVIDENCE IN PRACTICE |
|---|---|

**Research Summary**

Many patients with large chronic wounds or operative wounds that have delayed healing will be sent to a home setting after hospital discharge and will continue to need extensive wound care. Sterile wet-to-dry normal saline dressing changes are one traditional method of wound care. This treatment requires frequent home nursing visits. The dressing needs to stay moist to be effective. If the dressing becomes dry and adheres to the wound, disruption of the tissue occurs when removing the dry dressing. Wound care specialists prefer amorphous hydrogel dressings because they maintain a moist wound environment. However, the lack of scientific evidence of the effectiveness of amorphous hydrogel dressings in managing wounds has limited their clinical use. Capasso and Munro (2003) recently studied the cost and effectiveness of these two wound treatments. The nurse researchers performed a retrospective chart review and collected data from home care records of 150 patients who received wet-to-dry normal saline dressings and 150 who received amorphous hydrogel dressings. The researchers found no significant differences in the rate of wound closure between the two groups. There was no significant difference in the cost of wound care supplies. Interestingly, the total cost of wound care was $1,140 higher for patients in the normal saline group than for patients in the hydrogel group. The largest portion of the increased cost was attributed to charges for home nursing visits for dressing changes. The normal saline group required 33% more home nursing visits. The researches concluded that the amorphous hydrogel dressings are a better value for home treatment of some wounds.

**Application to Nursing Practice**

Demonstrating the value and cost-effectiveness of dressing choices enhances therapeutic decision making and guides treatment decisions. The results of this study validate many wound care nurse experiential observations. Nurses are concerned about cost and effectiveness when choosing therapies. Scientific data validate treatment choices, as well as enhance appropriate cost-effective care. This information helped Kathy plan her wound care therapy decisions for Jack's wound.

Data from Capasso VA, Munro BH: The cost and efficacy of two wound treatments, *AORN J* 77(5):984, 2003.

FIGURE **1-1** Maslow's hierarchy of needs. (From Maslow AH: *Motivation and personality*, ed 3, Upper Saddle River, NJ, 1987, Prentice Hall.)

The lowest level of needs on the hierarchy consists of very *basic physiological needs*, such as water, food, sleep, and sex. When these needs are not met, an individual feels sick, irritated, or complains of pain or discomfort. Those feelings motivate an individual to satisfy the need (Maslow, 1970). The second level on the hierarchy of needs consists of *safety needs*, which include establishing stability and consistency. These psychological needs include the security of a home and a family. For example, a woman living in an abusive home is unable to move to the next level of love and belongingness because she is constantly concerned for her safety. The third level on the hierarchy is *love and belongingness*, which is a desire to belong to groups. It consists of the need to feel love by others and to be accepted. The fourth level deals with the need for *self-esteem*. Self-esteem results from mastery of a task and also includes the recognition gained from others. The highest level of needs on the hierarchy is needs of *self-actualization*, which is the desire to become everything that one is capable of becoming. An individual at this level is concerned with maximizing his or her potential.

An understanding of Maslow's hierarchy of needs provides you with a framework to meet patient needs and specifically prioritize care for your patients. It is important that you understand that unless a patient's basic needs have been met, higher levels in the pyramid are not relevant (Benson and Dundis, 2003). You first ensure that basic needs of individuals are met. Also, all the levels have a varying element of depth for the individual (Benson and Dundis, 2003). The requirements to satisfy the needs of each level vary from person to person. Needs are greater or lesser for different persons. Therefore a thorough and indi-

tion of employees, and the social sciences use it to understand the needs of individuals. It is also effective in understanding what is important to individuals. You will use this model to better understand the needs of patients and families and their readiness to engage in health promotion activities. Maslow's model is in the shape of a pyramid divided into five levels. The bottom level, or physiological level, consists of the most basic needs for human survival: food, water, and shelter. As a person meets the needs of one level, the individual moves up to the next level. The premise of **Maslow's hierarchy of needs** (Figure 1-1) is that unsatisfied needs motivate human beings and that individuals have to meet certain lower level needs before they are able to satisfy higher level needs.

vidualized assessment of needs is an important aspect of patient care.

In addition, wellness activities involving health promotion and illness prevention strategies help patients achieve and maintain an optimal level of health. Nurses identify actual and potential risk factors that predispose a person or a group to illness. People have different attitudes and reactions to illness. Medical sociologists call the reaction to illness *illness behavior*. The nurse who understands how patients react to illness is able to minimize the effects of illness and assist patients and their families in maintaining or returning to the highest level of functioning.

## Definition of Health

Defining good health is difficult because each person has his or her own personal concept of health. The World Health Organization (WHO) defines health as a "state of complete physical, mental and social well-being, not merely the absence of disease or infirmity" (WHO, 1947). Individual views of health vary among different age-groups, genders, races, and cultures (Pender, 1996). Pender (1996) explains that "all people free of disease are not equally healthy." **Health** is a state of being that people define in relation to their own values, personality, and lifestyle. Pender (1996) suggests that for many people it is "conditions of life" rather than "pathological states" that define health. Nurses consider the total person, as well as the person's environment, to individualize nursing care and help patients identify and reach their health goals. Therefore health is a complex concept and means more than the absence of disease. Health is the manner in which people think about health and how they manage their lives in ways that are healthy or promote health (McGough, 2004).

## Models of Health and Illness

A model is a theoretical way of understanding a concept or an idea. Models represent various ways of approaching complex issues. Because health and illness are complex concepts, you use models to understand the relationships between these concepts and the patient's attitudes toward health and health practices. Models of health and illness contain a combination of biological characteristics (genetic predisposition), behavioral factors (lifestyle, stress, and health beliefs), and social conditions (cultural influences, family relationships, and social support) (McGough, 2004). Nurses develop and use a variety of health models to understand patients' attitudes and values about health and illness in order to provide effective health care. These models allow you to understand and predict patients' health behavior, including how they use health services, participate in recommended therapy, and care for themselves.

## Health Belief Model

**Health beliefs** are a person's ideas, convictions, and attitudes about health and illness. These beliefs are based on factual information or misinformation, common sense, or myths. Because health beliefs usually influence health behavior, they positively or negatively affect a patient's level of health. **Positive health behaviors** are activities related to maintaining, attaining, or regaining good health and preventing illness. Common positive health behaviors include immunizations, proper sleep patterns, adequate exercise, and good nutrition. Implementation of positive health behaviors is dependent on an individual's awareness of how to live a healthy life and the person's ability and willingness to carry out such behaviors in a healthy lifestyle. **Negative health behaviors** include activities that are actually or potentially harmful to health, such as smoking, drug or alcohol abuse, poor diet, and refusal to take necessary medications or to care for oneself.

Rosenstoch's (1974) and Becker and Maiman's (1975) **health belief model** (Figure 1-2) addresses the relationship between a person's beliefs and behaviors. It provides a way of understanding and predicting how patients will behave in relation to their health and how they will follow health care therapies or regimens.

The first component of this model involves the individual's perception of susceptibility to an illness. For example, a patient needs to recognize the familial link for coronary artery disease. After recognizing this link, the patient will perceive a personal risk of heart disease. The second component is the patient's perception of the seriousness of the illness. Demographic and sociopsychological variables, perceived threats of the illness, and cues to action (e.g., mass media campaigns and advice from family, friends, and medical professionals) all influence and modify this perception. The third component, the likelihood that the patient will take preventive action, results from the patient's perception of the benefits of and barriers to taking action. Preventive action includes lifestyle changes, increased participation in recommended medical therapies, or a search for medical advice or treatment.

The health belief model helps you to understand factors influencing patients' perceptions, beliefs, and behavior and to plan care that will most effectively assist patients in maintaining or restoring health and preventing illness. Understand that each patient's views of health and wellness, as well as individual belief systems, influence the ability to make lasting changes in a patient's health status. Be cautious not to make judgments when you encounter views and beliefs that differ from your own individual philosophies of health and wellness.

## Health Promotion Model

The **health promotion model** proposed by Pender (1982, 1993, 1996; Pender, Murdaugh, and Parsons, 2002) (Figure 1-3, p. 6) defines health as a positive, dynamic state, not merely the absence of disease. The model was proposed as a framework for integrating the perspectives of nursing

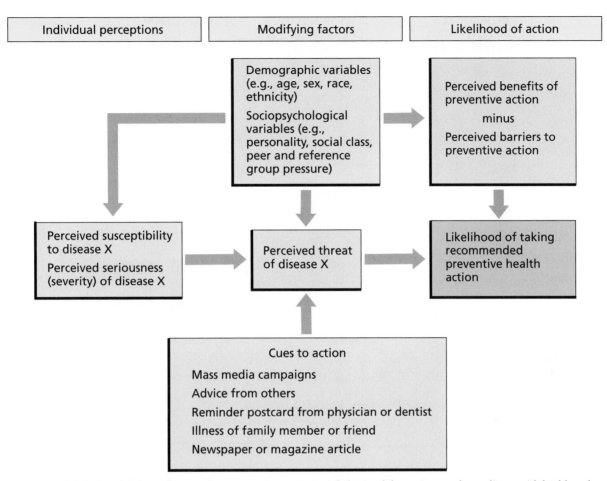

FIGURE **1-2** Health belief model. (Data from Becker MH, Maiman LA: Sociobehavioral determinants of compliance with health and medical care recommendations, *Med Care* 13[1]:10, 1975.)

and behavioral science and the factors that influence health behaviors (Pender and others, 2002). Health promotion is behavior motivated by the desire to increase well-being and actualize human health potential, whereas health protection is behavior that is motivated by a desire to avoid illness, detect it early, or maintain function within the constraints of an illness (Pender and others, 2002). The health promotion model describes the multidimensional nature of people as they interact within their environment to pursue health (Pender and others, 2002). This model focuses on the three functions of a patient's cognitive-perceptual factors (individual perceptions), modifying factors (demographic and social), and participation in health-promoting behaviors (likelihood of action). The model also organizes cues into a pattern to explain the likelihood of a patient developing health promotion behaviors (Pender, 1993, 1996). The focus of this model is to explain the reasons that individuals engage in health activities. It is not for use with families or communities. Revisions to the health promotion model were made in 1996 to increase its potential use for prediction and inter-

vention of health promotion. You will use this model to help implement health-promoting behaviors into the daily lives and health practices of patients.

## Holistic Health Model

The holistic health care movement comes from a variety of scientific, philosophical, and social bases that describe similar phenomenon (Mendel, 2003). Individual concepts of holistic health care, however, differ markedly among health care practitioners who use a holistic framework in practice (Mendel, 2003). **Holistic health,** sometimes called complementary or alternative medicine, is generally a comprehensive view of the person as a biopsychosocial and spiritual being (Edelman and Mandle, 2002). The intent of the holistic health model is to empower patients to engage in their own healing process (Edelman and Mandle, 2002). Holistic health consists of concepts of energy, holism, the mind-body connection, and balance in order to expand the definition of health. A broader definition of health is applicable to more patients in increasingly diverse populations and will optimize health outcomes (Saylor, 2003).

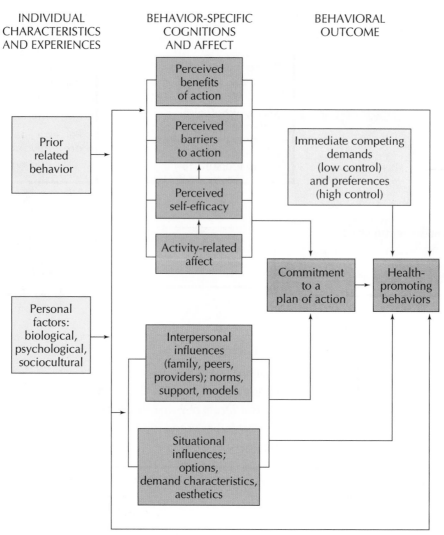

INDIVIDUAL CHARACTERISTICS AND EXPERIENCES

BEHAVIOR-SPECIFIC COGNITIONS AND AFFECT

BEHAVIORAL OUTCOME

FIGURE **1-3** Health promotion model. (From Pender NJ and others: *Health promotion in nursing practice,* ed 5, Upper Saddle River, NJ, 2005, Pearson Education.)

The holistic health model involves the use of a variety of techniques that in the past the health community viewed as "experimental" or "alternative." These techniques have recently gained popularity among most health care professionals, as we have begun to understand that personal health choices have a powerful impact on an individual's health. Some of the most widely used holistic interventions include aromatherapy, biofeedback, breathing exercises, massage therapy, meditation, music therapy, relaxation therapy, therapeutic touch, and guided imagery. Most holistic therapies are easy to learn and apply to almost any nursing setting and to all stages of health and illness. For example, health care providers use reminiscence in the geriatric population to help relieve anxiety for a patient dealing with memory loss or meditation for a cancer patient dealing with the difficult side effects of chemotherapy. Surgeons use music therapy in the operating room to create a soothing environment. Relaxation training is useful in any setting to distract a patient during a painful procedure, such as a dressing change. Breathing exer-

cises help patients deal with the shortness of breath that accompanies some chronic respiratory diseases. You will help patients recognize the many options available and assist them in making choices to enhance health. Know what strategies are effective in promoting health and giving patients more alternatives to be successful and satisfied (Saylor, 2003).

## Determinants of Health Status: *Healthy People 2010*

Since the 1970s there has been a nationally focused initiative toward better health for the American people. Researchers have established that changes in health risk factors and the timely receipt of clinical preventive services prevent premature deaths (Nelson and others, 2002). There are three influential documents that outline specific national goals for improving the physical health of Americans: *Healthy People: The Surgeon General's Report on Health Promotion and*

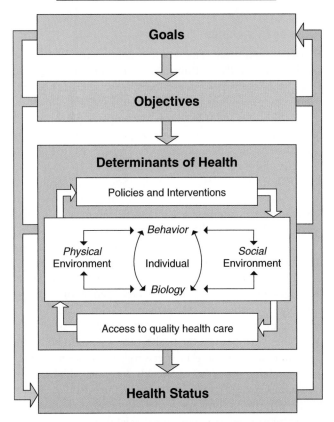

**Healthy People in Healthy Communities**
A Systematic Approach to Health Improvement

FIGURE **1-4** A model for a systematic approach to health improvement. (From U.S. Department of Health and Human Services, Public Health Service: *Healthy people 2010: understanding and improving health,* Washington, DC, 2000, U.S. Government Printing Office.)

*Disease Prevention* (U.S. Department of Health and Human Services [USDHHS], 1979); *Healthy People 2000: National Health Promotion and Disease Prevention Objectives* (USDHHS, 1990); and *Healthy People 2010: Understanding and Improving Health* (USDHHS, 2000). These reports serve as guidelines for government agencies, professional organizations, health care professionals, businesses, and individuals. Public health agencies monitor the progress toward health goals using objectives from the *Healthy People* documents. Widely cited by popular media, in professional journals, and at health conferences, *Healthy People* reports inspire health promotion programs throughout the country.

In *Healthy People 2010* (USDHHS, 2000), a model called a *systematic approach to health improvement* (Figure 1-4) describes four key elements of goals, objectives, determinants of health, and health status. The overall goals for *Healthy People 2010* are to increase the quality and years of life and to eliminate the nation's health disparities (USDHHS, 2000). In the *Healthy People 2010* document, there are 467 objectives written in 28 focus areas to provide direction for health care efforts on an individual, community, and national level.

These objectives focus either on interventions designed to reduce or eliminate illness, disability, and premature death or on broader issues, such as improving availability and distribution of health-related information. The goal is to achieve or make improvements for each objective by the year 2010 (USDHHS, 2000).

It is necessary to understand that many factors influence or determine the health of individuals and communities. These variables are called **determinants of health.** In the *Healthy People 2010* model (see Figure 1-4), individual biology (genetic makeup and physical and mental health) and individual behavior (responses, actions, and reactions to internal stimuli and external conditions) are able to influence health through their interaction with each other and with the person's social and physical environments. Social and physical environments include all factors, positive or negative, that affect a person's life. Numerous factors and situations influence the social and physical environment, any of which affect health. Policies and interventions also influence health. Some examples are disease prevention strategies, such as immunizations, or policies mandating child restraints and seat belts. There has been an increased concern regarding the issue of access to health care. The health of individuals and communities depends on access to quality health care services for all individuals (USDHHS, 2000).

**Health status** is a description of health that is measured by birth and death rates, life expectancy, quality of life, morbidity from specific diseases, risk factors, and many other factors. The information gathered from monitoring health status measures is used to report on the health of individuals and communities. Understanding that the determinants of health, as well as the status of the individual and community health, help to determine the health status of the nation is key to achieving the *Healthy People 2010* goals. The *Healthy People* initiatives have shown that physical health, and the improvement of physical health, is tangible, measurable, and objective (Hawks, 2004). In addition, health care professionals have become increasingly concerned with the multidimensional aspects of health, including emotional health, intellectual health, social health, and spiritual health (Hawks, 2004).

## Variables Influencing Health Beliefs and Health Practices

Persons' beliefs about their own health, as well as their health practices and the manner in which they care for themselves, will ultimately influence their health status. Health beliefs are a person's ideas and attitudes about health. A belief refers to the information or ideas that a person accepts as true, even if there is no supporting evidence (McGough, 2004). Beliefs play a very important role in health and lifestyle choices, because sometimes health choices are based solely on beliefs (McGough, 2004). Health practices are those activities that individuals do to care for themselves. Health practices include activities of daily living such as bathing and brushing teeth and formal activities such as taking medications and visiting the physician or health care provider for routine checkups. Health practices are related to self-care, or the process of taking care of oneself. It is well known that the manner in which persons care for themselves is an important determinant of their health status. In addition, there has been a shift in the approach to health care that focuses on the role of patients and their responsibility for self-care. The ability to care for oneself is as important for healthy living as it is for managing a complex medical regimen of a chronic illness. Many variables influence patients' health beliefs, health practices, and self-care. Internal and external variables influence how a person thinks and acts and how a person will deal with an illness. Consider the impact of these variables, and be able to incorporate appropriate interventions based on the person's unique characteristics. Internal variables include a person's developmental stage, intellectual background, and emotional and spiritual factors. External variables include family practices, socioeconomic factors, and cultural background.

## Internal Variables

**DEVELOPMENTAL STAGE.** A person's concept of illness is dependent on the person's developmental stage (see Chapter 19). Knowledge of the stages of growth and development will help you predict the patient's response to the present illness or the threat of future illness. Your educational interventions need to be age appropriate to be effective. For example, you use different techniques to teach contraception to an adolescent and to an adult.

**INTELLECTUAL BACKGROUND.** A person's beliefs about health are shaped in part by knowledge (or misinformation) about body functions and illnesses, educational background, and past experiences. Cognitive abilities shape the *way* a person thinks, including the ability to understand factors involved in illness and to apply knowledge of health and illness to personal health practices.

**EMOTIONAL FACTORS.** A person's degree of calm or stress influences health beliefs and practices. The manner in which a person handles stress throughout each phase of life influences the way the person reacts to illness. A person who generally is very calm often has little emotional response during illness, whereas a person normally unable to cope with stress either overreacts to illness or denies the presence of symptoms and does not take therapeutic action (see Chapter 22).

**SPIRITUAL FACTORS.** Spirituality is reflected in how a person lives his or her life, including the values and beliefs exercised, the relationships established with family and friends, and the ability to find hope and meaning in life. Spiritual health contributes to social and emotional health and additionally provides motivation for health behavior changes that determine physical and intellectual health (Hawks, 2004). Religious practices are one way people exer-

cise spirituality. You need to understand patients' spiritual beliefs to involve them effectively in nursing care (see Chapter 18).

## External Variables

**FAMILY PRATICES.** The way that families use health care services generally influences their health practices. Perceptions of the seriousness of diseases and history of preventive care behaviors (or lack of them) influence how patients will think about health. For example, a person raised in a family that believed in the importance of preventive care, such as dental checkups twice a year, is more likely to continue those health practices as an adult.

**SOCIOECONOMIC FACTORS.** Social and economic factors increase the risk for illness and influence the way that a person defines and reacts to illness. Social variables in part determine how the health care system provides medical care. Because the health care system is organized in certain ways, it determines how patients obtain care, the treatment method, the economic cost to the patient, and the potential reimbursement to the health care agency or patient. Economic variables affect a patient's level of health by increasing the risk for disease and influencing how or at what point the patient enters the health care system. In addition, economic status also affects a person's participation in treatment to maintain or improve health. A person who has high utility bills, a large family, and a low income tends to give a higher priority to food and shelter than to costly drugs or treatment or expensive foods for special diets.

**CULTURAL BACKGROUND.** A person's cultural background influences the beliefs, values, and customs of that person. It influences the approach to the health care system, personal health practices, and the nurse-patient relationship. You need to recognize and understand cultural patterns of behavior and beliefs to interact with the patient (see Chapter 17).

## Health Promotion, Wellness, and Illness Prevention

Health promotion activities are either passive or active. With **passive strategies of health promotion,** individuals gain from the activities of others without acting themselves. For example, the city decides to put fluoride in the municipal drinking water or milk manufacturers fortify homogenized milk with vitamin D. These are passive health promotion strategies. With **active strategies of health promotion,** individuals adopt specific health programs. Weight reduction and smoking cessation programs require patients to be actively involved in measures to improve their present and future levels of wellness while decreasing the risk of disease.

You need to emphasize health promotion, wellness strategies, and illness prevention activities as important forms of health care because they assist patients in maintaining and improving health. **Health promotion** activities, such as routine exercise and good nutrition, help patients maintain or enhance their present levels of health and reduce their risks of developing certain diseases. **Wellness education** teaches people how to care for themselves in a healthy way and includes topics such as physical awareness, stress management, and self-responsibility. **Illness prevention** activities, such as immunization programs, protect patients from actual or potential threats to health. The concepts of health promotion, wellness, and illness prevention are closely related and in practice overlap to some extent. All are focused on the future; the differences between them involve motivations and goals. Health promotion activities motivate people to act positively to reach more stable levels of health. Wellness strategies help patients achieve new understanding and control of their lives. Illness prevention activities motivate people to avoid declines in health or functional levels.

Illnesses, particularly chronic illnesses, contribute to much of the burden of health care costs. Therefore health care has become increasingly focused on health promotion, wellness, and illness prevention. The rapid rise of health care costs has motivated people to seek ways of decreasing the incidence and minimizing the results of illness or disability. Improving self-management, preventive services, and curative services reduces health care needs and costs. You have an important role in educating patients about improving their ability to manage their health. You do this by helping them recognize their responsibility in the health-related choices they make and also by helping them understand the impact this has on disease prevention. In the case study of Jack and the wound care specialist Kathy, there is an obvious need for greater education for Jack. Kathy teaches him to recognize alterations in skin integrity by doing more frequent skin inspections, and she teaches him the importance of seeking appropriate health care in a timely manner to avoid complications. Health promotion, wellness activities, and illness prevention are all strategies aimed at decreasing the incidence of illness and minimizing the deleterious results of that illness or disability.

## The Three Levels of Prevention

Health activities and nursing care occur at the primary, secondary, and tertiary levels of prevention (Table 1-1). Prevention includes all activities that limit the progression of a disease (Edelman and Mandle, 2002).

**Primary prevention** is true prevention. It precedes disease or dysfunction, and you apply it to patients considered physically and emotionally healthy. It is not therapeutic, does not use therapeutic treatments, and does not involve symptom identification (Edelman and Mandle, 2002). The purpose of primary prevention is to decrease the vulnerabil-

| TABLE 1-1 | The Three Levels of Prevention | | | |
|---|---|---|---|---|
| **Primary Prevention** | | **Secondary Prevention** | | **Tertiary Prevention** |
| Health Promotion | Specific Protection | Early Diagnosis and Prompt Treatment | Disability Limitations | Restoration and Rehabilitation |
| Health education | Use of specific immunizations | Case-finding measures: individual and mass | Adequate treatment to arrest disease process and prevent further complications | Provision of hospital and community facilities for training and education to maximize use of remaining capacities |
| Good standard of nutrition adjusted to developmental phases of life | Attention to personal hygiene | Screening surveys | Provision of facilities to limit disability and prevent death | Education of the public and industries to use rehabilitated persons to the fullest possible extent |
| Attention to personality development | Use of environmental sanitation | Selective examinations | | Selective placement |
| Provision of adequate housing and recreation and agreeable working conditions | Protection against occupational hazards | Cure and prevention of disease process to prevent spread of communicable disease, prevent complications, and shorten period of disability | | Work therapy in hospitals |
| Marriage counseling and sex education | Protection from accidents | | | |
| Genetic screening | Use of specific nutrients | | | |
| Periodic selective examinations | Protection from carcinogens | | | |
| | Avoidance of allergens | | | |

Modified from Leavell HR, Clark AE: *Preventive medicine for doctors in the community,* ed 3, New York, 1965, McGraw-Hill.

ity of the individual or population to an illness or dysfunction (Edelman and Mandle, 2002). Primary prevention includes passive and active strategies of health promotion. It is provided to an individual or to a general population or focuses on individuals at risk for developing specific diseases. Wellness activities (Edelman and Mandle, 2002) are synonymous with the activities identified for primary prevention by Leavell and Clark (1965) in Table 1-1. In our case study of Jack, primary prevention means simply wearing shoes at all times. Jack has diabetes and peripheral vascular disease. These conditions cause alterations in perception of pain in the extremities and alterations in circulation to the extremities. Both of these problems contribute to a risk for altered wound healing. Jack needs to make additional efforts to prevent injuries.

**Secondary prevention** focuses on persons who are experiencing health problems or illnesses and who are at risk for developing complications or worsening conditions. Activities are directed at diagnosis and prompt intervention, thereby reducing severity and enabling the patient to return to a normal level of health as early as possible (Edelman and Mandle, 2002). A large portion of secondary level nursing care is in homes, hospitals, or skilled nursing facilities. It includes screening techniques and treating early stages of disease to limit disability by delaying the consequences of advanced disease. If Jack had seen his primary care provider sooner, it is possible that earlier intervention would have prevented the progressive ulcer and the osteomyelitis. Then he could have avoided the surgical procedure and the lengthy course of IV antibiotics.

**Tertiary prevention** occurs when a defect or disability is permanent and irreversible. It involves minimizing the effects of long-term disease or disability by interventions directed at preventing complications and deterioration (Edelman and Mandle, 2002). Activities are for rehabilitation rather than diagnosis and treatment. Care at this level aims to help patients achieve as high a level of functioning as possible, despite the limitations caused by illness or impairment. This level of care is called *preventive care* because it involves preventing further disability or reduced functioning. Tertiary prevention for Jack includes continual monitoring and management of blood glucose levels and control of his diabetes. Tight control of blood glucose levels prevents further complications of his diabetes, such as diabetic ketoacidosis.

# Risk Factors

A **risk factor** is any situation, habit, environmental condition, physiological condition, or other variable that increases the vulnerability of an individual or group to an illness or accident. The presence of risk factors does not mean that a disease will develop, but risk factors increase the chances that the individual will experience a particular disease. Risk factors play a major role in how you identify a patient's health status. Risk factors also influence health beliefs and practices if a person is aware of their presence. Risk factors are in the following interrelated categories: genetic and physiological factors, age, physical environment, and lifestyle.

## Genetic and Physiological Factors

Physiological risk factors involve the physical functioning of the body. Certain physical conditions, such as being pregnant or overweight, place increased stress on physiological systems (e.g., the circulatory system), increasing susceptibility to illness in these areas. Heredity, or genetic predisposition to specific illness, is a major physical risk factor. For example, Jack has a family history of diabetes mellitus and therefore was at risk for developing the disease. Other documented genetic risk factors include family histories of cancer, heart disease, or kidney disease.

## Age

Age increases susceptibility to certain illnesses (e.g., the risk of heart disease increases with age for both genders). The risks of birth defects and complications of pregnancy increase in women bearing children after age 35. Many kinds of cancer pose a greater risk for persons over age 45 than for younger persons. Age risk factors are often closely associated with other risk factors, such as family history and personal habits. You need to educate patients about the importance of regularly scheduled checkups for their age-group (Figure 1-5).

## Physical

The physical environment in which a person works or lives increases the likelihood that certain illnesses will occur. A person's home environment often includes conditions that pose risks, such as unclean, poorly heated or cooled, or overcrowded dwellings. These conditions often increase the likelihood that a person will contract and spread infections and other diseases. Also, some kinds of cancer and other diseases are more likely to develop when industrial workers are exposed to certain chemicals or when people live near toxic waste disposal sites. Screening for these environmentally based risk factors is directed at the short-term effects of the exposure and the potential for long-term effects (Edelman and Mandle, 2002).

## Lifestyle

Lifestyle practices and behaviors have positive or negative effects on health. Practices with potential negative effects are risk factors. Examples of risk factors include overeating or poor nutrition, insufficient rest and sleep, and poor personal hygiene. Other habits that put a person at risk for illness include tobacco use, alcohol or drug abuse, and activities involving a threat of injury such as skydiving or mountain climbing. Some habits are risk factors for specific diseases. For example, excessive sunbathing increases the risk of skin

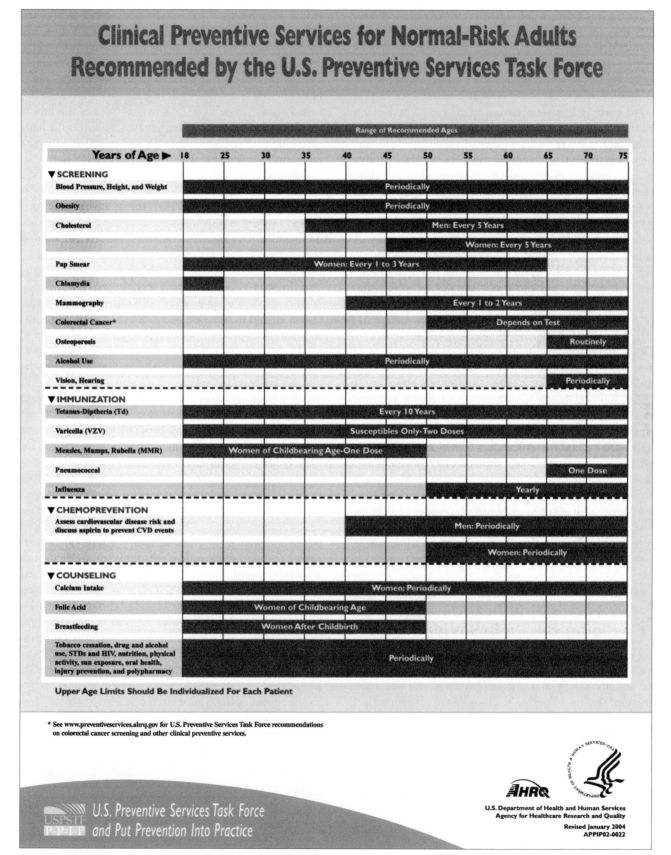

**FIGURE 1-5** Clinical preventive services for normal-risk adults recommended by the U.S Preventive Services Task Force. (From U.S. Department of Health and Human Services: *Put prevention into practice,* Rockville, Md, 2004, Agency for Health Care Research and Quality, http://www.ahrq.gov/ppip/adulttm.htm.)

cancer, and being overweight increases the risk of cardiovascular disease. These lifestyle risk factors have gained increased attention because many of the leading causes of death in the United States are related to lifestyle patterns or habits. This represents a huge impact on the economics of the health care system.

The effect of lifestyle behavior on the risk of developing disease has implications across the life span of a person. Understand that patients of all ages are vulnerable to the influences of unhealthy lifestyle patterns. You are able to influence the choices your patients make by preventing unhealthy behaviors and promoting healthy lifestyle patterns. Parents, caretakers, and teachers all influence the lifestyle practices of young children. Many adolescents encounter issues of seat belt use, gun possession, alcohol and drug use, and sexual promiscuity. Therefore it is important to understand the impact of lifestyle behaviors on health status. You need to educate your patients and the public on wellness-promoting lifestyle behaviors.

### Risk Factor Identification

The goal of risk factor identification is to assist patients in understanding those areas in their lives that they need to modify or even eliminate to promote wellness and prevent illness. You will perform comprehensive health risk appraisals, using a variety of available health risk appraisal forms, to estimate a person's specific health threats based on the presence of various risk factors (Edelman and Mandle, 2002). It is important to understand that implementation of a health risk appraisal needs to be linked with educational programs and other community resources to result in necessary lifestyle changes and risk reduction (Pender and others, 2002). You will often find risk factors in the patient's hospital record, which is from the data collected on admission to the hospital.

## Risk Factor Modification and Changing Health Behaviors

Identifying risk factors is the first step in health promotion, wellness education, and illness prevention activities. Once you identify risk factors, you implement health education programs that help a person to change a risky health behavior. This is called *risk factor modification*. Risk factor modification, health promotion, or any program that attempts to change unhealthy lifestyle behaviors is a wellness strategy in that it teaches patients to care for themselves in a healthier way. Wellness strategies need to be emphasized because they have the ability to decrease the potential high costs of unmanaged health problems.

Aim your attempts to change a behavior at stopping a health-damaging behavior (e.g., tobacco use or alcohol misuse) or adopting a healthy behavior (e.g., healthy diet or exercise) (Pender and others, 2002). When engaging an individual into health behavior change, use what you have learned from the health belief model. The health belief model is useful in analyzing the probability that a person will make changes for improving health or preventing disease (Edelman and Mandle, 2002). You need to influence the health beliefs of an individual in order to improve the individual's health. Assess what the patient believes and how the environment in which the patient lives reinforces the beliefs (McGough, 2004). Sometimes a person's beliefs and values maintain unhealthy behavior (McGough, 2004).

An understanding of the process of changing behaviors helps you support difficult health behavior change in your patients. Researchers believe that change involves movement through a series of stages. Five stages of change, ranging from no intention to change (precontemplation) to maintaining a changed behavior (maintenance stage), are in Table 1-2 (Norcross and Prochaska, 2002). Most people acting on their own do not successfully negotiate all the stages on their first attempt (Norcross and Prochaska, 2002). As an individual attempts change in behavior, relapse and recycling through the stages occurs frequently. When relapse occurs, the person will return to the contemplation or precontemplation stage before attempting change again. Relapse often feels like a failure, but the person needs to view it as a learning process. What the person learns from relapse can be applied to the next attempt to change. You need to be able to identify your patient's stage of change to implement appropriate care. Health promotion activities have a greater impact if you time them appropriately to match a specific stage of change.

The health care industry needs to do further work to design interventions and wellness strategies for people in all stages of health behavior change. A patient can maintain changes over time only if you integrate the health behavior changes into the patient's overall lifestyle. In addition, understand that true change comes from the patient's desire to change. Maintenance of healthy lifestyles prevents hospitalizations and potentially lowers the cost of health care. You assist your patients in adapting to a changed and healthier lifestyle. When health care professionals advise that a change in diet and an increase in exercise will prevent further problems, this sometimes motivates patients to adopt the needed health behaviors.

However, it is often not enough to warn people of the health risks of unhealthy behaviors. You will act as problem solver, educator, and counselor. You will help patients recognize health risks and make lifestyle changes, make informed choices, and manage their chosen lifestyle (McGough, 2004).

## Illness

**Illness** is a state in which a person's physical, emotional, intellectual, social, developmental, or spiritual functioning is diminished or impaired compared with previous experience. Cancer is a disease process, but some patients with leukemia who are responding to treatment continue to function as

| TABLE 1-2 | Stages of Health Behavior Change |
|---|---|
| | **Definition** |
| Precontemplation | Not intending to make changes within the next 6 months. |
| | Patient is unaware of the problem or underestimates it. |
| | "I guess I have faults, but there is nothing that I really need to change." |
| Contemplation | Considering a change within the next 6 months. Patient says he or she is seriously considering a change. |
| | "I have a problem and I really think I should work on it." |
| Preparation | Has tried to make changes, but without success. Intends to take action in the next month. |
| | "I have tried to quit smoking, but it didn't last long. I will probably try again in a few weeks." |
| Action | Actively engaged in strategies to change behavior. This stage sometimes lasts up to 6 months. This stage requires commitment of time and energy. |
| | "I am really working hard to change." |
| Maintenance | Sustained change over time. This stage begins 6 months after action has started and continues indefinitely. Important to avoid relapse. |
| | "I need to prevent myself from having a relapse of my problem." |

Exerpted from President and Fellows of Harvard College. *Harv Ment Health Lett* April 1 2004, http://www.health.harvard.edu/mental.

usual. Some patients with breast cancer preparing for surgery are affected in other ways than just physically. Interestingly, many patients find health within illness. An experience with illness sometimes motivates an individual to adopt more positive health behaviors. For example, Jack has likely learned the imperative nature of reducing his risk for injury by performing more frequent and better foot care.

Illness therefore is not synonymous with disease. Although you need to be familiar with different kinds of diseases and their treatments, be concerned more with illness, which includes not only disease but also the effects on functioning and well-being in all dimensions.

## Acute and Chronic Illness

Acute and chronic illnesses are two general classifications of illness used in this chapter. An **acute illness** is usually short term and severe. The symptoms appear abruptly, are intense, and often subside after a relatively short period. An acute illness affects functioning in any dimension. A **chronic illness** persists, usually longer than 6 months, and also affects functioning in any dimension. Patients fluctuate between maximal functioning and serious health relapses that are sometimes life threatening.

Because of successes in public health, medicine, and biomedical technology, acute and infectious diseases are no longer major causes of death, disease, and disability in the United States. Many health care analysts believe that the heaviest burden of illness today is due to chronic diseases that are largely preventable. Beyond the prevention of these diseases as previously discussed, a major role for nursing is to provide patient education aimed at helping patients manage their illness or disability to reduce the occurrence of symptoms and improve the tolerance of symptoms. You will also enhance wellness and improve quality of life for patients

living with chronic illnesses or disabilities. Kralik, Koch, and Price (2004) suggest that you use a holistic approach to establish a framework for assisting patients living with chronic illnesses in managing their care. In addition, self-management involves learning about responses to illnesses through daily life experiences and also as a result of trial and error. Taking responsibility for living well with illness strengthens patients. Therefore encourage patients to question the direction of their health care and to make choices about their health care (Kralik and others, 2004). The process of learning self-management skills is crucial to the transition of learning to live with a chronic illness (Kralik and others, 2004). The management of chronic illnesses promotes health within illness and also addresses human comfort and quality of life (Cumbie, Conley, and Burman, 2004). You, as a nurse, are able to reduce the impact of chronic illness on the individual, as well as on society, by providing quality, comprehensive, patient-centered care to patients living with chronic illness (Cumbie and others, 2004).

## Illness Behavior

People who are ill generally act in a way medical sociologists call **illness behavior.** It involves how people monitor their bodies, define and interpret their symptoms, take remedial actions, and use the health care system (Mechanic, 1982). Personal history, social situations, social norms, and the opportunities and constraints of community institutions all affect illness behavior (Mechanic, 1995). Although there is a large variability in the way people react to an illness, patients often use illness behavior displayed in sickness to manage life adversities (Mechanic, 1995). If people perceive themselves to be ill, illness behaviors act as coping mechanisms.

For example, illness behavior often results in patients being released from roles, social expectations, or responsibilities. For example, for Jack the foot wound and course of IV antibiotics are an added stressor or a temporary release from household and babysitting responsibilities. His wife, however, assumes the added responsibilities of caring for Jack and the grandchild.

## Variables Influencing Illness Behavior

Just as internal and external variables affect health behavior, they affect illness behavior as well. The influences of these variables affect the likelihood of seeking health care, the participation in therapy, and therefore health outcomes. Based on an understanding of these variables and behaviors, you individualize care to assist patients in coping with their illness at various stages. The goal of nursing is to promote optimal functioning in all dimensions throughout an illness.

**INTERNAL VARIABLES.** Internal variables influence the way patients behave when they are ill. These are the patient's perceptions of symptoms and the nature of the illness. If patients believe that the symptoms of their illnesses disrupt their normal routine, they are more likely to seek health care assistance than if they do not perceive the symptoms as disruptive. If patients believe that the symptoms are serious or perhaps life threatening, they are also more likely to seek assistance. Persons awakened by crushing chest pains in the middle of the night generally view this symptom as potentially serious and life threatening and will probably be motivated to seek assistance. However, sometimes such a perception also has the opposite effect. Some patients fear serious illness and react by denying it and not seeking medical assistance.

The nature of the illness, either acute or chronic, also affects a patient's illness behavior. Patients with acute illnesses are likely to seek health care and comply readily with therapy. On the other hand, a patient with a chronic illness, in which the symptoms are not curable but only partially relieved, is sometimes not motivated to comply with the therapy plan. Chronically ill patients often become less actively involved in their care, experience greater frustration, and comply less readily with care. You will generally spend more time than other health care professionals with chronically ill patients. You are in the unique position of being able to assist these patients in overcoming problems related to illness behavior.

**EXTERNAL VARIABLES.** External variables influencing a patient's illness behavior include the visibility of symptoms, social group, cultural background, economic variables, accessibility of the health care system, and social support. The visibility of the symptoms of an illness affects body image and illness behavior. A patient with a visible symptom is more likely to seek assistance than a patient who does not have visible symptoms.

Patients' social groups assist them in recognizing the threat of illness or support the denial of potential illness. Families, friends, and co-workers all influence patients' illness behavior. Patients often react positively to social support

while practicing positive health behaviors. Cultural and ethnic background teaches a person how to be healthy, how to recognize illness, and how to be ill. The effects of disease and its interpretation vary according to cultural circumstances.

Economic variables influence the way a patient reacts to illness. Because of economic constraints, a patient will delay treatment and in many cases continue to carry out daily activities. Patients' access to the health care system is closely related to economic factors. The health care system is a socioeconomic system that patients enter, interact within, and exit. For many patients, entry into the system is complex or confusing, and some patients seek nonemergency medical care in an emergency department because they do not know how to obtain health services otherwise. The physical proximity of patients to a health care agency often influences how soon they enter the system after deciding to seek care.

# Impact of Illness on Patient and Family

An illness of a family member affects the function of the entire family unit. The patient and family commonly experience behavioral and emotional changes and changes in body image, self-concept, family roles, and family dynamics.

## Behavioral and Emotional Changes

Individual behavioral and emotional reactions depend on the nature of the illness, the patient's attitude toward it, the reaction of others to it, and the variables of illness behavior. Short-term, non–life-threatening illnesses evoke few behavioral changes in the functioning of the patient or family. A husband and father who has a cold, for example, lacks the energy and patience to spend time in family activities and is irritable and prefers not to interact with his family. This is a behavioral change, but the change is subtle and does not last long. Some even consider such a change a normal response to illness.

Severe illness, particularly one that is life threatening, leads to more extensive emotional and behavioral changes, such as anxiety, shock, denial, anger, and withdrawal. These are common responses to the stress of illness. Jack and his wife, as well as the daughter who relied on her parents to care for her child, are experiencing behavioral changes in response to Jack's recovery and the knowledge of his vulnerability for further complications. You develop interventions to assist the patient and the family in coping with and adapting to this stress, because the stressor itself cannot usually be changed.

## Impact on Body Image

Body image is the subjective concept of physical appearance. Some illnesses result in changes in physical appearance, and patients and families react differently to these changes. These reactions of patients and families to changes in body image depend on the type of changes (e.g., the loss of a limb or an organ), the adaptive capacity of the family, the rate at which changes take place, and the support services available.

When a change in body image occurs, such as results from a leg amputation, the patient generally adjusts by experiencing phases of the grief process (see Chapter 23). Initially the change or impending change shocks the patient. As the patient and family recognize the reality of the change, they become anxious and sometimes withdraw. As the patient and family acknowledge the change, they gradually move toward accepting their loss. At the end of the acknowledgment phase, they accept the loss. During rehabilitation the patient is ready to learn how to adapt to the change in body image.

## Impact on Self-Concept

Self-concept is your mental self-image of all aspects of your personality. Self-concept depends in part on body image and roles but also includes other aspects of psychology and spirituality.

Self-concept is important in relationships with other family members. A patient whose self-concept changes because of illness is sometimes no longer able to meet family expectations, leading to tension or conflict. As a result, family members change their interactions with the patient. In the course of providing care, you are able to observe changes in the patient's self-concept (or in the self-concepts of family members) and develop a care plan to help the patient adjust to the changes resulting from the illness (see Chapter 20).

## Impact on Family Roles and Family Dynamics

People have many roles in life, such as wage earner, decision maker, professional, and parent. When an illness occurs, the roles of the patient and family change (see Chapter 21). Such a change is either subtle and short term or drastic and long term. Patients and their families generally adjust more easily to subtle, short-term changes. Long-term changes, however, require an adjustment process similar to the grief process (see Chapter 23). The patient and family often require specific counseling and guidance to assist them in coping with the role changes.

Family dynamics is the process by which the family functions, makes decisions, gives support to individual members, and copes with everyday changes and challenges. Because of the effects of illness, family dynamics often change. Role functions stop or are delayed. Another family member sometimes needs to assume the patient's usual roles and responsibilities. This often creates tension or anxiety in the family. Role reversal is also common. If a parent of an adult becomes ill and is unable to carry out usual activities, the adult child often assumes many of the parent's responsibilities. Such a reversal leads to conflicting responsibilities for the adult child or direct conflict over decision making. You will view the whole family and plan care to help the family regain the maximal level of functioning and well-being (see Chapter 21).

## KEY CONCEPTS

- Health and wellness are not merely the absence of disease and illness. Many variables determine the health status of an individual or community. A person's state of health, wellness, or illness depends on individual values, personality, and lifestyle.
- Unsatisfied needs motivate human beings. Basic human needs must be met before an individual is able to focus on higher level needs.
- The health belief model considers factors influencing health beliefs.
- The health promotion model increases individual well-being and self-actualization.
- Holistic health models of nursing promote optimal health by incorporating active participation of the patient in improving the health state. Holistic nursing interventions complement standard medical therapy.
- Internal and external variables influence health beliefs and practices, and you consider these when planning care.
- Health promotion activities help maintain or enhance health. Wellness education teaches patients how to care for

themselves. Illness prevention activities protect against health threats and thus maintain an optimal level of health.
- Nursing incorporates health promotion, wellness, and illness prevention activities rather than simply treating illness.
- The three levels of prevention are primary, secondary, and tertiary.
- Risk factors threaten health, influence health practices, and are important considerations in illness prevention activities. Risk factors involve genetic or physiological variables, age, physical environment, and lifestyle.
- Improvement in health often involves a change in health behaviors.
- Illness behavior, like health practices, is influenced by many variables, which you consider when you are planning care.
- Illness has many effects on the patient and family, including changes in behavior and emotions, family roles and dynamics, body image, and self-concept.

## CRITICAL THINKING IN PRACTICE

*Mr. Grow, 36 years old, is a financial adviser for a large company. He is married and has three small children. He is overweight and does not exercise. He often eats fast food at lunchtime in the car between appointments. His own father recently died from complications of a stroke. His wife is worried that he does not take care of himself.*

- - - - - - - - - - - - - - - - - -

1. a. Identify risk factors that increase Mr. Grow's susceptibility to disease.
   b. What risk factors need to be modified?
2. Based on Mr. Grow's risk factors for susceptibility to disease, what are important health promotion topics that you need to include while you provide education about health promotion to Mr. Grow?
3. Mr. Grow states, "I have tried to make changes in my diet and I tried to exercise every day, but I just never seem to be successful at making any healthy changes in my life.

I am thinking about trying to make some changes again after I get back from my vacation in about 2 weeks from now." Using the Stages of Change Model, which stage best describes Mr. Grow's desire to change.
4. Mr. Grow states that there are other people at work who are also overweight and who have stressful jobs. Therefore, you decide to implement a health promotion project at Mr. Grow's office. You provide education to the employees at the financial company about exercise and stress management. Then, you encourage the employees to walk over their lunch break and role play different stress management techniques. How would you evaluate the effectiveness of your health promotion program?

## NCLEX® REVIEW

1. Health is:
   1. The absence of illness
   2. The opposite of disease
   3. A condition between disease and good health
   4. A state of complete physical, mental, and social well-being
2. A person's state of health, wellness, or illness depends on an individual's:
   1. Self-concept
   2. Lifestyle only
   3. Known risk factors
   4. Values, personality, and lifestyle
3. According to the health belief model, health beliefs usually influence:
   1. Health status
   2. Health outcomes
   3. Health behaviors
   4. Health determinants
4. The health promotion model attempts to explain the:
   1. Effect of environment on an individual
   2. Effect of health activities on an individual
   3. Reasons individuals avoid health activities
   4. Reasons individuals engage in health activities
5. Holistic health interventions are used to:
   1. Replace standard medical therapy
   2. Improve standard medical therapy
   3. Complement standard medical therapy
   4. Compete with standard medical therapy
6. The health status of an individual or community is:
   1. Multifactorial
   2. One dimensional
   3. Determined by genetics
   4. Determined by environment

7. The internal variables that influence a patient's health beliefs and health practices are:
   1. Family practices, developmental stage, intellectual background, emotional factors
   2. Cultural background, emotional factors, spiritual factors, developmental stage
   3. Socioeconomic factors, intellectual background, spiritual factors, family practices
   4. Developmental stage, intellectual background, emotional factors, spiritual factors
8. Health promotion activities are activities that:
   1. Treat disease
   2. Prevent illness
   3. Help maintain or enhance health
   4. Aim at protecting against health threats
9. Primary prevention strategies:
   1. Identify disease problems
   2. Treat chronic disease states
   3. Reduce the severity of an illness
   4. Decrease vulnerability to an illness
10. The presence of certain risk factors:
    1. Has no role in health practices
    2. Suggests that a disease will definitely develop
    3. Increases the chance that disease will develop
    4. Decreases the chance that disease will progress
11. Changing health behaviors:
    1. Is easier for health care professionals
    2. Is difficult without guidance from a health care professional
    3. May be initiated regardless of the patient's stage in the change process
    4. May be either a cessation of health-damaging behavior or the adoption of a healthy behavior

12. External variables that influence a patient's illness behavior are:
    1. The nature of the illness and the perception of symptoms
    2. The perception of symptoms and the visibility of the symptoms
    3. The visibility of symptoms, social group, economics, and social support
    4. Dependent on the degree to which they disrupt the patient's normal routine
13. After reading the case study of Jack's hospitalization and illness, you understand that his illness is likely to affect the function of the:
    1. Siblings
    2. Parental dyad
    3. Individual only
    4. Entire family unit

14. You are a staff nurse working on a medical acute care unit. You are providing discharge teaching to a patient newly diagnosed with diabetes. You are trying to explain the dosage for the newly prescribed medications and the importance of follow-up visits in the clinic. The patient states: "I have not slept well for 3 days; I am tired, hungry, and uncomfortable. I will think about that later. I just want to go home." Understanding Maslow's hierarchy of needs, you understand that:
    1. The patient will not be able to listen to discharge instructions until his basic needs of sleep, comfort, and food have been met
    2. The patient should be forced to make a follow-up appointment immediately before he leaves your care in order to accomplish unresolved teaching
    3. You will need to make the appointment for him
    4. You should administer a quick examination to assess his knowledge level of the content you have taught

## REFERENCES

Becker MH, Maiman LA: Sociobehavioral determinants of compliance with health and medical care recommendations, *Med Care* 13(1):10, 1975.

Benson SG, Dundis SP: Understanding and motivating health care employees: integrating Maslow's hierarchy of needs, training and technology, *J Nurs Manag* 11:315, 2003.

Capasso VA, Munro BH: The cost and efficacy of two wound treatments, *AORN J* 77(5):984, 2003.

Cumbie SA, Conley VM, Burman ME: Advanced practice nursing models for comprehensive care with chronic illness: model for promoting process engagement, *Adv Nurs Sci* 27(1):70, 2004.

Edelman CL, Mandle CL: *Health promotion throughout the life span,* ed 5, St. Louis, 2002, Mosby.

Hawks S: Spiritual wellness, holistic health, and the practice of health education, *Am J Health Educ* 35(1):11, 2004.

Kralik D, Koch T, Price K: Chronic illness self-management: taking care to create order, *J Clin Nurs* 13(2):259, 2004.

Leavell HR, Clark AE: *Preventive medicine for doctors in the community,* ed 3, New York, 1965, McGraw-Hill.

Maslow AH: *Motivation and personality,* ed 3, New York, 1954, Harper & Row.

Maslow AH: *Motivation and personality,* ed 2, New York, 1970, Harper & Row.

Maslow AH: *Motivation and personality,* ed 3, Upper Saddle River, NJ, 1987, Prentice Hall.

McGough G: Using health psychology to support health education, *Nurs Stand* 18(39):46, 2004.

Mechanic D: The epidemiology of illness behavior and its relationship to physical and psychological distress. In Mechanic D: *Symptoms, illness behavior, and help seeking,* New York, 1982, Prodist.

Mechanic D: Sociological dimensions of illness behavior, *Soc Sci Med* 41(9):1207, 1995.

Mendel J: Scientific, philosophical and social informants of holistic health care, *Aust J Holist Nurs* 10(1):13, 2003.

Nelson DE and others: State trends in health risk factors and receipt of clinical preventive services among U.S. adults during the 1990s, *JAMA* 287(20):2659, 2002.

Norcross JC, Prochaska JO: Using the stages of change, *Harv Ment Health Lett* 18(11):5, 2002.

Pender NJ: *Health promotion and nursing practice,* Norwalk, Conn, 1982, Appleton-Century-Crofts.

Pender NJ: Health promotion and illness prevention. In Werley HH, Fitzpatrick JJ, editors: *Annual review of nursing research,* New York, 1993, Springer.

Pender NJ: *Health promotion and nursing practice,* ed 3, Stamford, Conn, 1996, Appleton & Lange.

Pender NJ, Murdaugh CL, Parsons MA: *Health promotion and nursing practice,* ed 4, Upper Saddle River, NJ, 2002, Prentice Hall.

Rosenstoch I: Historical origin of the health belief model, *Health Educ Monogr* 2:334, 1974.

Saylor C: Health redefined: a foundation for teaching nursing strategies, *Nurse Educ* 28(6):261, 2003.

U.S. Department of Health and Human Services: *Put prevention into practice,* Rockville, Md, 2004, Agency for Health Care Research and Quality, http://www.ahrq.gov/ppip/adulttm.htm.

U.S. Department of Health and Human Services, Public Health Service: *Healthy people: the Surgeon General's report on health promotion and disease prevention,* Washington, DC, 1979, U.S. Government Printing Office.

U.S. Department of Health and Human Services, Public Health Service: *Healthy people 2000: national health promotion and disease prevention objectives,* Washington, DC, 1990, U.S. Government Printing Office.

U.S. Department of Health and Human Services, Public Health Service: *Healthy people 2010: understanding and improving health,* Washington, DC, 2000, U.S. Government Printing Office.

U.S. Department of Health and Human Services, U.S. Preventive Services Task Force and Put Prevention Into Practice: *Clinical preventive services for normal-risk adults,* Washington, DC, 2004, U.S. Government Printing Office, http://www.ahrq.gov/ppip/pptools.htm.

World Health Organization Interim Commission: *Chronicle of WHO,* Geneva, 1947, The Organization.

# CHAPTER 2

# The Health Care Delivery System

## MEDIA RESOURCES

 **CD COMPANION** *evolve* **WEBSITE**

http://evolve.elsevier.com/Potter/basic

- **NCLEX® Review**
- **Audio Glossary**
- **English/Spanish Audio Glossary**

## OBJECTIVES

- Describe the six levels of health care.
- Explain the relationship between levels of care and levels of prevention.
- Discuss the types of settings where professionals provide various levels of health care.
- Discuss the role of nurses in different health care delivery settings.
- Differentiate primary care from primary health care.

- Explain the advantages and disadvantages of managed health care.
- Compare the various methods for financing health care.
- Discuss the implications that changes in the health care system have on nursing.
- Discuss opportunities for nursing within the changing health care delivery system.

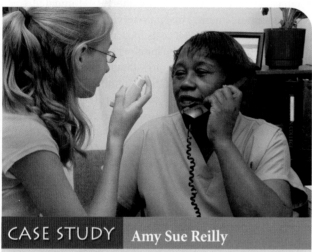

## CASE STUDY    Amy Sue Reilly

Amy Sue Reilly is a 15-year-old white female of Irish descent. She is a freshman at a Catholic high school. Her parents are divorced. Her mother, Anne, is a cashier at a local grocery store, and her father, Joseph, is a lawyer. She has two brothers and lives at home with her mother. Although her parents are divorced, Amy Sue reports that her family is very close and that her parents work together to meet all their children's needs.

Amy Sue has had asthma since she was 5 years old. Amy Sue has been able to control her asthma by taking oral medications and by using her inhalers when needed. However, she recently has had some difficulty breathing, especially during gym class.

Corrine is a 45-year-old African-American nurse. She recently accepted a job as a school nurse for the four Catholic schools in the area. Three of the schools are grade schools, and there is one high school. Before she took this job, Corrine worked at a pediatrician's office. Amy Sue's difficulty managing her asthma is significant for Corrine because Corrine's oldest daughter has asthma. In addition, because of her job in the pediatrician's office, Corrine has had experience with caring for children with asthma and with helping patients access the health care delivery system.

One day during gym class, Amy Sue enters Corrine's office. Amy Sue is having more problems breathing than usual. Corrine decides that Amy Sue needs to see to her physician today for treatment. After talking with Amy Sue, Corrine determines that Amy Sue is unsure of her insurance coverage. Corrine calls and notifies Anne of the change in Amy Sue's

health and the need for medical treatment. As they are on the phone, Anne states, "Our insurance company just switched from a preferred provider organization (PPO) to a health maintenance organization (HMO). As a result, we are in the middle of switching all our physicians because our HMO does not include the physicians we used to see for medical help. We have to see a new internal medicine physician in order to get a referral to a new pulmonary physician. Amy Sue is not scheduled to see the internal medicine physician for 3 more weeks! I am also not sure exactly what I need to do to make sure that our insurance will pay for Amy Sue's care and medications. I just do not know what to do right now. All these changes have made me so frustrated. I know that Amy Sue needs medical help, but I do not know where to send her. What do you think I should do?"

## KEY TERMS

acute care, p. 21
adult day care centers, p. 30
assisted living, p. 30
capitation, p. 20
case management, p. 25
critical pathway, p. 25
diagnosis-related groups (DRGs), p. 20
discharge planning, p. 25
evidence-based practice, p. 31
extended care facility, p. 29
globalization, p. 35
home care, p. 27
hospice, p. 31
independent practice association (IPA), p. 22

integrated delivery networks (IDNs), p. 21
managed care, p. 20
Medicaid, p. 28
Medicare, p. 28
Minimum Data Set (MDS), p. 29
nursing-sensitive outcomes, p. 32
outliers, p. 27
patient-centered care, p. 33
primary care, p. 22
professional standards review organizations (PSROs), p. 20
prospective payment system (PPS), p. 20
rehabilitation, p. 28
resource utilization groups (RUGs), p. 20

*Continued*

As you begin your career in nursing, you will quickly realize that the U.S. health care system is very complex and is constantly changing. Although health professionals from varied disciplines offer a broad variety of services to the public, gaining access to services is very difficult for those with limited health care insurance. The continuing emergence of new technologies and medications causes the costs of health care to skyrocket. Pressures to reduce costs come from declining reimbursement by third-party payers and from health care institutions being managed more as businesses than as service organizations. The challenges faced in reducing the costs of health care make it difficult for health care providers to maintain high-quality care for their patients. Many patients who would have been hospitalized for their condition 10 years ago are now treated in outpatient facilities, in part to reduce the costs resulting from lengthy hospitalization. As a result, hospitalized patients are sicker, and their treatment involves a higher level of technological care. Patients are discharged from hospitals sooner, often leaving families with the burden of providing care in the home setting. Nurses also face significant challenges of keeping individuals healthy and well within their own homes and communities.

Nursing is a caring discipline. The values of our profession are rooted in helping persons to regain, maintain, or improve their health; prevent illness; and find comfort and dignity. The health care system of the new millennium has become less service oriented and much more business oriented because of cost-saving initiatives. As a result, the practice of nursing is changing. Nursing needs to lead the way in change and retain its values for patient care while meeting the challenges of new roles and new responsibilities.

## Health Care Regulation and Competition

Through most of the twentieth century, there were few incentives for controlling health care costs. If a patient needed to be in the hospital a few extra days for a wound to heal or for the family to prepare to take care of him at home, there were few obstacles. Whatever a physician or health care provider chose to order for a patient's care and treatment, insurers (third-party payers) paid for. However, as health care costs continued to rise out of control, regulatory and competitive approaches have attempted to control health care spending. For example, **professional standards review organizations (PSROs)** were created to review the quality, quantity, and cost of hospital care provided through Medicare and Medicaid (Sultz and Young, 2004). Medicare-qualified hospitals are now required to have physician-supervised **utilization review (UR) committees** to review admissions, diagnostic testing, and treatments provided by physicians or health care providers to patients. The purpose is to identify and eliminate overuse of diagnostic and treatment services. Many hospitals have added nursing case managers to help meet the guidelines established by Medicare, Medicaid, and other payers.

One of the most significant factors that influenced how health care was paid for and that affected costs and competition was the **prospective payment system (PPS)**. Established by Congress in 1983, the PPS eliminated cost-based reimbursement. Hospitals serving Medicare patients were no longer paid for all costs incurred to deliver care to a patient. Instead, inpatient hospital services for Medicare patients were combined into 468 **diagnosis-related groups (DRGs)**. Each group has a fixed reimbursement amount with adjustments for case severity, rural/urban/regional costs, and teaching costs. Hospitals receive a set dollar amount for each patient based on the assigned DRG, regardless of the patient's length of stay or use of services in the hospital. Box 2-1 provides a hypothetical scenario, showing how the DRG PPS determines reimbursement for a patient's care. Most health care providers (e.g., health care networks or managed care organizations) now receive capitated payments. **Capitation** is the payment mechanism in which providers receive a fixed amount per patient or enrollee of a health care plan (Gosden and others, 2005). The purpose of capitation is to build a payment plan for select diagnoses or surgical procedures that includes the best standards of care, including essential diagnostic and treatment procedures, at the lowest cost.

Capitation and prospective payment have influenced the way care health care professionals deliver care in all types of settings. Rehabilitation settings now use DRGs, and long-term care settings use **resource utilization groups (RUGs)**. In all settings the health care industry makes an effort to manage costs so that the organizations will remain profitable. For example, when patients are hospitalized for lengthy periods, hospitals absorb the portion of costs not reimbursed. This simply adds more pressure to ensure that patients are managed effectively and discharged as soon as is reasonably possible. Soon after implementing prospective payment, hospitals began to increase discharge planning activities, and hospital lengths of stay began to shorten. Because patients are discharged home as soon as possible, home care agencies now provide complex technological care, including intravenous therapy, mechanical ventilation, and long-term parenteral nutrition.

The term **managed care** describes health care systems in which there is administrative control over primary health care services for a defined patient population. The provider or health care system receives a predetermined capitated

---

**BOX 2-1** | **Clinical Scenario of a DRG Example**

Mr. Truman, a 70-year-old man, went to his cardiologist because he was experiencing chest pain and shortness of breath. He had had cardiac surgery almost 10 years before but was beginning to have recurrent chest pain, even at rest. He has a history of hypertension and emphysema. Mr. Truman has smoked 1 pack of cigarettes a day for 54 years and does not follow a low-fat diet. He has been counseled to quit smoking, but he has been unwilling to stop. He was hospitalized late in the afternoon on November 1 after having a chest x-ray examination and laboratory work done at an outpatient testing center. He had an echocardiogram on November 2. Early in the morning on November 3, Mr. Truman had a cardiac catheterization, and the cardiologist determined he did not need surgery. He was discharged on the evening of November 3. During his hospital stay, Mr. Truman received usual and customary care and experienced no complications.

*Principal diagnosis:* Chest pain, not otherwise specified (NOS)

*Secondary diagnosis:* Hypertension NOS, hyperlipidemia, tobacco use disorder, other lung disease, history of past noncompliance
*Principal procedure:* Left heart cardiac catheterization
*DRG assigned:* DRG 125: Circulatory disorders except acute myocardial infarction with cardiac catheterization without complex diagnosis
*Average length of stay:* 2.8 days
*Actual length of stay:* 2 days
*Expected payment from Medicare (based on 2.8 days):* Estimated national average hospital base rate × relative weight for DRG = $4430 × 1.146 = $5077
*Actual hospital charges for Mr. Truman:* $11,700
*Actual reimbursement from Medicare:* $5300
*Loss for hospital:* $6400

Data from Ingenix and others: *DRG expert,* ed 21, Clifton Park, NY, 2005, Thomson Delmar Learning.

---

payment for each patient enrolled in the program. In this case, the managed care organization bears financial risk in addition to providing patient care. The organization's focus of care shifts from individual illness care to concern for the health of its covered population. If people stay healthy, the cost of medical care declines. Systems of managed care focus on containing or reducing costs, increasing patient satisfaction, and improving the health or functional status of the individual (Sultz and Young, 2004).

In theory, if people stay healthy, the cost of medical care declines. The purpose of managed care is to increase access to care while decreasing costs. However, health care spending continues to rise. The National Health Statistics Group reported that health care spending increased from $888 billion, or 13.4% of the gross domestic product (GDP), in 1993 to $1.679 trillion, or 15.3% of the GDP, in 2003. They project this amount will increase to $3.586 trillion, or 18.7% of the GDP, in the year 2014 (Heffler and others, 2005). Increases in health care spending are related to rising health care wages, increased costs of prescription drugs, higher insurance premiums, improved technology, and consumer demands.

You do not have to be a health care financing expert in your role as a nurse. However, it is important for you to understand the basics of health care financing to recognize the effects on employers and patients. Table 2-1 summarizes the most common types of health care plans.

## Levels of Health Care

The health care industry is moving toward health care practices that emphasize managing health rather than managing illness. The premise is that in the long term, health promotion reduces health care costs. A wellness perspective focuses on the health of populations and the communities in which they live rather than just on finding a cure for an individual's disease (Merzel and D'Afflitti, 2003). Larger health care systems have attempted to develop **integrated delivery networks (IDNs)** that include a set of providers and services organized to deliver a coordinated continuum of care to the population of patients served at a capitated cost (Oodyke, 2004). An integrated system reduces duplication of services, coordinates care across settings, and ensures that patients receive care in the most appropriate setting.

The health care system provides six levels of care (Figure 2-1): preventive, primary, secondary, tertiary, restorative, and continuing care. Levels of care describe the scope of services and settings where health care is offered to patients in all stages of health and illness. For example, the secondary level of care is the traditional **acute care** setting where patients who have signs and symptoms of disease are diagnosed and treated. **Restorative care** includes those settings and services where patients who are recovering from illness or disability receive rehabilitation and supportive care. Levels of care are not the same as levels of prevention (see Chapter 1). Levels of prevention describe the focus of health-related activities: avoiding disease (health promotion and disease prevention), curing disease (secondary prevention), and diminishing complications (tertiary prevention). At any level of care, nurses and other health care providers offer a variety of levels of prevention. For example, the nurse working in an acute care, tertiary setting, monitors the recovery of a patient who has had open heart surgery while also providing health promotion information to the family concerning diet and exercise.

It is important for you to understand how the health care industry organizes and delivers different levels of care. Each level creates different requirements and opportunities for

| TABLE 2-1 | Health Care Plans | |
|---|---|---|
| Type | Definition | Characteristics |
| Managed care organization (MCO) | Provides comprehensive, preventive, and treatment services to a specific group of voluntarily enrolled persons. Structures include a variety of models: *Staff model:* Physicians are salaried employees of the MCO. *Group model:* MCO contracts with single group practice. *Network model:* MCO contracts with multiple group practices and/or integrated organizations. **Independent practice association (IPA):** MCO contracts with physicians who usually are not members of groups and whose practices include fee-for-service and capitated patients. | Focus on health maintenance, primary care. All care provided by a primary care physician. Referral needed for access to specialist and hospitalization. |
| Medicare MCO | Program same as MCO but designed to cover health care costs of senior citizens. | Premium generally less than supplemental plans. |
| Preferred provider organization (PPO) | One that limits an enrollee's choice to a list of "preferred" hospitals, physicians, and providers. An enrollee pays more out-of-pocket expenses for using a provider not on the list. | Contractual agreement exists between a set of providers and one or more purchasers (self-insured employers or insurance plans). Comprehensive health services at a discount to companies under contract. Focus on health maintenance. |
| Exclusive provider organization (EPO) | One that limits an enrollee's choice to providers belonging to one organization. Sometimes able to use outside providers at additional expense. | Limited contractual agreement. Less access to select specialists. |
| Medicare | Federally funded national health insurance program in the United States for people over age 65. Part A provides basic protection for medical, surgical, and psychiatric care costs based on diagnosis-related groups (DRGs). Part B is a voluntary medical insurance; covers physician and certain outpatient services. | Payment for plan deducted from monthly individual Social Security check. Covers services of nurse practitioners. Does not pay full cost of certain services. Supplemental insurance is encouraged. |
| Medicaid | Federally funded, state-operated program of medical assistance to people with low incomes. Individual states determine eligibility and benefits. | Finances a large portion of maternal and child care for the poor. Reimburses for nurse midwifery and other advanced practice nurses (varies by state). Reimburses nursing home funding. |
| Private insurance | Traditional fee-for-service plan. Payment computed after services are provided on basis of number of services used. | Policies typically expensive. Most policies have deductibles that patients pay before insurance pays. |
| Long-term care insurance | Supplemental insurance for coverage of long-term care services. Policies provide a set amount of dollars for an unlimited time or for as little as 2 years. | Very expensive. Good policy has a minimum waiting period for eligibility, payment for skilled nursing, intermediate or custodial care, and home care. |

your role as a nurse. Box 2-2 highlights the types of services available to patients and families at each level of care. Changes unique to each level of care have developed as a result of health care reform. For example, the health care industry now places greater emphasis on wellness; thus the health care industry directs more resources towards primary and preventive care. Nursing has the chance to provide leadership to communities and health care systems that are coordinating resources to better serve their populations. The ability to find strategies that better address patient needs at all levels of care is critical to the success of improving the health care delivery system.

## Preventive and Primary Health Care Services

In the settings that deliver preventive and **primary care**, such as schools, physicians' or health care providers' offices, occupational health clinics, and nursing centers, health promotion is a major theme (Table 2-2). Health promotion is a key to quality health care. Successful programs help patients acquire healthier lifestyles and achieve a decent standard of living. The focus of health promotion is to keep people healthy through personal hygiene, good nutrition, clean living environments, regular exercise, rest, and the adoption of positive health attitudes. Health promotion programs lower the overall costs of health care by reducing the incidence of

Level of Care    Description

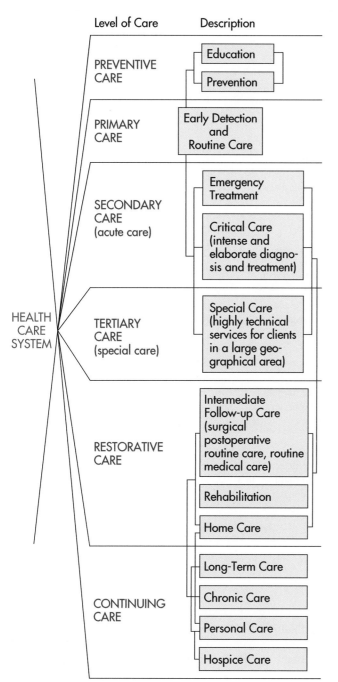

FIGURE **2-1** Spectrum of health services delivery. (Modified from Cambridge Research Institute: *Trends affecting the U.S. health care system,* 262, Health Planning Information Series, Human Resources Administration, Public Health Service, Department of Health, Education, and Welfare, Washington, DC, 1976, revised and updated 1992, U.S. Government Printing Office.)

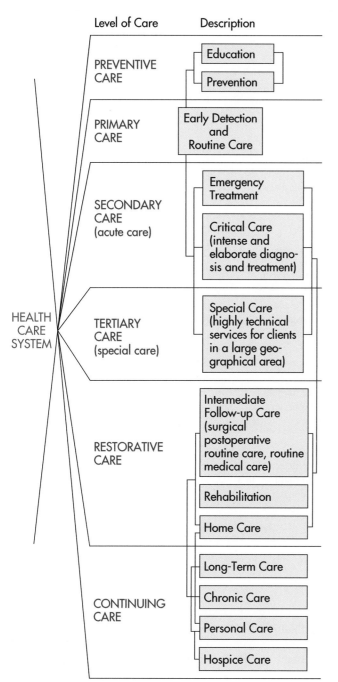

---

**BOX 2-2**    **Examples of Health Care Services**

**Preventive Care**

Blood pressure and cancer screening
Immunizations
Poison control information
Mental health counseling and crisis prevention
Community legislation (seat belts, air bags, bike helmets)

**Primary Care (Health Promotion)**

Prenatal care
Well-baby care
Nutrition counseling
Family planning
Exercise classes

**Secondary Acute Care**

Emergency care
Acute medical-surgical care
Radiological procedures

**Tertiary Care**

Intensive care
Subacute care

**Restorative Care**

Cardiovascular and pulmonary rehabilitation
Sports medicine
Spinal cord injury programs
Home care

**Continuing Care**

Assisted living
Psychiatric and older adult day care

disease and minimizing complications, thus reducing the need to use more expensive health care resources. In contrast, preventive care is more disease-oriented and focused on reducing and controlling risk factors for disease through activities such as immunization and occupational health programs.

Health care providers at the primary level of health care build interventions that lead to improved health outcomes for an entire population. The primary level of health care includes medical and health care services as well as health education, nutritional counseling, maternal/child health care, family planning, immunizations, and control of diseases. The primary health care model (Figure 2-2, p. 25) focuses on cooperation between health professionals and community members. This model emphasizes health promotion, the development of health polices, and the prevention of diseases within communities. The parts of the model are linked with each other and affect each other either positively or negatively. Successful community-based primary health care programs take societal and environmental factors into consideration when addressing the health needs of communities (Merzel and D'Afflitti, 2003). Chapter 3 provides a more comprehensive discussion of primary health care in the community.

## Secondary and Tertiary Care

The diagnosis and treatment of illness are traditionally the most commonly used services of the health care delivery sys-

## TABLE 2-2 Preventive and Primary Care Services

| Type of Service | Purpose | Available Programs/Services |
|---|---|---|
| School health | Comprehensive programs that integrate health promotion principles throughout a school's curriculum. Services stress program management, interdisciplinary collaboration, and community health principles. | Positive life skills<br>Nutritional planning<br>Health screening<br>Counseling<br>Communicable disease prevention<br>Crisis intervention |
| Occupational health | A comprehensive program geared to health promotion and accident or illness prevention. Goal is to increase worker productivity, decrease absenteeism, and reduce use of expensive medical care. | Environmental surveillance<br>Physical assessment<br>Health screening<br>Health education<br>Communicable disease control<br>Counseling |
| Physicians' offices | Provide primary health care (diagnosis and treatment). Beginning to focus more on health promotion practices. Advanced nurse practitioners often partner with a physician in managing patient population. | Routine physical examination<br>Health screening<br>Diagnostics<br>Treatment of acute and chronic ailments |
| Nursing centers | Nurse-managed clinics provide nursing services with a focus on health promotion and health education, chronic disease assessment management, and support for self-care and caregivers. | Day care<br>Physical and developmental<br>Health risk appraisal<br>Wellness counseling<br>Employment readiness<br>Acute and chronic care management |
| Block and parish nursing | Nurses living within a neighborhood provide services to older patients or those unable to leave their home. Provides services that are not available in traditional health care system. | Running errands<br>Transportation<br>Respite care<br>Homemaker aides<br>Spiritual health |
| Community Centers | Outpatient clinics that provide primary care to a specific patient population (e.g., well-baby, mental health, diabetes) that lives in a specific community. Sometimes affiliated with a hospital, medical school, church or other community organization. | Physical assessment<br>Health screening<br>Disease management<br>Health education<br>Counseling |

tem. With the arrival of managed care, these services are now often delivered at the primary level of care. For example, more physicians are performing simple surgeries in office surgical suites. However, if a patient develops a problem that the physician or health care provider is not able to care for, the patient will need a medical specialist. Care from a specialist sometimes requires hospitalization of the patient. Typically secondary care and tertiary care (also called *acute care*) are quite costly, particularly if patients wait to seek health care until after symptoms have developed.

**HOSPITALS.** Hospital emergency departments, urgent care centers, critical care units, and inpatient medical-surgical units are sites that provide secondary and tertiary levels of care. When you work in these settings, you will be challenged to work closely with all members of the health care team. Your ability to think critically and to identify patients' changing problems quickly and accurately will be essential. Planning and coordination of care are necessary to deliver services in a competent and timely manner. You will need to apply nursing research findings when selecting nursing interventions to improve patient outcomes. As a nurse you will constantly evaluate whether care is effective and how to improve it.

Customer service is the philosophy of most acute care organizations. Patient satisfaction becomes a priority in a busy, stressful location such as an inpatient nursing unit. Patients expect you to treat them courteously and respectfully and to involve them in daily care decisions. It is necessary for acute care nurses to be aware of patient needs and expectations early to form effective partnerships that ultimately enhance the level of nursing care given.

Managed care organizations expect patients who are hospitalized with a medical diagnosis or who enter the hospital to have a surgery to be cared for and discharged within a projected time period. Therefore, if you work in a hospital, you will need to use resources efficiently to help your patients

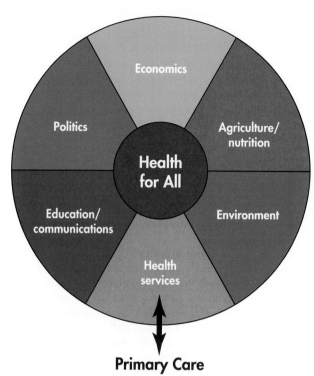

**Primary Care**

FIGURE **2-2** Primary health care model: a multisectoral or intersectoral approach. (© 1996 by P. Hatcher, J. Shoultz, W. Patrick; from Shoultz J, Hatcher PA: Looking beyond primary care to primary health care: an approach to community-based action, *Nurs Outlook* 45[1]:23, 1997.)

successfully recover and return home (Box 2-3). To contain costs, many hospitals have redesigned nursing units. Because of **work redesign,** more services are available on nursing units, thus minimizing the need to transfer and transport patients across multiple diagnostic and treatment areas.

Hospitalized patients are acutely ill and need comprehensive and specialized tertiary health care. The services provided by hospitals vary considerably. Some small rural hospitals offer only limited emergency and diagnostic services, as well as general inpatient services. In comparison, large urban medical centers offer comprehensive, state-of-the-art diagnostic services, trauma and emergency care, surgical intervention, intensive care units, inpatient services, and rehabilitation facilities. Larger hospitals hire professional staff from a variety of specialties such as social service, respiratory therapy, physical and occupational therapy, and speech therapy. The focus in hospitals is to provide the highest quality of care possible so that patients are discharged early but safely to the home or another health care facility that will adequately manage any remaining health care needs.

Because of the need to contain costs, many hospitals use a **case management** model of care. In this model a case manager, who is usually a nurse or a social worker, coordinates the efforts of all disciplines to achieve the most efficient and appropriate plan of care for the patient. Case management is particularly focused on discharge planning. The case manager advises nursing staff on specific nursing care issues and coordinates the referral of patients to services provided by other disciplines. The case manager also ensures that health care workers implement patient education and monitors the patient's progress through discharge. In many settings a case manager continues caring for patients after discharge from acute care facilities.

*Discharge planning begins the moment a patient is admitted to a health care facility.* You will play a large role in **discharge planning** if you choose to work in a hospital. Continuity of care is important in an acute care hospital. To achieve continuity of care, you use critical thinking skills and apply the nursing process (see Unit II). You anticipate and identify the patient's needs and work with all members of the multidisciplinary health care team to develop a plan of care that moves the patient from the hospital to another environment, such as the patient's home or a nursing home. Discharge planning is a centralized, coordinated, multidisciplinary process that ensures that the patient has a plan for continuing care after leaving a health care agency.

One tool you will use in an acute care setting to coordinate your patients' care is a critical pathway. A **critical pathway** is a multidisciplinary treatment plan that shows what treatments or interventions patients need to have while they are in the hospital for a specific reason. For example, some hospitals have critical pathways for patients who have pneumonia or congestive heart failure. The critical pathway helps ensure collaboration among different members of the health care team, which enables the patient to be discharged in an appropriate time frame.

Because patients leave hospitals as soon as their physical conditions allow, they often have continuing health care needs when they go home or to another facility. For example, a patient still requires wound care after surgery, or a patient who has had a stroke still requires ambulation training. Patients and families worry about how they will care for the patient's needs and manage illness over the long term. As the nurse, you will help by anticipating and identifying patients' continuing needs before the actual time of discharge and by coordinating health team members in achieving an appropriate discharge plan.

Some patients are more in need of discharge planning because of the risks they present (e.g., patients with limited financial resources or limited family support and patients with long-term disabilities or chronic illness). However, any patient who is being discharged from a health care facility with remaining functional limitations or who needs to follow certain restrictions or therapies for recovery needs discharge planning. All caregivers who care for a patient with a specific health problem participate in discharge planning. The process is truly multidisciplinary. For example, the patient with diabetes visiting a diabetes management center requires the collaboration of a nurse educator, dietitian, and physician or health care

| BOX 2-3 | USING EVIDENCE IN PRACTICE |
|---|---|

**Research Summary**

Older adults often experience fragmentation of health care because they see different physicians and health care providers and receive health care in multiple settings. This results in patients receiving conflicting information about medications and treatments. A large not-for-profit managed care delivery system in Colorado decided to study if interventions that encouraged older adults and their caregivers to assume a more active role in the hospital reduced the need for rehospitalization after discharge. The patients included in this study were age 65 and older and had a diagnosis that put them at risk for needing rehospitalization (e.g., congestive heart failure [CHF], chronic obstructive pulmonary disease [COPD], diabetes mellitus, and stroke). Researchers compared patients who received normal care with patients who received the special interventions.

The patients who received the special interventions had a transition coach who was a nurse practitioner (NP). The NP encouraged self-management of the illness and direct communication between the patient and the primary physician or health care provider during and after the hospital stay. The study investigators maintained a personal health record for each patient. After discharge from the hospital, the transition coach called or visited patients who went to a skilled nursing facility at least once a week. For the patients who were discharged to home, the transition coach scheduled a home visit within 24 to 72 hours of discharge. During the home visits the transition coach reviewed the patient's

medications and reconciled any inconsistencies. The transition coaches provided encouragement and support to facilitate management of the illness at home. The coaches also provided medication education and information about warning symptoms that required that the patient call the physician or health care provider immediately.

The patients who received the patient-centered interventions were half as likely to require rehospitalizations for their illnesses. Patients in this group also reported a high level of confidence about getting information needed to manage their illnesses. They felt more comfortable communicating with their physician or health care provider and better understood their medications.

**Application to Nursing Practice**

The results from this study support the benefits associated with following patients closely in all levels of health care. Although the managed care organization had to hire an NP, the reduction in hospitalizations probably outweighed the costs associated with this program. According to this study, nurses at the bedside are able to help patients avoid rehospitalizations by providing education about disease management and medications. Nurses also support and help patients maintain open, honest communication with their physicians or health care providers. Empowering patients to better manage their illnesses helps reduce health care costs and enhances patient satisfaction.

Data from Coleman EA and others: Preparing patients and caregivers to participate in care delivered across settings: the care transitions intervention, *J Am Geriatr Soc* 52(11):1817, 2004.

provider to ensure that the patient returns home with the right information to manage the condition. A patient who has experienced a stroke will not be discharged from a hospital until caregivers have established plans with physical and occupational therapists to begin a program of rehabilitation.

Effective discharge planning often requires referrals to various health care disciplines. In many agencies, patients need a physician's or health care provider's order for a referral, especially when specific therapies are planned (e.g., physical therapy). It is best to have patients and families participate in referral processes so that they are involved early in any necessary decision making. Some tips on making the referral process successful include the following:

• Make a referral as soon as possible.
• Inform the care provider receiving the referral of as much information about the patient as possible. This avoids duplication of effort and exclusion of important information.
• Involve the patient and family in the referral process, including selecting the necessary referral. Explain the service to be provided, the reason for the referral, and what to expect from the referral's services.

• Determine what the referral discipline recommends for the patient's care, and incorporate this into the treatment plan as soon as possible.

Successful discharge planning involves the patient from the beginning, uses the strengths of the patient in planning, provides resources to meet the patient's limitations, and focuses on improving the patient's long-term outcomes. Discharge planning depends on comprehensive patient and family education (see Chapter 10). Patients need to know what to do when they get home, how to do it, and what to watch for when problems develop. The Joint Commission on Accreditation of Healthcare Organizations (JCAHO) (2005) requires the following when patients are discharged from health care facilities or transferred to other levels of care:

• A process addresses the need for continuing care, treatment, and services after discharge or transfer.
• The transfer or discharge of a patient to another level of care, treatment, and services, different professionals, or different settings is based on the patient's assessed needs and the hospital's capabilities.

• When patients are transferred or discharged, appropriate information related to the care, treatment, and services provided is exchanged with other service providers.

**INTENSIVE CARE.** An intensive care unit (ICU) or critical care unit is a hospital unit in which patients receive close monitoring and intensive medical care. ICUs have advanced technologies, such as computerized cardiac monitors and mechanical ventilators. Although many of these devices are on regular nursing units, the patients hospitalized within ICUs are monitored and maintained on multiple devices. Nursing and medical staff within an ICU are educated on critical care principles and techniques. An ICU is the most expensive delivery site for medical care because each nurse is usually only assigned to care for one or two patients at a time and because of all the treatments and procedures the patients in the ICU require.

**SUBACUTE CARE. Subacute care** units are designated sites that provide medical specialty care for patients who need a greater intensity of care than generally provided in a skilled nursing facility but who no longer require acute care (Sultz and Young, 2004). Many of the patients who require subacute care are **outliers** (patients with extended lengths of stay, well beyond allowed inpatient DRG days). Thus a hospital transfers a patient to a subacute unit and reduces its financial burden, because the stay on the subacute unit meets different reimbursement guidelines. Subacute units are in hospitals and in skilled nursing and rehabilitation facilities. Managed care providers welcomed subacute units because patient care and treatment is provided at a fraction of the cost when compared with hospital care. However, the federal government and various state agencies have stopped the development of these units until their value is determined (Sultz and Young, 2004).

**PSYCHIATRIC FACILITIES.** Patients who suffer emotional and behavioral problems such as depression, violent behavior, and eating disorders often require special counseling and treatment in psychiatric facilities. Located in hospitals, independent outpatient clinics, or private mental health hospitals, psychiatric facilities offer inpatient and outpatient services, depending on the seriousness of the problem. Patients enter these facilities voluntarily or involuntarily. Hospitalization involves relatively short stays with the purpose of stabilizing patients before transfer to outpatient treatment centers. Patients with psychiatric problems receive a comprehensive multidisciplinary treatment plan that involves them and their families. Medicine, nursing, social work, and activity therapy collaborate to develop a plan of care that enables patients to return to functional states within the community. At discharge from inpatient facilities, patients are usually referred for follow-up care at clinics or with counselors.

**RURAL HOSPITALS.** Access to health care in rural areas has been a serious problem. Most rural hospitals have experienced a severe shortage of primary care providers. Many have been forced to close because of economic failure. In 1989 the Omnibus Budget Reconciliation Act (OBRA) directed the U.S. Department of Health and Human Services

(USDHHS) to create a new health care entity, the rural primary care hospital (RPCH). An RPCH provides 24-hour emergency care, with no more than six inpatient beds for providing temporary care for 72 hours or less to patients needing stabilization before transfer to a larger hospital. Physicians, nurse practitioners, or physician assistants staff the RPCH. The RPCH provides inpatient care to acutely ill or injured persons before transferring them to better-equipped facilities. Basic radiological and laboratory services are also available.

With health care reform, more big-city health care systems are branching out and establishing affiliations or mergers with rural hospitals. The rural hospitals provide a referral base to the larger tertiary care medical centers. Nurses who work in rural hospitals or clinics often function independently in the absence of a physician. Competence in physical assessment, clinical decision making, and emergency care are essential. Advanced practice nurses (e.g., nurse practitioners or clinical nurse specialists) use medical protocols and establish collaborative agreements with staff physicians.

## Restorative Care

Patients recovering from acute illnesses or who have chronic illnesses or disabilities usually require services designed to restore the patient's level of health. Care is necessary until patients return to their previous level of function or reach a new level of function limited by their illness or disability. The goal of restorative care is to assist an individual to regain maximal functional status, thereby enhancing the individual's quality of life. The goal is to promote patient independence and self-care. With the emphasis on early discharge from hospitals, most patients require some level of restorative care. For example, some surgical patients require ongoing wound care and activity and exercise management until they have recovered to a point at which they are able to resume normal activities of daily living independently.

The intensity of care has increased in restorative care settings, because patients leave hospitals earlier. It is common to have patients in a home or rehabilitation setting still receiving intravenous fluids (see Chapter 15), enteral nutrition (see Chapter 31), and pain control (see Chapter 30). The restorative health care team is an interdisciplinary group of health care professionals that includes the patient and family or significant others. In restorative settings, nurses recognize that success is dependent on effective and early partnering with patients and their families. Patients and families require a clear understanding of goals for physical recovery, the rationale for any physical limitations, and the purpose and potential risks associated with therapies. The more patients and families are involved in restorative care, the more likely that they will be motivated to follow treatment plans and that patients will be able to achieve optimal functioning.

**HOME CARE. Home care** is the provision of medically related professional and paraprofessional services and equipment to patients and families in their homes for health maintenance, education, illness prevention, diagnosis and treatment of disease, palliation, and rehabilitation. Patients in home care use nursing services more than any other service. However, home care might also include medical and social services; physical, occupational, speech, and respiratory therapy; and nutritional therapy. A home care service also coordinates the access to and delivery of home health equipment, or durable medical equipment (DME), which is any medically related product adapted for home use.

Home care agencies provide almost every type of health care service in the patient's home. Health promotion and education are traditionally the primary objectives of home care, yet at present, most patients receive professional services on the basis of some medically related need. The focus is on patient and family independence. Home care addresses recovery and stabilization of illness in the home, where problems related to lifestyle, safety, environment, family dynamics, and health care practices are identified.

Home care agencies provide skilled and intermittent professional services and home care aide services. These services usually are delivered once or twice a day, up to 7 days a week. Box 2-4 summarizes some of the services offered by home care agencies. Approved home care agencies usually receive reimbursement for services from the government (such as **Medicare** and **Medicaid** in the United States), private insurance, and private pay. The government has strict regulations that govern reimbursement for home care services. An agency cannot simply charge whatever it wants for a service and expect to receive full reimbursement. Government programs set the cost for reimbursement of most professional services.

If you choose to work as a home care nurse, you will provide individualized care and have one-on-one contact with patients and families. You will have your own caseload and help patients adapt to many permanent or temporary physical limitations so that they are able to assume a more normal daily home routine. Home care requires a strong knowledge base in many areas, such as family dynamics (see Chapter 21), cultural practices (see Chapter 17), spiritual values (see Chapter 18), and communication principles (see Chapter 9).

**REHABILITATION.** **Rehabilitation** is the restoration of a person to the fullest physical, mental, social, vocational, and economic usefulness possible (Clemen-Stone and others, 2002). Patients require rehabilitation after a physical or mental illness, injury, or chemical addiction. Rehabilitation was once available primarily for patients with illnesses or injury to the nervous or musculoskeletal system, but the health care delivery system has expanded its scope of such services. Today, specialized rehabilitation services, such as cardiovascular and pulmonary rehabilitation programs, help patients and families adjust to necessary changes in lifestyle and learn to function with the limitations of their disease. Drug rehabilitation centers help patients become free from drug dependence and return to the community.

Rehabilitation services include physical, occupational, speech therapy, and social services. Ideally rehabilitation begins the moment a patient enters a health care setting for treatment. For example, some orthopedic programs now have patients undergo physical therapy exercises before major joint repair to enhance their recovery postoperatively. Initially rehabilitation sometimes focuses on the prevention

---

| BOX 2-4 | **Home Care Services** |
| --- | --- |

**Wound Care**

Sterile dressing changes, debridement and irrigations, packing, and instructing patients and families in wound care techniques

**Respiratory Care**

Oxygen therapy, mechanical ventilation, suctioning, and care of tracheotomies

**Vital Signs**

Monitoring blood pressure and cardiopulmonary status; instructing patients and families in vital sign measurement

**Elimination**

Ostomy care, appliance application, skin care, and irrigation; insertion of indwelling and intermittent urinary catheters, irrigation, and instructing families in catheter management; home dialysis

**Nutrition**

Administration of tube feedings and enteral feedings; assessment of nutrition and hydration status; instructing patients and families in tube feedings

**Rehabilitation**

Ambulation and gait training, use of assistive devices, range-of-motion exercises, and instructing patients and families on transfer techniques

**Medications**

Monitoring compliance; administering injections; and instructing patients and families on drug information, medication preparation, and steps to take in the event of side effects

**Intravenous Therapy**

Administration of blood products, analgesic and chemotherapeutic agents, and long-term hydration

Instructing patients and families on use of intravenous devices, steps to take in the event of disconnection or accidental fluid infusion, and side effects

**Laboratory Studies**

Blood glucose monitoring (including patient and family instruction) and drawing blood for specific diagnostic purposes

of complications related to the illness or injury. As the condition stabilizes, rehabilitation maximizes the patient's functioning and level of independence.

Rehabilitation occurs in many health care settings, including specific rehabilitation institutions, outpatient settings, and the home. Frequently patients needing long-term rehabilitation (e.g., patients who have had strokes and spinal cord injuries) have severe disabilities affecting their ability to carry out the activities of daily living. When patients receive rehabilitation services in outpatient settings, patients get treatment at specified times during the week but remain at home the rest of the time. Specific rehabilitation strategies are applied to the home environment to help the patient achieve maximal levels of function and independence. Nurses and other members of the health care team visit homes and help patients and families learn to adapt to illness or injury.

**EXTENDED CARE FACILITIES.** An **extended care facility** provides intermediate medical, nursing, or custodial care for patients recovering from acute illness or patients with chronic illnesses or disabilities. Extended care facilities include intermediate care and skilled nursing facilities. Some include long-term care and assisted living facilities (see later discussion of continuing care). At one point, extended care facilities primarily cared for older adults. However, because hospitals discharge their patients sooner, there is a greater need for intermediate care settings for patients of all ages. For example, a young patient who has experienced a traumatic brain injury resulting from a car accident transfers to an extended care facility for rehabilitative or supportive care until discharge to the home becomes a safe option. The growth of extended care facilities will increase as the number of older adults grows.

An intermediate care or **skilled nursing facility** offers skilled care from a licensed nursing staff. This often includes administration of intravenous fluids, wound care, long-term ventilator management, and physical rehabilitation. Patients receive extensive supportive care until they are able to move back into the community or into residential care.

Extended care facilities provide around-the-clock nursing coverage. If you choose to work in this setting, you will need nursing expertise that is similar to that of nurses working in acute care inpatient settings along with a background in gerontological nursing principles (see Chapter 19).

## Continuing Care

Continuing care describes a variety of health, personal, and social services provided over a prolonged period to persons who are disabled, who never were functionally independent, or who suffer a terminal disease. The need for continuing health care services is growing in the United States. People are living longer, and many of those with continuing health care needs have no immediate family members to care for them. A decline in the number of children families choose to have, the aging of care providers, and the increasing rates of divorce and remarriage complicate this problem. Continuing care is available within institutional settings (e.g., nursing centers or nursing homes, group homes, and retirement com-

munities), communities (e.g., adult day care and senior centers), or the home (e.g., home care, home-delivered meals, and hospice) (Meiner and Lueckenotte, 2006).

**NURSING CENTERS OR FACILITIES.** The language of long-term care is confusing and constantly changing. The nursing home has been the dominant setting for long-term care (Meiner and Lueckenotte, 2006). With the Omnibus Budget Reconciliation Act of 1987, the term *nursing facility* became the term for nursing homes and other facilities that provide long-term care. Now, *nursing center* is the most appropriate term. A nursing center typically provides 24-hour intermediate and custodial care such as nursing, rehabilitation, dietary, recreational, social, and religious services for residents of any age with chronic or debilitating illnesses. In some cases, patients stay in nursing centers for room, food, and laundry services only. The majority of persons living in nursing centers are older adults. A nursing center is a resident's temporary or permanent home with surroundings made as homelike as possible (Sorrentino, 2003). The philosophy of care is to provide a planned, systematic, and interdisciplinary approach to nursing care to help residents reach and maintain their highest level of function (Resnick and Fleishell, 2002).

According to the U.S. Bureau of the Census, just over 5% of people 65 years and older live in nursing centers and other facilities (MissouriFamilies, 2005). Nursing centers have been under attack for years because of claims regarding inadequate care and abuse. Many of the claims are legitimate (Fleck, 2002). As a result, the nursing center industry has become one of the most highly regulated industries in the United States. The Omnibus Budget Reconciliation Act of 1987 (OBRA 1987), also known as the Nursing Home Reform Act, raised the standard of services provided by nursing centers. To receive payment from Medicare and Medicaid, nursing centers have to comply with OBRA 1987 and its minimal requirements for nursing homes. There currently are 18 requirements included in this law. Examples of the requirements include having sufficient nursing staff, developing a comprehensive plan of care for each resident, and providing services needed to maintain nutrition, grooming, and personal hygiene (Health Care Financing Administration [HCFA], 2004; Nursing Home Abuse and Neglect Resource Center, 2003).

Interdisciplinary functional assessment of residents is the cornerstone of clinical practice within nursing centers (Meiner and Lueckenotte, 2006). Government regulations require that staff in nursing centers assess each resident comprehensively, with care planning decisions made within a prescribed period. A resident's functional ability (e.g., ability to perform activities of daily living and instrumental activities of daily living) and long-term physical and psychosocial well-being are the focus. The facility needs to complete the Resident Assessment Instrument (RAI) on all residents. The RAI consists of the **Minimum Data Set (MDS)** (Box 2-5), Resident Assessment Protocols (RAPs), and utilization guidelines of each state. The RAI ultimately provides a na-

**BOX 2-5** **Minimum Data Set and Examples of Resident Assessment Protocols**

**Minimum Data Set**

Resident's background
Cognitive, communication/hearing, and vision patterns
Physical functioning and structural problems
Mood, behavior, and activity pursuit patterns
Psychosocial well-being
Bowel and bladder continence
Health conditions
Disease diagnoses
Oral/nutritional and dental status
Skin condition
Medication use
Special treatments and procedures

**Resident Assessment Protocols (Examples)**

Delirium
Falls
Pressure ulcers
Psychotropic drug use

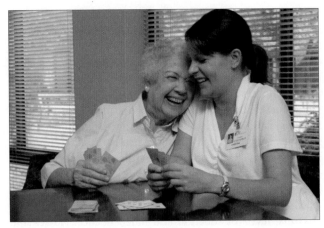

FIGURE **2-3** Providing nursing services in assisted living facilities promotes physical and psychosocial health.

tional database for nursing facilities so that policy makers will better understand the health care needs of the long-term care population. In addition, the MDS is a rich resource for nurses in determining the best type of interventions to support the health care needs of this growing population.

**ASSISTED LIVING.** **Assisted living** is one of the fastest growing industries within the United States. There are approximately 33,000 assisted living facilities that house about 88,000 people in the United States (National Center for Assisted Living [NCAL], 2001). Assisted living offers an attractive long-term care setting with a homier environment and greater resident autonomy. Patients require some assistance with activities of daily living but remain relatively independent within a partially protective setting. A group of residents live together, but each resident has his or her own room and shares dining and social activity areas. Usually people keep all of their personal possessions in their residences. Facilities range from hotel-like buildings with hundreds of units to modest group homes that house a handful of seniors. Assisted living provides independence, security, and privacy all at the same time (Ebersole and others, 2004). These facilities promote physical and psychosocial health (Figure 2-3). Services in an assisted living facility include laundry, assistance with meals and personal care, 24-hour oversight, and housekeeping (Sorrentino, 2003). Some facilities provide assistance with medication administration. Assisted living facilities do not directly provide nursing care services, although a home care nurse is able to visit a patient in an assisted living facility.

Unfortunately, most residents of assisted living facilities pay privately. The average monthly fee is $1873 (NCAL, 2001). With no government fee caps and little regulation, assisted living is not always an option for individuals with limited financial resources.

**RESPITE CARE.** The need to care for family members within the home creates great physical and emotional burdens for adult caregivers, especially when the family member is limited either physically or cognitively. The caregiver is usually an adult who not only has the responsibility for providing care to a loved one (e.g., spouse, parent, or sibling) but often maintains a full-time job, raises a family, and manages the routines of daily living as well. **Respite care** is a service that provides short-term relief or time off for persons providing home care to an ill, disabled, or frail older adult (Meiner and Lueckenotte, 2006). Adult day care is one form of respite care. Trained volunteers in the home also provide respite care. The family caregiver is able to leave the home for errands or some social time while a responsible person stays in the home to care for the loved one. Alternatively, some patients stay temporarily in a nursing center to provide the family relief.

**ADULT DAY CARE CENTERS.** **Adult day care centers** provide a variety of health and social services to specific patient populations who live alone or with family in the community. Services offered during the day allow family members to maintain their lifestyles and employment and still provide home care for their relatives (Meiner and Lueckenotte, 2006). Day care centers are associated with a hospital or nursing home or exist as independent centers. Frequently the patients of such centers do not require hospitalization but need continuous health care services while their families or support persons work. These patients include older adults needing daily physical rehabilitation, individuals with emotional illnesses needing daily counseling, and individuals with chemical dependence problems who are involved in rehabilitation programs. The centers usually operate 5 days per week during typical business hours and usually charge on a per diem basis. Adult day care centers allow patients to retain more independence by living at home, thus potentially reducing the costs of health care by avoiding or delaying an older adult's admission to a nursing center.

Services offered in day care settings include transportation to and from the facility, assistance with personal care, nursing and therapeutic services (e.g., counseling and rehabilitation), meals, and recreational activities (Lueckenotte, 2000). Nurses working in day care centers provide continuity between care delivered in the home and in the center. For example, nurses ensure that patients continue to take prescribed medication and administer specific treatments. Knowledge of community needs and resources is essential in providing adequate support of patients, who often spend only a few hours a week in the day care setting (Ebersole and others, 2004).

**HOSPICE.** A **hospice** is a system of family-centered care that allows patients to live and remain at home with comfort, independence, and dignity while alleviating the strains caused by terminal illness. The focus of hospice care is palliative care, not curative treatment (see Chapter 30). A hospice benefits patients in the terminal phase of any disease, such as cardiomyopathy, multiple sclerosis, acquired immunodeficiency syndrome (AIDS), or cancer.

A patient entering a hospice is at the terminal phase of illness, and the patient, family, and physician or health care provider agree that no further treatment will reverse the disease process. Staff members collaborate to provide care that ensures death with dignity in the patient's home. Hospice care is available 24 hours a day, 7 days a week, and services continue without interruption if the patient's care setting changes. Occasionally a patient is admitted to a hospice unit within a hospital. The patient and family need to accept the fact that the hospice will not use emergency measures such as cardiopulmonary resuscitation to prolong life. The focus is on symptom management and ensuring the patient's comfort. The hospice's multidisciplinary team works together continuously with the patient's physician or health care provider to develop and maintain a patient-directed individualized plan of care.

If you decide to be a hospice nurse, you will work in institutional and community settings. Hospice nurses are committed to the philosophy and objectives of the facilities for which they work. They provide care and support for the patient and family during the terminal phase and at the time of death and continue to offer bereavement counseling and follow-up to the family after the patient's death. Many hospice programs provide respite care, which is important in maintaining the health of the primary caregiver and family.

## Issues in Health Care Delivery

The climate in health care today influences health care professionals as well as consumers. In the midst of an evolving health care system, be prepared to participate fully and effectively within the managed care environment as a nurse. Those who provide patient care are the most qualified to make changes in the health care delivery system. As you face issues of how to maintain health care quality while reducing costs, you will need to acquire the knowledge, skills, and values necessary to practice competently and effectively. It will also become more important than ever before to collaborate with your colleagues in health care in designing new approaches for patient care delivery.

### Competency

The Pew Health Professions Commission, created in 1989, focuses on the health care work force. The Commission is a national and interdisciplinary group of health care leaders that helps policy makers and educators produce health care professionals who are able to meet the changing needs of Americans. The Commission (1998) recommended 21 competencies for health care professionals in the twenty-first century. The competencies emphasize the importance of public service, caring for the health of communities, and developing ethically responsible behaviors (Box 2-6). The health care practitioner competencies offer an excellent yardstick for gauging how well you practice nursing and provide guidance as you grow within the nursing profession. A consumer of health care expects that the standards of nursing care and practice in any health care setting are appropriate, safe, and effective. Ongoing competency is your responsibility. Health care organizations ensure quality care by establishing policies, procedures, and protocols that are scientifically valid and follow national accrediting standards. Your responsibility is to follow policies and procedures and to know the most current practice standards. As you progress in your career, it becomes your responsibility to obtain necessary continued education and to earn certifications when you choose to practice in specialty areas.

### Evidence-Based Practice

As you enter the nursing profession, it will be a challenge to stay familiar with new information in order to provide the highest quality of patient care. Nursing practice is dynamic and always changing because of new information coming from research studies, practice trends, technological development, and social issues affecting patients. Be able to analyze new knowledge to make valid and informed decisions about patient care (Barnsteiner and Prevost, 2002).

**Evidence-based practice** is defined as the integration of best knowledge, which includes clinical expertise, best research evidence, and patient values (Sackett and others, 2000). *Evidence-based practice, research-based practice,* and *best practice* are terms that are often used interchangeably. However, research-based practice refers to the use of knowledge based on the results of research studies, whereas evidence-based practice adds a nurse's clinical experience, practice trends, and patient preferences (Barnsteiner and Prevost, 2002). Thus, evidence-based practice is a broader concept than research-based practice.

---

| BOX 2-6 | Pew Health Professions Commission Twenty-One Competencies for the Twenty-First Century |

1. Embrace a personal ethic of social responsibility and service
2. Exhibit ethical behavior in all professional activities
3. Provide evidence-based, clinically competent care
4. Incorporate the multiple determinants of health in clinical care
5. Apply knowledge of the new sciences
6. Demonstrate critical thinking, reflection, and problem-solving skills
7. Understand the role of primary care
8. Rigorously practice preventive health care
9. Integrate population-based care and services into practice
10. Improve access to health care for those with unmet health needs
11. Practice relationship-centered care with individuals and families
12. Provide culturally sensitive care to a diverse society
13. Partner with communities in health care decisions
14. Use communication and information technology effectively and appropriately
15. Work in interdisciplinary teams
16. Ensure care that balances individual, professional, system, and societal needs
17. Practice leadership
18. Take responsibility for quality of care and health outcomes at all levels
19. Contribute to continuous improvement of the health care system
20. Advocate for public policy that promotes and protects the health of the public
21. Continue to learn and help others learn

From the Pew Health Professions Commission, The Fourth Report of the Pew Health Professions Commission: *Recreating health professional practice for a new century*, 1998, The Commission.

---

The goal of evidence-based practice is to provide evidence-based data to allow you to provide effective patient care by improving patient outcomes. Evidence-based practice will help you resolve problems that arise in the clinical setting. It will also help you provide innovative health care that exceeds quality standards. Using evidence-based practice will also help you provide consistent patient care using effective and efficient decision-making processes (Spector, 2005).

Using evidence-based practice requires you to review research and practice findings, critique research studies, investigate patients' values, and discuss the implications of choosing not to implement evidence-based practice changes with your colleagues. Many reliable web-based resources are available to provide you with information about evidenced-based education and practice. For example, the University of York Centre for Evidence-based Nursing provides links to evidence-based education and practice information (http://www.york.ac.uk/healthsciences/). The Cochrane Collaboration provides systematic reviews of the literature related to specific clinical topics (http://www.cochrane.org). Reviews from the Cochrane database are constantly updated as new research becomes available. The Agency for Healthcare Research and Quality (AHRQ) provides evidence-based information about health care outcomes, quality, and cost (http://www.AHRQ.gov/clinic/epcix.htm). Finally, the National Guidelines Clearinghouse is a U.S. government database for evidence-based clinical practice guidelines and related documents (http://www.guideline.gov/index.asp).

## Quality Health Care

Establishing health care goals on a national level facilitates research and enhances the quality of health care (McGlynn and others, 2003). Quality health care is difficult to define. What patients define as quality health care is not necessarily the same as what health professionals define as quality. Unless health care providers define quality, the purchasers of health care (e.g., employers, insurers, and health maintenance organizations [HMOs]) will buy services based on price alone. The health care system that delivers a given service (e.g., delivery of a baby and mother-infant care) for the cheapest price will become the primary provider of that service. Health care providers are trying to define how their services are better than their competitors by measuring health care outcomes. An outcome is a measure of what actually does or does not happen as a result of a process of care; it is the end result (desirable or undesirable) of care delivered (Donabedian, 1966). Examples of outcomes are readmission rates for patients who have had surgery, functional health status of patients after discharge (e.g., ability and time frame for returning to work), and the rate of infection after surgery. You will play an important role in gathering and analyzing quality outcome data as a nurse.

Health plans throughout the United States rely on the Health Plan Employer Data and Information Set (HEDIS) as a quality measure. The National Committee for Quality Assurance (NCQA) created HEDIS as a tool to collect various data to measure the quality of care and services provided by different health plans. It is the database of choice for the Health Care Financing Administration (HCFA). HEDIS compares how well health plans perform in three key areas: quality of care, access to care, and patient satisfaction with the health plan and physicians (HEDIS, 2004). The JCAHO (2005) requires health care organizations to determine how well an organization meets patient needs and expectations. Organizations are using outcomes such as patient satisfaction as a basis to redesign how to manage and deliver care to improve quality.

**NURSING-SENSITIVE OUTCOMES.** Nursing-sensitive outcomes are patient outcomes that are directly related to nursing care. They have a major effect on patient safety and quality of care (Stanton, 2004). Nurses assume accountability and responsibility for the consequences of these outcomes. Recently there has been a greater emphasis in health care and research on nursing-sensitive outcomes. The evaluation of patient outcomes remains important to nursing and the health care delivery system. However, nurses are just beginning to overcome the challenges associated with measuring the impact of these outcomes.

Nurses assume responsibility for a variety of outcomes that include individuals, family caregivers, the family, and the community. A research-based outcomes classification system, the Nursing Outcomes Classification (NOC), helps nurses better define and measure the impact of their interventions (Moorhead and others, 2004). NOC emphasizes patient outcomes that nursing interventions affect most. However, all health care disciplines are able to use this system.

The American Nurses Credentialing Center (ANCC) has established a Magnet Recognition Program to recognize health care organizations that achieve excellence in nursing practice (ANCC, 2005). Health care organizations that decide to apply for magnet status must demonstrate leadership in nursing. Magnet status also requires nurses to collect data on specific nursing-sensitive quality indicators or outcomes, such as pressure ulcer prevalence and patient falls, and to compare their outcomes against a national, state, or regional database to demonstrate quality of care.

There are many nursing-sensitive outcomes for nurses to measure. Examples of nursing-sensitive outcomes include the incidence of hospital-acquired pneumonia, the incidence of urinary tract infections, pain management, and failure to rescue (Stanton, 2004). Because of the importance of nursing-sensitive outcomes, the AHRQ recently funded several nursing research studies that looked at the relationship of nurse staffing levels to adverse patient outcomes. These studies found that higher levels of staffing by registered nurses (RNs) in hospitals were associated with fewer adverse patient outcomes. For example, the incidence of hospital-acquired pneumonia was highly sensitive to RN staffing levels. Adding just 30 minutes of RN staffing per patient day greatly reduced the incidence of pneumonia in patients following surgery. These studies also found that increased levels of nurse staffing positively impacted nurse satisfaction. Future studies will evaluate the impact of nurse workload on patient safety and the relationship between nurses' working conditions and patient outcomes. Other studies are investigating how nurses' workloads affect patient safety and how nurses' working conditions affect medication safety. Measuring and monitoring nursing-sensitive outcomes will help you improve your patients' outcomes. Nurses and health care facilities use nursing-sensitive outcomes to improve nurses' workloads, enhance patient safety, and develop sensible policies related to nursing practice and health care.

**PATIENT SATISFACTION.** Almost every major health care organization measures certain aspects of patient satis-

faction. The Picker Institute has identified eight dimensions of **patient-centered care** (Box 2-7) that most affect patients' experiences with health care (Picker Institute, n.d.). The eight dimensions cover much of the scope of nursing practice. This is no surprise because nurses are involved in almost every aspect of a patient's care in a hospital. A close look shows that most of the dimensions reflected in patient satisfaction apply to almost any health care setting.

The Picker Institute surveys patient satisfaction along the eight dimensions. The survey looks globally at patient perceptions of care in an attempt to understand how all hospital departments influence patient satisfaction. Like other companies that distribute patient satisfaction surveys, the Picker Institute mails surveys to patients. Staff involved in patient care receive the satisfaction scores as feedback regarding their success in meeting patient expectations. It is the responsibility of staff to identify the unique issues that influence patient satisfaction for their area. For example, nurses working on an oncology unit will have different patient satisfaction issues around physical comfort than nurses caring for new mothers. Patient satisfaction findings become the basis for many quality improvement studies.

It is important for you to recognize the need to identify patient expectations. The eight dimensions of care provide a useful guide. By learning early what a patient expects with regard to information, comfort, and availability of family and friends, you will plan better patient care. When do you ask about a patient's expectations? It will become a routine question when the patient first enters a health care setting, while care continues, and when a patient is ultimately discharged from your care. Patient expectations are an important measure of the evaluation of nursing care.

## Technology in Health Care

Technological advances are influencing where and how nurses provide care to patients. Sophisticated equipment such as electronic intravenous (IV) infusion devices, cardiac telemetry (a device that monitors a patient's heart rate wherever the patient is on a nursing unit), and computerized documentation patient information systems are just a few examples changing the way health care is delivered. In many ways, technological systems make your work easier, but they do not replace your judgment. For example, it is your responsibility when managing an intravenous infusion pump to monitor the infusion to be sure it infuses on time and without complications. An electronic infusion device provides a constant rate of infusion, but you must be sure you calculate the rate correctly. The device will set off an alarm if the infusion slows, making it important for you to respond to the alarm and to troubleshoot the problem. Technology does not replace a nurse's astute, critical eye and clinical judgment.

Computerized clinical information systems have replaced the traditional printed medical record. A comprehensive electronic record of a patient's medical problems, treatment, diagnostic procedures, and nursing care offers a rich source

---

| BOX 2-7 | **The Dimensions of Patient-Centered Care** |

### Access

Patients want to get to hospitals, clinics, and physicians' offices easily and without hassle.

Patients need to be able to find transportation when going to different health care settings.

Patients want to schedule appointments at convenient times without difficulty.

Patients want to be able to go see a specialist when a referral is made.

Patients expect to receive clear instructions on how to get referrals to other health care providers.

### Respect for Patient's Values, Preferences, and Expressed Needs

Patients expect you to treat them with dignity and respect.

Patients want you to inform and involve them in decisions about their care.

Patients' perceptions of needs should not be completely different from those identified by a care provider.

A setting that respects the patient focuses on quality of life.

### Coordination and Integration of Care

A competent and caring staff reduces patients' feelings of powerlessness.

Patients look for someone to be in charge of care and to communicate clearly with other health team members.

Patients look to have services and procedures well coordinated.

Patients need to know at all times whom to call for help.

### Information, Communication, and Education

Patients expect to receive accurate and timely information about their clinical status, progress, or prognosis.

Patients and families need to be informed of major changes in therapies or status.

Patients need tests and procedures explained clearly in language they understand.

Patients and family members want to know how to manage their own care.

### Physical Comfort

Physical care that comforts patients is one of the most elemental services caregivers provide.

Nurses need to respond in a timely and effective way to any request for pain medication, to explain the extent of pain for patients to expect, and to offer alternatives for pain management.

Patients expect privacy and to have their cultural values respected.

Patients often need help to complete activities of daily living.

The health care setting environment needs to be clean and comfortable.

### Emotional Support and Relief of Fear and Anxiety

Patients look to care providers to help reduce anxiety and concerns about health status, medical treatment, and prognosis of illness.

Patients need to understand the impact illness will have on their ability to care for themselves and their family.

Patients worry about their ability to pay for their medical care. Are there staff who will help with those worries?

### Involvement of Family and Friends

Care providers need to recognize, respect, and meet the needs of the patients' family and friends.

Patients have the right to determine if they want family members involved in decisions about their care.

Patients expect you to properly inform family or friends who will provide physical support and care after discharge.

### Transition and Continuity

Patients want information about medications to take, dietary or treatment plans to follow, and danger signals to look for after hospitalization or treatment.

Patients expect to have their continuing health care needs met after discharge with well-coordinated services.

Patients and family members expect access to any necessary health care resources (e.g., social, physical, financial) after discharge.

Data from National Research Corporation, Picker Institute: Eight dimensions of patient-centered care, 2005, http://www.nrcpicker.com/Default.aspx?DN =112,22,2,1,Documents; Picker Institute: Through the patient's eyes, n.d., http://www.pickerinstitute.org/about.htm.

---

of information to clinicians who provide patient care. An electronic database also provides valuable information for research and quality improvement activities. For example, a nurse researcher who wishes to track a nursing staff's progress in timely assessment of patients' pain is able to examine a database to review actual patient assessments and the time they occurred.

Documentation on a clinical information system minimizes free text entries and allows you to enter information quickly on specially designed flow sheets, pop-up screens, and nursing care plans. The computer displays important data in a way that allows you to follow your patient's progress and course easily. An electronic system does not make you less responsible for ensuring that you document clinical information about a patient accurately and completely in a timely manner. All members of the health care team usually are able to gain access to the electronic record; thus you have to make information accessible as soon as possible. Many hospitals have placed computers at the patient's bedside so you are able to document care as soon as you provide it. It is important to remember not to depersonalize your care when you use a bedside computer system. As you enter data, it often becomes easy to avoid interacting with the patient, who likely is interested in the type of information you are recording. The use of electronic information systems also requires rigorous confidentiality protocols. It is now easy for anyone to visit a nursing unit and try to gain access to a computer to obtain patient information. You will play a role in protecting patient rights and ensuring that information is accessible only to those directly involved in a patient's care. Chapter 8 reviews principles of nursing documentation.

## Globalization of Health Care

In today's society, many forces affect health care, continuously reshaping the health care delivery system. The advances in communication, primarily through the Internet, allow nurses, patients, and other health care providers to talk with others worldwide about health care issues. However, despite advances in technology and communication, the poorest areas in the world continue to be underserved (Simpson, 2004).

As a nurse you understand how worldwide communication and globalization of health care affect your practice. Health care consumers demand quality and service and have become more knowledgeable. They often search the Internet about their health concerns and medical conditions. They also use the Internet to select their health care providers. As a result of **globalization,** it is necessary for physicians and health care providers to make their services more accessible. Because of advances in communication, nurses and other health care providers practice across state and national boundaries. Furthermore, there is currently a nursing shortage in health care institutions across the United States. In an effort to provide quality care, health care institutions are recruiting nurses from around the world to work in the United States. The hiring of nurses from other nations has forced U.S. hospitals to better understand and work with nurses from different cultures who have different needs (Nash and Gremillion, 2004). For example, in the Philippines, nurses are not expected to take an active role in making decisions about patient care and strive to please physicians. They often put the needs of others before their own needs. However, in the United States, nurses are expected to think critically and be active participants in planning patient care. When nurses from the Philippines come to work in hospitals in the United States, the hospital staff need to teach the nurses from the Philippines how to be more assertive and take a more active role as a member of the health care team. The nurses from the Philippines need to learn how to use critical thinking and decision-making skills when providing patient care. They also need help in identifying and meeting their own personal needs.

Many problems affect the health status of people around the world. For example, poverty is still deadlier than any disease and is the most frequently cited reason for death in the world today. Nations and communities that experience poverty have limited access to vaccines, clean water, and standard medical care. The growth of urbanization also is currently affecting the world's health. As cities become more densely populated, problems with pollution, noise, crowding, inadequate water, improper waste disposal, and other environmental hazards become more apparent. Children, women, and older adults are **vulnerable populations** most threatened by urbanization. Although globalization of trade, travel, and culture improves the availability of health care services, the spread of communicable diseases such as tuberculosis and severe acute respiratory syndrome (SARS) has become more common. Finally, the results of global environmental changes and disasters affect health. Changes in climate and natural disasters threaten food supplies and often allow infectious diseases to spread more rapidly (Simpson, 2004).

As a leader in health care, remain aware of what is happening in your community, your nation, and around the world. There are more than 5 million nurses worldwide (Simpson 2004). Nursing's unique focus on caring helps nurses begin to address the issues presented by globalization. You and your fellow nurses will help overcome these issues by working together to improve nursing education throughout the world, by retaining nurses and recruiting people to be nurses, and by being an advocate for changes that will improve the delivery of health care (Simpson, 2004). Be prepared for your future in health care. Globalization has affected many other industries, and it is affecting the health care delivery system today. As a leader, you will need to take control of this situation and be proactive in developing solutions before someone outside of nursing takes control (Nash and Gremillion, 2004).

## The Future of Health Care

This discussion on the health care delivery system began with the issue of change. Change threatens many of us, but it also opens up opportunities for improvement. The ultimate issue in designing and delivering health care is the health and welfare of our population. Health care in the United States and around the world is not perfect. Many patients do not receive continuity of care when they see multiple health care providers. Many patients are uninsured or underinsured and are unable to gain access to necessary services. However, health care organizations are striving to become better prepared to deal with the challenges in health care. Many health care organizations are changing how they provide their services, reducing unnecessary costs, improving access to care, and trying to provide high-quality patient care. Professional nursing is an important player in the future of health care delivery. The solutions necessary to improve the quality of health care are not likely to be found without nursing's active participation.

## KEY CONCEPTS

- Increasing costs and decreasing of reimbursement are driving changes in health care, forcing health care institutions to deliver care more efficiently without sacrificing quality.
- In a managed care system, the provider of care receives a predetermined capitated payment regardless of services used by a patient.
- The Medicare prospective reimbursement system is based on payment calculated on the basis of DRG assignment.
- Levels of health care describe the scope of services and settings where health care is offered to patients in all stages of health and illness.
- Health promotion occurs in home, work, and community settings.
- Occupational health nursing includes reducing exposure to environmental hazards, health education, and helping workers return to work safely.
- Nurses are facing the challenge of keeping populations healthy and well within their own homes and communities.
- Successful community-based health programs involve building relationships with the community and incorporating cultural and environmental factors.
- Hospitalized patients are more acutely ill than in the past, requiring better coordination of services before discharge.
- Rehabilitation allows an individual to return to a level of normal or near-normal function after a physical or mental illness, injury, or chemical dependency.
- Nurse-managed clinics offer primary care delivered by advanced practice nurses with a focus on helping patients assume more responsibility for their health.
- Home care agencies provide almost every type of health care service with an emphasis on patient and family independence.
- Discharge planning begins at admission and helps in the transition of a patient's care from one environment to another.
- Health care organizations are being evaluated on the basis of outcomes such as prevention of complications, patients' functional outcomes, and patient satisfaction.
- Consumers of health care should be guaranteed competent health care professionals.
- Nurses need to remain knowledgeable and proactive about issues in the health care delivery system to provide quality patient care and positively impact health.

## CRITICAL THINKING IN PRACTICE

*Mrs. Yim is a 65-year-old widowed woman who lives at home. She came to the emergency department and was hospitalized this morning because she experienced a stroke. Currently she has lost movement on her left side but is able to speak clearly. You are a nurse on a neuroscience ICU, and you have just admitted Mrs. Yim to your unit.*

- - - - - - - - - - - - - - - - - - - -

1. Which level of health care is Mrs. Yim currently receiving?
   a. Preventive care
   b. Primary care
   c. Secondary care
   d. Tertiary care
   e. Restorative care
   f. Continuing care
2. When do you begin discharge planning for Mrs. Yim?
   a. Today
   b. When she is transferred to the general neurology unit
   c. Once her medical condition has stabilized
   d. When her family arrives to visit

3. Mrs. Yim is stabilized, and she is transferred to the general neurology unit. She is participating in occupational and physical therapy, but her left side continues to be weaker than the right, and she is having difficulty walking independently. The advanced practice nurse is hopeful that Mrs. Yim will overcome her impaired physical mobility. However, Mrs. Yim must be discharged from the hospital. What type of facility would best meet Mrs. Yim's needs at this time and why?
4. After several months, Mrs. Yim returns home. A home care nurse visits her every other week to monitor her safety and continued progress at home. Which of the following will help Mrs. Yim avoid future hospitalizations? (Mark all that apply.)
   a. Medication education
   b. Explaining symptoms that indicate Mrs. Yim should call her physician or health care provider immediately
   c. A pass to ride the city bus so Mrs. Yim can get to her daughter's house
   d. Verification of Mrs. Yim's current medication list and reconciliation of any discrepancies
   e. Food stamps

# NCLEX® REVIEW

1. A patient who is concerned about a family history of breast cancer makes an appointment for a routine screening mammography. This is an example of:
   1. Tertiary care
   2. Restorative care
   3. Secondary care
   4. Primary care

2. The greatest amount of health care resources will likely be used when a patient receives care in a:
   1. Secondary care setting
   2. Continuing care setting
   3. Restorative care setting
   4. Preventive care setting

3. You are caring for a hospitalized patient who requires transfer to a skilled nursing facility. Which of the following interventions **best** facilitates a referral to the skilled nursing facility?
   1. Provide instructions to the patient that will support the patient's independence and facilitate return to function.
   2. Provide options to the patient and family for possible skilled nursing facilities, and allow them to select the skilled nursing facility.
   3. Match the services provided at the skilled nursing facility with the patient's needs.
   4. Provide accurate information about the patient to the skilled nursing facility so the nurses at the facility will better understand the patient's needs.

4. A patient who is most likely to use the services of a subacute care unit is:
   1. An outlier
   2. A homeless person
   3. An acutely ill and unstable patient
   4. A patient assigned to a critical pathway

5. A patient who is most likely to be considered a member of a vulnerable patient population is:
   1. A single mother who is raising two children
   2. An older adult who is unable to pay for monthly drug prescription costs
   3. A patient who has suffered a traumatic spinal cord injury and is unable to walk
   4. A cancer patient who has decided to undergo experimental treatment for his tumor

6. Respite care is best described as:
   1. A transitional level of care provided between tertiary and restorative care
   2. A health promotion clinic designed to screen for health problems experienced by the homeless
   3. A service that offers short-term relief for persons who provide home care to ill family members
   4. Medical specialty care for patients with chronic illness and who require continued hospitalization

7. An example of a health care outcome is:
   1. The number of times patients seek health screening services
   2. The ability of patients to return to work following hip replacement
   3. The average length of time it takes to admit a patient to a hospital unit
   4. The total number of immunizations administered to well babies in a community

8. A patient is receiving health care by a health care provider who is a salaried employee. Which type of managed care organization (MCO) does the patient belong to?
   1. Group model
   2. Network model
   3. Independent practice association
   4. Staff model

# REFERENCES

American Nurses Credentialing Center: The magnet application and appraisal process, 2005, http://www.nursecredentialing.org/magnet/process.html.

Barnsteiner J, Provost S: How to implement evidence-based practice: some tried and true pointers, *Reflect Nurs Leadersh* 28(2):18, 2002.

Cambridge Research Institute: *Trends affecting the U.S. health care system,* 262, Health Planning Information Series, Human Resources Administration, Public Health Service, Department of Health, Education, and Welfare, Washington, DC, 1976, revised and updated 1992, U.S. Government Printing Office.

Clemen-Stone S and others: *Comprehensive community health nursing,* ed 6, St. Louis, 2002, Mosby.

Coleman EA and others: Preparing patients and caregivers to participate in care delivered across settings: the care transitions intervention, *J Am Geriatr Soc* 52(11):1817, 2004.

Donabedian A: Evaluating the quality of medical care, *Milbank Memorial Fund Q* 44:166, 1966.

Ebersole P and others: *Toward healthy aging: human needs and nursing response,* ed 6, St. Louis, 2004, Mosby.

Fleck C: Your health: nursing home care is found wanting, 2002, http://www.aarp.org/bulletin/yourhealth/Articles/a2003-06-23-nursinghome.html.

Gosden T and others: Capitation, salary, fee-for-service and mixed systems of payment: effects on the behaviour of primary care physicians, *Cochrane Database Syst Review* 3, 2005.

Health Care Financing Administration, Department of Health and Human Services (HCFA): Requirements for states and long term care facilities, 42 CFR 483 Subpart B (483.1-75), 2004, http://a257.g.akamaitech.net/7/257/2422/12feb20041500/edocket.access.gpo.gov/cfr_2004/octqtr/42cfr483.1.htm.

HEDIS: HEDIS reports home page, 2004, http://www.health.state.mn.us/divs/hpsc/mcs/hedishome.htm.

Heffler S and others: U.S. health spending projections for 2004-2014, 2005, http://content.healthaffairs.org/cgi/reprint/hlthaff.w5.74v1.

Ingenix and others: *DRG expert,* ed 21, Clifton Park, NY, 2005, Thomson Delmar Learning.

Joint Commission on Accreditation of Healthcare Organizations: *Hospital accreditation standards,* Oakbrook Terrace, Ill, 2005, The Commission.

McGlynn EA and others: Establishing national goals for quality improvement, *Med Care* 41(1):I16, 2003.

Meiner SE, Lueckenotte A: *Gerontologic nursing,* ed 3, St. Louis, 2006, Mosby.

Merzel C, D'Afflitti J: Reconsidering community-based health promotion: promise, performance and potential, *Am J Public Health* 93(4):557, 2003.

MissouriFamilies: Aging, 2005, http://missourifamilies.org/quick/agingqa/agingqa7.htm.

Moorhead S and others: *Nursing outcomes classification (NOC),* ed 3, St. Louis, 2004, Mosby.

Nash MG, Gremillion C: Globalization impacts the healthcare organization of the 21st century: demanding new ways to market product lines successfully, *Nurs Adm Q* 28(2):86, 2004.

National Center for Assisted Living: Assisted living facility profile, 2001, http://www.ncal.org/about/facility.htm.

National Research Corporation, Picker Institute: Eight dimensions of patient-centered care, 2005, http://nrcpicker.com/Default.aspx?DN=112,22,2,1,Documents.

Nursing Home Abuse and Neglect Resource Center: Federal regulations and nursing homes, 2003, http://www.nursinghomealert.com/stoppingabuse/federalregulations.html.

Oodyke RJ: Why is the integrated delivery network one of your keys to success in healthcare? 2004, http://www.hcfi.net/040504.pdf.

Pew Health Professions Commission, The Fourth Report of the Pew Health Professions Commission: *Recreating health professional practice for a new century,* 1998, The Commission.

Picker Institute: *Through the patient's eyes,* n.d., http://www.pickerinstitute.org/about.htm.

Resnick B, Fleishell A: Developing a restorative care program: a five step approach that involves the resident, *Am J Nurs* 102(7):95, 2002.

Sackett DL and others: Evidence-based medicine: how to practice and teach EBM, London, 2000, Churchill Livingstone.

Shoultz J, Hatcher PA: Looking beyond primary care to primary health care: an approach to community-based action, *Nurs Outlook* 45(1):23, 1997.

Simpson RL: No-borders nursing: how technology heals global ills, *Nurs Adm Q* 28(1):55, 2004.

Sorrentino S: *Mosby's textbook for nursing assistants,* ed 6, St. Louis, 2003, Mosby.

Spector N: Evidence-based health care in nursing regulation, 2005, http://www.ncsbn.org/pdfs/Evidencebased_NSpector.pdf.

Stanton MW: Hospital nurse staffing and quality of care, *Research in Action,* 2004, http://www.ahrq.gov/research/nursestaffing/nursestaff.pdf.

Sultz HA, Young KM: *Health care USA: understanding its organization and delivery,* ed 4, Sudbury, Mass, 2004, Jones & Bartlett.

# CHAPTER 3

# Community-Based Nursing Practice

## MEDIA RESOURCES

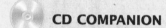 **CD COMPANION** 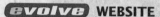 **WEBSITE**

http://evolve.elsevier.com/Potter/basic

- **NCLEX® Review**
- **Audio Glossary**
- **English/Spanish Audio Glossary**

## OBJECTIVES

- Explain the relationship between public health and community health nursing.
- Differentiate community health nursing from community-based nursing.
- Discuss the role of the community health nurse.
- Discuss the role of the nurse in community-based practice.

- Explain the characteristics of patients from vulnerable populations that influence a nurse's approach to care.
- Describe the competencies important for success in community-based nursing practice.
- Describe elements of a community assessment.

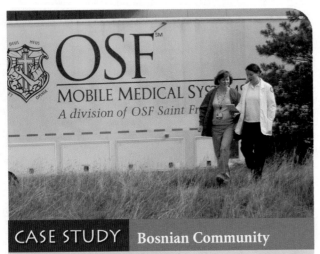

### CASE STUDY  Bosnian Community

Kim Callahan is a senior student in a community health nursing course. Her clinical experience comes from working in a community nursing service within a large city. The majority of patients receiving care from the agency are Bosnian immigrants. One major aspect of care the community nursing service provides is well-child examinations and immunizations to get the children ready to enter the public school system.

In addition, Kim and her classmates conducted an assessment of the community's health care needs and health care practices. This is a close community facing many challenges. Although there is an absence of chronic disease, there is a lack of general preventive health care practices. This includes routine immunizations, well-baby examinations, well-women examinations, and basic screenings for hypertension, cholesterol, etc. Many members of the community do not have adequate insurance and as a result do not receive proper medical care.

The community nursing service has funds to provide mobile primary prevention via a health care van that goes out to the community. Nurse practitioners and community health nurses are the primary care providers. Some services provided include well-baby examinations and immunizations. They also offer well-woman examinations such as Pap smears and mammography and screenings for hypertension, colorectal cancer, and cholesterol. However, many members of the community are suspicious of the free care and doubt that the examinations and results are confidential.

One of the priorities of the community agency is to reach out to the leaders within the community to create an environment of trust and safety, which will hopefully lead more people to increase their use of the services provided. Kim is working with her community nurse preceptor to develop community meetings. These meetings will explain the role of the community nurses in the delivery of care to the community, reinforce the privacy and confidentiality of the services, and describe the types of services they provide.

### KEY TERMS

community-based nursing, p. 43
community health nursing, p. 42
incident rates, p. 41
population, p. 42
public health nursing, p. 42
vulnerable populations, p. 44

Because of the rapid pace of today's health care climate, patients usually move quickly from acute care, hospital-based settings to community-based care that focuses on health promotion, disease prevention, or restorative care. There continues to be a growing need to organize health care delivery services where people live, work, and learn. One way to achieve this goal is through a community-based health care model (Flynn, 1998). Community-based health care organizations frequently spend resources on keeping individuals healthy and well, providing illness care in the patient's home environment and containing costs (U.S. Department of Health and Human Services [USDHHS], 2000a). With this new focus, nursing is in a position to play an important role in health care delivery. The focus of keeping individuals healthy and well has always been appropriate to the holistic practice of professional nursing.

Nursing's history documents the roles of nurses in establishing and meeting the public health goals of their patients and their families. Within the community health settings, nurses are leaders in assessing, implementing, and evaluating the types of public and community health services the community needs. Community health nursing and community-based nursing are components or parts of health care delivery necessary to improve the health of the general public.

## Community-Based Health Care

As a nurse it is important for you to gain an understanding of community-based health care. Historically, government-funded agencies support community health programs to improve the safety and adequacy of food supplies and to provide a safe water supply and adequate sewage disposal. Public health policy is largely responsible for the increase in life expectancy for Americans during the last century (Stanhope and Lancaster, 2004).

Today the challenges in community-based health care are many. Social lifestyles, political policy, and economic ambitions have all influenced some of the major public health problems, including the following: an increase in sexually transmitted diseases, environmental pollution, underimmunization of infants and children, and the appearance of new life-threatening diseases (e.g., acquired immunodeficiency syndrome [AIDS] and other emerging infections). More than ever before, the health care system needs a commitment to reform and bring attention to the health care needs of all communities.

### Achieving Healthy Populations and Communities

The U.S. Department of Health and Human Services, Public Health Service designed a program to improve the overall health status of people living in this country (see Chapter 1). The Healthy People Initiative was first created to establish health care goals for the year 2000. The Healthy People Initiative continually revises these goals. For example, the overall goals of *Healthy People 2010* are to increase the life expectancy and quality of life and to eliminate the inequality of health among populations (USDHHS, 2000b).

The current revision, *Healthy People 2010,* is designed to improve the delivery of health care services to the general public. There are many ways to accomplish this. Assessing the health care needs of individuals, families, or members of the community; developing and implementing public health policies; and improving access to care are ideas to improve delivery (Clark and others, 2003). For example, assessment sometimes includes the use of community meetings to identify and collect specific data about a population's health practices. The assessment also includes monitoring the population's health status, such as the commonness of communicable diseases or frequency of asthma. In addition, further community assessment occurs by accessing available information about the health of the community (Stanhope and Lancaster, 2004). Examples of assessment include, but are not limited to, the following: gathering information on **incident rates** for certain cancers, identifying and reporting emerging infections, determining adolescent pregnancy rates, and reporting the number of motor vehicle accidents by teenage drivers.

Public policy development and implementation refers to health professionals providing leadership in developing policies that support the population's health. Health professionals will use research-based findings in developing policies. For example, a health professional suggests the use of immunization to reduce infectious disease and suggests using seatbelts and initiating new driving restrictions for new teenage drivers to reduce disability due to motor vehicle accidents. Assurance refers to the role of public health in making sure that essential community-wide health services are available and accessible (Stanhope and Lancaster, 2004). Examples of assurance include the provision of prenatal care to the uninsured and beginning educational programs to ensure the competency of public health professionals. Population-based public health programs focus on disease prevention, health protection, and health promotion. This focus provides the foundation for health care services at all levels (see Chapter 2).

The five-level health services pyramid is an example of how to provide community-based services within the existing health care services in a community (Figure 3-1). For example, a rural community may have a hospital to meet the acute care needs of its patients. However, community assessment notes that there are few services to meet the needs of expectant mothers, to reduce teenage smoking, or to provide nutritional support for older adults. Community-based programs that provide these three services will improve the health of the specific populations, as well as the population of the community. When the lower-level services are accessible and effective, there is a greater likelihood that the higher tiers will contribute to the total health of the community (U.S. Public Health Service, 1995). For example, if there is inadequate mosquito control in a community, it becomes more difficult to enforce health promotion efforts and to prevent mosquito-borne diseases. On the other hand, when a community has the resources for providing childhood immunizations, primary preventive care services are able to focus on higher-tier services, such as child developmental problems and child safety.

The principles of public health practice aim at achieving a healthy environment for all individuals to live in. These principles apply to individuals, families, and the communities in which they live. Nursing plays a role in all levels of the health services pyramid. By using public health principles, you will be able to better understand the types of environments in which patients live and the types of interventions necessary to help keep patients healthy.

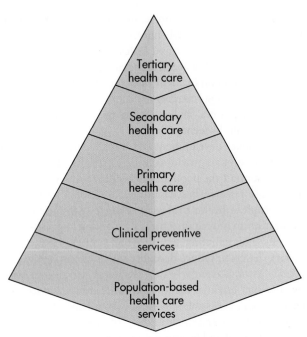

## SYNTHESIS IN PRACTICE

Kim meets with community leaders and members to assess the beliefs and concerns of the community. She identifies a lack of understanding in the community regarding health care practices in this country. In addition, the community has some misunderstandings and fear of health care services that the community agency and van provide.

Kim recognizes that members of this community came from a war-ravaged county where resources for health promotion were nonexistent. As a result, she understands the concerns and lack of understanding about community care and how this affects the use of services provided by the community health agency. She operates under the ethical principle of beneficence and wants to do the most good for the most people in this case. She respects the community's beliefs and their current level of health care knowledge. Kim wants to assist the community agency to meet the health care needs of the Bosnian community.

If she views the community as a patient, Kim will focus her care on the total community. She continually assesses the community's knowledge and acceptance of the health care services provided. In addition, Kim identifies community leaders to serve as "point persons" or contacts in educational programs designed to meet the health care needs of the community. These programs will also help to change the community's misconceptions and fear of the services provided.

## Community Health Nursing

Frequently you hear the terms *community health nursing* and *public health nursing* used interchangeably (SmithBattle, Diekemper, and Leander, 2004). There are some similarities. A **public health nursing** focus requires understanding the needs of a **population,** or a collection of individuals who have in common one or more personal or environmental characteristics (Stanhope and Lancaster, 2004). Examples of populations include high-risk infants, older adults, or a cultural group such as Native Americans.

A public health professional understands factors that influence health promotion and health maintenance of groups. They also understand the trends and patterns influencing the incidence of disease within populations, environmental factors contributing to health and illness, and the political processes used to affect public policy. A public health nurse requires preparation at the basic entry level. Sometimes a public health nurse requires a baccalaureate degree in nursing that includes educational preparation and clinical practice in public health nursing. A specialist in public health is prepared at the graduate level with a focus in the public health sciences (American Nurses Association [ANA], 1999).

**Community health nursing** is a nursing approach that combines knowledge from the public health sciences with professional nursing theories to safeguard and improve the health of populations in a community (ANA, 1999; Ayers, Bruno, and Langford, 1999). The focus of such nursing care is somewhat broader than that of public health, with an emphasis on the health of a community. In addition to considering the needs of populations, the community health nurse provides direct care services to subpopulations within a community. These subpopulations are occasionally a clinical focus in which the nurse has gained expertise. For example, a case manager follows older adults recovering from stroke and sees the need for community rehabilitation services, or a nurse practitioner gives immunizations to patients with the objective of managing communicable disease within the community. By focusing on subpopulations, the community health nurse cares for the community as a whole and considers the individual or family to be only one member of a group at risk.

Competence as a community health nurse requires the ability to use interventions. These interventions take into account how community problems resolve within the broad social and political context (Stanhope and Lancaster, 2004). The educational requirements for entry-level nurses practicing in community health nursing roles are not as clear-cut as those for public health nurses. A hiring agency does not always require an advanced degree. However, nurses with a graduate degree in nursing who practice in community settings are community health nurse specialists, regardless of their public health experience (Stanhope and Lancaster, 2004).

## Nursing Practice in Community Health

Community-focused nursing practice requires a unique set of skills and knowledge. In the health care delivery system, nurses who become expert in community health practice may have advanced nursing degrees, yet nurses with less education also become quite competent in formulating and applying population-focused assessments and interventions (Diekemper, SmithBattle, and Drake, 1999). The expert community health nurse comes to understand the needs of a population or community through experience with individual families and working through their social and health care issues. Critical thinking becomes important for the nurse who applies knowledge of public health principles, community health nursing, family theory, and communication in finding the best approaches in partnering with families. Diekemper and others (1999) interviewed community health nurses to hear their stories and to understand what population-focused practice involves. Often community health nurses see their practice evolve "naturally" as they serve families and communities. The best situation for this is when the working environment does not restrict the nurse's ability to work closely with members of the community.

A successful community health nursing practice involves building relationships with the community and responding to changes within the community (Diekemper and others, 1999). For example, you notice an increase in the number of grandparents assuming child care responsibilities. You, as a community nurse, establish an instructional program in cooperation with local schools to assist and support grandparents in this caregiving role. The community health nurse becomes an active part of a community. This means knowing the community's members, needs, and resources and then working to establish effective health promotion and disease prevention programs. This requires working with highly resistant systems (e.g., welfare system) and trying to encourage them to be more responsive to the needs of a population. Skills of patient advocacy, communicating people's concerns, and designing new systems in cooperation with existing systems help to make community-nursing practice effective.

## Community-Based Nursing

**Community-based nursing** involves the acute and chronic care of individuals and families to strengthen their capacity for self-care and promotes independence in decision making (Ayers and others, 1999). Care takes place in community settings such as the home or a clinic; however, the focus is nursing care of the individual or family (Feenstra, 2000). As with other practice settings, your community practice competence is based on critical thinking and decision making at the level of the individual patient—assessing health status, selecting nursing interventions, and evaluating outcomes of

care. Because direct care services are provided where patients live, work, and play, it is important that you know the diverse needs of the individual and family and appreciate the values of a multicultural community (Zotti, Brown, and Stotts, 1996). In so doing, community nursing practice provides a means to improve, protect, and enhance the quality of health of all who reside in a specific community (Sakamoto and Avilla, 2004).

The philosophical foundation for community-based nursing is a model that views human systems as open and interactive with the environment (Chalmers and others, 1998). In this model your patient exists within the larger systems of family, community, culture, and society. The social interaction units seen in Figure 3-2 depict four circles: the inner circle of the patient and the immediate family, the second circle of people and settings that have frequent contact with the patient and family, the third circle of the local community and its values and policies, and the outer circle of larger social systems such as government and church (Ayers and others, 1999).

As a nurse in a community-based practice setting, you need to understand the interaction of all of the units while caring for your patient and family. Usually you provide care for your patient in the area of the first three circles. For example, in your community practice clinical experience you are working with a home care nurse who has a patient newly diagnosed with diabetes. You work closely with the patient and family to create a comprehensive plan for the patient's health. As the nurse-patient relationship evolves, you begin to understand your patient's habits or lifestyle patterns. You learn how these change when the patient is with friends and co-workers. Together you anticipate ways to plan the patient's exercise schedule and meal routines. Knowing the resources available in the community (e.g., medical supply shops for glucose monitoring supplies and local diabetes association support groups) helps you to provide comprehensive support for the patient's needs.

Community-based nursing is family-centered care that takes place within the community (Ayers and others, 1999). This focus requires you to be knowledgeable about family theory (see Chapter 21), principles of communication (see Chapter 9), group dynamics, and cultural diversity (see Chapter 17). This knowledge helps you to partner with patients and families and to understand their health care needs. Ultimately you assist your patients and their families to assume responsibility for their health care decisions. The families become involved in planning, decision making, implementation, and evaluation of health care approaches.

### Vulnerable Populations

In the community you will care for patients from diverse cultures and backgrounds and with various health conditions. However, changes in the health care delivery system have made high-risk groups the community health nurse's principal patients. For example, it is unlikely that you will

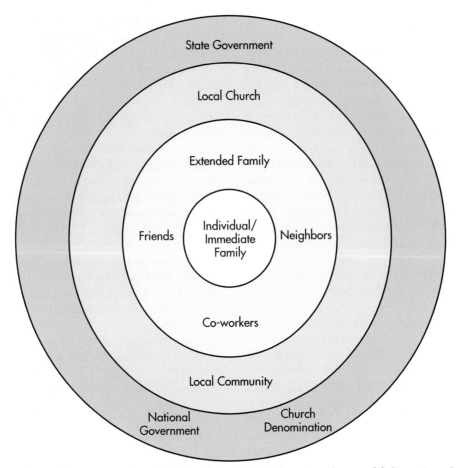

FIGURE **3-2**  These concentric circles represent the social interaction units of the human ecology model. (From Ayers M, Bruno AA, Lanford RW: *Community-based nursing care: making the transition,* St. Louis, 1999, Mosby.)

visit low-risk mothers and babies. Instead, you are more likely to make home visits to adolescent mothers or mothers with drug addiction.

**Vulnerable populations** of patients are those who are more likely to develop health problems as a result of excess risks, who have limits in access to health care services, or who are dependent on others for care. Individuals living in poverty, older adults, homeless persons, individuals in abusive relationships, substance abusers, severely mentally ill persons, and new immigrants are examples of vulnerable populations (Hwang, 2000). Vulnerable individuals and their families often belong to more than one of these groups. In addition, health care vulnerability affects all age-groups (Corrarino and others, 2000). Sometimes vulnerable individuals are a specific population with a unique health care problem. For example, the older adult who has received heart transplantation has unique health care needs (Baas and other, 2002).

Frequently, vulnerable patients come from varied cultures, have different beliefs and values, face language barriers, and have few sources of social support (Chalmers and others, 1998). Their special needs create challenges for nurses in caring for increasingly complex acute and chronic health conditions.

To become competent in the care of vulnerable populations, it is especially important for you to provide culturally appropriate care. Chapter 17 addresses factors influencing individual differences within cultural groups and the nurse's role in providing culturally appropriate care. To be culturally competent, you need to appraise and understand a patient and family's cultural beliefs, values, and practices. This is necessary to determine their specific needs and the interventions that will be successful in improving the patient's state of health. It is not enough for you to be sensitive to your patient's cultural uniqueness. Your communication skills and caring practices are critical in identifying and understanding your patient's perceptions of his or her problems and planning health care strategies that will be meaningful, culturally appropriate, and successful.

Vulnerable populations typically experience poorer outcomes than those patients with ready access to resources and health care services. Dramatically shorter life spans and higher death rates are real threats to members of ethnically and racially diverse minority groups (Barr and others, 2002; Hwang, 2000). Members of vulnerable groups frequently have cumulative risks or combinations of risk factors that make them more sensitive to the adverse effects of individ-

| BOX 3-1 | **Guidelines for Assessing Members of Vulnerable Population Groups** |

### Setting the Stage

- Create a comfortable, nonthreatening environment.
- Obtain information about the culture so you have an understanding of their practices, beliefs, and values that affect their health care.
- Provide a culturally competent assessment by understanding the meaning of the patient's language and nonverbal behavior.
- Be sensitive to the fact that your patients may have priorities other than their health care. These may include financial, legal, or social issues. You need to assist them with these concerns before you begin a health assessment.
- Work together with other health care and social need providers. If your patient needs financial assistance, consult a social worker. If there are legal issues, provide your patient with a resource. Do not attempt to provide financial or legal advice.

### Nursing History of an Individual or Family

- Because you often have only one opportunity to conduct a nursing history, obtain an organized history of all of the essential information you need to help the individual or family during that visit.
- Collect data on a comprehensive form that focuses on the specific needs of the vulnerable population with whom you work. However, remember to be flexible so that you do not overlook important health information. For example, if you are working with an adolescent mother, you are focusing on obtaining a nu-

tritional history on both the mother and baby. Be aware of the developmental needs of the adolescent mom and listen to her social needs as well.
- Identify the patient's developmental needs, as well as health care needs. Remember, your goal is to collect enough information to provide family-centered care.
- Identify any risks to the patient's immune system. This is especially important for vulnerable patients who are homeless and sleep in shelters.

### Physical Examination and Home Assessment

- It is important that you complete as thorough a physical and/or home assessment as possible. However, only collect data that you will use and is important to providing care to your patient and family.
- Be alert for signs of physical abuse or substance abuse (e.g., inadequately clothed to hide bruising, underweight, runny nose).
- Sharpen your observation skills when assessing your patient's home. Is there adequate water and plumbing? What is the status of the utilities? Are foods and perishables stored properly? Are there signs of insects or vermin? Look at the walls. Is the paint peeling? Are the windows and doors adequate? Are there water stains on the ceiling, evidence of a leaky rook? What is the temperature? Is it comfortable? What does the outside environment look like: Are there vacant houses/lots nearby? Is there a busy intersection? What is the crime level?

Modified from Stanhope M, Lancaster J: *Community and public health nursing*, ed 6, St. Louis, 2004, Mosby.

---

ual risk factors (Rew and others, 2001). When you assess members of vulnerable populations, it is important to take into account the multiple stressors that affect their lives. It is also important to learn your patients' strengths and resources for coping with stressors. Box 3-1 summarizes guidelines to follow when assessing members of vulnerable population groups.

**POOR AND HOMELESS PERSONS.** People who live in poverty are more likely to live in hazardous or dangerous environments, work at high-risk jobs, eat less nutritious diets, and have multiple stressors in their lives. When comparing the life expectancy of European Americans and African-Americans, researchers found the causes of the differences to be related to low socioeconomic status rather than race (Barr and others, 2002; Hwang, 2000). Patients with low income not only lack financial resources, but also may reside in poor living environments and face practical problems such as poor or unavailable transportation.

In general the homeless population has even fewer resources than the poor. They do not have the advantage of shelter and cope with finding a place to sleep at night and finding food. Chronic health problems worsen because the homeless have no place to store medications, if they can afford them, and do not get nutritious meals. In addition, they lack a healthy balance of rest and activity due to walking

throughout the day to meet basic needs and because of vagrancy laws that prohibit loitering (Hwang and Bugeja, 2000). There is a high incidence of mental illness, personality disorder, and substance abuse among the homeless population. Homeless adolescents are increasing, and this vulnerable population has more social, behavioral, physical, and health risks. Community-based nurses are frequently the only health care provider available to these youth (Rew and others, 2001).

In the community setting it is important that you help these patients to identify the available resources (e.g., mobile health care unit [Figure 3-3]), eligibility for assistance, and the interventions to improve their health status.

**ABUSED PATIENTS.** Physical, emotional, and sexual abuse, as well as neglect, are major public health problems affecting older adults, women, and children (Rew and others, 2001; Sebastian, 1996). Risk factors for abusive relationships include mental health problems, substance abuse, socioeconomic stressors, and dysfunctional family relationships. Sometimes there are not any risk factors present. It is important to provide protection for patients at risk for or who have suffered abuse. Interview patients at a time when their privacy is ensured and the individual suspected of being the abuser is not present. Victims of abuse fear retribution if they discuss their problems with a health care provider. Most

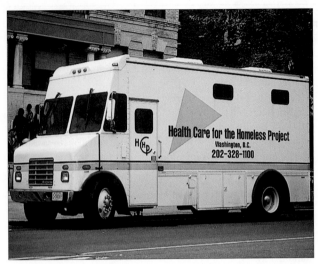

FIGURE **3-3** The homeless population has unique health care needs.

states have abuse hot lines and laws that require you to notify the hot lines if you suspect a patient is at risk.

**SUBSTANCE ABUSERS.** Substance abuse describes more than the use of illegal drugs. This term also includes the abuse of alcohol and prescribed medications, such as antianxiety agents and opioid analgesics. A patient with substance abuse has health and socioeconomic problems. The socioeconomic problems result from the financial strain of the cost of drugs, criminal convictions from illegal activities used to obtain drugs, communicable disease from sharing drug equipment, and family breakdown. For example, health problems for cocaine users include nasal and sinus disorders and cardiac alterations that are sometimes fatal (Stanhope and Lancaster, 2004).

You need to objectively assess substance use in terms of the amount, frequency, and type of substance used. It is important that you do not show any judgment or disapproval to your patient. Frequently these patients avoid health care for fear of judgmental attitudes by health care providers and concern over being turned in to the police.

**SEVERELY MENTALLY ILL PERSONS.** When a patient has a severe mental illness (e.g., depression or schizophrenia) or severe personality disorders (bipolar disorder), there are multiple health and socioeconomic problems you must explore. Many patients with pervasive mental illnesses are homeless or marginally housed. Others lack the ability to maintain employment or to even care for themselves on a daily basis. Patients suffering from pervasive mental illness require medication therapy, counseling, housing, and vocational assistance. In addition, mentally ill patients are at greater risk for abuse and assault (Eckert, Sugar, and Fine, 2002).

The mentally ill are no longer routinely hospitalized in long-term psychiatric institutions. Instead, the goal is to offer community resources; however, not all communities have

service networks to deal with this (Stanhope and Lancaster, 2004). Many patients have few or limited services and little skill in surviving and functioning within the community. There are an increased number of young mentally ill persons who have had only episodic hospital care. Collaboration with multiple community resources is a key to helping the pervasively mentally ill receive adequate health care.

**OLDER ADULTS.** Because people are living longer, there is an increase in the older adult population. This means more patients suffer from chronic disease and there is a greater demand for health care services provided in a community setting. Many associate old age with poor health and disease, not with health promotion and prevention (Barr and others, 2002). However, it is important that you view health promotion from a broad context. This begins with your understanding of what health means to older adults and the steps they can take to maintain their own health (Zahn and others, 1998). When people are able to control their own health, they are able to reduce disability from chronic disease (Baas and others, 2002). There is an opportunity to improve the lifestyle of older adults and their quality of life. Table 3-1 describes the major health problems older adults encounter and the role of community health nurses.

## Competency in Community-Based Nursing

As a nurse in community-based practice, you need a variety of skills and talents to be successful. You will assist patients with their health care needs and in developing relationships within the community. The Pew Health Professions Commission (1991) recommended competencies for health care professionals. One of the competencies they recommended is the practice of prevention and caring for the community's health (Dower, O'Neil, and Hough, 2001). You need to apply the nursing process (see Chapter 7) in a critical thinking approach to ensure good, individualized nursing care for specific patients and their families. Additional competencies discussed here will help you deliver care within the context of the patient's community, which will assist with long-term success of the care objectives.

### Case Manager

In community-based practice, case management is an important competency. Case management means making an appropriate plan of care based on assessment of patients and families and to coordinate needed resources and services for the patient's well-being across a continuum of care. Generally, in a community setting a nurse is responsible for the case management of more than one patient. This usually involves patients who need coordination of different health care services (e.g., patients with neurological disease, trauma victims, psychiatric patients, and pa-

| TABLE 3-1 | Major Health Problems in Older Adults and Community Health Nursing Roles and Interventions |
|---|---|
| **Problem** | **Community Health Nursing Roles and Interventions** |
| Hypertension | Monitor blood pressure and weight; educate about nutrition and antihypertensive drugs; teach stress management techniques; promote a good balance between rest and activity; establish blood pressure screening programs; assess patient's current lifestyle and promote lifestyle changes; promote dietary modifications by using techniques such as a diet diary. |
| Cancer | Obtain health history; promote monthly breast self-examinations and yearly Pap smears and mammograms for older women; promote regular physical examinations; encourage smokers to stop smoking; correct misconceptions about processes of aging; provide emotional support and quality of care during diagnostic and treatment procedures. |
| Arthritis | Help adult avoid the false hope and expense of arthritis fraud; educate adult about management of activities, correct body mechanics, availability of mechanical appliances, and adequate rest; promote stress management; counsel and assist the family to improve communication, role negotiation, and use of community resources. |
| Visual impairment (e.g., loss of visual acuity, eyelid disorders, opacity of the lens) | Provide support in a well-lighted, glare-free environment; use printed aids with large, well-spaced letters; assist adult with cleaning eyeglasses; help make arrangements for vision examinations and obtain necessary prostheses; teach adult to be cautious of false advertisements. |
| Hearing impairment (e.g., presbycusis) | Speak with clarity at a moderate volume and pace, and face audience when performing health teaching; help make arrangements for hearing examination and obtain necessary prostheses; teach adult to be cautious of false advertisements. |
| Cognitive impairment | Provide complete assessment; correct underlying causes of disease (if possible); provide for a protective environment; promote activities that reinforce reality; assist with personal hygiene, nutrition, and hydration; provide emotional support to the family; recommend applicable community resources such as adult day care, home care aides, and homemaker services. |
| Alzheimer's disease | Maintain high-level functioning, protection, and safety; encourage human dignity; demonstrate to the primary family caregiver techniques to dress, feed, and toilet adult; provide frequent encouragement and emotional support to caregiver; act as an advocate for patient when dealing with respite care and support groups; make sure to protect the patient's rights; provide support to maintain family members' physical and mental health; maintain family stability; recommend financial services if needed. |
| Dental problems | Perform oral assessment and refer as necessary; emphasize regular brushing and flossing, proper nutrition, and dental examinations; encourage patients with dentures to wear and take care of them; calm fears about dentist; help provide access to financial services (if necessary) and access to dental care facilities. |
| Drug use and abuse | Get drug use history; educate adult about safe storage, risks of drug, drug-drug, and drug-food interactions; give general information about drug (e.g., drug name, purpose, side effects, dosage); instruct adult about presorting techniques (using small containers with one dose of drug that are labeled with specific times to take drug). |
| Substance abuse | Arrange and monitor detoxification if appropriate; counsel adults about substance abuse; promote stress management to avoid need for drugs or alcohol; encourage adult to use self-help groups such as Alcoholics Anonymous and Al-Anon; educate public about dangers of substance abuse. |

Data from Stanhope M, Lancaster J: *Community and public health nursing*, ed 6, St. Louis, 2004, Mosby; Baas LD and others: The challenge of managing the care of older heart transplant recipients, *AACN Clin Issues* 13(1):114, 2002; Hwang SW: Mortality among men using homeless shelters in Toronto, Ontario, *JAMA* 283(16):2152, 2000; Hwang SW, Bugeja AL: Barriers to appropriate diabetes management among homeless people in Toronto, *Can Med Assoc J* 163(2):161, 2000.

tients with complex medical conditions). The greatest challenge for you is coordinating the activities of many different providers and payers, in different settings, throughout a patient's continuum of care. Although you may work in one location, you influence the selection and monitoring of care provided in other settings by formal and informal caregivers (Stanhope and Lancaster, 2004). To be an effective case manager you need to learn the roadblocks, shortages, and opportunities that exist within

the community to find solutions for patients' health care needs. Case management with individual patients and families reveals the big picture of health services and the health status of a community.

## Collaborator

When you practice in a community-based nursing setting, you competently work with individuals and their families and other related health care disciplines. Collaboration, or working with others to care for a patient, is important so that you make a mutually acceptable plan that will achieve common goals (Ayers and others, 1999). For example, when the hospital discharges your patient with terminal cancer, you collaborate with hospice staff, social workers, and pastoral or religious care to start a plan to support the patient and family. For collaboration to be effective, there needs to be mutual trust and respect for each professional's abilities and contributions. Similarly, patients need to trust the health care providers. Teamwork is central to serving the patient well. Together with other health care professionals you will explore patient issues, know the contributions each professional offers, and clarify roles. This will help you to develop a plan of care that patient and health care providers can accept and support.

## Educator

When working in a community setting you will need to be an educator, or teacher for your patients. You will have opportunities to work with single individuals and groups of patients. As an educator, you establish relationships with community service organizations. These organizations will help you to offer educational support to a wide range of patient groups. Some health education programs that occur in a community practice setting are perinatal classes, infant care, child safety, and cancer screening (Corrarino and others, 2000).

With the goal of helping patients assume responsibility for their own health care, the role of educator takes on greater importance in community-based nursing than in other types of care (Ayers and others, 1999). You expect patients and families to gain the skills and knowledge they need to learn how to care for themselves (see Chapter 10). In community-based practice you need to assess your patient's learning needs and readiness to learn as an individual, the systems the individual interacts with (e.g., family, business, and school), and the resources available for support. Likewise you adapt your teaching skills to instruct within the home setting and make the learning process meaningful. In this setting you have an opportunity to follow patients over time. As a result, you can plan to return for a review of skills, use follow-up phone calls, and refer the patient to community support and self-help groups. This follow-up gives you the opportunity to continue instruction and to reinforce important instructional topics. Evaluation of patient learning occurs over time, requiring patience and commitment.

## Counselor

As a counselor, you assist your patients in identifying and clarifying health problems and in choosing appropriate solutions for problems (Ayers and others, 1999). For example, if you work in employee assistance programs or women's shelters, a major amount of your patient interaction is through counseling. In this role you are responsible for providing information, listening objectively, and being supportive, caring, and trustworthy. Counselors do not make deci-

sions; they help patients reach decisions that best suit them (Stanhope and Lancaster, 2004). In a community-based practice setting you will face many situations where counseling is an important skill. Patients and families often need help first identifying or clarifying health problems. For example, you have a patient who repeatedly reports a problem in following a prescribed diet. After questioning the patient, you find that the problem is really that the patient cannot afford nutritious foods and has family members who do not support good eating habits. In this case, you may discuss with your patient factors that cause the problem, identify a range of solutions, and then discuss which solutions are most likely to be successful. As a counselor you encourage patients to make decisions and give them confidence in the choices they make.

To be an effective counselor you need to know what resources a community offers to patients. Frequently patients go outside their own family to obtain the support that is necessary to improve their health status. You need to know these resources well to direct your patients to appropriate resources. Be able to answer questions such as, What services do agencies provide? Is the staff accessible? What are the reimbursement limitations, and do these affect access? and Is there coordination between agencies within the community?

## Patient Advocate

Patient advocacy, or supporting patients, is perhaps even more important today in community-based practice because of the confusion surrounding access to health care services. Your patients often need someone to help them walk through the system. This means identifying where to go for services, how to reach the individuals with the appropriate authority, what services to request, and how to follow through with the information they received. You will be the one who presents the patient's point of view to obtain the appropriate resources. It is important that you provide patients necessary information to make informed decisions in choosing services appropriately.

## Change Agent

You will also act as a change agent, or someone who creates change, in a community-based setting. As a competent change agent, you will seek to implement new and more effective approaches to problems (Ayers and others, 1999). You act as a change agent within a family system or intercede with problems that reside within the patient's community. You use your assessment skills to identify any number of problems (e.g., quality of community child care services, availability of older adult day care services, or the status of neighborhood violence). It is important to empower individuals, their families, and their community to creatively solve problems or become instrumental in creating change within a health care agency.

To make changes you must be very familiar with the community itself. Many communities are resistant to change.

---

**BOX 3-2** | **Success Factors in Adopting Change**

- Patient perceives the change as more advantageous that other alternatives. The nature of the innovation determines what specific type of relative advantage (e.g., social, economic, community good) is important to those who adopt the change. *For example, a community health center wants to initiate a school-based exercise and nutrition program. The parents of the children and the school are equally concerned about the weight problem and lack of regular exercise programs.*
- The change is compatible with existing values, past experiences, and needs of potential adopters. A change agent will determine the needs of patients and recommend changes that fulfill those needs. *Before starting the school-based exercise and nutrition program, the organizers identified that 40% of the children in the school were at least 15 pounds overweight.*
- Try the innovation or change on a limited basis. Patients adopt new ideas more quickly when they can experiment with them.

Patients trying out a new technology can find out how it works in their own situation. *The school-based exercise and nutrition program was initiated for all third and fourth graders in the elementary school.*
- Simple innovations or changes are easier to adopt than complex ones. An innovation must be easy to understand and use. *These two grades were chosen because they have the same physical education teacher and eat lunch during the same period.*
- Communities adopt change when you communicate results clearly and when the results are visible. *At the end of a 10-week period, 10% of all overweight children lost at least 10 pounds, and 80% of all eligible children participated in the program. The school elected to phase in the program for all the elementary school children.*

Data from Rogers EM: *Diffusion of innovation,* ed 5, New York, 2004, Free Press.

---

They prefer to continue providing services as they always have. Before you can implement any change it is necessary to manage conflict between the health care providers involved in the patient's care, clarify their roles, and clearly identify the needs of the patients (Box 3-2). If the community has a history of poor problem solving, focus on developing problem-solving capabilities (Stanhope and Lancaster, 2004). For example, you have a patient who has trouble making routine health care visits. First, you help the patient find the source of the problem. In this case, the patient has limited access to transportation. You make the suggestion for the patient to visit an alternative site, such as a nursing clinic, because it is closer and its hours are more convenient for the patient.

## Community Assessment

When you practice in a community setting, it is important that you learn how to assess the community at large. This is the environment where your patients live and work. Without an adequate understanding of that environment, any effort to promote the patient's health and to institute necessary change is unlikely to be successful. The community has three components or parts: structure or locale, the people, and the social systems. A complete assessment involves a careful look at each component to begin to identify needs for health policy, health program development, and service provision (Box 3-3). When assessing the structure or locale, you travel around the neighborhood or community and observe its design, the location of services, and the locations where residents meet. A public library or the local health department is a great source for accessing statistics to assess the demographics of the community. To get information about existing social systems, such as schools or health care facilities, visit various sites and learn about their services.

Once you have a good understanding of the community, perform any individual patient assessment against that background. For example, you are assessing a patient's home for safety. Does the patient have secure locks on doors? Are windows secure and intact? Is lighting along walkways and entryways working? As you conduct the assessment, know the level of community violence and the resources that are available to the patient when help is necessary. No individual patient assessment should occur in isolation from the environment and conditions of the patient's community.

## Changing Patients' Health

In a community-based practice you will care for patients from diverse backgrounds and in diverse settings. It is relatively easy over time to become familiar with the resources that are available within a particular community practice setting. With practice you learn how to identify the unique needs of individual patients. However, the challenge is how to promote and protect a patient's health within the context of the community. Can a patient with lung disease, for example, have the quality of life necessary when the patient's community has a serious environmental pollution problem? Likewise, it is important to bring together the resources necessary to improve the continuity of care that patients receive. Be a leader in reducing the duplication of health care services and locating the best services for a patient's needs.

Perhaps the most important theme to consider to be an effective community-based nurse is to understand patients' lives. This begins when you are able to establish

---

**BOX 3-3** | **Community Assessment**

**Structure**

- Name of community or neighborhood
- Geographical boundaries
- Environment
- Water and sanitation
- Housing
- Economy

- Educational level
- Predominant cultural groups
- Predominant religious groups

**Population**

- Age distribution
- Sex distribution
- Growth trends
- Density

**Social System**

- Educational system
- Government
- Communication system
- Transportation system
- Welfare system
- Volunteer programs
- Health system

---

strong, caring relationships with patients and their families (see Chapter 16). This is a challenge when you have little time available to spend with patients. However, as your expertise grows, you are able to advise, counsel, and teach effectively. As you gain an understanding of the needs of the community, you also gain an awareness of what truly makes your patients unique. The day-to-day activities of family life are the variables that influence how you adapt your nursing interventions. Here are a few examples of factors you will consider in community-based practice: the time of day a patient goes to work, the availability of the spouse and patient's parents to provide child care, and the family values that shape views about health. Once you acquire a picture of a patient's life, you introduce interventions to promote health and prevent disease so that the picture becomes enhanced.

## EVALUATION

Kim has spent the last 12 weeks of her 14-week rotation working with the community agency and leaders in the Bosnian community. The goal is to provide educational programs to explain how the clinic provides services and the confidentiality of the services. The program will also explain that the services are free to patients who do not have adequate insurance or financial resources. Kim presented a series of three programs in the homes of four Bosnian leaders. Kim worked with the leaders on the design of the educational programs and continued to evaluate the community's response to the programs and health care needs. Throughout this period there was a gradual increase in the use of the services within the agency and the van. In addition, young women within the community have asked for some prenatal classes.

Kim also perceived a greater acceptance within the community. After the first 3 weeks following Kim's class, there are fewer "missed" appointments, and the members of the community share more relevant health care concerns with her. Finally, Kim feels a sense of confidence and competence in developing community health care programs. She has learned the importance of including the community and the community leaders in all aspects of program building from the assessment of needs through program development and evaluation.

As Kim prepares to finish her clinical experience she discusses the long-term health care goals of the community. In addition, she introduces the next student to the community and the community leaders to provide continuity in health care program development.

## KEY CONCEPTS

- The principles of public health nursing practice aim at assisting individuals with acquiring a healthy environment in which to live.
- Essential public health functions include assessment, policy development, and access to resources.
- When population-based health care services are effective, there is a greater likelihood of the higher tiers of services contributing efficiently to health improvement of the population.
- The community health nurse cares for the community as a whole and considers the individual or family to be only one member of a group at risk.
- A successful community health nursing practice involves building relationships with the community and being responsive to changes within the community.

- The community-based nurse's competence is based on decision making at the level of the individual patient.
- Vulnerable individuals and their families often belong to more than one vulnerable group.
- The special needs of vulnerable populations form the backdrop for the challenges nurses face in caring for these patients' increasingly complex acute and chronic health conditions.
- Chronic health problems are common and worsen among the homeless because they have few resources.
- An important principle in dealing with patients at risk or who have suffered abuse is protection of the patient.
- Patients who are substance abusers often avoid health care for fear of being turned in to criminal authorities.

- A community-based nurse is competent as a collaborator, educator, counselor, change agent, and patient advocate.
- Factors that increase the likelihood of a change being accepted and adopted include: that the change is advantageous, compatible, realistic, and easy to adopt.

- Assessment of a community includes three elements: structure or locale, the people, and the social systems.

## CRITICAL THINKING IN PRACTICE

*Within the Bosnian community, Katrina Dudek is a 30-year-old widow with two children. One is 3 years and the other is 6 months. She arrived in the community 5 months ago. Her husband was killed in a raid in their home in her native country. She is very fearful when anyone other than her close neighbors and friends enter her home. The community health nurse wants to work with Mrs. Dudek to determine the health care needs of her children and herself. The community health agency has not been successful in providing any care to Mrs. Dudek and her children.*

1. What key element would be helpful for initiating care for this family?
2. Mrs. Dudek is fearful about providing immunization history about her children. What is your action?
3. Although Mrs. Dudek is vulnerable to health care problems because she is new to this country, there are other factors that increase her vulnerability. What might some of these factors be?

## NCLEX® REVIEW

1. Community health nursing is a nursing approach that merges knowledge from professional nursing theories and the:
   1. Population sciences
   2. Public health sciences
   3. Environmental sciences
   4. Mental health sciences
2. A patient has a history of asthma with six hospitalizations over the past 2 years. She does try to control her illness and appropriately uses her inhalers and other prescribed medications. What level of prevention corresponds to her disease management?
   1. Primary prevention
   2. Secondary prevention
   3. Tertiary prevention
   4. Health promotion
3. Vulnerable populations are those who are more likely to develop health problems as a result of:

   1. Chronic diseases, homelessness, and poverty
   2. Lack of transportation, dependent on others for transportation
   3. Excess risks, limited access to health care
   4. Limited access to health care, lack of transportation
4. Major health care problems in older adults in community settings include:
   1. Polypharmacy, poverty, abuse, sensory loss, and chronic illness
   2. Acute illness and abandonment
   3. Poverty and inadequate support systems
   4. Acute illness, inadequate support systems, and poverty
5. Which of the following is not part of a community system?
   1. Information about the structure of the community
   2. Information about the population of the community
   3. Information about the social system of the community
   4. Information about building codes of the community

## REFERENCES

American Nurses Association: *Standards of public health nursing practice,* Washington, DC, 1999, The Association.

Ayers M, Bruno AA, Langford RW: *Community-based nursing care: making the transition,* St. Louis, 1999, Mosby.

Baas LD and others: The challenge of managing the care of older heart transplant recipients, *AACN Clin Issues* 13(1):114, 2002.

Barr RG and others: The national asthma education and prevention program (NAEPP), *Arch Intern Med* 162(15):1761, 2002.

Chalmers KI and others: The changing environment of community health practice and education: perceptions of staff nurses, administrators, and educators, *J Nurs Educ* 37:109, 1998.

Clark MJ and others: Involving communities in community assessment, *Public Health Nurs* 20(6):456, 2003.

Corrarino JE and others: The Cool Kids Coalition: a community effort to reduce scald burn risk in children. *MCN Am J Matern Child Nurs* 25(1):10, 2000.

Diekemper M, SmithBattle L, Drake MA: Bringing the population into focus: a natural development in community health nursing practice, part I, *Public Health Nurs* 16:3, 1999.

Dower C, O'Neil E, Hough H: Profiling the professions: a model for evaluating emerging health professions, San Francisco, 2001, Center for Health Professions, University of California, San Francisco.

Eckert LO, Sugar N, Fine D: Characteristics of sexual assault in women with a major psychiatric diagnosis, *Am J Obstet Gynecol* 186(6):1284, 2002.

Feenstra C: Community based and community focused: nursing education in community health, *Public Health Nurs* 17(3):165, 2000.

Flynn BC: Communicating with the public: community-based nursing research and practice, *Public Health Nurs* 15(3):155,1998.

Hwang SW: Mortality among men using homeless shelters in Toronto, Ontario, *JAMA* 283(16):2152, 2000.

Hwang SW, Bugeja AL: Barriers to appropriate diabetes management among homeless people in Toronto, *Can Med Assoc J* 163(2):161, 2000.

Pew Health Professions Commission: *Health America: practitioners for 2005,* Durham, NC, 1991, The Commission.

Rew L and others: Correlates of resilience in homeless adolescents, *J Nurs Scholarsh* 33(1):33, 2001.

Rogers EM: *Diffusion of innovations,* ed 5, New York, 2004, Free Press.

Sakamoto SD, Avilla A: The public health nursing practice manual: a tool for public health nurses, *Public Health Nurs* 21(2):179, 2004.

Sebastian JG: Vulnerability and vulnerable populations: an introduction. In Stanhope M, Lancaster J, editors: *Community health nursing: process and practice for promoting health,* ed 4, St. Louis, 1996, Mosby.

SmithBattle L, Diekemper M, Leander S: Moving upstream: becoming a public health nurse, part II. *Public Health Nurs* 21(2):95, 2004.

Stanhope M, Lancaster J: *Community and public health nursing,* ed 6, St. Louis, 2004, Mosby.

U.S. Department of Health and Human Services, Public Health Service: *Healthy People 2010,* ed 2, vol 1, part A focus area 7, Educational and community-based programs, Washington, DC, 2000a, U.S. Government Printing Office, www.healthypeople.gov.

U.S. Department of Health and Human Services, Public Health Service: *Healthy People 2010: A systematic approach to health improvement,* Washington, DC, 2000b, U.S. Government Printing Office, www.healthypeople.gov/implementation.

U.S. Public Health Service: *A time for partnership: prevention report,* Rockville, Md, December 1994/January 1995, Office of Disease Prevention and Health Promotion.

Zhan L and others: Promoting health: perspectives from ethnic elderly women, *J Community Health Nurs* 15:31, 1998.

Zotti ME, Brown P, Stotts RC: Community-based nursing versus community health nursing: what does it all mean? *Nurs Outlook* 44(5):211, 1996.

# CHAPTER 4

# Legal Principles in Nursing

## MEDIA RESOURCES

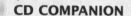 **CD COMPANION** 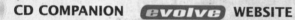 **WEBSITE**

http://evolve.elsevier.com/Potter/basic

- **NCLEX® Review**
- **Audio Glossary**
- **English/Spanish Audio Glossary**

OBJECTIVES

- Describe the legal obligations and role of nurses regarding federal and state laws that affect health care.
- Explain the legal concepts of standard of care and informed consent.
- List sources for standards of care for nurses.

- Explain the concept of negligence and identify the elements of professional negligence.
- Define the legal relationships of nurse-patient, nurse-health care provider, nurse-nurse, and nurse-employer.
- Identify nursing interventions to improve patient safety.

KEY TERMS

assault, p. 56
battery, p. 56
civil law, p. 54
common law, p. 54
crime, p. 54
criminal law, p. 54
defendant, p. 56
felony, p. 54
Good Samaritan laws, p. 58
informed consent, p. 57
living wills, p. 60
malpractice, p. 54
malpractice insurance, p. 56
misdemeanor, p. 54

negligence, p. 54
Nurse Practice Acts, p. 54
occurrence report, p. 61
plaintiff, p. 56
power of attorney for health care, p. 58
regulatory agencies, p. 54
risk management, p. 60
standard of care, p. 56
statutory law, p. 54
tort, p. 54

As a nurse it is important to have an understanding of the law and how it affects your nursing practice. You will be faced with many legal issues that will require the use of critical thinking abilities to practice safe nursing care. Safe and competent nursing care includes an understanding of the legal boundaries within which you will function. Frequently nurses function under several sources and jurisdictions of health care law simultaneously. Nurses' familiarity with the law enhances their ability to be patient advocates. In addition to understanding the federal laws that apply to health care, it is also important to know the law in your own state and the rules and regulations of your state's **regulatory agencies.** If you have specific questions, consult with your own attorney or with your employing institution's attorney.

## Legal Limits of Nursing

An understanding of the law coupled with sound judgment helps to ensure safe and appropriate nursing care. You need to understand the legal limits or standards that affect nurs-

ing practice to know your responsibilities as a nurse and to protect patients from harm.

### Sources of Law

Nursing practice is subject to several sources or types of law, specifically **statutory law,** administrative law, and common law. An example of a statute enacted by the U.S. Congress is the Americans With Disabilities Act (ADA), which protects the rights of handicapped individuals (ADA, 1995). Examples of statutes enacted by state legislatures are the **Nurse Practice Acts,** which are in all 50 states and the District of Columbia. Regulatory agencies, such as State Boards of Nursing, are created by statutes and function under administrative law. The State Board of Nursing regulates the practice of nursing through rules and regulations derived from the State Nurse Practice Act. Court decisions written by judges deciding a particular issue in litigated cases establish **common law.** An example of a common law is the doctrine of informed consent that is now an accepted standard of care.

Statutes are either criminal or civil. **Criminal law** is either a felony or a misdemeanor. A **felony** is a serious offense that has a penalty of imprisonment for greater than a year or possibly even death. A **misdemeanor** is a less serious **crime** that has a penalty of a fine or imprisonment for less than a year. An example of criminal conduct for nurses is misuse of a controlled substance.

**Civil laws** protect individual rights. A **tort** is a civil wrong or injury for which the court provides a remedy in the form of money damages (Black, 1999). Torts are intentional or unintentional. Intentional torts are willful acts that violate another person's rights. For example, assault and battery are intentional torts. Assault is an intentional threat to engage in harmful contact with another. Battery is unwanted touching. Unintentional torts include negligence. **Negligence** is conduct that falls below the standard of care. Malpractice is one example of negligence. **Malpractice** is defined as professional misconduct or unreasonable lack of skill (Black, 1999). In a malpractice lawsuit, the law uses nursing standards of care to measure nursing conduct and to determine whether the nurse acted as any reasonably prudent nurse would act under the same or similar circumstances. Box 4-1 describes the steps of a typical malpractice lawsuit.

---

**BOX 4-1** | **Anatomy of a Lawsuit**

*Petition—elements of the claim:* The plaintiff outlines what the defendant nurse did wrong and how as a result of that alleged negligence the plaintiff was injured.

*Answer:* The nurse admits or denies each allegation in the petition. Anything that is not admitted must be proved.

*Discovery:* The process of uncovering all the facts of the case. Involves using interrogatories, full access to the medical records in question, and depositions.

*Interrogatories:* Written questions requiring answers under oath. Usual questions concern witnesses, insurance experts, and which health care providers the plaintiff has seen before and after the event.

*Medical records:* The defendant obtains all of the plaintiff's relevant medical records for treatment before and after the incident.

*Witnesses' depositions:* Questions are posed to the witnesses under oath to obtain all relevant, nonprivileged information about the case.

*Parties' depositions:* The plaintiff and defendants (physician or health care provider, nurse, and hospital personnel) are almost always deposed.

*Other witnesses:* Factual witnesses, both neutral and biased, are deposed to obtain information and their version of the case. This may include family members on the plaintiff's side and other medical personnel (e.g., nurses) on the defendant's side.

*Treating physicians' or health care providers' depositions:* Before subsequent treating, physicians' or health care providers' depositions may be taken to establish issues such as those concerning preexisting conditions, causation, the nature and extent of injuries, and permanency.

*Experts:* The plaintiff selects experts to establish the essential legal elements of the case against the defendant. The defendant selects experts to establish the appropriateness of the nursing care.

*Trial:* The trial usually occurs at least 1 to 3 years after the filing of the petition. Approximately 5% of cases are actually tried before a judge. Most are dismissed or settled. Settlement means that compensation has been paid for the case to be dismissed.

**Proof of Negligence**

The nurse owed a duty to the patient.

The nurse did not carry out the duty or breached the duty (failed to use that degree of skill and learning ordinarily used under the same or similar circumstances by members of the profession).

The patient was injured.

The patient's injury was caused by the nurse's failure to carry out that duty.

The patient's injury resulted in compensable damages that can be quantified, such as medical bills, lost wages, pain and suffering.

---

## Standards of Care

Nursing standards of care are the legal guidelines for minimally safe and adequate nursing practice. The standards of care are defined in the Nurse Practice Acts of the State Board of Nursing of each state, the state and federal hospital licensing laws, professional and specialty organization standards, and the written policies and procedures of the employing institution (Mikos, 2004). There is also a body of law referred to as case law or common law, which consists of prior court rulings that affect nursing practice.

The Nurse Practice Acts of each state define the scope of nursing practice and expanded nursing roles, set educational requirements for nurses, and distinguish between nursing practice and medical practice. There are also rules and regulations enacted by the State Boards of Nursing that define the practice of nursing more specifically. For example, a State Board develops a rule regarding the administration of intravenous therapy.

Professional organizations also define standards of nursing care. The American Nurses Association (ANA) (2001) has developed standards for nursing practice, policy statements, and similar resolutions. The standards describe the scope, function, and role of the nurse and establish clinical practice standards. The Joint Commission on Accreditation of Healthcare Organizations (JCAHO) (2005c) requires that accredited hospitals fulfill certain standards with regard to nursing practice, such as having written policies and proce-

dures. Nursing specialty organizations define the standards of care for nurses to be certified in specialty areas, such as the operating room or critical care areas. These standards of care also determine whether a nurse is acting appropriately when performing professional duties.

The written policies and procedures of an employing institution define the standards of care for nurses at that institution. These policies are usually quite specific and are in policy and procedure manuals found on most nursing units. For example, a policy and procedure will outline the steps to take when changing a dressing or administering a medication. Know the policies and procedures of your employing institution because if you are involved in a lawsuit, this is one of the standards by which you will be measured.

If you are involved in a malpractice trial, the court will inform the jury about the standards of care and then the jury will determine whether you have acted the way a reasonable nurse would have acted in similar circumstances. If you are a specialized nurse, such as a nurse anesthetist, intensive care nurse, certified nurse midwife, or operating room nurse, you will be held to the standards of care and skill exercised by those in the same specialty area. In most cases a nursing expert will testify for the patient about the standards of care to establish that you were negligent. You will also most likely have a nursing expert testify on your behalf as to the appropriate standard of care and whether your actions were reasonable (Manson, 2002).

The best way to stay familiar with the current legal issues affecting your practice is to read the nursing literature in your practice area. Current nursing literature deals with the changing obligations and standards of care for nurses. It will also explain pertinent state and federal laws and will keep you up-to-date on any new rules, regulations, or case law.

## Civil Law

### Intentional Torts

ASSAULT. **Assault** is any intentional threat to bring about harmful or offensive contact with another individual. No actual contact is necessary. The law protects patients who are afraid of harmful contact. It is considered an assault to threaten to give a patient an injection or to threaten to restrain a patient for an x-ray procedure when the patient has refused consent.

BATTERY. **Battery** is any intentional touching without consent. The contact is harmful to the patient and causes an injury, or it is merely offensive to the patient's personal dignity. A battery always includes an assault, which is why the law commonly combines the two terms *assault* and *battery*. For example, you threaten to give a patient an injection without the patient's consent. If you actually give the injection, it is considered a battery. Another example of a battery is when a surgeon performs the wrong surgical procedure. For example, if a patient gives consent for a left knee repair but the surgeon performs right knee surgery, a battery has occurred.

### Unintentional Torts

NEGLIGENCE AND MALPRACTICE. Negligence is conduct that falls below the standard of care. The law has established the **standard of care** to protect people from the unreasonable risk of harm (Black, 1999). It is very simply the conduct of a "reasonable person." For example, if you are driving a car and fail to stop at a stop sign, your action is negligent. In general, courts define negligence as failure to use that degree of care that a reasonable person would use under the same or similar circumstances.

Malpractice is one type of negligence, called *professional negligence*. To establish the elements of negligence against you, the patient must allege the following: (1) you (**defendant**) owed a duty to the patient (**plaintiff**), (2) you breached that duty, (3) the patient was injured, and (4) the injury occurred as a result of your breach of duty (Cady, 2003). If you give nursing care that does not meet appropriate standards, a patient is able to make a claim for negligence or nursing malpractice against you. That negligence may involve your failure to check a patient's arm band and administering medication to the wrong patient. It may also involve your administering a medication to a patient even though there is documentation that the patient has an allergy to that medication. In general, the law defines nursing negligence as

---

| BOX 4-2 | **Common Sources of Negligence** |

Be aware of the common negligent acts that have resulted in lawsuits against hospitals and nurses:
1. Medication errors that result in injury to patients
2. Intravenous therapy errors resulting in infiltrations or phlebitis
3. Burns to patients caused by equipment, bathing, or spills of hot liquids and foods
4. Falls resulting in injury to patients
5. Failure to use aseptic technique where required
6. Errors in sponge, instrument, or needle counts in surgical cases
7. Failure to give a report, or giving an incomplete report, to an oncoming shift
8. Failure to adequately monitor a patient's condition
9. Failure to notify a physician or health care provider of a significant change in a patient's status

---

failure to use that degree of care that a reasonable nurse would use under the same or similar circumstances (Cady, 2003).

Certain common negligent acts have resulted in lawsuits against hospitals and nurses (Box 4-2). All of these acts have something in common. Carelessness or mistakes involving medications, intravenous (IV) therapy, equipment, or patient falls generally cause negligent acts. Failure to monitor the patient's condition appropriately and communicate that information to the physician or health care provider are also the cause of negligent acts.

The best way to avoid being liable for negligence is to follow standards of care, to give competent health care, and to communicate with other health care providers. It is also necessary to document patient assessments, interventions, and evaluations fully and to develop a caring rapport with the patient to avoid liability. Patient safety issues are the focus of attention by accrediting agencies such as the JCAHO (2005b) and public interest groups such as the Institute of Medicine. This interest is changing standards of care for patients and care delivery systems in the health care environment throughout the country (Mrayyan and Huber, 2003; Silver and Lusk, 2002). Become involved in developing and monitoring the policies and procedures of the institution in which you work. By being aware of common sources of patient injury, not only do you provide care designed to protect patient safety, but a system and a culture of patient safety develops in your health care institution, which leads to better prevention and protection overall (Mrayyan and Huber, 2003).

**Malpractice Insurance.** **Malpractice insurance** usually provides you with an attorney, the payment of attorney's fees, and the payment of any judgment or settlement if a patient sues you for medical malpractice. If you work for a health care institution, generally that institution's insurance will cover you during your employment. Usually you do not need to purchase any supplemental insurance unless you plan on practicing nursing outside of your employing insti-

---

**BOX 4-3  Statutory Guidelines for Legal Consent for Medical Treatment**

Those who may consent to medical treatment are governed by state law but generally include:

I. Adults
  A. Any competent individual 18 years of age or older for himself or herself
  B. Any parent for his or her unemancipated minor
  C. Any guardian for his or her ward
  D. Any adult for the treatment of his or her minor brother or sister (if an emergency and parents are not present)
  E. Any grandparent for a minor grandchild (if an emergency and parents are not present)

II. Minors (less than 18 years of age)
  A. Ordinarily minors may not consent for medical treatment without a parent. Emancipated minors, however, may consent to medical treatment without a parent. Emancipated minors include:
    1. Minors who are designated emancipated by a court order
    2. Minors who are married, divorced, or widowed
    3. Minors who are in active military service
  B. Unemancipated minors may consent to medical treatment if they have specific medical conditions:
    1. Pregnancy and pregnancy-related conditions (Various states differ in characterizing a pregnant minor as either emancipated or unemancipated. Know your state's rules in this matter.)
    2. A minor parent for his or her custodial child
    3. Sexually transmitted disease (STD) information and treatment
    4. Substance abuse treatment
    5. Outpatient and/or temporary sheltered mental health treatment
  C. The issue of emancipated or unemancipated minor does not relieve the health care provider's duty to attempt to obtain meaningful informed consent (Vukadinovich, 2004).

tution. For example, if your neighbors and friends called you to provide nursing care on a volunteer basis outside the health care institution, the hospital's insurance does not cover you if a neighbor or friend files suit against you.

## Consent

A signed consent form from your patient is necessary for all routine treatment, hazardous procedures such as surgery, some treatment programs such as chemotherapy, and participation in research studies (Cady, 2003). A patient will sign a general consent form for treatment when the patient is admitted to the hospital or other health care facility. A patient or the patient's representative has to sign separate special consent forms before anyone performs specialized procedures. Box 4-3 outlines the general guidelines for legal consent to medical treatments. Take special consideration and care regarding the patient who is deaf, illiterate, or

speaks a foreign language. In each instance, you will take steps to ensure that the patient understands the document being signed (Cady, 2003). It is also important to be sensitive to the cultural issues of consent and to understand the way in which patients and their families communicate to make important decisions. The cultural beliefs and values of your patients are sometimes very different from your own or the culture in which you are comfortable. Show respect by not imposing your own cultural values on your patients or their families.

**INFORMED CONSENT. Informed consent** is a patient's agreement to allow something to happen, such as surgery, based on a full disclosure of the risks, benefits, alternatives, and consequences of refusal (Black, 1999). Informed consent requires that you give the patient all relevant information required to make a decision, that the patient is capable of understanding the relevant information, and that the patient actually gives consent. If you perform a procedure on a patient without informed consent, you will possibly be liable for battery. Informed consent documentation includes the following:

- The patient's signature
- The witnesses' signatures
- The date and time of signing
- Verification that the patient voluntarily signed the consent, that the patient discussed the risks, benefits, alternatives, and the right to refuse the procedure with the physician or health care provider
- Verification that the patient understands the procedure and has had all questions answered satisfactorily (Cady, 2003)

Because nurses do not perform surgery or direct medical procedures, obtaining a patient's informed consent does not fall within a nurse's responsibility. Even though a nurse assumes the responsibility for witnessing the patient's signature on the consent form, the nurse does not legally assume the duty of obtaining informed consent. The physician assumes that responsibility. When you provide consent forms for patients to sign, ask them if they understand the procedures for which they are giving consent. If patients deny any understanding, or if you suspect that they do not understand, you notify the physician or health care provider and your nursing supervisor. A patient refusing surgery or other medical treatment must be informed about any harmful consequences of refusal. If the patient persists in refusing the treatment, make sure the rejection is written, signed, and witnessed (Cady, 2003).

Parents are normally the legal guardians of pediatric patients, and therefore they are the persons who will sign consent forms for treatment. If the parents are divorced, the parent with legal custody gives consent. When a parent refuses medically necessary treatment for a child, health care providers sometimes petition the court to intervene on the child's behalf.

If the patient is unconscious, you need to obtain consent from a person legally authorized to give consent on the patient's behalf. If the patient has executed a durable **power of attorney for health care,** the document will designate an individual who is able to give consent for medical treatment. A patient who is legally incompetent in a judicial proceeding needs to have the consent of the legal guardian. In emergency situations, if it is impossible to obtain consent from the patient or a legally authorized person, health care providers will give treatment because the law presumes the patient would wish to be treated (Cady, 2003).

You also need a patient's consent for voluntary psychiatric unit admission. They retain the right to refuse treatment until a court has determined that they are incompetent to decide for themselves (Cady, 2003).

## Statutory Laws

### Good Samaritan Laws

**Good Samaritan laws** have been enacted in almost every state to encourage nurses to assist in emergency situations. These laws limit liability and offer legal immunity if a nurse helps at the scene of an accident. For example, if you stop at the scene of an automobile accident and give appropriate emergency care such as applying pressure to stop hemorrhage, you are acting within accepted standards, even though proper equipment was not available. If the patient subsequently develops complications as a result of your actions, you are immune from liability as long as you acted without gross negligence (Good Samaritan Law, 1998). The statutes also provide that a nurse is able to assist a minor in an emergency at the scene of an accident or a competitive sports event before obtaining the parent's consent. However, although Good Samaritan Laws provide immunity to the nurse who does what is reasonable to save a person's life, if you perform a procedure for which you have no training, you will be liable for any injury resulting from that act. Therefore provide only care that is consistent with your level of expertise (Brooke, 2003). In addition, once you have committed to providing emergency care to a patient, you are responsible for following through, that is, to safely transfer the care of the patient to someone who can provide needed care, such as emergency medical technicians (EMTs) or emergency department staff. Otherwise, you will be liable for abandonment of the patient and responsible for any injury suffered after you left the patient (Brooke, 2003).

### Licensure

To practice nursing, you must be licensed by the Board of Nursing of the state in which you practice. All states require registered nurses (RNs) to have a passing score on the National Council Licensure Examination (NCLEX) to obtain an initial license. Some states require obtaining continuing education credits for relicensure.

The State Board of Nursing is able to suspend or revoke a nursing license if a nurse's conduct violates provisions of the licensing statute. For example, performance of an illegal act such as selling or taking controlled substances will jeopardize your license status. Because your license is a property right, the board will follow due process before suspending or revoking your license. Due process means that they will notify you of the charges against you and conduct a hearing so that you are able to present evidence to defend yourself. Usually a panel of members of the State Board of Nursing conducts the hearing rather than a judge in a courtroom. Some states allow you to file an appeal in court if you have tried and lost all other forms of appeal within the State Board of Nursing.

### Student Nurses

Student nurses are responsible for all of their actions that cause harm to patients. When a patient is injured as a direct result of your actions, you, your instructor, the staff nurses working with you, and the hospital or health care facility may all share the liability for the incorrect action. Faculty members are responsible for instructing and observing their students, but in some situations staff nurses also share these responsibilities. As a student nurse, no one should assign you to perform tasks for which you are unprepared. Your instructors should carefully supervise you as you learn new procedures. Every nursing school should provide clear definitions of student responsibility. During the clinical rotation, generally the school's liability insurance covers you; however, always check with your school as to the specific coverage.

Sometimes you will be employed as a nursing assistant or a nurse's aide when you are not attending classes. During the time when you work as an employee of a health care facility, perform only tasks that appear in a job description for a nurse's aide or nursing assistant. Your supervisor should not delegate the tasks of a licensed nurse to you (Whitman, 2004). For example, even if you have learned how to administer intramuscular medications as a student nurse, do not perform this task as a nurse's aide because it is outside the scope of your nurse's aide job description. When you are working at a health care facility, the health care facility's liability insurance will likely cover you. Any time that you are employed, however, always inquire about malpractice insurance coverage.

### Physician or Health Care Provider Orders

The physician or health care provider is responsible for directing the medical treatment of a patient. You are responsible for carrying out that medical treatment unless the physician's or health care provider's order is in error, violates hospital policy, or is harmful to the patient. Therefore you will assess all physician or health care provider orders, and if you determine they are erroneous or harmful, obtain further clarification from that physician or health care provider (Figure 4-1).

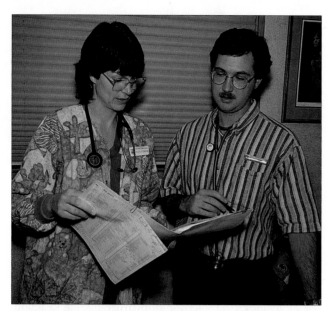

FIGURE **4-1** If an order creates questions, the nurse clarifies it with the physician or health care provider.

If the physician or health care provider confirms the order, but you still believe that it is inappropriate, inform the nurse manager or the nursing supervisor (Benner and others, 2002). Do not carry out the physician's or health care provider's order if there is a risk that harm will come to your patient. Your supervisor will help resolve the questionable order. If you carry out the questionable order, you are legally responsible for harm suffered by the patient (Benner and others, 2002).

Make sure all physician or health care provider orders are in writing and dated and timed appropriately. Make sure that they are transcribed correctly. Verbal orders or telephone orders are not recommended because they leave possibilities for error. If a verbal or telephone order is necessary in an emergency, make sure the physician or health care provider writes and signs it as soon as possible, usually within 24 hours (JCAHO, 2005b).

**RESTRAINTS.** You need to know when and how to use restraints correctly. The Resident's Rights section of the Medicaid Statute (1988) regulates the use of physical or chemical restraints in nursing facilities. In addition, the Food and Drug Administration (FDA) (U.S. Department of Health and Human Services, 1992) and JCAHO (2005a) have set guidelines for the use of restraints. These regulations set the standard that all patients have the right to be free from seclusion and physical or chemical restraints except to ensure the patient's safety in emergency situations. They further describe the procedures to follow in order to restrain any patient, including who orders restraints, when to write the order, and how often to renew the written order. The standards specifically prohibit restraining patients for staff convenience, punishment, or retaliation. The regulations also describe documentation of restraint use and

follow-up assessments. In particular, the documentation needs to describe all of the less restrictive interventions attempted before employing a physical or chemical restraint (Blank and others, 2004; Martin, 2002) (see Chapter 26). Liability for improper or unlawful restraint, as well as liability for patient injury from unprotected falls, lies with the nurse and the health care facility.

**CONFIDENTIALITY.** The Health Insurance Portability and Accountability Act of 1996 (HIPAA) sets standards regarding the electronic exchange of private and sensitive health information. Known as the Privacy Standards (Rosati, 2002), these rules create patient rights to consent to use and disclose protected health information, to inspect and copy one's medical record, and to amend mistaken or incomplete information. In addition, the standards require all hospitals and health agencies to have specific policies and procedures in place to ensure compliance with the standards. The policies and procedures need to provide reasonable safeguards to protect written and verbal communications about patients. Although HIPAA will not require such things as soundproof rooms in hospitals, it does mean that nurses and health care providers need to avoid discussing patients in public hallways and provide reasonable levels of privacy in communicating with and about patients in any matter. HIPAA violations have civil and criminal sanctions.

**DEATH AND DYING.** You also need to know your legal responsibilities concerning the process of death and dying. Carefully document all events that occur when you are caring for the dying patient. There are two standards for the determination of death: cardiopulmonary or whole brain (Uniform Determination of Death Act, 1980). The cardiopulmonary standard requires failure of a patient's circulatory and respiratory functions. The whole brain standard requires irreversible failure of all functions of the entire brain, including the brain stem. The reason for the development of the two definitions is to set the legal standard for determining death in all situations. The definitions are helpful when there is a question of whether to continue life support or when the discussion of organ donation is appropriate.

You are legally obligated to treat your deceased patient's remains with dignity and care. Wrongful handling causes emotional harm to survivors. In one litigated case, survivors sued when a mislabeling of bodies led to an Orthodox Jewish person being prepared for a Roman Catholic funeral and a Roman Catholic person being prepared for an Orthodox Jewish burial (*In re* Schiller, 1977).

**ORGAN AND TISSUE DONATION.** A signed consent is necessary before donating a patient's body, tissues, or organs for medical use. In some states a patient signs the back of his or her driver's license in the presence of witnesses, indicating consent to having his or her body donated. Consent is valid unless the driver's license is revoked, canceled, or suspended, and the person has to give consent each time the license is renewed. Generally a hospital is not liable for honoring a patient's consent for organ donation despite the family's objection. However, in practice, health care institutions will honor the family's wishes even if they conflict with the patient's organ donation consent. State laws provide whether a nurse is able to witness the consent of an individual donating his or her body, organs, or tissues for medical use. Be aware of the policies and procedures of your employing institution and your state's laws when someone asks you to serve as a witness for a person who is giving consent for organ donation.

In most states there is a law requiring that at the time of death a qualified health care provider ask the patient's family members to consider organ or tissue donation (National Organ Transplant Act, 1984). You approach individuals in the following order: (1) the spouse, (2) adult son or daughter, (3) parent, (4) adult brother or sister, (5) grandparent, and (6) guardian. The person in the highest class makes the donation unless he or she knows of a refusal or contrary indication by the decedent (Uniform Anatomical Gift Act, 1987). In addition, the law also provides that the physician or health care provider who certifies death shall not be involved in the removal or transplant of organs or tissues. The National Organ Transplant Act of 1984 prohibits selling or purchasing of organs and regulates this area of medical and nursing practice. Organ and tissue donation remains voluntary. Consent forms are available for this purpose.

**AUTOPSIES.** An autopsy requires consent by the patient before his or her death or by a close family member at the time of the patient's death (Autopsy Consent, 1998). The priority for giving consent for autopsies is (1) the patient, in writing before death; (2) durable power of attorney; (3) surviving spouse; and (4) surviving child, parent, brother, or sister in the order named. State statutes provide that when there are reasonable grounds to believe that a patient died as a result of violence, homicide, suicide, accident, or death occurring in any unusual or suspicious manner, you need to notify the coroner. You also notify the coroner if a patient's death is unforeseen and sudden and a physician or health care provider has not seen the patient in over 36 hours.

**ADVANCE DIRECTIVES.** You will encounter legal issues associated with caring for patients who are terminally ill, severely debilitated, or in a persistent vegetative state (permanently comatose). One of these legal issues involves the right to refuse medical treatment and the withholding of food and nutrition. The doctrine of informed consent ensures that the patient has the right to refuse treatment. The Supreme Court has held that a competent person has the right to refuse medical treatment, including lifesaving food and nutrition (*Cruzan v Director Missouri Department of Health*, 1990).

If a physician or health care provider has documented in the progress notes that the patient is deteriorating and the physician or health care provider and the patient have made the decision not to administer cardiopulmonary resuscitation, the physician or health care provider should write a "do not resuscitate" (DNR) order. A DNR order is written, not given verbally (Burns and others, 2003). Physicians or health care providers need to regularly review DNR orders in case the patient's condition warrants a change. Be familiar with your institution's policies and procedures concerning DNR orders.

Many times the decision regarding lifesaving treatment is in writing in the patient's living will or advance directive. **Living wills** are documents instructing the physician or health care provider to withhold or withdraw life-sustaining procedures in patients whose death is imminent. You will find that patients have completed living wills or advance directives that designate a health care power of attorney or a health care surrogate decision maker. The patient or state law designates a surrogate decision maker, who acts as a substitute. These individuals have the power to make health care decisions for the patient when the patient is no longer capable of making decisions for himself or herself (Scanlon, 2003). Each state providing for living wills or advance directives has its own requirements for executing them. In general, you need two witnesses, who are not a relative or the physician or health care provider, when the patient signs the document. Only a competent patient is able to revoke living wills, advance directives, and durable power of attorney for health care statements. Health care providers who ignore valid living wills, advance directives, or the directions of a health care power of attorney are subject to civil liability (Cady, 2003). The Patient Self-Determination Act (1991) requires health care institutions to inquire whether a patient has created an advance directive.

## Other Legal Issues in Nursing Practice

As a nurse you will be faced with nursing issues that will become liability concerns. It is important for you to anticipate these issues so you are better prepared to deal with any problems that arise.

### Quality Improvement, Risk Management, and Documentation

The underlying rationale for quality improvement and risk management programs is the development of an organizational system of ensuring appropriate, quality health care. **Risk management** involves several components, including identifying possible risks, analyzing them, acting to reduce the risks, and evaluating the measures taken to reduce the risks. The JCAHO (2005c) requires the use of quality improvement and risk management procedures. Both quality improvement and risk management require good documentation. Your documentation of your nursing care is your only memory of what actually was done for a patient and will serve as proof that you acted reasonably and safely. Make sure your documentation is thorough, accurate, and done in a timely manner.

Frequently the nursing notes are the first thing an attorney reviews when a lawsuit is filed. As a nurse you chart facts, not assumptions, about patient behavior. In addition, you document as fully as possible the physician or health care provider notifications made regarding the patient. Simply charting "physician notified" is insufficient information when presenting a chart in court. Your assessments and the reporting of significant changes in the assessments are very important factors in defending a lawsuit.

One tool used in risk management is the **occurrence report** or incident report. By reviewing occurrence reports, administrators determine areas of patient risk. For example, if a certain kind of problem has occurred repeatedly, such as patients falling when being transferred to stretchers, you use educational methods to help prevent the problem in the future. Complete occurrence reports when anything unusual happens that potentially causes harm to a patient, visitor, or employee, or when you make an error. For example, if a patient falls in the hospital, prepare an occurrence report. Most institutions provide specific forms for this purpose. Objectively record the details of the event and any statements the patient makes. An example is as follows: "Patient found lying on floor on right side. Abrasion on right forehead. Patient stated, 'I fell and hit my head.'" At the time of the event, always contact the physician or health care provider to examine the patient. After examining the patient, the physician or health care provider documents assessment findings and treatment plans in the progress notes. You document any problematic effects caused by the event. Do not include subjective assumptions and statements assigning blame or fault in the nursing notes or the occurrence report.

Occurrence reports are not in the patient's medical record, although they are evidence in lawsuits in some jurisdictions. Know your institution's policies and procedures regarding occurrence reports.

## Patient Privacy Rights

Issues of disclosure, privacy, and confidentiality are an important concern when working with patients or peers infected with human immunodeficiency virus (HIV) or acquired immunodeficiency virus (AIDS). You will care for patients with AIDS in every segment of your nursing practice. Use standard precautions as a standard of care to prevent the transmission of the HIV virus when caring for all patients. Persons with infectious diseases are protected under the handicapped and disabilities laws. The ADA (1995) protects the rights of disabled people and is the most extensive law on how employers will treat HIV-infected patients and health care workers. Co-workers who refuse to work with HIV-infected people will leave companies open to indirect charges of discrimination if the employer does not monitor the work environment. Several cases have held that the health care provider is obligated to disclose the fact that

he or she is infected with HIV. The ADA regulations protect the privacy of infected people by giving individuals the opportunity to decide whether to disclose their disability. As a health care worker, it is not a requirement for you to be tested for HIV as a condition of employment (Laughlin, 2002). If you are contaminated by a patient whose HIV status is unknown, you cannot check the patient's blood for HIV without the patient's consent.

## Patient Abandonment and Delegation Issues

You will encounter inadequate staffing during times of nursing shortages, staff downsizing periods, and cost containment. The JCAHO (2005c) requires institutions to have guidelines for the number of staff needed to care for patients. Legal problems will arise if an institution does not have enough registered nurses to provide competent and safe care. Liability issues occur if a patient is injured as a result of negligent care by any personnel (Mrayyan and Huber, 2003). Registered nurses are always responsible for performing the nursing process. Even though RNs delegate care to assistive personnel or licensed practical nurses, they maintain responsibility for patient outcomes.

If you are assigned to care for more patients than is reasonable for safe care, notify your nursing supervisor. If you are required to accept the assignment, document this information in writing and provide the document to nursing administrators. Although documentation does not relieve you of responsibility if patients suffer harm because of inattention, it shows that you attempted to act appropriately. Whenever you document information about short staffing, keep a copy of the document. Do not walk out when staffing is inadequate because you could be charged with abandonment. It is important to know your institution's policies and procedures on how to handle inadequate staffing before such a situation arises. The institution is ultimately responsible for staffing the hospital in order to provide safe care (Mrayyan and Huber, 2003).

Nurses within acute and long-term care facilities are often required to "float" from the area in which they normally practice to other nursing units. If you float, inform your supervisor if you lack experience in caring for the types of patients on the new nursing unit. Also, request an orientation to the unit. Even if you float to a nursing unit, you will be held to the same standard of care as nurses who regularly work in that area. A supervisor is liable if a staff nurse is assigned to a patient for whom he or she cannot safely care. In one case the court noted that if employers are going to float nurses out of their usual work area of practice, then the employers need to provide training and education to prepare the nurses to work in the other areas (*Winkelman v. Beloit Memorial Hospital*, 1992).

## Controlled Substances

In 1970 the Comprehensive Drug Abuse Prevention and Control Act was passed in the United States. The act controls and regulates hospital drug distribution systems of narcotics, antidepressants, hypnotics, sedatives, stimulants, and hallucinogens. You only administer controlled substances under the direction of a licensed physician. Several states allow advanced practice nurses to prescribe controlled substances.

Controlled substances are securely locked, and only authorized personnel have access to them. Maintain precise records regarding the dispensing, wasting, and storage of controlled substances. There are criminal penalties for the misuse of controlled substances. There have been cases in which physicians have illegally prescribed and dispensed controlled substances. If you are employed by such a physician and fail to report these activities, you are legally accountable for aiding and abetting the physician.

## Reporting Obligations

Health care providers are required to report incidents such as child, spousal, or elder abuse, rape, gunshot wounds, attempted suicide, and certain communicable diseases. In order to encourage reports of suspected cases, states provide legal immunity for the reporter if the person makes the report in good faith. Health care professionals who do not report suspected child abuse or neglect are liable for civil or criminal legal action. You are also required to report unsafe or impaired professionals. Because required reporting information varies among states, become familiar with the appropriate statutes in your state and the policies and procedures of your employing institution.

## KEY CONCEPTS

- Registered nurses are licensed by the state in which they practice.
- Under the law you are required to follow standards of care, which originate in Nurse Practice Acts, the guidelines of professional organizations, and written policies and procedures of employing institutions.
- You are responsible for performing procedures correctly and exercising professional judgment when you carry out physician or health care provider orders.
- All patients are entitled to confidential health care and freedom from unauthorized release of information.
- You will be liable for malpractice if the following are established: (1) you (defendant) owed a duty to the patient (plaintiff), (2) you did not carry out that duty or breached that duty, (3) the patient was injured, and (4) your failure to carry out that duty caused the patient's injury.
- Informed consent must meet the following criteria: (1) the person giving consent is competent and of legal age; (2) the consent is given voluntarily; (3) the person giving consent thoroughly understands the procedure, its risks and benefits, and alternative procedures; and (4) the person giving consent has a right to have all questions answered satisfactorily.

- You are obligated to follow the physician's order unless you believe that it is in error, violates hospital policy, or is possibly harmful to the patient, in which case you make a formal report explaining the refusal.
- You file an occurrence report in any unusual situation that will potentially cause harm to a patient; such reports are also for quality improvement and risk management.
- The civil law system is concerned with the protection of a person's private rights, and the criminal law system deals with the rights of individuals and society as defined by legislative statutes.
- Legal issues involving death include documenting all events surrounding the death, treating a deceased person with dignity, and obtaining timely consent for an autopsy from the decedent or close family member.
- A competent adult is able to legally give consent to donate specific organs, and nurses are sometimes able to serve as witnesses to this decision.
- You need to know the laws that apply to your specific area of practice.
- Depending on state laws, nurses are required to report possible criminal activities such as child abuse, as well as certain communicable diseases.

## CRITICAL THINKING IN PRACTICE

*You are taking care of Mr. Jones, a confused older adult patient with congestive heart failure. You and the orderly from the x-ray department are having a social conversation and not paying attention while transferring Mr. Jones from the bed to the x-ray cart. Mr. Jones falls and fractures his hip. You do not make an occurrence report because it was the orderly's fault.*

1. Identify the elements of negligence and how those elements will be applied to this fact situation.

*At one of your child's school sporting events, Tommy Brown, a 7-year-old, falls from the highest bleacher and stops breathing and is pulseless.*

2. What do you do?
3. Do you attempt cardiopulmonary resuscitation (CPR) on the child without his parent's consent?
4. Will your hospital malpractice insurance cover you if you are sued?
5. Which laws guide your nursing actions?

*As you are restarting Mr. Smith's IV line, you apply a soft wrist restraint to the opposite arm because he does not seem to know where he is or what time it is. He subsequently injures the restrained arm and loses the use of his hand due to nerve damage from the restraint. Mr. Smith files a lawsuit.*

- - - - - - - - - - - - - - - - - -

6. Identify the liability issues.
7. Identify the quality assurance and risk management issues.

*Two nurses are getting on the hospital elevator to go to the cafeteria. There are several visitors present in the elevator, as well as hospital personnel. The nurses are discussing a patient who*

*is in the intensive care unit (ICU) who has just tested positive for HIV. They identify the patient as the "guy in 514B." One of the visitors on the elevator who overhears this discussion is a woman who is engaged to the patient in 514B.*

- - - - - - - - - - - - - - - - - -

8. Have the nurses injured the patient in Room 514B?
9. Does the man in 514B have a legal cause of action against the nurses when his name was not shared?
10. Even though the patient's fiancée has a right to know the HIV status of her future husband, is there any obligation on the part of the nurses to disclose this information to her?

## NCLEX® REVIEW

1. The nurse understands that state law affects the way patient care is performed. Therefore he does an Internet search of which of the following on his state's website?
   1. HIPAA
   2. ADA
   3. Nurse Practice Act
   4. Uniform Anatomical Gift Act
2. When preparing an occurrence report, the nurse understands that:
   1. A copy should be put in the patient's record
   2. Subjective information should always be included
   3. Statements made by the patient should be included in the report
   4. If someone was at fault, that person should be blamed in the report
3. Even though you may witness the patient's signature on a form, obtaining informed consent is the responsibility of the:
   1. Patient
   2. Physician or health care provider
   3. Student nurse
   4. Supervising nurse
4. Your employer's malpractice insurance covers you for:
   1. Incidents that occur at your home
   2. Incident that occurs while you are driving to work
   3. Incidents that occur when you are driving home from work
   4. Incident that occurs while you are working within the scope of your employment
5. When you stop to help in an emergency at the scene of an accident, if the injured party files suit and your employing institution's insurance does not cover you, you will probably be covered by:
   1. Your automobile insurance
   2. Your homeowner's insurance
   3. *A Patient's Bill of Rights,* which may grant immunity from suit if the injured party consents

4. The Good Samaritan laws, which grant immunity from suit if there is no gross negligence
6. You are obligated to follow a physician's or health care provider's order unless:
   1. The order is a verbal order
   2. The physician's or health care provider's order is illegible
   3. The order has not been transcribed
   4. The order is in error, violates hospital policy, or would be detrimental to the patient
7. A 75-year-old Hispanic female patient is scheduled for a colon cancer surgery in the morning. You are the night nurse and discover that the patient has decided not to have the surgery even though the consent form has been signed. What is the best action for the nurse to take?
   1. Remind the patient that the consent is a legal document and once signed, remains in effect for 24 hours.
   2. Report the situation to the physician or health care provider, and record it in the nursing notes.
   3. Attempt to convince the patient that the procedure is necessary.
   4. Point out that without the procedure, the patient may die of cancer.
8. One of the elements of negligence is a breach of the standard of care or duty. Standard of care may best be defined as:
   1. Nursing competence as defined by the State Nurse Practice Act
   2. The degree of judgment and skill in nursing care given by a reasonable and prudent professional under similar circumstances
   3. Health services as prescribed by community ordinances
   4. Giving care to patients in good faith to the best of one's ability

## REFERENCES

American Nurses Association: *A new code of ethics,* Silver Spring, Md, 2001, The Association.

Benner P and others: Individual, practice, and system causes of errors in nursing: a taxonomy, *J Nurs Adm* 32(10):509, 2002.

Black HC: *Black's law dictionary,* ed 7, St. Paul, 1999, West Publishing.

Blank FS and others: A humane ED seclusion/restraint: legal requirements, a new policy, procedure, "psychiatric advocate" role, *J Emerg Nurs* 30(1):42, 2004.

Brooke PS: How good a Samaritan should you be? *Nursing* 33(6): 46, 2003.

Burns J and others: Do-not-resuscitate order after 25 years, *Crit Care Med* 31(5):1543, 2003.

Cady R: *The advanced practice nurse's legal handbook,* Philadelphia, 2003, Lippincott Williams & Wilkins.

Joint Commission on Accreditation of Healthcare Organizations: *Restraint and seclusion,* February 14, 2005, http://www.jcaho.org, 2005a.

Joint Commission on Accreditation of Healthcare Organizations: *Setting the Standard, International Center for Patient Safety: Patient Safety Goals,* 2006, May 31, 2005, http://www.jcipatientsafety.org, 2005b.

Joint Commission on Accreditation of Healthcare Organizations: *Comprehensive accreditation manual for hospitals: the official handbook,* 2005c, The Commission.

Laughlin S: Nurse immunity from liability, protection under the ADA, *J Nurs Law* 8(3):39, 2002.

Manson P: Nurse is expert on victim behavior, *Chicago Daily Law Bulletin,* 2002, http://web.lexis-nexis.com/universe/docu.

Martin B: Restraint use in acute and critical care settings: changing practice, *AACN Clin Issues* 13(2):294, 2002.

Mikos C: Legal checkpoints, *Nurs Manage* 35(9):20, 2004.

Mrayyan M, Huber D: The nurse's role in changing health policy related to patient safety, *JONAS Healthc Law Ethics Reg* 5(1):13, 2003.

Rosati K: HIPAA privacy: the compliance challenges ahead, *J Health Law* 35(1):45, 2002.

Scanlon C: Ethical concerns in end-of-life care: when questions about advance directives and the withdrawal of life-sustaining interventions arise, how should decisions be made? *Am J Nurs* 103(1):48, 2003.

Silver M, Lusk R: Patient safety: a tale of two systems, *Qual Manag Health Care* 10(2):12, 2002.

U.S. Department of Health and Human Services, Food and Drug Administration: *Safety alert,* Rockville, Md, 1992, U.S. Government Printing Office.

Vukadinovich DM: Minors' rights to consent to treatment: navigating the complexity of state laws, *J Health Law* 37(4):667, 2004.

Whitman M: Return and report: establishing accountability in delegation, *Am J Nur* 104(1):76, 2004.

## STATUTES

Americans With Disabilities Act, 42 USC §121.010-12213 (1995).

Autopsy Consent, Mo Rev Stat §194.115 (1998).

Good Samaritan Law, Mo Rev Stat §537.037 (1998).

Health Insurance Portability and Accountability Act of 1996, Pub L No. 104 (1996).

National Organ Transplant Act, Pub L No. 98-507 (1984).

Patient Self-Determination Act, 42 CFR 417 (1991).

Resident's Rights, Medicaid Statute, 42 USCA §1396R (1988).

Uniform Anatomical Gift Act (1987).

Uniform Determination of Death Act (1980).

## CASES

*Cruzan v. Director Missouri Department of Health,* 497 US 261 (1990).

*In re Schiller,* 148 NJ Super 168 (1977).

*Winkelman v. Beloit Memorial Hospital,* 484 NW2d 211 (1992).

# CHAPTER 5

# Ethics

## MEDIA RESOURCES

**CD COMPANION** *evolve* **WEBSITE**

http://evolve.elsevier.com/Potter/basic

- **NCLEX® Review**
- **Audio Glossary**
- **English/Spanish Audio Glossary**

## OBJECTIVES

- Explain the importance of accountability and responsibility in nursing practice.
- Discuss patient advocacy.
- Describe the role of ethics in nursing practice.
- Explain a process used to analyze an ethical dilemma.
- Describe ethical conflicts nurses experience in different clinical settings.

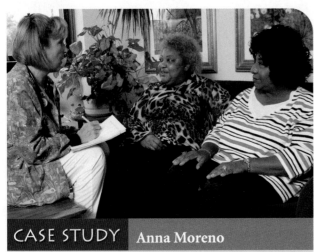

## CASE STUDY    Anna Moreno

Anna Moreno, an 82-year-old African-American retired school-teacher, lives with her 55-year-old daughter and three school-aged grandchildren. Her daughter, Lucille, is a single mother and a nurse. She works full time on the night shift at an intensive care unit. Anna Moreno assists with care of her grandchildren when her daughter is at work. She has been active in community life since retirement. She volunteers at the local library and contributes time and energy to the Altar Guild at the church where she has belonged for over 40 years. Her husband died about 5 years ago. She is ambulatory and able to drive herself to the library, the grocery store, and to pick up the grandchildren after school.

Anna Moreno is a breast cancer survivor. She has been cancer-free for 10 years. She has developed diabetes recently. Her hypertension is well controlled with medication.

A white home health nurse, Nancy LaCrosse, visits Anna Moreno about once a month to check on Ms. Moreno's blood glucose level and insulin compliance. During her last visit Ms. Moreno's daughter asked to speak to her privately and revealed the following concerns.

Last week Lucille received a call from the manager of the library where Anna Moreno volunteers. The manager reported finding Ms. Moreno seated on a stool in the janitor's closet, crying, confused, and with her clothes in disarray. She also described an increasing concern, shared by others at the library. Ms. Moreno was having problems finishing tasks at work. Library books were missing or turning up in odd locations, and phone messages were not legible. Lucille was defensive of her mother, and she accused the library manager of incompetence and age discrimination. Her mother was perfectly competent, she complained, and she could not help it if the library was al-

ways losing books. Under no circumstances would she consent to a physical or social evaluation for her mother because someone at the library had complaints. Nurse LaCrosse was a good listener, but this situation was complicated with many competing interests. As a home care nurse, she realizes she will need to find help from other health care disciplines. She also needs to sort out the competing interests in order to determine the most appropriate, and ethical, actions.

## KEY TERMS

accountability, p. 68
advocacy, p. 70
autonomy, p. 67
beneficence, p. 68
bioethics, p. 67
care, p. 71
code of ethics, p. 68
competence, p. 70
confidentiality, p. 69
deontology, p. 70
ethical dilemma, p. 70
ethical principles, p. 68
ethics, p. 67
ethics of care, p. 71

feminist ethics, p. 71
fidelity, p. 68
institutional ethics
  committee, p. 71
judgment, p. 70
justice, p. 67
law, p. 67
morals, p. 67
nonmaleficence,
  p. 68
point of view, p. 70
responsibility, p. 68
utilitarianism, p. 71
value, p. 67

Nursing practice involves care during all aspects of health, sickness, personal life, and community life. As a nurse you will play an important and often intimate role in the lives of your patients. Your relationship with patients and with others on the health care team will sometimes require participation in difficult or controversial decisions. Because we live in a nation of many different cultures, you will find yourself faced with complicated situations that arise from these differences. With the support of professional codes of practice and a commitment to critical thinking skills, you will contribute a vital and unique voice to the process of health care delivery.

The study of ethics has occupied the attention of civilization for thousands of years. When human beings gather in community, they turn to concerns about right living.

Whether you look to the ancient Chinese philosophers, the dialogues of the ancient Greeks, or traces of Mayan and Aztec culture, you will find evidence of a fundamental human effort to define right and wrong behavior. The term **ethics** refers to the consideration of standards of conduct or the study of philosophical ideals of right and wrong behavior (*American Heritage Dictionary,* 2001).

## Basic Definitions

Ethical issues differ from legal issues. Systems of government determine the content of the **law**. These same systems enforce laws (Harris, 1998). Breaking a law usually results in a public consequence, such as a ticket for speeding or jail time for stealing. The law guides public behavior that will affect others and that will preserve community. In the case study, age discrimination laws guide the behavior of the librarians. If Ms. Moreno is in fact experiencing age discrimination, the librarians will suffer the consequences of breaking a law. Ethics, on the other hand, has a broader base of interest and includes personal behavior and issues of character, such as kindness, tolerance, and generosity. In the case study, the nurse will use ethical standards of practice to guide her management of the complex health and social issues that this family currently faces.

A **value** is a personal belief about the worth you hold for an idea, a custom, or an object. The values you hold reflect cultural and social influences. For example, if your family makes a living in a rural place, you may value the environment differently from someone who visits rural areas for recreation. You use your values to shape your own point of view. Systems of ethics usually grow from shared values, negotiated and discussed over time by people who share values, such as religious groups, ethnic groups, or work groups.

As you enter the nursing profession, you will undergo socialization into the profession. You will learn professional values that help define your role as a nurse and that will influence your point of view. When you have a clear understanding of nursing values, as well as your personal values and your own point of view, you and the health care team will be able to make effective decisions regarding difficult ethical issues.

The terms *ethics* and *morals* sometimes are used interchangeably. **Morals** usually refer to judgment about behavior, and ethics is the study of the ideals of right and wrong behavior. Moral codes are more likely to reflect the character of the social setting from which they come (Davis and Aroskar, 1997).

The study of **bioethics** represents a particular branch of ethics, namely, the study of ethics within the field of health care. The bioethical field of study pertains to those who work in clinical settings, research, or education. Increasingly, the term clinical ethics is replacing the term bioethics (Chally and Hough, 2005).

The field of bioethics has become a prominent branch of the study of ethics, especially in the last 25 years. When researchers perfected kidney transplant technology in the early 1970s, the immediate ethical concern became the limited number of kidneys available compared with the greater number of patients in need of a transplant. The arrival of advanced medical technologies requires society to face difficult ethical questions. Who should get what resources? What constitutes quality of life? Who should decide? In the study of bioethics, health care professionals agree to negotiate these difficult and important questions.

Nursing professionals play an important role in the practice of bioethics. Skill and confidence in one's own point of view as a participant in the interdisciplinary process of ethics is critical to the successful resolution of ethical issues. As Chally and Hough (2005) explain, "When an ethical decision is made, everyone must respect and value the perspectives held by others. Through respectful collaboration, the best decision can be reached in even the most difficult dilemma." Nurses participate in bioethical discussion in two distinct ways: As professionals, nurses construct a professional code of ethics that reflects and defines practice; and as colleagues in the practice of health care delivery, nurses develop a specific point of view for contribution to ethical discussions about health care issues.

## Ethical Principles

Practitioners in health care delivery agree to a set of ethical principles that guide professional practice and decision making. These principles are common to all professions in health care. You will find these principles especially useful because they guide our commitment to advocacy, an important concept in caring for others (Table 5-1).

**Autonomy** refers to a person's independence. As a principle in bioethics, autonomy represents an agreement to respect the patient's right to determine a course of action. For example, the purpose of the preoperative consent is to assure in writing that the health care team respects the patient's independence by obtaining permission to proceed. The consent process implies that if a patient refuses treatment, in most cases the health care team will agree to abide by the patient's refusal.

**Justice** refers to the principle of fairness. You will often refer to this principle when discussing issues of health care resources. What constitutes a fair distribution of resources is not always clear. For example, approximately three times more candidates are on a waiting list for liver transplants than there are livers available for transplant in the United States. The just distribution of available organs is difficult to determine. In the United States a national multidisciplinary committee strives for fairness by ranking recipients according to need, rather than resorting to selling organs for profit or distributing them by lottery.

| TABLE 5-1 | Principles of Health Care Ethics |
|---|---|
| **Principle** | **Definition** |
| Autonomy | Independence; self-determination; self-reliance |
| Justice | Fairness or equity |
| Fidelity | Faithfulness; striving to keep promises |
| Beneficence | Actively seeking benefits; promotion of good |
| Nonmaleficence | Actively seeking to do no harm |

**Fidelity** refers to the agreement to keep promises. The principle of fidelity also promotes your obligation as a nurse to follow through with the care offered to patients. For example, if you assess a patient for pain and then offer a plan to manage the pain, the principle of fidelity encourages you to do your best to keep the promise to improve the patient's comfort.

The principle of **beneficence** promotes taking positive, active steps to help others. It encourages you to do good for the patient. It helps to guide decisions in which the benefits of a treatment pose a risk to the patient's well-being or dignity. A child's immunization causes discomfort during administration, but the benefits of protection from disease, both for the individual and for society, outweigh the temporary discomforts. The agreement to act with beneficence requires that the best interest of the patient remains more important than self-interest. For example, you will not simply practice obedience to medical orders, but you also will act thoughtfully to understand patient needs and then work actively to help meet those needs.

**Nonmaleficence** refers to the fundamental agreement to do no harm. It is closely related to the principle of beneficence. This principle will be helpful in guiding your discussions about new or controversial technologies. For example, a new bone marrow transplant procedure promises a chance at cure, but the long-term prognosis is uncertain, or the procedure requires long periods of pain or suffering. You will consider these risks in relationship to the potential good that may come of the procedure. The principle of nonmaleficence promotes a continuing effort to consider the potential for harm even when it is necessary to promote health.

## Codes of Ethics

A **code of ethics** is a set of **ethical principles** that all members of a profession generally accept. A profession's ethical code states the group's expectations and standards of behavior. Codes serve as guidelines to assist nurses and other professional groups when conflict or disagreement arises about correct practice or behavior. The code of ethics for nursing sets forth ideals of nursing conduct and provides a common foundation for nursing education. The American Nurses Association (ANA) and the International Council of Nurses (ICN) have established widely accepted codes that you as a

| BOX 5-1 | American Nurses Association Code of Ethics |
|---|---|

1. The nurse, in all professional relationships, practices with compassion and respect for the inherent dignity, worth, and uniqueness of every individual, unrestricted by considerations of social or economic status, personal attributes, or the nature of health problems.
2. The nurse's primary commitment is to the patient, whether an individual, family, group, or community.
3. The nurse promotes, advocates for, and strives to protect the health, safety, and rights of the patient.
4. The nurse is responsible and accountable for individual nursing practice and determines the appropriate delegation of tasks consistent with the nurse's obligation to provide optimum patient care.
5. The nurse owes the same duties to self as to others, including the responsibility to preserve integrity and safety, to maintain competence, and to continue personal and professional growth.
6. The nurse participates in establishing, maintaining, and improving health care environments and conditions of employment conducive to the provision of quality health care and consistent with the values of the profession through individual and collective action.
7. The nurse participates in the advancement of the profession through contributions to practice, education, administration, and knowledge development.
8. The nurse collaborates with other health professionals and the public in promoting community, national, and international efforts to meet health needs.
9. The profession of nursing, as represented by associations and their members, is responsible for articulating nursing values, for maintaining the integrity of the profession and its practice, and for shaping social policy.

Reprinted with permission from American Nurses Association, *Code of ethics for nurses with interpretive statements,* © 2001 American Nurses Publishing, American Nurses Foundation/American Nurses Association, Washington, DC.

nurse will follow. Although these codes differ in specific emphasis, they reflect the same underlying principles (Boxes 5-1 and 5-2), including responsibility, accountability, respect for confidentiality, competency, judgment, and advocacy.

A nurse assumes responsibility and accountability for all nursing care delivered. **Responsibility** refers to the execution of duties associated with a nurse's particular role. The responsible nurse demonstrates characteristics of reliability and dependability. For example, when administering a medication, you are responsible for assessing the patient's need for the drug, for giving it safely and correctly, and for evaluating the response to it. By agreeing to responsibility, you will gain trust from patients, colleagues, and society.

When nurses perform care, they are accountable. **Accountability** refers to the ability to answer for your actions. You are accountable to yourself most of all. You also

| BOX 5-2 | The ICN Code of Ethics for Nurses |

**Preamble**

Nurses have four fundamental responsibilities: to promote health, to prevent illness, to restore health, and to alleviate suffering. The need for nursing is universal.

Inherent in nursing is respect for human life, including the right to life, to dignity, and to be treated with respect. Considerations of age, color, creed, culture, disability or illness, gender, nationality, politics, race, and social status do not restrict nursing care.

Nurses render health services to the individual, the family, and the community and coordinate their services with those of related groups.

**The Code**

The *ICN Code of Ethics for Nurses* has four principal elements that outline the standards of ethical conduct.

**Elements of the Code**

**1. Nurses and People**

The nurse's primary professional responsibility is to people requiring nursing care.

In providing care, the nurse promotes an environment in which the human rights, values, customs, and spiritual beliefs of the individual, family, and community are respected.

The nurse ensures that the individual receives sufficient information on which to base consent for care and related treatment.

The nurse holds in confidence personal information and uses judgment in sharing this information.

The nurse shares with society the responsibility for initiating and supporting action to meet the health and social needs of the public, in particular those of vulnerable populations.

The nurse also shares responsibility to sustain and protect the natural environment from depletion, pollution, degradation, and destruction.

**2. Nurses and Practice**

The nurse carries personal responsibility and accountability for nursing practice and for maintaining competence by continual learning.

The nurse maintains a standard of personal health such that the ability to provide care is not compromised.

The nurse uses judgment regarding individual competence when accepting and delegating responsibility.

The nurse at all times maintains standards of personal conduct that reflect well on the profession and enhance public confidence.

The nurse, in providing care, ensures that use of technology and scientific advances are compatible with the safety, dignity, and rights of people.

**3. Nurses and the Profession**

The nurse assumes the major role in determining and implementing acceptable standards of clinical nursing practice, management, research, and education.

The nurse is active in developing a core of research-based professional knowledge.

The nurse, acting through the professional organization, participates in creating and maintaining equitable social and economic working conditions in nursing.

**4. Nurses and Co-workers**

The nurses sustains a cooperative relationship with co-workers in nursing and other fields.

The nurse takes appropriate action to safeguard individuals when a co-worker or any other person endangers their patient's care.

Modified from International Council of Nurses: *ICN code of ethics for nurses*, Geneva, 2000, 3, place Jean-Marteau, CH-1201, The Association.

---

balance accountability to the patient, the profession, the employing institution, and society. For example, you know that a patient who will be discharged soon remains confused about how to self-administer insulin. The professional commitment to accountability will guide the action that you take in response to this situation. In this case, you inquire about family members available to assist the patient and arrange home care to continue teaching at home. The goal is the prevention of injury to the patient. The principle that guides you is accountability.

The concept of **confidentiality** in health care has widespread acceptance in the United States. Federal legislation known as HIPAA (Health Insurance Portability and Accountability Act of 1996) requires that those with access to personal health information not disclose the information to a third party without patient consent. HIPAA legislation defines the rights and privileges of patients for protection of privacy without diminishing access to quality care and sets fines for violations (U.S. Department of Health and Human Services [USDHHS], 2002). You cannot copy or forward medical records without a patient's consent. Health care workers are not allowed to share health care information with others without specific patient consent. This includes laboratory results, diagnosis, and prognosis. In addition, family members or friends of the patient are not permitted access to the patient's personal health information without the patient's consent. Conflicting obligations arise when a patient wants to keep information from insurance companies to preserve coverage or from employers to preserve a job. The commitment to confidentiality is particularly challenging as medical records become computerized. Preservation of confidentiality is often in competition with the need to facilitate access to information. In the case of computer access, health care institutions work to protect confidentiality by using

family conferences, staff meetings, or even in one-on-one meetings. Many ethical problems begin when people feel misled or are not aware of their options and do not know when to speak up about their concerns. Patients and health care workers address such concerns in a variety of constructive settings. Ethics committees serve to complement relationships and offer a valuable resource for strengthening them.

Whether you resolve an ethical dilemma in a committee setting, at the bedside, or in a family conference, you will apply a careful, critical processing of the dilemma (Box 5-3). Resolving an ethical dilemma is similar to the nursing process because it requires deliberate, systematic thinking (Chally and Hough, 2005). The following offers details for processing an ethical dilemma.

**Step 1:** Is this an ethical dilemma?

The first step guides you to determine if the problem is an ethical one. Not all problems are ethical. You will learn to distinguish ethical problems from questions of procedure, legality, or medical diagnosis. Curtin and Flaherty (1982) suggest that a true ethical dilemma has one or more of the following characteristics:

1. Scientific data alone does not resolve the dilemma. To make this determination, it is necessary to gather detailed information about the situation from medical records, health care literature, or consultation with colleagues or with the patient and family. For example, what at first appears to be a dilemma might resolve after learning that a review of a diagnostic procedure reveals a different prognosis.
2. Dilemmas are perplexing. You cannot easily think logically or make a decision about the problem, or you may disagree with a decision that others are making, and the difference of opinion is perplexing.
3. The answer to the problem will have profound relevance for several areas of human concern.

In the case study, Nurse LaCrosse faces difficult decisions. She wants to secure a proper evaluation for Ms. Moreno, but the daughter seems adamantly against it at this point. Furthermore, Nurse LaCrosse does not want to completely dismiss the daughter's perceptions of discrimination at the library. Further information will help to determine a solution, but there are roadblocks to obtaining the information. The situation is frustrating, and the right course of action is not immediately clear.

**Step 2:** Gather all relevant information.

Accurate and complete information is essential for the ethical process to go forward.

For example, in the case study, Nurse LaCrosse already knows quite a bit about the health and the social situation of Ms. Moreno, but what about the grandchildren? What about the job situation of Lucille? Just what is the cognitive skill level of Anna Moreno, at least so far as Nurse LaCrosse is able to determine? What does Ms. Moreno want?

---

**BOX 5-3 How to Process an Ethical Dilemma**

**Step 1. Is this an ethical dilemma?**

If a review of scientific data does not resolve the question, the question is perplexing, and the answer will have profound relevance for several areas of human concern, then an ethical dilemma exists.

**Step 2. Gather all information relevant to the case.**

Complete assessment of the facts of the case is critical to an effective decision. An overlooked fact sometimes provides quick resolution, or deeply affects the options available. Patient, family, institutional, and social perspectives are important sources of relevant information.

**Step 3. Examine and determine your own values and opinions about the issues.**

Values clarification provides a foundation for clarity and for confidence during discussions that will be necessary for resolution of a dilemma. Taking this step ensures that you are able to distinguish between your personal values and those of the other participants and allows you to become a more open listener.

**Step 4. State the problem clearly.**

A clear, simple statement of the dilemma is not always easy, but it is essential for the next step to take place.

**Step 5. Consider possible courses of action.**

To respect all sides of an issue, it is helpful to list potential actions, especially when the list will reflect opinions that conflict.

**Step 6. Negotiate the outcome.**

Sometimes courses of action that seem unlikely at the beginning of the process take on new possibility as they are put to rational and respectful consideration. Negotiation requires a confidence in your own point of view and a deep respect for the opinions of others.

**Step 7. Evaluate the action.**

---

**Step 3:** Examine and determine your values and opinions about the issues.

A part of gathering information also will include a determination of your own opinion about the issues. The distinction between personal opinion and the facts of the case or the opinions of others is essential for resolution to proceed. People come to different conclusions about the same situation with no malice intended toward other people. Remembering this will help you to be an effective moderator in conversation.

Leaving room for the possibility that Lucille is correct in her accusations about the librarian will be an important part of the process. More likely, Lucille is overreacting to the situation and is in denial about her mother's health, because the loss of her mother's child care support will profoundly affect Lucille's ability to keep her full-time job. What if Nurse LaCrosse has strong opinions against single motherhood? The ability to process any dilemma requires that personal values be clear and that you respect the values of others.

**Step 4:** State the problem clearly.

After reviewing relevant information, develop a clear statement of the problem in language that all involved in the ethical discussion will understand. The statement lays the groundwork for the negotiations that follow. Discussions are more likely to remain focused and constructive when all parties agree on the statement of the dilemma.

In the case of Ms. Moreno, what is wrong with her, if anything, and who will best make that determination? Is Anna Moreno the best person to make the decision about her own well-being, or is the daughter, Lucille, the right person? What about Nurse LaCrosse: Is she able to make independent decisions regarding the health of Ms. Moreno?

**Step 5:** Consider possible courses of action.

You facilitate a discussion of ethical dilemmas by listing possible courses of action as they occur to the group. Possibilities occur at any time during the discussion.

A discussion with the librarian, Anna Moreno, Lucille, and Nurse LaCrosse will help to clarify the situation. Perhaps Nurse LaCrosse can bring in a social worker to evaluate the home setting, as well as to offer an independent opinion about the cognitive skills of Anna Moreno. The timing of the discussion is important because Lucille works nights. She will most likely function better if they schedule a meeting around her usual sleep times during the day. The children may or may not be a part of the meeting, depending on their ages. An important question remains: Is Ms. Moreno competent to give consent about her own health care issues?

**Step 6:** Negotiate the outcome.

Nurse LaCrosse consults with her manager at the home care agency. Together, they create a plan that involves multidisciplinary action. Ms. LaCrosse organizes a family conference where a nonthreatening discussion unfolds. Participants include a social worker with expertise in community resources and the pastor from Anna's church. Ms. LaCrosse also involves a nurse colleague from her agency with expertise in gerontological clinical issues. Anna Moreno and her daughter also attend. During the discussion Anna asks for her husband and becomes angry when Lucille reminds her that her husband died 5 years ago. As Lucille begins to realize that her mother's condition is worse than she realized, she begins crying. The team of people at the meeting recognizes that this family has suddenly become a vulnerable family, with issues of health and well-being at risk. They help Lucille take immediate action to obtain family leave from work, and they begin the long task of taking care of all the other issues that affect the situation: financial constraints, the care of the children, the care of Anna, confidentiality, and issues of consent (How much does Anna understand, and can she realistically consent to medical procedures?). The pastor helps to end the meeting with a prayer, which brings great comfort.

**Step 7:** Evaluate the action.

Make decisions and evaluate them in an ongoing manner.

Documentation of the ethical process takes a variety of forms. Whenever the process involves a family conference or results in a change in the management plan, you will document the process in the medical record. Some institutions use a formal consultation format whenever a request for discussion comes to the ethics committee. If the ethical dilemma does not directly affect patient care, however, documentation occurs by means of minutes from a meeting or in a memorandum to affected parties.

## Potential Ethical Problems in Nursing

In any practice setting you will be confronted with ethical issues unique to that practice. The following sections describe examples of ethical dilemmas common in health care settings today.

### Allocation of Scarce Resources: The Nursing Shortage

The nursing shortage in the United States is a real and a growing problem. The factors that contribute to the shortage are complex and numerous and include cultural, economic, and social elements. The shortage is due to a decline in the number of students entering nursing school, as well as the aging of the nursing workforce. The average age of registered nurses in 2000 was 45.2 years (Chitty, 2005). The statistics about the shortage are startling. For example, according to the Federal Bureau of Labor Statistics, the demand for nurses in 2000 was 2 million, and the supply was at 1.89 million, a 6% shortfall. Furthermore, researchers originally predicted a shortfall of this magnitude to occur much later, at around 2007 (Chitty, 2005).

The nursing shortage produces difficult working conditions, and affects patient outcomes (Needleman and others, 2001). The Institute of Medicine's report on the magnitude of medication errors includes discussion on the role of the nurse, and the role of inadequate staffing as a source of medication error (Kohn, Corrigan, and Donaldson, 2000).

You can also view the shortage in terms of ethical concerns. How does a nurse decide what is the best course to take when a patient care assignment feels too large to be safe? California is the first state in the United States to pass mandated staffing ratios. Laws limit the number of patients assigned to a nurse. Some hospitals in California have up to 25% of their nursing positions unfilled, however. The law stipulates that if a hospital does not have enough nurses to fulfill staffing requirements, then the hospital will "close beds." Hospitals will have to turn patients away. The nursing shortage and the mandated staffing ratios have created ethical dilemmas. For example, professional issues of advocacy and patient abandonment compete with ethical concerns about beneficence, maleficence, and justice. An obligation to participate in political solutions sometimes plays as important a role as the negotiation of personal concerns.

## Managed Care

In the acute care setting, managed care systems place a growing emphasis on decreasing hospitalization days. To safely accomplish a shorter hospitalization, a great deal of teaching and discharge planning falls to the bedside nurse. An ethical dilemma arises if you determine that the patient and the patient's family have not mastered a skill needed to provide safe care in the home, yet the patient's insurance will not cover further days in the hospital.

**Step 1:** Is this an ethical dilemma?

The situation is perplexing because it seems that whether the patient remains in the hospital or not, the consequences will be disastrous. A safe and affordable solution to this dilemma has relevance for the patient and for the acute care setting.

**Step 2:** Gather all the information relevant to the case.

Who pays for this patient's care, and who in this setting is responsible for negotiating with payers? What is the prognosis for this patient, and how long will home care be necessary? What will be the financial impact of unsafe care in the home? How much more time do you think the patient needs to learn the needed skill? Can a home care service provide the care and further teaching?

**Step 3:** Examine and determine your own values and opinions on the issues.

You have had some positive and some negative experiences with managed care in the past. It is important to separate personal responses in the past from this situation. The professional evaluation of the patient's readiness for discharge will play a critical role in the negotiations, so make sure you clearly understand your own opinion and the patient's situation.

**Step 4:** State the problem clearly.

What resources will provide the safest *and* most cost-effective care for this patient? How do you protect the principle of beneficence for this patient and yet remain accountable to the hospital and to the managed care plan?

**Step 5:** Consider possible courses of action.

You decide to take time to inform administrators and physicians or health care providers about the patient's lack of knowledge. You propose a solution by investigating the location and quality of home care services. You learn more from the patient about family resources.

**Step 6:** Negotiate the outcome.

Working with social workers, physicians or health care providers, and admission and utilization review personnel helps you to devise a safe plan for discharge. Certainly, working within the guidelines of the managed care plan will be essential for success. In addition, the patient responds to the dilemma by identifying other family members or community resources that facilitate a safe discharge. At the very least, you ensure that the physician or health care provider and others become aware of the potential for unsafe conditions after discharge.

**Step 7:** Evaluate the action.

The nature of the outcome will depend on your ability to pursue an option that protects this patient during and after discharge.

## End-of-Life Issues

Working with the chronically ill or disabled patient places you in contact with decisions about quality of life, such as the patient's ability to maintain independence and functional status (Tilden and others, 1996). The determination of measures of quality represents a relatively new field of study. For example, a patient who is profoundly disabled by a stroke begins to suffer from aspiration problems during feedings. Would a gastrostomy tube serve to prevent aspiration, or would it represent a surgical intervention that will prolong suffering?

**Step 1:** Is this an ethical dilemma?

Scientific data helps to predict improved nutrition and improved safety for this patient, but they do not help to address the ethical issues about quality of life. You are puzzled, as is the family, about the right decision. A decision that felt "right" to all parties would have profound relevance for this dilemma and influence similar clinical situations in a positive way.

**Step 2:** Gather all the information relevant to the case.

What is the prognosis for this patient? What are the surgical risks and benefits from placement of the gastrostomy tube? What is the medical risk of aspiration pneumonia in this patient before and after tube placement? Would pneumonia and the treatment represent an uncomfortable experience for the patient? Does the patient have a living will, advance directive, or identification of an individual with medical power of attorney?

**Step 3:** Examine and determine your own values and opinions on the issues.

Begin by exploring your personal feelings about the quality of this patient's life. Is the patient able to express an opinion? If yes, you will probably have personal opinions about the competence of the patient. These opinions are important to articulate. How do you feel about the competence of the family members and significant others? If the patient or health care workers made a decision with which you disagree, it is important to consider whether you could still participate in the care of the patient. Could you advocate for a position that was in conflict with your own values?

**Step 4:** State the problem clearly.

Will a gastrostomy tube improve the quality of this patient's life, or will a gastrostomy tube prolong suffering? How can the team best respect this patient's autonomy?

**Step 5:** Consider possible courses of action.

The patient could have the gastrostomy tube placed or perhaps have a nasogastric tube placed temporarily while the more difficult ethical issues are explored with the patient and the patient's family. The patient or the patient's significant others could decide against the insertion of a gastrostomy tube. If the patient decides against the gastrostomy tube, then you could make a referral to hospice care to ensure continued support for the patient and the family (Box 5-4).

**Step 6:** Negotiate the outcome.

If the patient is competent and an adult, the patient's decision will determine the outcome. If not, then the health

| BOX 5-4 | USING EVIDENCE IN PRACTICE |
|---|---|

### Research Summary

The hospice care movement has made great improvements possible in the understanding and provision of comfort at the end of life. However, research shows that the average length of time a patient spends in hospice care is 1 month or even less.

Referrals to hospice care depend on a provider's ability to predict when death is likely to occur for a particular patient. In an article that summarizes several investigations about physician accuracy in predicting death in their patients, the researchers concluded that in general physicians were accurate to within 2 weeks of the actual death about 25% of the time. In another study, researchers found that physicians predicted survival accurately in only 20% of cases. Of these, 63% were overly optimistic. Physicians often thought that patients had longer to live than proved to be the case. Of the physicians who made overly optimistic predictions, most were physicians who had longstanding relationships with their patients or who had seen their patients recently. The study described them as "surprisingly inaccurate." An editorial response to the study suggested that "Doctors may be reluctant to acknowledge that patients they know well are close to death."

### Application to Nursing Practice

Even though evidence shows that hospice care improves quality at the end of life, a reluctance to admit that the end is approaching delays an appropriate referral. The study described above suggests that one factor in this reluctance is that health care providers who are closest to the patient are least likely to recognize that the end is near.

Nurses are often in the position to affect decisions by patients, families, and even physicians or other health care providers. Your knowledge about the value of hospice care, the likely roadblocks to obtaining hospice care, and the commitment to patient advocacy will help to ensure that the option for hospice care remains a consideration.

Data from Christakis NA, Lamont EB: Extent and determinants of error in doctors' prognoses in terminally ill patients: prospective cohort study, *Br Med J* 320(7233):469, 2000; Glare P and others: A systematic review of physicians' survival predictions in terminally ill cancer patients, *Br Med J* 327(7408):195, 2003.

care team will have to rely on family members, significant others, or even legal documents that identify legal guardians to make the decision. In this last case the decision is sometimes more difficult to obtain. Your role in the negotiations includes patient advocacy and the contribution of the nursing perspective on quality of life for this individual. You also need to be honest and truthful with the family (Clark and Volker, 2003).

**Step 7:** Evaluate the action.

Regardless of the decision in this case, it is possible to reverse the decision if conditions or feelings changed. Continuing discussion with the patient and the family or significant others ensures a satisfactory conclusion to this dilemma.

## Cultural and Religious Sensitivity

The professional standards of justice and beneficence require respect for cultural differences in the health care setting, regardless of personal opinion or feeling (Davis and Koenig, 1996). Occasionally you will face a challenging situation in which cultural differences present an ethical dilemma. For example, a 15-year-old girl is admitted for management of her leukemia. You note that the child's religious beliefs do not allow her to receive blood transfusions, yet her condition will soon require a blood transfusion to prevent harmful consequences. Her parents share her religious convictions but are willing to compromise. The 15-year-old refuses to compromise.

**Step 1:** Is this an ethical dilemma?

Further review of the clinical situation will not change the dilemma. Scientific data will not affect the strong feelings of the child or of her parents. The case is perplexing because respecting the patient's autonomy will conflict with the health care team's wish to do no harm. The resolution of this dilemma will be difficult and will have profound relevance for several areas of concern, including the life of the patient.

**Step 2:** Gather all the information relevant to the case.

How soon does the patient need the transfusion? What are the legal definitions of "minor" in your state? Has the family agreed to transfusions in the past, and if so, how was the compromise reached? What are the specific religious constraints against blood transfusions that affect this case? Is the patient competent? Is she fully aware of the consequences of her decision to refuse the transfusion?

**Step 3:** Examine and determine your own values and opinions about the issues.

How do you feel about this patient's religious beliefs? How close or distant are the patient's beliefs from your personal beliefs? What is your personal opinion on the rights of minors to determine their medical course?

**Step 4:** State the problem clearly.

A patient, who is a minor, will refuse a lifesaving transfusion on the grounds of religious belief. If she is forced to receive the transfusion, she will consider herself violated in the eyes of her God. If she does not receive the transfusion, she will probably not survive.

**Step 5:** Consider possible courses of action.

The parents and health care team could force the patient to receive a transfusion, which will require restraints or use of physical force. You could respect the patient's wishes. You could encourage the patient and her family to explore this dilemma with the guidance of a religious leader from their faith.

**Step 6:** Negotiate the outcome.

In this case, your contribution consists of accurate documentation of the patient's state of mind. A patient care conference with the patient and her family is necessary. If the medical team decides to insist on the transfusion, then they will seek a court order. As advocate for the patient, even in the face of personal disagreement, you will ensure that the patient's voice is fairly represented to the judge.

7. Health care providers, including professional nurses, agree to "do no harm" to their patients. The point of this agreement is to reassure the public that in all ways the health care team will not only work to heal patients, they agree to do this in the least painful and harmful way possible. The principle that describes this agreement is called:
   1. Beneficence
   2. Accountability
   3. Nonmaleficence
   4. Respect for autonomy

8. Nurses and other providers agree to be advocates for their patients. Practice of advocacy calls for the nurse to:
   1. Seek out graduate education as soon as possible
   2. Work to understand the law as it applies to the patient's clinical condition
   3. Assess the patient's point of view and prepare to articulate this point of view
   4. Document all clinical changes in the medical record in a timely and legible way

# REFERENCES

*American Heritage Dictionary,* ed 4, Boston, 2001, Houghton Mifflin.

American Nurses Association: *Code of Ethics for nurses with interpretative statements,* Washington, DC, 2001, The Association.

Beauchamp T, Childress J: *Principles of biomedical ethics,* ed 5, New York, 2001, Oxford University Press.

Chally PS, Hough MC: Nursing ethics. In Chitty KK: *Professional nursing: concepts and challenges,* ed 4, St. Louis, 2005.

Chitty KK: *Professional nursing: concepts and challenges,* ed 4, St. Louis, 2005, Saunders.

Christakis NA, Lamont EB: Extent and determinants of error in doctors' prognoses in terminally ill patients: prospective cohort study, *Br Med J* 320(7233):469, 2000.

Clark AP, Volker DL: Truthfulness, *Clin Nurse Spec* 17(1):17, 2003.

Curtin L, Flaherty MJ: *Nursing ethics: theories and pragmatics,* Bowie, Md, 1982, Brady.

Davis A, Aroskar M: *Ethical dilemmas and nursing practice,* ed 4, Norwalk, Conn, 1997, Appleton & Lange.

Davis AJ, Koenig BA: A question of policy: bioethics in a multicultural society, *Nurs Policy Forum* 2(1):7, 1996.

Fry ST: The role of caring in a theory of nursing ethics, *Hypatia* 4(2):88, 1989.

Gilligan C: *In a different voice,* Cambridge, Mass, 1993, Harvard University Press.

Glare P and others: A systematic review of physicians' survival predictions in terminally ill cancer patients, *Br Med J* 327(7408):195, 2003.

Harris CH: Legal aspects of nursing. In Deloughery G: *Issues and trends in nursing,* ed 3, St. Louis, 1998, Mosby.

International Council of Nurses: *ICN code of ethics for nurses,* Geneva, 2000, 3, place Jean-Marteau, CH-1201, The Association.

Kohlberg L: *Essays on moral development,* vols 1-3, San Francisco, 1981, Harper & Row.

Kohn LT, Corrigan JM, Donaldson MS, editors: *To err is human,* Washington, DC, 2000, National Academy Press.

Leininger M: *Caring: an essential human need,* Detroit, 1988, Wayne State University Press.

Needleman J and others: *Nurse staffing and patient outcomes in hospitals: executive summary,* Boston, February 2001, Harvard School of Public Health, http://bhpr.hrsa.gov/nursing/staffstudy.htm.

O'Neil J: Ethical decision making and the role of nursing. In Deloughery G: *Issues and trends in nursing,* ed 3, St. Louis, 1998, Mosby.

Sherwin S: *No longer patient: feminist ethics and health care,* Philadelphia, 1992, Temple University Press.

Tilden V and others: Decisions about life-sustaining treatment, *Arch Intern Med* 155:633, 1996.

United States Department of Health and Human Services (USDHHS): HHS fact sheet: modifications to the standards for privacy of individually identifiable health information—final rule, August 9, 2002, http://www.hhs.gov/news/press/2002pres/20020809.html.

Watson J, editor: *Applying art and science of human caring,* New York, 1994, National League of Nursing Press.

# CHAPTER 6

# Critical Thinking and Nursing Judgment

## MEDIA RESOURCES

**CD COMPANION** *evolve* **WEBSITE**

http://evolve.elsevier.com/Potter/basic

- NCLEX® Review
- Audio Glossary
- English/Spanish Audio Glossary

## OBJECTIVES

- Describe characteristics of a critical thinker.
- Discuss the nurse's responsibility in making clinical decisions.
- Describe the components of a critical thinking model for clinical decision making.
- Discuss critical thinking skills used in nursing practice.
- Explain the relationship between clinical experience and critical thinking.

- Discuss the effect attitudes for critical thinking have on clinical decision making.
- Explain how professional standards influence a nurse's clinical decisions.
- Discuss how reflection can improve knowledge of nursing.
- Discuss the relationship of the nursing process to critical thinking.

## CASE STUDY    Mrs. Bryan

Mrs. Bryan is a 78-year-old widow who lives alone in a small rural community. Her daughter, Joyce, lives 100 miles away in a large urban city. Mrs. Bryan has always been a very independent woman. She loves music, art, bird-watching, and cooking. Over the last year Mrs. Bryan's health has declined. Doctors diagnosed her with stomach cancer over a year ago. For her condition, surgery is not a treatment option. She comes to the community clinic at least monthly to see her nurse practitioner for follow-up and recommendations for supportive care. Because of her condition, Mrs. Bryan has had a 10-lb weight loss, and she reports a poor appetite. She feels generally weaker but continues her usual routines in the home. She notices some breathlessness when she exerts herself. She receives Meals on Wheels for lunch and frequently has dinner with a close friend who lives down the street. Mrs. Bryan's daughter wants her mother to move closer to her so she will receive the appropriate care and attention she needs. This means that Mrs. Bryan will have to live in a nursing home, because Joyce has no room at home to care for her mother herself.

Inez Santiago is a 36-year-old married student nurse assigned to the community clinic Mrs. Bryan visits. Inez worked part-time as a schoolteacher while raising her two children. Now that her children are older, Inez has decided to become a nurse. When she first meets Mrs. Bryan, she finds the patient friendly, alert, and happy to have a student nurse. During their discussion, Inez and Mrs. Bryan discuss Mrs. Bryan's feelings about her health and the possibility of having to leave her home. Mrs. Bryan replies, "I love my home. I know Joyce knows what is best for me, but I cannot imagine never seeing my friends again."

## KEY TERMS

clinical decision making, p. 86
critical thinking, p. 81
decision making, p. 84
diagnostic reasoning, p. 84
evidenced-based knowledge, p. 81

inference, p. 86
intuition, p. 83
nursing process, p. 84
problem solving, p. 84
reflection, p. 82
scientific method, p. 84

As a professional nurse, you will face a variety of situations involving patients with uniquely different types of health care problems. Each situation will require critical thinking so that your patient receives the very best nursing care. Being a good critical thinker means that you are open to new ideas and able to focus on the circumstances surrounding a situation. Critical thinking skills allow you to make high-quality judgments about patient care. For example, when a patient's condition begins to change with a slowed response to questions, a grimace when turning to the side, a reluctance to move, and diaphoresis, critical thinking allows you to make clinical inferences. In this situation you guess that the patient is in pain. You assess the situation thoroughly and then act. Critical thinking is a process that you acquire through hard work, commitment, and an active curiosity about learning. This chapter introduces you to a model for critical thinking. You will learn to apply the elements of the model as you face patient situations and determine the type of nursing care each patient requires.

## Clinical Decisions in Nursing Practice

When caring for patients, you are responsible for making accurate and appropriate clinical decisions. Clinical decision making is a skill that separates professional nurses from unlicensed technical staff. To assist persons in maintaining, regaining, or improving their health you must think critically to problem solve and find solutions for patients' health problems. Many patients have problems a textbook cannot solve. Their clinical symptoms, the information about their health status, and how they present their situation may not immediately offer a clear picture of what actions you should take. Instead, you must learn to question, wonder, and explore different interpretations. Then find the set of actions that best help your patient.

No two patients have identical health problems. Because each patient is unique, nurses face challenges in making clinical decisions. You will observe each patient closely, search for and examine ideas, then make inferences or draw conclusions about patient problems. Then you will consider scientific principles relating to the problems, recognize the problems, and develop an approach to nursing care. You will learn to creatively seek new knowledge as needed, act quickly when events change, and make decisions that promote the patient's well-being. Although the responsibility for making clinical decisions seems challenging, it is what makes nursing a rewarding and challenging profession.

## Critical Thinking Defined

Thinking and learning are interrelated processes. Over time, your knowledge and practical experiences broaden your ability to make thoughtful observations, judgments, and choices. **Critical thinking** is both a process and a set of skills (Profetto-McGrath and others, 2003). Chaffee (2002) defined critical thinking as the active, organized, cognitive process used to carefully examine one's thinking and the thinking of others. It involves recognizing that an issue (e.g., patient problem) exists, analyzing information related to the issue (e.g., clinical data about a patient), evaluating information (including assumptions and evidence), and drawing conclusions (Settersten and Lauver, 2004). A critical thinker considers what is important in a situation, imagines and explores alternatives, considers ethical principles, and thus makes informed decisions. When you care for a patient, crit-

ical thinking begins by asking these questions: What do I really know about this nursing care situation? How do I know it? What are the options available to me? (Paul and Heaslip, 1995).

You can begin to learn critical thinking early in your practice. For example, as you learn about administering bed baths and other hygiene measures to your patients, take time to read nursing literature about the concept of comfort (Brock and Butts, 1998). What are the criteria for comfort? How do patients from other cultures perceive comfort? What are the different factors that contribute to comfort? The use of **evidence-based knowledge,** or knowledge based on research or clinical expertise, makes you an informed critical thinker. Thinking critically and learning about the concept of comfort will prepare you to better anticipate your patients' needs. You will also identify problems more quickly and provide appropriate care. Critical thinking involves a commitment to think clearly, precisely, and accurately and to act on what you know about a situation. When you direct your thinking toward understanding and assisting patients in finding solutions to their health problems, the process becomes purposeful and goal oriented.

Critical thinking requires not only cognitive skills but also a person's tendency to ask questions and to remain well informed. It is important to be honest in facing personal biases and always to be willing to reconsider and think clearly about issues (Facione, 1990). There are core critical thinking skills that, when applied to nursing, show the complex nature of clinical decision making (Table 6-1). Being able to apply all of these skills takes practice. You will need to have a sound knowledge base and thoughtfully consider the knowledge you gain during experiences with patients.

An effective critical thinker faces problems without forming a quick, single solution. Instead, a critical thinker focuses on the options for what to believe and do (Kataoka-Yahiro and Saylor, 1994). Learning to think critically will help you to care for patients as their advocate and to make informed

| TABLE 6-1 | Critical Thinking Skills |
|---|---|
| **Skill** | **Nursing Practice Application** |
| Interpretation | Be orderly in data collection. Look for patterns to categorize data (e.g., nursing diagnoses [see Chapter 7]). Clarify any data you are uncertain about. |
| Analysis | Be open-minded as you look at information about a patient. Do not make careless assumptions. Do the data reveal what you believe is true, or are there other options? |
| Inference | Look at the meaning and significance of findings. Are there relationships between findings? Do the data about the patient help you see that a problem exists? |
| Evaluation | Look at all situations objectively. Use criteria (e.g., expected outcomes, pain characteristics, learning objectives) to determine results of nursing actions (see Chapter 7). Reflect on your own behavior and how it affects the evaluation process. |
| Explanation | Support your findings and conclusions. Use scientific and experiential knowledge to select strategies you use in the care of patients. |
| Self-regulation | Reflect on your experiences. Identify how you will improve your own performance. |

Modified from Facione P: *Critical thinking: a statement of expert consensus for purposes of educational assessment and instruction. The Delphi report: research findings and recommendations prepared for the American Philosophical Association,* ERIC Doc No. ED 315-423, Washington, DC, 1990, ERIC.

| TABLE 6-2 | Concepts for a Critical Thinker |
|---|---|
| Concept | Component |
| Truth seeking | Seek the truth; be courageous about asking questions; be honest and objective about pursuing questions. |
| Open-mindedness | Be tolerant of different views; be sensitive to the possibility of your own biases; respect the right of others to have different opinions. |
| Analyticity | Be alert to potentially problematic situations; anticipate possible results or consequences; value reason; use evidence-based knowledge. |
| Systematicity | Be organized; focus; work hard in any inquiry. |
| Self-confidence | Trust in your own reasoning processes. |
| Inquisitiveness | Be eager to acquire knowledge and learn explanations even when applications of the knowledge are not immediately clear. Value learning for learning's sake. |
| Maturity | Multiple solutions are acceptable. Reflect upon your own judgments; have cognitive maturity. |

Modified from Facione N, Facione P: Externalizing the critical thinking in knowledge development and clinical judgement, *Nurs Outlook* 44:129, 1996.

## CLINICAL SCENARIO

Consider the situation involving Mrs. Bryan and Inez Santiago. Mrs. Bryan returns to the clinic with her friend. Inez observes the patient's slow, deliberate movements, unsteady gait, and facial expression of fatigue. Inez first concludes that Mrs. Bryan is "tired." She bases this on her experience with other patients and from noticing a change in Mrs. Bryan since the previous visit. When Mrs. Bryan provides more information on "feeling tired," Inez begins to consider the patient's health status and observes how Mrs. Bryan moves about or sits in the chair. Inez begins to ask the patient focused questions such as, "Tell me how you are feeling," "Have you been unable to sleep?" or "Are you having pain?" She measures the patient's pulse, blood pressure, and respiratory rate to get further information about Mrs. Bryan's status. Inez uses critical thinking to reason, to make inferences as to the meaning and significance of findings, and to form a mental picture of what is happening to Mrs. Bryan.

choices about their care. Facione and Facione (1996) have identified concepts for thinking critically (Table 6-2). Without these concepts, critical thinking skills are difficult to use. Critical thinking is more than just problem solving. It is an attempt to continually improve how you apply yourself when faced with patient care problems.

## Reflection

How often do you think back on a situation to consider How did I act? What could I have done differently? or What should I do if I have the same opportunity in the future? **Reflection** is the process of purposefully thinking back or recalling a situation to discover its purpose or meaning. For example, after caring for a patient who is suffering chronic pain from a bone tumor, you reflect on the patient's reaction to the approaches you used for pain relief.

What might you have done differently when the patient reported little benefit from using relaxation exercises? Was your response appropriate when the patient said, "I don't know, I feel like I will never get any relief." As a nurse it is helpful to think back on a patient situation to explore the factors that influenced how you handled the situation. Reflection is like rewinding a videotape. It involves playing back a situation in your head and taking time to honestly review everything you remember about the situation. Reflection requires adequate knowledge and is necessary for self-evaluation. By reviewing your actions you see successes and your opportunities for improvement. However, O'Neill and Dluhy (1997) caution you not to question or doubt every judgment that you make. Too much emphasis on reflection can block your thinking in a clinical situation because it creates second-guessing.

The process of reflection helps you to seek and understand the relationships between concepts learned in class and real-life clinical situations. It is a form of learning through investigational discovery (Kessler and Lund, 2004). Through reflection, you judge your personal performance and how closely you followed standards of nursing practice in your care. Reflection helps make sense out of an experience so that the next time a similar experience happens, you will use approaches that were successful or change an approach to achieve better patient outcomes.

Reflection is different for each individual. Learning to be reflective takes practice. Reflection involves connecting clinical content with thought processes and self-awareness. It is not simply describing what you observed or did for a patient (Kessler and Lund, 2004). When you choose to reflect on a clinical experience, be open to new information and look at the patient's perspective, as well as your own. Paget (2001) suggests that reflective practice improves a nurse's clinical practice, self-awareness, and how he or she interacts with patients. Learning from experience with patients can create an "aha" feeling, because reflection reveals an awareness of how well you are performing as a professional. Box 6-1 lists tips on how to use reflection in your practice.

---

**BOX 6-1  Tips on Facilitating Reflection**

- Stop and think about what is going on with your patient. What do your assessment findings mean? What physical or psychological changes are occurring? How does this compare to normal for the patient: always ask what could be happening (Fowler, 1998).
- Reflect carefully on any critical incidents (e.g., safety episodes, cardiac arrests, central events in the progression of a patient's disease, complex-care patients) (Bittner and Tobin, 1998). What occurred? What actions did you take? How did the patient respond? Were there any other options you thought of taking?
- At the end of each day after caring for a patient, take time to reflect. Ask yourself whether you achieved your original plan of care. If you did, why were you successful? If you did not, what were the barriers or problems? What would you do differently or the same?
- Keep a journal of your patient care experiences. A record of your experience will help you develop an awareness of how you use clinical decision-making skills (Kessler and Lund, 2004). Be sure to include the following: identification, description, significance, and implications (Baker, 1996). Telling a story and drawing a pic-

ture are two ways to identify the experience you wish to reflect on. Describe in detail what you felt, thought, and did. Analyze experience by considering feelings, thoughts, and possible meanings. It helps to look for themes in your entries. For example, if you have cared for several cardiac patients, what common themes do you see that will better prepare you for the next patient? Challenge any preconceived ideas you have when you look at actual situations. Describe the implications of the experience in terms of your own clinical practice or self-perceptions as a learner. Refer to the journal often when you care for patients that have similar situations.
- Talk with a close friend who works with you and has observed your clinical work. Ask if the friend's observations are the same as yours.
- Keep all written care plans or clinical papers. Use them frequently as a resource for future patients.
- Take time to reflect, both after having cared for a patient and before caring for new patients with similar conditions. How is your current patient similar to or different from previous patients?

---

## CLINICAL SCENARIO

After spending the day at the clinic, Inez spends time recalling her experience with Mrs. Bryan. Because she wanted to learn more about Mrs. Bryan's feelings toward nursing homes, Inez discussed the value of a nursing home as a safe environment. Mrs. Bryan immediately became less talkative. Inez reflects on why Mrs. Bryan's response concerned her. Mrs. Bryan's willingness to participate in the discussion had changed. Inez thinks that perhaps her explanation was not the best approach. If Mrs. Bryan has not yet accepted the idea of going to a nursing home, Inez reflects that asking open questions about Mrs. Bryan's feelings will be more useful next time. For example, Inez could ask, "Tell me what you think about your daughter's concerns for your safety." Inez thinks about how she will approach Mrs. Bryan differently during her next visit. Reflection allows Inez to be proactive and hopefully more effective.

## Language

Use of language is another important aspect of critical thinking. Thinking and language are closely related processes. Critical thinkers use language precisely and clearly. When language is unclear and inaccurate, it reflects sloppy thinking.

It is important to communicate clearly with patients, their families, and health care professionals. When you fail to use correct terminology and use jargon or vague descriptions, communication is ineffective. For example, when you are vague or unclear with your patient and the nursing team, then your patient is unable to cooperate with nursing therapies and members of the nursing team do not follow through on your recommendations because you did not communicate clearly. Critical thinking requires you to carefully frame your thoughts and to send a message that is clear.

## Intuition

**Intuition** is the inner sensing or "gut feeling" that something is so. In other words, you may walk into a patient's room and, by looking at the patient's appearance without the benefit of a thorough assessment, sense that he or she is about to worsen physically. Intuition is a common experience that many people have when interacting with their environments. Intuition in nursing develops through clinical experience. For example, an experienced home care nurse suspects that a patient is depressed by looking at the patient's expression, seeing disorder in the home environment, and making a quick assessment of the patient's mood. Intuition acts as a trigger, leading a nurse to consciously search for data that confirms the sense of a change in a patient's status (King and Clark, 2002).

Always remember that quality nursing practice does not depend solely on intuition. Just as it is critical for you to know what knowledge you have, it is even more critical to know what you do not know. Trust your intuition as a red flag that something is not quite right, but do not take your intuition as an automatic truth or fact. As soon as intuition strikes, look further to assess a patient's situation (Fowler, 1998). If you do not recognize how much you do not know about your patients, there is a risk of malpractice and even harming your patients. Learn to think carefully about each clinical situation. Thoughtful analysis of what you know, plus a review of the most current clinical data, allows you to make an accurate and sound clinical decision.

## Thinking and Learning

Learning is a lifelong process. Your intellectual and emotional growth involve gaining new knowledge and refining your ability to think, problem solve, and make judgments.

To learn, you must be flexible and always open to new information. The science of nursing is growing rapidly, and there will always be new information for nurses to apply in practice. As you have new experiences and apply the knowledge gained, you will become better at forming assumptions, presenting ideas, and making valid conclusions.

When you care for a patient, always think ahead and ask: What is the patient's status now? How might it change and why? What do I know to improve the patient's condition? In what way will a specific therapy affect the patient? Do not allow your thinking to become routine or standardized. Instead, learn to look beyond the obvious in any clinical situation, explore each patient's response to health alterations, and recognize what actions are needed to benefit the patient. Over time your experience with many patients will help you recognize patterns of behavior, see commonalities in signs and symptoms, and anticipate reactions to therapies. Thinking about those experiences will allow you to better anticipate each new patient's needs and recognize problems when they develop.

## Levels of Critical Thinking in Nursing

Your ability to think critically grows as you gain new knowledge and experience in nursing practice. Kataoka-Yahiro and Saylor (1994) developed a critical thinking model that includes three levels of critical thinking in nursing: basic, complex, and commitment.

### Basic Critical Thinking

At the basic level of critical thinking a learner trusts that experts have the right answers for every problem. Thinking is concrete and based on a set of rules or principles. For example, a student nurse uses a hospital procedure manual to confirm how to insert a feeding tube. The student follows the procedure step-by-step without adjusting the procedure to meet a patient's unique needs (e.g., positioning limitations or difficulty swallowing). At this level, answers to complex problems are either right or wrong (e.g., the tube will not advance because it is coiled in the throat), and one right answer usually exists for each problem. Basic critical thinking is an early step in the development of reasoning (Kataoka-Yahiro and Saylor, 1994). A basic critical thinker does learn to accept the diverse opinions and values of experts (e.g., instructors and staff nurses). However, weak competencies and inflexible attitudes can slow a person's ability to move to the next level of critical thinking.

### Complex Critical Thinking

Complex critical thinkers begin to detach themselves from authorities. They analyze and examine choices more independently. The person's thinking abilities and initiative to look beyond expert opinion begin to change. A nurse learns that alternative and perhaps conflicting solutions do exist.

Consider the case of Mr. Epstein, an 82-year-old patient who lives in a long-term care facility. His family is concerned about his unwillingness to exercise regularly. Physical therapy has scheduled routine walks. Although Mr. Epstein walks unsteadily, he can walk with a person at his side. Shawn, the nurse caring for Mr. Epstein, learns about his fear of falling and rather than trying to force the patient to walk, tries to understand the nature of his fears and to find ways that will make Mr. Epstein believe he can walk safely.

In complex critical thinking, you learn to synthesize knowledge. This means you develop a new thought or idea based on your experience and knowledge over time. When you choose therapies for patients, each option has benefits and risks that you weigh in making a decision. Thinking becomes more creative and innovative. There is a willingness to consider deviations from standard protocols or procedures and to provide more individualized care.

### Commitment

The third level of critical thinking is commitment (Kataoka-Yahiro and Saylor, 1994). A person anticipates the need to make choices without assistance from others. Whatever decision is made, the person accepts accountability for it. The nurse does more than consider the complex alternatives a problem poses. At the commitment level, a nurse chooses an action or belief based on the alternatives available and stands by it. Consider the situation of a 53-year-old woman recently diagnosed with breast cancer. At first she delayed seeking treatment because of her fear of hospitals and her family history of breast cancer. She skipped her last clinic appointment. Her nurse learns that the woman's daughter has been helpful in the past in aiding her mother to sort out decisions. The nurse discusses the woman's concerns and asks to involve the daughter in a group discussion. Then the nurse helps the mother sort out her worries with the daughter to make a decision about her treatment.

## Critical Thinking Competencies

Kataoka-Yahiro and Saylor (1994) have described critical thinking competencies as the cognitive processes a nurse uses to make judgments about the clinical care of patients. These include general critical thinking, specific critical thinking in clinical situations, and specific critical thinking in nursing (Kataoka-Yahiro and Saylor, 1994). General critical thinking processes are not unique to the nursing profession. They include the **scientific method, problem solving,** and **decision making.** Specific critical thinking competencies in clinical situations include **diagnostic reasoning,** clinical inferences, and clinical decision making. The specific critical thinking competency in nursing involves use of the **nursing process** (see Chapter 7).

## Scientific Method

The scientific method is a way to solve problems using reasoning. It is the systematic, ordered approach to gathering data and solving problems. The scientific method is used in nursing, medicine, and a variety of other disciplines. Nurse researchers use the scientific method when testing research questions in nursing practice situations. The steps of the scientific method are problem identification, collection of data, formulation of a research question or hypothesis, testing the question or hypothesis, and evaluating results of the study. The scientific method is one formal way to approach a problem, plan a solution, test the solution, and come to a conclusion. Table 6-3 provides an example of a nursing practice question solved using the scientific method.

## Problem Solving

We all face problems every day, whether it is how to help a child who has been rejected by friends to the ever-popular VCR that we cannot program correctly. When a problem arises, we obtain information and then use the information and what we already know to find a solution. As a nurse, patients will routinely present problems to you in practice. For example, you enter a patient's room and find the patient lying in a twisted manner. You know that the patient had back surgery and is supposed to remain in straight anatomical alignment to avoid stress on the surgical area. You suspect the patient is having pain but instead learn through questioning that he is uncomfortably cold. You reposition the patient and give him an additional blanket for warmth. When returning to the patient's room 30 minutes later, you find the patient asleep. You obtained information that correctly explained why the patient was uncomfortable. Then you tested a solution that was successful.

Effective problem solving also involves evaluating the solution over time to be sure that it is still effective. You return to the patient's room to ask whether the patient remains comfortable. If the problem recurs, it is necessary to try different options. Having solved a problem in one situation adds to your experience in your practice and allows you to apply that knowledge in future patient situations.

## Decision Making

When you face a problem or situation and choose a course of action from several options, you are making a decision. Decision making is an end point of critical thinking that is focused on resolving a problem. Following a set of criteria helps to make a thorough and thoughtful decision. For example, you use a decision-making process when you choose an elective course to take in your nursing program. First, you recognize and define the problem or situation (need to select a course that meets program requirements). Then you assess all the options (consider courses recommended by faculty and colleagues or choose one that is scheduled for a convenient time). Next, you weigh each option against a set of criteria (reputation of faculty, value of course for your career goals), and test possible options (talk directly with the faculty). Finally, you consider the consequences of the decision (examine pros and cons of selecting one course over another), and then make a final decision. Although the set of criteria seems to follow a sequence of steps, decision making involves moving back and forth in considering all criteria. The decision-making process leads to informed conclusions that are supported by evidence and by reason (Bandman and Bandman, 1995). In a clinical setting you learn to make sound decisions by approaching each clinical situation thoughtfully and systematically by using each step of the decision-making process mentioned above.

---

| TABLE 6-3 | **Using the Scientific Method to Solve Nursing Practice Questions** |

Clinical Problem: A group of hospice nurses discuss the problem of family members' often having difficulty communicating feelings to their dying loved ones. As a result, the family members have guilt and regret after their loved one has died. The nurses question that perhaps the family members have ineffective communication skills. They decide to study an approach designed to improve the family members' abilities to express their feelings more effectively. The hospice nurses use the scientific method.

| | |
|---|---|
| Problem identification | Family members have difficulty communicating with a dying loved one. |
| Data collection | Review previous studies about grieving families, especially in hospice settings. Review the literature on grief support and communication methods. Talk with dying patients about feelings they think are important to communicate. |
| Form a research question or hypothesis to study the problem | Family members will participate in a group class on communicating with dying loved ones. After this class, hospice patients will perceive family members as more supportive, as determined by an interview. |
| Test the hypothesis or answer the question | Include family members in a group class on communication skills. Have the family members use the learned approaches when they communicate with their loved ones. |
| Evaluate the results of the study. Is the research question answered or is the hypothesis supported? | Interview the dying patients to determine their perception of family support before and after the classes. Compare the results. |

## Diagnostic Reasoning

As soon as you receive information about a patient in a clinical situation, diagnostic reasoning begins. It is a process of determining a patient's health status after you assign meaning to the behaviors, physical signs, and reported patient symptoms that are presented (O'Neill and Dluhy, 1997). Part of diagnostic reasoning is **inference**, the process of drawing conclusions from related pieces of evidence (Smith Higuchi and Donald, 2002). An example of diagnostic reasoning is forming a nursing diagnosis (see Chapter 7). Diagnostic reasoning is a process of using the data you gather to logically explain a clinical judgment. For example, after turning a patient and observing an area of redness around the sacrum, you palpate the area and note that it is tender to touch and warm. You push on the area with your finger and after releasing pressure the area does not blanch or turn white. You think about what you know about normal skin integrity and the effects of pressure. The information you collect leads you to determine the patient has a pressure ulcer. Diagnostic reasoning provides a clear perspective of a patient's health status and whether or not the patient is progressing. Nurses do not make medical diagnoses, but they do assess and monitor patients to determine their level of progress. A nurse's diagnostic conclusions will help a physician or health care provider pinpoint the nature of a problem more quickly and select proper therapies.

## CLINICAL SCENARIO

In addition to stomach cancer, Mrs. Bryan had a myocardial infarction, a "heart attack," just 4 months ago. Her health care providers monitor her periodically for possible chest pain, shortness of breath, and/or irregular vital signs (signs and symptoms of recurrent cardiac problems). If Mrs. Bryan has a regular heart rate, denies discomfort, is breathing normally without difficulty, and has stable laboratory results, Inez makes the diagnostic decision that Mrs. Bryan's cardiac status is currently stable. Inez makes her diagnostic decision based on a thorough and comprehensive assessment. She critically analyzes any changes in Mrs. Bryan to determine her status. This allows Inez to begin the appropriate therapies, such as progressive monitored exercise, so that Mrs. Bryan can develop activity tolerance within her limitations. Any further diagnostic conclusions made by Inez during her visit with Mrs. Bryan help the physician or health care provider find the nature of a problem more quickly and select proper medical therapies.

## Clinical Decision Making

Clinical decision making is a problem-solving activity that focuses on defining patient problems and selecting appropriate treatment (Smith Higuchi and Donald, 2002). When you approach a clinical problem, such as a patient who has an area of redness over the sacrum, you make a decision that identifies the problem (a pressure ulcer), and then you choose the best nursing interventions (skin care and turning). Nurses make clinical decisions all the time in an attempt to improve a patient's health or to maintain wellness. This means minimizing the severity of the problem or resolving the problem completely. **Clinical decision making** requires careful reasoning so that the options for the best patient outcomes are chosen on the basis of the patient's condition and priority of the problem.

You improve your clinical decision making by knowing your patients. Nurse researchers have found that expert nurses develop a level of knowing that leads to pattern recognition of patient symptoms and responses (White, 2003). For example, an expert nurse who has worked on a general surgery unit for many years is more likely able to detect internal hemorrhage (fall in blood pressure, rapid pulse, change in consciousness) than a new nurse. Over time, a combination of experience, time spent in a specific clinical area, and the quality of relationships formed with patients allow nurses to know clinical situations and to quickly anticipate and select the right course of action. Spending more time during initial patient assessments to observe and measuring both normal and abnormal findings are both ways to improve knowing your patients. Also, consistently monitoring patients as problems develop, helps you to see how clinical changes evolve over time.

There are decision-making criteria that help nurses make appropriate decisions (Strader, 1992). Consider Mrs. Bryan and Inez. During a clinic visit Inez observes a bruised area of the skin over Mrs. Bryan's right hip. Mrs. Bryan says it is a scrape that happened when she fell against the edge of her bathtub. Inez considers her nursing knowledge and the unique situation of the patient when making a decision about the therapies that will promote healing and prevent further injury. Criteria that will help Inez make an appropriate clinical decision include the following:

- What needs to be achieved (healing of the skin, a safe home environment)?
- What needs to be preserved (mobility, nutrition, comfort, safety)?
- What needs to be avoided (further tissue injury, infection, further falls)?

Clinical decision-making criteria assist you in setting clinical care priorities (see Chapter 7). Because different patients bring different variables to a situation, an activity may be more of a priority in one situation and less of a priority in another. For example, if a patient is physically dependent, unable to eat, and incontinent of urine, skin integrity is a greater priority than if the patient is immobile but continent of urine and able to eat a normal diet. Do not assume that a certain condition is an automatic priority. For example, a patient immediately out of surgery is expected to experience a certain level of pain, which often becomes a priority of nursing care. However, if the patient is experiencing severe anxiety that heightens pain perception, it becomes necessary to focus on ways to relieve anxiety before pain-relief measures can be effective.

After you determine a patient's nursing care priorities, choose the nursing therapies most likely to relieve each problem. A wide range of choices may be available, from nurse-administered to patient self-care therapies. Collaborate with the patient, and then select, test, and evaluate each approach. Try to anticipate what might go wrong, and consider different approaches to minimize or prevent problems. For exam-

---

**BOX 6-2  USING EVIDENCE IN PRACTICE**

**Research Summary**

How can faculty create learning situations that promote students' ability to make good clinical decisions? One researcher went to the students and interviewed 17 fourth-year nursing students ranging in age from 21 to 27 years. The students had recently completed a 6-week clinical rotation in a critical care unit where they cared for one patient. The remaining 6 weeks were spent in a management rotation with the students caring for four patients. The researcher interviewed each student to discuss clinical decision-making situations in detail.

After interpreting each of the 17 interviews, the researcher identified five common themes that nursing students' associated with clinical decision making. These five themes are gaining confidence in their skills, building relationships with staff, connecting with patients, becoming comfortable as a nurse, and understanding the clinical picture. Technical and communication skills were most important to clinical decision making. Once a student feels confident in completing a technical skill or starting a conversation with a patient, he or she can then focus on the patient instead of the steps for performing the skill or the guidelines for communication. Students worked best with nurse preceptors who trusted them. Students learned from nurses who were willing to describe their thought processes they used in a clinical situation. Being able to connect with patients comes from "knowing the patient." When nurse and patient connect, the patient teaches the student the "how" of nursing. As students learn to recognize differences between patients, they begin to understand the rationale for different clinical decisions nurses make.

**Application to Nursing Practice**

The results of this study show the importance staff nurses play in a student nurse's clinical decision making. Students rely on staff nurses to support them and participate in the learning process. It is important for students to build good working relationships with nursing staff. In addition, clinical competence comes as students learn to form meaningful, connected relationships with their patients.

Data from White AH: Clinical decision making among fourth year nursing students: an interpretive study, *J Nurs Educ* 42(3):113, 2003.

---

ple, Inez will talk with Mrs. Bryan's daughter about checking the condition of Mrs. Bryan's bathroom to see if there are any obstacles creating a risk for falls. Based on the findings, Inez will recommend to Mrs. Bryan ways to minimize any hazards or obstacles in her home so that the risks for further injury are reduced.

You will make decisions about individual patients and about groups of patients. If you work on a busy hospital unit, you will likely care for several patients at one time. You will need to use decision-making criteria. These criteria include the clinical conditions of the patients, Maslow's hierarchy of needs (see Chapter 1), risks involved in treatment delays, and the patients' expectations of care to determine which patients have the greatest priorities for care. For example, a patient whose blood pressure drops suddenly and who faints requires attention immediately in contrast to the patient who needs assistance walking down the hallway. Visit the patient who has had no visitors and has recently been given a diagnosis of cancer before checking on the recovering surgical patient whose family has just arrived. Box 6-2 summarizes the essential components associated with nursing students' learning clinical decision-making.

## The Nursing Process as a Competency

Nurses apply the nursing process (see Chapter 7) as a competency when giving patient care (Kataoka-Yahiro and Saylor, 1994). The nursing process is a systematic five-step clinical decision-making approach that includes assessment, diagnosis, planning, implementation, and evaluation. The purpose of the process is to diagnose and treat human responses to actual or potential health problems (American Nurses Association, 2003). Use of the process allows nurses to help patients meet agreed-upon outcomes for better health. The process involves the general and specific critical thinking competencies, described earlier, in a way that focuses on a particular patient's unique needs. The format for the nursing process is unique to the discipline of nursing and offers a common language and way for nurses to "think through" patients' clinical problems (Kataoka-Yahiro and Saylor, 1994).

The nursing process is often called a blueprint or plan for patient care. It is flexible enough to be used in all settings and with all patients. When you use the nursing process, you identify a patient's health care needs, determine priorities, and establish goals and expected outcomes of care. Then you develop and communicate a patient-centered plan of care, deliver nursing interventions, and evaluate the effectiveness of your care (Table 6-4). When you become more competent in using the nursing process, you will be able to focus not only on a single patient problem but on multiple problems. As a nurse you must always be thinking and recognizing what step of the process is being used. Within each step of the process you will apply critical thinking to provide the very best professional care to your patients. The nursing process is described in Chapter 7.

| TABLE 6-4 | Summary of Nursing Process | |
|---|---|---|
| **Component** | **Purpose** | **Steps** |
| Assessment | To gather, verify, and communicate data about patient so that database is established | Collect nursing health history. |
| | | Perform physical examination. |
| | | Collect laboratory data. |
| | | Validate or confirm data is correct. |
| | | Cluster data by common themes or problem areas. |
| | | Document data. |
| Nursing diagnosis | To examine patient data to identify their health care needs to formulate nursing diagnoses | Analyze and interpret data. |
| | | Identify patient problems. |
| | | Form nursing diagnoses. |
| | | Document nursing diagnoses. |
| Planning | To identify patient's goals; to determine priorities of care; to determine expected outcomes; to design nursing strategies to achieve goals of care | Identify patient goals. |
| | | Establish expected outcomes. |
| | | Select nursing actions. |
| | | Delegate interventions. |
| | | Write nursing care plan. |
| | | Collaborate with other health care providers. |
| Implementation | To carry out nursing actions necessary for accomplishing plan of care | Perform nursing interventions. |
| | | Reassess patient. |
| | | Review and modify existing care plan. |
| Evaluation | To determine extent to which interventions helped achieve goals of care | Compare patient response to expected outcomes. |
| | | Analyze reasons for results and conclusions. |
| | | Modify care plan. |

## A Critical Thinking Model

Models help to explain concepts. Because critical thinking is complex, a model helps explain what is involved as you make clinical decisions and judgments about your patients. Kataoka-Yahiro and Saylor (1994) have developed a model of critical thinking for nursing judgment based in part on previous work by Paul (1993), Glaser (1941), and Miller and Malcolm (1990) (Figure 6-1). The model defines the outcome of critical thinking: nursing judgment that is relevant to nursing problems in a variety of settings. According to this model, there are five elements or parts of critical thinking: knowledge base, experience, competence, attitudes, and standards. Nurses perform critical thinking within the competency of the nursing process. The elements of the model combine to explain how nurses make clinical decisions that are necessary for safe, effective nursing care (Box 6-3).

### Specific Knowledge Base

The first component of critical thinking is a nurse's specific knowledge base. This varies according to your educational experience, including basic nursing education, continuing education courses, and additional college degrees. In addition, it includes reading the nursing literature to remain current in nursing science. Your knowledge base includes information and theory from the basic sciences, humanities, behavioral sciences, and nursing. You will use your knowledge base in a different way from other health care disciplines in regard to how you think about patient problems. The broad knowledge base gives you a more holistic view of patients and their health care needs. The depth and extent of knowledge influence your ability to think critically about nursing problems (Figure 6-2). Referring to the case study, Inez Santiago previously earned a degree in education. She is just starting her third year of study in nursing. She has successfully completed courses in anatomy and physiology, introduction to nursing concepts, and communication principles. Although she is new to nursing, her preparation and knowledge base will help her make the clinical decisions necessary to care for Mrs. Bryan.

### CLINICAL SCENARIO

As Inez Santiago thinks about her clinical experiences with patients, she recognizes she still has a lot to learn. However, each patient has given her valuable learning experiences. Specifically, she has been able to acquire good interviewing skills, and she understands the importance of the family in an individual's health. She has also learned the role nurses play as advocates for patients. Her time in the physical assessment laboratory and her first semester in a clinical area taught her to be a watchful observer. Inez also knows that her previous experience as a teacher will help her apply educational principles in her nursing role.

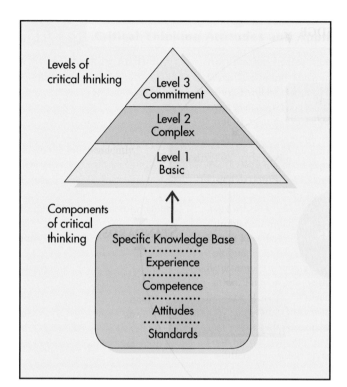

FIGURE 6-1 Critical thinking model for nursing judgment. (Redrawn from Kataoka-Yahiro M, Saylor C: A critical thinking model for nursing judgment, *J Nurs Educ* 33[8]:351, 1994. Modified from Glaser E: *An experiment in the development of critical thinking,* New York, 1941, Bureau of Publications, Teachers College, Columbia University; Miller M, Malcolm N: Critical thinking in the nursing curriculum, *Nurs Health Care* 11:67, 1990; and Paul R: The art of redesigning instruction. In Willsen J, Blinker AJA, editors: *Critical thinking: how to prepare students for a rapidly changing world,* Santa Rosa, Calif, 1993, Foundation for Critical Thinking.)

## Experience

The second component of the critical thinking model is experience in nursing. Nursing is a practice discipline. Clinical learning experiences are necessary for you to acquire clinical decision-making skills (Roche, 2002). You will learn from your experiences in observing, sensing, and talking with patients and then reflecting actively on your experiences alone and with fellow students. Clinical experience is the laboratory for testing nursing knowledge. You will learn that "textbook" approaches lay important groundwork for practice, but you must make adaptations to accommodate the setting, the unique qualities of each patient, and the experiences you have gained from caring for previous patients. Benner (1984) notes that the expert nurse understands the context of a clinical situation, recognizes signs suggesting patterns, and interprets them as relevant or irrelevant. This level of competency comes with experience and a commitment to learning. Perhaps the best lesson you can learn is to value all patient experiences. Each clinical experience serves as a stepping stone to building new knowledge and stimulating innovative thinking.

---

**BOX 6-3    Components of Critical Thinking in Nursing**

   I.  Specific knowledge base in nursing
  II.  Experience in nursing
 III.  Critical thinking competencies
      A.  General critical thinking competencies
      B.  Specific critical thinking competencies in clinical situations
      C.  Specific critical thinking competency in nursing—**The Nursing Process**
 IV.  Attitudes for critical thinking
      A.  Confidence
      B.  Independence
      C.  Fairness
      D.  Responsibility
      E.  Risk taking
      F.  Discipline
      G.  Perseverance
      H.  Creativity
      I.  Curiosity
      J.  Integrity
      K.  Humility
  V.  Standards for critical thinking
      A.  Intellectual standards
         1.  Clear
         2.  Precise
         3.  Specific
         4.  Accurate
         5.  Relevant
         6.  Plausible
         7.  Consistent
         8.  Logical
         9.  Deep
       10.  Broad
       11.  Complete
       12.  Significant
       13.  Adequate (for purpose)
       14.  Fair
      B.  Professional standards
         1.  Ethical criteria for nursing judgment
         2.  Criteria for evaluation
         3.  Professional responsibility

Modified from Kataoka-Yahiro M, Saylor C: A critical thinking model for nursing judgment, *J Nurs Educ* 33(8):351, 1994. Data from Paul RW: The art of redesigning instruction. In Willsen J, Blinker AJA, editors: *Critical thinking: how to prepare students for a rapidly changing world,* Santa Rosa, Calif, 1993, Foundation for Critical Thinking.

---

## Attitudes for Critical Thinking

The fourth component of the critical thinking model is attitudes. Paul (1993) identifies 11 attitudes that are central features of a critical thinker (see Box 6-3). These attitudes define how a successful critical thinker approaches a problem. For example, you are caring for a laryngectomy patient who needs help adjusting to permanent loss of speech. First, you must persevere to understand how the patient feels about the loss. Then you must think independently to find inter-

6. Tim completes his clinical day and discusses his experience with his best friend Joe. Tim is concerned about an error he made in setting up an IV infusion. He recalls being distracted when the charge nurse asked a question in the medication room. Tim states, "You know, so much was happening at the time, I should have stopped to answer the question and then double checked my IV infusion tubing." This is an example of:
   1. Risk taking
   2. Humility
   3. Reflection
   4. Problem solving

## REFERENCES

Agency for Health Care Policy and Research, Panel for Treatment of Pressure Ulcers in Adults: *Treatment of pressure ulcers,* Clinical Practice Guideline No. 15, AHCPR Pub No. 95-0653, Rockville, Md, 1994, Agency for Health Care Policy and Research, Public Health Service, U.S. Department of Health and Human Services.

American Nurses Association: *Nursing's social policy statement,* Washington, DC, 2003, The Association.

Baker CR: Reflective learning: a teaching strategy for critical thinking, *J Nurs Educ* 35(1):19, 1996.

Bandman EL, Bandman B: *Critical thinking in nursing,* ed 2, Norwalk, Conn, 1995, Appleton & Lange.

Benner P: *From novice to expert,* Menlo Park, Calif, 1984, Addison Wesley.

Bittner NP, Tobin E: Critical thinking: strategies for clinical practice, *J Nurs Staff Dev* 14(6):267, 1998.

Brock A, Butts JB: On target: a model to teach baccalaureate nursing students to apply critical thinking, *Nurs Forum* 33(3):5, 1998.

Chaffee J: *Thinking critically,* ed 7, Boston, 2002, Houghton Mifflin.

Facione N, Facione P: Externalizing the critical thinking in knowledge development and clinical judgment, *Nursing Outlook* 44:129, 1996.

Facione P: *Critical thinking: a statement of expert consensus for purposes of educational assessment and instruction. The Delphi report: research findings and recommendations prepared for the American Philosophical Association,* ERIC Doc No. ED 315-423, Washington, DC, 1990, ERIC.

Fowler LP: Improving critical thinking in nursing practice, *J Nurs Staff Dev* 14(4):183, 1998.

Glaser E: *An experiment in the development of critical thinking,* New York, 1941, Bureau of Publications, Teachers College, Columbia University.

Kataoka-Yahiro M, Saylor C: A critical thinking model for nursing judgment, *J Nurs Educ* 33(8):351, 1994.

Kessler PD, Lund CH: Reflective journaling: developing an online journal for distance education, *Nurse Educ* 29(1):20, 2004.

King L, Clark JM: Intuition and the development of expertise in surgical ward and intensive care nurses, *J Adv Nurs* 37(4):322, 2002.

Miller M, Malcolm N: Critical thinking in the nursing curriculum, *Nurs Health Care* 11:67, 1990.

O'Neill ES, Dluhy NM: A longitudinal framework for fostering critical thinking and diagnostic reasoning, *J Adv Nurs* 26:825, 1997.

Paget T: Reflective practice and clinical outcomes: practitioners' views on how reflective practice has influenced their clinical practice, *J Clin Nurs* 10(2):204, 2001.

Paul R: The art of redesigning instruction. In Willsen J, Blinker AJA, editors: *Critical thinking: how to prepare students for a rapidly changing world,* Santa Rosa, Calif, 1993, Foundation for Critical Thinking.

Paul RW, Heaslip P: Critical thinking and intuitive nursing practice, *J Adv Nurs* 22: 40, 1995.

Profetto-McGrath J , and others: A study of critical thinking and research utilization among nurses, *West J Nurs Res* 25(3):322, 2003.

Roche JP: A pilot study of teaching clinical decision making with the clinical educator model, *J Nurs Educ* 41(8):365, 2002.

Settersten L, Lauver D R: Critical thinking, perceived health status, and participation in health behaviors, *Nurs Res* 53(1):11, 2004.

Smith Higuchi KA, Donald JG: Thinking processes used by nurses in clinical decision making, *J Nurs Educ* 41(4),145, 2002.

Strader M: Critical thinking. In Sullivan EJ, Decker PJ: *Effective management in nursing,* ed 3, Redwood City, Calif, 1992, Addison-Wesley Nursing.

Watson G, Glaser E: *Watson-Glaser critical thinking appraisal manual,* New York, 1980, Macmillan.

White AH: Clinical decision making among fourth year nursing students: an interpretive study, *J Nurs Educ* 42(3):113, 2003.

# CHAPTER 7

# Nursing Process

## MEDIA RESOURCES

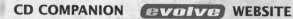

**CD COMPANION** *evolve* **WEBSITE**

http://evolve.elsevier.com/Potter/basic

- **NCLEX® Review**
- **Audio Glossary**
- **English/Spanish Audio Glossary**

## OBJECTIVES

- Describe each component of the nursing process.
- Explain the relationship between critical thinking and steps of the nursing process.
- Discuss the steps of nursing assessment.
- Explain the difference between comprehensive, problem-oriented, and focused assessments.
- Differentiate between subjective and objective data.
- Explain the type of conclusions that result from data analysis.
- List the steps of the nursing diagnostic process.
- Describe the way in which defining characteristics and the etiological process individualize a nursing diagnosis.
- Discuss the process of priority setting
- Describe goal setting.
- Discuss the difference between a goal and an expected outcome.
- Discuss the process of selecting nursing interventions.
- Develop a plan of care from a nursing assessment.
- Compare elements of a nursing care plan and a concept map.
- Evaluate nursing actions selected for a patient.
- Describe how evaluation leads to revision or modification of a plan of care.

## CASE STUDY   Mrs. Bryan

In Chapter 6 you read about Mrs. Bryan and her nurse, Inez Santiago. When Inez first met Mrs. Bryan, she learned about her patient's health status and began to identify her health problems. Mrs. Bryan had been diagnosed with stomach cancer a year ago and had a heart attack (myocardial infarction) 4 months ago. Mrs. Bryan's safety was a priority because she had fallen and bruised her hip. But she also was experiencing weight loss, fatigue, and a feeling of breathlessness during exertion. She was concerned that her daughter would try to place her in a nursing home. When Mrs. Bryan discussed her health problems with Inez, the two agreed that improving activity tolerance was an important issue because Mrs. Bryan wanted to remain independent. Inez selected progressive monitored exercise as an intervention to improve Mrs. Bryan's physical endurance. Once Inez proceeds with her intervention, she monitors Mrs. Bryan's heart rate, blood pressure, and self-report of fatigue to determine if her endurance improves. If it does, Inez will plan additional exercise sessions as part of her care. If not, Inez will need to think about other ways to manage her activity intolerance. Inez used the nursing process to care for Mrs. Bryan.

As you read this chapter, you will learn more about Mrs. Bryan and her clinical status. Use the case study as a guide to understanding each step of the nursing process. You will see how the critical thinking skills presented in Chapter 6 are essential to correctly using each step of the nursing process.

## KEY TERMS

actual nursing diagnosis, p. 108
adverse reaction, p. 129
assessment, p. 99
back-channeling, p. 105
clinical criteria, p. 108
closed-ended questions, p. 105
collaborative interventions, p. 118
collaborative problem, p. 107
concept map, p. 121
consultation, p. 123
counseling, p. 129
critical pathways, p. 122
cue, p. 100
data analysis, p. 106
data cluster, p. 106
database, p. 100
defining characteristics, p. 108
diagnostic process, p. 108
direct care interventions, p. 125
etiology, p. 111
evaluation, p. 130
expected outcome, p. 116
functional health patterns, p. 100
goal, p. 116
health care problems, p. 107
implementation, p. 125
indirect care interventions, p. 125
inference, p. 100
instrumental activities of daily living (IADLs), p. 129
interview, p. 102

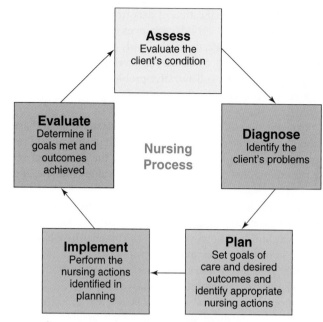

FIGURE **7-1** Five-step nursing process.

## Nursing Process Overview

The **nursing process** is a professional nurse's approach for selecting, organizing, and delivering appropriate nursing care to a patient. You will learn to integrate elements of critical thinking to form judgments and make good clinical decisions by successfully applying the nursing process. The nursing process is used to identify, diagnose, and treat human responses to health and illness (American Nurses Association, 2003). The process includes five steps: assessment, nursing diagnosis, planning, implementation, and evaluation (Figure 7-1). In practice you will use the nursing process continuously, allowing you to modify care as your patients' needs change. Using the nursing process promotes individualized nursing care. It also assists you in responding to patient needs in a timely and consistent manner to improve or maintain the patient's level of health.

The nursing process is simply one variation of scientific reasoning that allows you to organize care for your patients, whether the patient is an individual, family, or community. It is an approach that differentiates nursing practice from that of physicians and other health care professionals. A nurse collects data about a patient through assessment. This includes the use of observation, measurement techniques, record review, collaboration, and interview (Carpenito-Moyet, 2005). As the nurse thinks about the data, inferences begin to form and patterns appear. For example, when Mrs. Bryan reported feeling weak and tired, Inez gathered additional information. She measured Mrs. Bryan's pulse after she walked a distance and found that the pulse was abnor-

mally high. Mrs. Bryan also then reported feeling a bit more tired following exercise. Inez also learned that Mrs. Bryan had not exercised regularly for some time.

The combination of information allowed Inez to identify a nursing diagnosis of *activity intolerance related to sedentary lifestyle.* Once you choose a nursing diagnosis, you then determine what goals and outcomes are necessary to manage the patient's health problem. In Mrs. Bryan's case, Inez sets the goal of "Patient's activity tolerance will improve." For accuracy, Inez sets measurable outcomes in order to determine if Mrs. Bryan reaches the goal. For example, Inez selects the outcome, "Patient will report less fatigue after walking 100 feet within 2 weeks." With goals and outcomes selected, you then select nursing interventions most likely to be effective for the patient. After you administer interventions, you will then evaluate a patient's progress or success. After Mrs. Bryan participates in progressive monitored exercises, Inez will again obtain the patient's self-report regarding fatigue and measure the patient's vital signs.

The nursing process is central to your ability to provide timely and appropriate care to your patients. You will apply it when caring for a single patient, as well as with multiple patients at the same time.

## Assessment

**Assessment** is the deliberate and systematic collection of data to determine a patient's current and past health status, functional status, and present and past coping patterns (Carpenito-Moyet, 2005). There are two steps in nursing assessment:

- Collection and verification of data from a primary source (the patient) and secondary sources (e.g., family, friends, health professionals, medical record)
- Analysis of all data as a basis for developing nursing diagnoses, identifying collaborative problems, and developing a plan of individualized care

The purpose of the assessment is to establish a **database** about the patient's perceived needs, health problems, and responses to these problems. In addition, the data reveal related experiences, health practices, goals, values, lifestyle, and expectations about the health care system.

You will learn to apply principles of critical thinking (see Chapter 6) when conducing a patient assessment. Critical thinking allows you to see the big picture when you form conclusions or make decisions about a patient's health condition. While gathering data about a patient, you will synthesize relevant knowledge, recall prior clinical experiences, apply critical thinking standards and attitudes, and use standards of practice to direct assessment in a meaningful and purposeful way. Your knowledge from the physical, biological, and social sciences allows you to ask relevant questions and collect relevant history and physical assessment data related to a patient's clinical condition. For example, by knowing that Mrs. Bryan has a history of a myocardial infarction, you know to ask if she has chest pain or shortness of breath during exercise. You also know to question her about the location and character of any pain, because these are symptoms of heart disease. Good communication skills and critical thinking intellectual standards allow you to gather even more complete, accurate and relevant data.

Prior clinical experience contributes to assessment skills. For example, if you cared for a patient with heart disease in the past, you will know the type of factors that precipitate or signal chest pain. Thus you would assess thoroughly the types of factors that usually precede Mrs. Bryan's chest pain. You become competent in assessment through validation of abnormal assessment findings and personal observation of assessments performed by skilled nurses. You also learn to apply standards of practice and accepted standards of "normal" physical assessment data when assessing a patient. These standards help you to collect the right kind of information and ensure that you have a standard against which to compare your findings. The use of attitudes such as curiosity, perseverance, and risk taking then ensures that your database is thorough and complete.

## Data Collection

As you begin the assessment of a patient, it is important to think critically about what to assess. Determine what questions or measurements are appropriate based on your clinical knowledge and experience and your patient's re-

sponses. When you first meet a patient, make a quick observational overview or screening. Usually an overview is based on the treatment situation. For example, a community health nurse assesses the neighborhood and the community of the patient; an emergency department nurse uses the ABC (airway-breathing-circulation) approach; and a psychiatric nurse focuses on the patient's orientation to reality, anxiety level, and violence potential (Carnevali and Thomas, 1993). You need to differentiate important data from the total data collected. A **cue** is information that you obtain through use of the senses. An **inference** is your judgment or interpretation of those cues. For example the cue of a patient crying possibly implies fear or sadness. It is possible to miss important cues when you are conducting your initial overview. However, always try to interpret cues from the patient to know how in-depth your eventual comprehensive assessment is. Assessment is dynamic and allows you to freely explore relevant patient problems as you discover them.

After your observational overview, you will focus on assessment cues and patterns of information that suggest problem areas. There are two approaches for a comprehensive assessment. One involves use of a structured database format, based upon an accepted theoretical framework or practice standard. Gordon's 11 **functional health patterns** (1994) (Box 7-1), Pender's health promotion model (1996), and the Agency for Healthcare Research and Quality's (AHRQ's) standards for acute pain assessment (1992) are all examples of this. Gordon's functional health pattern assessment model provides a holistic framework for assessment and a database for deriving a broad range of nursing diagnoses (Gordon, 1994). For each of the health patterns there is a series of questions a nurse asks to understand how healthy each patient's pattern is. Theory and practice standards provide categories of information for you to assess a patient. The premise is that the categories will lead you to gather the most comprehensive assessment of the patient's health care problems.

The second approach for conducting a comprehensive assessment is the problem-focused approach. You focus on the patient's situation and begin with problematic areas, such as headache pain. Then you ask the patient follow-up questions to clarify and expand. For example, ask how the problem affects lifestyle, level of health, ability to function, and relationships with others (Table 7-1). Once you complete the initial assessment, you thoroughly analyze the extent and nature of the patient's pain. This allows you to develop a comprehensive plan for pain intervention.

Whatever approach you use to collect data, you will begin to cluster cues, make inferences, and identify emerging patterns and potential problems. To do this well, you anticipate critically, which means you always try to stay a step ahead of the assessment. When you make an inference about assessment information, it is important to have supporting cues. Sometimes it is necessary to explore further in order to have

BOX 7-1 **Typology of 11 Functional Health Patterns**

*Health perception–health management pattern:* Describes the patient's self-report of health and well-being; how health is managed (e.g., frequency of physician visits, adherence to prescribed therapies at home); knowledge of preventive health practices

*Nutritional-metabolic pattern:* Describes the patient's daily/weekly pattern of food and fluid intake (e.g., food preferences, special diet, food restrictions, appetite); actual weight, weight loss or gain

*Elimination pattern:* Describes patterns of excretory function (bowel, bladder, and skin)

*Activity-exercise pattern:* Describes patterns of exercise, activity, leisure, and recreation; ability to perform activities of daily living

*Sleep-rest pattern:* Describes patterns of sleep, rest, and relaxation

*Cognitive-perceptual pattern:* Describes sensory-perceptual patterns; language adequacy, memory, decision-making ability

*Self-perception–self-concept pattern:* Describes the patient's self-concept pattern and perceptions of self (e.g., self-concept/worth, emotional patterns, body image)

*Role-relationship pattern:* Describes the patient's pattern of role engagements and relationships

*Sexuality-reproductive pattern:* Describes the patient's patterns of satisfaction and dissatisfaction with sexuality pattern; patient's reproductive pattern; premenopausal and postmenopausal problems

*Coping–stress-tolerance pattern:* Describes the patient's ability to manage stress; sources of support; effectiveness of the pattern in terms of stress tolerance

*Value-belief pattern:* Describes patterns of values, beliefs (including spiritual practices), and goals that guide the patient's choices or decisions

Data from Gordon M: *Nursing diagnosis: process and application*, ed 3, St. Louis, 1994, Mosby; Carpenito-Moyet LJ: *Nursing diagnosis: application to clinical practice*, ed 11, Philadelphia, 2005, Lippincott Williams & Wilkins.

a clear picture of the patient's situation. Once you ask a question or make an observation of a patient, the information branches to additional questions or observations for you to examine (Figure 7-2). You take a risk when you do not anticipate assessment questions. This causes you to fail to recognize cues and to dismiss relevant problem areas. Knowing how to probe and frame questions is a skill that will grow with experience. You will learn to decide which questions are relevant to a situation while at the same time being sure the assessment is complete. Your thoughts about a patient will proceed from something revealed in the form of cues or data to a final conclusion that includes a nursing diagnosis and/or collaborative health problem. An accurate initial assessment is crucial to properly identifying patient needs and implementing the right course of action. Remember, assessment is an ongoing activity. Throughout each step of the nursing process you will continue to assess a patient's condition and needs. Patients change quickly, and your ability to be responsive and to assess in a timely way is very important.

## Types of Data

A nurse gathers data from or about a patient. **Subjective data** are your patients' perceptions about their health problems. Only patients provide this kind of information. For example, a patient's report of feeling fearful about impending surgery or reporting the occurrence of "terrible" headache pain are subjective findings. Subjective data usually include feelings of anxiety, physical discomfort, or mental stress. Although only patients provide subjective data relevant to their health condition, be aware that these problems sometimes result in physiological changes, which you can further explore through objective data collection.

**Objective data** are observations or measurements you make during assessment. Assessment of a patient's wound, a description of patient behavior, and identification of the size of a localized skin rash are examples of observed objective data. The measurement of objective data is based on an accepted standard, such as the Fahrenheit or Celsius measure on a thermometer, centimeters on a measuring tape, or known characteristics of behaviors. When you collect data during assessment, be descriptive, concise, and complete. Do not include your personal interpretive statements.

## Sources of Data

As a nurse, you will obtain data from a variety of sources. Each source of data provides information about the patient's level of wellness, anticipated prognosis, risk factors, health practices and goals, and patterns of health and illness.

**PATIENT.** A patient is usually your best source of information. A patient who is alert and answers questions appropriately, provides the most accurate information about health care needs, lifestyle patterns, present and past illnesses, perception of symptoms, and changes in activities of daily living. Always consider the setting for your assessment. A patient experiencing acute symptoms in an emergency department will not offer the same depth of information as one who comes to an outpatient clinic for a routine checkup. Always be attentive and show a caring presence with the patient (see Chapter 16). Patients are less likely to fully reveal the nature of their health care problems when nurses show little interest or are easily distracted by activities around them.

**FAMILY AND SIGNIFICANT OTHERS.** Family members and significant others are primary sources of information for infants or children, critically ill adults, mentally handicapped patients, or patients who are unconscious or have reduced cognitive function. In cases of severe illness, families may be the only available source of data needed by nurses and physicians or health care providers. The family and significant others are also good secondary sources of in-

## FOCUSED PATIENT ASSESSMENT

TABLE 7-1

| Factors to Assess | Questions and Approaches | Physical Assessment Strategies |
|---|---|---|
| Nature of pain | Ask patient to describe pain. Ask patient about location of pain. Ask patient to rate pain. | Observe patient's nonverbal cues, such as grimacing, irritability, as pain is described. Observe where patient points to pain, noting if it radiates or is localized. Use a 0-10 pain scale, and ask patient to numerically rate his or her pain. Following any pain relief measures, reassess using same 0-10 pain scale. |
| Precipitating factors | Ask if patient notices any activities, time of day, during which pain occurs or gets worse. Ask if pain is associated with any food or beverages. | Observe patient during activity, noting any occurrence or changes in pain associated with change of body position, posture, or activity. |
| Relieving factors | Ask patient about any measures he or she uses to reduce pain. | Observe patient during activities to relieve or avoid headaches such as medication, biofeedback, etc. |

formation. They can confirm findings a patient provides (e.g., does a patient take medications regularly at home, has the patient's appetite changed over time, or how well does the patient sleep?). Include them in assessment when appropriate. Remember, a patient does not always wish you to question the family. Often spouses or close friends will sit in during an assessment and provide the view of the patient's health problems or needs. Not only do they supply information about the patient's current health status, but they are also able to indicate when changes have occurred. Family members are frequently very well informed because of their experiences living with the patient and observing how health problems affect daily living activities.

**HEALTH CARE TEAM.** You will frequently communicate with other health care team members in gathering information about patients. In the acute care setting the change-of-shift report is the way for nurses from one shift to communicate information to nurses on the oncoming shift (see Chapter 8). Typically when nurses and other health care team members (e.g., physicians, dietitians, or social workers) consult on a patient's condition, they have information about the patient. This includes how the patient is interacting within the health care environment, the patient's reactions to treatment, the result of diagnostic procedures, needed therapies, and how the patient responds to visitors. Every member of the health care team is a source of information for identifying and verifying information about the patient.

**MEDICAL RECORDS.** The **medical record** is a source for the patient's medical history, laboratory and diagnostic test results, the physician's or health care provider's and therapists' treatment plan, and the patient's progress to date. Data in the records are baseline information about the patient's response to illness and the treatment plan. The Health

Insurance Portability and Accountability Act of 1996 (HIPAA) has a privacy rule that came into effect on April 14, 2003, to set standards for the protection of health information (HIPAAdvisory, 2003). Information in a patient's records is confidential. Each health care agency has policies governing how to share information between health care providers. A nurse can review a patient's medical record for assessment data, but be aware of agency policies governing how to share the information with other staff.

**OTHER RECORDS AND THE LITERATURE.** Educational, military, and employment records may contain pertinent health care information (e.g., immunizations or prior illnesses). If a patient received services at a community clinic or different hospital, the nurse first obtains written permission from the patient or guardian before seeing the records. New HIPAA (2003) regulations dictate specifically how you obtain an information release. Consult agency policies.

Reviewing nursing, medical, and pharmacological literature about a patient's illness helps you to complete your assessment database. This review increases your knowledge about expected signs and symptoms, treatment, and prognosis of specific illnesses and established standards of therapeutic practice. A knowledgeable nurse obtains pertinent, accurate, and complete information for the assessment database.

### Methods of Data Collection

As a nurse you will use the patient interview, nursing health history, physical examination, and results of laboratory and diagnostic tests to establish a patient's assessment database.

**INTERVIEW AND HEALTH HISTORY.** The first step in establishing a database is to collect subjective information by interviewing the patient. An **interview** is an organized conversation with the patient. The initial interview involves obtaining the patient's health history and information about

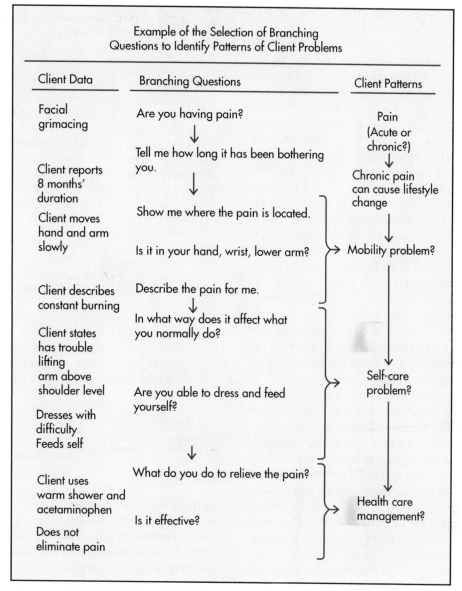

Example of the Selection of Branching
Questions to Identify Patterns of Client Problems

| Client Data | Branching Questions | Client Patterns |
|---|---|---|
| Facial grimacing | Are you having pain? ↓ Tell me how long it has been bothering you. ↓ | Pain (Acute or chronic?) ↓ Chronic pain can cause lifestyle change ↓ |
| Client reports 8 months' duration | | |
| Client moves hand and arm slowly | Show me where the pain is located. Is it in your hand, wrist, lower arm? | Mobility problem? |
| Client describes constant burning | Describe the pain for me. ↓ In what way does it affect what you normally do? | |
| Client states has trouble lifting arm above shoulder level | | |
| Dresses with difficulty Feeds self | Are you able to dress and feed yourself? ↓ | Self-care problem? |
| Client uses warm shower and acetaminophen | What do you do to relieve the pain? Is it effective? | Health care management? |
| Does not eliminate pain | | |

FIGURE 7-2 Example of branching logic for selecting assessment questions.

the current illness. During the initial interview you have the opportunity to:

1. Introduce yourself to the patient, explain your role, and the role of others during care
2. Establish a caring therapeutic relationship with the patient
3. Gain insight about the patient's concerns and worries
4. Determine the patient's goals and expectations of the health care delivery system
5. Obtain cues about which parts of the data collection phase require in-depth investigation

Subsequent interviews allow you to learn more about a patient's situation and to focus on specific problem areas. An interview helps a patient relate his or her own interpre-

tation and understanding of his or her condition. Therefore you and the patient will be partners during the interview rather than your controlling the interview. An interview consists of three phases: orientation, working, and termination.

A successful interview requires preparation. Collect any available information about the patient, and then create an environment conducive to the interview. The orientation phase begins with you introducing yourself and your position and explaining the purpose of the interview. Explain to the patient why you are collecting the data, and assure the patient that the information will remain confidential and will be used only by health care professionals who provide his or her care. Before personal health care data is collected, HIPAA regulations require patients to sign an authorization

(HIPAAdvisory, 2003). This usually occurs in admitting or screening areas before you meet the patient.

During the orientation phase you want to establish trust and confidence with a patient. One important goal for the initial interview is to lay the groundwork for understanding the patient's needs. Another is to begin a relationship that allows the patient to become an active partner in decisions about care. As the orientation phase proceeds, a patient should begin to feel more comfortable speaking with you. Initially you will gather demographic data (e.g., date of birth, gender, address, family members' names and addresses, marital status, religious preference and practices, and occupation), as specified by the facility. Because this information is the least personal, it helps initiate development of the therapeutic relationship and eases transition into the working portion of the interview.

During the working part of the interview you will gather information about the patient's health status. Remember to stay focused, orderly, and unhurried. Use a variety of communication strategies such as active listening, paraphrasing, and summarizing to promote a clear interaction (see Chapter 9). During the working part of the interview explore the patient's current illness, health history, and expectations of care. The general format for a **nursing health history** usually contains several basic components (Box 7-2).

The initial interview is normally the most extensive of all interviews. Major topics to cover include the progress of current illness and the health history. Ongoing interviews, which occur each time you interact with your patient, do not need to be as extensive. They update the patient's status and focus more toward changes in previously identified ongoing and new problems.

As in the other phases of the interview, the termination phase requires skill on the part of the interviewer. Give your patient a clue that the interview is coming to an end. For example, you say, "There are just two more questions" or "We'll be finished in 5 to 6 minutes." This helps the patient maintain direct attention without being distracted by wondering when the interview will end. This approach also gives the patient an opportunity to ask questions. When concluding the interview, summarize the important points and ask your patient if the summary is accurate. End the interview in a friendly manner, telling the patient when you will return to provide care. For example, "Thank you, Mr. Tenet. You have given me a good picture of your health and how you have been affected. You have told me you want to know more about the restrictions you will have after surgery. Is that correct? I will plan your care so that we have time to discuss your surgery and any restrictions. Do you have any questions?"

**Interviewing Techniques.** The manner in which you conduct the interview is just as important as the questions you ask. Pay attention to the environment, patient comfort, and communication techniques (see Chapter 9) to ensure a successful interview. During the interview you are responsible for directing the flow of the interview so that you obtain

---

| BOX 7-2 | **Basic Components for a Nursing Health History** |

*Reasons for seeking health care:* Goals of care, expectation of the services and care delivered, and expectations of the health care system

*Present illness or health concern:* Onset, symptoms, nature of symptoms (e.g., sudden or gradual), duration, precipitating factors, relief measures, and weight loss or gain

*Health history:* Prior illnesses throughout development, injuries and hospitalizations, surgeries, blood transfusions, allergies, immunizations, habits (e.g., smoking, caffeine intake, alcohol or drug abuse), prescribed and self-prescribed medications, work habits, relaxation activities, and sleep, exercise, and eating or nutritional patterns

*Family history:* Health status of the immediate family and living relatives, cause of death of relatives, and risk factor analyses for cancer, heart disease, diabetes mellitus, kidney disease, hypertension, or mental disorders

*Environmental history:* Hazards, pollutants, and physical safety

*Psychosocial and cultural history:* Primary language, cultural group, community resources, mood, attention span, and developmental stage

*Review of systems:* Head-to-toe review of all major body systems, as well as the patient's knowledge of and compliance with health care (e.g., frequency of breast or testicular self-examination or last visual acuity examination)

-or-

*Functional health patterns:* Method for organizing assessment data based on function

---

adequate information and your patient has the opportunity to contribute freely.

An interview may be focused or comprehensive. Listen and consider the information shared, because this will help you direct the patient to give more detail or discuss a topic that might reveal a possible problem. Because a patient's report will include subjective information, validate data from the interview later with objective data. For example, if the patient reports difficulty in breathing, you will later assess respiratory rate and lung sounds.

A good environment is free of distractions, unnecessary noise, and interruptions. The patient is more likely to be candid if the interview is private, out of earshot of other patients, visitors, and staff. Timing is important in avoiding interruptions. If possible, set aside a 15- to 30-minute period when no other activities are planned. Help the patient to feel relaxed and unhurried. Before you begin the interview, be sure the patient is comfortable. This includes adequate light, warmth, and positioning. If possible, sit facing the patient to facilitate eye contact. During the interview, observe your patient for signs of discomfort or fatigue.

When the interview involves a health history, it is helpful to begin by trying to find out, in the patient's own words, what the health problem is and what is likely causing it. Remember, patients are usually the best resources in relating their health history. You will begin by asking the patient a question to elicit the patient's story. For example, say, "So, for what reason did you come to the hospital today?" or "Tell me about the problems you are having." The use of such **open-ended questions** prompts patients to describe a situation in more than one or two words. This technique leads to a discussion in which patients actively describe their health status. The use of open-ended questions strengthens the nurse-patient relationship because it shows that you want to invest time in hearing the patient's thoughts. Encourage and let the patient tell the story all the way through. Listen for feelings as well as for words, and allow pauses in the conversation (Alfaro-LeFevre, 1998). The use of **back-channeling,** which includes active listening prompts such as "all right," "go on," or "uh-huh," indicates you have heard what the patient says and are attentive to hear the full story.

Once a patient has told his or her story, use a problem-seeking approach. This approach takes the information provided by the patient and then more fully describes and identifies specific problem areas. For example, focus on the symptoms the patient identifies and ask **closed-ended questions** that limit the patient's answers to one or two words such as "yes" or "no" or a number or frequency of a symptom. For example, ask "How often do you have the pain?" or "When you turn, is the pain worsened?" As closed-ended questions reveal more information, you need to have the patient discuss historical information in more detail. A good interviewer leaves with a complete story that contains enough details for understanding a patient's perceptions of his or her health status, as well as the information needed to help identify nursing diagnoses and/or collaborative health problems. Always clarify or validate any information you are unclear about.

**PHYSICAL EXAMINATION.** A physical examination is an investigation of the body to determine its state of health. A physical examination involves use of the techniques of inspection, palpation, percussion, auscultation, and smell (see Chapter 13). A complete examination includes a patient's height, weight, vital signs (see Chapter 12), general appearance and behavior, and a head-to-toe examination of all body systems. Perform actual hands-on physical assessment with sensitivity and competence to prevent your patient from becoming too anxious. Minimize anxiety by explaining each step of the examination and continuing throughout the examination to explain and ask about specific functions and discomforts. Always be sure to protect your patient's privacy and dignity.

**OBSERVATION OF PATIENT'S BEHAVIOR.** Throughout an interview and physical examination it is important for you to closely observe a patient's verbal and nonverbal behaviors. This information adds greater depth to the objective database. You learn to determine whether data obtained by observation matches what the patient verbally communicates. For example, if a patient expresses no concern about an upcoming diagnostic test but appears anxious and irritable, verbal and nonverbal data conflict. Observations lead you to gather the additional objective information to form accurate conclusions about a patient's condition.

An important aspect of observation includes a patient's level of function: the physical, developmental, psychological, and social aspects of everyday living. Observation of the level of function is different from observation during the interview. You observe what you see the patient doing, such as self-feeding or making a decision, rather than what the patient says he or she can do. Level of function differs from the physical assessment as well. The level of function is the degree of function at which the patient is operating, whereas the hands-on physical examination determines the greatest extent at which the person is able to function.

**DIAGNOSTIC AND LABORATORY DATA.** The results of diagnostic and laboratory tests can identify or verify alterations questioned or identified during the nursing health history and physical examination. For example, during the health history the patient reports having a bad cold for 6 days and at present has a productive cough with brown sputum and mild shortness of breath. On physical examination, you notice an elevated temperature, increased respirations, and decreased breath sounds in the right lower lobe. You review the results of an ordered complete blood count (CBC) and note the white blood cell count is elevated (indicating an infection). In addition, the radiologist's report of a chest x-ray examination shows the presence of a right lower lobe infiltrate. Such findings combined suggest the patient has the medical diagnosis of pneumonia and the associated nursing diagnosis of impaired gas exchange.

Some patients collect and monitor laboratory data in the home. This is true for patients with diabetes mellitus who often do daily blood glucose monitoring. Ask patients about their routine results to determine their response to illness and information about the effects of treatment measures. Compare laboratory data with the established norms for a particular test, age-group, and gender.

## Interpreting Assessment Data and Making Nursing Judgments

The successful analysis and interpretation of assessment data requires critical thinking. When you correctly analyze data, you will make necessary clinical decisions about your patient's care. These decisions are either in the form of nursing diagnoses or in the form of collaborative problems that require treatment from several disciplines (Carpenito-Moyet, 2005). Critically think about how to interpret assessment information to determine the presence of abnormal findings, to conduct further observations to clarify information, and then to identify the patient's problems. You begin by validating the data you have and then analyzing and interpreting the patient's clinical picture. You then cluster and document your findings.

**DATA VALIDATION.** After gathering assessment data, you validate the collected information to avoid making incorrect inferences (Carpenito-Moyet, 2005). **Validation** of assessment data is comparing the data with another source. For example, you observe a patient crying and logically infer it is related to hospitalization or a medical diagnosis. Making such an initial inference is not wrong, but problems result if you do not validate the inference with the patient. Instead say, "I notice that you have been crying, can you tell me about it?" By doing so you will discover the real reason for the crying. Ask your patient to validate the information obtained during the interview and health history. Validate findings from physical examination and observation of patient behavior by comparing data in the medical record and by consulting with other health team members or even family members.

Validation opens the door for gathering more assessment data because it often involves clarifying vague or ambiguous data. Occasionally you will need to reassess previously covered areas of the nursing history or gather further physical examination data. A nurse continually analyzes and thinks about a patient's database to make concise, accurate, and meaningful interpretations. Critical thinking enables you to fully understand the problems, to judge the extent of the problems more carefully, and to discover possible relationships between the problems.

**ANALYSIS AND INTERPRETATION.** After you collect extensive information about a patient, it becomes necessary to analyze and interpret the data. Patterns of meaning from your inferences begin to form. **Data analysis** involves recognizing patterns or trends, comparing them with standards, and then coming to a reasoned conclusion about the patient's response to a health problem (Box 7-3). Through reasoning and judgment you decide what information explains the patient's health status. Again, this will sometimes direct you to gather further information for clarification of your interpretation. For example, after interviewing a patient you begin to sort out the normal from abnormal findings. In the case of Mrs. Bryan, her data revealed several abnormalities, including a history of a 10-lb weight loss, poor appetite, and general weakness. Laboratory tests show a drop in the patient's total protein and albumen levels. She also reports feeling tired after walking and sometimes becomes breathless. Clarify this by asking how long her appetite has been reduced and what type of foods she is eating. As a nurse you look for patterns in the abnormal data. In Mrs. Bryan's case, she has nutritional and exercise problems. The patterns are formed from data clustering.

**DATA CLUSTERING.** As you interpret data, you organize the information into meaningful and usable clusters, keeping in mind your patient's response to illness. A **data cluster** is a set of signs or symptoms that are grouped together in a logical order. During data clustering, organize data and focus attention on patient functions needing support and assistance for recovery. Focused data clustering using a systems approach or functional health pattern approach assists you in correctly classifying and organizing data. This ultimately provides the framework for developing individualized nursing diagnoses and in identifying collaborative problems (Figure 7-3). Clustering also helps make documentation more concise and focused.

During data clustering, certain cues alert your thinking more than others. These cues help you to eventually identify

---

| BOX 7-3 | **Steps of Data Analysis** |

1. Recognize a pattern or trend.
   Example: 10-lb weight loss
   Poor appetite
   Weakness
   Feels tired after walking
   Notes dyspnea on exertion
2. Compare with standards for normal.
   No weight loss
   Adequate nutritional intake
   Walks without shortness of breath or abnormal increase in heart rate
3. Make a reasoned conclusion.
   Nutritional intake problem
   Problem with activity level

---

nursing diagnoses. You will become experienced in recognizing clusters that point to problems such as pain, anxiety, or immobility. Over time you will recall knowledge from previous experiences so that more complicated clusters become recognizable.

**DATA DOCUMENTATION.** Data documentation is the last part of a complete assessment. The timely, thorough, and accurate documentation of facts is necessary when recording patient data. If you do not record an assessment finding or problem interpretation, it is lost and unavailable to anyone else caring for the patient. If specific information is not given, the reader is left with only general impressions. Observation and recording of patient status is a legal and professional responsibility. The Nurse Practice Acts in all states and the American Nurses Association policy statement (2003) mandate, or require, accurate data collection and recording as independent functions essential to the role of a professional nurse. Review Chapter 8 for details on accurate documentation.

Thorough documentation ensures that information is available to those caring for the patient's needs. Record information even if it does not seem to indicate an abnormality. It may become important later, serving as baseline data for a change in status. A general rule of thumb is that if you assess it, record it.

## ✺ Nursing Diagnosis

After a nurse assesses a patient's database, the next step of the nursing process is to form diagnostic conclusions to determine the level of care the patient requires. Some of the conclusions lead to nursing diagnoses, but others do not. It is important to recognize that the outcome of the nursing diagnostic process includes problems treated primarily by nurses (nursing diagnoses) and problems requiring treatment by several disciplines (collaborative problems). Together, nursing diagnoses and collaborative problems represent the range of conditions that require nursing care (Carpenito-Moyet, 2005)

Nursing diagnosis is the second step of the nursing process that gives meaning to the data you collect and orga-

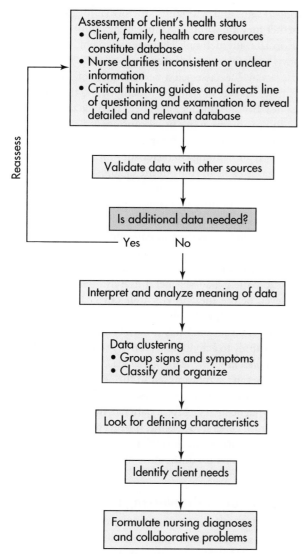

Assessment of client's health status
• Client, family, health care resources
  constitute database
• Nurse clarifies inconsistent or unclear
  information
• Critical thinking guides and directs line
  of questioning and examination to reveal
  detailed and relevant database

Reassess

Validate data with other sources

Is additional data needed?

Yes                No

Interpret and analyze meaning of data

Data clustering
• Group signs and symptoms
• Classify and organize

Look for defining characteristics

Identify client needs

Formulate nursing diagnoses
and collaborative problems

FIGURE **7-3** Nursing diagnostic process.

nize during assessment. The process of diagnosing is the result of your analysis of data and your resultant identification of specific patient responses to **health care problems.** The term *diagnosis* is derived from words meaning "to distinguish" or "to know." A **nursing diagnosis** is a clinical judgment about individual, family, or community responses to actual and potential health problems or life processes (NANDA International, 2005). It is a statement that describes the patient's actual or potential response to a health problem that the nurse is licensed and competent to treat.

A **medical diagnosis** is the identification of a disease condition based on a specific evaluation of physical signs, symptoms, history, diagnostic tests, and procedures. Physicians are licensed to treat diseases or pathological processes by performing surgery, prescribing medication, and ordering specific invasive and noninvasive therapies. The goal of a medical diagnosis is the identification, treatment, and cure of the disease or pathological process. A nurse is responsible

for safely and appropriately delivering the therapy ordered for a medical diagnosis.

A **collaborative problem** is a physiological complication that nurses monitor to detect the onset or changes in a patient's status (Carpenito-Moyet, 2005). Nurses manage collaborative problems such as bleeding, infection, and cardiac arrhythmia using physician-prescribed and nursing-prescribed interventions to minimize complications.

In Mrs. Bryan's case, Inez's assessment included the following information:

Functional Health Pattern (Activity and Exercise)
Patient states she feels tired and "worn out" when walking. Heart rate remained 15% higher than baseline for 5 minutes after walking up stairs. Patient becomes dyspneic when doing laundry and walking stairs; 2+ edema noted in both feet. Lung sounds reveal fine crackles in left and right lower lobes. Review of chest x-ray results shows an enlarged heart.

Inez clustered data from her assessment to reveal a problem in the area of activity and exercise. Her nursing diagnosis is *activity intolerance.* Further review of the medical record revealed that Mrs. Bryan has a previous medical diagnosis of a myocardial infarction 4 months ago and has been treated for congestive heart failure, which is likely contributing to the edema, dyspnea, and fluid buildup in her lungs. The patient's risk for circulatory edema or overload is a collaborative problem, which Inez will assist in managing.

Nursing diagnoses provide the basis for selection of nursing interventions to achieve outcomes for which the nurse is accountable (NANDA International, 2005). A nursing diagnosis focuses on the patient's actual or potential response to a health problem rather than on the physiological event, complication, or disease. As a nurse Inez introduces interventions to improve Mrs. Bryan's ability to exercise, such as progressive exercise and strengthening techniques.

A nurse cannot independently treat a medical diagnosis such as congestive heart failure. However, Inez manages the fluid administration and medication therapy prescribed for the associated collaborative problem of risk for circulatory edema or overload. Collaborative problems occur or probably will occur in association with a specific pathological condition or treatment (Carpenito-Moyet, 2005). You will need expert nursing knowledge to assess a patient's specific risk for these problems, identify the problems early, and then take preventive action.

Identification of nursing diagnoses leads to the development of an individualized plan of care so that your patient and family adapt well to changes resulting from health problems. For example, a patient with a medical diagnosis of appendicitis requires the physician to remove the infected appendix. After the appendectomy the patient has a nursing diagnosis of *impaired physical mobility related to painful incision.* In this case you direct nursing care at gradually increasing the patient's mobility to preoperative levels by decreasing incisional pain.

Critical thinking is necessary in formulating nursing diagnoses and identifying collaborative problems so that you can individualize care for your patient. The remainder of this section will focus on the accurate formulation of nursing diagnoses. During the diagnostic phase you will use your scientific and nursing knowledge and previous experience to analyze and interpret data about the patient and to select the correct diagnoses.

## NANDA International Diagnoses

Research in the field of nursing diagnosis continues to grow. As a result, new diagnostic labels are continually developed and added to the **NANDA International** listing (Box 7-4). The use of standard formal nursing diagnostic statements serves several purposes:

- Provides a precise definition that gives all members of the health care team a common language for understanding the patient's needs
- Distinguishes the nurse's role from that of the physician or health care provider
- Helps nurses focus on the scope of nursing practice

## Critical Thinking and the Nursing Diagnostic Process

Diagnostic reasoning is a process of using the data you gather about a patient to logically explain a clinical judgment, in this case a nursing diagnosis. The **diagnostic process** flows from the assessment process and includes decision-making steps. These steps include data clustering, identifying patient needs, and formulating the diagnosis or problem (see Figure 7-3).

Clusters and patterns of data often contain **defining characteristics,** the clinical criteria or assessment findings that support an actual nursing diagnosis. **Clinical criteria** are objective or subjective signs and symptoms, clusters of signs and symptoms, or risk factors. NANDA International–approved nursing diagnoses have identified sets of defining characteristics that support identification of a nursing diagnosis (NANDA International, 2005). Box 7-5 shows two examples of approved nursing diagnoses and their associated defining characteristics and related factors. As you analyze clusters of data, you begin to consider various diagnoses that might apply to your patient. It is important to recognize that the absence of certain defining characteristics suggest that you reject a diagnosis under consideration. Examine defining characteristics that either support or eliminate a nursing diagnosis carefully. To be more accurate, review all characteristics, eliminate nonrelevant ones, and confirm relevant ones.

While focusing on patterns of defining characteristics, you also compare a patient's pattern of data with data that are consistent with normal, healthful patterns. You will use accepted norms as the basis for comparison and judgment. This includes using laboratory and diagnostic test values, professional standards, and normal anatomical or physiological limits. When comparing patterns, you judge whether the grouped signs and symptoms are normal for the patient and whether they are within the range of healthful responses. You will isolate any defining characteristics not within healthy norms to allow you to identify a problem. In the example of Mrs. Bryan, Inez assessed a verbal report of fatigue, an abnormal heart rate in response to activity, and the symptom of dyspnea. In addition, her assessment revealed that Mrs. Bryan was still maintaining her usual routines at home and generally felt rested after sitting for several minutes. Recognizing the cluster of defining characteristics for *activity intolerance,* Inez was also able to rule out the diagnosis of *fatigue.*

Before finalizing a nursing diagnosis, identify the patient's general health care needs or problems. Identifying patient needs enables you to individualize nursing diagnoses, by considering all assessment data and focusing on the more relevant data. For example, after reviewing clusters of data from Mrs. Bryan's assessment, Inez was able to recognize that the patient had a general exercise tolerance problem. However, before Inez provided effective care, it was necessary to more specifically define Mrs. Bryan's problem. NANDA International has a variety of nursing diagnoses that can apply to activity (e.g., *activity intolerance, risk for activity intolerance, fatigue, impaired walking*). A careful review of Mrs. Bryan's symptoms led to the selection of *activity intolerance.* It is critical for a nurse to eventually arrive at the correct diagnostic label for a patient's need. A nurse usually moves from general to specific. It helps to think of the **problem identification** phase as the general health care problem and the formulation of the nursing diagnosis as the specific health problem.

## Formulation of the Nursing Diagnosis

NANDA International has identified three types of nursing diagnoses: actual diagnoses, at risk diagnoses, and wellness diagnoses (NANDA International, 2005). An **actual nursing diagnosis** describes human response to health conditions or life processes that exist in an individual, family, or community. It is a judgment supported by defining characteristics that cluster in patterns of related cues or inferences (NANDA International, 2005). The selection of an actual diagnosis indicates that sufficient assessment data are available to establish the nursing diagnosis. In the case of Mrs. Bryan, *activity intolerance* is an actual nursing diagnosis.

A **risk nursing diagnosis** describes human responses to health conditions or life processes that have a chance of developing in a vulnerable individual, family, or community (NANDA International, 2005). For example, an overweight patient with a spinal cord injury is at *risk for impaired skin integrity.* The key assessment for this type of diagnosis is the data that support the patient's vulnerability or risk. Such data include physiological, psychosocial, familial, lifestyle, and environmental factors that increase the patient's vulnerability to, or likelihood of developing, the condition. In the example above, the patient's vulnerability to skin breakdown is immobility, increased pressure on the skin, and reduced ability to sense pressure on the skin.

| BOX 7-4 | **NANDA International Nursing Diagnoses** |

**Activity** intolerance
Risk for **Activity** intolerance
Impaired **Adjustment**
Ineffective **Airway** clearance
Latex **Allergy** response
Risk for latex **Allergy** response
**Anxiety**
Death **Anxiety**
Risk for **Aspiration**
Risk for impaired parent/infant/child **Attachment**
**Autonomic** dysreflexia
Risk for **Autonomic** dysreflexia
Disturbed **Body** image
Risk for imbalanced **Body** temperature
**Bowel** incontinence
Effective **Breastfeeding**
Ineffective **Breastfeeding**
Interrupted **Breastfeeding**
Ineffective **Breathing** pattern
Decreased **Cardiac** output
**Caregiver** role strain
Risk for **Caregiver** role strain
Impaired **Comfort**
Impaired verbal **Communication**
Readiness for enhanced **Communication**
Decisional **Conflict**
Parental role **Conflict**
Acute **Confusion**
Chronic **Confusion**
**Constipation**
Perceived **Constipation**
Risk for **Constipation**
Ineffective **Coping**
Ineffective community **Coping**
Readiness for enhanced community **Coping**
Defensive **Coping**
Compromised family **Coping**
Disabled family **Coping**
Readiness for enhanced family **Coping**
Risk for Sudden Infant **Death** Syndrome
Ineffective **Denial**
Impaired **Dentition**
Risk for delayed **Development**
**Diarrhea**
Risk for **Disuse** syndrome
Deficient **Diversional** activity
Disturbed **Energy** field
Impaired **Environmental** interpretation syndrome
Adult **Failure** to thrive
Risk for **Falls**
Dysfunctional **Family** processes: alcoholism
Readiness for enhanced **Family** processes
Interrupted **Family** processes
**Fatigue**
**Fear**

Readiness for enhanced **Fluid** balance
Deficient **Fluid** volume
Excess **Fluid** volume
Risk for deficient **Fluid** volume
Risk for imbalanced **Fluid** volume
Impaired **Gas** exchange
Anticipatory **Grieving**
Risk for dysfunctional **Grieving**
Delayed **Growth** and development
Risk for disproportionate **Growth**
Ineffective **Health** maintenance
**Health-seeking** behaviors
Impaired **Home** maintenance
**Hopelessness**
**Hyperthermia**
**Hypothermia**
Disturbed personal **Identity**
Functional urinary **Incontinence**
Reflex urinary **Incontinence**
Stress urinary **Incontinence**
Total urinary **Incontinence**
Urge urinary **Incontinence**
Risk for urge urinary **Incontinence**
Disorganized **Infant** behavior
Risk for disorganized **Infant** behavior
Readiness for enhanced organized **Infant** behavior
Ineffective **Infant** feeding pattern
Risk for **Infection**
Risk for **Injury**
Risk for perioperative-positioning **Injury**
Decreased **Intracranial** adaptive capacity
Deficient **Knowledge**
Readiness for enhanced **Knowledge** (specify)
Sedentary **Lifestyle**
Risk for **Loneliness**
Impaired **Memory**
Impaired bed **Mobility**
Impaired physical **Mobility**
Impaired wheelchair **Mobility**
**Nausea**
Unilateral **Neglect**
**Noncompliance**
Imbalanced **Nutrition:** less than body requirements
Imbalanced **Nutrition:** more than body requirements
Readiness for enhanced **Nutrition**
Risk for imbalanced **Nutrition:** more than body requirements
Impaired **Oral** mucous membrane
Acute **Pain**
Chronic **Pain**
Readiness for enhanced **Parenting**
Impaired **Parenting**
Risk for impaired **Parenting**
Risk for **Peripheral** neurovascular dysfunction
Risk for **Poisoning**
**Post-trauma** syndrome

Used with permission from NANDA International: *NANDA nursing diagnoses: definitions and classification 2005-2006,* Philadelphia, 2005, NANDA International.

*Continued*

| BOX 7-4 | NANDA International Nursing Diagnoses—cont'd |

Risk for **Post-trauma** syndrome
**Powerlessness**
Risk for **Powerlessness**
Ineffective **Protection**
**Rape-trauma** syndrome
**Rape-trauma** syndrome: compound reaction
**Rape-trauma** syndrome: silent reaction
Impaired **Religiosity**
Readiness for enhanced **Religiosity**
Risk for impaired **Religiosity**
**Relocation** stress syndrome
Risk for **Relocation** stress syndrome
Ineffective **Role** performance
Bathing/hygiene **Self-care** deficit
Dressing/grooming **Self-care** deficit
Feeding **Self-care** deficit
Toileting **Self-care** deficit
Readiness for enhanced **Self-concept**
Chronic low **Self-esteem**
Situational low **Self-esteem**
Risk for situational low **Self-esteem**
**Self-mutilation**
Risk for **Self-mutilation**
Disturbed **Sensory** perception
**Sexual** dysfunction
Ineffective **Sexuality** patterns
Impaired **Skin** integrity
Risk for impaired **Skin** integrity
**Sleep** deprivation
Disturbed **Sleep** pattern
Readiness for enhanced **Sleep**

Impaired **Social** interaction
**Social** isolation
Chronic **Sorrow**
**Spiritual** distress
Risk for **Spiritual** distress
Readiness for enhanced **Spiritual** well-being
Risk for **Suffocation**
Risk for **Suicide**
Delayed **Surgical** recovery
Impaired **Swallowing**
Effective **Therapeutic** regimen management
Ineffective **Therapeutic** regimen management
Readiness for enhanced **Therapeutic** regimen management
Ineffective community **Therapeutic** regimen management
Ineffective family **Therapeutic** regimen management
Management of **Therapeutic** regimen
Ineffective **Thermoregulation**
Disturbed **Thought** processes
Impaired **Tissue** integrity
Ineffective **Tissue** perfusion
Impaired **Transfer** ability
Risk for **Trauma**
Impaired **Urinary** elimination
Readiness for enhanced **Urinary** elimination
**Urinary** retention
Impaired spontaneous **Ventilation**
Dysfunctional **Ventilatory** weaning response
Risk for other-directed **Violence**
Risk for self-directed **Violence**
Impaired **Walking**
**Wandering**

Used with permission from NANDA International: *NANDA nursing diagnoses: definitions and classification 2005-2006*, Philadelphia, 2005, NANDA International.

| BOX 7-5 | Examples of NANDA International–Approved Nursing Diagnoses With Defining Characteristics and Related Factors |

**Diagnosis: Activity Intolerance**

**Defining Characteristics:**

Verbal report of fatigue or weakness
Electrocardiographic changes reflecting arrhythmias or ischemia
Abnormal heart rate or blood pressure response to activity
Exertional discomfort or dyspnea

**Related Factors:**

Bed rest or immobility
Generalized weakness
Imbalance between oxygen supply/demand
Sedentary lifestyle

**Diagnosis: Diarrhea**

**Defining Characteristics:**

At least three loose, liquid stools a day
Hyperactive bowel sounds
Urgency
Abdominal pain
Cramping

**Related Factors:**

*Psychological:* High stress and anxiety
*Situational:* Alcohol abuse, toxins, laxative abuse, travel, radiation, tube feedings, adverse medication effects, contaminants
*Physiological:* Inflammation, irritation, malabsorption, infectious processes, parasites

Used with permission from NANDA International: *NANDA nursing diagnoses: definitions and classification 2005-2006*, Philadelphia, 2005, NANDA International.

A **wellness nursing diagnosis** describes human responses to levels of wellness in an individual, group, or community that have a readiness for enhancement or improvement (NANDA International, 2005). It is a clinical judgment about an individual, group, or community in transition from a specific level of wellness to a higher level of wellness. You will use this type of diagnosis when the patient wishes to or has achieved an optimal level of health. One example is *readiness for enhanced family coping related to unexpected birth of twins*. The nurse and the family unit work together to adapt to the stressors associated with twins and identify the family's strengths, resources, and needs. In doing so, the nurse incorporates the patient's strengths into a plan of care, with the outcome directed at an enhanced level of coping.

**COMPONENTS OF A NURSING DIAGNOSIS.** The nursing diagnosis flows from the assessment and diagnostic process. Throughout this book, the text states nursing diagnoses in a two-part format: the diagnostic label followed by a statement of a related factor (Table 7-2). It is this two-part format that provides a diagnosis with meaning and relevance for a particular patient.

**Diagnostic Label.** The diagnostic label is the name of the nursing diagnosis as approved by NANDA International. It describes the essence of a patient's response to health conditions in as few words as possible. Diagnostic labels include descriptors used to give additional meaning to the diagnosis. For example, the diagnosis *impaired physical mobility* includes the descriptor impaired. The term *impaired* describes the nature of or change in mobility that best describes the patient's response. Examples of other descriptors are compromised, decreased, delayed, or effective.

**Related Factor.** The **related factor** is a condition or etiology identified from the patient's assessment data. It is associated with the patient's actual or potential response to a health problem and can change by using nursing interventions. For example, a nursing diagnostic statement applicable to Mrs. Bryan includes the diagnostic label (e.g., *activity intolerance*) and the related factor (e.g., *related to generalized weakness*). Related factors include four categories: pathophysiological (biological or psychological), treatment-related, situational (environmental or personal), and maturational (Carpenito-Moyet, 2005). The "related to" phrase is not a cause-and-effect statement; rather, it indicates that the etiology contributes to or is associated with the problem (Figure 7-4). The inclusion of the "related to" phrase requires you to use critical thinking skills to individualize the nursing diagnosis and subsequent interventions.

The **etiology** or cause of the nursing diagnosis is always within the domain of nursing practice and a condition that responds to nursing interventions. Sometimes health care providers record medical diagnoses as the etiology of the nursing diagnosis. This is incorrect. Nursing interventions cannot change a medical diagnosis. However, you can direct nursing interventions at behavior or conditions that you can treat or manage. For example, the nursing diagnosis *acute pain related to breast cancer* is incorrect. Nursing actions cannot affect the medical diagnosis of breast cancer. Rewording the diagnosis to read *acute pain related to impaired skin integrity secondary to mastectomy incision* results in nursing interventions directed at reducing stress on the suture line and improving the patient's comfort.

Table 7-3 demonstrates the association between a nurse's assessment of a patient, the clustering of defining characteristics, and formulation of nursing diagnoses. The diagnostic

| TABLE 7-2 | NANDA Nursing Diagnosis Format |
|---|---|
| **Diagnostic Label** | **Related Factors** |
| Constipation | Insufficient fiber intake |
| | Effects of medications |
| | Inadequate fluid intake |
| | Insufficient physical activity |
| Imbalanced Nutrition: | Inability to ingest or digest food |
| Less than body | Inability to absorb nutrients |
| requirements | Inability to obtain food sources |
| Impaired skin integrity | Fluid retention |
| | Excessive secretions |
| | Immobilization |
| | Altered circulation |

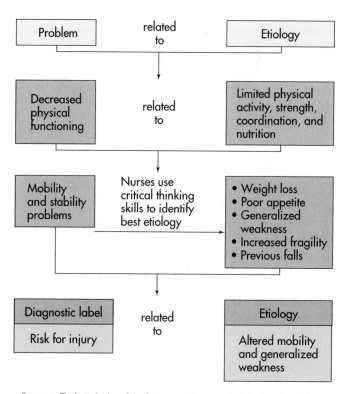

FIGURE **7-4** Relationship between diagnostic label and etiology (related factor). (Redrawn from Hickey P: *Nursing process handbook,* St. Louis, 1990, Mosby.)

| TABLE 7-3 | Formulation of Nursing Diagnoses | | |
|---|---|---|---|
| Assessment Activities | Defining Characteristics (Clustering Cues) | Nursing Diagnosis | Etiologies ("Related to") |
| Weigh patient. | Body weight is 20% under ideal. | Imbalanced nutrition: less than body requirements | Poor nutritional intake |
| Observe amount of food eaten during meals. | Eats only half of meals. Caloric intake is <1200 daily. | | |
| Ask patient to describe appetite and sense of taste. | Patient has less interest in eating. Sense of taste is reduced. | | |
| Measure patient's heart rate before and after walking. | Patient's heart rate remains 15% above baseline for over 5 minutes following exercise. | Activity intolerance | General weakness and sedentary life style |
| Ask patient to describe how she feels after walking or any strenuous activity. | Patient states feels weak after walking and notices sense of breathlessness. | | |
| Observe patient's normal activity pattern. | Patient performs daily living activities but does not regularly exercise. | | |
| Ask patient to discuss concerns about living in a residence. | Patient desires to remain independent. Patient fears nursing home placement. | Decisional conflict over patient's placement in nursing home | Threat of loss of independence |
| Observe interactions between mother and daughter. | Mother shows anxiety when discussing placement options with daughter. | | |
| Ask daughter to discuss concerns about her mother's care and supervision. | Daughter has concerns over mother's comfort and safety. | | |

process results in the formation of a total diagnostic label that will allow a nurse to develop an appropriate, patient-centered plan of care. The defining characteristics and relevant etiologies are from NANDA International (2005).

**Definition.** NANDA International approves a definition for each diagnosis following clinical use and testing. The definition describes the characteristics of the human response identified. For example, the definition of the diagnostic label *impaired physical mobility* is the "limitation in independent, purposeful physical movement of the body or of one or more extremities" (NANDA International, 2005). Refer to a definition to assist you in identifying a patient's diagnosis.

**Risk Factors.** Risk factors are environmental, physiological, psychological, genetic, or chemical elements that increase the vulnerability of an individual, family, or community to an unhealthful event (NANDA International, 2005). They are a component of all risk nursing diagnoses. The risk factors serve as cues to indicate a risk nursing diagnosis is applicable to a patient's condition. Examples of risk factors for the nursing diagnosis *risk for falls* include the following: a history of falls, age 65 or over, lives alone, presence of visual and or hearing limitations, and urinary urgency and/or incontinence. The risk factors help in selecting the correct risk diagnosis, just as defining characteristics help in the formulation of actual nursing diagnoses. In addition, risk factors are also useful when you plan nursing interventions.

**Support of the Diagnostic Statement.** Nursing assessment data must support the diagnostic label, and the related factors must support the etiology. To collect complete, rele-

vant, and correct assessment data it helps to identify assessment activities that produce specific kinds of data. For example, asking the patient about the quality and perception of pain results in subjective data. However, palpating an area, which sometimes elicits a painful expression, provides objective information. When you review your assessment data looking for clusters of defining characteristics, consider if you have probed and assessed the patient accurately and thoroughly to gather a complete database.

## Mind Mapping Nursing Diagnosis

When you care for a patient or groups of patients, it is a challenge to think about all patient needs and problems. This is especially true because of a nurse's holistic view of patients. Few patients that you care for will have only a single nursing diagnosis. Usually you will care for patients with multiple nursing diagnoses. There is a learning approach, mind mapping, to help you organize and link data about a patient's multiple diagnoses in a logical way. **Mind mapping** is a way to graphically represent the connections between concepts (e.g., nursing diagnoses) that are related to a central subject (e.g., a patient's health problems). A mind map forms a picture of each patient's diagnoses and the many interconnections between the assessment data associated with the patient problems (Mueller, Johnston, and Bligh, 2002).

The benefit of mind mapping is that it allows you to plot out associated thoughts, link together lines of reasoning, and see the relationship of one problem or nursing diagnosis with another. A mind map gives you a whole picture of a patient's

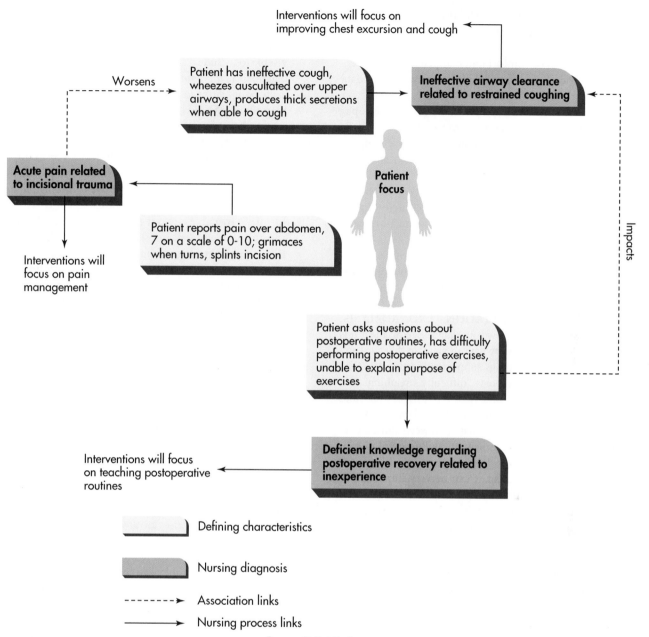

FIGURE **7-5** Mind map.

health situation with all of its interrelationships seen spatially. It is also a useful tool to help you identify patient priorities. As you develop a mind map for nursing diagnoses, eventually it expands and develops into a plan of care (see concept map, Figure 7-7). The mind map shown in Figure 7-5 demonstrates a surgical patient's three nursing diagnoses (*acute pain related to incisional trauma, ineffective airway clearance related to restrained coughing,* and *deficient knowledge regarding postoperative recovery related to inexperience*). The defining characteristics used to identify each diagnosis are shaded in blue. To draw a map you draw connecting arrows between diagnoses and defining characteristics that show a relationship between the diagnoses. For example, the patient's difficulty in performing postoperative exercises, a defining

characteristic for *deficient knowledge,* affects the patient's ability to cough and clear the airway. The mind map helps you to see the total picture and how to relate the diagnoses. The advantage of the mind map is its central focus on the patient and not just the patient's disease or health alteration.

## Sources of Diagnostic Errors

Errors can occur in the diagnostic process during data collection, data interpretation, clustering, and statement of the nursing diagnosis. You need methodical critical thinking for an accurate nursing diagnostic process.

**ERRORS IN DATA COLLECTION.** To avoid errors in data collection be knowledgeable and skilled in all assessment techniques. Avoid inaccurate or missing data, and collect data in an organized way. The following practice tips are essential to avoid data collection errors:

- Review your level of comfort and competence with interview and physical assessment skills before you begin data collection.
- Approach assessment in steps. Focus on completing a patient interview before starting an examination. Perhaps focus on only one body system to learn how to gather a complete assessment. Then move to a more complex head-to-toe examination.
- Review your clinical assessments in clinical or classroom settings. They will provide you with a constructive learning opportunity to determine how to revise an assessment or to gather additional information.
- Be organized in any examination. Have the appropriate forms and examination equipment ready to use. Be sure the environment is private, quiet, and comfortable for the patient.

**ERRORS IN INTERPRETATION AND ANALYSIS.** Following data collection, review your database to decide if it is accurate and complete. Review data to validate that measurable, objective physical findings support subjective data. For example, when a patient reports "difficulty breathing" you want to also listen to lung sounds, assess respiratory rate, and measure the patient's chest excursion. When data are not validated, this signals an inaccurate match between clinical cues and the nursing diagnosis (Lunney, 1998). Be careful to consider any conflicting cues or decide if there are insufficient cues to form a diagnosis. Also, it can be very important to consider a patient's cultural background or developmental stage when you interpret the meaning of cues. For example, a patient from the Middle East may express pain very differently than a patient from an Asian country. Misinterpreting how these patients expresses pain could easily lead to an inaccurate diagnosis.

**ERRORS IN DATA CLUSTERING.** Errors in data clustering occur when data are clustered prematurely, incorrectly, or not at all. Premature closure of clustering occurs when you make the nursing diagnosis before grouping all data. Incorrect clustering occurs when you try to make the nursing diagnosis fit the signs and symptoms obtained. The nursing diagnosis comes from the data, not the other way around. An incorrect nursing diagnosis affects quality of care.

**ERRORS IN THE DIAGNOSTIC STATEMENT.** The correct selection of a diagnostic statement is more likely to result in the appropriate selection of nursing interventions and outcomes (Dochterman and Jones, 2003). To reduce errors, word the diagnostic statement in appropriate, concise, and precise language. Use correct terminology reflecting the patient's response to the illness or condition. Use of standardized nursing language such as NANDA International diagnoses helps ensure accuracy. Be sure the etiology portion of the diagnosis is within the scope of nursing to diagnose and treat. Additional guidelines to reduce errors in the diagnostic statement follow:

1. Identify the patient's response, not the medical diagnosis (Carpenito-Moyet, 2005). Because the medical diagnosis requires medical interventions, it is legally inadvisable to include it in the nursing diagnosis. Change the diagnosis *acute pain related to myocardial infarction* to *acute pain related to physical exertion*.

2. Identify a NANDA International diagnostic statement rather than the symptom. Obtain nursing diagnoses from a cluster of defining characteristics; one symptom is insufficient for problem identification. For example, shortness of breath, pain on inspiration, and productive cough should be written as *ineffective breathing pattern related to increased airway secretions*.

3. Identify a treatable etiology rather than a clinical sign or chronic problem. A diagnostic test or a chronic dysfunction is not an etiology or one that can be treated with a nursing intervention. State altered respiratory function supported by abnormal arterial blood gases as *ineffective tissue perfusion related to inadequate oxygen intake*.

4. Identify the problem caused by the treatment or diagnostic study rather than the treatment or study itself. Patients experience many responses to diagnostic tests and medical treatment. These responses are the area of nursing concern. The patient who has angina and is scheduled for a cardiac catheterization may have a nursing diagnosis of *anxiety related to lack of knowledge about cardiac catheterization*.

5. Identify the patient response to the equipment rather than the equipment itself. Change the diagnosis *anxiety related to cardiac monitor* to *deficient knowledge regarding the need for cardiac monitoring*.

6. Identify the patient's problems rather than your problems. Nursing diagnoses are always patient centered and form the basis for goal-directed care. Potential intravenous complications related to poor vascular access indicates a nursing problem in initiating and maintaining intravenous therapy. The diagnosis *risk for infection related to presence of invasive lines* properly centers attention on patient needs.

7. Identify the patient problem rather than the nursing intervention. Plan nursing interventions later to alleviate patient problems. The statement *offer bedpan frequently because of altered elimination patterns* changes to *diarrhea related to food intolerance*. This corrects the misstatement and allows proper implementation of the nursing process.

8. Identify the patient problem rather than the goal. Goals are established in terms of patient problems. If you do not identify the problem, evaluation of problem resolution is difficult. Change *patient needs high-protein diet related to potential alteration in nutrition* to *imbalanced nutrition: less than body requirements related to inadequate protein intake* to allow for planning to correct the etiology.

9. Make professional rather than prejudicial judgments. Base nursing diagnoses on subjective and objective patient data, and do not include your personal beliefs and

values. Remove your judgment from *risk for impaired skin integrity related to poor hygiene habits* by changing the nursing diagnosis to *risk for impaired skin integrity related to knowledge about perineal care.*

10. Avoid legally inadvisable statements (Carpenito-Moyet, 2005). Statements that imply blame, negligence, or malpractice have the potential to result in litigation. The diagnosis *recurrent angina related to insufficient medication* implies that the physician or health care provider gave an inadequate prescription. Correct problem identification might read *chronic pain related to improper use of medications.*

11. Identify the problem and etiology so as to avoid a circular statement. Such statements are vague and give no direction to nursing care. Change *pain related to alteration in comfort* to identify the patient problem and the cause: *ineffective breathing pattern related to incisional pain.*

12. Identify only one patient problem in the diagnostic statement. Every problem has different specific expected outcomes. Confusion during the planning step occurs when you include multiple problems in a nursing diagnosis. It is, however, permissible to include multiple etiologies contributing to one patient problem. Restate *pain and anxiety related to difficulty in ambulating* as two nursing diagnoses, such as *impaired physical mobility related to pain in right knee* and *anxiety related to difficulty in ambulating.*

**DOCUMENTATION.** Once you identify the patient's nursing diagnoses, list them on the plan of care. In the clinical facility, list nursing diagnoses chronologically as you identify them. When initiating the original care plan, always place the highest priority nursing diagnoses first. Thereafter, add additional nursing diagnoses to the list. Date a nursing diagnosis at the time of entry. When caring for a patient always review the list and identify those nursing diagnoses with the greatest priority regardless of chronological order.

## Planning

Once you assess a patient's condition and identify appropriate nursing diagnoses, develop a plan of care. The nursing diagnoses, as well as any collaborative problems you identify, direct your selection of nursing interventions and the goals and outcomes you hope to achieve. **Planning** is the third step of the nursing process. During this step you identify a set of diagnoses, set patient-centered goals and expected outcomes, and prescribe nursing interventions (Carpenito-Moyet, 2005). Another aspect of planning is to set priorities for a patient. Remember, a single patient often has multiple diagnoses and collaborative problems. Eventually you will care for groups of patients. Being able to carefully and wisely set priorities for a single patient or group of patients ensures the most timely and effective care. Successful planning will require that you collaborate with the patient and family, consult with other members of the health care team, and review pertinent literature. Successful

planning also includes modifying care and recording relevant information about the patient's health care needs and clinical management.

### Establishing Priorities

Priority setting involves ranking nursing diagnoses in order of importance. This process allows you to attend to the patient's most important needs and to organize your ongoing care activities. Priorities help you to anticipate and sequence nursing interventions when a patient has multiple problems. Together with your patients, you will select mutually agreed-on priorities based on the urgency of the problem, the patient's safety and desires, the nature of the treatment indicated, and the relationship among the diagnoses. Establishing priorities is not just a matter of numbering the nursing diagnosis on the basis of severity or physiological importance.

You will classify priorities as high, intermediate, or low. Nursing diagnoses that, if untreated, result in harm to the patient or others have the highest priorities. For example, *risk for other-directed violence, impaired gas exchange,* and *acute pain* are typically high-priority nursing diagnoses that drive the priorities of safety, adequate oxygenation, and comfort. However, it is always important to consider each patient's unique case. High priorities are sometimes both psychological and physiological. Avoid classifying only physiological nursing diagnoses as high priority. Consider Mrs. Bryan's case study. Among Mrs. Bryan's nursing diagnoses are *risk for falls, imbalanced nutrition: less than body requirements, activity intolerance,* and *decisional conflict.* Mrs. Bryan's highest priorities are *risk for falls* and *decisional conflict.* Safety is the highest priority, because unless Mrs. Bryan has a safe home environment, there is a risk of additional falls. *Decisional conflict* is a high priority because of the issue of how to ensure a safe environment for Mrs. Bryan; she is no longer able to remain in her own home.

Intermediate-priority nursing diagnoses involve the nonemergent, non–life-threatening needs of the patient. In Mrs. Bryan's case, *imbalanced nutrition: less than body requirements* and *activity intolerance* are both intermediate diagnoses. Mrs. Bryan's nutritional problem is linked with her stomach cancer and will be an ongoing challenge. Similarly, her activity intolerance, which adds risk to her chances of falling, is associated with her past heart disease. Exercise therapies are important but not a life-threatening issue.

Low-priority nursing diagnoses are patient needs that are usually directly related to a specific illness or prognosis but may affect the patient's future well-being. Mrs. Bryan's nurse, Inez, knows that to ultimately resolve the decisional conflict between Mrs. Bryan and her daughter, they will need to learn more about nursing homes. Assessment of the Bryan family's knowledge reveals they have had no experience in selecting a nursing home and the two women share misinformation. *Deficient knowledge regarding nursing home resources or relocation related to inexperience and misinformation* is a relevant, but low-priority diagnosis for Mrs. Bryan.

The order of priorities changes as a patient's condition changes. Each time you begin a sequence of care such as the beginning of a hospital shift or a patient's clinic visit, it is important to reorder priorities. Ongoing patient assessment is critical to determine the status of the patient's nursing diagnoses.

Whenever possible, involve the patient in priority setting. In some situations you and the patient will assign different priority rankings to the nursing diagnoses. If you each place a different value on health care needs and treatments, resolve these differences through open communication. However, when the patient's physiological and emotional needs are at stake, you need to assume primary responsibility for setting priorities.

## Goals and Expected Outcomes

Once you identify a nursing diagnosis for a patient, ask yourself what the best approach to care is. Goals and expected outcomes are specific statements of patient behavior or physiological responses that you set to achieve as a result of your patient care. For example, in the case of Mrs. Bryan's *activity intolerance*, a goal of care includes "Patient's activity tolerance will improve in 1 month." In order for the nurse to monitor Mrs. Bryan's progress, it is necessary to use outcomes or measurable criteria to evaluate goal achievement. Some measurable outcomes for the activity goal are "Patient's heart rate will return to resting within 5 minutes following monitored progressive exercise" and "Patient will report less fatigue following walking within 2 weeks." After initiating appropriate exercise therapies the nurse will monitor Mrs. Bryan's exercise sessions (through patient self-report) and interview Mrs. Bryan about her tolerance to exercises to decide if Mrs. Bryan's activity tolerance improves. Goals and expected outcomes serve two purposes: to provide a clear focus for the type of interventions needed to care for the patient and to provide the focus for evaluation of the effectiveness of nursing interventions.

**GOALS OF CARE.** A patient-centered **goal** is a specific and measurable behavior or response that reflects the patient's highest possible level of wellness and independence in function. A goal is realistic and based on patient needs and resources. A patient goal represents predicted resolution of a problem, evidence of progress toward problem resolution, progress toward improved health status, or continued maintenance of good health or function (Carpenito-Moyet, 2005). A goal contains singular behaviors or responses. A goal written as "Patient will follow an exercise plan and understand exercise benefits" is incorrect because the statement includes two different patient behaviors, follow and understand. Instead, word the goal as "Patient will understand exercise benefits." The specific criteria used to measure success of the goal are the outcome statements. For example, "Patient will describe three benefits from progressive exercise."

Each goal is time-limited so that the health care team has a common time frame for problem resolution. The time frame depends on the nature of the problem, etiology, overall condition of the patient, and treatment setting. A

*short-term goal* is an objective behavior or response that you expect the patient to achieve in a short time, usually less than a week. In an acute care setting, you may set goals for over a course of just a few hours. For example, "Patient will maintain a balanced fluid status within the next 12 hours." A *long-term goal* is an objective behavior or response that you expect the patient to achieve over a longer period, usually over several days, weeks, or months. For example, "Patient will be tobacco free within 60 days." Goal setting establishes the framework for the nursing care plan. Table 7-4 shows the progression from nursing diagnoses to goals and expected outcomes, which you individualize to meet patient needs.

**Role of the Patient in Goal Setting.** Always partner with patients when setting goals. Mutual goal setting is an activity that includes the patient and family (when appropriate) in prioritizing the goals of care and in developing a plan of action to achieve those goals (McCloskey and Bulechek, 1994). Unless goals are mutually set and there is a clear plan of action, patients will fail to participate in the plan of care. Patients need to understand and see the value of nursing therapies, even though they are oftentimes totally dependent on you as the nurse. When developing goals, you act as an advocate or supporter for the patient to develop nursing interventions that promote the patient's return to health or prevent further deterioration when possible.

**EXPECTED OUTCOMES.** An **expected outcome** is a specific measurable change in a patient's status that you expect to occur in response to nursing care. An outcome is an objective criterion for measuring goal achievement and the resolution of the etiology for the nursing diagnosis (Table 7-5). Expected outcomes provide a focus or direction for nursing care because they are the desired physical, psychological, social, emotional, developmental, or spiritual responses that will resolve the patient's health problems. Taken from both short- and long-term goals, outcomes determine when a specific, patient-centered goal has been met.

Several expected outcomes are usually developed for each nursing diagnosis and goal. The reason for the multiple outcomes is that sometimes one nursing action is not always enough to resolve a patient problem. In addition, the listing of the step-by-step expected outcomes gives you practical guidance in planning interventions. Always write expected outcomes sequentially with time frames. Time frames give you progressive steps in which to move a patient toward recovery. They also give an order for when to perform the nursing interventions you select. In addition, time frames set limits for problem resolution.

There is much attention in the current health care environment to measuring outcomes sensitive to nursing interventions. The Iowa Intervention Project has published the *Nursing Outcomes Classification (NOC)* and has linked the outcomes to NANDA International nursing diagnoses (Moorhead, Johnson, and Maas, 2004). For any given NANDA International nursing diagnosis there are multiple NOC suggested outcomes. These outcomes have labels for describing the focus of nursing care and then include

| TABLE 7-4 | Examples of Goal Setting With Expected Outcomes for Mrs. Bryan | |
|---|---|---|
| **Nursing Diagnoses** | **Goals** | **Expected Outcomes** |
| Risk for falls related to weakness and barriers within home | Mrs. Bryan's home will be free of hazards within 1 month. | Modifiable hazards in kitchen and living room will be reduced within 1 week. Modifiable hazards in bathroom will be reduced within 1 month. |
| Decisional conflict over patient's placement in nursing home related to threat of loss of independence | Mrs. Bryan and daughter will decide on the mother's place of residence within 2 months. | Mrs. Bryan will express concerns to daughter about nursing home placement in 1 week. Daughter will express concerns over mother's safety in 1 week. Mother and daughter will visit three nursing homes together by 6/22. |
| Deficient knowledge regarding nursing home services related to inexperience and misinformation | Mrs. Bryan will understand the type of services to expect in a state-approved nursing home by 6/22. | Mrs. Bryan will describe five services of state-approved nursing homes within 2 weeks. Mrs. Bryan will explain what a nursing home provides for resident safety by 6/22. |

| TABLE 7-5 | Examples of NANDA International Nursing Diagnoses and Suggested NOC Linkages | |
|---|---|---|
| **Nursing Diagnosis** | **Suggested NOC Outcomes (Examples)** | **Outcome Indicators (Examples)** |
| Activity intolerance | Activity tolerance | Oxygen saturation with activity Pulse rate with activity Respiratory rate with activity Ease of breathing with activity |
| | Self-care status | Bathes self Dresses self Prepares food and fluid for eating |
| Decisional conflict | Decision making | Identifies relevant information Recognizes contradiction with others' desires |
| | Personal autonomy | Makes informed life decisions Considers other opinions when making choices |

indicators for use in measuring success with interventions (see Table 7-5). The NOC contains outcomes for individuals, family caregivers, the family, and the community for all types of health care settings. Efforts to measure outcomes and capture the changes in the status of patients over time allow nurses to improve patient care quality and add to the knowledge of nursing (Moorhead and others, 2004). The use of a common set of outcomes allows nurses to study the effects of nursing interventions over time and across settings. The 2004 edition of NOC includes 330 outcomes with definitions, indicators, and measurement scales. Use of the NOC outcomes in planning care for your patient provides a common nursing language for all nurses to use in measuring the success of your interventions.

**GUIDELINES FOR WRITING GOALS AND EXPECTED OUTCOMES.** There are seven guidelines for writing goals and expected outcomes: patient centered, singular, observable, measurable, time-limited, mutual factors, and realistic.

*Patient centered:* Outcomes and goals reflect the patient behavior and responses expected as a result of nursing inter-

ventions. Write the goal to reflect this, not to reflect your goals or interventions. A correct outcome statement is "Patient will ambulate in the hall 3 times a day." A common error is to write "Ambulate patient in the hall 3 times a day."

*Singular goal or outcome:* Be precise in evaluating a patient response to a nursing action. Each goal and outcome addresses only one behavior or response. If an outcome reads "Patient's lungs will be clear to auscultation and respiratory rate will be 22 breaths per minute by 8/22," consider the outcome when you evaluate that the lungs are clear but the respiratory rate is 28 breaths per minute. It will be difficult to determine whether the expected outcome has been achieved. By splitting the statement into two parts, "Lungs will be clear to auscultation by 8/22" and "Respiratory rate will be 22 breaths per minute by 8/22," you determine specifically if the patient achieves each outcome. Singularity allows you to decide if there is a need to modify the plan of care.

*Observable:* You must be able to determine through observation if change has taken place. Observable changes occur in physiological findings, the patient's knowledge, perceptions, and behaviors. Examples include "Lungs will be clear on auscultation by 8/22" and "Patient will prepare medication dose correctly by 9/12."

*Measurable:* You will learn to write goals and expected outcomes that set standards against which to measure the patient's response to nursing care. Examples such as "Body temperature will remain 98.6° F" and "Apical pulse will remain between 60 and 100 beats per minute" allow you to objectively measure changes in the patient's status. Do not use vague qualifiers such as "normal," "acceptable," "stable," or "sufficient" in the expected outcome statement. Vague terms result in guesswork in determining a patient's response to care. Terms describing quality, quantity, frequency, length, or weight allow you to evaluate if outcomes are met.

*Time limited:* The time frame for each goal and expected outcome indicates when you expect the response to occur. Time frames assist you and the patient in determining if progress is being made at a reasonable rate. If not, revision to the plan of care will be necessary. Time frames also promote accountability in the delivery and management of nursing care.

*Mutual factors:* Mutually set goals and expected outcomes ensure that the patient and nurse agree on the direction and time limits of care. Mutual goal setting increases the patient's motivation and cooperation. As a patient advocate, you will apply standards of practice, patient safety, and basic human needs when assisting patients with setting goals.

*Realistic:* Set goals and expected outcomes that the patient is able to reach. Achievable goals provide patients a sense of accomplishment. In turn, this sense of accomplishment further increases the patient's motivation and cooperation. When establishing realistic goals, you, through assessment, must know the resources of the health care facility, family, and patient. You should also be aware of the patient's physiological, emotional, cognitive, and sociocultural potential and the costs associated with treatment and resources available to reach expected outcomes in a timely manner.

## Critical Thinking in Planning Nursing Care

Nursing interventions are treatments or actions, based upon clinical judgment and knowledge, that nurses perform to meet patients' outcomes (Dochterman and Bulechek, 2004). During planning you make clinical decisions by choosing the interventions most appropriate to your patient's needs.

You will use critical thinking to select interventions that will successfully meet the patient's established goals and expected outcomes (Carnevali and Thomas, 1993). To select interventions you must be competent in three areas: (1) have knowledge of the **scientific rationale,** or reason, for the interventions, (2) possess the necessary psychomotor and interpersonal skills to perform the interventions, and (3) be able to function within a particular setting to use the available health care resources effectively.

**TYPES OF INTERVENTIONS.** There are three categories of nursing interventions: nurse-initiated, physician-initiated, and collaborative interventions. **Nurse-initiated interventions** are the independent responses of the nurse to a patient's nursing diagnoses and health care needs. A nurse

is able to act independently to intervene on a patient's behalf. Nurse-initiated interventions are autonomous actions based on scientific rationale. These interventions benefit the patient in a predicted way related to nursing diagnoses and patient goals (Dochterman and Bulechek, 2004). These interventions require no supervision or direction from others. Each state within the United States has developed Nurse Practice Acts that define the legal scope of nursing practice (see Chapter 4). According to the Nurse Practice Acts in a majority of states, nursing actions pertaining to activities of daily living, health education, health promotion, and counseling are in the domain of nursing practice. Specific examples include instructing patients on self-care activities, positioning patients for pressure relief, and communicating with patients about loss.

**Physician-initiated interventions** are based on the physician's response to treat or manage a medical diagnosis. Nurse practitioners working under collaborative agreements with physicians or who are licensed independently by state practice acts also write such interventions. As the nurse, you intervene by carrying out the independent provider's written orders and/or verbal orders. Administering a medication, implementing an invasive procedure, changing a dressing, and preparing a patient for diagnostic tests are examples of such interventions.

Each physician-initiated intervention involves specific nursing responsibilities and technical nursing knowledge. For example, when administering medications, you are responsible for knowing the classification of the drug, its physiological action, normal dosage, side effects, and nursing interventions related to its action or side effects (see Chapter 14). When a physician orders diagnostic testing, you are responsible for scheduling the test, preparing the patient, and knowing the normal findings and associated nursing implications.

**Collaborative interventions** are therapies that require the combined knowledge, skill, and expertise of multiple health care professionals. For example, in the case study introduced earlier, Mrs. Bryan is a 78-year-old widow, living alone in a rural community. She has inoperable stomach cancer and decides with the support of her daughter to move into the home of a friend. Mrs. Bryan's overall goal and health care need is to remain independent. Because of poor appetite and subsequent weight loss, she is very weak. She needs interventions developed by multiple health care professionals, as well as community resources. Inez Santiago, Mrs. Bryan's nurse, schedules a visit with a home care aide, an occupational therapist (OT), and a physical therapist (PT). During their visit the OT and PT evaluate Mrs. Bryan's safety and tolerance for certain activities of daily living, modify the home to remove risks to safety, establish an exercise program, and develop a schedule of interventions for the home care aide to complete. The weekly plan now includes one visit by the nurse, two visits from the home care aide, and one visit from the OT or PT, on alternating weeks. Thus in addition to Mrs. Bryan living with a friend, there is a total of four visits a week to Mrs. Bryan's new home. Her daughter is more accepting of her mother's recent move. The care for this patient requires the coordination of collaborative interventions all directed toward the long-term goal of maintaining Mrs. Bryan's independence and safety, as well as supporting her level of health.

**Selection of Interventions.** You must learn to not select interventions randomly. Patients with the diagnosis of *anxiety,* for example, do not always need care in the same way with the same interventions. You treat *anxiety* related to the uncertainty of results from a diagnostic test differently than *anxiety* related to a threat to loss of a loved one. When choosing interventions, you should consider six factors: (1) characteristics of the nursing diagnosis, (2) expected outcomes and goals, (3) evidence base (research or proven practice guidelines) for the intervention, (4) feasibility of the intervention, (5) acceptability to the patient, and (6) your own competency (Dochterman and Bulechek, 2004; McCloskey and Bulechek, 1998) (Box 7-6). Review resources such as standardized care plans, the *Nursing Interventions Classification (NIC),* critical pathways, nursing policies, textbooks, and nursing literature when choosing interventions. Collaboration with other health professionals is also useful. As you select interventions, review your patient's needs, priorities, and previous experiences to select those nursing interventions that have the best potential for achieving the expected outcomes.

**Nursing Interventions Classification.** The Iowa Intervention Project has developed a set of nursing interventions that provides a level of standardization to enhance communication of nursing care across settings and to compare outcomes (Dochterman and Bulechek, 2004; Iowa Intervention

Project, 1993). The NIC taxonomy includes 486 interventions grouped into 30 classes and 7 domains for ease of use (Table 7-6). Each class includes interventions that will improve the condition of a patient who has an alteration within the class (Box 7-7). Each intervention then has a variety of nursing activities from which to choose (Box 7-8). The NIC interventions are linked with NANDA International nursing diagnoses. For example, if a patient has a problem with activity and exercise management, e.g., *activity intolerance,* there are a variety of interventions from which to choose (e.g., body mechanics promotion or exercise promotion). NIC is a valuable resource for you to select interventions for your patients. The classification is comprehensive, including independent and collaborative interventions. It remains your decision to determine which interventions best suit your patient's needs and situation.

## Nursing Care Plan

In any health care setting, you as the nurse are responsible for providing a written plan of care for your patients. The plan of care may take several forms (e.g., nursing Kardex, standardized care plans, and computerized plans). Generally a written nursing care plan includes nursing diagnoses, goals and/or expected outcomes, and specific nursing activities and interventions. Design a written care plan to direct clinical nursing care and to decrease the risk of incomplete, incorrect, or inaccurate care. A nursing care plan is a written guideline for coordinating nursing care, promoting continuity of care, and listing outcome criteria to be used in the evaluation of nursing care. In addition, the written care plan communicates nursing care priorities to other health care

---

| BOX 7-6 | Choosing Nursing Interventions |

### Characteristics of the Nursing Diagnosis

Interventions should alter the etiological factor or signs and symptoms associated with the diagnostic label.

When an etiological factor cannot change, direct interventions toward treating the signs and symptoms (e.g., defining characteristics).

For potential or high-risk diagnoses, direct interventions at altering or eliminating risk factors for the nursing diagnoses.

### Expected Outcomes

Because an outcome is stated in terms used to evaluate the effect of an intervention, this language can assist in selecting the intervention.

*Nursing Interventions Classification (NIC)* is designed to show the link to *Nursing Outcomes Classification (NOC)* (Moorhead, Johnson, and Maas, 2004).

### Research Base

Research in support of a nursing intervention will indicate the effectiveness of using the intervention with certain patients.

Refer to research articles or evidence-based practice protocols that describe the use of research findings in similar clinical situations.

When research is not available, use scientific principles (e.g., infection control).

### Feasibility of the Intervention

A specific intervention has the potential for interacting with other interventions.

Be knowledgeable of the total plan of care.

Consider cost: Is the intervention clinically effective and cost efficient?

Consider time: Are time and personnel resources available?

### Acceptability to the Patient

Treatment plan must be acceptable to patient and family and match patient's goals, health care values, and culture.

Promote informed choice, help a patient know how to participate and anticipate the effect of interventions.

### Capability

Be prepared to carry out the intervention.

Know the scientific rationale for the intervention.

Have the necessary psychosocial and psychomotor skills to complete the intervention.

Be able to function within a particular setting and effectively and efficiently use health care resources.

Modified from Dochterman JM, Bulechek GM: *Nursing interventions classification (NIC),* ed 4, Mosby, 2004, St. Louis.

| TABLE 7-6 | Nursing Interventions Classification (NIC) Taxonomy |

| 1. **Physiological: Basic** Care that supports physical functioning | 2. **Physiological: Complex** Care that supports homeostatic regulation | 3. **Behavioral** Care that supports psychosocial functioning and facilitates life-style changes |
|---|---|---|

**Level 2 Classes**

| | | |
|---|---|---|
| A *Activity and Exercise Management:* Interventions to organize or assist with physical activity and energy conservation and expenditure | G *Electrolyte and Acid-Base Management:* Interventions to regulate electrolyte/acid-base balance and prevent complications | O *Behavior Therapy:* Interventions to reinforce or promote desirable behaviors or alter undesirable behaviors |
| B *Elimination Management:* Interventions to establish and maintain regular bowel and urinary elimination patterns and manage complications due to altered patterns | H *Drug Management:* Interventions to facilitate desired effects of pharmacological agents | P *Cognitive Therapy:* Interventions to reinforce or promote desirable cognitive functioning or alter undesirable cognitive functioning |
| C *Immobility Management:* Interventions to manage restricted body movement and the sequelae | I *Neurologic Management:* Interventions to optimize neurologic functions | Q *Communication Enhancement:* Interventions to facilitate delivering and receiving verbal and nonverbal messages |
| D *Nutrition Support:* Interventions to modify or maintain nutritional status | J *Perioperative Care:* Interventions to provide care before, during, and immediately after surgery | R *Coping Assistance:* Interventions to assist another to build on own strengths, to adapt to a change in function, or to achieve a higher level of function |
| E *Physical Comfort Promotion:* Interventions to promote comfort using physical techniques | K *Respiratory Management:* Interventions to promote airway patency and gas exchange | S *Patient Education:* Interventions to facilitate learning |
| F *Self-Care Facilitation:* Interventions to provide or assist with routine activities of daily living | L *Skin/Wound Management:* Interventions to maintain or restore tissue integrity | T *Psychological Comfort Promotion:* Interventions to promote comfort using psychological techniques |
| | M *Thermoregulation:* Interventions to maintain body temperature within a normal range | |
| | N *Tissue Perfusion Management:* Interventions to optimize circulation of blood and fluids to the tissue | |

From Dochterman JM, Bulechek GM: *Nursing interventions classification (NIC)*, ed 4, St. Louis, 2004, Mosby.

professionals. The care plan also identifies and coordinates resources used to deliver nursing care. For example, in the plan you list the specific equipment and supplies necessary for nursing treatments (e.g., dressing change).

Written care plans organize information exchanged by nurses in change-of-shift reports (see Chapter 8). You will learn to focus your reports on the nursing care and treatments and expected outcomes documented in your care plans. At the end of a shift, you will discuss care plans and the patient's overall progress with the next caregiver. Thus all nurses are able to discuss current and pertinent information about the patient's plan of care.

The nursing care plan enhances the continuity of nursing care by listing specific nursing actions necessary to achieve the goals of care. You are able to carry out these nursing activities throughout the day and from day to day. A correctly formulated nursing care plan makes it easy to continue care from one nurse to another. As a result, all nurses have the opportunity to deliver the same high-quality care.

The written care plan includes the patient's long-term needs. Incorporating the goals of the care plan into discharge planning is important. This is especially true for a patient undergoing long-term rehabilitation in the community or who will require ongoing home care. Same-day surgeries and earlier discharges from hospitals require you as the nurse to begin planning discharge needs from the moment the patient enters a health care agency. The adaptation of the care plan enhances the continuity of nursing care between

| TABLE 7-6 | Nursing Interventions Classification (NIC) Taxonomy—cont'd |
|---|---|

| Domain 4 | Domain 5 | Domain 6 | Domain 7 |
|---|---|---|---|
| **4. Safety** Care that supports protection against harm | **5. Family** Care that supports the family unit | **6. Health System** Care that supports effective use of the health care delivery system | **7. Community** Care that supports the health of the community |
| U *Crisis Management:* Interventions to provide immediate short-term help in both psychological and physiological crises<br><br>V *Risk Management:* Interventions to initiate risk-reduction activities and continue monitoring risks over time | W *Childbearing Care:* Interventions to assist in understanding and coping with the psychological and physiological changes during the childbearing period<br><br>Z *Childrearing Care:* Interventions to assist in rearing children<br><br>X *Lifespan Care:* Interventions to facilitate family unit functioning and promote the health and welfare of family members throughout the lifespan | Y *Health System Mediation:* Interventions to facilitate the interface between patient/family and the health care system<br><br>a *Health System Management:* Interventions to provide and enhance support services for the delivery of care<br><br>b *Information Management:* Interventions to facilitate communication among health care providers | c *Community Health Promotion:* Interventions that promote the health of the whole community<br><br>d *Community Risk Management:* Interventions that assist in detecting or preventing health risks to the whole community |

From Dochterman JM, Bulechek GM: *Nursing interventions classification (NIC)*, ed 4, St. Louis, 2004, Mosby.

nurses working in hospital settings and those working in community agencies. Figure 7-6 provides an example of the care plan format used throughout this text.

**STUDENT CARE PLANS.** Student care plans are useful for learning the problem-solving technique, the nursing process, skills of written communication, and organizational skills needed for nursing care. Most important, your use of the nursing care plan helps you apply knowledge gained from the nursing and medical literature and the classroom to a practice situation. Students typically write care plans for each nursing diagnosis, using a columnar format that includes assessment findings, goals, expected outcomes, nursing interventions with supporting rationales, and evaluative outcome criteria. The student care plan is more elaborate than a care plan in a hospital or community health care agency because its purpose is to teach the process of planning care. Each school uses a different format for student care plans. Some schools model the student care plan on what their related health care agencies use.

**CONCEPT MAPS.** You will care for patients who present multiple health problems and related nursing diagnoses. It is often not realistic to have a written columnar plan developed for each nursing diagnosis. Plus the columnar plans have no way to show the association between different nursing diagnoses and different nursing interventions. A **concept map** is a visual representation of patient problems and interventions that shows their relationships to one another (Schuster, 2003). The concept map is an ex-

---

**BOX 7-7** | **Examples of Level 3 Interventions for Activity and Exercise Management**

**A. Activity and Exercise Management**

Interventions to organize or assist with physical activity and energy conservation and expenditure.

**Level 3 Interventions**

Body Mechanics Promotion
Energy Management
Exercise Promotion
Exercise Promotion: Strength Training
Exercise Promotion: Stretching
Exercise Therapy: Ambulation
Exercise Therapy: Balance
Exercise Therapy: Joint Mobility
Exercise Therapy: Muscle Control
Teaching Prescribed Activity/Exercise
Examples of Linked Nursing Diagnoses:
Activity Intolerance
Fatigue
Mobility, Impaired Physical

From Dochterman JM, Bulechek GM: *Nursing interventions classification (NIC)*, ed 4, St. Louis, 2004, Mosby.

---

**BOX 7-8** | **Examples of Nursing Activities for Level 3 Interventions**

**Body Mechanics Promotion**

Instruct to use a firm mattress
Assist to demonstrate appropriate sleeping positions
Assist to avoid sitting in the same position for prolonged periods
Assist patient to identify appropriate posture exercises

**Exercise Therapy: Joint Mobility**

Initiate pain control measures before beginning joint exercise
Encourage active range-of-motion (ROM) exercises, according to regular planned schedule
Encourage patient to visualize body motion before beginning movement
Encourage ambulation, if appropriate

From Dochterman JM, Bulechek GM: *Nursing interventions classification (NIC)*, ed 4, St. Louis, 2004, Mosby.

---

tension of mind mapping, which you read about earlier. With a concept map you are able to group and categorize nursing concepts to give you a holistic perspective about your patient's health care needs and to help make clinical decisions (King and Shell, 2002).

There are different approaches to writing concept maps. Schuster (2000) suggests these simple steps in developing a clinical plan of care:

1. Before you care for a patient, gather the clinical assessment database.
2. Review all information about the patient's health problems, treatments, and medications in course textbooks, pharmacology texts and other related resources.
3. Review on the nursing unit any standardized nursing care plans, clinical pathways, protocols, or patient education materials appropriate for patient care preparation.
4. Prepare the map by first developing a skeleton diagram of the patient's health problems. Write the patient's major medical diagnoses in the middle of the map, then add associated nursing care needs like spokes on a wheel. Don't worry if you have difficulty labeling nursing diagnoses at first. It is important to recognize the major nursing care focus for the patient. Add diagnostic labels later.
5. Identify and group clinical assessment data, treatments, medications, and medical history data related to the nursing diagnoses. Remember, sometimes symptoms apply to more than one nursing diagnosis. Repeat symptoms under different categories when appropriate. For example,

place lethargy and fatigue under "activity intolerance" and "imbalanced nutrition."

6. Analyze relationships among the nursing diagnoses. Draw lines between nursing diagnoses to show relationships. The links must be accurate, meaningful and complete. You must be able to explain why nursing diagnoses are related (Figure 7-7).
7. On the map itself or a separate sheet of paper, list nursing interventions to attain the outcomes for each nursing diagnosis.
8. While caring for your patient, write down the patient's responses to each nursing activity. Also write your clinical impressions and inferences regarding the patient's progress toward expected outcomes and the effectiveness of interventions.
9. Keep the concept map with you throughout the clinical day. As you revise the plan, take notes and add or delete nursing interventions.

The concept map is very useful because it provides a deeper and more complete understanding of the patient's needs, problems, strengths, and weaknesses (King and Shell, 2002).

**CRITICAL PATHWAYS.** **Critical pathways** allow staff from all disciplines, such as medicine, nursing, and pharmacy, to develop integrated care plans for a projected length of stay or number of visits for patients with a specific case type (Zander and McGill, 1994). For example, a pathway for a surgical procedure will recommend on a day-by-day basis the patient's activities, consults, procedures, discharge planning activities, and educational topics expected for the patient's progression to discharge. A pathway ensures continuity of care because it maps out clearly the responsibility of each health care discipline. Well developed, pathways incorporate evidence-based protocols used in the care of the spe-

## CARE PLAN   Activity Tolerance

### ASSESSMENT

Mrs. Bryan has been participating in progressive exercises for only about 1 week. Inez makes a visit to Mrs. Bryan's home for a follow-up visit. Mrs. Bryan is cheerful but continues to report feeling tired. Mrs. Bryan explains, **"I think I am feeling a little stronger, but I still become breathless when I go up and down the stairs."** Mrs. Bryan notes that she wishes she had started regular exercise sooner. She has been doing exercises 3 times a day for a week. Inez walks with Mrs. Bryan back and forth down her bedroom hall. Mrs. Bryan's **pulse before walking was 88 beats per minute but increased to 100 beats minute after walking** and **remained at that level for 3 minutes before falling to the low 90s.** Mrs. Bryan is able to walk with a steady gait. She occasionally holds on to furniture and the walls when she walks for any distance. Inez notes that Mrs. Bryan **walked a farther distance (approximately 20 feet)** during this visit than a week ago.

*Defining characteristics are shown in bold type.

---

### NURSING DIAGNOSIS  Activity intolerance related to sedentary lifestyle

---

### PLANNING

**GOAL**

• Patient's activity tolerance will improve.

**EXPECTED OUTCOMES***
**Activity Tolerance***

• Patient will report less fatigue after walking 100 feet within 2 weeks.
• Patient's heart rate will return to baseline within 5 minutes of exercise.

*Outcomes classification label from Moorhead S, Johnson M, Maas M: *Nursing outcomes classification (NOC)*, ed 3, St. Louis, 2004, Mosby.

---

| INTERVENTIONS† | RATIONALE |
|---|---|
| **Activity Therapy** | |
| • Perform progressive walking exercise plan. | Adults should accumulate 30 minutes or more a day of moderate-intensity activity (Konradi and Anglin, 2003). |
| • Walk up and down hallway to kitchen (for 10 minutes) 3 times per day, increase to two cycles in 2 weeks. | |
| • Have patient maintain an exercise log (pulse, feelings, breathlessness, distance). | Provides positive reinforcement and may increase adherence to exercise prescription. |
| • Have patient perform flexibility exercises in AM after awakening. | Stretches all muscle groups and joints. Improves flexibility, circulation, and posture. |
| **Energy Management** | |
| • Increase number of uninterrupted rest periods to 20 minutes twice a day. | Improves patient's energy reserve. |
| • Plan walking at times when patient feels most rested (1 hour after breakfast, just before lunch, 1 hour before dinner). | |

†Intervention classification labels from Dochterman JM, Bulechek GM, editors: *Nursing interventions classification (NIC)*, ed 4, St. Louis, 2004.

---

### EVALUATION

• Measure patient's heart rate before and after walking, then again 3 and 5 minutes after exercise.
• Ask patient to describe how she feels and whether she is comfortable with breathing before and after exercise.

• Review Mrs. Bryan's exercise log.

FIGURE **7-6**  Care plan.

cific case type. You can use the pathway to monitor a patient's progress and as a documentation tool.

## Consulting Other Health Care Professionals

Consultation occurs at any step in the nursing process, but you will do this most often during planning and intervention. During these times you are more likely to identify a problem requiring additional knowledge or skills or a need

to obtain community or agency resources. **Consultation** is a process in which you seek another health care provider's (such as a dietitian, physical therapist, or clinical nurse specialist) help to identify ways to handle problems in patient care management or problems related to the planning and implementation of programs. Consultation is based on the problem-solving approach, and the consultant is the motivator for change. Oftentimes a senior nurse is a valuable con-

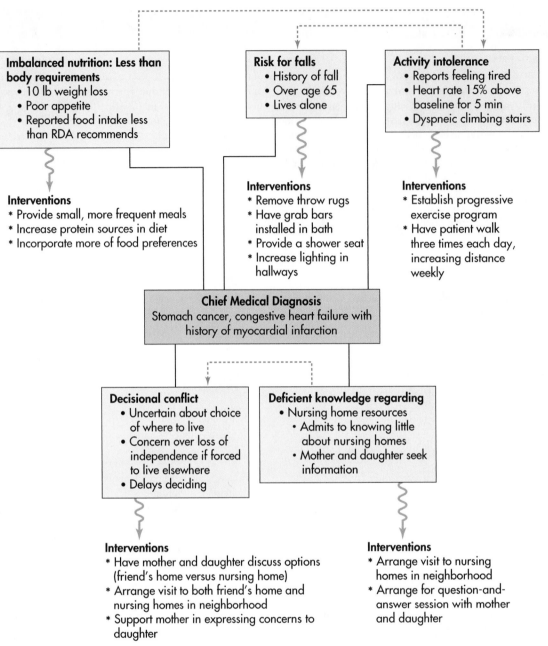

**Imbalanced nutrition: Less than body requirements**
• 10 lb weight loss
• Poor appetite
• Reported food intake less than RDA recommends

**Interventions**
* Provide small, more frequent meals
* Increase protein sources in diet
* Incorporate more of food preferences

**Risk for falls**
• History of fall
• Over age 65
• Lives alone

**Interventions**
* Remove throw rugs
* Have grab bars installed in bath
* Provide a shower seat
* Increase lighting in hallways

**Activity intolerance**
• Reports feeling tired
• Heart rate 15% above baseline for 5 min
• Dyspneic climbing stairs

**Interventions**
* Establish progressive exercise program
* Have patient walk three times each day, increasing distance weekly

**Chief Medical Diagnosis**
Stomach cancer, congestive heart failure with history of myocardial infarction

**Decisional conflict**
• Uncertain about choice of where to live
• Concern over loss of independence if forced to live elsewhere
• Delays deciding

**Deficient knowledge regarding**
• Nursing home resources
• Admits to knowing little about nursing homes
• Mother and daughter seek information

**Interventions**
* Have mother and daughter discuss options (friend's home versus nursing home)
* Arrange visit to both friend's home and nursing homes in neighborhood
* Support mother in expressing concerns to daughter

**Interventions**
* Arrange visit to nursing homes in neighborhood
* Arrange for question-and-answer session with mother and daughter

FIGURE **7-7** Concept map.

sult when you face an unfamiliar patient care situation. Through consultation and collaboration you are able to use the best resources to individualize nursing actions to meet expected outcomes.

**WHEN TO CONSULT.** Consultation occurs when you identify a problem that you cannot solve using personal knowledge, skills, and resources. Consultation with other care providers increases your knowledge about the patient's problem and helps you to learn skills and obtain the resources you need to solve the problem. A good time to consult with another health care professional is when the exact problem remains unclear.

**HOW TO CONSULT.** Begin with your own understanding of a patient's clinical problems. The first step in making

a consult is to identify the general problem area. Second, direct the consultation to the appropriate professional, such as another nurse, a social worker, or another member of the health care team.

Third, provide the consultant with relevant information and resources about the problem area. Include a pertinent, brief summary of the problem, methods used to resolve the problem, and outcomes of those methods. Other resources may include the patient's medical record and conversations with nurses, other members of the health team, and the patient's family.

Fourth, do not prejudice or influence consultants. Consultants are in the clinical setting to help identify and resolve a nursing problem, and biasing or prejudicing them can block problem resolution. Avoid bias by not overloading consultants with subjective and emotional conclusions about the patient and problem.

Fifth, be available to discuss the consultant's findings and recommendations. When you request a consultation, provide a private, comfortable atmosphere for the consultant and patient to meet. However, this does not mean that you leave the environment. A common mistake is turning the whole problem over to the consultant. The consultant is not there to take over the problem but to assist you in resolving the problem. When possible, request the consultation for a day when both you and the consultant are scheduled to work and during a time when there are few distractions.

Finally, incorporate the consultant's recommendations into the care plan. The success of the advice depends on the implementation of the problem-solving techniques suggested.

## Implementation

**Implementation,** the fourth step of the nursing process, begins after you develop the care plan. It involves the provision of care to patients. Implementation describes the performance of nursing interventions necessary for achieving the goals and expected outcomes of nursing care. A **nursing intervention** is any treatment, based upon clinical judgment and knowledge, that a nurse performs to enhance patient outcomes (Dochterman and Bulechek, 2004). Interventions include both direct and indirect care; those aimed at individuals, families, and the community.

**Direct care interventions** are treatments performed through interaction with the patient. For example, a patient may require medication administration, insertion of an intravenous infusion, or counseling during a time of grief. **Indirect care interventions** are treatments performed away from the patient but on behalf of the patient or group of patients (Dochterman and Bulechek, 2004). Examples include action aimed at managing the patient's environment (safety and infection control), documentation, and interdisciplinary collaboration. Implementation is continuous with all steps of the nursing process. As you carry out an intervention, the patient's condition can change, requiring further assessment, or the patient may respond to the intervention as expected based on your evaluation.

### Types of Nursing Interventions

Direct and indirect care interventions include those you read about earlier: nurse-initiated, physician-initiated, and collaborative. At times you develop, communicate, and organize nursing interventions on the basis of protocols or preprinted (standing) orders. An understanding of these guidelines is necessary for safe nursing practice.

**PROTOCOLS AND STANDING ORDERS.** A **protocol** is a written plan specifying the procedures to be followed during care of patients with a select clinical condition or situation, such as the administration of chemotherapy. A protocol provides a standard of care or clinical guideline, which you individualize for a specific patient, depending on institutional policy. Nurses, who provide primary care for pa-

tients in outpatient settings, frequently follow diagnostic and treatment protocols. The established protocols describe the conditions that nurses are permitted to treat, such as controlled hypertension, and the recommended treatment plan. This includes therapies the nurse is permitted to administer, such as diet counseling, stress management, and prescriptions for antihypertensives. Protocols are nursing, medical, or interdisciplinary.

A **standing order** is a preprinted document containing orders for the conduct of routine therapies, monitoring guidelines, and/or diagnostic procedures for specific patients with identified clinical problems. The orders direct the conduct of patient care in various clinical settings. Licensed, prescribing physicians or health care providers in charge of care at the time of implementation approve and sign standing orders. These orders are commonly found in critical care settings and other specialized practice settings where patients' needs can change rapidly and require immediate attention. Standing orders are also common in the community health setting, when the nurse encounters situations that do not permit immediate contact with a physician or health care provider. Thus protocols and standing orders give you the legal protection to intervene appropriately in the patient's best interest.

Before implementing any intervention use sound judgment in determining whether an intervention is correct and appropriate. You also have the responsibility to obtain correct theoretical knowledge and develop the clinical competencies necessary to safely perform the intervention. Nursing responsibility is equally great for all types of interventions.

### Critical Thinking in Implementation

The selection of nursing interventions for a patient is part of clinical decision making. The critical thinking model discussed in Chapter 6 provides a framework for how to make decisions when implementing nursing care. You will learn how to implement a care plan using appropriate knowledge. For example, an important knowledge base is the NIC. The interventions found within NIC help to differentiate nursing practice from the practice of other health care professionals. NIC interventions include 514 nursing interventions such as anxiety reduction, infection control, and postmortem care, along with over 12,000 nursing activities (Dochterman and Bulechek, 2004). Each intervention has a list of nursing activities from which you can choose to individualize for a particular patient. In addition, NIC is linked to NANDA International diagnoses and NOC outcomes, which helps to show the relationship between a patient's diagnoses, outcomes, and selected interventions.

You will also apply prior clinical experiences in performing specific interventions. Consider what interventions have worked before and what have not worked in previous clinical situations. Be aware of both professional and agency standards of practice. The standards of practice offer guidelines for selection of interventions, their frequency, and the determination of whether the procedures may be delegated. As you perform any nursing intervention, apply intellectual standards. For example, a patient instruction should be relevant, clear, logical, and complete to promote patient learning. All critical thinking attitudes, such as confidence, creativity, and self-discipline apply to the implementation process. A beginning student will need supervision from an instructor or experienced nurse to guide the decision-making process for implementation.

## Implementation Process

Preparation for implementation ensures efficient, safe, and effective nursing care. Follow these five preparatory activities: reassess the patient, review and revise the existing nursing care plan, organize resources and care delivery, anticipate and prevent complications, and implement nursing interventions.

**REASSESSING THE PATIENT.** Assessment is a continuous process that occurs each time you interact with a patient. When you gather new data and identify a new patient need, you modify the care plan. You also modify a plan when you resolve a patient's health care need. During the initial phase of implementation, reassess the patient. This is a partial assessment and sometimes focuses on one dimension of the patient, such as level of comfort, or on one system, such as the cardiovascular system. The reassessment helps you to decide if the proposed nursing action is still appropriate for the patient's level of wellness. For example, you planned to ambulate a patient following lunch; however, a reassessment reveals shortness of breath and increased fatigue, which require you to assist the patient back to bed.

**REVIEWING AND REVISING THE CARE PLAN.** After reassessing a patient, review the care plan, compare assessment data to validate the stated nursing diagnoses, and determine whether the nursing interventions remain the most appropriate. If the patient's status has changed and the nursing diagnosis and related interventions are no longer appropriate, modify the nursing care plan. An out-of-date or incorrect care plan compromises the quality of nursing care. Review and modification enable you to provide timely nursing interventions to best meet the patient's needs. There are four steps to modifying the written care plan:

1. Revise data in the assessment section to reflect the patient's current status. Date any new data to inform other health team members of the time that the change occurred.
2. Revise the nursing diagnoses. Delete diagnoses that are no longer relevant, and add any new diagnoses. It is necessary to revise related factors, as well as the patient's goals, outcomes, and priorities. Date any revisions.
3. Revise specific interventions that correspond to the new nursing diagnoses and goals. This revision should reflect the patient's present status.
4. Determine the method of evaluation to achieve outcomes.

In the case study for Mrs. Bryan, her plan of care required multiple collaborative interventions. As her fatigue and weight loss progressed, she became weaker and her nursing needs changed. Mrs. Bryan moved in with a friend, and more community, friends, and family resources were used to safely maintain Mrs. Bryan's independence. Table 7-7 illustrates another example of a revised care plan.

**ORGANIZING RESOURCES AND CARE DELIVERY.** A facility's resources include equipment and skilled personnel. Organization of equipment and personnel makes timely, efficient, skilled patient care possible. Preparation for care delivery also involves preparing the environment and patient for the nursing intervention.

**Equipment.** Most nursing procedures require some equipment or supplies. Before delivering an intervention, decide what supplies are necessary and determine their availability. Equipment should be in working order to ensure safe use. Place supplies in a convenient location to provide easy access during the procedure. Extra supplies should be available in case of errors or accidents, but do not open extra supplies unless they are needed. This controls health care costs. After a procedure, return any unopened supplies.

**Personnel.** The model of care (e.g., primary nursing versus total patient care) used by nursing varies among health care facilities and determines the way in which personnel are designated for patient care delivery. For example, a primary nurse is accountable for the nursing care a patient receives during his or her length of stay. A team nurse is accountable for the specific shift in which he or she works. It is the nurse's responsibility to determine whether to perform an intervention or to delegate it to another member of the nursing team. Your assessment of a patient directs the decision about delegation and not the intervention alone. For example, you know assistive personnel can competently ambulate patients. However, you learn that a patient experienced cardiac irregularities during the previous shift, so you decide to personally assist the patient with ambulation and evaluate the patient's cardiac status. In this case, you use the assistive personnel to perform an intervention for a more stable patient.

Nursing staff work together when patient needs demand it. If a patient makes a request, such as use of a bedpan, position the patient on the pan if you have time rather than trying to find the technician who is in a different room. When interventions are complex or physically difficult, you may need assistance from colleagues. You will be more effective in performing procedures when a technician assists with patient positioning and handing off supplies.

**Environment.** A patient's care environment should be safe and conducive to the implementation of therapies. Patient safety is your first concern. If the patient has sensory deficits, physical disability, or an alteration in level of consciousness, arrange the environment to prevent injury. Provide assistive devices (e.g., walkers or eyeglasses), rearrange furniture and equipment, and make rooms free of clutter.

The patient benefits most from nursing interventions when surroundings are compatible with activities. When you need to expose a patient's body parts, do so privately because the patient will be more relaxed. Reducing distractions enhances learning opportunities. Make sure the lighting is adequate to perform procedures correctly.

| TABLE 7-7 | A Revised Nursing Care Plan |

**Nursing diagnosis:** Ineffective airway clearance related to pain of abdominal incision
**Definition:** Ineffective airway clearance is the state in which an individual is unable to clear secretions or obstructions from the respiratory tract to maintain airway patency.

| Assessment | Goals | Implementation | Evaluation (Achieved Outcomes) |
|---|---|---|---|
| Smoked two packs/day for 20 years; chest x-ray film showing slight change of emphysema; crackles auscultated in RRL; scheduled for abdominal surgery | Airway will remain clear (11/8) as evidenced by: *Lungs clear to auscultation (11/8)* *Patient coughs productively (11/8)* | Demonstrate turn, cough, and deep breathing to patient. Patient demonstrates turning, coughing, and deep breathing exercises. | Patient able to cough productively *11/8*. Airway is clear to auscultation in all lobes (*not met 11/8*). |

**Modified 24 Hours After Surgery**

**Nursing diagnosis:** Ineffective airway clearance related to decreased inspiratory effort secondary to pain of abdominal incision

| | | | |
|---|---|---|---|
| Decreased chest wall movements; crackles bilateral in bases that do not clear with coughing; elevated temperature (39° C [102.2 ° F]); reports incisional pain 6 on scale of 0 to 10 | Airways will remain clear (11/9) as evidenced by: *Lungs clear to auscultation (11/10)* *Temperature <100° F (11/9)* *Pain intensity less than baseline by 11/9* | Administer chest physiotherapy to all lobes of the lung: 08-12-16-20-24-04. Have patient perform incentive spirometry every 2 hours around the clock. Teach patient to splint incision with pillow before and during coughing. Administer analgesics as ordered for incisional pain. | Lung fields are clear on auscultation. Patient becomes afebrile *11/9*. Chest x-ray film demonstrates atelectasis resolving *11/10*. |

**Patient.** Before you begin to perform interventions, be sure the patient is as physically and psychologically comfortable as possible. Symptoms such as nausea, dizziness, or pain, for example, frequently interfere with a patient's full concentration and cooperation. Offer comfort measures before initiating interventions to help the patient participate more fully. If you need a patient to be alert, administer a dose of pain medication to relieve discomfort but not impair mental faculties (e.g., ability to follow instruction, reasoning, and communication).

Even if symptoms are not a factor, make the patient physically comfortable during interventions. Start any intervention by controlling environmental factors, positioning, and taking care of other physical needs (e.g., elimination). Also consider the patient's level of endurance, and plan only the amount of activity the patient can comfortably tolerate.

Awareness of the patient's psychosocial needs helps you create a favorable emotional climate. Some patients feel reassured by having a significant other present for encouragement and moral support. Other strategies include planning sufficient time or multiple opportunities for the patient to work through and ventilate feelings and anxieties. Adequate preparation allows the patient to obtain maximal benefit from each intervention.

**ANTICIPATING AND PREVENTING COMPLICATIONS.** Risks to patients come from both illness and treatment. As the nurse, you must identify these risks, evaluate the relative benefit of the treatment versus the risk, and initiate risk prevention measures. Many conditions place the patient at risk for complications. For example, the patient with preexisting chronic lung disease is at risk for developing pneumonia following abdominal surgery. Your knowledge of pathophysiology helps to identify possible complications that can occur. A thorough assessment reveals the level of the patient's current risk. Scientific rationales for how certain interventions (e.g., coughing techniques and postural drainage) prevent or minimize complications help you plan useful preventive measures.

Some nursing procedures also pose risks for the patient. You need to be aware of potential complications and take precautionary measures. For instance, the patient using a feeding tube is at risk for aspiration. In this situation, elevate the head of the bed and have pharyngeal suction equipment at the bedside before initiating the feedings.

**Identifying Areas of Assistance.** Certain nursing situations require you to obtain assistance by seeking additional personnel, knowledge, and/or nursing skills. Before beginning care, review the plan to determine the need for assistance and the type required. You may need assistance in performing a procedure, comforting a patient, or preparing the patient for a procedure. For example, when you are assigned to care for an overweight immobilized patient, you may require additional personnel to help to turn and position the patient. Be sure to determine the number of additional personnel in advance and when you need them. Discuss your need for assistance with potential resources, such as other nurses or assistive personnel.

You will require additional knowledge and skills in situations in which you are less familiar or experienced. You need additional knowledge when administering a new medication or implementing a new procedure. You find such information in a hospital's formulary or procedure book. If you are still uncertain about the new medication or procedure, ask other members of the health care team.

Because of the continual growth in health care technology, you may lack the skills needed to perform a new procedure. When this occurs, first locate information about the procedure in the literature and the agency's procedures book. Next, collect all equipment necessary for the procedure. Finally, ask another nurse who has completed the procedure correctly and safely to provide assistance and guidance. The assistance can come from another staff nurse, a supervisor, educator, or a nurse specialist. Requesting assistance occurs frequently in practice and is a learning process that continues throughout educational experiences and into professional development.

## Implementation Skills

Nursing practice includes cognitive, interpersonal, and psychomotor (technical) skills. You need each type of skill to implement direct and indirect nursing interventions. You are responsible for knowing when one type of implementation skill is preferred over another and for having the necessary knowledge and skill to perform each.

**COGNITIVE SKILLS.** Cognitive skills involve application of knowledge from nursing and other disciplines. Use good judgment and make sound clinical decisions during any nursing intervention. This ensures that no nursing action is automatic. Always think and anticipate so that patient care is appropriate and individualized. Know the rationale for therapeutic interventions, and understand normal and abnormal physiological and psychological responses. Know nursing science, be able to identify patient learning and discharge needs, and recognize the patient's health promotion and illness prevention needs.

**INTERPERSONAL SKILLS.** Interpersonal skills are essential for effective nursing action. Develop a trusting relationship, express a level of caring, and communicate clearly with the patient and family. Good communication is critical for keeping patients informed, providing effective teaching, and effectively supporting patients who have challenging emotional needs. Proper use of interpersonal skills enables you to be perceptive of the patient's verbal and nonverbal communication.

**PSYCHOMOTOR SKILLS.** Psychomotor skills require the integration of cognitive and motor activities, such as learning to give an injection. You must understand anatomy and pharmacology (cognitive) and use good coordination and precision to administer the injection correctly (motor). With time and practice you will learn to perform skills correctly, smoothly, and confidently. This is critical in establishing patient trust. You are responsible for acquiring necessary psychomotor skills. In the case of a new skill, assess your level of competency and obtain the necessary resources to ensure the patient receives safe treatment.

## Direct Care

As a nurse you will provide a wide variety of direct care measures. Always remember that any care activity involves patient interaction. Remain sensitive to a patient's clinical condition, values and beliefs, expectations, and cultural views. This will ensure an individualized approach to care.

**ACTIVITIES OF DAILY LIVING.** Activities of daily living (ADLs) are activities usually performed during a normal day; including ambulation, eating, dressing, bathing and grooming. A patient's need for assistance with ADLs may be temporary, as in the case of an acute illness, permanent, or rehabilitative. A patient with impaired mobility because of bilateral arm casts has a temporary need for assistance. After the casts are removed, the patient will gradually regain the strength and range of motion needed to perform ADLs. A patient with an irreversible injury to the cervical spinal cord is paralyzed and thus has a permanent need for assistance. It would be unrealistic to plan rehabilitation with the goal of the patient becoming independent with ADLs. Instead, through restorative care, the patient will learn new ways to perform ADLs, becoming more independent.

There are patients who will likely require ADL assistance. When your assessment reveals a patient is experiencing fatigue, a limitation in mobility, confusion, and pain, assistance with ADLs is likely. Assistance can range from partial to complete care. Always consider a patient's preferences when assisting with ADLs. Involving the patient in planning the timing and types of interventions boosts the patient's self-esteem and willingness to become more independent.

**INSTRUMENTAL ACTIVITIES OF DAILY LIVING.** Illness or disability sometimes alters a patient's ability to be independent in society. **Instrumental activities of daily living (IADLs)** include skills such as shopping, preparing meals, writing checks, and taking medications. Nurses in home care and community nursing frequently assist patients in adapting ways to perform IADLs. Often family and friends are excellent resources for assisting patients. In acute care it is important for you to anticipate how a patient's illness might affect the ability to perform IADLs so that you make the appropriate referrals.

**PHYSICAL CARE.** You will routinely perform a variety of physical care techniques when caring for a patient. Examples include turning and positioning, performing invasive procedures, and administering medications. Physical care techniques involve the safe and competent administration of nursing procedures. The specific knowledge and skills needed to perform these procedures are found in subsequent clinical chapters of this text. Common methods for administering physical care techniques appropriately include protecting you and the patient from injury, using proper infection control practices, staying organized, and positioning patients correctly.

**COUNSELING. Counseling** is a direct care method that helps the patient use a problem-solving process to recognize and manage stress and to facilitate interpersonal relationships. As a nurse you will counsel patients to accept actual or impending changes resulting from stress. Counseling involves emotional, intellectual, spiritual, and psychological support. A patient and family who need nursing counseling have normal adjustment difficulties and are upset or frustrated, but they are not necessarily psychologically disabled. A good example is the stress a young woman may face when caring for her aging mother. However, patients with psychiatric diagnoses require therapy by nurses specializing in psychiatric nursing or by social workers, psychologists, or psychiatrists.

Nurse counseling encourages patients to examine available alternatives and decide which choices are useful and appropriate. When patients are able to examine alternatives, they develop a sense of control and are able to better manage stress.

**TEACHING.** Teaching is an important nursing responsibility. In teaching, the focus of change is intellectual growth, learning new knowledge or psychomotor skills (Redman, 2001). Teaching is used to present correct principles, procedures, and techniques of health care to patients and to inform patients about their health status (see Chapter 10). Teaching takes place in all health care settings (Figure 7-8). As a nurse you are responsible for assessing the learning needs and readiness of patients and you are accountable for the quality of education you deliver. The teaching-learning process is an interaction between the teacher and learner in which you address specific learning objectives. This process offers an organizational structure and framework for patient education.

**CONTROLLING FOR ADVERSE REACTIONS.** An **adverse reaction** is a harmful or unintended effect of a medication, diagnostic test, or therapeutic intervention. Adverse reactions can follow any nursing intervention, so learn to anticipate and know the adverse reactions to expect. For example, the patient receiving a tube feeding is at risk for aspiration. Steps to take to prevent aspiration are to elevate the head of the bed and have pharyngeal suction at the bedside before starting the feeding. Controlling for adverse reactions involves reducing risk or counteracting the effect. When administering a medication, understand the known and potential side effects of the drug. After administration of the medication, evaluate the patient's response for adverse effects. Also know the drugs available to counteract any side effects.

**PREVENTIVE MEASURES. Preventive nursing actions** promote health and prevent illness to avoid the need for acute or rehabilitative health care. Prevention includes assessment and promotion of the patient's health potential, application of prescribed measures (e.g., immunizations), health teaching, and identification of risks for illness and/or trauma. Consider the situation of Mrs. Bryan, who has had a fall in the past and has experienced continued weakness. Inez implements preventive measures to make Mrs. Bryan's home setting safer. With Mrs. Bryan's deciding to live with a friend, Inez will conduct a home environment assessment and choose the interventions (e.g., installing grab bars in the bath and arranging furniture) that will ensure Mrs. Bryan's safety and ability to move about comfortably in her new home.

All patients need preventive nursing interventions aimed at promoting health and preventing illness. As changes in the health care system continue, there is and will be greater emphasis on health promotion and illness prevention.

## Indirect Care

Indirect care measures are actions that support the effectiveness of direct care measures (Dochterman and Bulechek, 2004). Many indirect measures are managerial in nature, such as emergency cart maintenance. Others are environmental, such as specimen and supply management. A good amount of a nurse's time is spent in indirect care activities. Communication of information about patients (e.g., change of shift report and consultation) is critical to ensuring that direct care activities are planned and coordinated with proper resources. Delegation of care to assistive personnel is another indirect care activity. Proper delegation ensures that the right care providers perform the right tasks so that an RN and assistive personnel work most efficiently for the patient.

**DELEGATING, SUPERVISING, AND EVALUATING THE WORK OF OTHER STAFF MEMBERS.** Depending on the system of health care delivery, the nurse who develops the care plan frequently does not perform all of the nursing interventions. Some activities you will coordinate and delegate to other members of the health care team (see Chapter 24). Noninvasive and frequently repetitive interventions such as skin care, ambulation, grooming, and hygiene measures are examples of care activities that you will assign to assistive personnel such as certified nurse assistants. Licensed practical nurses perform these measures in addition to medication administration and many invasive tasks (e.g., dressing care and catheterization). When you delegate aspects of care to another staff member, you are responsible for assigning the

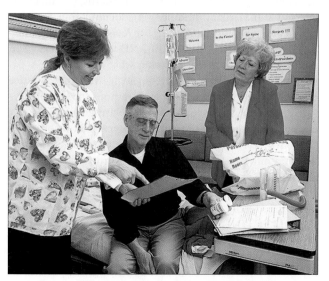

FIGURE **7-8** Teaching patient discharge instructions.

task and making sure the staff member completes the task according to the standard of care. You are also responsible for delegating direct care interventions to personnel competent to provide the care (McCloskey and others, 1996).

## ✳ Evaluation

When a repairman comes to a home to fix a leaking faucet, he turns the faucet on, observes the flow of water, and determines the problem. Then he changes parts to the faucet and turns the faucet on once again to see if the leak is fixed. After a patient diagnosed with pneumonia has completed a 5-day dose pack of antibiotics, the physician or health care provider has the patient return to the office to have a chest x-ray examination to determine if the pneumonia has cleared. When a nurse on a surgical unit provides wound care, he or she first assesses the appearance of the wound, applies the appropriate dressing, and then returns later to determine if the wound has healed. These three scenarios depict what ultimately occurs during the process of evaluation, the last step of the nursing process. The repairman rechecks the faucet, the physician or health care provider orders a chest x-ray examination, and the nurse reinspects the wound. Evaluation involves an examination of a condition or situation and then a judgment as to whether change has occurred. Ideally, after an intervention takes place, evaluation should reveal improvement.

**Evaluation** is crucial to determine whether after application of the nursing process, a patient's condition or well-being improves. The nurse applies all that is known about a patient and the patient's condition, as well as experience with previous patients, to evaluate if nursing care was effective. The nurse conducts evaluation to determine if expected outcomes are met, not if nursing interventions were completed. The expected outcomes are the standards against which you judge if goals have been met and if care is successful.

### Critical Thinking and Evaluation

Evaluation is an ongoing process whenever you have contact with a patient. Once you deliver an intervention, you gather subjective and objective data from the patient, family, and health care team members. You also review knowledge regarding the patient's current condition, treatment, resources available for recovery, and the expected outcomes. By referring to previous experiences caring for similar patients, you are in a better position to know how to evaluate your patient. You also apply critical thinking attitudes and standards to determine whether outcomes of care are achieved. If outcomes are met, the overall goals for the patient are also met. You compare patient behavior and responses assessed before delivering nursing interventions with behavior and responses that occur after administering nursing care. Critical thinking directs you to analyze the findings from evaluation. Has the patient's condition improved? Can the patient improve, or are there physical factors preventing recovery? To what degree does this patient's motivation or willingness to pursue healthier behavior influence response to therapies?

In evaluation you make clinical decisions and continually redirect nursing care. For example, when evaluating your patient for a change in vital signs, you apply knowledge of disease processes, physiological responses to interventions, and the correct procedure for vital sign measurement to interpret whether a change has occurred and whether the change is desirable. A patient in acute pain may have an increased heart rate, blood pressure, and increased muscle tension. You know that this is a sympathetic nervous system response to painful stimuli. You administer a pain medication, help the patient try a relaxation exercise, and reposition the patient. Then you return to evaluate if the patient's perception of pain has decreased and if the vital signs have returned either to a more acceptable level or to the patient's baseline before pain.

Positive evaluations occur when you meet desired results and lead you to conclude that the nursing intervention effectively met the patient's goal of improved comfort. Negative evaluations or undesired results indicate that the intervention was not effective in minimizing or resolving the actual problem or avoiding a potential problem. Possibly new data about the patient's condition have altered the patient's ability to meet the established outcome. As a result, change the care plan and try different therapies or a different approach in administering existing therapies.

This sequence of critically evaluating and revising therapies continues until you and the patient appropriately resolve the problems. Outcomes must be realistic and adjusted based on the patient's prognosis and nursing diagnoses. Remember that evaluation is dynamic and ever changing, depending on the patient's nursing diagnoses and condition. A patient whose health status continuously changes requires more frequent evaluation. In addition, priority diagnoses are usually evaluated first. For example, you might evaluate a patient's *acute pain* before evaluating the status of *deficient knowledge*.

### The Evaluation Process

The evaluation process includes five elements: (1) identifying evaluative criteria and standards, (2) collecting data to determine if you met the criteria or standards, (3) interpreting and summarizing findings, (4) documenting findings, and (5) terminating, continuing, or revising the care plan.

**IDENTIFYING CRITERIA AND STANDARDS.** You evaluate nursing care by knowing what to look for. A patient's goals and expected outcomes give you the objective criteria needed to judge a patient's response to care. In the case of Mrs. Bryan, she has the goal of "Patient's activity tolerance will improve in 1 month." The expected outcomes are "Patient's heart rate will return to the normal resting rate within 5 minutes following monitored progressive exercise" and "Patient will report less fatigue following walking within 2 weeks." The patient's heart rate and self-report of fatigue following exercise are your criteria for evaluation.

**COLLECTING EVALUATIVE DATA.** Remember that proper evaluation will allow you to answer the following questions: What is the patient's response to nursing care? Was the therapy effective in improving the patient's physical or emotional health? Evaluative measures are simply the assessment skills and techniques you use to collect data for evaluation. Examples of evaluative measures include auscultation of lung sounds, observation of a patient's skill performance, or inspection of the skin. In Mrs. Bryan's case, evaluative measures used for improving activity tolerance include measuring heart rate following exercise and comparing the rate with baseline. A second evaluative measure is to ask the patient to describe or rate her level of fatigue after exercise.

In many clinical situations it is important to collect evaluative measures over a period of time to determine if a pattern of improvement or change exists. A one-time observation of a pressure ulcer is insufficient to determine that the ulcer is healing. You want to see a consistency in change. For example, over a period of 2 days is the pressure ulcer decreasing in size? Is the amount of drainage declining? Recognizing a pattern of improvement or decline allows you to reason and decide if the patient's problems are resolved (Table 7-8).

**INTERPRETING AND SUMMARIZING FINDINGS.** An expert nurse recognizes relevant evidence, even evidence that sometimes does not match clinical expectations, and makes judgments about a patient's condition. To develop clinical judgment you learn to match the results of evaluative measures with expected outcomes to determine if a patient's status is improving or not. When interpreting findings, you compare the patient's behavioral responses and physiological signs and symptoms you expect to see with those actually seen during evaluation. In the case of Mrs. Bryan you compare the patient's heart rate 5 minutes after exercise with her normal resting heart rate. If the heart rate is higher than resting baseline, you determine that the patient did not tolerate exercise and you need a change in the plan. If the heart rate returned to baseline, the plan of care could continue or you might decide the patient's activity intolerance was resolved.

Evaluation is easier to perform after you care for a patient over a period of time. You can then make subtle comparisons of patient responses and behaviors. When you have not had the chance to care for a patient over an extended time, evaluation improves by referring to previous experiences and asking colleagues, familiar with the patient, to confirm evaluation findings.

Remember to evaluate each expected outcome and its place in the sequence of care. If not, it will be difficult to determine which outcome in the sequence faltered. This prevents you from revising and redirecting the plan of care at the most appropriate time.

**DOCUMENTING FINDINGS.** Documentation and reporting are an important part of evaluation. Accurate information must be present in a patient's medical record for nurses to make ongoing clinical decisions. When documenting the patient's response to interventions, always describe the same evaluative measures. Your aim is to present a clear argument from the evaluative data as to whether a patient is progressing or not. Written nursing progress notes, assessment flow sheets, and information shared between nurses during change-of-shift reports (see Chapter 8) communicate a patient's progress toward meeting expected outcomes and goals for the nursing plan of care.

**CARE PLAN REVISION.** As you evaluate expected outcomes, you determine if the goals of care have been met. You then decide if you need to adjust the plan of care. If you meet a goal successfully, discontinue that portion of the care plan. Unmet and partially met goals require you to continue intervention. After you evaluate a patient, you may want to modify or add nursing diagnoses with appropriate goals and expected outcomes, and establish interventions. You must also redefine priorities. This is an important step in critical thinking—knowing how the patient is progressing and how problems either resolve or worsen.

Careful monitoring and early detection of problems are a patient's first line of defense (Benner, Stannard, and Hooper, 1996). Base clinical judgments on your observations of what is occurring with a specific patient and not merely what happens to patients in general. Frequently changes are not very obvious. Evaluations are patient specific, based on a close familiarity with each patient's behavior, physical status, and reaction to caregivers.

**Discontinuing a Care Plan.** After you determine that expected outcomes and goals have been met, you confirm this evaluation with the patient when possible. If you and the patient agree, then you discontinue that portion of the care plan. Documentation of a discontinued plan ensures that other

| TABLE 7-8 | **Evaluation Measures to Determine the Success of Goals and Expected Outcomes** | |
| --- | --- | --- |
| **Goals** | **Evaluation Measures** | **Expected Outcomes** |
| Patient's pressure ulcer will demonstrate signs of healing within 7 days. | Inspect color, condition, and location of pressure ulcer. | Erythema will be reduced in 2 days. |
| | Note odor and color of drainage from ulcer. | Ulcer will have no drainage in 2 days. |
| | Measure diameter of ulcer daily. | Skin overlying ulcer will begin to close in 7 days. |
| | | Diameter of ulcer will decrease in 5 days. |
| Patient will tolerate ambulation to end of hall by 11/20. | Palpate patient's radial pulse before exercise. | Pulse will remain below 110 beats per minute during exercise. |
| | Palpate patient's radial pulse 5 minutes after exercise. | Pulse rate will return to resting baseline within 10 minutes after exercise. |
| | Assess respiratory rate during exercise. | Respiratory rate will remain within two breaths of patient's baseline rate. |
| | Observe patient for dyspnea or breathlessness during exercise. | Patient will deny feeling of breathlessness. |

nurses will not unnecessarily continue interventions for that portion of the plan of care. Continuity of care assumes that care provided to patients is relevant and timely. You will waste much time when you do not communicate achieved goals.

**Modifying a Care Plan.** When goals are not met, you identify the factors that interfere with goal achievement. Usually a change in the patient's condition, needs, or abilities makes alteration of the care plan necessary. For example, while monitoring Mrs. Bryan's ability to walk up and down steps, the nurse notices a grimace in Mrs. Bryan's expression and asks if she is having discomfort. The patient acknowledges she is having pain in her left hip. Her ability to tolerate exercise lessens, not as a result of activity intolerance but because of the onset of acute pain. As a result, the nurse considers adding a diagnosis of acute pain, but first assesses the extent of pain and its effects on Mrs. Bryan's mobility. Ultimately Inez will establish a new diagnosis, *impaired physical mobility related to right-sided hip pain.* Inez introduces new interventions for pain relief before attempts at having Mrs. Bryan walk.

Occasionally a lack of goal achievement results from an error in nursing judgment or failure to follow each step of the nursing process. Patients often have multiple problems. Always remember the possibility of overlooking or misjudging something. When there is failure to achieve a goal, no matter what the reason, repeat the entire nursing process sequence for that nursing diagnosis to discover changes the plan needs. You then will reassess the patient, determine accuracy of the nursing diagnosis, establish new goals and expected outcomes, and select new interventions.

A complete reassessment of all patient factors relating to the nursing diagnosis and etiology is necessary when modifying a plan. You will compare new data about the patient's condition with previously assessed information. Knowledge from previous experiences helps you direct the reassessment process. Caring for patients who have had similar health problems gives you a strong background of knowledge to use for anticipating patient needs and knowing what to assess.

After reassessment, determine what nursing diagnoses are accurate for the situation. Ask whether you selected the correct diagnosis and whether it and the etiological factor is current. Then revise the problem list to reflect the patient's changed status. You may make a new diagnosis. Nursing care is based on an accurate list of nursing diagnoses. Accuracy is more important than the number of diagnoses selected. As the patient's condition changes, the diagnoses do as well. For example, you find that a patient with diabetes has a serious visual impairment. It is unlikely that the patient will be able to self-administer insulin. Assessment reveals that a family member is available as a resource. To develop a plan designed to educate an alternate caregiver about the administration of insulin, establish a new diagnosis, *ineffective health maintenance related to inability to self-administer insulin secondary to visual impairment.*

**Goals and Expected Outcomes.** When you revise care plans, review the goals and expected outcomes for needed changes. Examine the goals for unchanged nursing diagnoses. Are they still appropriate? A change in one diagnosis may affect others. It is also important to determine that each goal and expected outcome is realistic for the problem, etiology, and time frame. Unrealistic expected outcomes and time frames make goal achievement difficult.

Clearly document goals and expected outcomes for new or revised nursing diagnoses so that all team members are aware of the revised care plan. When the goal is still appropriate but has not yet been met, you may change the evaluation date to allow more time. You may also decide at this time to change interventions. For example, when a patient's wound does not heal with a wet-to-moist dressing, you may choose a different dressing material such as a colloid dressing instead. All goals and expected outcomes are patient centered, with realistic expectations for patient achievement.

The evaluation of interventions examines two factors: the appropriateness of the interventions selected and the correct application of the intervention. The appropriateness of an intervention may be based on the standard of care for a patient's health problem. A **standard of care** is the minimum level of care accepted to ensure high quality of care to patients. Standards of care define the types of therapies typically administered to patients with defined problems or needs. If the patient has a specific nursing diagnosis such as *acute pain,* the nursing department's established standard of care for this problem includes pain control measures. Review the standard of care to determine if you chose the right interventions or if additional ones are required.

You may only need to increase or decrease the frequency of interventions. Use clinical judgment based on previous experience and the patient's actual response to therapy. For example, if a patient continues to have congested lung sounds, you increase the frequency of coughing and deep breathing exercises to remove secretions.

During evaluation, you may find that some planned interventions are designed for an inappropriate level of nursing care. If you need to change the level of care, substitute a different action verb, such as *assist* in place of *provide.* Sometimes the level of care is appropriate, but the interventions are unsuitable because of a change in the expected outcome. In this case, discontinue the interventions and plan new ones.

Make any changes in the plan of care based on the nature of the patient's unfavorable response. Consulting with other nurses often yields suggestions for improving the approach to care delivery. Senior nurses are often excellent resources because of their experience. Simply changing the care plan is not enough. Implement the new plan, and reevaluate the patient's response to the nursing actions. *Evaluation is continuous.*

Occasionally during evaluation you may discover unmet patient needs. This is normal. The nursing process is a systematic, problem-solving approach to individualized patient care, but there are many variables affecting each patient with health care problems. Patients with the same health care problem are not treated the same way. As a result, you will sometimes make errors in judgment. The systematic use of evaluation provides a way for you to catch these errors. By consistently incorporating evaluation into practice you will minimize errors and ensure that the patient's plan of care is appropriate and relevant.

## KEY CONCEPTS

- The nursing process has five steps: assessment, nursing diagnosis, planning, implementation, and evaluation.
- Use of the nursing process is the foundation for clinical decision making.
- The assessment step of the nursing process involves collection and verification of data from a primary and/or secondary source and analysis of the data.
- When you first meet a patient, you will conduct an initial assessment screening and then focus on cues and patterns of information to make a more comprehensive assessment.
- Attention to the environment, patient comfort, and communication techniques ensures a successful assessment interview.
- Data validation involves comparing data with another source to ensure accuracy of the assessment.
- Data analysis involves recognizing patterns or trends, comparing data with standards, and then forming a reasoned conclusion about the data's meaning.
- Data clustering organizes the assessed information into meaningful clusters or sets of signs and symptoms.
- The diagnostic process includes analysis and interpretation of data, identification of patient and family needs, and formulation of nursing diagnoses and collaborative problems.
- Nursing diagnoses provide the basis for selection of nursing interventions to achieve outcomes for which a nurse is accountable.
- NANDA International defines three types of nursing diagnoses: actual, at risk, and wellness.
- Defining characteristics are the clinical criteria or assessment findings that support an actual nursing diagnosis.
- Nursing diagnostic errors may lead to inappropriate and/or inadequate nursing care.
- A correctly written nursing diagnosis is within the domain of nursing practice and contains a NANDA International–approved diagnostic problem statement and a precise

- statement of the influencing factors contributing to the problem, connected by the phrase *related to.*
- During the planning component, you determine patient goals, establish priorities, develop expected outcomes of nursing care, and write a nursing care plan.
- Nursing Outcomes Classification (NOC) outcomes have labels for describing the focus of nursing care and then include indicators for use in measuring success with interventions
- The nurse begins the nursing care plan by first addressing the nursing diagnoses that have the highest priority.
- The care plan is a written guideline for patient care so that all members of the health care team can quickly understand the care given.
- A mind map offers a graphic representation of the connections between nursing diagnoses and how they relate to the patient's health problems.
- There are three types of nursing interventions: nurse-initiated, physician-initiated, and collaborative.
- The Nursing Interventions Classification (NIC) is a comprehensive standardized classification of the interventions that nurses use in the care of patients.
- Select interventions based on characteristics of a nursing diagnosis, goals and expected outcomes, evidence base for the intervention, feasibility, acceptability, and nurse competency.
- Direct care interventions include activities of daily living, instrumental activities of daily living, physical care, counseling, teaching, controlling for adverse reactions, and preventive measures.
- Evaluation determines a patient's response to nursing actions and the extent to which goals of care have been met.
- You evaluate by comparing the patient's response to nursing actions with expected outcomes established during planning.
- When goals of care are not met, you identify factors that interfere with goal achievement, reassess the patient's condition, revise existing or develop new nursing diagnoses, and select appropriate interventions.

## CRITICAL THINKING IN PRACTICE

*Mr. Vacaro is a 72-year-old patient who has been visiting the clinic for over a month. He visits weekly for follow-up care for a chronic venous stasis ulcer of the left leg. He is also diagnosed with hypertension and takes six different medications. Mr. Vacaro lives alone and has a parish nurse who visits only once a week. The clinic nurse's note at the time of his first visit contained the following information: "Ulcer with irregular margins, 4 cm wide by 5 cm long and approximately 0.5 cm deep, and foul-smelling purulent yellowish drainage. Brownish rust-colored skin around ulcer. Zinc oxide and calamine gauze applied to ulcer. Ace bandage applied to gauze. Patient instructed to return in 2 weeks. Discussed medication schedule with patient. Patient reports having difficulty obtaining medications from pharmacy because he has no regular transportation. Has not taken one of his blood pressure medications for 3 days. When discussing options for ways to obtain medications, he shows limited problem-solving skills."*

1. After reviewing the nurse's note, what additional assessment information might you like to have on Mr. Vacaro?
2. The clinic nurse decides to contact the parish nurse and asks the nurse to describe what she knows about Mr. Vacaro's ability to obtain medications. This is an example of what type of assessment activity?
3. Identify two nursing diagnoses that would apply to Mr. Vacaro's case.
4. As the nurse caring for the patient on the follow-up visit, what expected outcomes do you anticipate for the goal of "Wound will demonstrate healing within 4 weeks"? What evaluative measures do you use to determine if the wound is healing?
5. Among the nursing diagnoses that apply to Mr. Vacaro, what would be his priority and why?

## NCLEX® REVIEW

1. The identification of your patient's health care needs occurs in the nursing process step of:
   1. Planning
   2. Evaluation
   3. Assessment
   4. Implementation
2. Before formulating a list of nursing diagnoses you must first:
   1. Establish a list of priorities
   2. Document your assessment findings
   3. Review your assessment with other health team members
   4. Validate the interpretation of the data with your patient and physical examination findings
3. Establishing priorities for your patient's care occurs in the nursing process step of:
   1. Planning
   2. Evaluation
   3. Assessment
   4. Implementation
4. Expected outcomes are needed in a plan of care to:
   1. Identify the anticipated patient response to care
   2. Determine that the nursing care was delivered
   3. Provide documentation of the type of care given
   4. Support the need for additional health care personnel
5. Evaluation is an important part of nursing care. During this process you best determine the effectiveness of a specific nursing action by:
   1. Reassessing the patient for new problems
   2. Determining that the specific nursing action was completed
   3. Comparing the patient's response to the nursing action with other patients who received the same nursing action
   4. Comparing the patient's response to the nursing action with the expected outcomes established during planning

## REFERENCES

Agency for Health Care Policy and Research, Acute Pain Management Guideline Panel: *Acute pain management: operative or medical procedures and trauma,* Clinical Practice Guideline, AHCPR Pub No. 92-0032, Rockville, Md, 1992, Agency for Health Care Policy and Research, Public Health Service, U.S. Department of Health and Human Services.

Alfaro-LeFevre R: *Applying nursing diagnosis and nursing process: a step-by-step guide,* ed 4, Philadelphia, 1998, Lippincott.

American Nurses Association: *Nursing: a social policy statement,* ed 2, Washington, DC, 2003: The Association.

Benner P, Stannard D, Hooper PL: A "thinking-in-action" approach to teaching clinical judgment: a classroom innovation for acute care advanced practice nurses, *Adv Pract Nurs Q* 1(4):70, 1996.

Carnevali DL, Thomas MD: *Diagnostic reasoning and treatment decision making in nursing,* Philadelphia, 1993, Lippincott.

Carpenito-Moyet LJ: *Nursing diagnosis application to clinical practice,* ed 11, Philadelphia, 2005, Lippincott Williams & Wilkins.

Dochterman JM, Bulechek GM: *Nursing interventions classification (NIC),* ed 4, St. Louis, 2004, Mosby.

Dochterman JM, Jones, DA: *Unifying nursing languages: the harmonization of NANDA, NIC, NOC,* Washington DC, 2003, American Nurses Association.

Gordon M: *Nursing diagnosis: process and application,* ed 3, St. Louis, 1994, Mosby.

Hickey P: *Nursing process handbook,* St. Louis, 1990, Mosby.

HIPAAdvisory, OCR guidance explaining significant aspects of the privacy rule, 2003, http://www.hipaadvisory.com/regs/finalprivacymod/guidance.htm

Iowa Intervention Project: The NIC taxonomy structure, *Image J Nurs Sch* 25:1816, 1993.

King M, Shell R: Teaching and evaluating critical thinking with concept maps, *Nurse Educ* 27(5):214, 2002.

Konradi DB, Anglin LT: Walking for exercise self-efficacy appraisal process: use of a focus group methodology, *J Gerontol Nurs* 29(5):29, 2003.

Lunney M: Accuracy of nurses' diagnoses: foundation of NANDA, NIC, and NOC, *Nurs Diagn* 9(2):83, 1998.

McCloskey JC, Bulechek GM: Standardizing the language for nursing treatments: an overview of the issues, *Nurs Outlook* 42:56, 1994.

McCloskey JC, Bulechek GM: Nursing interventions core to specialty practice, *Nurs Outlook* 46(2):61, 1998.

McCloskey JC and others: Nurses' use and delegation of indirect care interventions, *Nurs Econ* 14(1):22, 1996.

Moorhead S, Johnson M, Maas M: *Nursing outcomes classification (NOC),* ed 3, St. Louis, 2004, Mosby.

Mueller A, Johnston M, Bligh D: Joining mind mapping and care planning to enhance student critical thinking and achieve holistic nursing care, *Nurs Diagn* 13(1):24, 2002.

NANDA International: *NANDA nursing diagnoses: definitions and classifications, 2005-2006,* Philadelphia, 2005, NANDA International.

Pender NJ: *Health promotion and nursing practice,* ed 3, Stamford, Conn, 1996, Appleton & Lange.

Redman BK: *The practice of patient education,* ed 9, St. Louis, 2001, Mosby.

Schuster PM: Concept mapping: reducing clinical care plan paperwork and increasing learning, *Nurse Educ* 25(2):76, 2000.

Schuster PM: *Concept mapping: a critical thinking approach to care planning,* St. Louis, 2003, Mosby.

Zander K, McGill R: Critical and anticipated recovery paths: only the beginning, *Nurs Manage* 25(8):34, 1994.

# CHAPTER 8

# Documentation and Reporting

## MEDIA RESOURCES

**CD COMPANION** *evolve* **WEBSITE**

http://evolve.elsevier.com/Potter/basic

- **NCLEX® Review**
- **Audio Glossary**
- **English/Spanish Audio Glossary**

## OBJECTIVES

- Describe guidelines for effective documentation and reporting in a variety of health care settings.
- Describe methods for multidisciplinary communication within the health care team.
- Compare different methods used in documentation.

- Discuss the advantages of using a critical path as a documentation tool.
- Identify common record-keeping forms.
- Discuss advantages and disadvantages of standardized documentation forms.
- Discuss advantages of computerized documentation.

### KEY TERMS

accreditation, p. 137
acuity recording, p. 145
case management plan, p. 144
change-of-shift report, p. 147
charting by exception (CBE), p. 143
computer-based patient record, p. 146
critical pathways, p. 144
DAR (data, action, patient response), p. 142
diagnosis-related groups (DRGs), p. 139
documentation, p. 136

flow sheets, p. 144
focus charting, p. 142
graphic records, p. 144
incident report, p. 149
Kardex, p. 144
PIE note, p. 142
problem-oriented medical record (POMR), p. 141
record, p. 137
reports, p. 137
SOAP note, p. 142
source record, p. 143
standardized care plans, p. 146
transfer report, p. 148
variances, p. 144

Documentation is a vital aspect of nursing practice, and it is defined as anything written or printed within a patient record. The information you communicate about patient care reflects the quality of your care and provides accountability for each health care team member's care. You will document expected outcomes and the nursing care you provide for a patient (e.g., assessments and interventions) in the medical record. Effective documentation ensures continuity of care, saves time, and minimizes the risk of errors (Yocum, 2002).

The health care environment creates many challenges for accurately documenting and reporting the care delivered to patients. The quality of nursing care depends on your ability to communicate effectively verbally and in writing, and you are held accountable for the accuracy of documentation you enter into the patient's record. Regulations from agencies such as the Joint Commission on Accreditation of Healthcare Organizations (JCAHO) and the Centers for Medicare and Medicaid Services require health care institutions to monitor and evaluate the quality and appropriateness of patient care (see Chapters 2 and 6). Typically, such monitoring and evaluations occur through the auditing of information health care providers document in patient records.

## Confidentiality

You do not disclose information about patients' status to other patients, family members (unless granted by the patient), or to health care staff not involved in their care. Legal and ethical obligations require you to keep information about patients strictly confidential. In 2003 legislation to protect patient privacy for health information in the form of the Health Insurance Portability and Accountability Act (HIPAA) was finalized (U.S. Department of Health and Human Services [USDHSS], 2003). This legislation governs all areas of health information management, which includes, for example, reimbursement, medical record coding, security, and patient record management. Previously the rule required written consent for disclosure of all patient information. Under new regulations, in order to eliminate barriers that could delay access to care, providers are required only to notify patients of their privacy policy and to make a reasonable effort to get written acknowledgement of this notification. As a result, patients have more control over their personal health care information and who has access to this information (USDHHS, 2003).

Sometimes you have a reason for using health care records for data gathering, research, or continuing education. This is permitted if you use the records as specified and permission is granted. When you are a student in a clinical setting, confidentiality and compliance with HIPAA legislation are part of professional practice. You may only review the medical record for information needed to provide safe, efficient care. For example, when you are assigned to provide complete care for a patient, you need to review the current medical record and plan of care.

However, you do not share this information with other classmates. In addition, you should never access the medical records of other patients on the specific clinical area. To further maintain confidentiality and protect patient privacy, written materials used in your student clinical practice should not have patient identifiers, such as room number, date of birth, medical record number, or other identifiable demographic information.

## Standards

Within a health care organization there are standards that govern the type of information you document. Institutional standards or policies often dictate the frequency of documentation, such as how often a nursing assessment is recorded or how often a nurse records a patient's level of pain. Know the standards of your health care organization to ensure complete and accurate documentation.

In addition, your documentation needs to conform to the standards of the Joint Commission for Accreditation of Healthcare Organizations (JCAHO) to maintain institutional **accreditation** and to minimize liability. Usually an organization incorporates JCAHO standards into its policies and revises documentation forms to suit those standards. Current documentation standards require that all patients admitted to a health care facility have an assessment of physical, psychosocial, environmental, self-care, knowledge level, and discharge planning needs (JCAHO, 2005a). JCAHO standards require that your documentation be within the context of the nursing process, including evidence of patient and family teaching and discharge planning.

The documentation of care and patient information is vital in ensuring patient safety in health care organizations. Electronic records and information create complexities in information management. The goal of information management is to support decision making and to improve patient outcomes, improve health care documentation, ensure patient safety, and improve performance in patient care, treatment and services, governance, management, and support processes (JCAHO, 2005a).

## Multidisciplinary Communication Within the Health Care Team

Patient care requires effective communication among all members of the health care team. A documentation system that reflects multidisciplinary plans of care for a patient is an effective, efficient means of communication. Multidisciplinary communication is a concise method to document and verify patient progress (Davidson and others, 2004). Effective communication takes place along two approaches, the patient's record and reports. A patient's **record** or chart is a confidential, permanent legal documentation of

information relevant to a patient's health care. Information about the patient's health care is recorded after each patient contact. The record is a continuing account of the patient's health care status and is available to all members of the health care team.

**Reports** are oral, written, or audiotaped exchanges of information between members of the health care team. Common reports given by nurses include change-of-shift reports, telephone reports, transfer reports, and incident reports. A physician or health care provider may call a nursing unit to receive a verbal report on a patient's condition and progress. The laboratory submits a written report providing the results of diagnostic tests. A transfer report informs the staff of a receiving health care setting about the type of care a patient will require.

## Purpose of Records

Documentation serves multiple purposes: it facilitates communication with health care providers for continuity of patient care, it maintains a legal and financial record of care, it aids in clinical research, and it guides professional and organizational performance improvement (JCAHO, 2005a). Although often each agency uses a different record format, records contain the same information. Each page of the record includes the current date and patient identification, including basic demographic data (age, birth date), physician or health care provider, date admitted, and medical record number. Each patient record includes the following:

- Admission data
- A signed consent for treatment
- Physician's or health care provider's orders
- Medical history and physician's or health care provider's physical examination
- Nurses' documentation of ongoing assessments, a plan of care, interventions, and evaluation.
- Medication records
- Physician's or health care provider's progress notes
- Progress notes from other disciplines such as respiratory therapy and physical therapy
- Results of laboratory tests
- Discharge information

### Communication

The record is a way for health care team members to provide continuity of care and to communicate patient needs and progress toward meeting desired patient outcomes. For example, Mr. Kleinschmidt had a stroke a week ago. Currently he has left-sided paralysis and some problems with verbal expression. He is able to understand information, and he participates in his care. He lives with his wife, who is also active in his care. Mr. Kleinschmidt's overall plan of care focuses on activities of daily living. Participants in multidisciplinary conference develop an extensive rehabilitation plan.

In his medical record is a summary of the multidisciplinary conference, which focuses on activities of daily living, patient education, and discharge planning. Including such precise information in the medical record provides for continuity of care as Mr. Kleinschmidt is transferred from the acute care facility to the rehabilitation institute.

The record also includes the patient's responses to interventions and consequent modifications in the plan of care. The record is the most current and accurate source of information about a patient's health care status. The information communicated in a record prepares you to know a patient thoroughly so that you can make timely and appropriate care decisions.

## Legal Documentation

Effective documentation is one of the best defenses for legal claims associated with health care (Table 8-1). To limit nursing liability, your documentation must follow organizational standards for documentation, which include a clear indication of the individualized and goal-directed nursing care you

| TABLE 8-1 | Legal Guidelines for Recording | |
|---|---|---|
| **Guidelines** | **Rationale** | **Correct Action** |
| Do not erase, apply correction fluid, or scratch out errors made while recording. | Charting becomes illegible: it may appear as if you were attempting to hide information or deface record. | Draw single line through error, write word *error* above it, and sign your name or initials. Then record note correctly. Check agency policy. |
| Do not write retaliatory or critical comments about patient or care by other health care professionals. | Statements can be used as evidence for nonprofessional behavior or poor quality of care. | Enter only objective descriptions of patient's behavior; patient comments should be quoted. |
| Need to add additional patient information. | New information is acquired. | If additional information is to be added to an existing entry, write the date and time of the new entry on the next available space and include "Addendum to note of [date and time of prior note]" (Sullivan 2000). |
| | Forgot to chart during a shift. | Write the current date and time in the next available space, and write "Late entry for [date and time/shift missed] (Sullivan, 2000). |
| Correct all errors promptly. | Errors in recording can lead to errors in treatment. | Avoid rushing to complete charting; be sure information is accurate. |
| Record all facts. | Record must be accurate and reliable. | Be certain entry is factual; do not speculate or guess. |
| Do not leave blank spaces in nurses' notes. | Another person can add incorrect information in space. | Chart consecutively, line by line; if space is left, draw line horizontally through it and sign your name at end. |
| Record all entries legibly and in black ink. | Illegible entries can be misinterpreted, causing errors and lawsuits; ink cannot be erased; black ink is more legible when records are photocopied or transferred to microfilm. | Never erase entries or use correction fluid, and never use pencil. |
| If order is questioned, record that clarification was sought. | If you perform order known to be incorrect, you are just as liable for prosecution as the physician or health care provider is. | Do not record "physician made error." Instead, chart that "Dr. Smith was called to clarify order for analgesic." |
| Chart only for yourself. | You are accountable for information you enter into chart. | Never chart for someone else. **Exception:** If caregiver has left unit for day and calls with information that needs to be documented, include the name of the source of information in the entry and include that the information was provided via telephone. |
| Avoid using generalized, empty phrases such as "status unchanged" or "had good day." | Specific information about patient's condition or case can be accidentally deleted if information is too generalized. | Use complete, concise descriptions of care. |
| Begin each entry with time, and end with your signature and title. | This guideline ensures that correct sequence of events is recorded; signature documents who is accountable for care delivered. | Do not wait until end of shift to record important changes that occurred several hours earlier; be sure to sign each entry. |
| For computer documentation keep your password to yourself. | Maintains security and confidentiality. | Once logged onto the computer, do not leave the computer screen unattended. |

provide. The best way to ensure documentation meets legal standards is to record information as you provide care. This increases the likelihood of your documentation being accurate and most current. It is important to avoid recording data that is routine, superficial, or not relevant.

## Financial Billing

**Diagnosis-related groups (DRGs)** are the basis for establishing reimbursement for patient care. A DRG is a classification based on patients' primary and secondary medical diagnoses. Under the prospective payment system (PPS), Medicare reimburses hospitals a set dollar amount for each DRG (see Chapter 2). Your nursing documentation verifies the specific nursing care provided and thus supports the reimbursement your health care agency receives.

Your patient's medical record is also audited to review financial charges of equipment and services used in the patient's care. Private insurance carriers and auditors from federal agencies review records to determine the reimbursement that a patient or a health care agency receives. Your timely and accurate documentation of supplies and equipment used assists in determining the patient's financial charges.

## Education

A patient's record contains a variety of information (e.g., medical and nursing diagnoses, signs and symptoms of disease, successful and unsuccessful therapies, diagnostic findings, and patient behaviors). Reading the patient care record is an effective way to learn the nature of an illness and the patient's response to the illness. Review of patients with similar medical problems allows you to identify patterns and trends. Such information builds your clinical knowledge. As you identify patterns associated with specific diseases and conditions, you are able to anticipate the type of care your patient will require.

## Research

Statistical data are important elements of patient records, including the frequency of clinical disorders, complications, use of specific medical and nursing therapies, recoveries from illness, and mortality. After you obtain appropriate agency approvals, you review patients' records in a research study to collect information on a particular health problem. For example, if you suspect that early ambulation decreases the complications in postoperative patients, you would review the records of select surgical patients to evaluate the rate of postoperative complications with early versus late ambulation.

## Auditing and Monitoring

The JCAHO requires hospitals to establish performance improvement programs to conduct objective, ongoing reviews of patient care and asks institutions to establish standards for quality care. Nurses monitor or review records throughout the year to determine the degree to which performance improvement standards are met. For example, nurses may monitor records to determine their success in documenting institution of fall precautions or evaluation of pain measures. Deficiencies identified during monitoring are shared with all members of the nursing staff so that corrections in policy or practice can be made. Performance improvement programs keep you informed of the extent to which you meet standards of nursing practice (see Chapter 2).

## Guidelines for Quality Documentation and Reporting

High-quality recording and reporting are necessary to enhance efficient, safe, individualized patient care. Accurate documentation is one of the best defenses of legal claims associated with nursing care (Martin, 2001; Sullivan, 2004). There are five common issues in malpractice caused by inadequate or incorrect documentation: (1) failing to document the correct time of events, (2) failing to record verbal orders or failing to have them signed, (3) charting actions in advance to save time, (4) documenting incorrect data, and (5) failing to give a report, or giving an incomplete report, to an ongoing shift (see Table 8-1). Problems arise when a record is reviewed in a malpractice suit and time gaps are found, information is squeezed between lines or crossed out, or key facts were omitted (Ladebauche, 1995).

In some settings, agency policy requires a registered nurse to co-sign documentation completed by licensed practical or vocational nurses or assistive personnel. A co-signature indicates that the supervising nurse reviewed the record entry and was aware of the care and patient status even though others delivered the care.

To limit liability, nursing documentation must clearly indicate that individualized, goal-directed nursing care was provided to a patient based on the nursing assessment. The recorded information in the patient's record must describe exactly what happened to a patient. This is best achieved when the nurse charts immediately after care was provided (Sullivan, 2000). Quality documentation and reporting have six important characteristics: they are factual, accurate, complete, current, organized, and confidential.

### Factual

A record contains descriptive, objective information about what you see, hear, feel, and smell. Objective data are data that are measurable and observable, such as a patient's report of pain severity on a scale of 0 to 10, the size of a wound, or a patient's pulse oximetry reading. To be factual, avoid words such as *appears, seems,* or *apparently* because they are vague and lead to conclusions that you cannot support by objective information.

The only subjective data included in a record are what the patient says. Write subjective information with quotation marks, using the patient's own words. For example, a patient's statement of *"My lower back hurts"* is subjective and acceptable documentation. Another example is stated as follows: The patient reports feeling a pressure in his chest. It is acceptable not to use quotation marks when you paraphrase the patient's words. Remember, when documenting subjective information, it is also important to include complementary objective findings so that your database is as descriptive as possible.

## Accurate

The use of precise measurements makes documentation more accurate. For example, documenting that "Patient voided 450 ml clear urine" is more accurate than "Voided an adequate amount." Maintain accuracy by using an institution's accepted abbreviations, symbols, and system of measurement. To avoid misunderstandings, write out any abbreviations that are possibly confusing. JCAHO National Patient Safety Goals 2004 require that health care institutions standardize abbreviations, acronyms, and symbols throughout their system (JCAHO, 2005b). They also require institutions to identify a list of unacceptable abbreviations, acronyms, and symbols that the agency will not use (see Chapter 14). It is important for you to know an institution's acceptable and unacceptable abbreviation list to keep your documentation accurate and compliant with requirements. For example, *the abbreviation for every day (qd)* **should no longer be used.** *If a treatment or medication is needed daily, the written order or care plan should use the term "daily" or "every day." The abbreviation qd (every day) can be misinterpreted to mean O.D. (right eye).*

Correct spelling demonstrates a level of competency and attention to detail. Misspelled words lead to confusion. For example, often words sound the same but have different meanings, such as *accept* and *except* or *dysphagia* and *dysphasia.* Incorrect use of terms confuses the intended meaning.

JCAHO standards (2005) require that "all entries in medical records be dated and there is a method to identify all authors of entries." Therefore any descriptive entry in a patient's record ends with the caregiver's full name and status. Occasionally you will include observations reported to another caregiver or interventions performed by someone else. For example, "Patient suctioned by Judith Hill, RN." As a nursing student, you need to enter full name, student nurse abbreviation, and educational institution, such as "Marianne Smith, SN [student nurse], CMTC [Central Maine Technical College]." The abbreviation for *student nurse* sometimes differs regionally, being either *NS,* which stands for *nursing student,* or *SN,* which stands for *student nurse.* The signature holds this person accountable for information recorded.

## Complete

The information within a recorded entry or a report needs to be complete, containing appropriate and essential information. Criteria for thorough communication exist for certain health problems or nursing activities (Table 8-2). You make written entries in the patient's medical record, de-

| TABLE 8-2 | Examples of Criteria for Reporting and Recording |
|---|---|
| **Topic** | **Criteria to Report or Record** |
| **Assessment** | |
| Subjective data (patient behavior [e.g., anxiety, confusion, hostility]) | • Description of episode in quotation marks<br>• Onset, location, description of condition (severity, duration, frequency; precipitating, aggravating, and relieving factors)<br>• Onset, behaviors exhibited, precipitating factors |
| Objective data (e.g., rash, tenderness, breath sounds) | • Onset, location, description of condition (severity, duration, frequency; precipitating, aggravating, and relieving factors) |
| **Nursing Interventions and Evaluation** | |
| Treatments (e.g., enema, bath, dressing change) | • Time administered, equipment used (if appropriate), patient's response (objective and subjective changes) compared with previous treatment; for example, rated pain 0 on a scale of 0-10 during dressing change or reported "severe abdominal cramping during enema" |
| Medication administration | • Immediately after administration, document: time medication given, dose, route, any preliminary assessments (e.g., pain level, vital signs), patient response or effect of medication, for example:<br>  ◦ 1500 Pain reported at 6 (scale 0-10). Tylenol 500 mg given PO 1530: patient reports pain level 2 (scale 0-10)<br>  ◦ Pruritus and hives developed over lower abdomen 1 hour after penicillin was given |
| Patient teaching | • Information presented, method of instruction (e.g., discussion, demonstration, videotape, booklet), patient response, including questions and evidence of understanding such as return demonstration or change in behavior |
| Discharge planning | • Measurable patient goals or expected outcomes, progress toward goals, need for referrals |

scribing nursing care that you administer and the patient's response. For example:

> 0845 Reports continuous throbbing pain on lateral aspect of left fractured femur increased with movement of the leg with a severity of 8 (scale 0-10). B/P = 132/74, T = 37°, P = 92, R = 18. Morphine 10 mg IV given for pain. Sue Jacobs, RN.
> 0915 Reports pain at 2 (scale 0-10) and able to turn in bed independently. Sue Jacobs, RN.

You include routine activities such as daily hygiene measures, vital signs, and pain assessment in flow sheets or graphic records. Describe these activities in greater detail when it is relevant because of a change in functional ability or status. For example, you have a patient who has previously required a total bath and now the patient has improved and is able to wash his or her face, hands, and upper body. This warrants additional documentation.

## Current

Making entries promptly is essential in effective documentation (JCAHO, 2005a). Delays in documentation result in serious omissions and untimely delays in patient care. To increase currency and decrease unnecessary duplication, many health care agencies keep records near the patient's bedside to facilitate immediate documentation of care activities. You need to communicate the following nursing care at the time of occurrence:

1. Vital signs
2. Pain assessment
3. Administration of medications and treatments
4. Preparation for diagnostic tests or surgery
5. Change in patient status and who was notified
6. Treatment for sudden changes in patient status

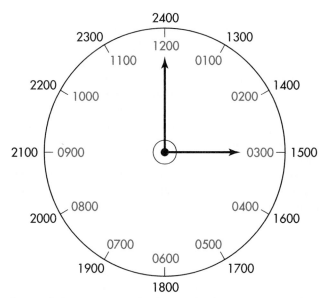

FIGURE **8-1** Comparison of 24 hours of military time and civilian time.

7. Patient response to intervention
8. Admission, transfer, discharge, or death of patient

Many agencies use military time, a 24-hour time cycle. The military clock ends with midnight at 2400 and begins at 1 minute after midnight as 0001. For example, 10:22 AM is 1022 military time; 1:00 PM is 1300 military time. Figure 8-1 compares military and corresponding civilian times.

## Organized

Written communication is easier to understand when written in a logical order. For example, an organized note describes your assessment, interventions, and patient's response in a sequence. It is also more effective when concise, clear, and to the point. To make clear and organized entries it is often helpful to make a list of what you need to include before beginning to write in the permanent legal record. Once you have identified the pertinent content, you will often delete unnecessary words. This process becomes easier with practice.

## Methods of Recording

The documentation system selected by a nursing service reflects the philosophy of the department. Staff use the same documentation system throughout an agency. There are several acceptable methods for recording health care information (Table 8-3).

### Narrative Documentation

Narrative documentation is the traditional method for recording nursing care. However, in many settings other methods have replaced narrative charting. Narrative charting uses a storylike format to document information specific to patient conditions and nursing care. Narrative charting is beneficial in emergency situations in which a chronological order of events is important. However, narrative charting does have some disadvantages, including the tendency to be repetitive and time consuming, and it requires the reader to sort through much information to locate the desired patient information.

### Problem-Oriented Medical Records

The **problem-oriented medical record (POMR)** is a structured method of documentation that emphasizes the patient's problems. The method is organized in a way to correspond to the nursing process and facilitates communication of patient needs. Organization of data is by problem or diagnosis. Ideally, each member of the health care team contributes to a single list of identified patient problems. The POMR has the following major sections: database, problem list, care plan, and progress notes.

**DATABASE.** The database contains all available assessment information pertaining to the patient. This section is the foundation for identifying patient problems and planning care. The database remains active and current, and you make revisions as new data are available.

| TABLE 8-3 | Formats for Recording |
|---|---|
| Narrative note | Patient stated: "I'm dreading surgery. Last time I had such pain when I got out of bed." Discussed alternatives for pain control and importance of postoperative activity. Encouraged to ask for pain medication before pain is severe. Patient stated: "I feel better prepared now." Able to verbalize that activity enhances circulation and healing. |
| SOAP | S (subjective data): "I'm dreading surgery. Last time I had such pain when I got out of bed."<br>O (objective data): Noted muscle tension and loud voice.<br>A (assessment/analysis): Fear of postoperative pain.<br>P (plan): Assess pain level every 2 hours. Provide comfort measures, and give analgesics as needed. |
| PIE charting | P (problem): "I'm dreading surgery. Last time I had such pain when I got out of bed."<br>I (intervention): Discussed alternatives for pain control and importance of postoperative activity. Encouraged to ask for pain medication before pain is severe.<br>E (evaluation): "I feel better prepared now." Able to verbalize that activity enhances circulation and healing. |
| Focus charting | D (data): "I'm dreading surgery. Last time I had such pain when I got out of bed."<br>A (action): Discussed alternatives for pain control and importance of postoperative activity. Encouraged to ask for pain medication before pain is severe.<br>R (response): "I feel better prepared now." Able to verbalize that activity enhances circulation and healing.<br>NOTE: Some agencies add P (plan). Example: P (plan): Assess pain level every 2 hours. Provide comfort measures, and give analgesics as needed. |

**PROBLEM LIST.** The problem list develops after a review of the patient data. Priority problems are identified, and all problems are listed in chronological order to serve as an organizing guide for the patient's care. You add new problems to the list as they are identified on the basis of your ongoing nursing assessment. After you have resolved a problem, record the data, and draw a line through the problem and its number.

**CARE PLAN.** Disciplines involved in the patient's care develop a care plan for each problem listed. For example, a physical therapist might communicate a plan for increasing a patient's ambulation, a speech therapist might communicate a plan to improve the patient's swallowing. Nurses document a plan of care in a variety of formats. Current JCAHO standards require that a plan of care be developed for all patients on admission to acute, subacute, rehabilitation, or extended care agencies (JCAHO, 2005a). Generally these plans of care include nursing diagnoses, expected outcomes, and interventions (see Chapter 7).

**PROGRESS NOTES.** Health care team members use progress notes to monitor and record the progress of a patient's problems. Narrative notes, flow sheets, discharge summaries, and structured notes are formats you use to document the patient's progress.

**SOAP Documentation.** One format for entering a progress note is the **SOAP note.** SOAP is an acronym for the following :

S: Subjective data (verbalizations of the patient)
O: Objective data (data that are measured and observed)
A: Assessment (diagnosis based on the subjective and objective data)
P: Plan (what the caregiver plans to do)

An I and E are sometimes added (i.e., SOAPIE) in various institutions. The I stands for intervention, and the E represents evaluation. The logic for SOAP(IE) notes is similar to that of the nursing process: Collect data about each of your patient's problems, draw conclusions, and develop a plan of care. Number each SOAP note, and title it according to the problem on the list.

**PIE Documentation.** The **PIE note** documentation format is similar to SOAP charting in its problem-oriented nature. However, it differs from the SOAP method in that PIE charting has a nursing origin, whereas SOAP originated from the medical model. PIE is an acronym for problem, interventions, evaluation as follows:

P: Problem or nursing diagnosis applicable to patient
I: Interventions or actions taken
E: Evaluation of the outcomes of nursing interventions

The PIE format simplifies documentation by unifying the care plan and progress notes into a complete record. The PIE format also differs from SOAP because the narrative note does not include assessment information. Your daily assessment data appear on special flow sheets, thus preventing duplication of information. You number or label the PIE notes according to the patient's problems. Then, once a patient's problem becomes resolved, you drop the problem from daily documentation. Continuing problems are documented daily.

**Focus Charting.** A third narrative format is **focus charting.** It is a unique narrative format in that it places less emphasis on patient problems and instead focuses on patient concerns such as a sign or symptom, a condition, a behavior, or a significant event. Each entry includes **data, actions,** and **patient response (DAR)** for the particular patient situation. This allows for greater flexibility in patient documentation and encourages nurses to broaden their thinking to include any patient concerns (Allen and Englebright, 2000). Focus

| TABLE 8-4 | Components of a Source Record |
|---|---|
| Admission sheet | Specific demographic data about patient: legal name, identification number, sex, age, birth date, marital status, occupation and employer, health insurance, nearest relative to notify in an emergency, religious preference, name of attending physician or health care provider, date and time of admission |
| Physician's or health care provider's order sheet | Record of physician's or health care provider's orders for treatment and medications, with date, time, and physician's or health care provider's signature |
| Nurse's admission assessment | Summary of nursing history and physical examination |
| Graphic record and flow sheet | Record of repeated observations and numerical measurements such as vital signs, pain assessment, daily weights, and intake and output |
| Medical history and examination | Results of initial examination performed by physician or health care provider, including findings, family history, confirmed diagnoses, and medical plan of care |
| Nurses' notes | Record of nursing assessment, planning, implementation, and evaluation of care |
| Medication records | Accurate documentation of all medications administered to patient: date, time, dose, route, and nurse's signature |
| Patient education record | Documentation of patient's or significant other's response to educational needs and level of understanding of diagnosis and treatment plan |
| Physician's or health care provider's progress notes | Ongoing record of patient's progress and response to medical therapy and review of disease process |
| Health care discipline's records | Entries made into record by all health-related disciplines (e.g., respiratory therapy, radiology, social work, laboratories) |
| Discharge summary | Summary of patient's condition, progress, prognosis, rehabilitation, and teaching needs at time of dismissal from hospital or health care agency |

charting combines a shorthand approach to documenting normal assessments and routine care with a concise longhand method for documenting exceptions to predetermined norms. Focus charting avoids some of the pitfalls of charting by exception (Allen and Englebright, 2000). In addition, focus charting saves time because it is easily understood by multiple caregivers, it is adaptable to most health care settings, and it enables all caregivers to track the patient's condition and progress toward the outcomes of care.

## Source Records

In a **source record,** the patient's chart is organized so that each discipline (e.g., nursing, medicine, social work, and respiratory therapy) has a separate section in which to record data. Unlike the POMR, this format does not organize the information by patient problems. The advantage of a source record is that caregivers are able to easily locate the proper section of the record in which to make entries. Table 8-4 lists a summary of the components of a source record.

A disadvantage of source records is fragmented data. Information is well organized but not according to the patient's problems. Details about a particular problem appear in multiple areas throughout the record. For example, in the case of a wound infection, the nurse describes the appearance of the wound in the nurses' notes. The physician or health care provider notes in a separate section the progress of the wound's healing and the proposed course of therapy. The results of tests measuring growth of bacteria from the wound are in the laboratory test section. Thus any

data relevant to a single problem requires careful investigation to locate.

In the source record, you chart a narrative description of nursing care delivered. In a hospital, entries in the patient's record occur during each shift of duty. If you see a patient in a clinic or at home, you document the care provided during each visit or telephone contact, including a description that summarizes important observations relating to the patient's condition, nursing care, and evaluation of response.

## Charting by Exception

**Charting by exception (CBE)** is an innovative approach to reduce the time required to complete documentation. In a CBE system an agency defines criteria for nursing assessments and standards of practice for nursing interventions. Thus CBE simply involves completing a flow sheet that incorporates those standard assessment criteria and interventions. As a result, you simply use a check mark on the flow sheet to indicate normal findings or routine interventions. A narrative note becomes necessary when there are abnormal findings or variances in the use of interventions. You write a narrative note *only* when the standardized statement on the form does not match the patient's status or abnormal data are present (Murphy, 2003). Therefore, when you see any entries in the chart, you know that something out of the ordinary has occurred. This makes it easier to track unexpected changes in a patient's condition as they develop. This charting system helps eliminate repetition, decreases subjective data, and decreases documentation time (Cummins, 1999).

## Case Management Plan and Critical Pathways

The case management model of delivering care uses a multidisciplinary approach to documenting patient care. **Critical pathways** (or care maps) summarize the standardized plan of care within a **case management plan.** These standardized documents include one- to two-page care plans for the problems, key interventions, and expected outcomes for patients with a specific disease or condition (see Figure 7-6). These pathways provide an optimal sequencing and timing of interventions by physicians or health care providers, nurses, and other members of the multidisciplinary health care team. Use of critical pathways minimizes delays, optimizes resource utilization, maximizes quality care, and monitors and documents the patient's progress (Coffey and others, 2005). Critical pathways incorporated into documentation tools eliminate other nursing forms and thus reduce duplication and the amount of charting (Lavin and Enright, 1996).

The critical pathways direct and monitor the flow of patient care by defining patient-focused outcomes and specifying those interventions provided for each given day of care. Because of the nature of human response, there are **variances** in the patient outcomes when the patient deviates from the critical path plan. These variances are deviations or detours from the pathway and refer to either positive or negative changes, depending on the clinical situation. A positive variance occurs when a patient progresses more rapidly than the case management plan expected (e.g., discontinuation of a nasogastric tube a day early). A negative variance occurs when the activities on the clinical pathway do not occur as predicted or the patient does not meet the expected outcomes. An example of a negative variance is the addition of oxygen therapy for a postoperative patient experiencing breathing problems. You classify deviations from the case management plan into operational-, community-, practitioner-, or patient-caused variances. Your responsibility is to determine why the problem arose and to implement changes to eliminate the variance or to justify the actions taken to manage the critical path deviation (Iyer and Camp, 1999).

## Common Record-Keeping Forms

The patient chart includes a variety of forms to make documentation easy, quick, and comprehensive. When possible, avoid duplication within the record.

### Admission Nursing History Forms

Admission nursing history forms provide baseline data for later comparisons with changes in the patient's condition. The form allows the admitting nurse to make a thorough assessment (e.g., biographical data, holistic assessment, and review of health risk factors) and to identify relevant nursing diagnoses or problems for the patient's care plan. Each institution designs nursing history forms based on its standards of practice and philosophy of nursing care.

## Flow Sheets and Graphic Records

**Flow sheets** and **graphic records** allow documentation of certain routine observations or specific measurements made repeatedly, such as the bath, vital signs, pain assessment, and intake and output. Flow sheets provide a quick and easy reference for assessing changes in a patient's status. Critical care units commonly use flow sheets for many types of data. The flow sheets are an effective way to record information so that you are able to observe trends over time. Flow sheets are part of the permanent record. Figure 8-2 is an example of a nursing assessment flow sheet.

When documenting a significant change on a flow sheet, you describe this in the progress notes and describe nursing measures implemented in response to the change. For example, if a patient's blood pressure becomes dangerously high, record in the progress note the blood pressure; related assessments, such as flushing, headache; and the medication administered to lower the pressure. Also, include evaluation of the interventions, for example, serial blood pressure and other pertinent evaluation measures.

## Patient Education Record

Patient teaching is an essential part of nursing interventions. Many hospitals have an education record that identifies patients' level of knowledge related to their diagnosis, treatment, and medications. The goal of patient and family education is to improve health care outcomes by promoting healthy behavior and self-care and involving the patient and/or family in care decisions. Education supports recovery and a rapid return to function (see Chapter 10). Standards for patient education include assessment of needs, abilities, learning preferences, and readiness to learn. Based on the patient assessment, patient education needs usually include safe and effective use of medications, nutrition and diet modifications, safety and safe use of medical equipment, pain management, and rehabilitation techniques to promote functional independence and self-care activities, and available resources (JCAHO, 2005a).

## Patient Care Summary or Kardex

Many hospitals now have computerized systems that provide certain basic information in the form of a patient care summary. This summary prints for each patient during each shift. Data automatically updates as orders enter the system and as nurses make decisions. In some settings a **Kardex** (flip-over card file) kept at the nurses' station provides information for the daily care of a patient. It often has two parts: an activity and treatment section and a nursing care plan section. The updated information in the Kardex eliminates the need for you to refer repeatedly to the patient's chart. Information commonly found in the Kardex or patient care summary includes the following:

1. Basic demographic data (name, age, sex)
2. Primary medical diagnosis
3. Current physician's or health care provider's orders (e.g., diet, activity, vital signs)

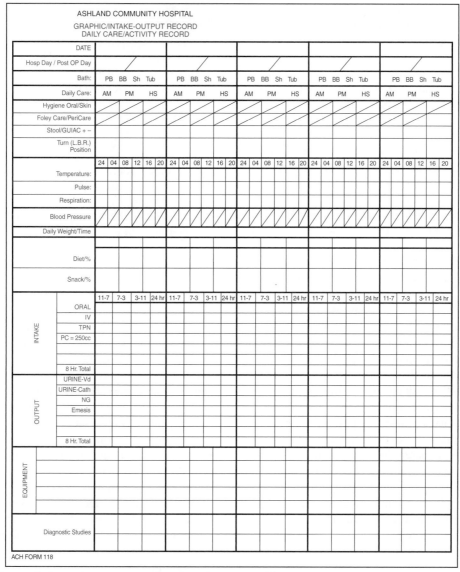

FIGURE 8-2 Nursing assessment flow sheet. (Courtesy Ashland Community Hospital, Ashland, Ore.)

4. A nursing care plan
5. Nursing orders or nursing interventions (e.g., intake and output, positioning, comfort measures, teaching)
6. Scheduled tests and procedures
7. Safety precautions used in the patient's care
8. Factors related to activities of daily living
9. Nearest relative/guardian or person to contact in an emergency
10. Emergency code status
11. Allergies

## Acuity Recording

Most hospitals use a patient acuity system to rank the intensity of nursing care required for each patient on a nursing unit. The combined acuity measurements for all patients on a unit offers a useful guide in determining ongoing staffing needs. An **acuity recording** system determines the hours of care for a nursing unit and the number of staff required to care for a given group of patients.

Each morning staff nurses are typically required to enter the acuity scores of each of their patients into a computerized documentation system. The acuity data is then gathered electronically by managerial and administrative staff to make staffing decisions.

The acuity level allows the nursing staff to compare patients with one another. For example, an acuity system rates a patient from 1 to 5 (1 requires the most time, 5 requires the least amount of time). A patient returning from surgery who requires many assessments and interventions rates as an acuity level 2. On the same continuum, another patient awaiting discharge after a very successful recovery from surgery rates as an acuity level 5. Staffing assignments are then determined by examining the total acuity points of the patients on a particular nursing unit. For example, more experienced nurses may care for patients with higher acuity.

## Standardized Care Plans

Some institutions use **standardized care plans** to make documentation more efficient. The plans, based on the institution's standards of nursing practice, are preprinted established guidelines used to care for patients with similar health problems. After completing a nursing assessment, place the appropriate standard care plans in your patient's record. It is very important that you make necessary modifications to individualize each care plan. Most standardized plans also allow the addition of specific desired outcomes and the target dates of achievement of these outcomes (see Chapter 7).

## Discharge Summary Forms

There is much emphasis placed on preparing a patient for a timely discharge from a health care institution. Discharge planning and case management are complementary aspects of patient care (Birmingham, 2003). Ideally, you begin discharge planning on admission and in some cases even before admission, as is necessary with same-day surgery admissions and childbirth. When doing discharge planning, be responsive to changes in the patient's condition and involve the patient and family in the discharge planning process (see Chapter 2).

A discharge summary provides important information pertaining to the patient's unresolved problems and continued health care after discharge. Discharge planning achieves specific outcomes that include identifying patients who without discharge planning would suffer adverse consequences; collaboratively determining the proper level of care with appropriate health care professionals; matching the patient to the most appropriate postacute services; and ensuring a smooth transition of patients to the next level of care (Birmingham, 2004). You will need to include in a summary the reason for hospitalization, significant findings, patient's status, and any specific teaching plan given to the patient and/or family (JCAHO, 2005a). Discharge summary forms make the summary concise and instructive. Many forms include copies that you give to the patient, family members, or home care nurses. Discharge summaries involve multiple disciplines and help to ensure that your patient leaves the hospital in a timely manner with the appropriate health care resources (Box 8-1).

## Computerized Documentation

The technology that exists for computerization in the health care delivery system is virtually unlimited and holds potential for improving the accuracy and efficiency of documentation. It is estimated that the majority of health care facilities have some type of electronic health record (EHR) and documentation system (Moody and others, 2004). Computerized documentation systems are designed to minimize repetitive

---

> **BOX 8-1   Discharge Summary Information**
>
> Use clear, concise descriptions in patient's own language.
> Provide step-by-step description of how to perform a procedure (e.g., home medication administration).
> Reinforce explanation with printed instructions.
> Identify precautions to follow when performing self-care or administering medications.
> Review signs and symptoms of complications the patient needs to report to his or her physician or health care provider.
> List names and phone numbers of health care providers and community resources for the patient to contact.
> Identify any unresolved problem, including plans for follow-up and continuous treatment.
> List actual time of discharge, mode of transportation, and who accompanied the patient.

---

clerical and monitoring tasks and increase your time for direct patient care. There are many benefits to computerized documentation. When properly used, the systems improve documentation accuracy, timeliness, completeness, and communication across health care disciplines (Smith and others, 2005). Computers also help you reduce errors (e.g., better legibility than handwritten notations), standardize nursing care plans, increase your job satisfaction and productivity, and document all areas of patient care.

In addition, the computerized system assists nurses in retrieving data about nursing care outcomes. This information can enhance quality improvement and increase quality of patient care (Keenan and others, 2002). The software programs allow access to specific assessment data quickly, and the information automatically transfers to different reports.

Computerized documentation will potentially change drastically with the increased use of new technology. Therefore in the future, nursing will potentially use either pen-based or voice recognition computers in documentation. A notebook-size computer with handwriting recognition capabilities will allow you to document with ease and flexibility at a level that is not possible in the current systems.

A form of computerized documentation is a complete **computer-based patient record**. The record is a comprehensive system that uses many components of data collection and has a much broader scope than current charting systems. Know the legal risks of computerized documentation. Address confidentiality issues because there is an increased risk of unauthorized individuals gaining access to information. Consequently, the American Nurses Association, the American Medical Record Association, and the Canadian Nurses Association developed guidelines for safe computer charting (Moody, 2004):

1. Do not share the password used to enter and sign off computer files with other caregivers. A good system requires frequent changes in personal passwords to prevent unauthorized persons from accessing and tampering with records (Eggland, 1997).

2. Avoid leaving the computer terminal unattended when logged on.

3. Follow the correct protocol for correcting errors according to agency policy.

4. Software systems have a system for backup files. If you inadvertently delete part of the permanent record, follow agency policy. It is necessary to type an explanation into the computer file with the date, time, and your initials and to submit an explanation in writing to your manager (Smith, 2000).

5. Avoid leaving information about a patient displayed on a monitor where others see it. Keep a log that accounts for every copy of a computerized file that you have generated from the system.

6. Follow the agency's confidentiality procedures for documenting sensitive material, such as a diagnosis of human immunodeficiency virus (HIV) infection.

7. Protection of printouts from computerized records is important. Shredding of printouts and the logging of the number of copies generated by each caregiver are ways to minimize duplicate records and protect the confidentiality of patient information.

## Home Care Documentation

Home care continues to grow as increasing numbers of older adults use home care services. Medicare has specific guidelines for establishing eligibility for home care reimbursement. Skilled home nursing care falls into one of four categories: observation and assessment, teaching and training, skilled treatments and procedures, and management and evaluation of a care plan (Carusa and others, 2004). When you provide home care, your documentation must specifically address the category of care and your patient's response to care. Documentation in the home care system has different implications than in other areas of nursing. The documentation is both the quality control and the justification for reimbursement from Medicare, Medicaid, or private insurance companies (Carusa and others, 2004). Document all of your services for payment (e.g., direct skilled care, patient instructions, skilled observation, and evaluation visits) (JCAHO, 2005a).

## Long-Term Care Documentation

Increasing numbers of older adults and disabled people in the United States are requiring care in long-term health care facilities. Nursing personnel often face documentation challenges much different from those in the acute care setting. Changes in the Medicare program in the form of the PPS determine the standards and policies for reimbursement and documentation in long-term health care. The federally mandated Long Term Care Facility Resident Assessment Instrument (version 2.0) provides standardized protocols for assessment and care planning, as well as a minimum data set to promote quality improvement within and across facilities (Taunton and others, 2004). When residents' records are reviewed for reimbursement, there is an expectation that these protocols, such as skin assessments, wound care, and assisted ambulation, are carried out.

You assess each resident in long-term care by using the Long Term Care Facility Resident Assessment Instrument, an eight-page tool mandated by the Omnibus Budget Reconciliation Act of 1989 (OBRA) and updated in 1995 (Health Care Financing Administration [HCFA], 1995). Documentation supports a multidisciplinary approach to the assessment and planning process for patients. Communication among nurses, social workers, recreational therapists, and dietitians is essential in the regulated documentation process. The fiscal support for long-term care residents hinges on the justification of nursing care as demonstrated in sound documentation of the services rendered. The ultimate goal is to provide the highest quality care at the lowest cost per resident (Boroughs, 1999).

## Reporting

Reports are an exchange of information among health care team members. A report reflects a summary of activities or observations seen, performed, or heard by the health care provider. For example, after completing a work shift, you give a verbal report to nurses on the next shift and the laboratory submits written reports describing the results of diagnostic tests for inclusion in the permanent medical record.

### Change-of-Shift Report

The **change-of-shift report** occurs at the end of each shift. You will report information about your assigned patients to nurses working on the next shift. The purpose of the report is to provide better continuity and individualized care for patients. For example, if you find that a certain position increases a patient's breathing, you relay that information to the next nurse caring for the patient.

Change-of-shift reports involve transfer of information from nurses who have completed a shift of care to nurses about to begin a shift of care. Such reports are given orally, by audiotape recordings, or during walking rounds at the patient's bedside. Oral reports occur in person, with staff members from both shifts participating. You will complete audiotaped reports before the end of the shift and then make the recording available to incoming staff. This will increase efficiency and minimize social interactions. In the case of recorded reports, it is essential for staff to have an opportunity for last-minute updates, to clarify information, or to receive information on care events or changes in the patient's condition that occur after taping.

Walking reports given in person or during rounds allow you to obtain immediate feedback when questions arise about a patient's care. When you make rounds, the patient and family members also have the opportunity to participate in any discussions and care decisions.

An effective change-of-shift report is quick and efficient. A good report provides a baseline for comparisons and indicates the kind of care anticipated for the next shift. An organized and concise approach helps you set goals and anticipate patient needs and lessens the chance of overlooking important information. A sample format is as follows: background information (name, age, and medical diagnosis), primary health problem, nursing diagnoses, observations of the patient's condition and response to therapies, progress with teaching, interventions, and family involvement. It is especially important to report any recent changes or priority situations concerning the patient's condition.

When giving a report, maintain a professional manner. Describe interactions in objective terms, avoiding such judgmental labels as "uncooperative," "difficult," or "bad" when describing patient behaviors. This kind of language will contribute to prejudicial opinions about the patient. Judgmental statements overheard by the patient or family will possibly also lead to legal charges.

## Telephone Reports and Orders

**TELEPHONE REPORTS.** When significant events or changes in a patient's condition have occurred, a telephone report needs to include clear, accurate, and concise information. When documenting the phone call, include when the call was made, who made it (if you did not make the call), who was called, to whom information was given, what information was given, what information was received, and verification of the information with the provider (Figure 8-3). JCAHO standards (2005b) require that health care institutions identify a process for a verification "read-back" when taking critical test results. An example follows: "Laboratory technician J. Ignacio reported a potassium level of 5.9. Information was transcribed and read back for verification. Dr. Wade notified at 2030. D. Markle, RN."

**TELEPHONE ORDERS AND VERBAL ORDERS.** A telephone order (TO) involves a physician's or health care provider's stating a prescribed therapy over the phone to a registered nurse, whereas a verbal order (VO) involves the physician's or health care provider's stating orders for a nurse to write down. Telephone and verbal orders frequently occur at night or during an emergency. It is important to verify the order by writing the order completely and then reading it back to the prescriber. This "read-back" is a requirement by the JCAHO National Patient Safety Goals 2004 (JCAHO, 2005b). An example follows: "10/16/2007: 0815, Tylenol #3 tabs 2 every 6 hours for incisional pain. T.O. Dr. Knight/J. Woods, RN." The physician or health care provider later verifies the telephone or verbal order legally by signing it within a set time (e.g., 24 hours) as set by hospital policy. Telephone and verbal orders are used only when absolutely necessary and not for the sake of convenience. Box 8-2 provides guidelines that promote accuracy when receiving telephone orders.

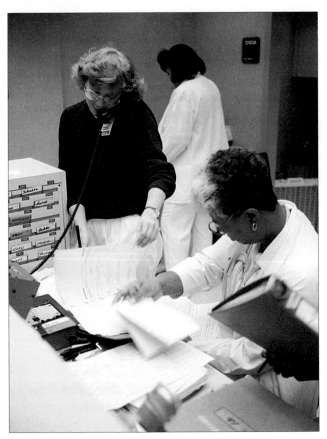

FIGURE **8-3** Persons involved with telephone reports must verify that information is accurate.

## Transfer Reports

Patients frequently transfer from one unit to another or to another facility to receive different levels of care. For example, patients transfer from intensive care units to general nursing units when the level of care no longer requires intense monitoring. A **transfer report** involves communication of information about patients from the nurse on the sending unit to the nurse on the receiving unit. Transfer reports are by phone or in person. When giving a transfer report, include the following information:

1. Patient's name, age, primary physician or health care provider, and medical diagnosis
2. Summary of medical progress up to the time of transfer
3. Current health status (physical and psychosocial)
4. Allergies
5. Emergency code status
6. Family support
7. Current nursing diagnoses or problems and care plan
8. Any critical assessments or interventions to be completed shortly after transfer (helps receiving nurse to establish priorities of care)
9. Need for any special equipment

<table>
<tr><td>

**BOX 8-2** **Guidelines for Telephone Orders and Verbal Orders**

Clearly identify the patient's name, room number, and diagnosis.
Read back all orders to the physician or health care provider (JCAHO, 2005b).
Use clarification questions to avoid misunderstandings.
Write "TO" (telephone order) or "VO" (verbal order), including date and time, name of patient, complete order; sign the name of the physician or health care provider and nurse.
Follow agency policies; some institutions require documentation of the "read-back" or require two nurses to review and sign telephone (and verbal) orders.
The physician or health care provider co-signs the order within the time frame required by the institution (usually 24 hours, verify agency policy).

</td></tr>
</table>

At the completion of the transfer report the receiving nurse will clarify any information by asking questions about the patient's status.

## Incident Reports

An incident is any event not consistent with the routine operation of a health care unit or routine care of a patient. Examples include patient falls, needle-stick injuries, a visitor becoming ill, and medication errors. Completion of an **incident report** occurs when there is an actual or potential injury and is not a part of the patient record (see Chapter 4). Therefore document an objective description of what you observed and follow-up actions taken in the patient's medical record without reference to the existence of the incident report. For example, a visitor to the agency faints. You should objectively record the details of the event and any statements made by the visitor. "Patient's husband complained of becoming dizzy and then began to fall to the floor. Nurse assisted visitor to the floor and turned him to his left side. His pulse was 62, and respirations were present. He remained unconscious for less than 2 minutes and gradually resumed consciousness. No abrasions observed. Visitor stated, 'I felt dizzy and light-headed, and I don't remember anything else.'"

At the time of the event, always contact the physician or health care provider to examine the patient. In the above example, follow the agency policy when a visitor is injured or becomes ill. In this example the patient's physician or health care provider should also be notified. Incident reports are an important part of quality improvement. Analysis of incident reports helps with the identification of trends within an organization that provide justification for changes in policies and procedures or for in-service programs (see Chapter 4 for other examples and further discussion).

## KEY CONCEPTS

- A patient's health care record is a confidential, written legal documentation of the care received.
- The record is a continuing account of the patient's health care status and is available to all members of the health care team. It facilitates communication with health care providers for continuity of patient care, maintains a legal and financial record of care, aids in clinical research, and guides professional and organizational performance improvement.
- Your signature on an entry in a record designates accountability for the contents of that entry.
- Accurate record keeping requires an objective interpretation of data with precise measurements, correct spelling, and proper use of abbreviations.
- Effective documentation verifies the specific nursing care provided, use of services and equipment, and medications and thus supports the reimbursement your health care agency receives.
- Document changes in a patient's condition to keep a record current.
- The case management model of delivering care uses a multidisciplinary approach to documenting patient care.

- Critical pathways (or care maps) summarize the standardized plan of care within a case management plan. These pathways direct and monitor the flow of patient care by defining patient-focused outcomes and specifying those interventions provided.
- To limit liability, nursing documentation exactly describes what happened to a patient and must clearly indicate that individualized, goal-directed nursing care was provided based on the nursing assessment.
- You organize problem-oriented medical records by the patient's health care problems.
- Medicare guidelines for establishing a patient's home care reimbursement are the basis for documentation by home care nurses.
- Long-term care documentation is multidisciplinary and closely linked with fiscal requirements of outside agencies.
- Computerized information systems provide information about patients in an organized and easily accessible fashion.
- The major purpose of the change-of-shift report is to maintain continuity of care.
- When information relevant to care is communicated by telephone, verify the information.
- Incident reports objectively describe any event not consistent with the routine care of a patient.

## CRITICAL THINKING IN PRACTICE

*Mr. Smith is a 65-year-old patient with a history of diabetes admitted with the diagnosis of pneumonia. Mr. Smith is in room 10, bed A. During your shift, Mr. Smith has started an antibiotic and is placed on oxygen. While you were at lunch, Mr. Jones, the patient in room 10, bed B, requested pain medication. The nurse covering for you incorrectly administered the medication to Mr. Smith instead of Mr. Jones. When you return from lunch, you discover the medication error. Mr. Smith is complaining of nausea from the codeine in the pain medication. You immediately notify the physician, who gives you an order for an antiemetic to treat Mr. Smith's nausea.*

- - - - - - - - - - - - - - - - - - - -

1. When taking a telephone order from the physician or health care provider, it is common for most organizations to require you to:
   a. Photocopy the order for your records
   b. Write the order in its entirety and read it back to the prescriber for verification
   c. Write the order but do not implement until it has been signed by the prescriber
   d. Take the order from the prescriber but insist that the prescriber come to the patient care division to write the order himself or herself

2. When a medication error occurs, what documentation should occur in the medical record?
   a. Document a note describing the incident, the patient's reaction, who was notified, and any actions taken.
   b. Document who made the error and why it occurred.
   c. Document a note describing the incident, the patient's reaction, who was notified, any actions taken, and that an incident report was completed.
   d. Document only the patient symptoms and what you did to relieve them.

3. What information about Mr. Smith do you include in your end-of-shift report?

## NCLEX® REVIEW

1. An advantage of CBE is that:
   1. Entries follow the format of the nursing process
   2. It originates from a nursing model rather than a medical model
   3. It moves away from charting only problems
   4. Narrative descriptions are used only when there are abnormal findings

2. The advantage of focus charting is that:
   1. It focuses on tracking the patient problems
   2. It enables all caregivers to track the patient's condition and progress toward the outcomes of care
   3. It uses check marks in a flow sheet
   4. It details the use of services and equipment on a spreadsheet

3. When comparing documentation for acute care in hospitals with documentation for long-term care, major differences are related to:
   1. The goal of the highest quality care at the lowest cost
   2. Using a multidisciplinary approach for assessment and planning
   3. The prospective payment system's determining the standards for reimbursement
   4. Increasing numbers of older adults and disabled people requiring long-term care

4. When giving a change-of-shift report, you are expected to:
   1. Include community resources that the patient can contact
   2. Include a step-by-step description of how to perform procedures
   3. Provide an organized and concise description of patient status and anticipated needs
   4. Review sign and symptoms of complications that should be reported to the physician or health care provider

5. When you receive telephone orders from a physician or health care provider you must:
   1. Make a photocopy of the order to avoid errors
   2. Read back the order to the prescriber
   3. Wait until the prescriber signs the order
   4. Include why the telephone order was needed

6. Incident reports are an important part of quality improvement programs. The intended goal of the incident report is:
   1. To provide information in the medical record
   2. To reprimand individuals involved in the incident
   3. To identify changes needed to prevent reoccurrences
   4. To document actual injury and follow-up actions taken

7. A nurse makes the following documentation in the patient record: "0830 Patient appears to be in severe pain and refuses to ambulate. Blood pressure and pulse are elevated. Physician notified and analgesic administered as ordered with adequate response. J Cass, RN." The most significant statement about the documentation would be that it is:
   1. Acceptable because it includes assessment, interventions, and evaluation
   2. Good because it showed immediate responsiveness to the problem
   3. Inadequate because pain is not described on a scale of 0 to 10
   4. Unacceptable because it is vague subjective data

**8.** Documentation of assessment of a patient recovering from surgery included the following information: complete bath; level of pain 6 (scale 0-10); turning in bed with assist of one; and dressing clean, dry, and intact. The least appropriate information is:
1. Complete bath
2. Level of pain
3. Turning in bed with assistance
4. Status of the dressing

**9.** A nurse documents an assessment completed at 5 PM. In military time this is:
1. 0500
2. 1300
3. 1700
4. 2100

## REFERENCES

Allen J, Englebright J: Patient-centered documentation: an effective and efficient use of clinical information systems, *J Nurs Adm* 32(2):90, 2000.

Birmingham J: Discharge planning: the old/new wave, *Inside Case Management* 19(5):1, 2003.

Birmingham J: Discharge planning: collaboration between provider and payer case managers using Medicare's conditions of participation, *Lippincotts Case Manag* 9(3):147, 2004.

Boroughs DS: Documentation in the long-term care setting, *J Nurs Adm* 29(12):46, 1999.

Carusa JT and others: Making sense of Medicare: a Medicare house call, *Am J Nurs* 104(7):71, 2004.

Coffey RJ and others: An introduction to critical paths, *Qual Manag Health Care* 14(1):46, 2005.

Cummins KM: Charting by exception, a timely format for you? *Am J Nurs* 99(3):24G, 1999.

Davidson N and others: An interdisciplinary documentation performance improvement project, *J Nurses Staff Dev* 20(5):236, 2004.

Eggland ET: Using computers to document, *Nursing* 27(1):17, 1997.

Health Care Financing Administration: Long term care facility resident assessment instrument (RAI) user's manual for use with version 2.0 of the Health Care Financing Administration's Minimum Data Set, resident assessment protocols, and utilization guidelines, Baltimore, Md, 1995, Health Care Financing Administration.

Iyer P, Camp NH: *Nursing documentation: a nursing process approach,* St. Louis, 1999, Mosby.

Joint Commission on Accreditation of Healthcare Organizations: *Comprehensive accreditation manual for hospitals (CAMH),* update 2, Chicago, 2005a, The Commission.

Joint Commission on Accreditation of Healthcare Organizations: *Setting the standard: the Joint Commission and healthcare safety and quality,* http://www.jcaho.org/general+public/patient+safety, accessed Sept 2005, 2005b, The Commission.

Keenan GM and others: The HANDS project: studying and refining the automated collection of a cross-setting clinical data set, *Comput Nurs* 20(3):89, 2002.

Ladebauche P: Limiting liability to avoid malpractice litigation, *MCN Am J Matern Child Nurs* 20(5):243, 1995.

Lavin J, Enright B: Charting with managed care in mind, *RN* 59(8):47, 1996.

Martin BA: Torts-r-us, *Vermont Nurse Connection* 4(1):4, 2001.

Moody LE and others: Electronic health records documentation in nursing, *Comput Nurs* 22(6):337, 2004.

Murphy EK: Charting by exception, *AORN J* 78(5):821, 2003.

Omnibus Budget Reconciliation Act of 1989, Pub L No. 101-239, 103 Stat 2106.

Smith K and others: Evaluating the impact of computerized clinical documentation, *Comput Nurs* 23(3):132, 2005.

Smith LS: Safe computer charting, *Nursing* 30(9):85, 2000.

Sullivan GH: Keep your charting on course, *RN* 63(5):74, 2000.

Sullivan GH: Legally speaking, does your charting measure up? *RN* 67(3):61, 2004.

Taunton RE and others: Care planning for nursing home residents: incorporating the minimum data set requirements into practice, *J Gerontol Nurs* 30(12):40, 2004.

United States Department of Health and Human Services: Standards for privacy of individuals, Health Insurance Portability and Accountability Act of 1996, 64 *Federal Register* 60053 (1999), Identifiable health information, August 2003, http://www.os.dhhs.gov/ocr/hipaa/finalreg.htm.

Yocum RF: Documenting for quality patient care, *Nursing* 32(8):58, 2002.

# CHAPTER 9

# Communication

## MEDIA RESOURCES

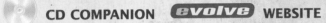

**CD COMPANION** *evolve* **WEBSITE**

http://evolve.elsevier.com/Potter/basic

- **NCLEX® Review**
- **Audio Glossary**
- **English/Spanish Audio Glossary**

## OBJECTIVES

- Identify situations that require careful communication.
- Describe the elements of the communication process.
- Describe the three levels of communication and their uses in nursing.
- Differentiate aspects of verbal and nonverbal communication.
- Identify features and expected outcomes of the nurse-patient helping relationship.
- List nursing focus areas within each phase of a therapeutic nurse-patient helping relationship.

- Describe behaviors and techniques that affect communication.
- Explain the focus of communication within each phase of the nursing process.
- Discuss effective communication for patients of varying developmental levels.
- Identify patient health states or responses that contribute to impaired communication.
- Explain techniques used to assist patients with special communication needs.

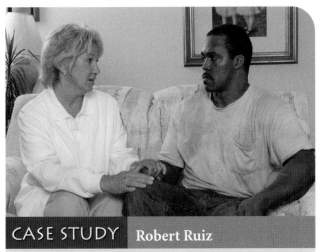

## CASE STUDY — Robert Ruiz

Roberto Ruiz is a 44-year-old man of Puerto Rican descent referred to hospice because he suffers human immunodeficiency (HIV) virus/acquired immunodeficiency syndrome (AIDS). After being near death, Roberto has gotten better and is at home. He is weak and stays in most of the time because of his compromised immune system. He gave his beloved dog to a friend in case he did not survive his last hospitalization. Hospice goals were to support the medication regimen, manage his pain, and promote quality of life.

Roberto lives alone and has an extensive network of friends, having lived and worked in the community for over 10 years. His home is full of special art objects that he has collected. Roberto appears tired, speaks softly, and smiles frequently. He talks about how his quality of life is better now than it has ever been. His home is a haven or sanctuary, and he feels peaceful.

Suzanne is a 54-year-old nurse whose mother died 10 years ago and had received hospice care. This was a brief but significant experience that gave her a dedication to hospice and a commitment to quality of life in end-of-life care.

As they work to manage Roberto's pain, he says, "I can stand some pain. I don't want to be 'out of it.' I want to feel alive."

Suzanne sees Roberto as a courageous man. His passion for life inspires Suzanne and the other members of the hospice team. From her coursework in end-of-life care (ELNEC, 2000) she knows that posing questions for the patient's reflection helps her assess his needs and support his self-care strategies.

"What are your needs at this time?" "What are your concerns at this time and for the future?" Roberto talks about wanting to get strong enough to have his dog again. He wants to make a trip home to New York to visit his family and make peace.

## KEY TERMS

active listening, p. 164
assertive communication, p. 167
channel, p. 155
communication, p. 154
connotative meaning, p. 156
denotative meaning, p. 156
empathy, p. 164
environment, p. 155
feedback, p. 155
humor, p. 167
interpersonal communication, p. 155
intrapersonal communication, p. 155

language, p. 156
message, p. 155
metacommunication, p. 156
nonverbal communication, p. 156
public communication, p. 156
receiver, p. 155
referent, p. 154
sender, p. 155
socializing, p. 166
sympathy, p. 164
therapeutic communication, p. 157
touch, p. 167
verbal communication, p. 156

ommunication in nursing is a journey to a destination of clear meaning. Nurses travel this road to help patients and families heal and promote health and wholeness. Communication is the heart of nursing and essential in conveying caring and applying nursing skills and knowledge as part of a health care team of patients, families, and colleagues. Relax! Clear, caring communication takes a lifetime to master and begins one moment at a time. Yet, be alert! Start today to pay attention to communication in your life. Watch what you and others say, how it is said, the nonverbal messages, and what words people choose in written and electronic communication. Consider what is not said, but implied by posture or tone of voice or a "look." Think of yourself as an explorer. You will mine treasures from every interaction. Sometimes these treasures are lessons you learn from awkward moments or missed opportunities. Sometimes these treasures are when a patient shows gratitude for your gentle touch by comfortable silence and eye contact. Hagerty and Patusky (2003) conclude that having less time with patients in the current health care environment does not have to be a barrier to connections with patients. When you are focused on the patient, you can make a difference, learn from every interaction, and build competency in therapeutic, interpersonal communication.

Nurses building caring relationships demonstrate their caring through what Watson (1985) identified as "carative factors"(see Chapter 16). These factors include instilling faith and hope, cultivating sensitivity to self and to others, and developing a helping-trust relationship. Promoting and accepting the expression of positive and negative feelings, using scientific problem solving for decision making, and promoting interpersonal teaching-learning are also factors. It is important to provide a supportive environment, assist with gratification of human needs, and allow for spiritual forces and phenomena. These aspects of caring within interpersonal relationships are intimately connected to your ability to communicate effectively.

You will use nonverbal, verbal, and technological skills to communicate in both personal and impersonal situations. You send and receive information through many different channels. You will communicate in person, in writing, over the telephone, through fax and electronic mail, and through the Internet. Communication in all these modes is an ongoing, dynamic, and often complex process.

## The Power of Communication

Like any therapy, communication can result in both harm and good. Your posture, your expressions and gestures, every word you choose, and every phrase you speak can hurt or heal through the messages they send. Even techniques meant to be therapeutic can have unexpected negative effects. Failure to communicate leads to serious problems, increases liability, and threatens professional credibility. Inappropriate

or missing communication causes delays in health care delivery, adding cost to the patient and agency. Respect communication for its potential power and do not misuse it to manipulate or bully others. Good communication empowers others and enables people to know themselves and to make their own choices. As you grow in self-awareness and learn from situations that did not go as well as you had planned, celebrate the joy of being part of helping relationships. Consider the case study on p. 153, with the patient Roberto Ruiz.

Taylor (2004) suggests a thinking process called practical reflection to improve communication. The three steps to practical reflection are experiencing, interpreting, and learning. To experience you journal or talk about the details of an interaction that did not go well. You answer questions such as, What happened? Who was involved? What went wrong and how did you feel about it? To interpret, you answer, What did I hope or expect to happen? What interfered with the outcome? What factors were involved? To learn you reflect on what the story tells you about yourself and the lessons you learned.

In a team meeting Suzanne reflects on her initial fears about working with patients who have HIV/AIDS. Now Suzanne and other nurses who visit Roberto call him their favorite patient. She has begun to see Roberto as a person and not as a fearful disease. Roberto has introduced her to the healing power of music, and they chat about favorite movies. She begins to pay more attention to appreciating her own life, adding music, and seeing how Roberto savors moments of his day.

## Decision Making and Communication

As a nurse you constantly make decisions about what, when, where, why, and how to send messages to others. Deciding which techniques best fit each unique nursing scenario is challenging. Situations that challenge your decision-making skills and call for careful use of therapeutic techniques often involve persons such as those described in Box 9-1. Practice helps, so take the initiative to discuss and role-play these scenarios before facing them in the clinical setting.

## Basic Elements of the Communication Process

Examine Figure 9-1, the basic elements of the communication process. Although this model oversimplifies, it helps you identify essential components of communication. People in conversation rarely analyze the meaning of every gesture or word. In your professional role you will learn to pay attention to each aspect so that interactions are purposeful and effective.

The **referent** motivates one person to communicate with another. In a health care environment, sights, sounds, odors,

| BOX 9-1 | Challenging Communication Situations |

The *silent, withdrawn* person who does not express any feelings or needs

The *sad, depressed* person who has slow mental and motor responses

The *angry, hostile* person who does not listen to explanations

The *sullen, uncooperative* person who resents being asked to do something

The *talkative, lonely* person who wants someone with him or her all the time

The *demanding* person who wants someone to wait on him or her or meet his or her requests

The *ranting and raving* person who blames nursing staff unfairly

The *sensory impaired* person who cannot hear or see well

The *verbally impaired* person who cannot articulate words

The *gossiping, catty* person who violates confidentiality and stirs up trouble

The *bitter, complaining* person who is negative about everything

The *mentally handicapped* person who is frightened and distrustful

The *confused, disoriented* person who is bewildered and uncooperative

The *anxious, nervous* person who cannot cope with what is happening

The *grieving, crying* person who has had a major loss

The *unresponsive, comatose* person who cannot communicate at all

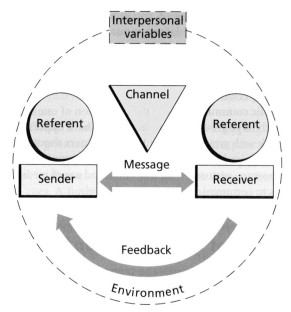

FIGURE **9-1** Communication as active process between sender and receiver.

time schedules, messages, objects, emotions, sensations, perceptions, ideas, and other cues initiate communication. Considering the referent during an interaction helps the sender develop and organize the message.

The **sender** is the person who delivers the message. The roles of sender and receiver change back and forth as two persons interact.

The **message** is the content of the conversation. It includes verbal and nonverbal information the sender expresses. The most effective message is clear, organized, and expressed in a manner familiar to both the sender and the receiver.

The **channel** is the means of conveying and receiving the message through visual, auditory, and tactile senses. Your facial expression sends a visual message. Your spoken words travel through auditory channels. Placing your hand on another person uses the channel of touch. Usually, the more channels the sender uses to convey a message, the more clearly the receiver will understand the message.

You send the message to the **receiver.** The message then acts as one of the receiver's referents, prompting a response. The more the sender and receiver have in common and the closer the relationship, the more likely the receiver will accurately perceive the sender's meaning and respond appropriately.

The **environment** is the physical and emotional climate in which the interaction takes place. For effective communication, make the environment comfortable and suit the participants' needs. The more positive an environment the sender and receiver can create, the more successful the exchange.

The message the receiver returns to the original sender is **feedback.** Feedback indicates whether the receiver understood the meaning of the sender's message. Your positive intent is not enough to ensure accurate reception of a message. Seek verbal and nonverbal feedback from the receiver to be sure the receiver understands the message.

## Levels of Communication

There are three levels of communication, each important in nursing. **Intrapersonal communication** is a powerful form of communication that occurs within an individual. Intrapersonal communication is also called *self-talk, self-verbalization,* and *inner thought* (Balzer Riley, 2004). People "talk to themselves" by forming thoughts internally that strongly influence perceptions, feelings, behavior, and self-concept. Be aware of the nature and content of your own thinking, and try to replace negative, self-defeating thoughts with positive ones. Use positive self-talk as a tool to improve health and self-esteem. In forms such as imagery or meditation, you use it to enhance coping and reduce stress. Self-instruction provides a mental rehearsal for difficult tasks or situations so individuals deal with them more effectively. During interactions, participants engage in both intrapersonal and interpersonal or public communication.

**Interpersonal communication** is interaction that occurs between two people or within a small group. It refers to nonverbal and verbal behavior within a social context and includes symbols and cues used to give and receive meaning.

---

**BOX 9-5** | **Communication Through the Nursing Process**

**Assessment**

Interviewing and history taking

Physical examination (use of visual, auditory, and tactile channels)

Observation of nonverbal behavior

Review of medical records, literature, diagnostic tests

**Nursing Diagnosis**

Written analysis of assessment findings

Discussion of health care needs and priorities with patient and family

**Planning**

Written care plans

Health team planning sessions

Discussions with patient and family to determine methods of implementation

Making referrals

**Implementation**

Discussion with other health professionals

Health teaching

Provision of therapeutic support

Contact with other health resources

Record of patient's progress in care plan and nurse's notes

**Evaluation**

Acquisition of verbal and nonverbal feedback

Written results of expected outcomes

Update of written care plan

Explanation of revisions to patient

---

record. Opiates, antidepressants, neuroleptics, hypnotics, or sedatives cause patients to slur words or use incomplete sentences. Communicate directly with the patient and family members to fully assess communication difficulties and build a plan to enhance communication.

## Developmental Factors

Consider the patient's developmental level in assessment of communication. An infant's self-expression is limited to crying, body movement, and facial expression. Older children express their needs more directly. Pay attention to your nonverbal behavior when working with children. Sudden movements, threatening gestures, and loud noises can be frightening. Include the parents as sources of information about the child's health.

Age also influences communication. Problems with hearing or speech are barriers to communication. Assess the hearing ability of older adults (see Chapter 13). Get an older adult's attention before you begin your assessment questions. Face the patient, and stand or sit on the same level so the patient can read your lips. Speak slowly and clearly. Give older adults enough time to ask questions. Do not assume an older adult has communication impairments.

## Sociocultural Factors

When caring for patients from diverse cultures, recognize how to adapt your communication approach. Green-Hernandez (2004) describes behaviors that demonstrate cultural competence. To be culturally competent, show respect for all persons whatever their age, gender, religion, socioeconomic group, sexual orientation, or ethnicity. Accept patients' rights. Recognize and attend to any personal biases or prejudices that might interfere with patients' care. Take cultural issues into account, and work to be culturally sensitive.

There may be language barriers with a foreign-born patient. Persons of different cultures use different types of verbal and nonverbal cues to convey meaning. Make a conscious effort not to interpret messages through your own cultural perspective; instead consider the context of the other individual's background. Avoid stereotyping persons from other cultures or making jokes about them (see Chapter 17). Consider the cultural sensitivity the nurse demonstrates in the following example (Jambunathan and Stewart, 1995).

> Carrie Barton is caring for Huan Mi, a young female refugee from Vietnam's Hmong Delta who has just delivered a small baby boy. Carrie understands that childbirth in different cultures is treated as a traumatic life crisis and a time of vulnerability for the mother and infant. She knows that Ms. Huan's lack of prenatal care was related to the woman's fear of miscarriage if touched by doctors or nurses. She is careful in how she touches Ms. Huan. Carrie has learned that touching the head is considered dangerous. Carrie did not try to argue with Ms. Huan's refusal of an episiotomy because she preferred to tear and heal naturally. She also respected Ms. Huan's decision not to have the baby circumcised, because it is "unnatural" to her. When teaching her about birth control, Carrie was aware that Ms. Huan might have difficulties practicing the techniques because of male/female role expectations. She was careful in how she sought feedback about Ms. Huan's understanding of the information. She knows that Asian persons often agree with the speaker to be polite rather than to indicate agreement or understanding.

Cultural insensitivity in communication takes many forms, including making fun of another's culture, ethnicity, language, or dress. Telling jokes that make fun of specific cultures, stereotyping, patronizing, and incorrectly interpreting culturally based behavior are culturally insensitive. This also includes behaving in ways that offend the cultural practices of others. In the example above, Carrie simply avoided touching Mrs. Huan's head. She did not laugh at her fears.

## Gender

Gender influences how we think, act, feel, and communicate. There are differences in male and female communication patterns. Males grow up using communication to achieve goals, establish individual status and authority, and compete for attention and power. Females grow up using communication to build connections and cooperate with others. Females also communicate to respond to, show interest in, and support others. Men typically prefer to talk about topics that do not expose personal feelings, whereas women enjoy discussing feelings and personal issues. Men tend to speak directly when giving criticism or orders. Women speak indirectly, couching criticism and commands in praise or vagueness to avoid causing offense or hurt feelings. A male nurse might say to his colleague, "Help me turn Jeremy." A female nurse might say, "Jeremy needs to be turned," expecting her colleague to understand the implied request for help. Men use more banter, teasing, and playful "put-downs." They sometimes hesitate to ask questions for fear of appearing unknowledgeable, whereas women ask questions to elicit information. Men usually want others to know of their accomplishments; women tend to downplay their achievements (Beebe and others, 2004).

It is important for you to recognize a patient's gender communication pattern. Gender-insensitive communication means a nurse of one gender misinterprets or reacts to messages differently than the other gender intends. Being insensitive can block any attempt at forming a therapeutic nurse-patient relationship.

## Nursing Diagnosis

After collecting assessment data from a patient, cluster pertinent defining characteristics for patterns and problems. Success in accurately identifying the patient's communication problem ensures the formulation of an accurate nursing diagnosis. Nursing diagnoses for patients with communication difficulties include the following:

- Anxiety
- Communication, impaired verbal
- Coping, compromised family
- Coping, ineffective
- Coping, readiness for enhanced family
- Powerlessness
- Social interaction, impaired

*Impaired verbal communication* is the nursing diagnostic label to describe the patient who has limited or no ability to communicate verbally. This diagnosis is useful for a wide variety of patients with special problems and needs related to communication. It is defined as "decreased, delayed, or absent ability to receive, process, transmit, and use a system of symbols" (NANDA International, 2005). A patient with this diagnosis will have defining characteristics such as the inability to articulate words, difficulty forming words, and difficulty in understanding. The related factor for a diagnosis should focus on the cause of the communication disorder. In the case of impaired verbal communication, a related factor might be physiological, mechanical, anatomical, psychological, cultural, or developmental. Be accurate in choosing a related factor so that the interventions you select will effectively resolve the patient's problem.

## Planning

Once you identify the nature of a patient's communication problem, you must consider several factors to design a plan of care. Motivation improves communication. Patients often need encouragement to try different communication strategies. Select interventions and communication techniques appropriate for the patient's age, cultural beliefs, and practices. Plan for adequate time that allows patients to practice new communication approaches. It also helps to plan practice sessions in a quiet, private environment. When possible, involve the family in selecting approaches that will foster communication with the patient.

## Goals and Outcomes

If you effectively communicate with a patient, your ultimate goal is having the patient experience a sense of trust in you and the health care team. Select expected outcomes that are specific and measurable. Outcomes allow you to determine if your goal has been met, once interventions are tried. For example, outcomes for the patient might include the following:

- Patient initiates conversation about diagnosis or health care problem.
- Patient understands messages from family members and the health care team.
- Patient expresses increased satisfaction with the communication process.

Sometimes you will care for patients who have difficulty in sending, receiving, and interpreting messages. This interferes with healthy interpersonal relationships. In this case, impaired communication is a contributing factor to other nursing diagnoses such as *impaired social interaction* or *ineffective coping*. Plan interventions to help such patients improve their communication skills. For example, role play helps patients rehearse situations in which they have difficulty communicating.

## Setting Priorities

Always maintain an open line of communication so that the patient can express any emergent needs or problems. Keep a call light in reach for the patient restricted to bed, or provide appropriate alternative communication devices such as a message board or Braille computer. If you plan to have a lengthy discussion with a patient, be sure to take care of the patient's physical needs first to avoid interruptions. Make the patient comfortable by ensuring that any symptoms are under control and that elimination needs have been met.

## Continuity of Care

Remember to include family caregivers during the planning and intervention phases of the nursing process. This collaboration offers support to the family and patient. When you use collaboration, patients are more likely to comply with plans. Collaboration also promotes communication among family members to facilitate positive patient-family relationships. Encourage collaboration by asking others for ideas and suggestions about how to reach goals. It gives others the opportunity to express themselves and strengthens problem-solving ability.

Also collaborate with other health care providers who have expertise in communication strategies. Speech therapists help patients with aphasia. Interpreters are invaluable when a patient speaks a foreign language. Psychiatric nurse specialists help in communicating with angry or highly anxious patients.

## Implementation

To effectively carry out a plan of care, nurses need to use communication techniques to meet the patient's individual needs. Nurses need to understand communication techniques that create barriers to effective interaction. Before you adapt communication to help patients with special needs, you need to learn the basics of therapeutic communication, which are the foundation for professional communication. Learning therapeutic communication techniques provides you with an awareness of the variety of nursing responses possible in different situations. As you practice these skills, you will become more comfortable with them and experience great satisfaction from the outcomes that you achieve through therapeutic relationships.

## Empathy

**Empathy** is the ability to understand and accept another person's reality, to accurately perceive feelings, and to communicate this understanding to the other. Balzer Riley (2004) writes, "When patients or colleagues are hurting, confused, troubled, anxious, doubtful of self-worth, or uncertain as to identity, then understanding is called for." Such empathetic understanding requires sensitivity and imagination, especially if you have not had similar experiences. You cannot be empathetic in all situations, but it is an important goal—a key to unlocking concern and communicating emotional support for others.

Empathy statements reflect an understanding of what has been communicated and tell the person that you heard both the feeling and the factual content of the communication. They foster shared respect and goals. Empathy statements are neutral and nonjudgmental. You will use them to establish trust in very difficult situations. For example, a patient has just received bad news:

> Nurse: "That must have been a difficult thing to hear."
> Nurse to family member: "It sounds like you're really afraid of what might happen to your husband."

## Sympathy

**Sympathy** is the concern, sorrow, or pity you feel for the patient, when you personally identify with the patient's needs. Sympathy is a subjective look at another person's world that prevents a clear perspective of all sides of the issues confronting that person. Sharing sympathy with another feels good, creates a bond, and minimizes differences. Although sympathy is a compassionate response to another's situation, it is not as therapeutic as empathy because your own emotional issues prevent effective problem solving and impair good judgment. Stuart and Laraia (2005) explain that sympathy causes problems in a helping relationship. This is because helpers who share the patient's needs are unable to help the patient select realistic solutions for problems and assume the patient's feelings are similar to their own. For example, a patient is grieving over an amputation.

> Nurse: "I'm so sorry about your amputation. I know just how you feel."
> A better empathic response is, "I can only imagine how hard it is to lose a leg."

## Listening and Responding

**Active listening** means listening attentively with the whole person—mind, body, and spirit. To be an active listener, listen for main and supportive ideas, acknowledge and respond, and give appropriate feedback. Pay attention to the other person's total communication, including the content, the intent, and the feelings expressed. Attentive listening allows you to better understand the message others communicate to you and is an excellent way to build trust. In many situations, the person just wants someone to listen.

Examine the following description of skills for attentive listening identified by the acronym SOLER (Townsend, 2003).

**S**—Sit facing the patient. This posture gives the message that you are there to listen and interested in what the patient is saying.

**O**—Offer an open posture (i.e., keeps arms and legs uncrossed). This posture suggests that you are "open" to what the patient says. A "closed" position conveys a defensive stance, possibly involving a similar response in the patient.

**L**—Lean toward the patient. This posture conveys that you are involved and interested in the interaction.

**E**—Establish and maintain intermittent eye contact. This behavior conveys your involvement and willingness to listen to what the patient is saying. Absence of eye contact or shifting of the eyes gives the message that you are not interested in what is being said.

**R**—Relax. It is important to communicate a sense of being relaxed and comfortable with the patient. Restlessness communicates a lack of interest and also conveys a feeling of discomfort that you transfer to the patient.

**PROVIDE INFORMATION.** Giving information, whether factual information or professional advice, helps the other person make decisions. Informing patients helps reduce anxiety and meet patient needs for safety and security. When offering suggestions, stress that the patient has the right to make decisions about options so that patient autonomy is maintained. Speak in simple language, and translate medical terms.

> *Nurse:* "Mr. Valdez, this new medicine is called Lanoxin. It acts as a cardiotonic and antidysrhythmic—that means it will help your heart have a stronger and more regular beat."

**PARAPHRASE COMMUNICATION.** *Paraphrasing* is restating the receiver's own words to make sure you have received information accurately. Be careful not to change the meaning when you paraphrase.

**CLARIFY COMMUNICATION.** *Clarifying* is used to validate whether the person interprets the message correctly. Try to restate an unclear or ambiguous message, or ask the other person to restate it, explain further, or give an example of what they mean.

**FOCUS COMMUNICATION.** *Focusing* directs conversation to a specific topic or issue when a discussion becomes unclear. Focusing limits the area to which the sender can respond. Use it when the sender rambles or introduces many unrelated topics in the same conversation.

> *Patient to nurse:* "I've come today to talk about how to lose weight again. I saw a picture of myself taken on New Year's Eve. I had an extra chin. I was wearing a blouse I thought was so attractive. I got it at that plus-size consignment shop. You might tell other patients about it. They have such good prices and stylish clothes. . . ."
> *Nurse to patient:* "I hear your concern about your weight. Tell me, what you have done in the past to lose weight?"

**SUMMARIZE COMMUNICATION.** *Summarizing* provides a concise review of main ideas from a discussion. It brings a sense of satisfaction and closure to an individual conversation, or it is used during the termination phase of a nurse-patient relationship. By reviewing a conversation, you focus on key issues and obtain additional relevant information as needed.

> *Nurse to patient:* "We've talked about what to expect when you go home and the self-care you'll need to do. You feel like you're ready, but you still need to make arrangements for a leave of absence from work."
> *Patient to nurse:* "Yes, and I also have to fill out workers' compensation papers."

**USE APPROPRIATE SELF-DISCLOSURE.** *Self-disclosure* is used during the working phase of a helping relationship.

Self-disclosures are personal statements, intentionally revealed to the other person. The purpose is to model and educate, foster a therapeutic alliance, validate reality, and encourage autonomy (Stuart and Laraia, 2005). Keep self-disclosures relevant and appropriate. Make these statements to benefit the patient, not you, and use them sparingly so that the patient remains the focus of the interaction. Tie your comments back to the patient focus (Balzer Riley, 2004). An inappropriate response to a patient is, "My mother had cancer, too. It was so long and drawn out. I was so sad for so long. Even taking care of my children was hard." A more appropriate response is, "When my mother was dying, I was torn between wanting to stay with her every moment and trying to meet the needs of my small children. Is that how it is for you?"

**AVOID INATTENTIVE LISTENING.** Fidgeting, breaking eye contact, daydreaming during conversation, and "pseudo listening"—pretending to listen when one really is not—convey the message that what the sender has to say is not important. These behaviors discourage conversation and damage trust. Examples of this are looking at your watch, tapping your foot impatiently, and gazing out the window as the patient talks.

**AVOID MEDICAL VOCABULARY.** Technical words can cause confusion and anxiety. Avoid use of such terms, or translate them into lay terms.

> *Nurse to patient:* "Sit up while your lungs are auscultated."
>      A better response is, "Let me help you sit up while I listen to your lungs."
> *Nurse to young child:* "Do you need to urinate?"
>      A better response is, "Do you need to use the potty?"

**AVOID GIVING PERSONAL OPINIONS.** When you give a personal opinion, it takes decision making away from the patient. Instead, offer options that are available to the patient. The problem and its solution belong to the patient, not the nurse.

> *Patient:* "I don't know how much longer I'll be able to take care of my husband. I just don't know what to do."
> *Nurse:* "If I were you, I'd put my husband in a nursing home."
>      A better response is, "Sounds like that's a difficult decision. Let's talk about what choices are available for someone like your husband who needs a lot of care."

**AVOID PRYING.** Asking irrelevant personal questions to satisfy your curiosity is inappropriate and invasive. If patients wish to share private information, they will.

**AVOID CHANGING THE SUBJECT.** Changing the subject is insensitive and tends to block further communication. If changing the subject is necessary, explain why.

> *Patient:* "I really miss my kids. I cry every time I think of them."
> *Nurse:* "Dr. Marcus will be here in a minute to take out your chest tube."
>      A better response is, "It must be hard to be apart from your children. Maybe we can talk about it after Dr. Marcus takes out your chest tube." ▪

## Acceptance and Respect

Conveying acceptance is an important part of therapeutic communication. It means you are nonjudgmental. As a nurse you are expected to provide high-quality care regardless of social or economic status, personal attributes, or the nature of the illness. Acceptance is a willingness to hear a message or to acknowledge feelings. This does not mean that you agree or approve. Acceptance includes giving positive feedback, making sure verbal and nonverbal cues match, and using touch. Being empathetic, restating, and avoiding arguments also show acceptance and respect.

**ASKING FOR EXPLANATIONS.** Sometimes asking "why" implies an accusation and results in resentment, insecurity, and mistrust. Try to phrase questions without using "why."

*Patient:* "I don't follow the diabetic diet the doctor talked about."
*Nurse:* "Tell me what problems you have had with the eating plan."

**AVOID APPROVAL OR DISAPPROVAL.** Do not impose your own attitudes, values, beliefs, and moral standards on others while in the professional helping role. People have the right to be themselves and make their own decisions. Avoid using terms such as *should, ought, good, bad, right,* or *wrong.* Agreeing or disagreeing sends the subtle message that you have the right to make value judgments about patient decisions. Instead, help the other person anticipate the consequences of decisions.

**AVOID ARGUING.** Challenging or arguing with someone's perceptions denies that their perceptions are real and implies that they are lying, misinformed, or uneducated. You should present information or reality in a way that avoids argument.

*Patient:* "My husband does not like it when I complain to the doctor about side effects of my drugs. He says the doctor is too busy."
*Nurse:* "It is true that the physicians here have many patients and your husband is thoughtful to be concerned, but that information helps the doctor prescribe the best medication for you and save everyone time."

**AVOID BEING DEFENSIVE.** Defensiveness in the face of criticism implies the sender has no right to an opinion. When you focus on the need for self-defense, defense of the health care team, or defense of others, you ignore the sender's concerns.

*Patient:* "The other nurse did the bandage differently. Don't you know what you are doing?"
*Nurse:* "I would appreciate it if you would tell me in what way the dressing is different so we can work together to get it just right for you."

## Silence

Give a new meaning to the word *listen* by rearranging the letters to read *silent.* Dyer (2002) says when you are silent you hear at a new level. It takes time and experience to become comfortable with silence. We fill empty spaces with words, but quiet can serve as time for you to observe, sort out feelings, think how to say things, and consider what has been communicated. Sometimes interrupting a meaningful silence is seen as disrespectful. Silence is therapeutic in times of profound sadness, deep thought, or grief when there are no "right" words. Relax your body, slow your breathing, and concentrate on offering your presence rather than words. Silence is a gift you give.

Mrs. Hartz, who is dying of renal failure, has just voiced feelings of deep grief about having to leave her family and friends behind. The nurse sits quietly while they both wipe away tears, think about love and loss, and appreciate the sharing that is taking place between them.

## Hope and Encouragement

Hope is essential for healing and communicates a "sense of possibility" to others (Benner, 1984). Encouragement and positive feedback are important in fostering hope and self-confidence. This helps people achieve their potential and reach their goals. You can give hope and encouragement by commenting on the positive aspects of the other person's behavior, performance, or response. Strengthen hope by sharing a vision of the future and reminding others of their resources and strengths. Suzanne encourages Roberto to make his home a sacred place, a sacred space, for his own healing. She knows that he is healing, although he is not cured from the physical illness. Cohen (2003) speaks of the healing influence of special places in nature, in sacred sites, and in hospitals' creation of healing environments. For example, an intensive care unit with a window overlooking a beautiful garden creates a positive mood.

**AVOID FALSE REASSURANCE THAT CAN DO MORE HARM THAN GOOD.** Although false reassurance might be intended kindly and helps you to avoid distress, you tend to block conversation and discourage further expression of feelings.

*Patient:* "I don't think I'm going to beat this lupus."
*Nurse:* "Don't worry, I'm sure everything will be all right."
A better response is, "Tell me more about what you're thinking," or "What's it like to feel that way?"

## Socializing

**Socializing** is an important component of your communication as a nurse. You use it as a tool to get to know one another and to help people relax. At the beginning of an interaction use social conversation that is easy and superficial to make connections. This helps the patient feel comfortable in sharing feelings and concerns. A friendly, informal, and warm communication style helps establish trust.

*Nurse:* "It certainly is a lovely day, Mrs. Spier."
*Patient:* "Yes, isn't it? If I were home and feeling better, I'd be planting my garden."
*Nurse:* "You're a gardener? What types of plants do you grow?"
*Patient:* "Oh, a little of everything. I like some tomatoes, lettuce, radishes, and maybe some squash."

**AVOID INAPPROPRIATE SOCIALIZING.** Move beyond social conversation to talk about issues or concerns affecting the patient's health.

## Assertiveness and Autonomy

**Assertive communication** is based on a philosophy of protecting individual rights and responsibilities. It includes the ability to be self-directive in acting to accomplish goals and advocate for others. Assertive responses promote self-esteem and uphold personal and professional rights. Feelings of security, competence, power, and professionalism characterize assertive responses. Assertive statements convey a message without resorting to sarcasm, whining, anger, blaming, or manipulation. Assertive responses are good tools to deal with criticism, change, negative conditions in personal or professional life, and conflict or stress in relationships.

Assertive responses often contain "I" messages, such as "I want," "I need," "I think," or "I feel." Simple assertive messages are usually stated in three parts, referencing the nurse, the other individual's behavior, and its effect.

> *Nurse to nurse:* "When you are late for work, I have to stay late and am late picking up my children from the babysitter."

You can state a more complex assertive message by using the ASSERT formula (Berko and others, 1997):

*Action:* Describe the action that prompted the need for the message.
*Subjective:* Express a subjective interpretation of the action.
*Sensations:* Express sensations related to the action.
*Effects:* Indicate the effects of the action.
*Request:* Make a request of the other person.
*Tell:* Tell your intentions if the request is not met.

> *Nurse to supervisor:* "When you say I'm not performing well, that sounds serious. I feel surprised and confused, because I had a sense that I was doing a good job. Please give me some examples of what you mean. If there are none, I'll discuss this evaluation with the director of nursing."

**AVOID PASSIVE RESPONSES.** Passive responses avoid issues or conflict. Some characteristics are feelings of sadness, depression, anxiety, and hopelessness.

> *Nurse to co-worker, hopelessly:* "I guess there's nothing we can do about it."
> *Nurse to spouse during argument:* "Whatever you say."
> A better response is: "What can we do to make things better?"

**AVOID AGGRESSIVE RESPONSES.** Aggressive responses provoke confrontation at the other person's expense. Some characteristics of aggression are feelings of anger, frustration, resentment, and stress.

> *Nurse to angry patient:* "Who do you think you are? You can't talk to me that way."

A better response is: "I want to hear your concerns and help you have positive experience. Can we take a deep breath and talk about them now, or should I come back later?"

## Humor

**Humor** is a coping strategy that adds perspective and helps you and the patient adjust to stress. The Association for Applied and Therapeutic Humor (2004) defines therapeutic humor as any intervention that promotes health and wellness by stimulating expression or appreciation of the silliness of life's inconsistencies. Laughter is a diversion from stress-related tension. It provides a sense of well-being and more of a feeling of control or mastery. Humor helps provide emotional support to patients and humanizes the illness experience. Laughter provides both a psychological and physical release for you and the patient, promotes open, relaxed interaction, and illustrates our shared experience in being human.

You assess whether humor is appropriate by noticing if patients use humor in their conversations. Start with small doses to see if this is helpful. To offer positive humor, share humorous incidents or situations, offer a clown nose to someone who could use a laugh, or share puns or simple jokes that are not offensive. Positive humor is associated with hope and love and joy with the intent to bring people closer. Avoid negative humor, which is inappropriate. Ethnic, religious, sexist, ageist, or put-down humor creates distance. Realize that humor sometimes backfires; not everyone will appreciate a humorous approach because of negative moods, stress, or physical discomfort. Humor is often a signal for closer attention. When a patient preparing for surgery quips, "Well, I won't die from it," gently explore concerns of the patient.

Sometimes health care staff use dark, negative humor after difficult or traumatic situations to survive a situation intact and to relieve tension and stress. This "coping humor" seems callous or uncaring by those not involved in the situation. Avoid using "coping humor" within earshot of patients or their loved ones. Understand that humor is a release, but timing, content, and receptivity are important in the use of therapeutic humor (Balzer Riley, 2004).

## Touch

**Touch** is a powerful form of communication (see Chapter 16). It is an integral part of human behavior; from birth until death, people need to be touched and to touch others. You are privileged to experience more of this intimate form of personal contact than almost any other professional. Through touch you can convey affection, emotional support, encouragement, and tenderness. Benner (2004) writes about a colleague's experience as a critical care patient. A nurse rubbed her shoulders to soothe and comfort her. The nurse enjoyed providing this comfort and savored this moment of caring connection. She valued this as part of the art of nursing, which is sometimes left out due to the emphasis on the high-tech nature of our work.

- Southeast Asians consider the head as the seat of life, which should not be touched except by close kin (Miller, 1995).
- Amish patients consider touching taboo between unrelated males and females.
- Use same-gender caregivers for female and older Asian, Middle Eastern, Hispanic, and African cultures, especially when touch is involved.
- Among Africans and Southeast Asians touching the head of the patient by a nonrelative may predispose loss of one's spirit and power (Orque, 1983).

Inappropriate touch: In a cancer support group, the wife of a patient had her arms wrapped around herself as if she were "holding herself together." The nurse moved too quickly and attempted to hug the patient without permission. The patient backed off and struggled to hold back tears.

Better approach: The nurse says, "I see you are distressed. Would a hug help?" The woman is then free to decline this well-intended act that might trigger tears that would embarrass this very private person.

Another concern is the confusion about the use of touch with culturally diverse patients (Box 9-6). Some risk is involved, yet nurses continue to observe for cues that a patient would welcome touch. Comfort touch is important for vulnerable patients experiencing severe illness with its accompanying physical and emotional losses. We use touch to awaken patients, to get their attention, to tease, or to add emphasis to explanations. Gleeson and Timmins (2004) report that patients with dementia are less anxious and eat better when touched. Touch may also convey understanding better than words or gestures. Therapeutic Touch is a special form of alternative touch therapy, a body energy field technique, used by nurses to achieve health assessment, pain reduction, and relaxation by influencing a patient's energy fields. In Therapeutic Touch, you pass the hands over the body without actually touching to "recreate and change proposed 'energy imbalances'" to restore innate healing forces (Spencer and Jacobs, 2003).

Because much of what you do involves touching, learn to use touch wisely. The zones of touch are described in Box 9-2. Touch delivered in the social or consent zones is less anxiety producing than touch delivered in the vulnerable or intimate zones. Students initially find giving intimate care stressful, especially with patients of the opposite sex. Shift your focus from personal discomfort to your role as a caregiver with the intent to provide sensitive nursing care. Trust that you will become more comfortable with experience. Remember that the patient who is ill and dependent must permit closer physical contact than is normally tolerated and may be uncomfortable with touch. Remain sensitive to your own responses and to patients' feelings. If a patient refuses to hold your hand during an episode of pain or pulls away from physical contact, this signals that the patient is uncomfortable with being touched. People perceive touch negatively when it is given without consent; used within a hostile or mistrusting relationship; and delivered to a vulnerable, intimate, or painful area of the body. Your touch should never be angry, rough, violent, overly stimulating, threatening, overly tentative, sexual, or unnecessarily painful.

## Communicating With Patients With Special Needs

Many health problems and human responses contribute to impaired communication. This includes the infant whose self-expression is limited to crying, body movement, and facial expression. Others with special needs are patients who are hearing and visually impaired, persons suffering from a stroke or late-stage Alzheimer's disease, and persons with autism or schizophrenia who respond to internal stimuli and misinterpret external stimuli. The person who does not speak or understand English and the patient with learning disabilities and limited vocal skills who uses gaze and body orientation to display a readiness to communicate will challenge you to accommodate their special needs. Also, unresponsive or heavily sedated patients are sometimes unable to send or receive verbal messages. Research suggests that nurses have difficulty communicating with patients with severe communication impairments because of a breakdown in understanding. This is the result of a lack of an understandable communication system (Box 9-7).

The patient who cannot communicate effectively has difficulty expressing needs and responding appropriately to the environment and requires special thought and sensitivity. Such persons benefit greatly when you adapt communication techniques to their circumstances (Box 9-8). When caring for a patient with impaired verbal communication related to cultural difference, you may provide a table of simple words in the patient's language to meet the expected outcome that the patient will communicate basic needs such as food, water, toileting, rest, sleep, and pain relief. Collaborate with team members to design the best communication strategies. A speech therapist can help the patient with aphasia, an interpreter (translator) may be needed for the patient who speaks a foreign language, and a psychiatric nurse specialist might help an angry or highly anxious patient to communicate.

Good communication will improve the quality of your patient's interpersonal relationships and well-being. If the patient uses ineffective communication techniques that interfere with coping or interpersonal relationships, intervene to help your patient send, receive, and interpret messages more effectively. Serve as a communication role model and teacher to help patients express needs, feelings, and concerns. Help patients develop social interaction skills and communicate thoughts and feelings clearly. This will help them interpret messages sent from others, increasing their autonomy and assertiveness. Methods such as role-playing allow patients to practice situations in which they have difficulty communicating.

BOX 9-7 USING EVIDENCE IN PRACTICE

**Research Summary**

Because nurses care for a variety of patients with communication problems, nurse researchers study the effects this has on nurses in practice. One group of researchers interviewed 20 nurses who cared for patients with severe communication impairment. The patients suffered from cerebral palsy and traumatic brain injury. In the interviews the researchers explored nurses' positive and negative experiences in providing care to these patients. The researchers analyzed the major themes from all 20 interviews and learned that nurse-patient communication is difficult when patients have severe communication impairment. Some nurses discovered ways to facilitate communication with such patients. Many of the communication difficulties were breakdowns in understanding. The nurses lacked a readily interpretable communication system for them and patients to use.

**Application in Nursing Practice**

Results from this study offer recommendations for ways nurses can communicate more effectively. Nurses would benefit from receiving training in the use of alternative communication modes, such as sign language. Nurses should have easy access to simple alternative communication devices when caring for patients who cannot speak. The researchers recommend collaboration with speech pathologists, who provide bedside training for patients with severe communication impairment.

Data from Hemsley B and others: Nursing the patient with severe communication impairment, *J Adv Nurs* 35(6):827, 2001.

**PROVIDING ALTERNATIVE COMMUNICATION METHODS.** Patients with physical communication barriers (e.g., those with a laryngectomy or endotracheal tube) may be unable to speak, or the clarity of speech may be so poor that they need alternative methods of communication (see Box 9-8). For these patients, provide simple communication methods to decrease frustration. Remember to be patient as the patient tries to communicate. The patient must be physically able to use the method you provide (e.g., communication boards or pencil and pad). Patients who are unable to speak are at risk for injury unless they are able to communicate personal needs quickly.

**COMMUNICATING WITH CHILDREN.** Communication with a child requires special considerations to develop a working relationship with the child and family. Because contact between parent and child is usually close, assume the information communicated by parents is reliable, although some parents may exaggerate. Offer a child toys or materials so the parent gives full attention to your information gathering. Give periodic attention to infants and younger children as they play to include them. An older child can be actively involved in communication. Consider the influence of development on language and thought processes.

Children, particularly the young, are especially responsive to nonverbal messages. Sudden movements or gestures can be frightening. Remain calm and gentle, and, if possible, let the child make the first move. Use a quiet, friendly, confident tone of voice. The child feels helpless in most situations involving health care personnel. When it is necessary to give explanations or directions, use simple, direct language and be honest. To minimize fear and anxiety, prepare the child by explaining what to expect. Avoid staring, and meet the child at eye level.

Drawing and playing with young children allow the child to communicate nonverbally (making the drawing) and verbally (explaining the picture) (Figure 9-2). Use a child's drawing as a basis for beginning a conversation.

**COMMUNICATING WITH OLDER ADULT PATIENTS.** Sensory alterations prevent receiving messages clearly. Motor disturbances such as dysarthria interfere with speech clarity. Many older adults adapt to sensory losses and learn to communicate effectively. When obvious deficits exist, maximize existing motor and sensory function to help the patient communicate more effectively (see Box 9-8). Ebersole and Hess (2003) indicate that older adults often suffer from other sensory deprivations (elimination of order or meaning and restricting the environment to dull monotony) and sensory overload (Box 9-9). Identify these challenges, and work with the patient to enhance effective communication. Attend to wisdom these patients have to offer you, and think of them as teachers about living.

## Evaluation

Together, you and the patient determine the success of the plan of care by evaluating the patient communication outcomes.

### Patient Care

Evaluate whether communication interventions were effective. Compare the expected outcomes you established in the plan of care with the actual outcomes you observe when interacting with patients. If you meet your outcomes, you have resolved the goals of care and the nursing diagnosis. When outcomes remain unmet, you may revise the existing plan with new goals, outcomes, and/or interventions. For example, if using a pen and paper proves frustrating for a nonverbal patient whose handwriting is shaky, you revise the care plan to include use of a picture board instead. In this case, observing the patient's handwriting and asking other caregivers about the patient's success in communicating needs would be your evaluation measures. Remember, careful evaluation requires you to make observations similar to those in your original assessment. For example, after initially assessing the extent of a patient's ability to hear the spoken word and providing various interventions to promote hearing, you would then return to evaluate the patient's ability to hear any interaction or instruction. It is also helpful to question the patient about whether needs were adequately met.

You can evaluate the effectiveness of your own communication by making process recordings, written records of your

| BOX 9-8 | **Communicating With Patients Who Have Special Needs** |

### Patients With Difficulty Hearing

Avoid shouting.
Use simple sentences.
Punctuate speech with facial expression and gestures.

### Patients With Difficulty Seeing

Communicate verbally before touching the patient.
Orient the patient to sounds in the environment.
Inform the patient when the conversation is over and when you are leaving the room.

### Patients Who Are Mute or Cannot Speak Clearly

Place sign by unit call system to answer call light in person.
Listen attentively, be patient, and do not interrupt.
Do not finish patients' sentences for them.
Ask simple questions that require "yes" or "no" answers.
Allow time for understanding and responses.
Use visual cues (e.g., words, pictures, objects) when possible.
Allow only one person to speak at time.
Do not shout or speak too loudly.
Encourage the patient to converse.
Let the patient know if you do not understand.
Use communication aids as needed:
  Pad and felt-tipped pen or Magic Slate
  Flash cards
  Communication board with words, letters, or pictures denoting basic needs
  Computer toy ("speak and spell" type)
  Call bells or alarms
  Sign language
  Use of eye blinks or movement of fingers for simple responses ("yes" or "no")

### Patients Who Are Cognitively Impaired

Reduce environmental distractions while conversing.
Get the patient's attention before speaking.
Use simple sentences and avoid long explanations.
Avoid shifting from subject to subject.
Ask one question at a time.
Allow time for the patient to respond.
Include family and friends to conversations, especially in subjects known to the patient.

### Patients Who Are Unresponsive

Call the patient by name during interactions.
Communicate both verbally and by touch.
Speak to the patient as though he or she could hear.
Explain all procedures and sensations.

### Patients Who Do Not Speak English

Speak to the patient in a normal tone of voice (shouting may be interpreted as anger).
Establish a method for the patient to signal the desire to communicate (call light or bell).
Provide a professional interpreter/translator as needed:
  Use a person familiar with the patient's culture and with biomedicine if possible.
  Allow plenty of time for the interpreter to transmit messages.
  Communicate directly to the patient and family rather than the interpreter.
  Ask one question at a time.
  Avoid making comments to the interpreter about the patient or family (they may understand some English).
Develop a communication board, pictures, or cards using words translated into English for the patient to make basic requests (e.g., pain medication, water, elimination).
Have a dictionary (English/Spanish or appropriate) available if the patient can read.

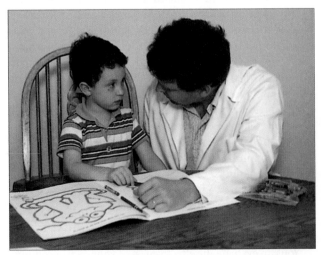

FIGURE **9-2** Drawing helps children communicate.

verbal and nonverbal interactions with patients. These recordings are useful in reflecting about how your communication style might improve.

## Patient Expectations

Review the patient's expectations of care and determine if the patient achieved expectations. This is an important part of the evaluation process. Ask patients and their families for input about goal achievement, factors that affected outcomes, and suggestions for changes that might be made in the plan of care. Suzanne consistently asked Roberto if the pain medications were relieving his discomfort. He was pleased that she was open to working with him to balance pain management with the clarity of his thinking.

Avoiding patient input during evaluation and its resultant care plan modification leads to a task-oriented rather than a critical thinking, patient-centered approach to nurs-

| BOX 9-9 | CARE OF THE OLDER ADULT |
|---|---|

In dealing with impaired communications with older adults, the primary goal is to establish a reliable communication system that all health care team members easily understand. Ideally, an inter-disciplinary model delivers effective care for older adults. Communication with older adults requires special attention. Be aware of the physical, psychological, and social changes of aging.

Use the following interventions to assist with impaired communication with older adults:

- During conversation, maintain a quiet environment that is free from background noise.
- Avoid shifting from subject to subject; allow time for conversation.
- Be an attentive listener. Use explorative questions to facilitate conversation (e.g., "How do you feel?").

- Avoid long sentences to explain the subject. Try to keep it short, simple, and to the point.
- Allow the older adult the opportunity to reminisce. Reminiscing has therapeutic properties that increase the sense of well-being.
- If you are experiencing problems understanding the patient (e.g., dysarthria), let the patient know and facilitate methods that help the patient speak more clearly. Consult with a speech therapist if necessary.
- Include the patient's family and friends in conversations, particularly in subjects known to the patient.
- Be aware of cultural differences among patients.

---

ing. It denies the patient's right to see the total picture of care and to be involved in all phases of the nursing process. A goal of total pain relief for Roberto was incompatible with his own goals of being alert enough to care for his dog and make art. Suzanne's willingness to consistently reevaluate the plan of care affected Roberto's quality of life. She used her therapeutic communication skills to engage the team in holistic care to address his goals for body, mind, and spiritual well-being. They focused on helping Roberto live every moment of his life the way he wanted to live it.

## KEY CONCEPTS

- Communication is a powerful therapeutic tool and an essential nursing skill used to influence others and achieve positive health outcomes.
- Nurses consider many contexts and factors influencing communication when making decisions about what, when, where, how, why, and with whom to communicate.
- Communication is most effective when the receiver and sender accurately perceive the meaning of one another's messages.
- The sender's and receiver's physical and developmental status, perceptions, values, emotions, knowledge, socio-cultural background, roles, and environment influence message transmission.
- Effective verbal communication requires appropriate intonation, clear and concise phrasing, proper pacing of statements, and proper timing and relevance of a message.
- Effective nonverbal communication complements and strengthens the message conveyed by verbal communication.
- Nurses use intrapersonal, interpersonal, and public interaction to achieve positive change and health goals.
- Strengthen helping relationships by establishing trust, empathy, autonomy, confidentiality, and professional competence.
- Effective communication techniques are facilitative and tend to encourage the other person to openly express ideas, feelings, or concerns.

- Ineffective communication techniques are inhibiting and tend to block the other person's willingness to openly express ideas, feelings, or concerns.
- The nurse must blend social and informational interactions with therapeutic communication techniques so that others explore feelings and manage health issues.
- When using therapeutic humor, consider timing, receptivity, and content of the humorous intervention.
- Methods that facilitate communication with children include sitting at eye level; interacting with parents; using simple, direct language; and incorporating play activities.
- Older adult patients with sensory, motor, or cognitive impairments require the adaptation of communication techniques to make up for their loss of function and special needs.
- Patients with impaired verbal communication require special consideration and alterations in communication techniques to facilitate the sending, receiving, and interpreting of messages.
- Desired outcomes for patients with impaired verbal communication include increased satisfaction with interpersonal interactions, the ability to send and receive clear messages, and attendance to and accurate interpretation of verbal and nonverbal cues.

## CRITICAL THINKING IN PRACTICE

*Walter Jordan is a 34-year-old man brought to the emergency department with crushing chest pain, shortness of breath, and exercise intolerance. His wife is at his side, in tears, moaning, "He's dying."*

1. What factors influencing communication are present in this scenario, and how would they affect your communication?
2. You take Mrs. Jordan's arm to escort her to the waiting room. She reacts angrily, wrenching her arm out of your grasp. What should you do now?

3. The couple's 4-year-old son is in the emergency department. His eyes are wide open, his skin is pale, and his eyes are tearing. How would you explain to him what is happening with his father?
4. The Jordans' 16-year-old daughter is pacing and picking at her nails. Construct a way to establish a helping-trust relationship with her.
5. You notice Emily, a team member, going into the bathroom in tears. How can you offer help without invading privacy?

## NCLEX® REVIEW

1. "Communication is not the message that was intended but rather the message that was received." The statement that best helps explain this is:
   1. Clear communication can ensure the patient will receive the message intended.
   2. Sincerity in communication is the responsibility of the sender and the receiver.
   3. Attention to personal space can minimize misinterpretation of communication.
   4. Contextual factors such as attitudes, values, beliefs, and self-concept influence communication.
2. You demonstrate active listening by:
   1. Agreeing with the patient
   2. Repeating everything the patient says to clarify
   3. Assuming a relaxed posture and leaning toward the patient
   4. Smiling and nodding continuously throughout the interview
3. As a nurse you build helping, caring relationships by:
   1. Using touch for calming and comfort
   2. Not asking the patient to do anything painful
   3. Establishing trust and demonstrating empathy
   4. Being sympathetic and protective of the patient
4. Gender influences how we think, act, feel, and communicate. In Western culture, when you are trying to be sensitive to gender in communication, it is important to remember that:
   1. Males use indirect communication to meet their needs, whereas females communicate directly
   2. Males grow up using aggressive communication, whereas females use passive communication
   3. Males and females should be treated equally; therefore it serves no purpose to distinguish between genders in communication
   4. Males grow up using communication to achieve goals, whereas females use communication to build connections with others

5. A nursing assistant comes to you to complain about a nurse on the unit where you work. The most effective response would be:
   1. To call the supervisor to ask for advice
   2. To tell him it is none of your business
   3. To listen sympathetically to help build team spirit
   4. To suggest he talk with the nurse to resolve the issue
6. The statement that best explains the role of collaboration with others for the patient's plan of care is:
   1. The professional nurse consults the physician or health care provider for direction in establishing goals for patients.
   2. The professional nurse depends on the latest literature to complete an excellent plan of care for patients.
   3. The professional nurse works independently to plan and deliver care and does not depend on other staff for assistance.
   4. The professional nurse collaborates with colleagues and the patient's family to provide combined expertise in planning care.
7. When working with an older adult, you should remember to:
   1. Avoid touching the patient
   2. Avoid shifting from subject to subject
   3. Avoid allowing the patient to reminisce
   4. Avoid asking the patient how he or she feels
8. When giving nursing care to a patient who is unresponsive, remember to:
   1. Speak loudly
   2. Use touch sparingly to avoid startling the patient
   3. Use the patient's name and explain procedures as if the patient can hear
   4. Spend as little time as possible with the patient to minimize stimulation

## REFERENCES

Applied Association for Therapeutic Humor, 2004, www.AATH.org.

Aucoin J, Lane PL: Space invasion, *Nursing,* p 32, Feb 2004.

Balzer Riley J: *Communication in nursing,* ed 4, St. Louis, 2004, Mosby.

Beebe SA and others: *Interpersonal communication: relating to others,* ed 4, Boston, 2004, Allyn & Bacon.

Benner P: *From novice to expert: excellence and power in clinical nursing practice,* Englewood Cliffs, NJ, 1984, Prentice Hall.

Benner P: Relational ethics of comfort, touch, and solace: endangered arts? *Am J Crit Care* 13(4):346, 2004.

Berko MR and others: *Connecting: a culture-sensitive approach to interpersonal communication competency,* ed 2, Philadelphia, 1997, Harcourt Brace.

Cohen K: Where healing dwells: the importance of sacred space, *Altern Ther Health Med* 9(4):68, 2003.

Dossey BM, Keegan L, Guzetta CE: *Holistic nursing: a handbook for practice,* ed 6, Boston, 2005, Jones & Bartlett.

Dyer W: *Getting into the gap: making conscious contact with God through meditation,* Carlsbad, Calif, 2002, Hay House.

Ebersole P, Hess P: *Toward healthy aging: human needs and nursing response,* ed 6, St. Louis, 2003, Mosby.

Edelman CL, Mandle CL: *Health promotion throughout the lifespan,* ed 5, St. Louis, 2002, Mosby.

ELNEC: Module 6, Communication, *End-of Life Nursing Education Consortium Training Program,* 2000, Washington, DC, 2003, American Association of Colleges of Nursing and Duarte, Calif, City of Hope.

Faas A: A personal reflection, *Dimens Crit Care Nurs* 23(4):176, 2004.

Gleeson M, Timmins F: Touch: a fundamental aspect of communication with older people experiencing dementia, *Nurs Older People* 16(2):18, 2004.

Green-Hernandez C, and others: Making your nursing care culturally competent, *Holist Nurs Pract* 18(4):215, 2004.

Haggerty BM, Patusky KL: Reconceptualizing the nurse-patient relationship, *J Nurs Scholarsh* 35(2):145, 2003.

Helmsley B and others: Nursing the patient with severe communication impairment, *J Adv Nurs* 35(6):827, 2001.

Horrigan B: Pamela Miles Reiki vibrational healing, *Altern Ther Health Med* 9(4):74, 2003.

Jambunathan J, Stewart S: Among women in Wisconsin: what are their concerns in pregnancy and childbirth? *Birth* 22(4):204, 1995.

King I: *Toward a theory for nursing,* New York, 1971, John Wiley & Sons.

Miller JA: Caring for Cambodian refugees in the emergency department, *J Emerg Nurs* 21(6):498, 1995.

NANDA International: *Nursing diagnoses: definitions and classifications, 2005-2006,* Philadelphia, 2005, NANDA International.

Orque MS: Nursing care of the South Vietnamese patients. In Orque MS, Bloch R, Monrroy LSA, editors: *Ethnic nursing care,* St. Louis, 1983, Mosby.

Spencer JW, Jacobs JJ: *Complementary and alternative medicine: an evidence-based approach,* St Louis, 2003, Mosby.

Stuart GW, Laraia MT: *Principles and practice of psychiatric nursing,* ed 7, St. Louis, 2005, Mosby.

Taylor BJ: Improving communication through practical reflection, *Reflect Nurs Leadersh* 30(2):28, 2004.

Townsend M: *Psychiatric mental health nursing: concepts of care,* ed 4, Philadelphia, 2003, FA Davis.

Watson J: *Nursing: human science and health care,* Norwalk, Conn, 1985, Appleton-Century-Crofts.

# CHAPTER 10

# Patient Education

## MEDIA RESOURCES

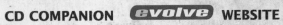

CD COMPANION **evolve** WEBSITE

http://evolve.elsevier.com/Potter/basic

- **NCLEX® Review**
- **Audio Glossary**
- **English/Spanish Audio Glossary**

## OBJECTIVES

- Identify appropriate topics for a patient's health education needs.
- Describe the similarities and differences between teaching and learning.
- Identify the purposes of patient education.
- Compare the communication and teaching processes.
- Describe the domains of learning.
- Differentiate factors that determine readiness to learn from those that determine ability to learn.
- Compare the nursing and teaching processes.

- Write learning objectives for a teaching plan.
- Describe the characteristics of a good learning environment.
- Identify the principles of effective teaching.
- Describe ways to adapt teaching for patients with different learning needs.
- Use the nursing process to make a teaching plan of care.
- Describe ways to incorporate teaching with routine nursing care.
- Identify the methods for evaluating learning.
- Describe appropriate documentation of teaching.

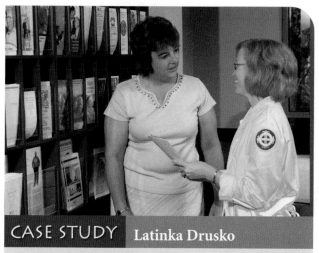

## CASE STUDY    Latinka Drusko

Latinka Drusko is a 55-year-old accountant. She immigrated to the United States from Bosnia in 1991 and has two grown sons who live close to her. Latinka's husband recently died. Latinka is overweight and smokes 1 to 1½ packs of cigarettes a day. She is visiting the local public health department for information to improve her health status.

Ashley is a 23-year-old nursing student who is completing her community health clinical rotation. Ashley meets Latinka in the health education section of the health department. After Ashley introduces herself, Latinka states, "I am interested in getting some information to help me become healthier. I would like to stop smoking and lose some weight. Do you think you can help me?" Ashley gives Latinka some written material and sets up a time when they can meet later.

### KEY TERMS

affective learning, p. 179
analogies, p. 190
attentional set, p. 179
cognitive learning, p. 179
functional health illiteracy, p. 191
health beliefs, p. 180

learning, p. 177
learning objective, p. 178
motivation, p. 179
psychomotor learning, p. 179
reinforcement, p. 189
return demonstration, p. 179
teaching, p. 177

Patient education will be one of your most important roles as a nurse practicing in any health care setting. Factors such as shorter hospital stays and the increased demand on nurses' time complicate your ability to provide quality patient education. As nurses try to find the most effective way to educate patients, health care consumers have become more assertive in seeking knowledge and understanding of their health and the resources available within the health care system. Providing your patients with needed information for self-care is necessary to ensure continuity of care from the hospital to the home (Falvo, 2004). Patient education is important because the patient has a right to know and to be informed about diagnosis and prognosis of illness, as well as treatment options and risks associated with treatments. Creating a well-designed, comprehensive teaching plan that fits your patient's unique learning needs reduces health care costs, improves the quality of care, and provides information about treatments. Ultimately, this will help the patient make informed decisions about health care. Effective patient education also helps patients become healthier and more independent.

## Standards for Patient Education

Accrediting agencies set guidelines for providing patient education in health care institutions. These guidelines ensure that patients and their families receive information necessary to maintain the patient's optimal level of health. In the United States, the Joint Commission on Accreditation of Healthcare Organizations (JCAHO) (2005) sets standards for patient and family education (Box 10-1). All health care professionals must participate in patient education to meet these standards. It is important to document evidence of successful patient education in your patient's medical record.

## Purposes of Patient Education

The goal of patient education is to assist individuals, families, or communities in achieving optimal levels of health (Edelman and Mandle, 2002). In today's health care arena, patients know more about health and want to be involved in health maintenance. To meet this need, you provide education to patients in convenient and familiar places (e.g., in their homes, churches, or schools). Comprehensive patient education includes three important purposes, each involving a separate phase of health care.

## Maintenance and Promotion of Health and Illness Prevention

Health care consumers are health conscious (Falvo, 2004). People participate in healthy activities, such as regular exercise and health screening programs, to maintain their health. Many places, such as the school, home, clinics, and workplace, provide information and skills to patients to help them take on healthier behaviors (Box 10-2). For example, in childbearing classes, expectant parents learn about physical and psychological changes in the woman and about fetal development. After learning about normal childbearing, the mother is more likely to engage in physical exercise, and the father is more likely to support the mother during her pregnancy.

The Internet has a tremendous affect on the importance of patient education. Today your patients have more access to information about their health. Regardless of the source of information, promoting healthy behavior through education increases self-esteem by encouraging your patients to assume more responsibility for health. When patients become more health conscious, they are more likely to seek early diagnosis of health problems (Redman, 2001).

### Restoration of Health

Injured or ill patients need information or skills that will help them improve or restore their level of health (see Box 10-2). Patients recovering from or adapting to illness or in-

---

| BOX 10-1 | JCAHO Education Standards for Hospitals |
| --- | --- |

**Standard PC.6.10** The patient receives education and training specific to the patient's needs and as appropriate to the care, treatment, and services provided.

**Elements of Performance for PC.6.10**
1. Education provided is appropriate to the patient's needs.
2. The assessment of learning needs addresses cultural and religious beliefs, emotional barriers, desire and motivation to learn, physical or cognitive limitations, and barriers to communication as appropriate.
3. As appropriate to the patient's condition and assessed needs and the hospital's scope of services, the patient is educated about the following:
   - The plan for care, treatment, and services
   - Basic health practices and safety
   - The safe and effective use of medications
   - Nutrition interventions, modified diets, or oral health
   - Safe and effective use of medical equipment or supplies when provided by the hospital
   - Understanding pain, the risk for pain, the importance of effective pain management, the pain assessment process, and methods for pain management

- Habilitation or rehabilitation to help them reach maximum independence possible

**Standard PC.6.30** The patient receives education and training specific to the patient's abilities as appropriate to the care, treatment, and services provided by the hospital.

**Elements of Performance for PC.6.30**
1. Education provided is appropriate to the patient's abilities.
2. Education is coordinated among the disciplines providing care, treatment, and services.
3. The content is presented in an understandable manner.
4. Teaching methods accommodate various learning styles.
5. Comprehension is evaluated.

**Standard PC.6.50** The hospital provides academic education to children and youth as needed.

**Elements of Performance for PC.6.50**
1. The hospital defines the length of stay and absence from school that would require providing educational services in accordance with applicable law and regulation.
2. The hospital addresses the specific academic educational needs of children and youth.

jury seek information about their health. However, patients who find it difficult to adapt to illness may become passive and uninterested in learning. Identify the patient's willingness to learn, and motivate the patient to learn.

Family or friends often positively contribute to your patient's return to health and often need to know as much as the patient. When you exclude these individuals from the patient's teaching plan, conflicts may arise. However, for education to be successful, do not assume the family should be involved. Assess the patient-family relationship before including the family in patient education.

## Coping With Impaired Functioning

Not all patients fully recover from illness or injury. Many learn to cope with permanent health changes. In these cases, patients need new knowledge and skills to continue activities of daily living (see Box 10-2). For example, the patient who loses the ability to speak after surgery of the larynx learns new ways of communicating. The patient with heart disease learns about diet, medication, and exercise to reduce further heart damage.

Patient education often focuses on helping patients manage their health care needs. This includes giving medications and applying dressings. You also teach patients to adapt to the additional emotional effects of chronic conditions. If the patient has no family or friends or if no one is willing to help the patient, you will need to make other arrangements for the patient's continuing care. Base care on the patient's needs, such as referring the patient to a long-term care facility. In the case of serious disability, the patient's role in the family or community may change. In these cases, family members and friends need to be supportive and accepting. The ability to provide support results from education, which begins as soon as you identify the patient's needs and determine family and friends are willing to help.

## Teaching and Learning

It is impossible to separate **teaching** from **learning**. Teaching is an interactive process that promotes learning. It consists of a conscious and deliberate set of actions that helps individuals gain new knowledge or perform new skills (Bastable, 2003; Redman, 2001). A teacher provides information that encourages the learner to engage in activities that lead to a desired change or health behavior. You use teaching and learning principles when developing teaching plans.

Learning is the acquisition of new knowledge or skills through reinforced practice and experience (Bastable, 2003). Generally teaching and learning begin when a person identifies a need for knowing or acquiring an ability to do something. Teaching is most effective when it responds to a learner's immediate needs. The teacher identifies these needs by asking questions and determining the learner's interests.

---

| **BOX 10-2** | **Topics for Health Education** |
| --- | --- |

**Health Maintenance and Promotion and Illness Prevention**

First aid
Avoidance of risk factors (e.g., smoking, alcohol)
Growth and development
Hygiene
Immunizations
Prenatal care and normal childbearing
Nutrition
Exercise
Safety (e.g., in home, car, workplace, hospital)
Screening (e.g., blood pressure, vision, cholesterol level)

**Restoration of Health**

Patient's disease or condition
  Anatomy and physiology of body system affected
  Cause of disease
  Origin of symptoms
  Expected effects on other body systems
  Prognosis
  Limitations on function
  Rationale for treatment
  Medications

Tests and therapies
Nursing measures
Surgical intervention
Expected duration of care
Hospital or clinic environment
Hospital or clinic staff
Long-term care
Methods for patient participation in care

**Coping With Impaired Function**

Home care
  Medications
  Diet
  Activity
  Self-help devices
Rehabilitation of remaining function
  Physical therapy
  Occupational therapy
  Speech therapy
Prevention of complications
  Knowledge of risk factors
  Implications of noncompliance with therapy
  Environmental alterations

| TABLE 10-1 | Comparison of Terms Used in Communication and Teaching | |
|---|---|
| **Communication** | **Teaching** |
| **Referent** | |
| Idea that initiates reason for communication | Perceived need to provide person with information, establishment of relevant learning objectives by teacher |
| **Sender** | |
| Person who conveys message to another | Teacher who performs activities aimed at assisting other person to learn |
| **Intrapersonal Variables (Sender)** | |
| Knowledge, values, emotions, and sociocultural influences that affect sender's thoughts | Teacher's philosophy of education (based on learning theory), knowledge of teaching content, teaching approach, experiences in teaching, emotions, and values |
| **Message** | |
| Information expressed or transmitted by sender | Content or information taught |
| **Channels** | |
| Methods used to transmit message (visual, auditory, touch) | Methods used to present content (visual and auditory materials, touch, taste, smell) |
| **Receiver** | |
| Person to whom message is sent | Learner |
| **Intrapersonal Variables (Receiver)** | |
| Knowledge, values, emotions, and sociocultural influences that affect receiver's thoughts | Willingness and ability to learn (physical and emotional health, education, experience, developmental level) |
| **Feedback** | |
| Information revealing that true meaning of message was received | Determination of whether the learner achieved learning objectives |

Interpersonal communication is essential for successful teaching (Falvo, 2004) (see Chapter 9).

## Role of the Nurse in Teaching and Learning

You have many roles in the teaching and learning process:

- Answering your patient's questions
- Providing information based on your patient's health needs or treatment plans
- Clarifying information from a variety of sources (e.g., physicians or health care providers, newspapers, television, the Internet)

To be an effective educator, you must engage the patient as a partner in learning and not merely pass on facts (Falvo, 2004). Carefully determine what your patients need to know and find the time when they are ready to learn. When you value and implement patient education, patients are better prepared to assume health care responsibilities. It is important to provide effective patient education to achieve desired patient outcomes. For example, children with asthma need to learn to use inhalers correctly to prevent respiratory distress. By including the child and by individualizing your ed-

ucational approach based on the child's developmental level and previous experience with inhalers, you help the child control the disease, have improved self-esteem, and stay out of the acute care setting.

## Teaching as Communication

The teaching process closely parallels the communication process (see Chapter 9). Effective teaching depends in part on the effectiveness of your communication skills. A teacher applies each element of the communication process while giving information to learners. Thus the teacher and learner become involved in a teaching process that increases the learner's knowledge and skills.

Compare the steps of the teaching process with those of the communication process (Table 10-1). In teaching, you need to provide the patient with information. Either you or the patient identifies the educational need. Then, identify specific learning objectives. A **learning objective** describes what the patient will be able to do after successful instruction.

You are the sender who wants to communicate a message to the patient. Promote learning by communicating in a language recognized by the patient. Many interpersonal variables influence your style and approach. Attitudes, values, cultural preferences, emotions, and knowledge influence the way you send messages (Falvo, 2004). Evaluating past experiences with teaching will help you choose the best way to present information.

To teach effectively, deliver the content clearly and precisely. Organize your information in a logical sequence so that your patient will easily understand the skills or ideas. Each lesson progresses from simple to more complex skills or ideas.

You can teach your patient in a variety of ways. All the senses are channels for presenting information. The auditory channel is the simplest, as in a lecture or discussion. The learning process becomes more active and stimulating when you use visual and psychomotor channels as well.

The receiver in the teaching-learning process is the learner. Interpersonal variables affect your patient's willingness and ability to learn. Language, attitudes, anxiety, cultural preferences, and values influence the ability to understand a message. The ability to learn depends on emotional and physical health, stage of development, and previous knowledge.

To be an effective teacher, have a method to evaluate the success of a teaching plan. A good form of feedback is **return demonstration**. The learner restates the received information or demonstrates learned skills, which allows you to assess the success of learning.

## Domains of Learning

Learning occurs in three domains or areas: (1) cognitive (understanding), (2) affective (values), and (3) psychomotor (motor skills). A topic to be learned sometimes involves all domains or only one. You will work with patients who need to learn in each domain.

**Cognitive learning** includes what the patient actually knows and understands. All intellectual behaviors are in the cognitive domain. This includes:

- Acquisition of knowledge
- Comprehension (ability to understand)
- Application (using abstract ideas in concrete situations)
- Analysis (relating ideas in an organized way)
- Synthesis (recognizing parts of information as a whole)
- Evaluation (judging the worth of a body of information)

**Affective learning** encompasses or includes the patient's feelings, attitudes, opinions and values. Although the affective domain is sometimes hard to identify, it greatly affects the success of education, either positively or negatively.

**Psychomotor learning** occurs when patients acquire skills that require the integration of knowledge and physical skills. Examples of psychomotor learning include learning to walk with a walker or giving an insulin injection. As patients

are able to complete psychomotor skills with more confidence, they are able to perform the behaviors in more complex or different situations. Adaptation occurs when your patient changes a response when unexpected problems arise. This results in originating, which involves creating new patterns of behavior.

Teaching your patient often involves incorporating behaviors from all three learning domains. Before you teach patients the proper method of giving an injection, they must first understand the reasons why they need the injections. Then they must know the proper location for administering the injection and the importance of using sterile technique (cognitive). The techniques of locating an acceptable area on the skin and introducing the needle use the senses of touch and vision (psychomotor). In addition, the patient must be willing to accept the need for injections and must overcome any fear of or distaste for injections (affective).

## Basic Learning Principles

To teach effectively and efficiently, you first need to understand how people learn. Learning depends on the motivation to learn, the ability to learn, and the learning environment. The ability to learn depends on physical and cognitive characteristics, one's developmental level, physical wellness, and intellectual thought processes.

### Motivation to Learn

**Motivation** is an internal impulse (e.g., an idea, an emotion, or a physical need) that causes a person to take action and addresses a person's desire to learn (Redman, 2001). Previous knowledge, attitudes, and sociocultural factors influence motivation. If a person does not want to learn, it is unlikely that learning will occur. Often patient motives are physical. Physical changes in function motivate a patient to learn strategies to help adapt to the functional change. For example, a patient with a lower limb amputation is motivated to learn to walk with a prosthesis.

An **attentional set** is the mental state that allows the learner to focus on and understand the material. People often use mental pictures to visualize ideas. Before learning anything, patients must pay attention to or concentrate on the information to be learned. Physical discomfort, anxiety, and environmental distractions make it more difficult for the patient to concentrate. Any physical condition that impairs your patient's ability to concentrate (e.g., pain, fatigue, or hunger) interferes with learning. Assess your patient for factors that reduce attention before beginning a teaching plan. Verbal and nonverbal cues reveal that your patient is not ready to learn.

Anxiety either increases or decreases the ability of a person to pay attention. Anxiety is uneasiness or uncertainty resulting from anticipating a threat or danger. Patients feel anxious when faced with change or the need to act differently. Learning requires a change in behavior and thus pro-

**BOX 10-3** CULTURAL FOCUS

Ashley recognizes that she knows very little about Bosnian culture. Therefore, before she meets with Latinka, Ashley takes some time to read about Bosnian culture. Ashley finds that during the 1990s, about 300,000 people from Bosnia immigrated to the United States as a result of the Balkan wars. The immigrants were older and had experienced significant trauma related to the war. They also came from a society that provided universal insurance coverage. People from Bosnia tend to have strong ties with their families and communities. Common values include hospitality, spontaneity, owning a home, and telling stories. Bosnians have unique health concerns. There is a high prevalence of smoking that worsened during and after the war. In Bosnia walking and bicycling are common, but in the United States this type of exercise is less common because places are further apart from each other and there is more traffic. Folk and family remedies are passed down from mother to daughter. Common treatments include using herbal teas for colds or the flu. Bosnians are often disappointed with health care in America, and many do not comply with medical prescriptions. Ashley uses this information about Bosnian culture to develop a culturally competent plan that focuses on helping Latinka lose weight and stop smoking.

**Implications for Practice**

- Ashley has a better understanding of Bosnian culture, but she recognizes that not all Bosnian people are the same. Therefore Ashley assesses Latinka's values and her beliefs about the American health care system.
- Ashley asks Latinka about her experiences with the war in Bosnia.
- Ashley asks Latinka to describe the coping strategies used to deal with the war and immigration to the United States.
- Ashley helps Latinka develop healthy coping strategies to deal with her feelings and fears.
- Latinka shares that she is very close to her children and her neighbors. Many times, people who are successful at sticking to an exercise plan exercise with other people. Therefore Ashley helps Latinka develop an exercise routine that includes her children and friends.

Data from Flowers DL: Culturally competent nursing care: a challenge for the 21st century, *Crit Care Nurse* 24(4):48, 2004; Lipson JG and others: Bosnian and Soviet refugees' experiences with health care, *West J Nurs Res* 25(7):854, 2003; MapZones: *Bosnia and Herzegovina Culture*, 2002, http://www.mapzones.com/world/europe/bosnia_hercegovina/cultureindex.php; and Searight HR: Bosnian immigrants' perceptions of the United States health care system: a qualitative interview study, *J Immigr Health* 5(2):87:2003.

duces anxiety. A mild level of anxiety may motivate learning. However, a high level of anxiety prevents learning from taking place. It disables a person, creating an inability to attend to anything other than relieving the anxiety.

Your patient's **health beliefs** are powerful motivators, and a number of variables influence this (see Chapter 1). Know your patient's health beliefs to determine the factors that will

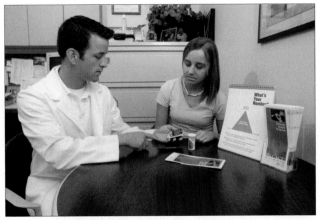

FIGURE **10-1** Nurse instructing a patient with a glucose meter.

motivate learning (Box 10-3). Do not assume that you know what your patient believes; your patient's view of health may not match your view of health (Falvo, 2004).

In addition, health teaching often involves changing attitudes and values. Simply teaching facts does not alter this. Therefore you compare how the patient views health and the patient's motivation to learn in relation to what knowledge they need to stick to prescribed therapy. You include beliefs that motivate your patient to learn in the teaching plan. For example, if your patient is a busy executive with high blood pressure, use the patient's desire to succeed and the concern that illness will impair work to motivate behavioral change. To facilitate successful teaching, stress and encourage the motivating factor for several months after the initial teaching intervention.

Learning is enhanced when patients are actively involved in the educational session (Edelman and Mandle, 2002). A patient's involvement in learning implies an eagerness to acquire knowledge or skills and allows the patient to make decisions during teaching sessions. For example, to help a patient with diabetes learn to monitor blood glucose levels, you assist the patient in choosing a blood glucose meter. You incorporate the patient's lifestyle into a schedule for blood glucose testing (Figure 10-1).

**READINESS TO LEARN.** Readiness to learn is significant. Your patients cannot learn when they are unwilling or unable to accept the reality of illness. A temporary or permanent loss of health is difficult for patients to accept. The stages of grieving (see Chapter 23) encompass a series of responses patients experience during illness. People experience these stages at different rates. It is important for you to properly time patient teaching to ease your patient's adjustment to illness or disability (Table 10-2). Introduce the teaching plan when your patient enters the stage of acceptance, which is most compatible with learning.

## Ability to Learn

The ability to learn is influenced by your patient's developmental level and physical capabilities. You must consider these important factors in developing an effective teaching plan.

| TABLE 10-2 | Relationship Between Psychosocial Adaptation to Illness and Learning | | |
|---|---|---|---|
| Stage | Patient's Behavior | Learning Implications | Rationale |
| Denial or disbelief | Patient avoids discussion of illness ("There's nothing wrong with me") and disregards physical restrictions. Patient suppresses and distorts information that has not been presented clearly. | Provide support, empathy, and careful explanations of all procedures while they are being done. Let patient know you are available for discussion. Explain situation to family. Teach in present tense (explain current therapy). | Patient is not prepared to deal with problem. Any attempt to convince or tell patient about illness will result in further anger or withdrawal. Provide only information patient pursues or absolutely requires. |
| Anger | Patient blames and complains and often directs anger at nurse. | Do not argue with patient, but listen to concerns. Teach in present tense. Reassure family of patient's normality. | Patient needs opportunity to express feelings and anger. Patient is still not prepared to face future. |
| Bargaining | Patient offers to live better life in exchange for promise of better health ("If God lets me live, I promise to be more careful"). | Continue to introduce only reality. Teach only in present tense. | Patient is still unwilling to accept limitations. |
| Resolution | Patient begins to express emotions openly, realizes that illness has created changes, and begins to ask questions. | Encourage expression of feelings. Begin to share information needed for future, and set aside formal times for discussion. | Patient begins to perceive need for assistance and is ready to accept responsibility for learning. |
| Acceptance | Patient recognizes reality of condition, actively pursues information, and strives for independence. | Focus teaching on future skills and knowledge required. Continue to teach about present occurrences. Involve family in teaching information for discharge. | Patient is more easily motivated to learn. Acceptance of illness reflects willingness to deal with its implications. |

**DEVELOPMENTAL CAPABILITY.** Cognitive development influences your patient's ability to learn. Learning occurs more readily when new information complements existing knowledge. Therefore, for teaching to be successful, consider your patient's stage of development and intellectual abilities. For example, if you give teaching booklets and brochures to a patient who cannot read, the information provided is not helpful to the patient. Learning, like developmental growth, is an evolving process. Assess the patient's level of knowledge and intellectual skills before beginning a teaching plan. For example, reading a medication label or instructions in a teaching booklet requires reading and comprehension skills.

**AGE-GROUP.** Age reflects the developmental capability for learning and learning behaviors that the patient is able to acquire. Without proper biological, motor, language, and personal-social development, many types of learning cannot take place (see Chapter 19). Learning occurs when behavior changes as a result of experience or growth (Hockenberry and others, 2003). Box 10-4 summarizes teaching methods to adapt based on a patient's developmental level.

**PHYSICAL CAPABILITY.** The ability to learn often depends on a person's level of physical development and overall physical health. To learn psychomotor skills, your patient needs to have the necessary level of strength, coor-

dination, and sensory acuity. For example, it is useless for you to teach your patient to transfer from a bed to a wheelchair if the patient has insufficient upper body strength. Therefore do not overestimate the patient's physical abilities. To learn psychomotor skills, your patient requires the following characteristics:

1. Size (height and weight that match the task to be performed or the equipment to be used [e.g., crutch walking])
2. Strength (ability of the patient to follow strenuous exercise program)
3. Coordination (dexterity needed for complicated motor skills such as using utensils or changing a bandage)
4. Sensory acuity (visual, auditory, tactile, gustatory, and olfactory: sensory resources needed to receive and respond to messages taught)

Any condition (e.g., pain, breathing difficulty) that drains a person's energy will also impair the ability to learn. For example, when an illness becomes aggravated by complications such as a high fever or respiratory difficulty, postpone teaching. After working with your patient, assess the patient's energy level by noting the patient's willingness to communicate, amount of activity initiated, and responsiveness toward questions. You may stop teaching temporarily

---

**BOX 10-4** **Teaching Methods Based on Patient's Developmental Capacity**

**Infant**

Keep routines (e.g., feeding, bathing) consistent.

Hold infant firmly while smiling and speaking softly to convey sense of trust.

Have infant touch different textures (e.g., soft fabric, hard plastic).

**Toddler**

Use play to teach procedure or activity (e.g., handling examination equipment, applying bandage to doll).

Offer picture books that describe story of children in hospital or clinic.

Use simple words such as *cut* instead of *laceration* to promote understanding.

**Preschooler**

Use role-playing, imitation, and play to make it fun for preschoolers to learn.

Encourage questions and offer explanations. Use simple explanations and demonstrations.

Encourage children to learn together through pictures and short stories about how to perform hygiene.

**School-Age Child**

Teach psychomotor skills needed to maintain health. (Complicated skills, such as learning to use a syringe, take considerable practice.)

Offer opportunities to discuss health problems and answer questions.

**Adolescent**

Help adolescent learn about feelings and need for self-expression.

Use teaching as collaborative activity.

Allow adolescents to make decisions about health and health promotion (safety, sex education, substance abuse).

Use problem solving to help adolescents make choices.

**Young or Middle Adult**

Encourage participation in teaching plan by setting mutual goals.

Encourage independent learning.

Offer information so that adult understands effects of health problem.

**Older Adult**

Teach when patient is alert and rested.

Involve adult in discussion or activity.

Focus on wellness and the person's strength.

Use approaches that enhance reception of stimuli for patients with sensory alterations (see Chapter 36).

Keep teaching sessions short.

---

when your patient needs rest. Resume teaching when your patient feels better.

## Learning Environment

Factors in the physical environment where teaching takes place make learning a pleasant or difficult experience. Choose a setting that helps your patient focus attention on the learning task. The number of people you are teaching, need for privacy, room temperature, room lighting, noise, room ventilation, and room furniture are important considerations when choosing the setting.

The ideal environment that promotes learning is a room that has good lighting and ventilation, appropriate furniture, and a comfortable temperature (Figure 10-2). A darkened room interferes with the patient's ability to see the demonstration of a skill or visual aids such as posters or pamphlets. A room that is too cold, hot, or stuffy will make the patient too uncomfortable to pay attention to you. Comfortable furniture eliminates distractions such as the need to change position or shift body weight.

It is also important for you to choose a quiet setting that offers privacy and where interruptions are infrequent. If your patient desires, family members might share in discussions. However, the patient may be reluctant to discuss the nature of the illness when other persons, even family members, are in the room.

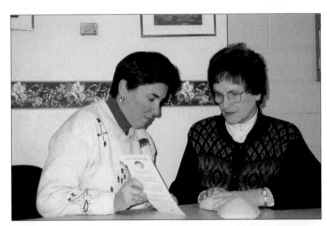

FIGURE **10-2** Choosing comfortable, pleasant environments enhances the learning experience. The nurse is explaining the breast self-examination procedure to the patient.

Teaching a group of patients requires a room that allows everyone to be seated comfortably and within hearing distance of the teacher. The size of the room should not be too big for the group. This tempts participants to sit outside the group along the perimeter. Arranging the group to allow participants to observe one another further enhances learning. More effective communication occurs as learners observe the verbal and nonverbal interactions of others.

| TABLE 10-3 | Comparison of the Nursing and Teaching Processes | |
|---|---|---|
| **Basic Steps** | **Nursing Process** | **Teaching Process** |
| Assessment | Collect data about patient's physical, psychological, social, cultural, developmental, and spiritual needs from patient, family, and all databases, medical record, nursing history, and literature. | Gather data about patient's learning needs, motivation, ability to learn, and teaching resources from patient, family, learning environment, and all databases. |
| Nursing diagnosis | Identify appropriate nursing diagnoses. | Identify patient's learning needs on basis of three domains of learning. |
| Planning | Develop individualized care plan. Set diagnosis priorities based on patient's immediate needs. | Establish learning objectives, stated in behavioral terms. Identify priorities regarding learning needs. Collaborate with patient on teaching plan. |
| Implementation | Collaborate with patient on care plan. Perform nursing care therapies. Include patient as active participant in care. Involve family in care as appropriate. | Identify type of teaching method to use. Implement teaching methods. Actively involve patient in learning activities. Include family participation as appropriate. |
| Evaluation | Identify success in meeting desired outcomes and goals of nursing care. | Determine outcomes of teaching-learning process. Measure patient's ability to achieve learning objectives. Reteach as needed. |

# Integrating the Nursing and Teaching Processes

There are distinct comparisons between the nursing process (see Chapter 7) and the teaching process. During the nursing process, assessment reveals your patient's health care needs. The nursing diagnoses you identify are unique to your patient's situation. You develop an individualized plan of care with appropriate interventions that you implement. Evaluation determines the level of success in meeting goals of care.

Assess and diagnose your patient's health care problems, any needs for education. When education becomes a part of the care plan, the teaching process begins. The teaching process requires you to analyze the patient's need, motivation, and ability to learn (Table 10-3). Learning needs specify the information or skills your patient requires. You set specific learning objectives and implement the teaching plan, using teaching and learning principles to ensure that your patient acquires knowledge and skills (Table 10-4). Finally, the teaching process requires an evaluation of learning based on learning objectives.

## Assessment

Successful patient teaching requires that you assess the patient's learning needs to determine teaching content (Redman, 2001). Other factors that influence the content you need to teach include learning resources and the patient's ability and willingness to learn. A thorough assessment will help you choose the best teaching methods and ensures a more individualized approach toward patient education (see Synthesis in Practice Box) (Table 10-5).

**LEARNING NEEDS.** Together, you and your patient identify information critical for the patient to learn. Questions such as "What do you think is important for you to know to take care of yourself?" allow the patient to be an active participant in planning self-care. Learning needs change depending on where your patient is in the recovery process. Assessment of learning needs is an ongoing activity. Examples of key areas of assessment are (1) questions raised by the patient or family about health issues; (2) the patient's understanding of current health status, implications of illness, types of therapy, and prognosis; (3) information or skills needed to perform self-care; (4) experiences that influence the patient's need to learn; and (5) information necessary for family members to meet the patient's needs.

**MOTIVATION TO LEARN.** Ask questions that identify your patient's motivation to learn. These questions help determine whether the patient is prepared and willing to learn. Ask questions that relate to the patient's learning behaviors, health beliefs, attitudes about health care providers, knowledge of information to be learned, physical symptoms that interfere with learning (e.g., fatigue, pain, or dizziness), and sociocultural background and learning-style preference.

**ABILITY TO LEARN.** Determine the patient's physical and cognitive levels. Many factors can impair the ability to learn. You need to assess the patient's physical strength and coordination, any sensory deficits, the patient's reading and developmental level (see Box 10-4), and the patient's level of cognitive functioning (see Chapter 19).

**TEACHING ENVIRONMENT.** Create an environment for a teaching session that is favorable to learning. Assess for distractions, noise, the patient's comfort level, and the availability of rooms and equipment. In the home setting, lighting, space, and the availability of equipment are especially important to assess.

**RESOURCES FOR LEARNING.** Identify resources for learning, which often include the support of family members or significant others. If you include family or signifi-

| TABLE 10-4 | Teaching and Learning Principles and Related Nursing Interventions |
|---|---|

| Teaching and Learning Principles | Related Nursing Interventions |
|---|---|
| • Beliefs about illness, the health care delivery system, and health care providers affect learners. | • Carefully assess the patient's beliefs and attitudes before planning teaching sessions. |
| • Learning styles vary from one patient to another. | • Determine how the patient learns best, and use this learning style while you teach the patient. |
| | • Do not assume you know what the patient is thinking or feeling. |
| • Beliefs about illness or health problems are based on a combination of physiological, psychosocial, and cultural factors, as well as personal experiences. Not all patients adapt or react to illness in the same way. | • Individualize teaching interventions, and match information with the patient's needs. |
| • Learners must be ready and motivated to learn. | • Acknowledge patient's fears, frustrations, and readiness to learn. |
| | • Provide education when the patient is ready to learn. |
| • Effective communication is necessary for teaching to be effective. | • Establish rapport with the patient. |
| | • Recognize the stressors the patient is feeling, and support the patient's effective coping strategies. |
| | • Do not agree with negative beliefs. |
| | • Provide prompt and accurate feedback. |
| • Enforce learning by repetition, reinforcement, and success. | • Build on the patient's previous knowledge and experiences. |
| | • Help the patient apply information in different settings and situations. |
| | • Keep the patient actively involved in learning (e.g., ask questions, have patient perform return demonstrations). |
| | • Provide positive reinforcement. |
| • Learning is enhanced when information is presented using words and language that the learner understands. | • Provide verbal and printed information at the fifth-grade reading level. |
| | • If the patient's first language is not English, provide instructions written in the language the patient understands. |
| | • Use interpreters when necessary to provide information to the patient who does not understand English. |

Modified from Falvo DR: *Effective patient education: a guide to increased compliance,* ed 3, Sudbury, Mass, 2004, Jones & Bartlett; and Lubkin IM, Larsen PD: *Chronic illness: impact and interventions,* ed 5, Sudbury, Mass, 2002, Jones & Bartlett.

## FOCUSED PATIENT ASSESSMENT                                    TABLE 10-5

| Factors to Assess | Questions and Approaches | Physical Assessment Strategies |
|---|---|---|
| Learning needs | Determine what the patient understands about the topic. | Observe for a puzzled expression on the patient's face. |
| | Ask what the patient wants to know about the topic. | Observe for restlessness as evidenced by multiple position changes. |
| Resources for learning | Determine if the patient has someone who can help him or her at home. | Observe for signs of anxiety when discussing home and transportation issues. |
| | Ask if the patient can get to the local health department or wellness center to obtain teaching materials. | |
| Ability to learn | Ask if the patient wears glasses or contacts or seems to have trouble seeing to read the newspaper. | Observe where the patient holds the reading material and for squinting of eyes when reading. |
| | Ask if the patient has trouble hearing when someone speaks to him or her. | Observe whether the patient turns his or her head when attempting to listen. |

## SYNTHESIS IN PRACTICE

Ashley decides to continue to care for Latinka during the rest of her community health clinical rotation. As Ashley begins to assess Latinka's educational needs, she reviews Latinka's health concerns and request for information. Ashley knows that people learn best when you provide the information they want. Ashley also wants to provide culturally competent patient education. Therefore Ashley knows that assessing Latinka's perceptions of the American health care system and concerns related to immigrating to the United States is a priority before she begins teaching about losing weight and smoking cessation.

Ashley's parents decided to stop smoking and have not smoked for 6 months. Ashley talks with her parents to find out what strategies helped them best to quit smoking. Ashley recalls that her mother gained about 10 lb when she quit smoking. Because Latinka expressed an interest in losing weight and quitting smoking, Ashley decides she needs to help Latinka develop healthy strategies that do not involve food to cope with nicotine withdrawal symptoms.

Ashley knows that she has the ethical responsibility to provide culturally sensitive patient teaching. She must accept Latinka and respect her culture when providing patient teaching. The health department has patient handouts that Ashley can use, but the handouts were designed for Caucasians and African-Americans, not for Bosnians. Therefore Ashley decides to take the printed information home with her and revises it so it reflects Latinka's culture. Ashley also makes sure that the information is written in words that are easy to understand. She realizes that if Latinka cannot read English well, she will need the printed information translated into Bosnian. Ashley is excited to learn more about Latinka and her culture. After establishing a caring relationship with Latinka, Ashley begins to assess Latinka's health needs and learning styles so she can put together an effective individualized teaching plan.

cant others, assess the readiness of family and friends to learn any information necessary to help care for the patient. Determine the family perceptions of the patient's illness, the patient's willingness to involve family members in care, and the family's willingness to help provide care. Also determine the resources available in the home and the teaching tools needed. Ensure that available teaching resources such as brochures, audiovisual materials, and posters are available when needed. Select the most appropriate teaching tool for the patient's needs and ability to learn. Assess written materials for reading level. There are computer programs designed to assess reading level. Also, organizations such as a literacy council can be of great assistance.

**CULTURAL CONSIDERATIONS.** Assess the language the patient most commonly uses. Make sure brochures are in your patient's native language. Determine the patient's role in the family and how the patient's culture influences the patient's perception of illness. You also explore the significance of prescribed medications and therapies in the patient's culture and explore alternative therapies the patient uses (Box 10-5). Teaching that does not include cultural considerations is ineffective (Falvo, 2004).

**PATIENT EXPECTATIONS.** Complete your assessment by understanding what your patient expects to learn. For example, if your patient is newly diagnosed with insulin dependent diabetes mellitus, what are the expectations regarding self-management? Does the patient expect to self-administer the insulin, or is the expectation that a spouse will give the injection? Assess your patient's expectations in all three learning domains.

### Nursing Diagnosis

After assessing information related to your patient's ability and need to learn, interpret the data to form diagnoses that reflect the patient's specific learning needs. This ensures that teaching will be goal directed and individualized. If a patient has several learning needs, nursing diagnoses allow for priority setting.

Several nursing diagnoses apply to learning needs. Each diagnostic statement describes the specific type of learning need and its cause. Classifying diagnoses by the three learning domains helps you focus specifically on the subject matter and teaching methods. Nursing diagnoses you might use with patients who have learning needs include the following:

- Ineffective health maintenance
- Health-seeking behaviors
- Deficient knowledge (affective, cognitive, psychomotor)
- Noncompliance (with medications)
- Ineffective therapeutic regimen management
- Ineffective community therapeutic regimen management
- Ineffective family therapeutic regimen management

You are able to manage or eliminate some health care problems through education. In these situations, the related factor of the diagnostic statement is *deficient knowledge.* For example, your patient is not taking a medication at the appropriate time because the patient does not understand how the medication works. Your focus becomes explaining the action of the medication and its purpose.

Some nursing diagnoses indicate that barriers to learning exist (e.g., *pain* and *fatigue*). In these cases, delay teaching until you resolve the nursing diagnosis.

### Planning

After determining nursing diagnoses, identify your patient's learning needs and develop a teaching plan. The plan includes topics for instruction, teaching resources (e.g., equipment or booklets), recommendations for involving family, and teaching objectives. The setting influences the complexity of the

To help Latinka modify her diet to make it healthier, Ashley investigates what Latinka normally eats. The Bosnian diet is high in animal fats and has a Turkish influence. Meat, bread, vegetables, stews, cheese, legumes, fish, eggs, coffee, sweetened fruit juices, and sweet cakes are common in the Bosnian diet. Using this information, Ashley develops the following teaching plan for Latinka:

**Outcome**
At the end of the teaching session, Latinka will verbalize understanding of three ways to make her diet lower in fat and calories.

**Teaching Strategies**
- Complete a diet history to explore what foods Latinka prepares at home.
- Review Latinka's favorite recipes and meals, and make suggestions of food substitutions that will make meals healthier (e.g., eat fruit instead of drinking sweetened fruit juice; use lean ground beef, low-fat cheese, margarine or vegetable oil, and decrease number of eggs used in recipes).
- Encourage Latinka to increase the number of legumes and fresh vegetables in her diet while decreasing the amount of sweet bread she eats.
- Provide Latinka with culturally sensitive teaching handouts on healthy food choices.
- Summarize what was taught.
- Make a follow-up appointment to reinforce teaching.

**Evaluation Strategies**
- Have Latinka complete a 3-day food diary, and evaluate her food choices on her follow-up appointment.
- Ask Latinka to describe what substitutions to make in her favorite recipes to make them healthier.
- Ask Latinka to make a healthy menu for 2 days.

Data from Flowers DL: Culturally competent nursing care: a challenge for the 21st century, *Crit Care Nurse* 24(4):48, 2004; Jonsson IM and others: Choice of food and food traditions in pre-war Bosnia-Herzegovina: focus group interviews with immigrant women in Sweden, *Ethn Health* 7(3):149, 2002; and Lipson JG and others: Bosnian and Soviet refugees' experiences with health care, *West J Nurs Res* 25(7):854, 2003.

plan. No matter what the length, the teaching plan provides continuity of instruction, especially when several nurses or disciplines share teaching responsibilities.

It is very important that you set clear goals and measurable outcomes so you can effectively evaluate and change the teaching plan as needed. Expected outcomes guide the choice of teaching strategies and who is involved in the plan. Patient participation ensures a more relevant and meaningful plan (see care plan). In many situations you will include the patient's family in the teaching plan. For example, if a patient with a spinal cord injury needs to perform self-urinary catheterization and needs help with this skill at home, it would be appropriate to include family members and other possible caregivers in the educational plan.

Patients receive education in almost every health care setting. Your responsibility is to refer the patient to appropriate multidisciplinary health care providers if indicated. For example, you refer a patient with a new diagnosis of chronic renal failure to a dietitian for dietary considerations. Patients in acute care settings often require assistance from discharge planners, case managers, and community agencies to be successfully discharged to home. It is your responsibility to collaborate with and include these multidisciplinary health care team members in the teaching plan.

Patients are also members of communities. Teaching plans often include information needed to help patients return to their communities as functioning members. Therefore you consider the patient's community when planning an educational session. For example, when teaching transfer techniques to the patient with the spinal cord injury, you need to include how the patient will transfer onto and off public transportation that is available in the patient's community.

**SETTING PRIORITIES.** Learning objectives identify the expected outcomes of a planned learning experience, which help establish priorities for learning. Prioritize learning needs based on your patient's needs, nursing diagnoses, and previous knowledge. In most situations it is not appropriate to delegate educational interventions to assistive personnel. You are ultimately responsible for ensuring that all teaching needs have been met. Therefore you will need to find out and prioritize what the patient needs to know. Usually, teaching needs focused on patient safety issues are the most important (Kiger, 2004). For example, a patient with newly diagnosed hypertension and angina needs to learn about newly prescribed medications, which include nitroglycerine spray for angina and a calcium channel blocker. In this situation, knowledge regarding the early identification of chest pain and appropriate use of the nitroglycerine spray is the learning priority.

Learning objectives are either short term (relating to immediate learning needs) or long term (relating to permanent adaptation to a health problem). Always develop learning objectives with the patient. Each objective is a statement of a single behavior that identifies the patient's ability to do something after a learning experience. The objective contains an active verb describing what the learner will do after the objective is met, such as walk with crutches, administer an injection, or identify drug doses. Use a verb that has few

## CARE PLAN    Patient Education for Smoking Cessation

### ASSESSMENT

Latinka Drusko states that she currently smokes 1 to 1½ packs of cigarettes a day. Her husband recently died of bladder cancer. Latinka states that she is **concerned about how smoking is affecting her health.** She began smoking before she immigrated to the United States. She knows that cigarette smoking is a risk factor for cancer. Latinka tried to quit smoking once before, but she states, "When my husband was diagnosed with cancer, the stress became too much, so I started smoking again. **I want to get control of my health. I just don't know how to do it. Can you help me quit smoking for good?**"

*Defining characteristics are shown in bold type.

### NURSING DIAGNOSIS Health seeking behaviors related to lack of knowledge of smoking cessation.

### PLANNING

**GOAL**

- Latinka will quit smoking through the use of a smoking cessation plan within 6 months.

**EXPECTED OUTCOMES***

**Health Seeking Behavior (Smoking Cessation)**

- Latinka will seek assistance from the nurses in the health department to develop a smoking cessation plan.
- Latinka will describe strategies to eliminate her unhealthy behavior.
- Latinka will follow self-developed strategies for smoking cessation to maximize her health.

*Outcomes classification label from Moorhead S, Johnson M, Maas M: *Nursing outcomes classification (NOC)*, ed 3, St. Louis, 2004, Mosby.

| INTERVENTIONS† | RATIONALE |
| --- | --- |
| **Health Education** | |
| • Determine Latinka's current knowledge about smoking cessation, her health beliefs, and her learning needs. | Patient demonstrates readiness to learn and perceives information as important to learn effectively (Falvo, 2004). |
| • Emphasize immediate or short-term positive health benefits associated with smoking cessation instead of emphasizing the negative long-term effects of smoking. | Emphasizing the short-term benefits of smoking is effective with older adults. Short-term benefits of smoking cessation include enhanced self-esteem, blood pressure and pulse return to normal, walking becomes easier, lung function improves, energy increases, and breathing becomes easier (Sheahan, 2002). |
| • Use group discussions and role-playing to influence health beliefs, attitudes, and values. | Using role-playing and having the patient perform behaviors enhances healthy behaviors (Bandura, 1997). |
| • Plan long-term follow-up to reinforce healthy behavior. | People who have quit smoking for more than 2 weeks still crave nicotine, but the withdrawal symptoms related to nicotine have diminished (Sheahan, 2002). They need continued praise and reinforcement for at least 2 years to keep from smoking. |
| **Self-Modification Assistance** | |
| • Evaluate Latinka's social environment for level of support for smoking cessation. | Older women tend to experience social isolation and a change in income when their spouse dies. Therefore they are less likely to attempt smoking cessation. Older adults are more likely to be successful with smoking cessation when their family and friends are supportive and do not smoke (Sheahan, 2002). |
| • Encourage Latinka to identify small successes. | Relapses in smoking cessation are common in older adults. Helping them see their successes provides encouragement (Sheahan, 2002). |
| **Smoking Cessation Assistance** | |
| • Help Latinka set a definite quit date within the next 2 weeks. | A special date, like a birthday, and sharing this date with supportive significant others can boost the commitment to quit smoking (Sheahan, 2002). |
| • Manage nicotine replacement therapy. | Older smokers do not tend to participate in formal smoking cessation programs. Using nicotine replacement therapy, such as a transdermal nicotine patch, helps minimize nicotine withdrawal symptoms (Sheahan, 2002). |

†Intervention classification labels from Dochterman JM, Bulechek GM, editors: *Nursing interventions classification (NIC)*, ed 4, St. Louis, 2004, Mosby.

*Continued*

**CARE PLAN** | Patient Education for Smoking Cessation—cont'd

**EVALUATION**

- Have Latinka describe the steps she has identified in the smoking cessation plan she developed during the educational session.
- Ask Latinka to describe strategies to implement whenever she is tempted to start smoking again.
- Have Latinka keep a log that records when she was tempted to smoke and what she did to avoid smoking during these times.

Have Latinka bring this log in with her, and evaluate it when she returns for follow-up care.

- Observe Latinka's respiratory status, activity tolerance, and energy level. Ask Latinka to compare these symptoms before and after she stopped smoking.

---

interpretations and state the verb in terms of how the patient is to demonstrate learning (Redman, 2001).

Behavioral objectives are measurable and observable, indicating how learning is evidenced (e.g., to perform the three-point crutch gait) and describing the conditions or timing under which the behavior occurs. Conditions or time frames should be realistic and designed for the learner's needs. It helps to consider the conditions under which the patient or family will typically perform the learned behavior (e.g., to walk from bedroom to bath using crutches).

Determine achievement of the objective when the patient meets acceptable criteria you select. Set criteria on the basis of a desired level of accuracy, success, or satisfaction. For example, a patient undergoing therapy for a fractured leg will walk on crutches to the end of the hall within 3 days.

### Implementation

Implementation of a teaching plan involves applying all teaching and learning principles. Implementation involves believing that each interaction with a patient is an opportunity to teach. Maximize opportunities for effective learning, and create an active learning environment. Because learning situations vary, there is no single correct way to teach. The principles of teaching are in effect techniques that incorporate the principles of learning.

**TIMING.** When is the right time to teach? When a patient first enters a clinic or hospital? At discharge? At home? Each is appropriate because patients have learning needs and opportunities as long as they stay in the health care system. Plan to teach when the patient is most attentive, receptive, and alert. The frequency of sessions depends on the learner's abilities and the complexity of the material (Falvo, 2004).

The length of teaching sessions also affects learning. Prolonged sessions cause patients to lose concentration and attentiveness, especially older adult patients. Patients tolerate frequent sessions lasting 20 to 30 minutes better, and this keeps their interest in the material. Nonverbal cues, such as poor eye contact or slumped posture, indicate a patient has lost concentration. If you note a loss of concentration, stop the session.

**ORGANIZING TEACHING MATERIAL.** Give careful consideration to the order of information presented. An outline of content helps to organize information into a logical se-

quence. Material should progress from simple to complex ideas because a person learns simple facts and concepts before learning how to make associations or complex interpretations of ideas. For example, to teach a woman how to feed her husband who has a gastric tube, first teach the wife how to measure the tube feeding and how to manipulate the equipment. Once you accomplish this, teach her how to administer the feeding.

Because patients are more likely to remember information taught in the beginning of a teaching session, present essential information first. Informative but less critical content follows the essential information. Other interventions that reinforce learning include using repetition and summarizing key points (Kiger, 2004).

**TEACHING APPROACHES.** To be a successful teacher, choose a teaching approach that matches your patient's needs. A patient's learning needs change over time. Therefore teaching approaches need to be modified as you care for the patient over time.

**Telling.** The telling approach is useful when teaching limited information (e.g., when preparing the patient for an emergent diagnostic procedure). Outline the task the patient needs to do and give explicit instructions. There is no time for feedback with this method.

**Selling.** The selling approach uses two-way communication. Instruction is based on the patient's response. You give specific feedback to the patient who shows success at learning. For example, the patient learns a step-by-step procedure for changing a dressing. Information from the patient is used to adapt the teaching approach.

**Participating.** The participating approach involves you and the patient in setting objectives and participating in the learning process together. The patient helps decide content, and you guide and counsel the patient. For example, a parent with a child diagnosed with sickle cell disease works with you to manage the child's pain. In this method there is opportunity for discussion, feedback, and revision of the teaching plan.

**Entrusting.** The entrusting approach provides the patient the opportunity to manage self-care. The patient accepts responsibilities and performs the tasks well, while you observe the patient's progress and remain available for assistance. For example, a patient who is receiving continuous intravenous pain medication at home for end-stage cancer requires a higher dose of pain medication. The patient understands the dosage of the medication and how the medication pump works. You help the patient determine an appropriate new pain medication dosage and allow the patient to adjust the settings on the medication pump.

**Reinforcing.** The principle of **reinforcement** applies to the process of learning. The teacher is often the source of reinforcement. Reinforcement is using a stimulus that increases the probability of a response. A learner who receives reinforcement before or after a desired learning behavior will likely repeat the behavior. Feedback is a common form of reinforcement.

Reinforcers are positive or negative. Positive reinforcement, such as a smile or praise and support, produces the desired responses. Although negative reinforcement (e.g., frowning) may work, people usually respond better to positive reinforcement.

Three types of reinforcers are social, material, and activity. Most reinforcers are social (e.g., smiles, compliments, words of encouragement, or physical contact), which are used to acknowledge a learned behavior. Examples of material reinforcers are food, toys, and music. These work best with young children. Activity reinforcers (e.g., physical therapy) rely on the principle that a person is motivated to engage in an activity if promised that, after its completion, the opportunity to participate in more desirable activity will be available.

Choosing an appropriate reinforcer involves careful thought and attention to individual preferences. Never use reinforcers as threats. Reinforcement is not effective with every patient.

**INCORPORATING TEACHING WITH NURSING CARE.** You can teach effectively while delivering nursing care. For example, educate your patient on the actions of medications while you are administering them. When you follow a teaching plan informally, your patient feels less pressure to perform and learning becomes more of a shared activity. Teaching during routine care is efficient and cost-effective.

**TEACHING METHODS.** Active participation is a key to learning. By actively experiencing a learning event, the person is more likely to retain knowledge. A teaching method is the way you deliver information and is based on the patient's learning needs (Box 10-6). The instructional method you choose depends on the time available for teaching, the setting, the resources available, and your comfort level with teaching. Skilled teachers are flexible and combine more than one method into a teaching plan.

**One-on-One Discussion.** Whenever you teach a patient at the bedside, in a physician's or health care provider's office, or in the home, you share information through one-on-one discussion. You provide information informally, allowing the patient to ask questions or share concerns. Use various teaching aids during the discussion, depending on the patient's learning needs.

**Group Instruction.** Group instruction offers an economical way to teach a number of patients at one time, and often the experience of being part of a group may provide the support necessary for patients to meet learning objectives (Redman, 2001). Group instruction sometimes involves both lecture and discussion. Lectures are efficient in helping groups of patients learn about a subject. After hearing information from a lecture, learners need the opportunity to share ideas and seek clarification. Group discussions allow patients and families to learn from each other as they share common experiences.

**Preparatory Instruction.** Patients frequently face unfamiliar tests or procedures that create anxiety. Providing information about procedures helps patients understand what to expect during the procedure. The following are guidelines for giving preparatory explanations:

1. Describe physical sensations during the procedure, but do not evaluate them. When drawing a blood specimen, explain that the patient will feel a sticking sensation as the needle punctures the skin.
2. Describe the cause of the sensation, preventing false impressions of the experience. Explain that a needle insertion burns because alcohol used to cleanse the skin enters the puncture site.
3. Patients are prepared only for aspects of the experience that have commonly been noticed by other patients. Explain that it is normal for a tight tourniquet to cause a person's hand to tingle and feel numb.

The patient finds comfort in knowing what to expect. When preparatory instructions accurately describe the actual experience, the patient is able to cope more effectively with the stress from procedures and therapies (Redman, 2001).

**Demonstrations.** Demonstrations are useful methods for teaching psychomotor skills. An effective demonstration requires advance planning. When using a demonstration, include the following steps:

1. Assemble and organize equipment.
2. Perform each step in sequence while analyzing the knowledge and skills involved.
3. Determine when to give explanations, considering the patient's learning needs.
4. Judge the proper speed and timing of the demonstration, based on the patient's cognitive abilities and anxiety level.

Demonstrate the procedure or skill in the same order in which the patient will perform it. Encourage the patient to ask questions so that the patient clearly understands each step. To enable the patient to easily observe each step of the procedure, perform demonstrations slowly, avoiding a hurried approach. Give the patient the opportunity to practice the procedure under supervision. At the end of the demonstration have the patient complete the procedure independently to ensure competece. This demonstration occurs under the same conditions that the patient will experience at home.

---

**BOX 10-6** | **Teaching Methods Based on Patient's Learning Needs**

**Cognitive**

**Discussion (One-on-One or Group)**

Involves nurse and patient or nurse with several patients
Promotes active participation and focuses on topics of interest to patient
Allows peer support
Enhances application and analysis of new information

**Lecture**

More formal method of instruction because teacher controls it
Helps learner acquire new knowledge and gain comprehension

**Question-and-Answer Session**

Designed specifically to address patient's concerns
Assists patient in applying knowledge

**Role Play, Discovery**

Allows patient to actively apply knowledge in controlled situation
Promotes synthesis of information and problem solving

**Independent Project (Computer-Assisted Instruction), Field Experience**

Allows patient to assume responsibility for completing learning activities at own pace
Promotes analysis, synthesis, and evaluation of new information and skills

**Affective**

**Role Play**

Allows expression of values, feelings, and attitudes

**Discussion (Group)**

Allows patient to acquire support from others in group
Permits patient to learn from others' experiences
Promotes responding, valuing, and organization

**Discussion (One-on-One)**

Allows discussion of personal, sensitive topics of interest or concern

**Psychomotor**

**Demonstration**

Provides presentation of procedures or skills by nurse
Permits patient to incorporate modeling of nurse's behavior
Allows nurse to control questioning during demonstration

**Practice**

Gives patient opportunity to perform skills using equipment
Provides repetition

**Return Demonstration**

Permits patient to perform skills as nurse observes
Is excellent source of feedback and reinforcement

**Independent Project, Game**

Requires teaching method that promotes adaptation and origination of psychomotor learning
Permits learner to use new skills

---

**Analogies.** Learning occurs when a teacher translates complex language or ideas into words or concepts that the patient understands. **Analogies** add to verbal instruction by providing familiar images that make complex information more real and understandable (Redman, 2001). For example, comparing arterial blood pressure to the flow of water through a hose is an analogy that is useful when explaining hypertension to a patient. When using analogies, know the concept; be aware of the patient's background, experience, and culture; and keep the analogy simple and clear.

**Role-Playing.** Role-playing is used to teach ideas and attitudes. An example includes teaching family caregivers better ways of communicating with older adult parents. The technique involves rehearsing a desired behavior. As a result, patients learn required skills and feel more confident in performing them independently.

**Discovery.** Discovery is a useful technique for teaching problem solving, application, and independent thinking. During individual or group discussion, you present a problem or situation pertaining to the patients' learning for patients to solve. For example, you ask patients with heart disease to plan a meal low in cholesterol.

**MAINTAINING ATTENTION AND PARTICIPATION.** Your actions can also increase learner attention and partici-pation. When conducting a discussion with a patient, change the tone and intensity of your voice, make eye contact, and use gestures that accentuate key points of discussion. A learner remains interested in a teacher who is actively enthusiastic about the subject under discussion (Kiger, 2004).

**THE PROBLEM OF ILLITERACY.** The National Adult Literacy Survey, conducted in the United States in 1992, found that 40 to 44 million Americans could not read or write and another 50 million Americans had only marginal reading skills. Although illiteracy existed among all races, African-American, American Indian/Alaska Native, Hispanic, and Asian/Pacific Islander adults were more likely to be illiterate than white adults. In 2003 the National Assessment of Adult Literacy Survey was completed. Although the results are not final yet, it is expected that these statistics will not change much when compared with the data from 1992 (National Center for Education Statistics, 2003). Two other national reports concluded that almost 50% of the adults in the United States have difficulty reading and understanding health information (Vastag, 2004). The ability to read and understand health information is called health literacy. Low health literacy is more common in adults over 65 years of age and in low-income populations (Cashen and others, 2004). Low health literacy is a risk factor for decreased compliance with health instructions, interferes with the ability to provide informed consent, increases the frequency of hospitalizations, and has a negative impact on the patient's health status (Baker and others, 2002).

A significant problem for health care providers is **functional health illiteracy.** Functional health illiteracy decreases your patient's self-worth and self-respect. Often these patients are ashamed of not being able to understand you, so they find ways to hide their inability to read health information and understand patient teaching (Erlen, 2004). Therefore carefully assess your patient's ability to read before providing patient education. For example, have a patient read a medication label and explain how often to take a drug or have the patient answer questions after reading a teaching brochure.

The readability of health education material ranges from a sixth- to eighth-grade reading level or higher (Erlen, 2004; Wilson and others, 2003). Thus it appears that written health information available to a patient often exceeds the patient's reading ability. Box 10-7 provides interventions for teaching illiterate patients.

**CULTURAL VARIABLES.** Health education materials often fail to recognize cultural beliefs, values, language, perceptions, and attitudes held by patients and families. Be aware of the patient's cultural background, beliefs, and ability to understand instructions not written in the patient's native language (Cashen and others, 2004; Watts and others, 2004). Cultural diversity is widespread and poses a great challenge to provide culturally sensitive health care and patient education. Meeting the educational needs of culturally diverse patients is a current topic frequently researched by nurses (Box 10-8). When educating patients of different ethnic groups, do the following (Edelman and Mandle, 2002):

1. Become aware of each culture's distinctive aspects.
2. Collaborate with other nurses and educators to assist in dealing with cultural diversity.
3. Enlist the help of people in the cultural group to share values and beliefs.
4. Use input and experiences of ethnic nurses in providing care to members of their community.

**SPECIAL NEEDS OF CHILDREN AND OLDER ADULTS.** The choice of instructional methods and application of teaching-learning principles is based on a patient's age. Children, adults, and older adults learn differently. You adapt teaching strategies to each learner's abilities and developmental stage.

Children pass through several developmental stages (see Chapter 19). In each stage, children gain new cognitive and psychomotor abilities that respond to different types of learning. You will need parental input and participation when providing health education to children.

Older adults experience numerous physical and psychological changes as they age. These changes can create barriers to learning. Sensory changes require teaching methods that enhance the patient's functioning (Lubkin and Larsen,

---

| BOX 10-7 | **Patient Teaching Strategies for the Illiterate Patient** |
|---|---|

- Make teaching materials visually appealing.
- Use simple words the patient can understand.
- Use the active voice when providing instructions (e.g., tell patient to "take medication before bedtime" instead of "medication should be taken at bedtime").
- Use examples to keep the patient an active participant in learning.
- Present the most important information first, and summarize it at the end of the session.
- Use teaching materials that reflect the reading level of the patient, and space out information to decrease intimidation.
- Use pictures or illustrations when possible.
- Ask specific questions and address what you have taught (e.g., "When will you take this medication?"). Just asking if the patient has any questions is not helpful because the illiterate patient often does not have the ability to process information.
- Observe the patient's ability to perform desired behaviors.

Modified from Erlen JA: Functional health illiteracy: ethical concerns, *Orthop Nurs* 23(2):150, 2004.

---

2002). For example, changes in visual acuity may require the use of large-print materials. Older adults learn and remember effectively if you pace the learning properly and if the material is relevant to the learner's needs and abilities (Ebersole and others, 2004). Educational strategies for gerontological nursing practice are highlighted in Box 10-9.

## Evaluation

**PATIENT CARE.** Patient education is not complete until you evaluate the outcomes of the teaching-learning process (see Evaluation box) (Table 10-6). Success depends on the patient's ability to meet learning objectives.

You will use return demonstrations, questions, observation of patient behaviors, role-playing, and discussions to evaluate your patient's learning. For example, the patient who will use a three-point crutch gait while walking to the end of the hall must demonstrate the actual crutch-walking technique.

If evaluation indicates a knowledge or skill deficit still exists, modify the teaching plan. Alternative teaching methods often help to clarify information or strengthen skills that the patient was unable to comprehend or perform originally. Evaluation also reveals new learning needs or new factors that may interfere with the patient's ability to learn. Use this information to update the teaching plan and make it relevant to patient needs. Like the nursing process, the teaching process is continuous and ever changing.

**PATIENT EXPECTATIONS.** After you educate patients to manage their health promotion activities, disease process, and their physical and functional limitations, you send them back to their home and community. It is important to have a method for evaluating your patient's expectations regarding patient education. Did your patient and family receive the education they expected? Were the expectations regarding self-

---

**BOX 10-8   USING EVIDENCE IN PRACTICE**

**Research Summary**

Anticoagulation therapy is used when patients need to avoid the development of blood clots in conditions such as atrial fibrillation, atherosclerosis. Warfarin (Coumadin) is the most commonly used oral anticoagulant. Patients need to know about the action, dose, side effects and food-drug interactions of warfarin so their anticoagulation therapy will be successful. This research study assessed the readability and cultural sensitivity of printed information about anticoagulation therapy used at an outpatient clinic. The study also evaluated the reading skills of the patients at the clinic and compared the patients' reading skills with the readability level of the written instructions. Finally, the study evaluated the patients' knowledge about warfarin and its food-drug interactions.

The participants in this study were African-Americans who were 50 years old or older. They all spoke English and had an average educational level of eleventh grade. However, their actual reading levels were between the seventh- and eighth-grade levels. Those with higher levels of education were more literate, whereas those who were older were less literate. The readability of the printed materials ranged from ninth grade to thirteenth grade,

and none of the information contained information about the beliefs or attitudes of African-Americans. More than 50% of the participants were not able to read the printed educational materials about warfarin. Those who did not understand their medication tended to be older. Overall, the patients had only a moderate level of understanding about their medications, and 66% of them did not understand the side effects of warfarin or food-drug interactions.

**Application to Nursing Practice**

The results from this study show how nurses can better meet the educational needs of their patients. Nurses need to assess the reading level of their patients before handing out written information. Patient education materials need to be written at a level that matches the readability level of the patient. Educational materials also need to include information that takes cultural beliefs, values, and language into consideration. Nurses have an ethical responsibility to provide patient education that is culturally sensitive to help reduce barriers experienced by minority groups in health care.

Data from Wilson FL and others: Literacy, readability and cultural barriers: critical factors to consider when educating older African Americans about anticoagulation therapy, *J Clin Nurs* 12(2):275, 2003.

---

**BOX 10-9   CARE OF THE OLDER ADULT**

- Provide individualized information that is based on what the patient needs to know.
- Present information slowly in frequent sessions.
- Include family members when necessary.
- Repeat information frequently.
- Reinforce teaching with audiovisual material, written exercises, and practice.
- Emphasize the older adult's current concerns and past positive coping strategies.
- Allow more time for learners to express themselves, demonstrate learning, and ask questions.
- Establish reachable short-term goals.
- Establish follow-up sessions.
- Base new information on patients' previous level of learning.

Data from Edelman CL, Mandle CL: *Health promotion throughout the lifespan*, ed 5, St. Louis, 2002, Mosby; and Falvo DR: *Effective patient education: a guide to increased compliance*, ed 3, Sudbury, Mass, 2004, Jones & Bartlett.

care met? Are there some education expectations remaining? Did the educational program increase your patients' comfort in managing their health status in their home? If your patients' expectations are not met, then you increase the risk that your patients will not continue following the prescribed treatment plan, will be less independent, and perhaps will ig-

nore signs and/or symptoms indicating a need to make an appointment with their health care provider.

## Documentation of Patient Teaching

Because patient teaching often occurs informally (e.g., during medication administration or physical examination), it is difficult to document patient education consistently. However, because you are legally responsible for providing accurate and timely information to patients, quality documentation is essential. Documentation also helps members of the health care team coordinate patient education. Document the following information about patient education:

1. *Assessment data and related nursing diagnoses:* Provide information and support for goals and outcomes.
2. *Interventions planned and used:* Planned education provides continuity of care. Specifically describe subject matter so that other nurses can follow up and reinforce teaching (e.g., "verbalized side effects of digoxin").
3. *Evaluation of learning:* Document evidence of learning (e.g., a return demonstration of coughing and deep breathing). This informs staff about the patient's progress and determines material that you still need to teach.
4. *Ability of patient and/or family to manage care:* Identify needs for outpatient or home care follow-up after discharge. Appropriate referrals better meet the patient's needs.

## EVALUATION

After Ashley and Latinka met the first time, Latinka decided to quit smoking on her birthday, which was in 1½ weeks. During that time Ashley made an appointment for Latinka to see the advanced practice nurse at the health department so Latinka could get a prescription for nicotine patches. Ashley and Latinka decided to meet together 2 weeks after Latinka started her smoking cessation plan. In the meantime Ashley called Latinka on her birthday to provide encouragement and support.

Today Ashley and Latinka meet to evaluate how the teaching plan is going. Ashley completes a physical assessment and asks Latinka questions about her progress to date. Latinka states she is less short of breath and has more energy now that she is not smoking. She feels better about herself and likes that her house does not smell like cigarette smoke as much any more. Latinka's sons, who also smoked, decided to quit with their mom as a birthday present. Latinka states, "If one of us feels like smoking, we call each other for help. It is really nice that we can support each other together." Ashley reinforces that having a good support system at home will help Latinka continue not to smoke. Latinka also relates that the nicotine patch is working well. She still suffers from nicotine withdrawal symptoms, but Latinka says, "They aren't that bad as long as I use my patches."

Because Ashley is also concerned about Latinka's weight management plan, she asks Latinka about her level of exercise and diet choices since the last time they met. Latinka says that she walks with her sons 2 days a week, and she walks with her neighbor another 2 days a week. She has been experimenting with her recipes also. She made her famous *burek,* which is a Bosnian meat pie. She used egg whites instead of egg yolks and ground sirloin instead of ground beef. She added more vegetables to her recipe and decreased the amount of butter she used. Latinka said, "I thought it was good, but I wasn't sure if it matched up to my old recipe. So, I served it to my boys, and they didn't even notice the difference.

Ashley reviews healthy coping strategies with Latinka and provides reinforcement for all the positive changes made so far. They decide to meet again in 3 weeks. Ashley asks Latinka if there is anything that Latinka would like to review at their next appointment. Latinka says, "I think I would like to review all the good things that will happen to me now that I am not smoking. I also want to talk about what I am going to do with all the money I am saving now that I don't smoke. I might even bring you a sample from my new stew recipe." Latinka tells Ashley she is so glad that Ashley is her nurse. Ashley feels a sense of satisfaction. She has helped Latinka make healthy changes, and she looks forward to learning more about Bosnian culture.

### Documentation Note

Ashley documents her visit with Latinka.

"Outcomes of education plan assessed. Pt reports quit smoking about 4 weeks ago on her birthday. Her sons have quit smoking also, providing support for each other. Has symptoms of nicotine withdrawal, but reports the nicotine replacement patch is helpful in minimizing symptoms. Verbalized increased feelings of energy and less shortness of breath. Walking 4 days a week with sons and neighbor. Has begun to successfully experiment with healthy substitutions in family recipes. Has requested to review short-term benefits associated with smoking cessation and will review diet information at next visit."

## OUTCOME EVALUATION

**TABLE 10-6**

| Nursing Action | Patient Response/Finding | Achievement of Outcome |
|---|---|---|
| Determine Latinka's current knowledge about smoking cessation, her health beliefs, and her learning needs. | Latinka has seen the nurse at the health department twice in the last week to get help in developing her smoking cessation plan. Latinka posted the smoking cessation plan on her refrigerator to be able to read it daily. | Latinka has a well-developed written plan that she helped develop to stop smoking. |
| Help Latinka set a definite quit date within the next 2 weeks. | Latinka states that the inclusion of her sons in the plan makes it easier to follow. Latinka's son calls her every other day to encourage her to quit smoking on her birthday. | Latinka's plan has identified her birthday in 10 days as her quit date. |
| Provide encouragement to maintain a smoke-free lifestyle (e.g., encourage Latinka to save the money used previously to buy cigarettes to buy a special reward). | Latinka called her friends to plan a lunch and shopping trip to celebrate her quitting smoking. Latinka puts the money she saves each week from not buying cigarettes into a jar to use to go shopping. | Latinka bought a new dress with the money she saved after quitting smoking. |

## KEY CONCEPTS

- Ensure that patients, families, and communities receive information needed to maintain optimal health.
- Health education is aimed at the promotion, restoration, and maintenance of health.
- Teaching is most effective when it is responsive to the learner's needs.
- Teaching is a form of interpersonal communication, with teacher and student actively involved in a process that increases the student's knowledge and skills.
- Teaching a patient a specific behavior involves incorporation of behaviors from all three learning domains.
- A person's health beliefs influence the willingness to gain the knowledge and skills necessary to maintain health.
- Patients of different age-groups require different teaching strategies as a result of developmental capabilities.
- Presentation of teaching content progresses from simple to more complex ideas.

- Assess the reading ability and the ability of the patient to understand health information before providing patient education.
- Patient teaching is culturally sensitive and individualized to meet the needs of the patient.
- The patient is an active participant in a teaching plan, agreeing to the plan, helping to choose instructional methods, and recommending times for instruction.
- A combination of teaching methods improves the learner's attentiveness and involvement.
- Make sure teaching methodologies match the patient's learning need.
- Learning objectives describe what a person is to learn in behavioral terms.
- Evaluate a patient's learning by observing the performance of expected learning behaviors under desired conditions.

## CRITICAL THINKING IN PRACTICE

*Mr. Green, an African-American older adult, was diagnosed with type 2 diabetes 1 week ago. Mr. Green and his wife are at an outpatient diabetes management clinic to learn diabetes management skills. You need to teach Mr. Green about his oral hypoglycemic agent, how to test his blood glucose, and how to recognize and treat low blood glucose levels (hypoglycemia).*

1. Using basic learning principles, explain what you will need to assess or determine before you begin teaching Mr. Green.
2. When you teach Mr. Green how to test his blood glucose, which of the domains of learning are involved?
   a. Cognitive learning
   b. Psychomotor learning
   c. Affective learning
   d. All the above
3. As you are teaching Mr. Green, you suspect that he is unable to read and comprehend the information about his medications and signs, symptoms, and treatment of hypoglycemia in the printed handouts you have given him. Describe the interventions you employ in developing a teaching plan for this patient.

4. Mr. Green is having a hard time dealing with his diagnosis. You assess that he is in the anger stage of adaptation to illness. It is important to match your timing of education with how the patient adapts to an illness. Match the stages of adaptation listed below with the appropriate nursing interventions.

| Stage | Nursing Intervention |
|---|---|
| 1. Denial or disbelief | a. Focus on what the patient will need to know in the future, and involve the family in learning. |
| 2. Anger | b. Encourage the patient to express feelings, and set aside times for teaching sessions. |
| 3. Bargaining | c. Let the patient know you are ready to talk whenever he is ready to talk, and provide emotional support. |
| 4. Resolution | d. Do not argue with the patient, and assure the family that this is a normal response. |
| 5. Acceptance | e. Teach in present tense, and discuss the reality of the illness. |

## NCLEX® REVIEW

1. A patient must learn to use a walker. Acquisition of this skill will require learning in the:
   1. Cognitive domain
   2. Affective domain
   3. Psychomotor domain
   4. Attentional domain
2. Place a check next to all the accurate teaching-learning principles a nurse applies when teaching a postsurgical patient about the importance of exercise (there may be more than one correct answer).

1. Provide patient education when there are visitors in the room.
2. Time teaching sessions to coincide with times when the patient's pain medications are working.
3. Provide patient teaching when the patient is most awake and alert.
4. Teach the patient how to cough and deep breathe when the patient is talking about current stressors in his or her life.
5. Assess the patient's feelings about the surgery and beliefs about exercise before beginning to teach.

3. The school nurse is about to teach a freshman-level health class about nutrition. To achieve the best learning outcomes, the nurse:
   1. Provides information using a lecture
   2. Uses simple words to promote understanding
   3. Develops topics for discussion that require problem solving
   4. Completes an extensive literature search focusing on eating disorders

4. A patient's priority nursing diagnosis is *deficient knowledge related to lack of understanding about breast self-examination (BSE)*. The nurse teaches the patient how to do BSE. The nurse knows the patient understands BSE when the patient:
   1. States that she needs to perform BSE at least once a year
   2. Needs reinforcement of how to perform BSE
   3. Performs BSE correctly on herself before the end of the teaching session
   4. Calls the American Cancer Association for more information about BSE

5. A patient who is having chest pain is going for an emergency cardiac catheterization. The most appropriate teaching approach in this situation is the:
   1. Telling approach
   2. Selling approach
   3. Entrusting approach
   4. Participating approach

6. An older adult is started on a new antihypertensive medication. In teaching the patient about the medication, you should:
   1. Speak loudly
   2. Present the information once
   3. Expect the patient to understand the information quickly
   4. Allow the patient time to express himself or herself and ask questions

7. A patient must learn how to administer a subcutaneous injection. You know the patient is ready to learn when the patient:
   1. Has walked 400 feet
   2. Expresses the importance of learning the skill
   3. Can see and understand the markings on the syringe
   4. Has the physical skill needed to prepare and inject the medication

## REFERENCES

Baker DW and others: Functional health literacy and the risk of hospital admission among Medicare managed care enrollees, *Am J Public Health* 92(8):1278, 2002.

Bandura A: *Self-efficacy: the exercise of control,* New York, 1997, WH Freeman.

Bastable S: *Nurse as educator: principles of teaching and learning for nursing practice,* Sudbury, Mass, 2003, Jones & Bartlett.

Cashen MS and others: eHealth technology and Internet resources: barriers for vulnerable populations, *J Cardiovasc Nurs* 19(3):209, 2004.

Dochterman JM, Bulechek GM, editors: *Nursing interventions classification (NIC),* ed 4, St. Louis, 2004, Mosby.

Ebersole P and others: *Toward healthy aging,* ed 6, St. Louis, 2004, Mosby.

Edelman CL, Mandle CL: *Health promotion throughout the lifespan,* ed 5, St. Louis, 2002, Mosby.

Erlen JA: Functional health illiteracy: ethical concerns, *Orthop Nurs* 23(2):150, 2004.

Falvo DR: *Effective patient education: a guide to increased compliance,* ed 3, Sudbury, Mass, 2004, Jones & Bartlett.

Flowers DL: Culturally competent nursing care: a challenge for the 21st century, *Crit Care Nurse* 24(4):48, 2004.

Hockenberry MJ and others: *Wong's nursing care of infants and children,* ed 7, St. Louis, 2003, Mosby.

Joint Commission on Accreditation of Healthcare Organizations: *Hospital accreditation standards,* Oakbrook Terrace, Ill, 2005, The Commission.

Jonsson IM and others: Choice of food and food traditions in pre-war Bosnia-Herzegovina: focus group interviews with immigrant women in Sweden, *Ethn Health* 7(3):149, 2002.

Kiger AM: *Teaching for health,* ed 3, New York, 2004, Churchill Livingstone.

Lipson JG and others: Bosnian and Soviet refugees' experiences with health care, *West J Nurs Res* 25(7):854, 2003.

Lubkin IM, Larsen PD: *Chronic illness: impact and interventions,* ed 5, Sudbury, Mass, 2002, Jones & Bartlett.

MapZones: *Bosnia and Herzegovina culture,* 2002, http://www.mapzones.com/world/europe/bosnia_hercegovina/cultureindex.php.

Moorhead S, Johnson M, Maas M: *Nursing outcomes classification (NOC),* ed 3, St. Louis, 2004, Mosby.

National Center for Education Statistics: *National assessments of adult literacy,* 2003, http://www.nces.ed.gov/naal/.

Redman B: *The practice of patient education,* ed 9, St. Louis, 2001, Mosby.

Searight HR: Bosnian immigrants' perceptions of the United States health care system: a qualitative interview study, *J Immigr Health* 5(2):87:2003.

Sheahan SL: How to help older adults quit smoking, *Nurse Pract* 27(12):27, 2002.

Vastag B: Low health literacy called a major problem, *JAMA* 291(18):2181, 2004.

Watts T and others: Breast health information needs of women from minority ethnic groups, *J Adv Nurs* 47(5):526, 2004.

Wilson FL and others: Literacy, readability and cultural barriers: critical factors to consider when educating older African Americans about anticoagulation therapy, *J Clin Nurs* 12(2):275, 2003.

# CHAPTER 11

# Infection Control

## MEDIA RESOURCES

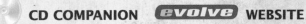

CD COMPANION  *evolve* WEBSITE

http://evolve.elsevier.com/Potter/basic

- **NCLEX® Review**
- **Audio Glossary**
- **English/Spanish Audio Glossary**
- **Video Clips**

## OBJECTIVES

- Identify the body's normal defenses against infection.
- Discuss the events in the inflammatory response.
- Describe the signs and symptoms of a localized and a systemic infection.
- Describe characteristics of each link of the infection chain.
- Assess patients at risk for acquiring an infection.

- Explain conditions that promote development of health care–associated infections.
- Describe strategies for standard precautions.
- Identify principles of surgical asepsis.
- Describe nursing interventions designed to break each link in the infection chain.
- Perform proper barrier isolation techniques.
- Perform proper procedures for hand hygiene.
- Apply and remove a surgical mask and gloves using correct technique.

## KEY TERMS

Current trends and rising costs in health care delivery have increased the importance of infection prevention and control. Increases in drug-resistant microorganisms and concern about occupational exposure to tuberculosis (TB), human immunodeficiency virus (HIV), and hepatitis have increased concern about transmission of infections. As a nurse you will participate in cost-effective quality health care by using strategies that prevent and control infections.

Infection prevention and control are some of the most important functions you will perform. This chapter emphasizes techniques for prevention and control of infections and the critical thinking skills necessary to achieve these goals.

## Scientific Knowledge Base

### Nature of Infection

An **infection** is the invasion of a susceptible host by pathogens or **microorganisms,** resulting in disease. The principal infecting agents are bacteria, viruses, fungi, and protozoa (Table 11-1). It is important to know the difference between an infection and colonization. If a microorganism is present or invades a host, grows, and/or multiplies but does not cause disease or infection, this is referred to as **colonization.** Disease or infections result only if the **pathogens** multiply and alter normal tissue function. An infectious disease transmitted directly from one person to another is considered a contagious or **communicable disease** (Tweeten, 2005).

### Chain of Infection

The presence of a pathogen does not mean that an infection will begin. Development of an infection requires the presence of the following elements: the infectious agent or pathogen, reservoir or place for pathogen growth, portal of exit from the reservoir, mode of transmission or vehicle, portal of entry, and a susceptible host (Figure 11-1). Infection develops if this chain stays intact. Your efforts to control and prevent infections are directed at breaking this chain.

**INFECTIOUS AGENT.** The development of an infectious disease depends on the number of infectious agents or microorganisms present; their **virulence,** or ability to produce disease; their ability to enter and survive in the host; and the susceptibility of the host.

**RESERVOIR.** A place where microorganisms survive, multiply, and await transfer to a susceptible host is called a **reservoir.** Common reservoirs are humans and animals (hosts), insects, food, water, and organic matter on inanimate surfaces (fomites). Frequent reservoirs for health care–associated infections include health care workers, patients, equipment, and the environment. Human reservoirs are divided into two types: those with acute or symptomatic disease and those who show no signs of disease but are

| TABLE 11-1 | Common Pathogens and Some Infections or Diseases They Produce | |
|---|---|---|
| **Organism** | **Major Reservoir(s)** | **Major Diseases/Infections** |
| **Bacteria** | | |
| *Staphylococcus aureus* | Skin, hair, upper respiratory | Wound infection, abscess, cellulitis, osteomyelitis, pneumonia, food poisoning |
| *Staphylococcus epidermidis* | Skin | IV line infection, bacteremia, endocarditis |
| *Streptococcus pyogenes* | Skin, upper respiratory, perianal | Wound infection, impetigo, strep throat, puerperal sepsis (postpartum sepsis) |
| *Escherichia coli* | Colon | Gastroenteritis, urinary tract infection |
| *Pseudomonas aeruginosa* | Water, soil | Wound or burn infections, urinary tract infection, pneumonia |
| *Neisseria gonorrhoeae* | Genitourinary tract, rectum, mouth | Sexually transmitted disease (gonorrhea), pelvic inflammatory disease, septic arthritis |
| *Chlamydia trachomatis* | Genitourinary tract, rectum | Sexually transmitted disease (chlamydia), pelvic inflammatory disease, neonatal eye and lung infections |
| *Mycobacterium tuberculosis* | Droplet nuclei from lungs | Tuberculosis |
| **Viruses** | | |
| Hepatitis A virus | Feces | Hepatitis A |
| Hepatitis B virus | Blood and some body fluids | Hepatitis B |
| Hepatitis C virus | Blood | Hepatitis C |
| Herpes simplex virus (Types I and II) | Lesions of mouth, skin, genitals | Cold sores, herpetic whitlow, sexually transmitted disease |
| Varicella-zoster virus | Vesicle fluid, respiratory tract infection | Varicella (chickenpox) primary infection, herpes zoster (shingles) reactivation |
| **Fungi** | | |
| *Candida albicans* | Skin, mouth, genital tract | Bacteremia, pneumonia, wound infection |
| **Protozoa** | | |
| *Plasmodium falciparum* | Blood, infected female Anopheles mosquito | Malaria |

From Ritter H: Clinical microbiology. In Carrico R, editor: *APIC text of infection control and epidemiology,* Washington, DC, 2005, Association for Professionals in Infection Control and Epidemiology, Inc.

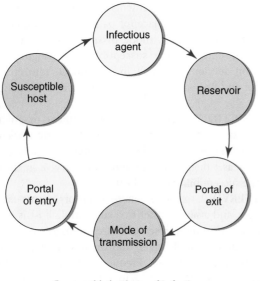

Figure **11-1** Chain of infection.

**carriers** of the disease. Humans can transmit microorganisms or disease in either case.

**PORTAL OF EXIT.** After microorganisms find a site in which to grow and multiply, they must find a portal of exit if they are to enter another host and cause disease. Microorganisms exit through a variety of sites such as skin and mucous membranes, respiratory tract, gastrointestinal tract, reproductive tract, and blood.

**MODE OF TRANSMISSION.** Many times there is little that you are able to do about the infectious agent or the susceptible host, but by practicing infection prevention and control techniques, such as hand hygiene, you will interrupt the mode of transmission (Box 11-1). The same microorganism is sometimes transmitted by more than one route. For example, the virus that causes chickenpox spreads by airborne route in droplet nuclei and also by direct contact with vesicle fluid.

**PORTAL OF ENTRY.** Organisms are able to enter the body through the same routes they use for exiting. Common portals of entry include nonintact skin, mucous membranes, genitourinary (GU) tract, gastrointestinal (GI) tract, and

## BOX 11-1 Modes of Transmission

**Routes and Means**

**Contact**

*Direct.* Person-to-person (fecal-oral) or physical contact between source and susceptible host (e.g., touching patient)

*Indirect.* Personal contact of susceptible host with contaminated inanimate object (e.g., needles or sharps, dressings)

*Droplet.* Large particles that travel up to 3 feet and come in contact with susceptible host (e.g., coughing, sneezing, talking)

**Air**

Droplet nuclei suspended in air (e.g., coughing, sneezing, talking)

**Vehicles**

Contaminated items
Water
Drugs, solutions
Blood
Food (improperly handled, stored, cooked)

**Vector**

External mechanical transfer (flies)
Internal transmission such as parasitic conditions between vector and host, for example:
Mosquito
Tick
Flea

Modified from Tweeten S: General principles of epidemiology. In Carrico R, editor: *APIC text of infection control and epidemiology,* Washington, DC, 2005, Association for Professionals in Infection Control and Epidemiology, Inc.

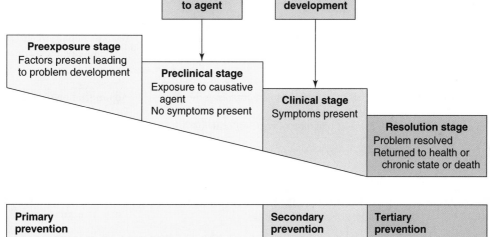

FIGURE **11-2** Stages of the natural history of a condition and their relationship to primary, secondary, and tertiary levels of prevention. (From Clark MJ: *Community health nursing: caring for populations,* ed 4, Upper Saddle River, NJ, 2003, Pearson Education.)

respiratory tract. For example, obstruction to the flow of urine due to the presence of a urinary catheter allows organisms to ascend the urethra.

**SUSCEPTIBLE HOST.** Susceptibility to an infectious agent depends on the individual's degree of resistance to pathogens. Although everyone is constantly in contact with large numbers of microorganisms, an infection does not develop until an individual becomes susceptible to the strength and numbers of those microorganisms. A person's natural defenses against infection and certain risk factors (see Assessment section) affect susceptibility.

A host is no longer considered susceptible if it has acquired **immunity** from either a natural or artificially induced event. Natural active immunity results from having a certain disease, such as measles, and mounting an immune response that usually lasts a lifetime. Natural passive immunity is the acquisition of an **antibody** by one person from another, such as a baby born with its mother's antibodies. The baby acquires these antibodies through the placenta during the last months of pregnancy. This type of immunity is of short duration, usually lasting only a few weeks to months.

## Course of Infection

Infections follow a progressive course (Figure 11-2). The severity depends on the extent of the infection, the **pathogenicity** and virulence of the causative microorganisms, and

| TABLE 11-2 | Normal Body System Defense Mechanisms Against Infection |
|---|---|

| Defense Mechanisms | Action | Factors That May Alter Defense |
|---|---|---|
| **Skin** | | |
| Intact multilayered surface, body's first line of defense against infection | Provides mechanical barrier to microorganisms | Cuts, abrasions, puncture wounds, areas of maceration |
| Shedding of outer layer of skin cells | Removes organisms that stick to skin's outer layers | Failure to bathe regularly |
| Sebum | Contains fatty acid that kills some bacteria | Excessive bathing |
| **Mouth** | | |
| Intact multilayered mucosa | Provides mechanical barrier to microorganisms | Lacerations, trauma, extracted teeth |
| Saliva | Washes away particles containing microorganisms | Poor oral hygiene, dehydration |
| | Contains microbial inhibitors (e.g., lysozyme) | |
| **Respiratory Tract** | | |
| Cilia lining upper airways, coated by sticky mucous blanket | Trap inhaled microbes and sweep them outward in mucus to be expectorated or swallowed | Smoking, high concentration of oxygen and carbon dioxide, decreased humidity, cold air |
| Macrophages | Engulf and destroy microorganisms that reach lung's alveoli | Smoking |
| | | Immunosuppression |
| **Urinary Tract** | | |
| Flushing action of urine flow | Washes away microorganisms on lining of bladder and urethra | Obstruction to normal flow by urinary catheter placement, obstruction from growth or tumor, or delayed micturition |
| Intact multilayered epithelium | Provides barrier to microorganisms | Introduction of urinary catheter, continual movement of catheter in urethra |
| **Gastrointestinal Tract** | | |
| Acidity of gastric secretions | Chemically destroys microorganisms incapable of surviving low pH | Administration of antacids |
| | | $H_2$ blockers |
| Rapid peristalsis in small intestine | Prevents retention of bacterial contents | Delayed motility from impaction of fecal contents in large bowel or mechanical obstruction by masses |
| **Vagina** | | |
| At puberty, normal flora cause vaginal secretions to achieve low pH | Acidic secretions reduce growth of many microorganisms | Antibiotics and birth control pills that disrupt normal flora |

the host's susceptibility. If infection is localized, such as in a wound, antibiotic therapy and proper wound care controls the infection's spread and minimizes the illness. The patient will experience only localized symptoms such as pain, tenderness, and swelling at the wound site. An infection that affects the entire body instead of just a single organ or part is systemic and often potentially fatal.

## Defenses Against Infection

The body has normal defenses against infection. Normal flora, body system defenses, and inflammation are nonspecific defenses that protect against microorganisms, regardless of prior exposure. The immune system is composed of separate cells and molecules, some of which fight specific pathogens.

**NORMAL FLORA.** The body usually contains normal **flora,** or large numbers of microorganisms that reside on

the surface and deep layers of the skin, in the saliva and oral mucosa, and in the intestinal walls. Normal flora usually does not cause disease but instead help to maintain health. For example, the skin's flora reduces multiplication of organisms landing on the skin. The number of flora maintains a sensitive balance with other microorganisms to prevent infection. Any factor that disrupts this balance places a person at serious risk for infection. For example, the use of broad-spectrum antibiotics for the treatment of infection eliminates or changes normal bacterial flora, leading to **suprainfection.** Microorganisms resistant to antibiotics then cause serious infection (Williams and Peterson, 2000).

**BODY SYSTEM DEFENSES.** Microorganisms are able to easily enter the skin, respiratory tract, and gastrointestinal tract. However, these body systems also have unique defenses against infection, physiologically suited to their structure

| BOX 11-2 | CARE OF THE OLDER ADULT |
|---|---|

The older adult experiences a number of age-associated physiological changes that influence susceptibility to infection. These changes include the following:

- There are fewer tears to flush and remove debris from the eye and a decrease in lysozymes that affect certain microorganisms. A decreased blink reflex leads to corneal dryness. Caution patients and families to observe for eye infections and use artificial tears when necessary.
- Drying of the oral mucosa and recession and weakening of gingival tissues require frequent oral hygiene and regular dental care.
- An increased chest diameter and rigidity, weakened cough, decreased ability to swallow, and decreased elastic tissue surrounding alveoli predispose older adults to ventilatory problems. Aspiration and postoperative pneumonia are common complications. When caring for older adult patients, elevate the

head of the bed and encourage the patient to ambulate as soon as possible (unless contraindicated). Instruct and assist patient in deep breathing and coughing techniques.
- A decrease in production of digestive juices and a reduction in intestinal motility affect removal of potential pathogens in the bowel. Patients and families should learn about safe food preparation and eat foods that are nutritionally good and easy to digest.
- A thinning of the dermal and epidermal skin layers, along with a decrease in skin elasticity predisposes older adults to skin tearing. Rigorous nursing care is necessary to prevent pressure ulcers in bedridden patients (see Chapter 35).
- With aging there is a decreased production of T-lymphocytes and B-lymphocytes. With reduced immunity it is important for older adults to receive regular immunizations and medical checkups.

Modified from Gantz M and others: Geriatrics. In Carrico R, editor: *APIC text of infection control and epidemiology,* Washington, DC, 2005, Association for Professionals in Infection Control and Epidemiology, Inc.

| TABLE 11-3 | Inflammation | |
|---|---|---|
| **Physiological Response** | | **Signs and Symptoms** |
| **Vascular and Cellular Response** | | |
| Arterioles supplying infected or injured area dilate, delivering blood and leukocytes. | | Redness |
| Tissue necrosis causes release of histamine, bradykinin, prostaglandin, and serotonin, which increase blood vessel permeability. | | Warmth |
| Fluid, protein, and cells enter interstitial spaces to cause swelling. | | Edema |
| | | Pain |
| White blood cells (WBCs) enter tissues and phagocytose microorganisms. More WBCs are released into bloodstream. | | WBC count normally 5000 to 11,000/mm$^3$; 15,000 to 20,000/mm$^3$ common with inflammation |
| Phagocytic release of pyrogens from bacteria occurs. | | Fever |
| **Inflammatory Exudate** | | |
| Fluid, dead cells, and WBCs form exudate at inflammatory site that later clears with lymphatic drainage. | | Purulent drainage  Serous or sanguineous exudate |
| **Tissue Repair** | | |
| Healthy new cells replace damaged cells. Cells mature to take on structural characteristics and appearance of injured cells. | | Tissue defects heal and close |

and function (Table 11-2). Any condition that impairs an organ's specialized defenses increases susceptibility to infection. When a person ages, there are normal physiological changes that influence susceptibility to infection (Box 11-2).

**INFLAMMATION.** The body's cellular response to injury or infection is **inflammation.** Inflammation is a protective vascular reaction that delivers fluid, blood products, and nutrients to interstitial tissues in an area of injury. This process neutralizes and eliminates pathogens or **necrotic** tissues and establishes a means of repairing body cells and tissues (Table 11-3). Signs of inflammation include swelling, redness, heat, pain or tenderness, and loss of function in the

affected body part. When inflammation becomes systemic, signs and symptoms include fever, leukocytosis (increased number of white blood cells), malaise, anorexia, nausea, vomiting, and lymph node enlargement. Many physical agents (e.g., temperature extremes and radiation), chemical agents (e.g., gastric acid or poisons), and microorganisms trigger the inflammatory response.

**IMMUNE RESPONSE.** When a foreign material (**antigen**) enters the body, a series of responses changes the body's biological makeup. The next time that antigen enters the body, antibodies bind to antigens they find and neutralize, destroy, or eliminate the antigen.

**BOX 11-8** PROCEDURAL GUIDELINES FOR

## Hand Hygiene

**Delegation Considerations:** The skill of hand hygiene is performed by all caregivers.

**Equipment:** alcohol-based waterless antiseptic containing emollients, easy-to-reach sink with warm running water, antimicrobial or regular lotion soap, paper towels or air dryer and clean orangewood stick (optional)

1. Inspect surface of hands for breaks or cuts in skin or cuticles.
2. Note condition of nails. Nail tips should be less than ¼-inch long and free of artificial nails or extenders. Avoid artificial nails and long or unkempt nails that harbor microbial loads (CDC, 2002). Your agency may ban these depending upon their policy. Report and cover any skin lesions before providing patient care.
3. Inspect hands for visible soiling.
4. Push wristwatch and long uniform sleeves above wrists. Avoid wearing rings. If worn, remove during washing.
5. Hand antisepsis using an instant alcohol waterless antiseptic rub
   A. Dispense ample amount of product into palm of one hand (see illustration).
   B. Rub hands together, covering all surfaces of hands and fingers with antiseptic (see illustration).
   C. Rub hands together until the alcohol is dry. Allow hands to completely dry before applying gloves.

6. Hand washing using regular lotion soap or antimicrobial soap and water
   A. Be sure fingernails are short, filed, and smooth.
   B. Stand in front of sink, keeping hands and uniform away from sink surface. (If hands touch sink during hand washing, repeat.)
   C. Turn faucet on (see illustration) or push knee pedals laterally or press pedals with foot to regulate flow and temperature.
   D. Avoid splashing water against uniform.
   E. Regulate flow of water so that temperature is warm.
   F. Wet hands and wrists thoroughly under running water. Keep hands and forearms lower than elbows during washing.
   G. Apply a small amount of lotion soap or antiseptic, lathering thoroughly (see illustrations). Soap granules and leaflet preparations are also an option.

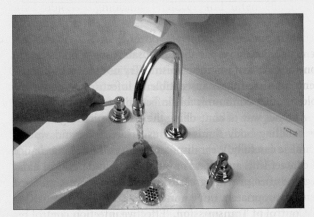

STEP **6C** Regulate flow of water.

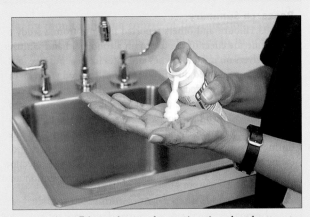

STEP **5A** Apply waterless antiseptic to hands.

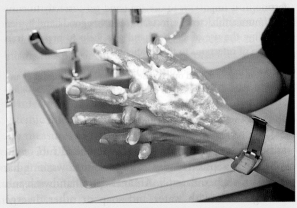

STEP **5B** Rub hands thoroughly.

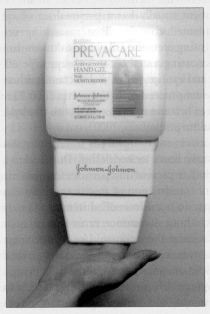

STEP **6G**

**BOX 11-8** PROCEDURAL GUIDELINES FOR

## Hand Hygiene—cont'd

- *Critical Decision Point:* Antimicrobial-impregnated wipes (towelettes) are not a substitute for an alcohol-based hand rub or an antimicrobial soap. They may not adequately remove proteinaceous material (Underwood, 2005).

- *Critical Decision Point:* The decision whether to use an antiseptic or handwash or not is dependent on the procedure you will perform and the patient's immune status.

H. Perform hand hygiene using plenty of lather and friction for at least 15 seconds. Interlace fingers, and rub palms and back of hands with circular motion at least 5 times each. Keep fingertips down to facilitate removal of microorganisms.

I. Areas under fingernails are often soiled. Clean them with the fingernails of other hand and additional soap, or clean with an orangewood stick.

J. Rinse hands and wrists thoroughly, keeping hands down and elbows up (see illustration).

K. Dry hands thoroughly from fingers to wrists and forearms with paper towel, single-use cloth, or warm air dryer.

L. If used, discard paper towel in proper receptacle.

M. To turn off hand faucet, use clean, dry paper towel, avoiding touching handles with hands (see illustration). Turn off water with foot or knee pedals (if applicable).

N. Apply lotion to hands. Use the facility-provided lotion if available.

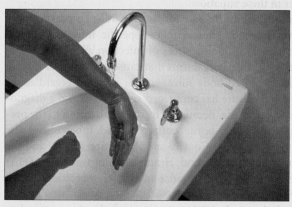

STEP **6J** Rinsing hands.

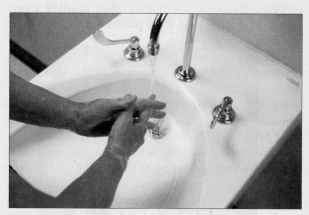

STEP **6G** Lather hands thoroughly.

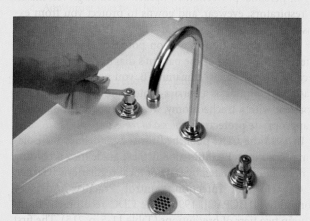

STEP **6M** Turning off faucet with clean, dry paper towel.

---

faces of the hands to reduce the number of microorganisms present. Surgical hand antisepsis is an antiseptic handwash or antiseptic hand rub that surgical personnel perform preoperatively to eliminate transient and reduce resident hand flora. Antiseptic detergent preparations often have persistent antimicrobial activity (Centers for Disease Control and Prevention [CDC], 2002).

When hands are visibly dirty or contaminated with proteinaceous material or visibly soiled with blood or other body fluids, wash them with either a nonantimicrobial soap and water or an antimicrobial soap and water. Handwashing is also indicated before eating, after using the restroom, and

if you become exposed to spore-forming organisms (e.g., *Clostridium difficile*) (Underwood, 2005). You may use an alcohol-based hand rub for routinely decontaminating hands in the following situations:

1. Before having direct contact with patients
2. Before putting on sterile gloves and before inserting indwelling urinary catheters, peripheral vascular catheters, or other invasive devices
3. After contact with a patient's intact skin (for example, when taking a pulse or blood pressure and when lifting a patient)

**BOX 11-9    PROCEDURAL GUIDELINES FOR**

**Caring for a Patient on Isolation Precautions—cont'd**

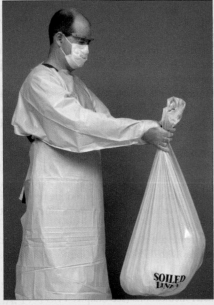

STEP **12b** Secure soiled linen in a waterproof bag.

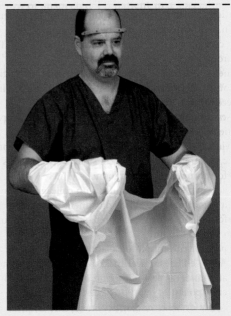

STEP **14c** Nurse removes gown.

A 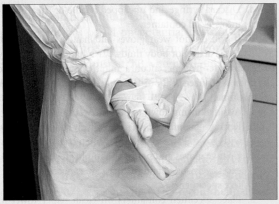    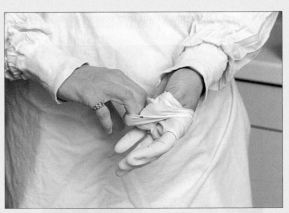 B

STEP **14a** Removing disposable gloves. **A,** Nurse places gloved finger inside cuff to pull first glove off hand. **B,** Nurse removes second glove by sliding fingers inside glove cuff and pulling.

    b. Remove eyewear or goggles.
    c. Untie waist and neck strings of gown. Allow gown to fall from shoulders (see illustration). Remove hands from sleeves without touching outside of gown. Hold gown inside at shoulder seams and fold inside out; discard disposable gown in trash receptacle or linen gown in laundry bag.
    d. Untie *top* mask strings, then hold strings while untying bottom strings, pull mask away from face and drop into trash receptacle. (Do not touch outer surface of mask.)

    e. Perform hand hygiene.
    f. Explain to patient when you plan to return to room. Ask whether patient requires any personal care items, books, or magazines.
    g. Leave room and close door, if necessary. (Close door if patient is on airborne precautions.)
    h. Dispose of all contaminated supplies and equipment in a manner that prevents spread of microorganisms to other persons (see agency policy).

| TABLE 11-5 | CDC Isolation Guidelines |
|---|---|

**Standard Precautions (Tier One)**

Standard precautions apply to blood, all body fluids, secretions, excretions (except sweat), nonintact skin, and mucous membranes.

Perform hand hygiene between patient contacts; after contact with blood, body fluids, secretions, and excretions and after contact with equipment or articles contaminated by them; and immediately after removing gloves.

Wear gloves when touching blood, body fluids, secretions, excretions, nonintact skin, mucous membranes, or contaminated items. Remove gloves and perform hand hygiene between patient care.

Wear masks, eye protection, or face shields if patient care activities generate splashes or sprays of blood or body fluid.

Wear gowns if soiling of clothing is likely from blood or body fluid. Perform hand hygiene after removing gown.

Clean and reprocess patient care equipment properly, and discard single-use items.

Place contaminated linen in a leakproof bag, and handle to prevent skin and mucous membrane exposure.

Discard all sharp instruments and needles in a puncture-resistant container. CDC recommends that you dispose of needles uncapped or that you use a mechanical device for recapping.

A private room is unnecessary unless the patient's hygiene is unacceptable. Check with an infection control professional.

Respiratory hygiene/cough etiquette contains respiratory secretions in patients exhibiting signs and symptoms of respiratory infection. Ensure that patients cover mouth/nose when coughing or sneezing; use tissues to contain respiratory secretions and dispose of tissues in nearest waste receptacle. Perform hand hygiene after having contact with respiratory secretions and contaminated objects; contain respiratory secretions with procedure mask or surgical mask. Sit at least 3 feet away from others if coughing.

**Transmission Categories (Tier Two)**

| Category | Disease | Barrier Protection |
|---|---|---|
| Airborne precautions | Droplet nuclei smaller than 5 microns; measles; chickenpox (varicella); disseminated varicella zoster; pulmonary or laryngeal TB | Private room, negative airflow of 6 to 12 exchanges per hour, mask or respiratory protection device (see CDC TB guidelines) |
| Droplet precautions | Droplets larger than 5 microns; diphtheria (pharyngeal); rubella; streptococcal pharyngitis, pneumonia, or scarlet fever in infants and young children; pertussis; mumps; mycoplasma pneumonia; meningococcal pneumonia or sepsis; pneumonic plague | Private room or cohort patients; mask |
| Contact precautions | Direct patient or environmental contact; colonization or infection with multidrug-resistant organism; respiratory syncytial virus; shigella and other enteric pathogens; major wound infections; herpes simplex; scabies, varicella zoster (disseminated) | Private room or cohort patients; gloves, gowns |
| Protective environment | Recommended only for allergenic hematopoietic stem cell transplants | Private room, positive airflow with 12 or more exchanges per hour, gloves, gown |

Modified from Garner JS: Guidelines for isolation precautions for hospitals, *Infect Control Hosp Epidemiol* 17(1):54, 1996; Siegel J: *APIC text of infection control and epidemiology*, Washington, DC, 2005, Association of Professionals in Infection Control and Epidemiology.

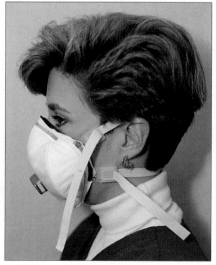

FIGURE **11-3** Disposable HEPA air-purifying respirator.

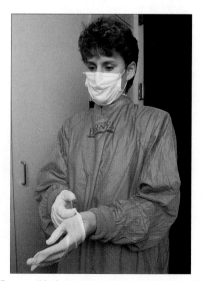

FIGURE **11-4** Nurse wearing an N-95 mask.

plant recipients. When a private room is recommended, post a card on the patient's room door, listing the precautions for the isolation category (check agency policy). The card is a handy reference for health care workers and visitors and alerts all who enter the room of any special precautions.

The isolation room or an adjoining anteroom will need to contain hand hygiene, bathing, and toilet facilities. Make soap and antiseptic solutions available. Personnel and visitors wash their hands before coming to the patient's bedside and again before leaving the room. If toilet facilities are unavailable, there are special procedures for handling portable commodes, bedpans, or urinals (check agency policy). Store PPE in an anteroom between the room and hallway or in a convenient location close to the point of use. Resupply PPE as needed.

Each patient care room, including those used for isolation, contains a special impervious bag for soiled or contaminated linen and a trash container with plastic liners. These receptacles prevent transmission of microorganisms by preventing seepage to and soiling of the outside surface. Have a disposable, rigid container available in the room to discard used needles, sharps, and syringes.

Depending on the microorganisms and mode of transmission, critically evaluate what articles or equipment to take into an isolation room. For example, the Hospital Infection Control Practices Advisory Committee (HICPAC) of CDC recommends taking only dedicated articles into an isolation room of a patient infected or colonized with vancomycin-resistant enterococci (HICPAC, 1995).

***Personal Protective Equipment (PPE).*** Gowns or coverups protect health care workers from coming in contact with infected blood and body fluids or materials. You will use gowns used for barrier protection made of a fluid-resistant material, and you need to change the gown immediately if it is damaged or heavily contaminated.

Isolation gowns usually open at the back and have ties or snaps at the neck and waist to keep the gown closed and secure. A gown is long enough to cover all outer garments. Long sleeves with tight-fitting cuffs provide added protection.

Wear a mask or respirator if you anticipate splashing or spraying of blood or body fluids. The mask also protects you from inhaling microorganisms from a patient's respiratory tract and prevents the transmission of pathogens from your respiratory tract. Occasionally a patient who is susceptible to infection will wear a mask to prevent inhalation of pathogens. Patients requiring respiratory precautions wear masks when ambulating or being transported outside of their room to protect other patients and personnel.

Masks prevent the transmission of infections caused by direct contact with mucous membranes. A mask discourages

---

**BOX 11-10** PROCEDURAL GUIDELINES FOR

## Donning a Surgical Type of Mask

**Delegation Considerations:** The skill of applying a surgical mask may be delegated when personnel are trained in required procedure.

**Equipment:** disposable mask

1. Find top edge of mask (usually has thin metal strip along edge). Pliable metal fits snugly against bridge of nose
2. Hold mask by top two strings or loops. Tie two top ties at top of back of head (see illustration), with ties above ears. (*Alternative:* slip loops over each ear.)

3. Tie two lower ties snugly around neck with mask well under chin (see illustration).
4. Gently pinch upper metal band around bridge of nose. NOTE: Change mask if wet, moist, or contaminated.

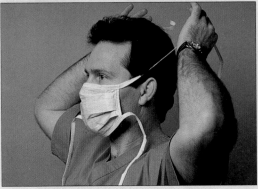

STEP 2

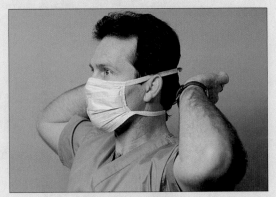

STEP 3

the wearer from touching the nose or mouth. A properly applied mask fits snugly over the mouth and nose so that the pathogens and body fluids cannot enter or escape through the sides (Box 11-10). If a person wears glasses, the top edge of the mask fits below the glasses so they will not cloud over as the person exhales. Keep talking to a minimum while wearing a mask. Discard a mask that has become moist because it is ineffective. Warn patients and family members that a mask causes a sensation of smothering. If family members become uncomfortable, have them leave the room and discard the mask.

Apply gloves when there is a risk of exposing the hands to blood, body fluids, or potentially infectious material. In addition, use gloves when you have scratches or breaks in the skin and when performing venipuncture or finger or heel sticks. In most cases you will wear disposable, single-use gloves. You wear gloves alone or in combination with other PPE. When other PPE is necessary, first put on a mask and eyewear (if required), apply a gown (if required), and then apply gloves. Pull the glove cuffs up over the wrists or cuffs of a gown.

After contacting infectious material, change gloves and perform hand hygiene if you have not finished caring for the patient. If your actions do not involve more patient contact, it is unnecessary to reapply gloves. Teach patients and their families the reasons for wearing gloves and the correct method for applying gloves.

Many gloves used for barrier protection or surgical asepsis are made of latex. Before applying latex gloves, assess the potential for latex allergies. The symptoms range from mild dermatitis to severe anaphylactic shock. Latex sensitivity results from repeated contact or by inhaling aerosolized latex allergens contained in the glove powder.

The American Nurses Association (ANA) (1996) provides the following suggestions for nurses to avoid becoming latex allergic:

1. Whenever possible, wear powder-free gloves (they are lower in protein allergens).
2. Wear gloves only when indicated.
3. Wash with a pH-balanced soap immediately after removing gloves.
4. Apply only non–oil-based hand care products (oil-based products break down latex allergens).
5. If a reaction or dermatitis occurs, report to employee health and/or seek medical treatment immediately.

Wear eyewear and face shields, properly fitted, during procedures where it is possible to splatter the eyes or face with blood or other infectious material (Figure 11-5). In many instances caregivers purchase their own eyewear with prescription lenses. Regular glasses are insufficient. Glasses need to have side shields to prevent material from entering the eye between the glasses and face.

***Specimen Collection.*** A patient with a suspected or actual infectious disease sometimes undergoes many laboratory studies. Body fluids and materials suspected of containing infectious organisms are collected for culture and sensitivity tests. A laboratory technician places the specimen in a special medium that promotes the growth of organisms. A laboratory technologist then identifies the type of microorganisms growing in the culture. Additional sensitivity test results indicate the antibiotics to which the organisms are resistant or sensitive. This helps the health care workers to choose the proper medications to use in the patient's treatment.

Obtain all culture specimens with sterile equipment. Collecting fresh material from the site of infection, as in the case of wound drainage, ensures that resident flora does not contaminate the specimen. Seal all specimen containers tightly to prevent spillage and contamination of the outside of the container (Box 11-11). After you transfer the specimens to containers, label each specimen properly with the patient's name, patient identifier, date and time, and type of specimen. Place the specimen containers in labeled leakproof bags before transporting them to the laboratory if required by facility policy.

***Bagging.*** Bagging articles generally is the same for all patient's rooms regardless of whether the room is an isolation room. Bagging articles prevents accidental exposure of personnel to contaminated articles and prevents contamination of the surrounding environment. Garner (1996b) recommends a single bag for discarding or wrapping items if the bag is leakproof and sturdy and if you place the article in the bag without contaminating the outside of the bag. Typically you place reusable equipment such as stethoscopes, forceps, or suction bottles in single bags according to agency policy.

Place all soiled linen in a designated waterproof impervious bag in the patient's room. Do not overfill the bag. Handle, transport, and process linen soiled with blood or

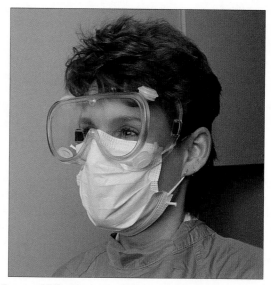

FIGURE **11-5** Nurse wearing protective goggles and mask.

---

**BOX 11-11** | **Specimen Collection Techniques***

**Wound Specimen**

Clean site with sterile water or saline before wound specimen collection. Wear gloves, and use cotton-tipped swab or syringe to collect as much drainage as possible. Have clean test tube or culture tube on clean paper towel. After swabbing center of wound site, grasp collection tube by holding it with paper towel. Carefully insert swab without touching outside of tube. After securing tube's top, transfer tube into bag for transport and then perform hand hygiene.

**Blood Specimen**

Wearing gloves, use syringe and culture media bottles to collect up to 11 ml of blood per culture bottle (check agency policy). After prepping, perform venipuncture at two different sites to decrease likelihood of both specimens being contaminated with skin flora. Place blood culture bottles on bedside table or other surface; swab off bottle tops with alcohol. Inject appropriate amount of blood into each bottle. Remove gloves, and transfer specimen into clean, labeled bag for transport. Perform hand hygiene.

**Stool Specimen**

Wearing gloves, use clean cup with seal top (need not be sterile) and tongue blade to collect small amount of stool, approximately the size of a walnut. Place cup on clean paper towel in patient's bathroom. Using tongue blade, collect needed amount of feces from patient's bedpan. Transfer feces to cup without touching cup's outside surface. Dispose of tongue blade, and place seal on cup. Transfer specimen into clean bag for transport. Remove gloves, and perform hand hygiene.

**Urine Specimen**

Wearing gloves, use syringe and sterile cup to collect 1 to 5 ml of urine. Place cup or specimen tube on clean towel in patient's bathroom. If patient has a urinary catheter, use syringe to collect specimen from specimen port. Have patient follow procedure to obtain a clean-voided specimen from catheter port (see Chapter 32) if not catheterized. Transfer urine into sterile container by injecting urine from syringe or pouring it from used collection cup. Secure top of container and transfer specimen into clean, labeled bag for transport. Remove gloves, and perform hand hygiene.

Data from Ritter H: Clinical microbiology. In Carrico R, editor: *APIC text of infection control and epidemiology,* Washington, DC, 2005, Association for Professionals in Infection Control and Epidemiology, Inc.
*Agency policies may differ on type of containers and amount of specimen material required.

---

body fluids in a way that will prevent exposure of skin or mucous membrane and/or contamination of the health care worker's clothing. Some hospitals still require double bagging. A standard-size linen bag, not overfilled, tied securely and intact is adequate to prevent infection transmission. Consult agency policy and any applicable regulations for the proper procedure.

Biohazardous waste includes both infectious and medical waste that must be disposed of in special red bags. These dis-

posal procedures are a high expense for health care facilities. Consider the following waste materials as infectious or medical waste (Hedrick and Wideman, 2005):

1. Cultures, including discarded cultures of infectious organisms
2. Pathological waste, such as discarded human tissue, organs, and body parts
3. Blood and blood products, including discarded serum or plasma and materials containing free-flowing blood
4. Sharps, including discarded needles, syringes, scalpels, blood vials, broken or unbroken glass, and pipettes
5. Selected isolation material, discarded waste material from patients with highly communicable diseases

***Removal of Protective Equipment.*** The method of removing protective clothing, gloves, mask, eyewear, and gown before leaving an isolation room depends on the protective equipment worn at the time. If you wear all four protective items, first remove the gloves because they are most likely to be contaminated. If you untie a gown with gloves still on, there is a chance of contaminating your hair or a portion of the uniform. The procedural guidelines for isolation precautions (see Box 11-9) reviews steps for removing PPE.

***Transporting Patients.*** Patients infected with highly communicable organisms, such as TB, leave their rooms only for essential purposes such as diagnostic procedures or surgery. Before transferring the patient to a wheelchair or stretcher, give the patient the appropriate barrier protection. For example, a patient infected by an organism transmitted by the respiratory tract needs to wear a mask. Personnel transporting the patient practice the appropriate precautions while in the patient's room. Notify personnel in diagnostic areas or the operating room that the patient is on isolation precautions. Record the type of isolation on the patient's chart, and explain ways to avoid transmitting infection during transport.

**Control of Portals of Entry.** Many measures that control the exit of microorganisms also control the entrance of pathogens. Evaluate the patient, and provide interventions to control and prevent organisms from gaining a portal of entry (Box 11-12).

**Protection of the Susceptible Host.** A patient's resistance to infection improves by initiating measures that protect normal body defense mechanisms. In the acute care setting, many of the interventions either promote existing body defense mechanisms or control exposure to microorganisms. Regular bathing removes transient microorganisms from the skin. Lubrication helps to keep the skin hydrated and intact. Regular oral hygiene removes proteins in the saliva that attract microorganisms. Flossing removes tartar and plaque that cause infection. An adequate fluid intake promotes normal urine formation and a resultant outflow of urine to flush the bladder and urethra of microorganisms. For immobilized or dependent patients, regular coughing and deep breathing exercises remove mucus from lower airways.

**Infection Control of Portals of Entry**

**Intact Skin and Mucosa**

Keep skin clean and well lubricated.
Avoid positioning patients on tubes or objects that might cause breaks in skin.
Use dry, wrinkle-free linen.
Offer frequent oral hygiene (see Chapter 27).
Provide frequent position changes for patients with impaired mobility.
Clean skin of incontinent patients with nonabrasive agent; avoid drying with abrasive towel or tissue.

**Urinary Tract**

Teach women to clean rectum and perineum by wiping from area of least contamination (urinary meatus) toward area of most contamination (rectum).
Do not allow urine in drainage bags and tubes to flow back into the bladder. Never raise a drainage system above the level of the bladder.
Keep points of connection between catheter or drain and tubing closed.

**Invasive Tubes and Lines**

When obtaining specimens from drainage tubes or inserting needles into intravenous lines, disinfect tubes and ports by wiping them liberally with a disinfectant solution before entering the system.

**Wound Care**

Keep draining wounds covered to contain drainage.
Clean outward from a wound site using a clean swab for each application.

**Role of the Infection Prevention and Control Department.** Most health care facilities employ health professionals who are specially trained in the area of infection control. Their responsibilities include collection and analysis of data on health care–associated infections and providing consultation and education to staff and others on infection control and prevention.

**Health Promotion in Health Care Workers and Patients.** A health care worker who becomes ill exposes susceptible patients to infectious diseases. An institution's employee health service provides programs to assist in infection control, such as immunization programs, recommendations for work restrictions, and protocols for management of job-related exposures to infectious diseases.

**Surgical Asepsis.** Surgical asepsis, or aseptic technique, is designed to eliminate all microorganisms, including spores and pathogens, from an object and to protect an area from these microorganisms. Surgical asepsis requires more precautions than medical asepsis. Breaks in technique will result in contamination, thus increasing the patient's risk for infection (Church, 2005).

Although you commonly practice surgical asepsis in the operating room, labor and delivery area, and major diagnostic or procedural areas, you will also use surgical aseptic techniques at the patient's bedside (e.g., when inserting intravenous catheters). Use surgical asepsis during procedures that require intentional perforation of the patient's skin (e.g., surgical incision), when the skin's integrity is broken related to trauma or burns, and during procedures that involve insertion of a catheter or surgical instruments into sterile body cavities (Church, 2005).

A series of steps involving sterile technique are used in the operating room, such as applying a mask, protective eyewear, and a cap; performing a surgical scrub; and applying a sterile gown and gloves. In contrast, performing a sterile dressing change at a patient's bedside sometimes only requires hand hygiene and donning sterile gloves (Box 11-13). Regardless of the procedures followed in different settings, the use of surgical asepsis depends on developing an aseptic conscience. Always recognize the importance of strict adherence to aseptic principles. Also, be an excellent role model and patient advocate, reinforcing proper practice for other caregivers.

**Preparation for Sterile Procedures.** In the operating room it is easy to enforce the control of aseptic technique. In treatment rooms and at the bedside it is important to have a patient's full cooperation. Therefore assess the patient's understanding of sterile procedure and the reasons for not moving or interfering with the procedure. Special precautions, such as masking the patient or changing the patient's position, are sometimes necessary to prevent contamination during procedures. Determine whether a patient has undergone a sterile procedure in the past. Explain how you will perform the procedure and what the patient can do to avoid contaminating sterile objects:

1. Avoid sudden movements of body parts covered by sterile drapes.
2. Do not touch sterile supplies, drapes, or your sterile gloves and gown.
3. Avoid coughing, sneezing, or talking over a sterile area.

Certain sterile procedures last for an extended time. Assess the patient's needs (e.g., pain control or elimination) in advance, and anticipate factors that will disrupt a procedure. If a patient is in pain, try to administer analgesics no more than 30 minutes before a sterile procedure begins. Patients often assume relatively uncomfortable positions during sterile procedures. Help the patient to assume the most comfortable position possible. Finally, the patient's condition sometimes results in events that contaminate a sterile field (e.g., the patient with a respiratory infection who transmits organisms by coughing or breathing). Anticipate such a problem (e.g., offering a mask to the patient before the procedure begins).

**Principles of Surgical Asepsis.** When beginning a surgically aseptic procedure, explain that the patient needs to follow principles to ensure maintenance of asepsis. Failure to

**BOX 11-13    PROCEDURAL GUIDELINES FOR**

## Putting on Sterile Gloves

**Delegation Considerations:** The skill of sterile glove application may be delegated if personnel are qualified to perform sterile glove procedure.

**Equipment:** pair of sterile gloves.

1. Consider the procedure you will perform, and consult agency policy on use of gloves.
2. Inspect hands for cuts, open lesions, or abrasions. Cover with an occlusive dressing before gloving.
3. Assess if the patient or health care worker has a known allergy to latex.
4. Determine correct glove size and type of glove material you will use.
5. Examine glove package to ensure package is not wet, torn, or discolored.
6. Perform thorough hand hygiene.
7. Remove outer glove package wrapper by carefully separating and peeling apart sides.
8. Grasp inner package, and lay it on clean, flat surface just above waist level. Open package, keeping gloves on wrapper's inside surface.
9. Identify right and left glove. Each glove has cuff approximately 5 cm (2 inches) wide. Glove dominant hand first.
10. With thumb and first two fingers of nondominant hand, grasp edge of cuff of the glove for the dominant hand. Touch only glove's inside surface.

11. Carefully pull glove over dominant hand (see illustration) leaving a cuff and being sure the cuff does not roll up wrist. Be sure thumb and fingers are in proper spaces (see illustration).
12. With gloved dominant hand, slip fingers underneath second glove's cuff (see illustration).
   Carefully pull second glove over nondominant hand (see illustration). Do not allow fingers and thumb of gloved dominant hand to touch any part of exposed nondominant hand. Keep thumb of dominant hand abducted.
13. After second glove is on, interlock hands (see illustration). Cuffs usually fall down after application. Be sure to touch only sterile sides.

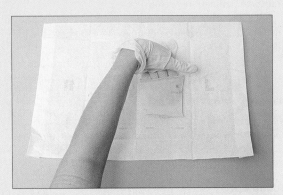

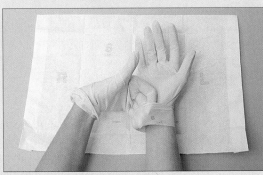

STEP **12** Using gloved dominant hand to pull glove onto nondominant hand.

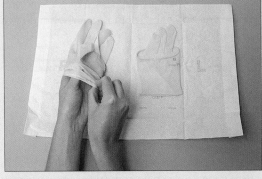

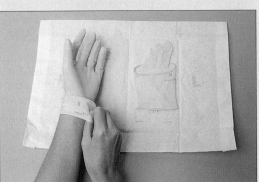

STEP **11** Pulling glove over dominant hand.

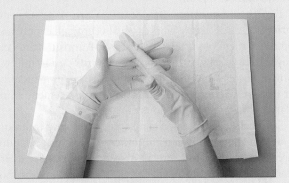

STEP **13** Interlock hands, touching only sterile sides.

follow each principle conscientiously endangers patients, placing them at risk for an infection. Principles of surgical asepsis include the following:

1. *A sterile object remains sterile only when touched by another sterile object.* The following principles guide you in placement and handling of sterile objects:
   - Sterile touching sterile remains sterile; for example, wear sterile gloves to handle objects on a sterile field.
   - Sterile touching clean becomes contaminated; for example, if the sterile tip of a syringe touches the surface of a clean disposable glove, the syringe is contaminated.
   - Sterile touching contaminated becomes contaminated; for example, when you touch a sterile object with an ungloved hand, the object is contaminated.
   - Sterile touching questionable is contaminated; for example, when you find a tear or break in the covering of a sterile object, discard or reprocess it regardless of whether the object appears untouched.
2. *Only place sterile objects on a sterile field.* Be sure item is sterile before use. The package or container holding a sterile object must be intact and dry. A package that is torn, punctured, wet, or open is unsterile. Place sterile items on sterile field (e.g., sterile drape) by not reaching over field (Figures 11-6 and 11-7).
3. *A sterile object or field out of the range of vision or an object held below a person's waist is contaminated.* Never turn your back on a sterile tray or leave it unattended. Any object held below waist level is considered contaminated because you cannot view it at all times. Keep sterile objects either on or out over the sterile field.
4. *A sterile object or field becomes contaminated by prolonged exposure to the air.* Avoid activities that create air currents, such as excessive movements or rearranging linen after a sterile object or field becomes exposed. When opening sterile packages, minimize the number of people walking into the area. Microorganisms also travel by droplet through the air. No one should talk, laugh, sneeze, or cough over a sterile field or when gathering and using sterile equipment. When opening a tray and adding sterile equipment, wear a mask. Microorganisms traveling through the air can fall on sterile items or fields if you reach over the work area (Box 11-14).
5. *A sterile object or field becomes contaminated by capillary action when a sterile surface comes in contact with a wet contaminated surface.* Moisture seeps through a sterile package's protective covering, allowing microorganisms to travel to the sterile object. When stored sterile packages become wet, discard the objects immediately or send the equipment for resterilization. Spilling solution over a sterile drape contaminates the field unless the drape cannot be penetrated by moisture.
6. *Because fluid flows in the direction of gravity, a sterile object becomes contaminated if gravity causes a contaminated liquid to flow over the object's surface.* To avoid contami-

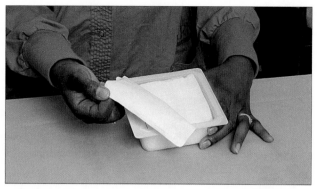

FIGURE **11-6** Opening a commercially packaged sterile item.

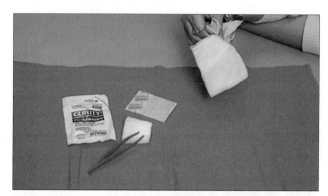

FIGURE **11-7** Adding item to a sterile field.

nation during a surgical hand scrub, hold your hands above the elbows. This allows water to flow downward without contaminating your hands and fingers. Because gravity makes water flow downward, this is also the reason for drying from fingers to elbows with the hands held up, after the scrub.

7. *The edges of a sterile field or container are contaminated.* A 2.5-cm (1-inch) border around a sterile towel or drape is considered contaminated (Box 11-15). The edges of sterile containers become exposed to air after they are open and are thus contaminated. After you remove a sterile needle from its protective cap or after you remove forceps from a container, the objects must not touch the container's edge. The lip of an opened bottle of solution also becomes contaminated after it is exposed to air. When pouring a sterile liquid, first pour a small amount of solution and discard it. The solution washes away any microorganisms on the bottle lip. Then pour the liquid a second time to fill a sterile container with the amount of solution you need.

**RESTORATIVE CARE.** The need for infection control is also present when patients are in the restorative phase of their care. Nurses in long-term care settings contribute to quality health care by practicing skills and techniques necessary to prevent infections.

**BOX 11-14** PROCEDURAL GUIDELINES FOR

## Opening Wrapped Sterile Items

**Delegation Considerations:** The skill of opening wrapped sterile items may be delegated if personnel are qualified to perform the procedure.

**Equipment:** sterile kit or package.

1. Place sterile kit or package containing sterile items on clean, dry, flat work surface above waist level.
2. Open outside cover, and remove kit from dust cover. Place on work surface.
3. Grasp outer surface of tip of outermost flap.
4. Open outermost flap away from body, keeping arm outstretched and away from sterile field (see illustration).
5. Grasp outside surface of edge of first side flap.
6. Open side flap, pulling to side, allowing it to lie flat on table surface. Keep your arm to side and not over sterile surface (see illustration). Do not allow flaps to spring back over sterile contents.
7. Repeat steps for second side flap (see illustration).
8. Grasp outside border of last and innermost flap.
9. Stand away from sterile package, and pull flap back, allowing it to fall flat on table (see illustration).
10. Use the inner surface of the package (except for the 1-inch border around the edges) as a field to add additional items because it is sterile. Grasp the 1-inch border to move the field over the work surface.

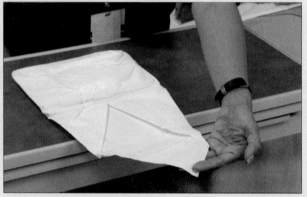

STEP **4** Open outermost flap of sterile kit away from body.

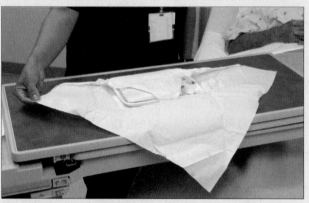

STEP **7** Open second side flap, pulling to side.

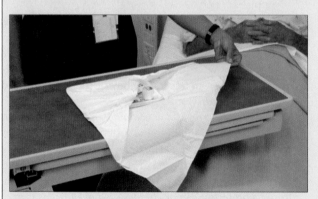

STEP **6** Open first side flap, pulling to side.

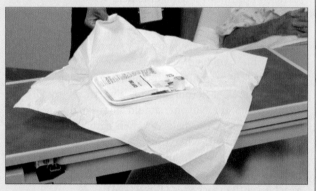

STEP **9** Open last and innermost flap.

**Long-Term Care.** Some of the same risks for infections that are present in acute care apply in long-term care facilities, such as skilled nursing homes (Gantz and others, 2000). Certain risks of health care–associated infections increase because of the usual age of patients seen in long-term care facilities. For example, in older adults several age-associated physical changes alter the natural barriers to infections (see Box 11-2).

Some major infections in long-term care are urinary tract infections, pressure ulcer infections, and pneumonia. These are the three most common infections in long-term care facilities. You will play an important role in the control of these infections by using critical thinking skills and knowledge of how to prevent these infections. See Chapters 28, 32, and 35 for additional information on approaches for preventing and managing these infections.

| BOX 11-15 | PROCEDURAL GUIDELINES FOR |
| --- | --- |

## Preparation of a Sterile Field

**Delegation Considerations:** The skill of preparing a sterile field may be delegated to personnel qualified to perform the procedure.
**Equipment:** sterile pack, sterile gloves (optional)
1. Perform hand hygiene.
2. Place pack containing sterile drape on work surface, and open as described under "Opening Wrapped Sterile Items, Box 11-13."
3. Apply sterile gloves (optional, see agency policy).
4. With fingertips of one hand, pick up the folded top edge of the sterile drape along the 1-inch border.
5. Gently lift the drape up from its outer cover, and let it unfold by itself without touching any object. Keep it above the waist. Discard the outer cover with the other hand.

6. With the other hand, grasp an adjacent corner of the drape and hold it straight up and away from the body (see illustration).
7. Holding the drape, first position and lay the bottom half over the intended work surface (see illustration).
8. Allow the top half of the drape to be placed over the work surface last (see illustration).
9. Grasp the 1-inch border around the edge to position as needed.

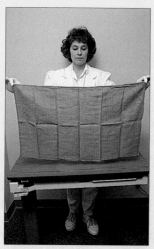

STEP **6** Hold corners of sterile drape up and away from body.

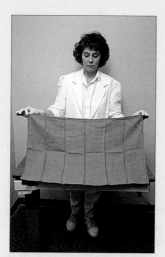

STEP **7** Position bottom half of sterile drape over top half of work surface.

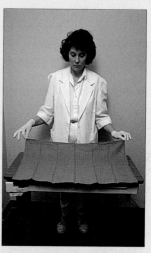

STEP **8** Allow top half of drape to be placed over bottom half of work surface.

## KEY CONCEPTS

- Normal body flora help the body resist infection by reducing the reproduction of pathogenic microorganisms.
- Immunity to infection is measured by the capacity to produce antibodies in response to exposure to an antigen.
- An infection can develop if the six elements of the infection chain are present and uninterrupted.
- A microorganism's virulence depends on its ability to resist attack by the body's normal defenses.
- Increasing age, poor nutrition, stress, inherited conditions, chronic disease, and treatments or conditions that compromise the immune response increase susceptibility to infection.
- Wear gloves, gowns, and masks in combination with eye protection devices such as goggles or glasses with solid side shields when in contact with blood or potentially infectious material or whenever you anticipate splashes or spray of blood or potentially infectious material.

- Invasive procedures, medical therapies, long hospitalization, and contact with health care personnel increase a hospitalized patient's risk for acquiring a health care–associated infection.
- Surgical asepsis requires more stringent techniques than medical asepsis.
- The CDC recommends that you consider all patients as potentially infected with HIV and other blood-borne pathogens; therefore health care workers will reduce the risk of exposure to blood and body fluids.
- Standard precautions involve using appropriate barrier protection with all patients regardless of presence of infection.
- Following aseptic principles is the key to your success in preventing patients from acquiring infections.
- A patient in isolation precautions is subject to sensory deprivation because of the restricted environment.

- Lack of hand hygiene is the main cause of health care–associated infections.
- An infection control professional provides educational and consultative services to maintain aseptic practices.
- If the skin is broken or if you perform an invasive procedure into a body cavity normally free of microorganisms, enforce surgical aseptic practices.

- A sterile object becomes contaminated by direct contact with a clean or contaminated object, by exposure to airborne microorganisms, or by contact with a wet surface containing microorganisms.

## CRITICAL THINKING IN PRACTICE

*In the case study, Mrs. Eldredge was readmitted to the hospital with a surgical site infection. She received diagnostic tests, local wound care, treatment with antibiotics, and supportive care, including nutrition and progressive exercise.*

1. List three signs and symptoms of a surgical site infection.
2. Mrs. Eldredge's wound culture grew a resistant strain of *S. aureus*. You checked your facility's policy for isolation precautions and found that Mrs. Eldredge needed to be in contact precautions. What are your next steps?
3. You are preparing to change Mrs. Eldredge's dressing. What personal protective equipment do you wear to perform this procedure? Explain your answer.
4. Explain why a nutritional assessment is important for Mrs. Eldredge.

## NCLEX® REVIEW

1. The **most** effective way to break the chain of infection is by:
   1. Using hand hygiene
   2. Wearing gloves
   3. Placing patients in isolation
   4. Providing private rooms for all patients
2. A patient's surgical wound has become swollen, red, and tender. You note that the patient has a new fever and leukocytosis. Your best immediate intervention is to:
   1. Use surgical technique to change the dressing
   2. Reassure the patient and recheck the wound later
   3. Notify the physician or health care provider and support the patient's fluid and nutritional needs
   4. Alert the patient and caregivers to the presence of an infection to ensure care after discharge
3. A patient has an indwelling urinary catheter. You recognize that the catheter represents a risk for urinary tract infection because:
   1. It keeps an incontinent patient's skin dry
   2. It can get caught in the linens or equipment
   3. It obstructs the normal flushing action of urine flow
   4. It allows the patient to remain hydrated without having to urinate

4. You have redressed a patient's wound and now plan to administer a medication to the patient. It is important to:
   1. Remove gloves and use hand hygiene before leaving the room
   2. Remove gloves and use hand hygiene before administering the medication
   3. Leave the gloves on to administer the medication
   4. Leave the medication on the bedside table to avoid having to remove gloves
5. You need to wear a gown when working with a patient:
   1. If the patient's hygiene is poor
   2. If the patient has AIDS or hepatitis
   3. If you are assisting with medication administration
   4. If blood or body fluids may get on your clothing from a task you plan to perform
6. Remove gloves and perform hand hygiene:
   1. Only after wound care
   2. When leaving the room
   3. When you have completed all tasks for the patient
   4. When the specific task you put them on for is completed

## REFERENCES

Advisory Committee on Immunization Practices, Centers for Disease Control and Prevention: *MMWR Morb Mortal Wkly Rep* May 17, 1998, Jan 12, 2001.

American Nurses Association: *Latex allergy, WP-70M, 1996,* Washington, DC, 1996, The Association.

Arnold F, McDonald LC: Antimicrobials and resistance. In Carrico R, editor: *APIC text of infection control and epidemiology,* Washington, DC, 2005, Association for Professionals in Infection Control and Epidemiology, Inc.

Centers for Disease Control and Prevention: Update: universal precautions for prevention of transmission of human immunodeficiency virus, hepatitis B, and other bloodborne pathogens in health care setting, *MMWR Morb Mortal Wkly Rep* 37(24):377, 1988.

Centers for Disease Control and Prevention: Guidelines for preventing the transmission of tuberculosis in health care facilities, *MMWR Morb Mortal Wkly Rep* 43(RR-13):1, 1994.

Centers for Disease Control and Prevention, Hospital Infection Control Practice Advisory Committee and the HICPAC/SHEA/APIC/IDSA Hand Hygiene Task Force: Guideline for hand hygiene in health-care settings, *MMWR Morbid Mortal Wkly Rep: Recommendations and Reports* 51(RR16), 2002.

Church NB: Surgical services. In Carrico R, editor: *APIC text of infection control and epidemiology,* Washington, DC, 2005, Association for Professionals in Infection Control and Epidemiology, Inc.

Clark MJ: *Nursing in the community,* Norwalk, Conn, 1992, Appleton & Lange.

Fauerbach L: Risk factors for infection transmission. In Carrico R, editor: *APIC text of infection control and epidemiology,* Washington, DC, 2005, Association for Professionals in Infection Control and Epidemiology, Inc.

Gantz M: Geriatrics. In Carrico R, editor: *APIC text of infection control and epidemiology,* Washington, DC, 2005, Association for Professionals in Infection Control and Epidemiology, Inc.

Garner JS: Guidelines for isolation precautions for hospitals, *Infect Control Hosp Epidemiol* 17(1):54, 1996a.

Garner J: Isolation systems. In Olmsted R, editor: *APIC infection control and applied epidemiology,* St. Louis, 1996b, Mosby.

Guinto CH and others: Evaluation of dedicated stethoscopes as a potential source of nosocomial pathogens, *Am J Infect Control* 30(8):499, 2002.

Hedrick E, Wideman JM: Waste management. In Carrico R, editor: *APIC text of infection control and epidemiology,* Washington, DC, 2005, Association for Professionals in Infection Control and Epidemiology, Inc.

Hilburn J and others: Use of alcohol hand sanitizer as an infection control strategy in an acute care facility, *Am J Infect Control* 31:119, 2003.

Hospital Infection Control Practices Advisory Committee: Recommendations for preventing the spread of vancomycin resistant organisms, *Am J Infect Control* 23:87, 1995.

Hospital Infection Control Practices Advisory Committee: Guidelines for isolation precautions in hospitals, *Am J Infect Control* 24:24, 1996.

Occupational Safety and Health Administration: Occupational exposure to blood borne pathogens: final rule, 29 CFR 1919:1130, *Federal Register* 56:64175, 1991.

Occupational Safety and Health Administration: Respiratory protective devices: final rules and notice, *Federal Register* 60:30336, 1995.

Ritter H: Clinical microbiology. In Carrico R, editor: *APIC text of infection control and epidemiology,* Washington, DC, 2005, Association for Professionals in Infection Control and Epidemiology, Inc.

Russell ML, Henderson EA: The measurement of influenza vaccine coverage among health care workers, *Am J Infect Control* 31:457, 2003.

Rutala WA, Weber, DJ: Cleaning, disinfection, and sterilization in healthcare facilities. In Carrico R, editor: *APIC text of infection control and epidemiology,* Washington, DC, 2005, Association for Professionals in Infection Control and Epidemiology, Inc.

Stricof RL: Endoscopy. In Carrico R, editor: *APIC text of infection control and epidemiology,* Washington, DC, 2005, Association for Professionals in Infection Control and Epidemiology, Inc.

Tweeten S: General principles of epidemiology. In Carrico R, editor: *APIC text of infection control and epidemiology,* Washington, DC, 2005, Association for Professionals in Infection Control and Epidemiology, Inc.

Underwood M: Hand hygiene. In Carrico R, editor: *APIC text of infection control and epidemiology,* Washington, DC, 2005, Association for Professionals in Infection Control and Epidemiology.

Williams D, Peterson P: Antimicrobial use and development of resistance. In Pfeiffer J, editor: *APIC text of infection control and epidemiology,* Washington, DC, 2000, Association for Professionals in Infection Control and Epidemiology, Inc.

# CHAPTER 12

# Vital Signs

## MEDIA RESOURCES

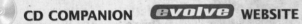

**CD COMPANION** *evolve* **WEBSITE**

http://evolve.elsevier.com/Potter/basic

- **NCLEX® Review**
- **Audio Glossary**
- **English/Spanish Audio Glossary**
- **Video Clips**

## OBJECTIVES

- Explain the principles and mechanisms of thermoregulation.
- Describe nursing interventions that promote heat loss and heat conservation.
- Discuss physiological changes associated with fever.
- Accurately assess body temperature, pulse, respiration, oxygen saturation, and blood pressure.

- Describe factors that cause variations in vital signs.
- Identify ranges of acceptable vital sign values for an adult, child, and infant.
- Explain variations in techniques used to assess an infant's, a child's, and an adult's vital signs.
- Delegate vital sign measurement to assistive personnel.

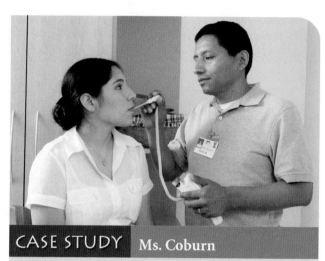

## CASE STUDY  Ms. Coburn

Ms. Coburn is a 26-year-old school teacher. Her maternal grandparents immigrated to America from Brazil. She lives alone in an apartment building. She smokes one pack of cigarettes a day. She has smoked since she was 16 years old, and she is 20 lb overweight. She made an appointment at the neighborhood clinic because she started having headaches and frequently felt tired.

Miguel is a 42-year-old Hispanic nurse who works in the neighborhood clinic. He enjoys providing health-related teaching to the patients at the clinic and has provided nursing care for Ms. Coburn for the past 2 years. Miguel relates to Ms. Coburn well because his younger sister is also unmarried. In addition, his sister is a teacher, and she smokes. He wonders if his sister kept her promise to quit smoking last week.

During Ms. Coburn's office visit, Miguel assesses Ms. Coburn's symptoms. He asks her about her headache and her fatigue. After interviewing Ms. Coburn, Miguel takes her vital signs. Her temperature is 98° F, her respiratory rate is 14 breaths per minute, her pulse is 86 beats per minute, and her blood pressure is 164/98 mm Hg. Ms. Coburn asks Miguel, "So, does this mean I am healthy?" Miguel responds, "Ms. Coburn, your blood pressure is pretty high right now. After you see the nurse practitioner today, I am going to take your blood pressure again. We are also going to talk about the changes you can begin to make to help you be healthier and feel better."

After Ms. Coburn sees the nurse practitioner, Miguel begins providing health teaching to Ms. Coburn and then retakes her blood pressure. Ms. Coburn's blood pressure this time is 146/94.

Ms. Coburn states, "The nurse practitioner told me that I will have to start taking medicine for my high blood pressure if it does not come down on its own." Miguel replies, "We need to watch your blood pressure closely over the next few weeks. In the meantime, remember you decided that you are going to walk for at least 15 minutes 3 days a week, try to eat foods with less salt, and think about not smoking anymore."

## KEY TERMS

afebrile, p. 228
antipyretic, p. 239
apical pulse, p. 247
apnea, p. 260
auscultatory gap, p. 258
basal metabolic rate (BMR), p. 227
bradycardia, p. 247
bradypnea, p. 260
cardiac output (CO), p. 240
centigrade, p. 229
core temperature, p. 227
diaphoresis, p. 227
diastolic, p. 248
diffusion, p. 260
dysrhythmia, p. 247
eupnea, p. 260
Fahrenheit, p. 229
febrile, p. 228
fever, p. 228
heat stroke, p. 228
hypertension, p. 248
hyperthermia, p. 228
hypotension, p. 249
hypothermia, p. 228
Korotkoff sound, p. 256

malignant hyperthermia, p. 228
nonshivering thermogenesis, p. 227
orthostatic hypotension, p. 249
oxygen saturation, p. 261
perfusion, p. 260
postural hypotension, p. 249
pulse deficit, p. 247
pulse pressure, p. 248
pyrexia, p. 228
pyrogens, p. 228
sphygmomanometer, p. 250
stroke volume (SV), p. 240
systolic, p. 248
tachycardia, p. 247
tachypnea, p. 260
thermoregulation, p. 227
vasoconstriction, p. 227
vasodilation, p. 227
ventilation, p. 260
vital signs, p. 226

The cardinal **vital signs** are temperature, pulse, respiration, blood pressure (BP), and oxygen saturation. A sixth vital sign, assessment of pain, is a standard of care in health care settings. Frequently pain and discomfort are the signs that lead a patient to seek health care. Therefore assessing your patient's pain helps you understand the patient's clinical status and progress. Many factors such as the temperature of the environment, physical exertion, and the effects of illness cause vital signs to change, sometimes outside the acceptable range. Measurement of vital signs and the assessment of pain (see Chapter 30) provide data to determine a patient's usual state of health (baseline data) and response to physical and psychological stress and medical and nursing therapy. A change in vital signs indicates a change in physiological functioning or a change in comfort, signaling the need for medical or nursing intervention.

Measurement of vital signs is a quick and efficient way of monitoring a patient's condition or identifying problems and evaluating the patient's response to intervention. The basic skills required to measure vital signs are simple, but do not take them for granted. Vital signs and other physiological measurements are the basis for clinical problem solving.

## Guidelines for Measuring Vital Signs

You assess vital signs whenever a patient enters a health care agency. Vital signs are included in a complete physical assessment (see Chapter 13) or obtained individually to assess a patient's condition. The patient's needs and condition determine when, where, how, and by whom vital signs are measured. It is important that you are able to measure vital signs correctly, understand and interpret the values, communicate findings appropriately, and begin interventions as needed. The following guidelines will help you incorporate vital sign measurement into nursing practice:

1. When caring for the patient, you are responsible for vital sign measurement. You may delegate the measurement of selected vital signs to assistive personnel. However, it is your responsibility to review vital sign measurements, interpret their significance, and make decisions about interventions.
2. Make sure equipment is in working order and appropriate to ensure accurate findings.
3. Select equipment based on the patient's condition and characteristics (e.g., do not use an adult-size blood pressure cuff for a child).
4. Know the patient's usual range of vital signs. A patient's usual values sometimes differ from the standard range for that age or physical state. You use the patient's usual values as a baseline for comparison with findings taken later.
5. Know the patient's medical history, therapies, and prescribed medications. Some illnesses or treatments cause predictable vital sign changes.

---

| BOX 12-1 | **When to Measure Vital Signs** |

- On admission to a health care facility
- When assessing the patient during home health visits
- In a hospital on a routine schedule according to a physician's or health care provider's order or hospital standards of practice
- Before and after a surgical procedure or invasive diagnostic procedure
- Before, during, and after a transfusion of blood products
- Before, during, and after the administration of medications or applications of therapies that affect cardiovascular, respiratory, or temperature-control functions
- When the patient's general physical condition changes (e.g., loss of consciousness or increased intensity of pain)
- Before and after nursing interventions that influence a vital sign (e.g., before and after a patient currently on bed rest ambulates, before and after a patient performs range-of-motion exercises)
- When the patient reports nonspecific symptoms of physical distress (e.g., feeling "funny" or "different")

---

6. Control or minimize environmental factors that affect vital signs. Measuring the pulse after the patient exercises will yield a value that is not a true indicator of the patient's condition.
7. Use an organized, systematic approach when measuring vital signs.
8. Based on the patient's condition, collaborate with the physician or health care provider to decide the frequency of vital sign assessment. In the hospital the physician or health care provider orders a minimum frequency of vital sign measurements for each patient. After surgery or treatment intervention, you will measure vital signs frequently to detect complications. As a patient's physical condition worsens, it is sometimes necessary to monitor vital signs as often as every 5 to 10 minutes. You will use vital sign assessment during medication administration as well. For example, the physician or health care provider orders you to give certain cardiac drugs only within a range of pulse or blood pressure values. Outside of the hospital, vital sign assessment occurs whenever the patient seeks care from a health care provider. In either environment you are responsible for judging whether your patients need more frequent assessments (Box 12-1).

Analyze the significance of vital sign measurement. Do not interpret vital signs without knowing your patient's other physical signs or symptoms and ongoing health status.

Verify and communicate significant changes in vital signs. Baseline measurements will allow you to identify and interpret changes in vital signs. When vital signs appear abnormal, it helps to have another nurse, physician, or health care provider repeat the measurement. Inform the physician or health care provider of abnormal vital signs, document findings in the patient's chart, and report vital sign changes to nurses working the next shift.

# Body Temperature

Body temperature is the difference between the amount of heat produced by body processes and the amount of heat lost to the external environment.

$$\text{Heat produced} - \text{Heat lost} = \text{Body temperature}$$

Despite environmental temperature extremes and physical activity, temperature-control mechanisms of human beings keep the body's core temperature or temperature of deep tissues relatively constant within a range as low as 35° C (95° F) during sleep and cold exposure to 40° C (104° F) during strenuous exercise. However, surface temperature fluctuates, depending on blood flow to the skin and the amount of heat lost to the external environment. Because of these surface temperature fluctuations, the acceptable temperature of human beings ranges from 36° to 38° C (96.8° to 100.4° F) (Thibodeau and Patton, 2003). The body's tissues and cells function best within this relatively narrow temperature range. For healthy young adults the average oral temperature is 37° C (98.6° F). No single temperature is normal for all people. An acceptable temperature range for adults depends on age, gender, range of physical activity, and state of health. You take the measurement of body temperature to obtain a representative average temperature of core body tissues.

Average normal temperatures vary depending on the measurement site. Sites reflecting **core temperature,** such as the pulmonary artery, are more reliable indicators of body temperature than sites reflecting surface temperature. The pulmonary artery offers accurate readings because of the blood mix from all regions of the body and is the standard used when determining the accuracy of all other sites used to measure body temperature.

## Body Temperature Regulation

Physiological and behavioral mechanisms act to precisely regulate and control body temperature mechanisms. For the body temperature to stay constant and within an acceptable range, the body has to maintain the relationship between heat production and heat loss.

**NEURAL AND VASCULAR CONTROL.** The hypothalamus, located between the cerebral hemispheres of the brain, controls body temperature. The hypothalamus attempts to maintain a comfortable temperature or "set point." When the hypothalamus senses an increase in body temperature, it sends impulses out to reduce body temperature by sweating and **vasodilation** (widening of blood vessels). If the hypothalamus senses the body's temperature is lower than set point, it sends signals out to increase heat production by muscle shivering or heat conservation by **vasoconstriction** (narrowing of surface blood vessels). Disease or trauma to the hypothalamus or spinal cord, which carries hypothalamic messages, decreases the body's ability to control body temperature.

**HEAT PRODUCTION. Thermoregulation** requires normal heat production processes. Heat is produced as a by-product of metabolism. As metabolism increases, the body produces additional heat. When metabolism decreases, the body produces less heat. Heat production occurs during rest, voluntary movements, involuntary shivering, and **nonshivering thermogenesis.** Basal metabolism accounts for the heat produced by the body at absolute rest. The average **basal metabolic rate (BMR)** depends on the body surface area. Voluntary movements such as muscular activity during exercise require additional energy. The metabolic rate increases during activity, sometimes causing heat production to increase up to 50 times normal. Shivering is an involuntary skeletal muscle response to temperature differences in the body. Shivering sometimes increases heat production to four to five times normal. Nonshivering thermogenesis occurs primarily in neonates, or newborn infants. Because neonates cannot shiver, a limited amount of vascular brown adipose tissue present at birth is metabolized for heat production.

**HEAT LOSS.** Heat loss and heat production occur at the same time. The skin's structure and exposure to the environment result in constant, normal heat loss through radiation, conduction, convection, and evaporation. Infants and young children who have a larger ratio of surface area to body weight lose more heat to the environment than adults.

Radiation is the transfer of heat between two objects without physical contact. Heat radiates from the skin to any surrounding cooler object. Up to 85% of the human body's surface area radiates heat to the environment.

Conduction is the transfer of heat from one object to another with direct contact. When the warm skin touches a cooler object, heat transfers from the skin to the object until their temperatures are similar. Heat conducts through solids, gases, and liquids. Conduction normally accounts for a small amount of heat loss. You increase a patient's conductive heat loss by applying an ice pack or bathing a patient with tepid water. Applying several layers of clothing reduces conductive loss. The body gains heat by conduction when it makes contact with materials warmer than skin temperature (e.g., prewarmed blankets).

Convection is the transfer of heat away by air movement. An electric fan promotes heat loss through convection. Convective heat loss increases when moistened skin comes into contact with slightly moving air.

Evaporation is the transfer of heat energy when a liquid is changed to a gas. The body continuously loses heat by evaporation. About 600 to 900 ml of water a day evaporates from the skin and lungs, resulting in water and heat loss. By regulating perspiration or sweating, the body promotes additional evaporative heat loss. **Diaphoresis** is visual perspiration of the forehead and upper thorax. When diaphoresis occurs, the body temperature is reduced.

**BEHAVIORAL CONTROL.** When the environmental temperature falls, a person adds clothing, moves to a warmer place, raises the thermostat setting on a furnace, increases muscular activity by running in place, or sits with arms and legs tightly wrapped together. In contrast, when the temperature becomes hot, a person removes clothing, stops activity, lowers the thermostat setting on an air conditioner, seeks a cooler place, or takes a cool shower.

## Temperature Alterations

Changes in body temperature are related to excess heat production, heat loss, minimal heat production, or any combination of these alterations. The nature of the change affects the type of clinical problems experienced by the patient.

**FEVER.** Pyrexia, or **fever,** occurs because heat loss mechanisms are unable to keep pace with excess heat production, resulting in an abnormal rise in body temperature. A fever is usually not harmful if it stays below 39° C (102.2° F) in adults or 40° C (104° F) in children. A single temperature reading does not always indicate a fever. You determine if a patient has a fever by taking several temperature readings at different times of the day and comparing these with the usual value for that patient at that time.

A true fever results from an alteration in the hypothalamic set point. Substances that trigger the immune system, or **pyrogens,** stimulate the release of hormones in an effort to promote the body's defense against infection. These hormones also trigger the hypothalamus to raise the set point, inducing a **febrile** episode. To meet the new set point, the body produces and conserves heat. The patient experiences chills, shivers, and feels cold, even though the body temperature is rising. If the set point has been "overshot" or the pyrogens are removed, the skin becomes warm and flushed because of vasodilation. Diaphoresis leads to evaporative heat loss. When the fever "breaks," the temperature returns to an acceptable range and the patient becomes **afebrile.**

Fever, or **pyrexia,** is an important defense mechanism. Mild temperature elevations up to 39° C (102.2° F) enhance the body's immune system by stimulating white blood cell production. Increased temperature reduces the concentration of iron in the blood plasma, causing the growth of bacteria to slow. Fever also fights viral infections by stimulating interferon, the body's natural virus-fighting substance.

Fevers also serve a diagnostic purpose. Fever patterns differ depending on the causative pyrogen (Box 12-2). The duration and degree of fever depend on the pyrogen's strength and the ability of the individual to respond. The term *fever of unknown origin* (FUO) refers to a fever whose etiology or cause health care providers cannot determine.

**HYPERTHERMIA.** An elevated body temperature related to the body's inability to promote heat loss or reduce heat production is **hyperthermia.** Any disease or trauma to the hypothalamus impairs heat loss mechanisms. **Malignant hyperthermia** is a hereditary condition of uncontrolled heat production. Malignant hyperthermia occurs when patients with this condition receive certain anesthetic drugs.

Prolonged exposure to the sun or high environmental temperatures overwhelm the body's heat loss mechanisms. Heat also depresses hypothalamic function. These conditions cause **heat stroke,** a dangerous heat emergency. Signs and symptoms of heat stroke include giddiness, confusion,

---

| BOX 12-2 | Patterns of Fever |
|---|---|
| Sustained | A constant body temperature continuously above 38° C (100.4° F) that demonstrates little fluctuation |
| Intermittent | Fever spikes mixed with usual temperature levels; temperature returns to acceptable value at least once in 24 hours |
| Remittent | Fever spikes and falls without a return to normal temperature levels |
| Relapsing | Periods of febrile episodes mixed with acceptable temperature values; febrile episodes and periods of normothermia are sometimes longer than 24 hours |

---

| TABLE 12-1 | Classification of Hypothermia | |
|---|---|---|
| | C | F |
| Mild | 34°-36° | 93.2°-96.8° |
| Moderate | 30°-34° | 86.0°-93.2° |
| Severe | <30° | <86.0° |

---

delirium, excess thirst, nausea, muscle cramps, visual disturbances, and even incontinence. The most important sign of heat stroke is hot, dry skin.

**HYPOTHERMIA.** Heat loss during prolonged exposure to cold overwhelms the body's ability to produce heat, causing **hypothermia.** Hypothermia is classified by core temperature measurements (Table 12-1). Hypothermia can be intentional or accidental. During prolonged neurological or cardiac surgery, surgeons use intentional hypothermia to reduce the body's needs for oxygenated blood.

Accidental hypothermia develops gradually and may go unnoticed for several hours. The hypothermic patient suffers uncontrolled shivering, loss of memory, depression, and poor judgment. As the body temperature falls below 34° C (93.2° F), heart and respiratory rates and blood pressure fall.

## Nursing Process

Knowledge of body temperature physiology assists you when assessing your patient's response to temperature alterations and helps you intervene safely.

### Assessment

Assessment of thermoregulation requires you to make judgments about the site for temperature measurement, type of thermometer, and frequency of measurement. Table 12-2 presents a focused patient assessment for temperature measurement.

## FOCUSED PATIENT ASSESSMENT

**TABLE 12-2**

| Factors to Assess | Questions and Approaches | Physical Assessment Strategies |
|---|---|---|
| Temperature measurement site | Ask Ms. Coburn's preferred route. Ask Ms. Coburn if hearing aids are in use. Ask Ms. Coburn if she has recently ingested liquid or smoked. Inquire about Ms. Coburn's recent physical activity. | Assess Ms. Coburn's ability to position herself. Identify any signs of trauma to oral mucosa, aural drainage, diaphoresis. Assess Ms. Coburn's level of consciousness. Assess for dyspnea. Assess for presence of perspiration or diaphoresis. Assess for flushed, warm, dry skin. Note shivering or diaphoresis. |
| Frequency of temperature measurement | Note physician or health care provider order for temperature monitoring in chart. Note Ms. Coburn's previous health status, temperature, onset and duration of febrile episode. Assess Ms. Coburn's comfort and well-being. Assess environmental comfort. | |

**SITES.** There are several sites for measuring core and surface body temperature. The core temperatures of the pulmonary artery, esophagus, and urinary bladder are often used in intensive care settings and require continuous invasive monitoring devices placed in body cavities or organs.

You obtain intermittent temperature measurements routinely from the tympanic membrane, temporal artery, mouth, rectum, and axilla. In some health care settings, you are also able to apply special chemically prepared thermometer patches to the skin.

To ensure accurate temperature readings, measure each site correctly (Skill 12-1). Depending on the site you use, temperatures will vary between 36.0° C (96.8° F) and 38.0° C (100.4° F). Research findings from numerous studies are contradictory; however, it is generally accepted that rectal temperatures are usually 0.5° C (0.9° F) higher than oral temperatures, and tympanic and axillary temperatures are usually 0.5° C (0.9° F) lower than oral temperatures. Sites reflecting core temperatures are more reliable than sites reflecting surface temperature. Each temperature measurement site has advantages and disadvantages (Box 12-3). You will select the safest and most accurate site for the patient. Use the same site if possible when repeated measurements are necessary.

**THERMOMETERS.** Two types of thermometers are commonly available for measuring body temperature: electronic and single-use or reusable chemical dot. The mercury-in-glass thermometer, a third type of device used for over 100 years, is not used in most health care facilities because of the environmental hazards of mercury. However, some patients use mercury-in-glass thermometers at home.

Each device measures temperature in either the **centigrade** or **Fahrenheit** scale. Electronic thermometers allow you to convert scales by activating a switch. When it is necessary to manually convert temperature readings, use the following formulas:

To convert Fahrenheit to centigrade, subtract 32 from the Fahrenheit reading and multiply the result by $\frac{5}{9}$.

Example: $(104° F - 32° F) \times 5/9 = 40° C$

To convert centigrade to Fahrenheit, multiply the centigrade reading by $\frac{9}{5}$ and add 32 to the product.

Example: $(9/5 \times 40° C) + 32 = 104° F$

**Electronic Thermometers.** All electronic thermometers consists of a rechargeable battery–powered display unit and a temperature-processing probe or sensor (Figure 12-1). One form of electronic thermometer uses a pencil-like, unbreakable probe connected by a thin wire to the display unit. Separate probes are available for oral (blue tip) and rectal (red tip) use. You obtain axillary temperatures with the oral probe. Electronic thermometers provide 4-second predictive temperatures and 3-minute standard temperatures. In day-to-day clinical situations, most nurses use the 4-second predictive.

Another form of electronic thermometer is used exclusively for tympanic temperature measurement. An otoscope-like speculum with an infrared sensor tip detects heat radiated from the tympanic membrane of the ear. Within 2 to 5 seconds of placement in the auditory canal and pressing the scan button, a reading appears on the display unit, and an audible signal indicates that the thermometer has measured the peak temperature reading.

The newest type of electronic thermometer measures the temperature of the superficial temporal artery. A handheld scanner with an infrared sensor detects the temperature of cutaneous blood flow by sweeping the sensor across the forehead and just behind the ear (Figure 12-2). After scanning is complete, a reading appears on the display unit. Temporal artery temperature is considered a reliable noninvasive measure of core temperature (Sidberry and others, 2002) (Box 12-4).

*Text continued on p. 236*

------------------------------------------------------

## SKILL 12-1 ¦ Measuring Body Temperature

### Delegation Considerations

You can delegate the skill of temperature measurement to assistive personnel. Before delegation, instruct the assistive personnel about:

- Appropriate route and device to measure temperature
- Any precautions needed to properly position patient for rectal temperature measurement
- Specific factors related to patient that will falsely raise or lower temperature
- Frequency of temperature measurement for the patient
- Usual temperature values for the patient

- The need to report any abnormal temperatures that you will need to confirm

### Equipment

- Appropriate thermometer
- Tissue or soft wipe
- Lubricant (for rectal measurements only)
- Pen, vital sign flow sheet or record form
- Disposable gloves, plastic thermometer sleeve or disposable probe or sensor cover when needed
- Towel

| STEP | RATIONALE |
|------|-----------|
| **ASSESSMENT** | |
| 1. Assess for signs and symptoms of temperature alterations and for factors that influence body temperature. | Physical signs and symptoms indicate abnormal temperature. You accurately assess nature of variations. |
| 2. Determine any previous activity that will interfere with accuracy of temperature measurement. When taking oral temperature, wait 20 to 30 minutes before measuring temperature if patient has smoked or ingested hot or cold liquid or food. | Smoking and hot or cold substances cause false temperature readings in oral cavity. |
| 3. Determine appropriate site and measurement device you will use. | Chosen on basis of preferred site for temperature measurement and any patient contraindications (see Box 12-3). |
| **PLANNING** | |
| 1. Explain route by which you will take temperature and importance of maintaining proper position until reading is complete. | Patients are often curious about such measurements and often prematurely remove thermometer to read results. |
| **IMPLEMENTATION** | |
| 1. Perform hand hygiene. | Reduces transmission of microorganisms. |
| 2. Assist patient in assuming comfortable position that provides easy access to route through which you will measure temperature. | Ensures comfort and accuracy of temperature reading. |
| 3. Obtain temperature reading. | |
| **A. Oral Temperature Measurement With Electronic Thermometer:** | |
| (1) Apply gloves *(optional)*. | Use of oral probe cover, which is removable without physical contact, minimizes need to wear gloves. |
| (2) Remove thermometer pack from charging unit. Attach oral thermometer probe stem (blue tip) to thermometer unit. Grasp top of probe stem, being careful not to apply pressure on the ejection button. | Charging provides battery power. Ejection button releases plastic cover from probe stem. |
| (3) Slide disposable plastic probe cover over thermometer probe stem until cover locks in place (see illustration). | Soft plastic cover will not break in patient's mouth and prevents transmission of microorganisms between patients. |
| (4) Ask patient to open mouth; then gently place thermometer probe under tongue in posterior sublingual pocket lateral to center of lower jaw. | Heat from superficial blood vessels in sublingual pocket produces temperature reading. With electronic thermometer, temperatures in right and left posterior sublingual pocket are significantly higher than in area under front of tongue. |

| STEP | RATIONALE |
|------|-----------|

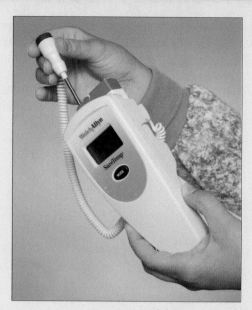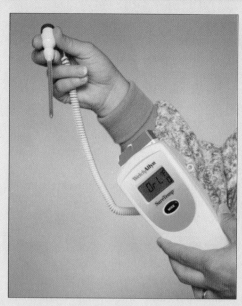

STEP **3A(3)** Disposable plastic cover is placed over the probe.

| | |
|---|---|
| (5) Ask patient to hold thermometer probe with lips closed. | Maintains proper position of thermometer during recording. |
| (6) Leave thermometer probe in place until audible signal indicates completion and patient's temperature appears on digital display; remove thermometer probe from under patient's tongue. | Makes sure probe stays in place until signal occurs to ensure accurate reading. |
| (7) Push ejection button on thermometer probe stem to discard plastic probe cover into appropriate receptacle. | Reduces transmission of microorganisms. |
| (8) Return thermometer probe stem to storage position of recording unit. | Returning probe stem automatically causes digital reading to disappear. Storage position protects stem. |
| (9) If gloves are worn, remove and dispose of in appropriate receptacle. Perform hand hygiene. | Reduces transmission of microorganisms. |
| (10) Return thermometer to charger. | Maintains battery charge of thermometer unit. |

**B. Rectal Temperature Measurement With Electronic Thermometer:**

| | |
|---|---|
| (1) Draw curtain around bed, and/or close room door. Assist patient to Sims' position with upper leg flexed. Move aside bed linen to expose only anal area. Keep patient's upper body and lower extremities covered with sheet or blanket. | Maintains patient's privacy, minimizes embarrassment, and promotes comfort. |
| (2) Apply gloves. | Maintains standard precautions when exposed to items soiled with body fluids (e.g., feces). |
| (3) Remove thermometer pack from charging unit. Attach rectal probe stem (red tip) to thermometer unit. Grasp top of probe stem, being careful not to apply pressure on the ejection button. | Charging provides battery power. Ejection button releases plastic cover from probe stem. |

| SKILL 12-1 | Measuring Body Temperature—cont'd |
| --- | --- |

| STEP | RATIONALE |
| --- | --- |
| (4) Slide disposable plastic probe cover over thermometer probe stem until cover locks in place. | Probe cover prevents transmission of microorganisms between patients. |
| (5) Squeeze liberal portion of lubricant onto tissue. Dip probe cover's end into lubricant, covering 2.5 to 3.5 cm (1 to 1½ inches) for adult. | Lubrication minimizes trauma to rectal mucosa during insertion. Tissue avoids contamination of remaining lubricant in container. |
| (6) With nondominant hand, separate patient's buttocks to expose anus. Ask patient to breathe slowly and relax. | Fully exposes anus for thermometer insertion. Relaxes anal sphincter for easier thermometer insertion. |
| (7) Gently insert thermometer probe into anus in direction of umbilicus 3.5 cm (1½ inches) for adult. Do not force thermometer. | Ensures adequate exposure against blood vessels in rectal wall. |

---

• *Critical Decision Point:* If you cannot adequately insert thermometer into rectum, remove thermometer and consider alternative method for obtaining temperature.

---

| STEP | RATIONALE |
| --- | --- |
| (8) Once positioned, hold thermometer probe in place until audible signal indicates completion and patient's temperature appears on digital display; remove thermometer probe from anus (see illustration). | Probe needs to stay in place until signal occurs to ensure accurate reading. |
| (9) Push ejection button on thermometer stem to discard plastic probe cover into an appropriate receptacle. | Reduces transmission of microorganisms. |
| (10) Return thermometer stem to storage position of recording unit. | Returning probe automatically causes digital reading to disappear. Storage position protects stem. |
| (11) Wipe patient's anal area with tissue or soft wipe to remove lubricant or feces, and discard tissue. Assist patient in assuming a comfortable position. | Provides for comfort and hygiene. |
| (12) Remove and dispose of gloves in appropriate receptacle. Perform hand hygiene. | Reduces transmission of microorganisms. |
| (13) Return thermometer to charger. | Maintains battery charge of thermometer unit. |
| C. **Axillary Temperature Measurement With Electronic Thermometer:** | |
| (1) Draw curtain around bed, and/or close room door. Assist patient to supine or sitting position. Move clothing or gown away from shoulder and arm. | Maintains patient's privacy, minimizes embarrassment, and promotes comfort. Exposes axilla for correct thermometer placement. |

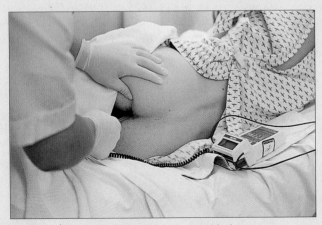

STEP **3B(8)** Probe removed smoothly from anus.

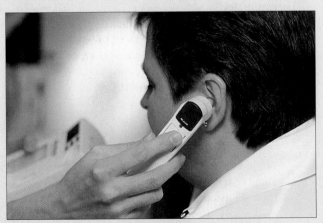

STEP **3D(6)** Tympanic membrane thermometer with probe cover placed in patient's ear.

| STEP | RATIONALE |
|---|---|
| (2) Remove thermometer pack from charging unit. Attach oral thermometer probe stem (blue tip) to thermometer unit. Grasp top of thermometer probe stem, being careful not to apply pressure on ejection button. | Ejection button releases plastic cover from probe. |
| (3) Slide disposable plastic probe cover over thermometer stem until cover locks in place. | Probe cover prevents transmission of microorganisms between patients. |
| (4) Raise patient's arm away from torso. Inspect for skin lesions and excessive perspiration. Insert thermometer probe into center of axilla, lower arm over probe, and place arm across patient's chest. | Maintains proper position of probe against blood vessels in axilla. |

• *Critical Decision Point:* Do not use axilla if skin lesions are present because this alters local temperature and area is sometimes painful to touch.

| STEP | RATIONALE |
|---|---|
| (5) Once positioned, hold thermometer probe in place until audible signal indicates completion and patient's temperature appears on digital display; remove thermometer probe from axilla. | Thermometer probe needs to stay in place until signal occurs to ensure accurate reading. |
| (6) Push ejection button on thermometer stem to discard plastic probe cover into appropriate receptacle. | Reduces transmission of microorganisms. |
| (7) Return thermometer stem to storage position of recording unit. | Returning probe automatically causes digital reading to disappear. Storage position protects stem. |
| (8) Assist patient in assuming a comfortable position, replacing linen or gown. | Restores comfort and sense of well-being. |
| (9) Perform hand hygiene. | Reduces transmission of microorganisms. |
| (10) Return thermometer to charger. | Maintains battery charge of thermometer unit. |

**D. Tympanic Membrane Temperature With Electronic Tympanic Thermometer:**

| STEP | RATIONALE |
|---|---|
| (1) Assist patient in assuming comfortable position with head turned toward side, away from you. If patient has been lying on one side, use upper ear. | Ensures comfort and exposes auditory canal for accurate temperature measurement. Heat trapped in lower ear will cause false high temperature readings. |
| (2) Note if there is obvious earwax in the patient's ear canal. | Makes sure earwax does not block lens cover of speculum. This ensures clear optical pathway. Switch to other ear, or select alternative measurement site. |
| (3) Remove thermometer handheld unit from charging base, being careful not to apply pressure to the ejection button. | Base provides battery power. Removal of handheld unit from base prepares it to measure temperature. Ejection button releases plastic probe cover from thermometer tip. |
| (4) Slide disposable speculum cover over otoscope-like tip until it locks into place. Be careful not to touch lens cover. | Soft plastic probe cover prevents transmission of microorganisms between patients. Ensures clear optical pathway by making sure lens cover is clean and ear canal is clear of earwax. |
| (5) If holding handheld unit with right hand, obtain temperature from patient's right ear; left-handed persons obtain temperature from patient's left ear. | The less acute angle of approach, the better the probe will seal inside the auditory canal. |
| (6) Insert speculum into ear canal following manufacturer's instructions for tympanic probe positioning (see illustration): | Correct positioning of the speculum tip with respect to ear canal ensures accurate readings. |
| (a) Pull ear pinna backward, up and out for an adult. For children younger than 2 years of age, point covered probe toward midpoint between eyebrow and sideburns (Hockenberry and other, 2003). | The ear tug straightens the external auditory canal, allowing maximum exposure of the tympanic membrane. |

## SKILL 12-1 ｜ Measuring Body Temperature—cont'd

| STEP | RATIONALE |
|---|---|
| (b) Move thermometer in a figure-eight pattern. | Some manufacturers recommend movement of the speculum tip in a figure-eight pattern; that allows the sensor to detect maximum tympanic membrane heat radiation. |
| (c) Fit speculum tip snugly into canal and do not move, pointing speculum tip toward nose. | Gentle pressure seals ear canal from ambient air temperature, which alters readings as much as 2.8° C (5° F). Operator error will lead to false low temperatures. |
| (7) Once positioned, press scan button on handheld unit. Leave speculum in place until audible signal indicates completion and patient's temperature appears on digital display. | Pressing scan button causes detection of infrared energy. Speculum needs to stay in place until signal occurs to ensure accurate reading. Signal indicates device has detected infrared energy. |
| (8) Carefully remove speculum from auditory canal. | Prevents rubbing of sensitive outer ear lining. |
| (9) Push ejection button on handheld unit to discard speculum cover into appropriate receptacle. | Reduces transmission of microorganisms. Automatically causes digital reading to disappear. |
| (10) If temperature is abnormal or a second reading is necessary, replace speculum cover and wait 2 minutes before repeating the measurement in the same ear. Also you can repeat measurement in other ear, or try an alternative temperature site or instrument. | Time allows ear canal to regain usual temperature. |
| (11) Return handheld unit to thermometer base. | Protects sensor tip from damage. |
| (12) Assist patient in assuming a comfortable position. | Restores comfort and sense of well-being. |
| (13) Perform hand hygiene. | Reduces transmission of microorganisms. |

## EVALUATION

| | |
|---|---|
| 1. Inform patient of temperature reading and record measurement. | Promotes participation in care and understanding of health status. |
| 2. If you are assessing temperature for the first time, establish temperature as baseline if it is within normal range. | Used to compare future temperature measurements. |
| 3. Compare temperature reading with patient's previous temperature and normal temperature range for patient's age-group. | Body temperature fluctuates within narrow range; comparison reveals presence of abnormality. Improper placement or movement of thermometer causes inaccuracies. |

## RECORDING AND REPORTING

■ Record temperature and route in nurses' notes or vital sign flow sheet. Document measurement of temperature after administration of specific therapies in narrative form in nurses' notes.

■ Record in nurses' notes any signs or symptoms of temperature alterations.

■ Report abnormal findings to nurse in charge, physician, or health care provider.

## UNEXPECTED OUTCOMES
## AND RELATED INTERVENTIONS

■ Temperature 1° C above usual range.
  • Assess possible sites for localized infection and for related data suggesting systemic infection.

• Follow interventions listed in Box 12-7.
• If fever persists or reaches unacceptable level as defined by physician or health care provider, administer antipyretics and antibiotics as ordered.

■ Temperature 1° C below usual range.
  • Initiate measures to increase body temperature.
  • Remove any wet clothing or linen, and cover patient with warm blankets.
  • Close room doors to eliminate drafts.
  • Encourage warm liquids.
  • Monitor apical pulse rate and rhythm (see Skill 12-2) because hypothermia causes bradycardia and dysrhythmias.

**BOX 12-3** | **Advantages and Limitations of Select Temperature Measurement Sites**

**Site Advantages**

**Oral**

Easily accessible—requires no position change.
Comfortable for patient.
Provides accurate surface temperature reading.
Reflects rapid change in core temperature.
Reliable route to measure temperature in intubated patients.

**Tympanic Membrane**

Easily accessible site.
Minimal patient repositioning required.
Obtained without disturbing, waking, or repositioning patients.
Used for patients with tachypnea without affecting breathing.
Provides accurate core reading because eardrum is close to hypothalamus; sensitive to core temperature changes.
Very rapid measurement (2 to 5 seconds).
Unaffected by oral intake of food or fluids or smoking.
Used in newborns to reduce infant handling and heat loss.

**Rectal**

Argued to be more reliable when oral temperature is difficult or impossible to obtain.

**Axilla**

Safe and inexpensive.
Used with newborns and unconscious patients.

**Skin**

Inexpensive.
Provides continuous reading.
Safe and noninvasive.
Used for neonates.

**Temporal Artery**

Easy to access without position change.
Very rapid measurement.
No risk of injury to patient or nurse.
Eliminates need to disrobe or unbundle.
Comfortable for patient.
Used in premature infants, newborns, and children (Sidberry and others, 2002).
Reflects rapid change in core temperature.
Sensor cover not required.

**Site Limitations**

Causes delay in measurement if patient recently ingested hot/cold fluids or foods, smoked, or receive oxygen by mask/cannula.
Not used with patients who have had oral surgery, trauma, shaking or chills, or history of epilepsy.
Not used with infants, small children, or confused, unconscious, or uncooperative patients.
Risk of body fluid exposure.

More variability of measurement than with other core temperature devices.
Requires removal of hearing aids before measurement.
Requires disposable sensor cover with only one size available.
Otitis media and cerumen impaction will distort readings.
Not used with patients who have had surgery of the ear or tympanic membrane.
Does not accurately measure core temperature changes during and after exercise.
Does not obtain continuous measurement.
Affected by ambient temperature devices such as incubators, radiant warmers, and facial fans.
Anatomy of ear canal makes it difficult to position correctly in neonates, infants, and children under 3 years old (Holtzclaw, 2003).
Inaccuracies reported due to incorrect positioning of handheld unit (Maxton and others, 2004).

Lags behind core temperature during rapid temperature changes (Maxton and others, 2004).
Not used for patients with diarrhea, patients who have had rectal surgery, rectal disorders, bleeding tendencies, or neutropenia.
Requires positioning and is a source of patient embarrassment and anxiety.
Risk of body fluid exposure.
Requires lubrication.
Not used for routine vital signs in newborns.
Readings sometimes influenced by impacted stool (Maxton and others, 2004).

Long measurement time.
Requires continuous positioning by nurse.
Measurement lags behind core temperature during rapid temperature changes.
Not recommended to detect fever in infants and young children.
Requires exposure of thorax, which results in temperature loss, especially in newborns.

Measurement lags behind other sites during temperature changes, especially during hyperthermia.
Diaphoresis or sweat impairs adhesion.
Sometimes affected by environmental temperature.

Inaccurate with head covering or hair on forehead.
Affected by skin moisture such as diaphoresis or sweating.
Not used if continuous measurement is required.

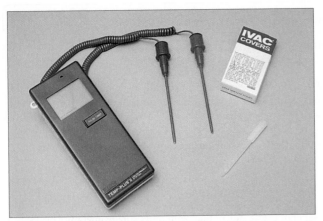

FIGURE **12-1** Electronic thermometer used for oral, rectal, or axillary measurements.

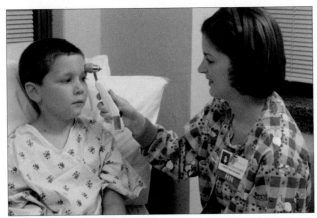

FIGURE **12-2** Temporal artery thermometer scanning forehead.

BOX 12-4   PROCEDURAL GUIDELINES FOR

## Measurement of Temporal Artery Temperature

**Delegation Considerations:** You can delegate this skill to assistive personnel. Instruct the assistive personnel to report the finding to the nurse. It is the nurse's responsibility to assess the significance of the findings.

**Equipment:** temporal artery thermometer, alcohol wipes or probe cover (optional)

1. Perform hand hygiene.
2. Ensure that forehead is dry; wipe with towel if needed.
3. Place probe flush on patient's forehead to avoid measuring ambient temperature.
4. Press the red scan button with your thumb. Continuous scanning for the highest temperature will occur until you release the scan button (see Figure 12-2).
5. Slowly slide thermometer straight across forehead while keeping probe flush on skin.
6. Keeping the scan button pressed, lift probe from forehead and touch probe to neck just behind earlobe (the area where perfume is typically applied).
7. While scanning, a clicking sound occurs and stops when peak temperature is reached.
8. Release the scan button, read and record temperature. The reading remains on for 15 seconds after you release the button.
9. Clean probe with alcohol wipe, or remove and dispose of probe cover if used.

**Chemical Dot Thermometers.** Single-use or reusable chemical dot thermometers are thin strips of plastic with a temperature sensor at one end. The sensor consists of a matrix of chemically impregnated dots that are formulated to change color at different temperatures. In the Celsius version, there are 50 dots, each representing temperature increments of 0.1° C over a range of 35.5° C to 40.4° C. The Fahrenheit version has 45 dots with increments of 0.2° F and a range of 96.0° F to 104.8° F. Chemical dots on the thermometer change color to reflect temperature reading, usually within 60 seconds. Most are designed for single use (Figure 12-3). Therefore they are useful when caring for patients on protective isolation (see Chapter 11). In one brand that is reusable for a single patient, the chemical dots return to the original color within a few seconds. You usually use the chemical dots for oral temperatures. You also use them at axillary or rectal sites, covered by a plastic sheath at the latter site, with a placement time of 3 minutes. Chemical dot thermometers are useful for screening temperatures, especially in infants and young children. Research has also demonstrated the ability of oral chemical dot thermometers

to screen temperatures in orally intubated critical care patients (Potter and others, 2003). You use electronic thermometers to confirm measurements made with a chemical dot thermometer when treatment decisions are involved.

Another form of disposable thermometer is a temperature-sensitive patch or tape. Applied to the forehead or abdomen, chemical sensitive areas of the patch change color at different temperatures.

**Glass Thermometers.** The mercury-in-glass thermometer is a glass tube sealed at one end, with a mercury-filled bulb at the other. Exposure of the bulb to heat causes the mercury to expand and rise in the enclosed tube. The length of the thermometer is marked with Fahrenheit or centigrade calibrations.

Obtaining a temperature with a mercury-in-glass thermometer requires careful preparation of the device (Box 12-5). In addition to proper positioning of the thermometer using the oral, rectal, or axillary site, you maintain this position for at least 3 minutes to obtain an accurate reading. In addition to the time delay, the mercury-in-glass device is easily breakable, and when broken, releases hazardous mercury. If you break a thermometer or suspect a mercury spill, you are required to take immediate action (Box 12-6). It is also important that you teach your patients and their families what to do in the event of breakage of a mercury-in-glass thermometer.

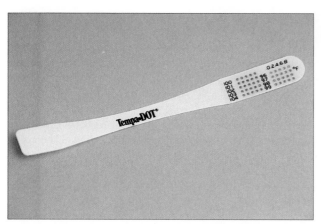

FIGURE 12-3 Disposable, single-use thermometer strip.

---

**BOX 12-5** PROCEDURAL GUIDELINES FOR

## Preparation of Mercury-in-Glass Thermometer

**Equipment:** mercury-in-glass thermometer (rectal or oral), plastic sleeve, lubricating jelly (rectal only), disposable gloves

1. Perform hand hygiene. Apply gloves to avoid contact with body fluids (e.g., saliva, stool).
2. Hold end (if color-coded, tip will be blue or red) of glass thermometer with fingertips to reduce contamination of bulb.
3. Read mercury level while gently rotating thermometer at eye level. If mercury is above desired level, grasp tip of thermometer securely, stand away from solid objects, and sharply flick wrist downward. Brisk shaking lowers mercury level in glass tube. Continue shaking until reading is below 35.5° C (96° F). Make sure thermometer reading is below patient's actual temperature before use.
4. Insert thermometer into plastic sleeve cover to protect from body secretions (e.g., saliva, stool). Apply lubricant to cover 2.5 to 3.5 cm (1 to 1½ inches) on rectal thermometer.
5. Place thermometer using technique appropriate to oral, rectal, or axillary site.
6. Leave thermometer in place 3 minutes for oral or rectal temperatures, 2 minutes for axillary temperature, or according to agency policy.
7. Remove the thermometer. Carefully discard the plastic sleeve. Wipe off secretions with clean tissue, moving toward the bulb.
8. Read thermometer at eye level, read findings, store thermometer in storage container. Remove gloves, and perform hand hygiene.

---

### 🌑 Nursing Diagnosis

After assessment, review all of the available data and look for patterns and trends that are suggestive of a health problem relating to temperature imbalance. For example, an increase in body temperature, flushed skin, skin that is warm to

---

**BOX 12-6** | **Steps to Take in the Event of a Mercury Spill**

1. Do NOT touch spilled mercury droplets. If skin contact occurs, immediately flush area with water for 15 minutes.
2. If possible, remove patient and visitors from immediate impacted environment; shut door of impacted environment; turn off ventilation system to enclosed area.
3. Using rubber gloves, remove any clothing, linen, or shoes contaminated with mercury and place in plastic trash bag. Contaminated clothing, including shoes, will spread mercury.
4. Using rubber gloves, wipe off visible mercury beads with moistened paper towels and put into plastic trash bag.
5. Notify agency's environmental services department, or obtain a mercury spill kit if available.
6. Follow procedures for mercury removal as directed by Material Safety Data Sheet (MSDS). Remove spills using special absorbent materials. Seal everything contaminated with mercury in a plastic bag, and discard.
7. After impacted area is clean, keep area well ventilated to the outside for at least 24 hours.
8. Complete occurrence report as directed by agency's procedure.

Data from: United States Environmental Protection Agency: *What should I do if I have a mercury spill?*, 2005, http://www.epa.gov/epaoswer/hazwaste/mercury/spills.htm.

---

touch, and tachycardia are defining characteristics for the diagnosis of *hyperthermia.* You will validate findings to ensure the accuracy of the diagnosis. Nursing diagnoses for patients with body temperature alterations include:

- Risk for imbalanced body temperature
- Hyperthermia
- Hypothermia
- Ineffective thermoregulation

Once you determine a diagnosis, you decide which factor likely caused the patient's health problem. The related factor allows the nurse to select appropriate nursing interventions. In the example of *hyperthermia,* the related factor of vigorous activity will result in much different interventions than the related factor of exposure to a hot environment.

### 🌑 Planning

The plan of care (see care plan) depends on your assessment of the patient's perception and acceptance of the body temperature alteration. It also depends on the extent to which the patient's internal compensatory mechanisms and behavior have adjusted to the temperature alteration. Make sure the patient actively participates in choosing therapies for the care plan when able.

You set the priorities of care based on the extent the temperature alteration affects the patient. Safety is a top priority.

## CARE PLAN Hyperthermia

### ASSESSMENT

Ms. Coburn is a 26-year-old schoolteacher who lives alone on the eighth floor of an apartment building. On a hot August day, she calls 911, unable to breathe. She is taken to the emergency department, where upon arrival her skin is **warm and dry to touch.** Her face is **flushed,** and she appears to have **labored breathing.** She states that she has not been drinking much lately because she has become nauseated from the heat. Her apartment is not air-conditioned, and one of her two windows does not open. She complains of being very tired and irritable. Vital signs obtained are as follows: BP right arm 116/62, left arm 114/64; right radial **pulse 128**, regular and bounding; **respiratory rate 26;** SpO$_2$ 98% on room air; temporal artery **temperature 39.2° C (102.6° F).**

*Defining characteristics are shown in bold type.

### NURSING DIAGNOSIS Hyperthermia related to prolonged exposure to hot environment.

### PLANNING

#### GOAL
**Thermoregulation**
- Patient will regain normal range of body temperature within next 24 hours.
- Pulse will return to normal range.

- Patient will not be drowsy or irritable.

- Patient will maintain fluid and electrolyte balance during next 3 days.

#### EXPECTED OUTCOMES*

- Body temperature will decline at least 1° C (1.8° F) within the next 8 hours.
- Within the next 8 hours, heart rate will be less than 100 beats per minute.
- Patient will report a sense of comfort and rest within next 48 hours.
- Patient will report increase in energy level within next 3 days.
- Intake will equal output within next 24 hours.
- Postural hypotension will not be evident during ambulation.

*Outcomes classification label from Moorhead S, Johnson M, Mass M: *Nursing outcomes classification (NOC),* ed 3, St. Louis, 2004, Mosby.

### INTERVENTIONS

**Temperature Regulation**
- Monitor temperature every 2 hours and as appropriate
- Administer antipyretic medication as appropriate

- Monitor skin color and temperature
- Instruct patient to increase caffeine-free oral fluids of choice.
- Instruct patient to limit physical activity and increase frequency of rest periods over next 2 days.
- Initiate social services consult to access resources to provide temporary air-conditioning for home environment.

### RATIONALE

Frequent temperature readings during febrile episodes are needed.
Antipyretics reduce set point (Holtzclaw, 2003) and promote comfort.
Indicates signs and symptoms of fever.
Fluids lost through insensible water loss require replacement.
Activity and stress increase metabolic rate, contributing to heat production. Hyperthermia leads to heatstroke and death.
Air-conditioning will prevent future episodes of hyperthermia.

†Intervention classification labels from Dochterman JM, Bulechek GM, editors: *Nursing interventions classification (NIC),* ed 4, St. Louis, 2004, Mosby.

### EVALUATION
- Ms. Coburn's body temperature is within normal limits within 4 hours of admission.
- Ms. Coburn reports that she does not feel nauseated. Her lips and mucous membranes are now moist.
- Ms. Coburn reports that she is breathing easier and feels rested.

## ✳ Implementation

**HEALTH PROMOTION.** You direct health promotion for patients at risk for altered body temperature toward promoting balance between heat production and heat loss. You consider patient activity, temperature of the environment, and clothing. Teach patients at risk from hyperthermia to:

- Avoid strenuous exercise in hot, humid weather
- Avoid exercising in areas with poor ventilation

- Drink fluids such as water and clear fruit juices before, during, and after exercise
- Wear light, loose-fitting, light-colored clothing
- Wear a protective covering over the head when outdoors
- Expose themselves to hot climates gradually

Prevention is the key for patients at risk for hypothermia. Prevention involves educating patients, family members, and friends. Patients most at risk include the very young and the very old and persons debilitated by trauma, stroke, diabetes, drug or alcohol intoxication, sepsis, and Raynaud's disease. Mentally ill or handicapped patients often fall victim to hypothermia because they are unaware of the dangers of cold conditions. Persons without adequate home heating, shelter, diet, or clothing are also at risk.

### ACUTE CARE

**Hyperthermia.** Treatment for an elevated temperature depends on the fever's cause, any adverse effects, and the strength, intensity, and duration of the fever. You play a key role in assessing fever and implementing temperature-reducing strategies (Box 12-7). The goal is a "safe" rather than a "low" temperature (Holtzclaw, 2003). The physician or health care provider may try to determine the cause of the fever by isolating the causative pyrogen. In this case you will get the necessary culture specimens for laboratory analysis, such as urine, blood, sputum, and from wound sites. The physician or health care provider will order appropriate antibiotics to be given after obtaining the cultures. Antibiotics destroy pyrogenic bacteria and eliminate the body's stimulus for fever.

The objective of fever therapy is to increase heat loss, reduce heat production, and prevent complications. Nonpharmacological therapy for fever uses methods that increase heat loss by evaporation, conduction, convection, or radiation.

When you use nursing measures to enhance body cooling, make sure to avoid stimulating shivering. Shivering is counter-productive because of the heat produced by muscle activity. Physical cooling, including the use of water-cooled blankets, is appropriate when the patient's own thermoregulation fails or in patients with neurological damage (e.g., spinal cord injury) (Holtzclaw, 2003).

**Antipyretics** are drugs that reduce fever. Nonsteroidal drugs such as acetaminophen, salicylates, indomethacin, ibuprofen, and ketorolac reduce fever by increasing heat loss. Antipyretics are generally ordered if a fever is over 102.2° F (39° C) (Holtzclaw, 2003). Corticosteroids reduce heat production by interfering with the hypothalamic response. These drugs mask signs of infection by suppressing the immune system. Corticosteroids are not used to treat a fever. However, it is important to be aware of their effect on suppressing the ability of the patient to develop a fever in response to a pyrogen.

**Heat Stroke.** First aid treatment for victims of heat stroke includes moving the patient to a cooler environment, reducing clothing covering the body, placing wet towels over the skin, and using oscillating fans to increase convective heat loss. Emergency medical treatment includes hypothermia blankets, intravenous (IV) fluids, and irrigating the stomach and lower bowel with cool solutions.

**Hypothermia.** The priority treatment for hypothermia is to prevent a further decrease in body temperature. Removing wet clothes, replacing them with dry ones, and wrapping the patient in blankets are key nursing interventions. In emergencies away from a health care setting, the patient lies under blankets next to a warm person. A conscious patient benefits from drinking hot liquids such as soup,

---

### BOX 12-7 Nursing Interventions for Patients With a Fever

#### Assessment

Obtain frequent core temperature readings (i.e., temporal, tympanic, rectal) during the febrile episode.

Assess for contributing factors such as dehydration, infection, or environmental temperature.

Identify physiological response to fever (e.g., diaphoresis, tachycardia, hypotension).

Obtain all vital signs.

Assess skin color and temperature, presence of thirst, anorexia, and malaise; observe for shivering and diaphoresis.

Assess patient comfort and well-being.

#### Interventions (Unless Contraindicated)

Obtain blood cultures when ordered (see Chapter 11). Blood specimens are obtained to coincide with temperature spikes when the antigen-producing organism is most prevalent.

Minimize heat production: reduce the frequency of activities that increase oxygen demand such as excessive turning and ambulation; allow rest periods; limit physical activity.

Maximize heat loss: reduce external covering on patient's body without causing shivering; keep clothing and bed linen dry.

Satisfy requirements for increased metabolic rate: provide supplemental oxygen therapy as ordered to improve oxygen delivery to body cells; provide measures to stimulate appetite, and offer well-balanced meals; provide fluids (at least 3 L/day for a patient with normal cardiac and renal function) to replace fluids lost through insensible water loss and sweating.

Promote patient comfort: encourage oral hygiene because oral mucous membranes dry easily from dehydration; control temperature of the environment without inducing shivering; apply damp cloth to patient forehead.

Identify onset and duration of febrile episode phases: examine previous temperature measurements for trends.

Initiate health teaching as indicated.

Control environmental temperature to 21° to 27° C (70° to 80° F).

---

while avoiding alcohol and caffeinated fluids. Keeping the head covered, placing the patient near a fire or in a warm room, or placing heating pads next to areas of the body (head and neck) that lose heat the quickest helps.

**RESTORATIVE AND CONTINUING CARE.** Educate patients about the importance of taking and continuing any antibiotics as directed until the course of treatment is completed.

Children and older adults are especially at risk for a fluid volume deficit because they quickly lose large amounts of fluids in proportion to their body weight. Identifying preferred fluids and encouraging oral fluid intake is an important nursing intervention.

## Evaluation

You evaluate all nursing interventions by comparing the patient's actual response with the outcomes of the care plan (Table 12-3). This reveals whether you have met goals of care.

## OUTCOME EVALUATION

TABLE 12-3

| Nursing Action | Patient Response/Finding | Achievement of Outcome |
|---|---|---|
| Ask Ms. Coburn to keep a diary of temperature and acetaminophen use for next 24 hours. | Diary completed. | Temperature between 98° F and 100.8° F; four doses of acetaminophen taken appropriately |
| Ask Ms. Coburn to implement rest periods over next 48 hours. | Ms. Coburn remained home from work, reports less malaise. | Energy level returning to baseline |
| Ask Ms. Coburn to describe fluid intake for past 24 hours. | Fluids increased to 8 oz water or fruit juice every 4 hours while awake. | Adequate fluid intake |

After any intervention you measure the patient's temperature to evaluate for change. In addition, you use other evaluative measures such as palpation of the skin and assessment of pulse and respiration. If therapies are effective, body temperature will return to an acceptable range, other vital signs will stabilize, and the patient will report a sense of comfort.

## Pulse

The pulse is the palpable bounding of the blood flow in a peripheral artery. Blood flows through the body in a continuous circuit. Electrical impulses from the sinoatrial (SA) node travel through heart muscle to stimulate cardiac contraction. Approximately 60 to 70 ml of blood enter the aorta with each contraction (**stroke volume [SV]**). The pulse feels like a tap when palpating an artery lightly against underlying bone or muscle. The number of pulsing sensations occurring in 1 minute is the pulse rate.

The volume of blood pumped by the heart during 1 minute is the **cardiac output (CO),** the product of heart rate and the ventricle's SV (see Chapter 28). The cause of an abnormally slow, rapid, or irregular pulse sometimes alters cardiac output. Although cardiac output depends on heart rate, a change in heart rate alone does not alter cardiac output.

### Locating the Peripheral Pulse

You can assess any accessible artery for pulse rate (Figure 12-4), but you will frequently use the radial artery because it is easy to palpate. When a patient's condition suddenly deteriorates, use the carotid site for finding a pulse quickly.

The radial and apical locations are the most common sites for pulse rate assessment. Persons learning to monitor their own heart rates (e.g., athletes or patients using heart medications) usually use these sites. If the radial pulse is abnormal, difficult to palpate, or inaccessible because of a dressing or cast, assess the apical pulse. When a patient takes a medication that affects the heart rate, the apical pulse provides a more accurate assessment of heart rate. Table 12-4 summarizes pulse sites and criteria for measurement. Skill 12-2 outlines radial and apical pulse rate assessment.

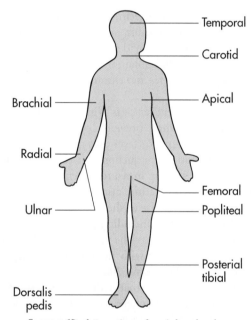

FIGURE **12-4** Location of peripheral pulses.

### Stethoscope

You will need a stethoscope to auscultate the apical sound waves that create the pulse (Figure 12-5). The five major parts of the stethoscope are the earpieces, binaurals, tubing, bell chestpiece, and diaphragm chestpiece.

Make sure the plastic or rubber earpieces fit snugly and comfortably in your ears. Also, make sure the binaurals are angled and strong enough so the earpieces stay firmly in place without causing discomfort. The earpieces follow the contour of the ear canal, pointing toward your face when the stethoscope is in place.

The polyvinyl tubing is flexible and 30 to 45 cm (12 to 18 inches) in length. Longer tubing decreases the transmission of sound waves. The tubing is thick walled and moderately rigid to eliminate transmission of environmental noise and prevent the tubing from kinking, which distorts sound wave transmission. Stethoscopes have single or dual tubes.

*Text continued on p. 246*

| TABLE 12-4 | Pulse Sites | |
| --- | --- | --- |
| **Site** | **Location** | **Assessment Criteria** |
| Temporal | Over temporal bone of head, above and lateral to eye | Easily accessible site used to assess pulse in children |
| Carotid | Along medial edge of sternocleidomastoid muscle in neck | Easily accessible site used during physiological shock or cardiac arrest when other sites are not palpable; site to assess character of peripheral pulse |
| Apical | Fourth to fifth intercostal space at left midclavicular line | Site used to auscultate for heart sounds; site used for infants and young children |
| Brachial | Groove between biceps and triceps muscles at antecubital fossa | Site used to assess upper extremity blood pressure; used during cardiac arrest in infants |
| Radial | Radial or thumb side of forearm at the wrist | Common site used to assess character of pulse peripherally; assesses status of circulation to hand |
| Ulnar | Ulnar side of forearm at wrist | Site used to assess status of circulation to ulnar side of hand; used to perform Allen's test |
| Femoral | Below inguinal ligament, midway between symphysis pubis and anterior superior iliac spine | Site used to assess character of pulse during physiological shock or cardiac arrest when other pulses are not palpable; assesses status of circulation to the leg |
| Popliteal | Behind knee in popliteal fossa | Site used to auscultate lower extremity blood pressure; assess status of circulation to the leg |
| Posterior tibial | Inner side of ankle, below medial malleolus | Site used to assess status of circulation to the foot |
| Dorsalis pedis | Along top of foot, between extension tendons of great and first toe | Site used to assess status of circulation to the foot |

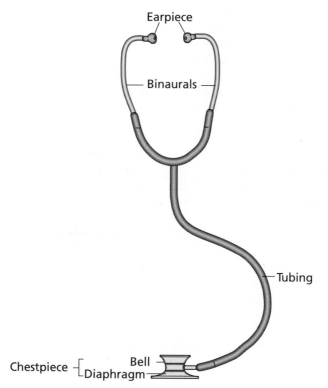

FIGURE **12-5** Parts of a single tubing stethoscope.

## SKILL 12-2 ┆ Assessing the Radial and Apical Pulses

### Delegation Considerations

You can delegate the skill of pulse measurement to assistive personnel if the patient is stable and not at high risk for cardiac irregularity. Before delegation, instruct the assistive personnel about:
- Patient history or risk for irregular pulse.
- Frequency of pulse measurements.
- Appropriate patient position when obtaining apical pulse measurement.
- Usual values for the patient.
- Need to report any abnormalities that you will confirm.

### Equipment

- Stethoscope (apical pulse only)
- Wristwatch with second hand or digital display
- Pen, pencil, vital sign flow sheet or record form
- Alcohol swab

| STEP | RATIONALE |
|------|-----------|

### ASSESSMENT

1. Determine need to obtain radial and/or apical pulse:
   a. Assess for any risk factors for pulse alterations.

   Certain conditions place patients at risk for pulse alterations: a history of heart disease, cardiac dysrhythmia, onset of sudden chest pain or acute pain from any site, invasive cardiovascular diagnostic tests, surgery, sudden infusion of large volume of IV fluid, internal or external hemorrhage, dehydration, or administration of medications that alter cardiac function. A history of peripheral vascular disease alters pulse rate and quality.

   b. Assess for signs and symptoms of altered SV and CO, such as dyspnea, fatigue, chest pain, orthopnea, syncope, palpitations (person's unpleasant awareness of heartbeat), jugular venous distention, edema of dependent body parts, cyanosis or pallor of skin (see Chapter 28).

   Physical signs and symptoms indicate alteration in cardiac function, which affects pulse rate and rhythm.

   c. Assess for signs and symptoms of peripheral vascular disease such as pale, cool extremities; thin, shiny skin with decreased hair growth; thickened nails.

   Physical signs and symptoms indicate alteration in local arterial blood flow.

2. Assess for factors that influence pulse rate and rhythm: age, exercise, position changes, fluid balance, medications, temperature, sympathetic stimulation.

   Allows you to accurately assess presence and significance of pulse alterations. Acceptable range of pulse rate changes with age (see Table 12-5).

3. Determine patient's previous baseline pulse rate (if available) from patient's record.

   Allows you to assess for change in condition. Provides comparison with future pulse measurements.

### PLANNING

1. Explain to patient that you will assess pulse or heart rate. Encourage patient to relax and not speak. If patient has been active, wait 5 to 10 minutes before assessing pulse.

   Activity and anxiety elevate heart rate. Patient's voice interferes with your ability to hear sound when measuring apical pulse. Obtaining pulse rates at rest allows for objective comparison of values.

### IMPLEMENTATION

1. Perform hand hygiene.

   Reduces transmission of microorganisms.

2. If necessary, draw curtain around bed and/or close door.

   Maintains privacy.

3. Obtain pulse measurement.

**A. Radial Pulse:**
   (1) Assist patient to assume a supine or sitting position.

   Provides easy access to pulse sites.

| STEP | RATIONALE |
|---|---|
| (2) If supine, place patient's forearm straight alongside or across lower chest or upper abdomen with wrist extended straight (see illustration). If sitting, bend patient's elbow 90 degrees and support lower arm on chair or on your arm. Slightly extend the wrist with palm down until you note the strongest pulse. | Relaxed position of lower arm and extension of wrist permit full exposure of artery to palpation. |
| (3) Place tips of first two or middle three fingers of your hand over groove along radial or thumb side of patient's inner wrist (see illustration). | Fingertips are most sensitive parts of hand to palpate arterial pulsation. Nurse's thumb has pulsation that will interfere with accuracy. |
| (4) Lightly compress against radius, obliterate pulse initially, and then relax pressure so pulse becomes easily palpable. | Pulse is more accurately assessed with moderate pressure. Too much pressure occludes pulse and impairs blood flow. |
| (5) Determine strength of pulse. Note whether thrust of vessel against fingertips is bounding (+4), normal (+3), weak (+2), thready (+1), or absent (0). | Strength reflects volume of blood ejected against arterial wall with each heart contraction. Accurate description of strength improves communication among nurses and other health care providers. |
| (6) After you feel pulse regularly, look at watch's second hand and begin to count rate: when sweep hand hits number on dial, start counting with zero, then one, two, and so on. | Rate is accurate only after you are sure pulse can be palpated. Timing begins with zero. Count of one is first beat palpated after timing begins. |
| (7) If pulse is regular, count rate for 30 seconds and multiply total by 2. | A 30-second count is accurate for rapid, slow, or regular pulse rates. |
| (8) If pulse is irregular, count rate for 60 seconds. Assess frequency and pattern of irregularity. | Inefficient contraction of heart fails to transmit pulse wave, interfering with CO, resulting in irregular pulse. Longer time ensures accurate count. |
| (9) When pulse is irregular, compare radial pulses bilaterally. | A marked inequality indicates compromised arterial flow to one extremity, and you need to take action. |

• **_Critical Decision Point:_** If pulse is irregular, assess for pulse deficit. Count apical pulse (step 3B) while a colleague counts radial pulse. Begin pulse count by calling out loud simultaneously when to begin measuring pulses. If pulse count differs by more than 2, a pulse deficit exists, which sometimes indicates alterations in CO.

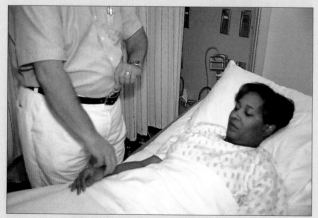

STEP **3A(2)** Pulse check with patient's forearm at side with wrist extended.

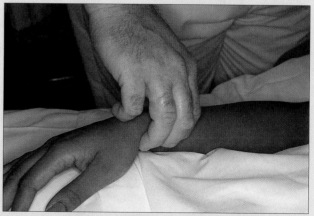

STEP **3A(3)** Hand placement for pulse checks.

## SKILL 12-2 | Assessing the Radial and Apical Pulses—cont'd

| STEP | RATIONALE |
|---|---|

**B. Apical Pulse:**

(1) Perform hand hygiene, and clean earpieces and diaphragm of stethoscope with alcohol swab.

Reduces transmission of microorganisms.

(2) Draw curtain around bed, and/or close door.

Maintains privacy and minimizes embarrassment.

(3) Assist patient to supine or sitting position. Move bed linen and gown to uncover sternum and left side of chest.

Exposes portion of chest wall for selection of auscultatory site.

(4) Locate anatomical landmarks to identify the point of maximal impulse (PMI), also called the apical impulse (see illustration for step 3B[4]A to D). The heart is located behind and to left of sternum with base at top and apex at bottom. Find the angle of Louis just below the suprasternal notch between the sternal body and manubrium; feels like a bony prominence. Slip fingers down each side of angle to find the second intercostal space (ICS). Carefully move fingers down the left side of the sternum to fifth ICS and laterally to the left midclavicular line (MCL). A light tap felt within an area 1 to 2 cm (½ to 1 inch) of the PMI is reflected from the apex of the heart.

Use of anatomical landmarks allows correct placement of stethoscope over apex of heart. This position enhances ability to hear heart sounds clearly. If unable to palpate the PMI, reposition patient on left side. In the presence of serious heart disease, locate the PMI to the left of the MCL or at the sixth ICS.

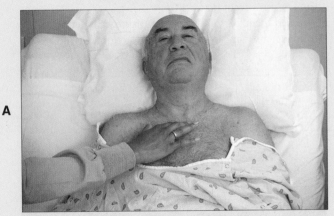

STEP **3B(4)A** Locating the angle of Louis.

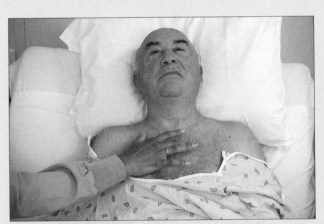

STEP **3B(4)B** Locating the left second intercostal space (2ICS).

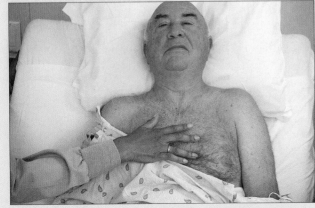

STEP **3B(4)C** Moving down the left side of the sternum to fifth intercostal space (5ICS).

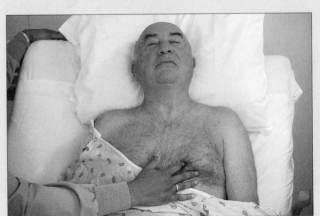

STEP **3B(4)D** Locating the PMI.

| STEP | RATIONALE |
|---|---|
| (5) Place diaphragm of stethoscope in palm of hand for 5 to 10 seconds. | Warming of metal or plastic diaphragm prevents patient from being startled and promotes comfort. |
| (6) Place diaphragm of stethoscope over PMI at the fifth ICS, at left MCL, and auscultate for normal $S_1$ and $S_2$ heart sounds (heard as "lub dub") (see illustrations). | Allow stethoscope tubing to extend straight without kinks, which distort sound transmission. Normal sounds $S_1$ and $S_2$ are high pitched and best heard with the diaphragm. |
| (7) When $S_1$ and $S_2$ are heard with regularity, use watch's second hand and begin to count rate: when sweep hand hits number on dial, start counting with zero, then one, two, and so on. | Apical rate is accurate only after you are able to hear sounds clearly. Timing begins with zero. Count of one is first sound heard after timing begins. |
| (8) If apical rate is regular, count for 30 seconds and multiply by 2. | You assess regular apical rate within 30 seconds. |

---

• *Critical Decision Point:* If heart rate is irregular or patient is receiving cardiovascular medication, count for 1 minute (60 seconds). Irregular rate is more accurately assessed when measured over longer interval.

---

| | |
|---|---|
| (9) Note if heart rate is irregular, and describe pattern of irregularity ($S_1$ and $S_2$ occurring early or later after previous sequence of sounds; for example, every third or every fourth beat is skipped). | Irregular heart rate indicates dysrhythmia. Regular occurrence of dysrhythmia within 1 minute indicates inefficient contraction of heart and alteration in CO. |
| (10) Replace patient's gown and bed linen; assist patient in returning to comfortable position. | Restores comfort and promotes sense of well-being. |
| (11) Perform hand hygiene. | Reduces transmission of microorganisms. |
| (12) Clean earpieces and diaphragm of stethoscope with alcohol swab routinely after each use. | Stethoscopes are frequently contaminated with microorganisms. Regular disinfection controls nosocomial infections. |

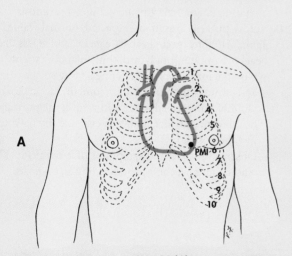
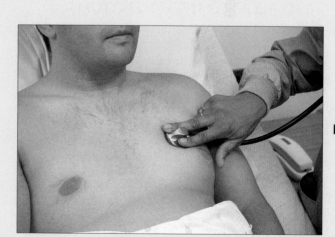

STEP **3B(6) A,** Location of PMI in adults. **B,** Stethoscope over the PMI.

## SKILL 12-2 ┊ Assessing the Radial and Apical Pulses—cont'd

| STEP | RATIONALE |
|------|-----------|

### EVALUATION

1. Discuss findings with patient as needed, and record measurement.

   Promotes participation in care and understanding of health status.

2. Compare readings with previous baseline and/or acceptable range of heart rate for patient's age (see Table 12-5).

   Evaluates for change in condition and presence of cardiac alterations.

3. Compare peripheral pulse rate with apical rate, and note discrepancy.

   Differences between measurements indicate pulse deficit and warn of cardiovascular compromise. Some abnormalities require therapy.

4. Compare radial pulse equality, and note discrepancy.

   Differences between radial arteries indicate compromised peripheral vascular system.

5. Correlate pulse rate with data obtained from blood pressure and related signs and symptoms (palpitations, dizziness).

   Pulse rate and blood pressure are interrelated.

### RECORDING AND REPORTING

■ Record pulse rate with assessment site in nurses' notes or vital signs flow sheet.

■ Record pulse rate after administration of specific therapies, and document in narrative in nurses' notes.

■ Report any signs and symptoms of alteration in cardiac output in nurses' notes.

■ Report abnormal findings to nurse in charge and physician or health care provider

### UNEXPECTED OUTCOMES AND RELATED INTERVENTIONS

■ Radial pulse is weak, thready, or difficult to palpate.
  • Assess both radial pulses, and compare findings. Local obstruction to one extremity (e.g., blood clot, edema) decreases peripheral blood flow.
  • Assess for swelling in surrounding tissues or any encumbrance (e.g., dressing or cast) that impedes blood flow.
  • Perform complete assessment of all peripheral pulses (see Chapter 13).
  • Obtain Doppler or ultrasound stethoscope to detect low-velocity blood flow.
  • Observe for symptoms associated with altered tissue perfusion, including pallor and cool skin temperature of tissue distal to the weak pulse.

  • Auscultate apical pulse to determine pulse rate and identify pulse deficit.
  • Have a second nurse assess pulses.

■ Apical pulse is greater than expected normal value. (See Table 12-5 for expected values, e.g., heart rate greater than 100 beats per minute [tachycardia] in an adult patient.)
  • Identify related data, including pain, fear, anxiety, recent exercise, hypotension, blood loss, fever, or inadequate oxygenation.
  • Observe for signs and symptoms of inadequate CO, including fatigue, chest pain, orthopnea, cyanosis.

■ Apical pulse is less than expected normal value. (See Table 12-5 for expected values, e.g., heart rate less than 60 beats per minute [bradycardia] in an adult patient.)
  • Observe for factors that alter heart rate such as digoxin and antidysrhythmics; it is sometimes necessary to withhold prescribed medications until the physician or health care provider is able to evaluate the need to adjust the dosage.
  • Observe for signs and symptoms of inadequate CO, including fatigue, chest pain, orthopnea, cyanosis.

The chestpiece consists of a bell and a diaphragm that you rotate into position. The diaphragm or bell needs to be in proper position during use to hear sounds through the stethoscope. To test the position of the chestpiece, tap lightly on the diaphragm to determine which side is functioning. The diaphragm is the circular, flat-surfaced portion of the chestpiece covered with a thin plastic disk. It transmits high-pitched sounds created by the high-velocity movement of air and blood. You auscultate bowel, lung, and heart sounds using the diaphragm. Always place the stethoscope directly on the skin, because clothing obscures the sound. Position the diaphragm to make a tight seal against the patient's skin (Figure 12-6).

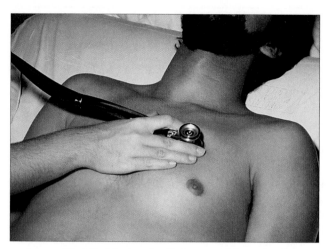

FIGURE **12-6** Positioning the diaphragm of the stethoscope.

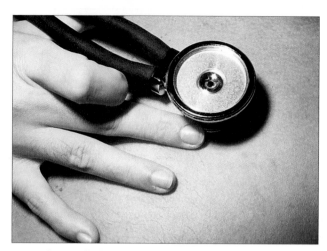

FIGURE **12-7** Positioning the bell of the stethoscope.

Exert enough pressure on the diaphragm to leave a temporary red ring on the patient's skin when the diaphragm is removed.

The bell is the bowl-shaped chestpiece usually surrounded by a rubber ring. The ring avoids chilling the patient with cold metal when you place the bell on the skin. The bell transmits low-pitched sounds created by the low-velocity movement of blood. You auscultate heart and vascular sounds using the bell. Apply the bell lightly, resting the chestpiece on the skin (Figure 12-7). Compressing the bell against the skin reduces low-pitched sound amplification and creates a "diaphragm of skin."

The size of the stethoscope chestpiece varies from small, used for infants and young children, to large. You determine the appropriate size chestpiece by assessing the surface area you will auscultate.

The stethoscope is a delicate instrument and requires proper care for optimal function. Remove the earpieces regularly, and clean them of cerumen (earwax). Inspect the bell and diaphragm for dust, lint, and body oils, and clean with mild soap and water.

## Assessment of Pulse

**PULSE RATE.** Before measuring a pulse, review your patient's record to obtain a baseline rate for comparison (Table 12-5). When assessing the pulse, consider the variety of factors influencing pulse rate (Table 12-6). A combination of these factors sometimes causes significant changes. If you detect an abnormal rate while palpating a peripheral pulse, the next step is to assess the apical rate. The apical rate requires auscultation of the heart sounds, which provides a more accurate assessment of cardiac contraction.

You assess the **apical pulse** by listening for heart sounds (see Chapter 13). After properly positioning the bell or the diaphragm of the stethoscope on the chest, try to identify the first and second heart sounds ($S_1$ and $S_2$). At normal slow rates, $S_1$ is low pitched and dull, sounding like a "lub." $S_2$ is a higher-pitched and shorter sound and creates the sound

| TABLE 12-5 | Acceptable Ranges of Heart Rate for Age |
|---|---|
| **Age** | **Heart Rate (beats/min)** |
| Infants | 120-160 |
| Toddlers | 90-140 |
| Preschoolers | 80-110 |
| School-agers | 75-100 |
| Adolescent | 60-90 |
| Adult | 60-100 |

"dub." You count each set of "lub-dub" as one heartbeat. Count the number of "lub-dubs" occurring in 1 minute.

Pulse rate assessment reveals variations in heart rate. Two common abnormalities in pulse rate are **tachycardia** and **bradycardia.** Tachycardia is an abnormally elevated heart rate, more than 100 beats per minute in adults. Bradycardia is a slow rate, less than 60 beats per minute in adults.

**PULSE RHYTHM.** Normally a regular interval of time occurs between each pulse or heartbeat. An interval interrupted by an early or late beat or a missed beat indicates an abnormal rhythm or **dysrhythmia.** A dysrhythmia alters cardiac output, particularly if it occurs repetitively. If a dysrhythmia is present, you need to assess the regularity of its occurrence. Dysrhythmias are regularly irregular or irregularly irregular. The physician or health care provider sometimes orders additional tests to evaluate the occurrence of dysrhythmias (see Chapter 25).

An inefficient contraction of the heart that fails to transmit a pulse wave to the peripheral pulse site creates a **pulse deficit.** To assess a pulse deficit, ask a colleague to assess the radial pulse rate while you assess the apical rate. When you compare rates and find a difference between the apical and radial pulse rates, a pulse deficit exists. Pulse deficits are frequently associated with dysrhythmias.

| TABLE 12-6 | Factors Influencing Pulse Rates | |
|---|---|---|
| Factor | Increase Pulse Rate | Decrease Pulse Rate |
| Exercise | Short-term exercise | Long-term exercise conditions the heart, resulting in lower rate at rest and quicker return to resting level after exercise |
| Temperature | Fever and heat | Hypothermia |
| Emotions | Acute pain and anxiety increase sympathetic stimulation, affecting heart rate | Unrelieved severe pain increases parasympathetic stimulation, affecting heart rate; relaxation |
| Drugs | Positive chronotropic drugs such as epinephrine | Negative chronotropic drugs such as digitalis, beta-adrenergic blockers |
| Hemorrhage | Loss of blood increases sympathetic stimulation | |
| Postural changes | Standing or sitting | Lying down |
| Pulmonary conditions | Diseases causing poor oxygenation, such as asthma, chronic obstructive pulmonary disease (COPD) | |

**STRENGTH AND EQUALITY.** The strength or amplitude of a pulse reflects the volume and pressure of the blood ejected against the arterial wall with each heart contraction and the condition of the arterial vascular system leading to the pulse site. Normally the pulse strength remains the same with each heartbeat. Assess both radial pulses to compare the characteristics of each. A pulse in one arm is sometimes unequal in strength or absent in many disease states. Pulse strength is assigned a number grade and described as bounding (+4), full (+3), normal (+2), diminished (+1), or absent (0). Evaluating pulse strength and equality is included during assessment of the vascular system (see Chapter 13).

## Blood Pressure

Blood pressure is the force exerted on the walls of an artery created by the pulsing blood under pressure from the heart. Blood flows throughout the circulatory system because of pressure changes, moving from an area of high pressure to an area of low pressure. The heart's contraction ejects blood under high pressure into the aorta. The peak of maximum pressure when ejection occurs is the **systolic** blood pressure. When the heart relaxes, the blood remaining in the arteries exerts a minimum or **diastolic** pressure. Diastolic pressure is the lowest pressure exerted against the arterial walls at all times.

The standard unit for measuring BP is millimeters of mercury (mm Hg). The measurement indicates the height to which the BP raises a column of mercury. You record blood pressure as a ratio with the systolic reading before the diastolic (e.g., 120/80). The difference between systolic and diastolic pressure is the **pulse pressure.** For a BP of 120/80, the pulse pressure is 40.

### Physiology of Arterial Blood Pressure

Blood pressure reflects the interrelationships of cardiac output, peripheral vascular resistance, blood volume, blood viscosity, and artery elasticity. An increase in cardiac output is sometimes the result of greater heart muscle contractility, an increase in heart rate, or an increase in blood volume. When peripheral arteries constrict, such as during periods of stress, peripheral vascular resistance increases, which results in an increase in BP. As vessels dilate and resistance falls, BP drops. When blood is forced through the rigid arteries, BP rises. If the blood volume decreases, such as during dehydration or hemorrhage, there is less pressure exerted against arterial walls and BP falls. When the hematocrit rises, the percentage of red blood cells in the blood increases, causing an increase in blood viscosity. The heart then contracts more forcefully to move the viscous blood through the circulatory system, resulting in an increased BP.

### Blood Pressure Variations

Many factors during the day continually influence blood pressure. A single measurement does not adequately reflect a patient's BP. Blood pressure trends, not individual measurements, guide nursing interventions. Your understanding of the factors that influence BP results in a more accurate interpretation of BP readings. Box 12-8 summarizes factors affecting blood pressure.

**HYPERTENSION.** The most common alteration in BP is **hypertension,** an often asymptomatic disorder characterized by persistently elevated BP. The Joint National Committee on Prevention, Detection, Evaluation, and Treatment of High Blood Pressure (JNC) (NHBPEP, 2003) has set criteria for determining categories of hypertension (Table 12-7). Prehypertension is a designation for patients at high risk of developing hypertension. In these patients, adopting healthy lifestyles reduces the risk or prevents hypertension. Hypertension is defined as systolic blood pressure (SBP) of 140 mm Hg or greater, diastolic blood pressure (DBP) of 90 mm Hg or greater, or taking antihypertensive medication (NHBPEP, 2003). The diagnosis of hypertension in adults is made on the average of two or more readings taken at each of two or more visits after an initial screening. One BP recording revealing a high SBP or DBP does not qualify as a diagnosis of hyperten-

| BOX 12-8 | Factors Influencing Blood Pressure |
| --- | --- |

### Age

Blood pressure tends to rise with advancing age:

| Age | Arterial Pressure (mm Hg) |
| --- | --- |
| Newborn (3000 g [6.6 lb]) | 40 (mean) |
| 1 month | 85/54 |
| 1 year | 95/65 |
| 6 years | 105/65 |
| 10-13 years | 110/65 |
| 14-17 years | 120/75 |
| Adult | 120/80 |

You assess the level of a child's or adolescent's blood pressure with respect to body size and age. Larger children have higher blood pressures than smaller children of the same age. Older adults have a rise in systolic pressure related to decreased elasticity.

### Sympathetic Stimulation

Anxiety, fear, and pain stimulates the sympathetic nervous system to increase heart rate, increase cardiac output, and vascular resistance, causing BP to rise. Anxiety raises BP as much as 30 mm Hg.

### Gender

There is no clinically significant difference in blood pressure levels between boys and girls before puberty.
After puberty, males have higher readings.
During and after menopause, women have higher blood pressures than men of the same age.

### Ethnicity

The incidence of hypertension is higher in urban African-Americans than European-Americans.
African-Americans tend to develop more severe hypertension at an earlier age and have twice the risk for complications of hypertension such as stroke and heart attack. Hypertension-related deaths are also higher among African-Americans.

### Daily Variation

Blood pressure varies throughout the day with lower blood pressure during sleep, highest blood pressure in the afternoon, a decrease in the evening, and an increase beginning at 4 to 6 AM. Blood pressure drops 10% to 20% during nighttime sleep.

### Medication

Some medications directly or indirectly affect blood pressure. Antihypertensive medications lower blood pressure. Narcotic analgesics lower blood pressure. Vasoconstrictors and intravenous fluids such as normal saline increase blood pressure.

### Activity

Older adults often experience a 5- to 10-mm Hg fall in blood pressure about 1 hour after eating.
Blood pressure is sometimes reduced for several hours after a period of vigorous exercise.
Blood pressure falls as a person moves from lying to sitting or standing position; normal postural variations are minimal.
Increase in oxygen demand by the body for activity increase BP.

### Weight

Obesity is an independent predictor of hypertension (Thomas and others, 2002).

### Smoking

Smoking results in vasoconstriction, a narrowing of blood vessels. BP rises when a person smokes and returns to baseline in about 15 minutes after stopping smoking (NHBPEP, 2003).

Modified from Thomas SA, DeKeyser F: Blood pressure, *Annu Rev Nurs Res* 14:3, 1996; The sixth report of the Joint National Committee on Detection, Evaluation, and treatment of High Blood Pressure, *Arch Intern Med* 157:2413, 1997; Brashers VL: *Clinical application of pathophysiology,* St. Louis, 1998, Mosby; Whaley LF, Wong DL: *Nursing care of infants and children,* ed 6, St. Louis, 1999, Mosby.

sion. However, if you assess a high reading (for example, 150/90 mm Hg), encourage the patient to return for another checkup within 2 months (Table 12-8).

Persons with a family history of hypertension are at significant risk. Obesity, cigarette smoking, heavy alcohol consumption, high blood cholesterol levels, and continued exposure to stress are also linked to hypertension.

HYPOTENSION. **Hypotension** is present when the systolic blood pressure falls to 90 mm Hg or below. Although some adults have low blood pressure normally, hypotension is an abnormal finding associated with an illness (e.g., hemorrhage or myocardial infarction). Hypotension occurs when arteries dilate, the peripheral vascular resistance decreases, the circulating blood volume decreases, or the heart fails to provide adequate cardiac output. Signs and symptoms associated with hypotension include pallor, skin mottling, clamminess, confusion, dizziness, chest pain, increased heart rate, and decreased urine output. Hypotension is life threatening and needs to be reported to the physician or health care provider immediately.

**Orthostatic hypotension,** also referred to as **postural hypotension,** occurs when a patient with a normal blood pressure develops symptoms (e.g., light-headedness or dizziness) and low blood pressure when rising to an upright position. In severe cases, loss of consciousness occurs. When a healthy person changes from a lying to sitting to standing position, the peripheral blood vessels in the legs constrict, preventing the pooling of blood in the legs caused by grav-

| TABLE 12-7 | Classification of Blood Pressure for Adults Age 18 Years and Older | | |
|---|---|---|---|
| Category | Systolic (mm Hg)* | | Diastolic (mm Hg)* |
| Normal | <120 | | <80 |
| Prehypertension† | 120-139 | or | 80-89 |
| Stage 1 Hypertension | 140-159 | or | 90-99 |
| Stage 2 Hypertension | >160 | or | >100 |

Data from National High Blood Pressure Education Program (NHBPEP); National Heart, Lung, and Blood Institute; National Institutes of Health: The seventh report of the Joint National Committee on Detection, Evaluation and Treatment of High Blood Pressure, *JAMA* 289(19):2560, 2003.
*Based on the average of two or more readings taken at each of two or more visits after an initial screening. Patient should not be taking antihypertensive drugs and not be acutely ill. When systolic and diastolic blood pressures fall into different categories, select the higher category to classify the individual's blood pressure status. For example, classify 160/92 mm Hg as Stage 2 hypertension.
†Based on average of two or more readings.

| TABLE 12-8 | Recommendations for Blood Pressure Follow-up |
|---|---|
| Initial Blood Pressure | Follow-up Recommended* |
| Normal | Recheck in 2 years. |
| Prehypertension | Recheck in 1 year.† |
| Stage 1 hypertension | Confirm within 2 months.† |
| Stage 2 hypertension | Evaluate or refer to source of care within 1 month. For those with higher pressure (e.g., >180/110 mm Hg), evaluate and treat immediately or within 1 week depending on clinical situation and complications. |

Data from National High Blood Pressure Education Program (NHBPEP); National Heart, Lung, and Blood Institute; National Institutes of Health: The seventh report of the Joint National Committee on Detection, Evaluation and Treatment of High Blood Pressure, *JAMA* 289(19):2560, 2003.
*Modify the scheduling of follow-up according to reliable information about past BP measurements, other cardiovascular risk factors, or target organ damage.
†Provide advice about lifestyle modifications.

ity. Orthostatic hypotension occurs when the peripheral blood vessels in the legs are already constricted or are unable to constrict in response to a change in position. Patients with a decreased blood volume, anemia, dehydration, experiencing prolonged bed rest, with recent blood loss, or taking antihypertensive medications are at risk for orthostatic hypotension. Assess for orthostatic hypotension by obtaining pulse and blood pressure readings with the patient supine, sitting, and standing (Box 12-9).

| BOX 12-9 | PROCEDURAL GUIDELINES FOR |
|---|---|

## Measuring Orthostatic Blood Pressure

**Delegation Considerations:** You cannot delegate this skill.
**Equipment:** sphygmomanometer, stethoscope

1. With patient supine, take blood pressure in each arm. Select arm with highest systolic reading for subsequent measurements.
2. Leaving blood pressure cuff in place, help patient to sitting position. After 1 to 3 minutes with patient in sitting position, take blood pressure. If orthostatic symptoms occur such as dizziness, weakness, light-headedness, feeling faint, or sudden pallor, stop blood pressure measurement and help patient to a supine position.
3. Leaving blood pressure cuff in place, help patient to standing position. After 1 to 3 minutes with patient in standing position, take blood pressure. If orthostatic symptoms occur (see above), stop blood pressure measurement and help patient to a supine position. In most cases, you will detect orthostatic hypotension within 1 minute of standing.
4. Record patient's blood pressure in each position; for example: "140/80 supine, 132/72 sitting, 108/60 standing." Note any additional symptoms or complaints.
5. Report findings of orthostatic hypotension or orthostatic symptoms to nurse in charge and physician or health care provider. Instruct patient to ask for assistance when getting out of bed if orthostatic hypotension is present or orthostatic symptoms occur.

## Assessment of Blood Pressure

You measure arterial blood pressure either directly (invasively) or indirectly (noninvasively). The direct method requires the insertion of a thin catheter into an artery. The more common noninvasive method requires use of the **sphygmomanometer** and stethoscope. You measure blood pressure indirectly by auscultation or palpation. Most use the auscultation technique (Skill 12-3).

**BLOOD PRESSURE EQUIPMENT.** Before assessing blood pressure, you need to be comfortable using a sphygmomanometer and stethoscope. A sphygmomanometer includes a pressure manometer, an occlusive cloth or vinyl cuff that encloses an inflatable rubber bladder, and a pressure bulb with a release valve that inflates the bladder. The two types of sphygmomanometers are the aneroid and the mercury (Figure 12-8, p. 256). The aneroid manometer has a glass-enclosed circular gauge containing a needle that registers millimeter calibrations. Before using the aneroid model, be sure that the needle points to zero. Metal parts in the aneroid manometer are subjects to temperature variations and need to be checked every 6 months to verify their accuracy (Jones and others, 2003). Aneroid manometers have the advantages of being safe, lightweight, portable, and compact.

Mercury manometers, once the gold standard, are less common because they contain mercury, a dangerous substance. Many cities have prohibited the sale or use of devices

*Text continued on p. 256*

# SKILL 12-3 | Measuring Blood Pressure

## Delegation Considerations

You can delegate the skill of blood pressure measurement to assistive personnel unless the patient is considered unstable. Before delegation, instruct the assistive personnel about:

- Frequency of blood pressure measurements for the patient
- Usual values for the patient
- Any patient alterations affecting the appropriate limb for blood pressure measurement
- Appropriate-size blood pressure cuff for designated extremity
- Patient's risk for orthostatic hypotension
- Need to report any abnormalities that you will confirm

## Equipment

- Aneroid sphygmomanometer
- Cloth or disposable vinyl pressure cuff of appropriate size for patient's extremity
- Stethoscope
- Alcohol swab
- Pen, vital sign flow sheet or record form

| STEP | RATIONALE |
|---|---|

### ASSESSMENT

1. Determine need to assess patient's BP:
   a. Note risk factors for alterations in BP.

   Certain conditions place patients at risk for BP alterations: history of cardiovascular disease, renal disease, diabetes, circulatory shock (hypovolemic, septic, cardiogenic, or neurogenic), acute or chronic pain, rapid IV infusion of fluids or blood products, increased intracranial pressure, postoperative conditions, toxemia of pregnancy.

   b. Assess for signs and symptoms of BP alterations:
      (1) High BP (hypertension) is often asymptomatic until pressure is very high. Assess for headache (usually occipital), flushing of face, nosebleed, and fatigue in older adults.
      (2) Low BP (hypotension) is associated with dizziness; confusion; restlessness; pale, dusky, or cyanotic skin and mucous membranes; cool, mottled skin over extremities.

   Physical signs and symptoms sometimes indicate alterations in BP.

2. Determine best site for BP assessment. Avoid applying cuff to extremity when: intravenous fluids infusing; an arteriovenous shunt or fistula is present; breast or axillary surgery has been performed on that side; extremity has been traumatized, diseased, or requires a cast or bulky bandage. Use the lower extremities when the brachial arteries are inaccessible.

   Inappropriate site selection results in poor amplification of sounds, causing inaccurate readings. Application of pressure from inflated bladder temporarily impairs blood flow and will further compromise circulation in extremity that already has impaired blood flow.

3. Determine previous baseline BP (if available) from patient's record.

   Allows you to assess for change in condition. Provides comparison with future BP measurements.

### PLANNING

1. Explain to patient that you will assess BP. Have patient rest at least 5 minutes before measuring lying or sitting BP and 1 minute when standing (NHBPEP, 2003). Ask patient not to speak while measuring BP (NHBPEP, 2003).

   Reduces anxiety that falsely elevates readings. Blood pressure readings taken at different times are more objective to compare when assessed with patient at rest. Exercise causes false elevations in BP. Talking to a patient when assessing the BP increases readings 10% to 40% (Thomas and others, 2002).

2. Be sure patient has not ingested caffeine or smoked for 30 minutes before BP assessment (NHBPEP, 2003).

   Caffeine or nicotine causes false elevations in BP. Smoking increases BP immediately and lasts up to 15 minutes. Caffeine increases BP up to 3 hours.

| STEP | RATIONALE |
| --- | --- |
| 3. Have patient assume sitting or lying position. Be sure room is warm, quiet, and relaxing. | Maintains patient's comfort during measurement. The patient's perceptions that the physical or interpersonal environment is stressful affect the BP measurement (Thomas and others, 2002). |
| 4. Select appropriate cuff size. | Improper cuff size results in inaccurate readings (see Table 12-9). If cuff is too small, it tends to come loose as inflated or results in false-high readings. If the cuff is too large, false-low readings result. |
| 5. Perform hand hygiene, and clean stethoscope earpieces and diaphragm with alcohol swab. | |

## IMPLEMENTATION

| | |
| --- | --- |
| 1. With patient sitting or lying, position patient's forearm or thigh, supported at heart level, if needed, with palm turned up (see illustration); for thigh, position with knee slightly flexed. If sitting, instruct patient to keep feel flat on floor without legs crossed. | If arm is extended and not supported, patient will perform isometric exercise that increases diastolic pressure 10%. Placement of arm above the level of the heart causes false low reading. Even in the supine position a diastolic pressure effort up to 3 to 4 mm Hg occurs for each 5 cm change in heart level (Netea and others, 2003). Leg crossing falsely increases systolic and diastolic BP. |
| 2. Expose extremity (arm or leg) fully by removing constricting clothing. | Ensures proper cuff application. Do not place BP cuff over clothing. |
| 3. Palpate brachial artery (arm) or popliteal artery (leg). With cuff fully deflated, apply bladder of cuff above artery by centering arrows marked on cuff over artery. If there are no center arrows on cuff, estimate the center of the bladder and place this center over artery. Position cuff 2.5 cm (1 inch) above site of pulsation (antecubital or popliteal space). Wrap cuff evenly and snugly around extremity (see illustrations). | Inflating bladder directly over artery ensures proper pressure is applied during inflation. Loose-fitting cuff causes false-high readings. |
| 4. Position manometer vertically at eye level. Make sure observer is no farther than 1 m (approximately 1 yard) away. | You obtain accurate readings by looking at the aneroid needle or meniscus of the mercury at eye level. The meniscus is the point where the crescent-shaped top of the mercury column lines up with the manometer scale. Looking up or down results in inaccurate readings. |
| 5. Measure blood pressure. | |

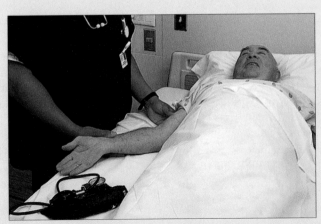

STEP **1** Patient's forearm supported in bed.

| STEP | RATIONALE |
|------|-----------|

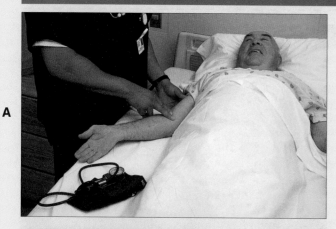

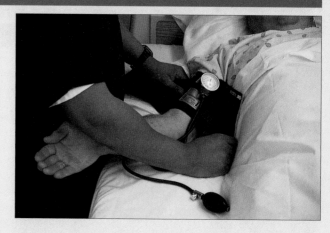

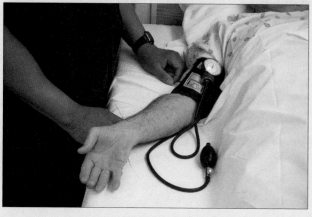

Step **3 A,** Nurse palpating patient's brachial artery. **B,** Center bladder of cuff above artery. **C,** Blood pressure cuff wrapped around upper arm.

**A. Two-Step Method:**

(1) Relocate brachial pulse. Palpate artery distal to the cuff with fingertips of nondominant hand while inflating cuff. Note point at which pulse disappears and continue to inflate cuff to a pressure 30 mm Hg above that point. Note the pressure reading. Slowly deflate cuff, and note point when pulse reappears. Deflate cuff fully and wait 30 seconds.

Estimating systolic pressure prevents false-low readings, which result in the presence of an auscultatory gap. Palpation determines maximal inflation point for accurate reading. If unable to palpate artery because of weakened pulse, use an ultrasonic stethoscope (see Chapter 13). Completely deflating cuff prevents venous congestion and false-high readings.

(2) Place stethoscope earpieces in ears, and be sure sounds are clear, not muffled.

Ensures each earpiece follows angle of ear canal to facilitate hearing.

(3) Relocate brachial artery, and place bell or diaphragm of stethoscope over it. Do not allow chestpiece to touch cuff or clothing (see illustration).

Proper stethoscope placement ensures the best sound reception. The bell will give better sound reproduction, while the diaphragm is easier to secure with fingers and covers a larger area. Stethoscope improperly positioned causes muffled sounds that often result in false-low systolic and false-high diastolic readings.

(4) Close valve of pressure bulb clockwise until tight.

Tightening of valve prevents air leak during inflation.

(5) Quickly inflate cuff to 30 mm Hg above patient's estimated systolic pressure (see illustration).

Rapid inflation ensures accurate measurement of systolic pressure.

(6) Slowly release pressure bulb valve, and allow manometer needle gauge to fall at rate of 2 to 3 mm Hg/sec. Make sure there are no extraneous sounds.

Too rapid or slow a decline in pressure release causes inaccurate readings. Noise interferes with precise determination of Korotkoff phases.

## SKILL 12-3 ▏ Measuring Blood Pressure—cont'd

| STEP | RATIONALE |
|---|---|

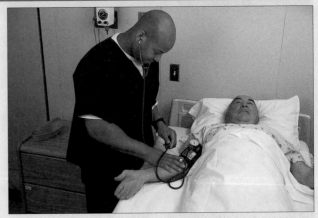

STEP **5A(3)** Stethoscope over brachial artery to measure BP.

STEP **5A(5)** Inflating the BP cuff.

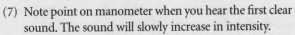

(7) Note point on manometer when you hear the first clear sound. The sound will slowly increase in intensity.

First Korotkoff sound reflects systolic blood pressure.

(8) Continue to deflate cuff gradually, noting point at which sound disappears in adults. Note pressure to nearest 2 mm Hg. Listen for 20 to 30 mm Hg after the last sound, and then allow remaining air to escape quickly.

Beginning of the fifth Korotkoff sound is an indication of diastolic pressure in adults (NHBPEP, 2003). Fourth Korotkoff sound involves distinct muffling of sounds and is an indication of diastolic pressure in children (NHBPEP, 2003).

**B. One-Step Method:**

(1) Place stethoscope earpieces in ears, and be sure sounds are clear, not muffled.

Ensures each earpiece follows angle of ear canal to facilitate hearing.

(2) Relocate brachial artery, and place diaphragm of stethoscope over it. Do not allow chestpiece to touch cuff or clothing.

Proper stethoscope placement ensures optimal sound reception.

(3) Close valve of pressure bulb clockwise until tight.

Tightening of valve prevents air leak during inflation.

(4) Quickly inflate cuff to 30 mm Hg above patient's usual systolic pressure.

Inflation above systolic level ensures accurate measurement of systolic pressure.

(5) Slowly release pressure bulb valve, and allow manometer needle to fall at rate of 2 to 3 mm Hg/sec. Note point on manometer when you hear the first clear sound. The sound will slowly increase in intensity.

Too rapid or slow a decline in pressure release causes inaccurate readings. The first Korotkoff sounds reflect systolic pressure.

(6) Continue to deflate cuff gradually, noting point at which sound disappears in adults. Note pressure to nearest 2 mm Hg. Listen for 20 to 30 mm Hg after the last sound, and then allow remaining air to escape quickly.

Beginning of the fifth Korotkoff sound is an indication of diastolic pressure in adults (NHBPEP, 2003). Fourth Korotkoff sound involves distinct muffling of sounds and is an indication of diastolic pressure in children (NHBPEP, 2003).

**6.** The JNC recommends the average of two sets of BP measurements, 2 minutes apart. Use the second set of BP measurements as your baseline.

Two sets of BP measurements help to prevent false positives based on a patient's sympathetic response (alert reaction). Averaging minimizes the effect of anxiety, which often causes a first reading to be higher than subsequent measurements (NHBPEP, 2003).

**7.** Remove cuff from extremity unless you need to repeat measurement. If this is the first assessment of patient, repeat procedure on the other extremity.

Comparison of BP in both extremities detects circulatory problems. (Normal difference of 5 to 10 mm Hg exists between extremities.)

**8.** Assist patient in returning to comfortable position, and cover arm or leg if previously clothed.

Restores comfort and promotes sense of well-being.

| STEP | RATIONALE |
|------|-----------|
| 9. Discuss findings with patient as needed. | Promotes participation in care and understanding of health status. Makes patient accountable for follow-up assessment. |
| 10. Perform hand hygiene. Clean earpieces, bell, and diaphragm of stethoscope with alcohol swab. | Reduces transmission of microorganisms when nurses share stethoscopes. |

## EVALUATION

1. Compare reading with previous baseline and/or acceptable value of blood pressure for patient's age.

Evaluates for change in condition and alterations.

2. Compare blood pressure in both arms or both legs.

If using upper extremities, use the arm with higher pressure for subsequent assessments unless contraindicated.

3. Correlate blood pressure with data obtained from pulse assessment and related cardiovascular signs and symptoms.

Blood pressure and heart rate are interrelated.

## RECORDING AND REPORTING

■ Record BP and site assessed on vital sign flow sheet or nurses' notes.

■ Record any signs and symptoms of BP alterations in narrative form in nurses' notes.

■ Document measurement of BP after administration of specific therapies in narrative form in nurses' notes.

■ Inform patient of value and need for periodic reassessment.

■ Report any abnormal findings to nurse in charge, physician, or health care provider.

## UNEXPECTED OUTCOMES AND RELATED INTERVENTIONS

■ Unable to obtain BP reading.
   • Determine that no immediate crisis is present by obtaining pulse and respiratory rate.
   • Assess for signs and symptoms of decreased CO; if present, notify nurse in charge, physician, or health care provider immediately.
   • Use alternative sites or procedures to obtain BP: auscultate BP in lower extremity, use a Doppler ultrasonic instrument, implement palpation method to obtain systolic blood pressure.
   • Repeat BP measurement with sphygmomanometer. Electronic BP measurements are less accurate in low blood flow conditions.

■ Blood pressure is above acceptable range.
   • Repeat BP measurement in other arm, and compare findings. Verify correct selection and placement of cuff.

   • Ask nurse colleague to repeat measurement in 1 to 2 minutes.
   • Observe for related symptoms, though symptoms are sometimes not apparent until blood pressure is extremely elevated.
   • Report elevated BP to nurse in charge, physician, or health care provider to initiate appropriate evaluation and treatment.
   • Administer antihypertensive medications as ordered.

■ Patient is hypotensive, and BP is not sufficient for adequate perfusion and oxygenation of tissues.
   • Compare BP value to baseline. A systolic reading of 90 mm Hg is an acceptable value for some patients.
   • Position patient in supine position to enhance circulation, and restrict activity if it is decreasing BP.
   • Assess for signs and symptoms of decreased CO; if present, notify nurse in charge, physician, or health care provider.
   • Increase rate of IV infusion, or administer vasoconstricting drugs if ordered.

■ Patient has a difference of more than 20 mm Hg systolic or diastolic when comparing BP measurements on upper extremities.
   • Report abnormal findings to nurse in charge, physician, or health care provider.

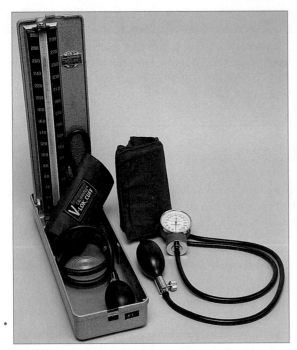

<small>FIGURE **12-8** Sphygmomanometers. *Left,* Mercury; *right,* aneroid.</small>

### TABLE 12-9  Common Mistakes in Blood Pressure Assessment

| Error | Effect |
| --- | --- |
| Bladder or cuff too wide | False-low reading |
| Bladder or cuff too narrow or too short | False-high reading |
| Cuff wrapped too loosely or unevenly | False-high reading |
| Deflating cuff too slowly | False-high diastolic reading |
| Deflating cuff too quickly | False-low systolic and false-high diastolic reading |
| Arm below heart level | False-high reading |
| Arm above heart level | False-low reading |
| Arm not supported | False-high reading |
| Stethoscope that fits poorly or impairment of the examiner's hearing, causing sounds to be muffled | False-low systolic and false-high diastolic reading |
| Stethoscope applied too firmly against antecubital fossa | False-low diastolic reading |
| Inflating too slowly | False-high diastolic reading |
| Repeating assessments too quickly | False-high systolic reading |
| Inadequate inflation level | False-low systolic reading |
| Multiple examiners using different Korotkoff sounds for diastolic readings | False-high systolic and low diastolic reading |

containing mercury. However, some facilities or nursing units still have mercury manometers. Pressure created by inflating the bladder cuff moves the column of mercury up the tube against the force of gravity. Millimeter calibrations mark the height of the mercury column. To ensure accurate readings, the mercury column falls freely as pressure is released and is always at zero when the cuff is deflated

The release valves of both aneroid and mercury sphygmomanometers need to be clean and freely moveable in either direction. The valve, when closed, holds the mercury or pressure constant. A sticky valve makes pressure cuff deflation hard to regulate. The pressure bulb and tubing is airtight.

Cloth or disposable vinyl compression cuffs contain an inflatable bladder and come in different sizes. The size selected is proportional to the circumference of the limb being assessed. Ideally, you select a cuff that is 40% of the circumference (or 20% wider than the diameter) of the midpoint of the limb that you use to measure the blood pressure. The bladder, enclosed by the cuff, encircles at least 80% of the arm of an adult and the entire arm of a child (NHBPEP, 2003). Many adults require a large adult cuff. The lower edge of the cuff is above the antecubital fossa, allowing room for placement of the stethoscope. An improperly fitting cuff causes inaccurate BP measurement (Table 12-9).

**AUSCULTATION.** The best method for BP measurement by auscultation is in a quiet room at a comfortable temperature. Although the patient is able to lie or stand, sitting is the best position. The patient's position is the same during each BP measurement to permit a meaningful comparison of values. Before assessment, you attempt to control factors responsible for artificially high readings such as pain, anxiety, or exertion. The patient's perception that the physical or interpersonal environment is stressful will affect the BP. Measurements taken at home are sometimes different than those taken at the patient's place of employment or in a physician's or health care provider's office.

During the initial assessment, obtain and record the BP in both arms. Normally there is a difference of 5 to 10 mm Hg between the right and left arms. In subsequent assessments, measure the BP in the arm with the higher pressure. Pressure differences between extremities greater than 20 mm Hg indicate vascular problems. You need to report these differences to the physician or health care provider.

Indirect measurement of arterial BP works on a basic principle of pressure. Blood flows freely through an artery until an inflated cuff applies pressure to tissues and causes the artery to collapse. After the cuff pressure is released, the point at which blood flow returns and sound appears through auscultation is the systolic pressure.

In 1905 Korotkoff, a Russian surgeon, first described the sounds heard over an artery during cuff deflation. The first **Korotkoff sound** is a clear, rhythmic tapping that corresponds to the pulse rate and gradually increases in intensity. Onset of the sound corresponds to the systolic pressure.

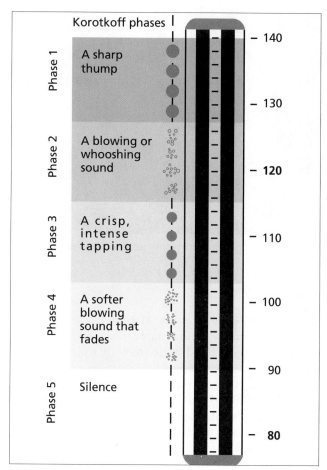

Korotkoff phases

Phase 1 — A sharp thump
Phase 2 — A blowing or whooshing sound
Phase 3 — A crisp, intense tapping
Phase 4 — A softer blowing sound that fades
Phase 5 — Silence

FIGURE 12-9 The sounds auscultated during blood pressure measurement can be differentiated into five Korotkoff phases. In this example, the blood pressure is 140/90.

A murmur or swishing sound appears as the cuff continues to deflate, which is the second Korotkoff sound. As the artery distends, there is a turbulence in blood flow. The third Korotkoff sound is a crisper and more intense tapping. The fourth Korotkoff sound becomes muffled and low pitched as the cuff is further deflated. The onset of the fourth Korotkoff sound is the diastolic pressure in infants and children, pregnant women, and patients with elevated cardiac output or peripheral vasodilation. The fifth Korotkoff sound is the disappearance of sound; in adolescents and most adults, this sound corresponds with the diastolic pressure (Figure 12-9). In some patients the sounds are clear and distinct. In other patients you hear only the beginning and the ending sounds.

The JNC recommends recording two numbers for a BP measurement: the point on the manometer when you hear the first sound for systolic and the point on the manometer when you hear the fifth sound for diastolic. Some institutions recommend recording the point when you hear the fourth sound as well, especially for patients with hypertension. You divide

the numbers by slashed lines (e.g., 120/80, 120/100/80), and note the arm used to measure the BP (e.g., RA 130/70).

You will make many decisions about a patient's care and implement nursing interventions on the basis of blood pressure findings in conjunction with other findings. The importance of obtaining an accurate blood pressure cannot be overemphasized (Box 12-10). There are several possibilities for error if you do not follow the auscultation procedure correctly (see Table 12-9). If you are unsure of a reading, ask a colleague to reassess the BP.

PROCEDURAL GUIDELINES FOR

## Palpating the Systolic Blood Pressure

**Delegation Considerations:** You cannot delegate this skill.
**Equipment:** sphygmomanometer

1. Perform hand hygiene.
2. Apply BP cuff to the extremity selected for measurement.
3. Continually palpate the brachial, radial, or popliteal artery with fingertips of one hand.
4. Inflate the BP cuff 30 mm Hg above the point at which you no longer palpate the pulse.
5. Slowly release valve and deflate cuff, allowing manometer needle to fall at rate of 2 mm Hg per second.
6. Note point on manometer when pulse is again palpable; this is the systolic blood pressure.
7. Deflate cuff rapidly and completely. Remove cuff from patient's extremity unless you need to repeat the measurement.
8. Perform hand hygiene.

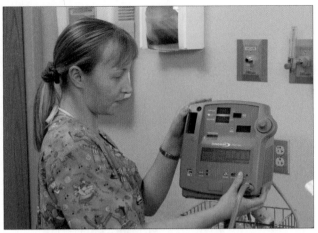

FIGURE **12-10** Electronic blood pressure machines vary in appearance.

**ULTRASONIC STETHOSCOPE.** If you are unable to auscultate sounds because of a weakened arterial pulse, use an ultrasonic stethoscope (see Chapter 13). This stethoscope allows the nurse to hear low-frequency systolic sounds and is commonly used when measuring the BP of infants and children and low BP in adults.

**PALPATATION.** Indirect measurement of BP by palpation is useful for patients whose arterial pulsations are too weak to create Korotkoff sounds. Severe blood loss and weakened heart contractility are examples of conditions that result in blood pressures too low to auscultate accurately. In this case, you assess the systolic blood pressure by palpation (Box 12-11). The diastolic pressure is difficult to determine by palpation. A subtle change in sensation, usually in the form of a thin, snapping vibration, marks the diastolic level. When you use the palpation technique, you record the systolic value and the manner in which you measured it (e.g., RA 78/−, palpated).

You will use the palpation technique along with auscultation in some instances. In some hypertensive patients the sounds usually heard over the brachial artery when the cuff pressure is high disappear as pressure is reduced and then reappear at a lower level. This temporary disappearance of sound is the **auscultatory gap.** It typically occurs between the first and second Korotkoff sounds. The gap in sound sometimes covers a range of 40 mm Hg, possibly causing an underestimation of systolic pressure or overestimation of diastolic pressure. You need to inflate the cuff high enough to hear the true systolic pressure before the auscultatory gap. Palpation of the radial artery helps to determine how high to inflate the cuff. You inflate the cuff 30 mm Hg above the pressure at which you palpate the radial pulse. You then record the range of pressures in which the auscultatory gap occurs (e.g., "BP RA 180/94 with an auscultatory gap from 180 to 160").

**Electronic Blood Pressure Machines.** Many different styles of electronic BP machines are available to determine BP automatically (Figure 12-10). Electronic BP machines rely on an electronic sensor to detect the vibrations caused by the rush of blood through an artery. When the cuff deflates, one style of BP machine determines the initial burst of oscillations and translates the information in a systolic pressure reading. The machine makes the diastolic measurement when the oscillations are lowest, just before they stop. Although electronic BP machines are fast and free the care provider for other activities, consider the advantages and limitations of electronic BP machines (Box 12-12). Use the devices when you need frequent assessments, such as in critically ill or potentially unstable patients, during or after invasive procedures, or when therapies require frequent monitoring (Box 12-13).

**BLOOD PRESSURE ASSESSMENT IN LOWER EXTREMITIES.** If the patient has dressings, casts, intravenous catheters, or arteriovenous fistulas or shunts in the upper extremities, you need to measure blood pressure in the lower extremities. Comparing upper extremity BP with the blood pressure in the legs is also necessary for patients with certain cardiac and BP abnormalities. The popliteal artery, palpable behind the knee in the popliteal space, is the site for auscultation. Position the cuff with the bladder over the posterior aspect of the midthigh, 2.5 cm (1 inch) above the popliteal artery. Make sure the cuff is wide and long enough to allow for the larger girth of the thigh. For most measurements, place the patient in a prone position. If such a position is impossible, flex the knee slightly for easier access to the artery (Figure 12-11). The procedure is identical to brachial artery auscultation. Systolic pressure in the legs is usually higher by 10 to 40 mm Hg than in the brachial artery, but the diastolic pressure is the same.

**ASSESSMENT OF BLOOD PRESSURE IN CHILDREN.** All children 3 years of age through adolescence should have BP checked at least yearly. Blood pressure in children changes with growth and development. You will help parents under-

## BOX 12-12 | Advantages and Limitations of Automatic Blood Pressure Machines

**Advantages**

- Ease of use.
- Efficient when frequent repeated measurements are indicated.
- Ability to use a stethoscope not required.
- Allows you to record BP more frequently, as often as every 15 seconds with accuracy (Yarrows and others, 2001).

**Limitations**

- Expensive.
- Requires source of electricity.
- Requires space to position machine.
- Sensitive to outside motion interference and not used in patients with seizures, tremors, or shivers.
- Not accurate for hypotensive patients or in conditions with reduced blood flow (e.g., hypothermia) (Anwar and White, 2001)
- Accuracy standards for electronic blood pressure machine manufacturers are voluntary (Jones and others, 2003).
- Vulnerable to error in clinical circumstances (Jones and others, 2003):
  - Arrhythmias
  - Older adults
  - Obese extremity

## BOX 12-13 | PROCEDURAL GUIDELINES FOR

# Automatic Blood Pressure Measurement

**Delegation Considerations:** You can delegate the skill of blood pressure measurement to assistive personnel unless the patient is considered unstable. Instruct the assistive personnel to report the findings to the nurse. It is the nurse's responsibility to assess the significance of the findings.

**Equipment:** electronic BP machine, BP cuff of appropriate size as recommended by manufacturer, source of electricity

1. Determine the appropriateness of using electronic BP measurement. Patients with irregular heart rate, peripheral vascular disease, seizures, tremors, and shivering are not candidates for this device.
2. Determine best site for cuff placement (see Skill 12-3, step 3).
3. Assist patient to comfortable position, either lying or sitting. Plug in device, and place device near patient, ensuring that connector hose, between cuff and machine, will reach.
4. Locate on/off switch, and turn on machine to enable device to self-test computer systems.
5. Select appropriate cuff size for patient extremity and appropriate cuff for machine. Electronic BP cuff and machine are matched by manufacturer and are not interchangeable.
6. Expose extremity for measurement by removing constricting clothing to ensure proper cuff application. Do not place BP cuff over clothing.
7. Prepare BP cuff by manually squeezing all the air out of the cuff and connecting cuff to connector hose.
8. Wrap flattened cuff snugly around extremity, verifying that only one finger fits between cuff and patient's skin. Make sure the "artery" arrow marked on the outside of the cuff is correctly placed (see illustration for Skill 12-3, step 3, *B*).
9. Verify that connector hose between cuff and machine is not kinked. Kinking prevents proper inflation and deflation of cuff.
10. Following manufacturer's directions, set the frequency control of automatic or manual, then press start button. The first BP measurement will pump the cuff to a peak pressure of about 180 mm Hg. After this pressure is reached, the machine

begins a deflation sequence that determines the BP. The first reading determines the peak pressure inflation for additional measurements.

11. When deflation is complete, digital display will provide the most recent values and flash time in minutes that has elapsed since the measurement occurred.

- *Critical Decision Point:* If unable to obtain BP with electronic device, verify machine connections (e.g., plugged into working electrical outlet, hose-cuff connections tight, machine on, correct cuff). Repeat electronic BP; if unable to obtain, use auscultatory technique (see Skill 12-3).

12. Set frequency of BP measurements, upper and lower alarm limits for systolic, diastolic, and mean BP readings. Intervals between BP measurements are set from 1 to 90 minutes. The nurse determines frequency and alarm limits based on patient's acceptable range of BP, nursing judgment, and physician or health care provider order.
13. You are able to obtain additional readings at any time by pressing the start button. (Sometimes you will need these for unstable patients.) Pressing the cancel button immediately deflates the cuff.
14. If frequent BP measurements are required, leave the cuff in place. Remove cuff every 2 hours to assess underlying skin integrity and if possible, alternate BP sites. Patients with abnormal bleeding tendencies are at risk for microvascular rupture from repeated inflations. When you are finished using the electronic BP machine, clean BP cuff according to facility policy to reduce transmission of microorganisms.
15. Compare electronic BP readings with auscultatory BP measurements to verify accuracy of electronic BP device.
16. Record BP and site assessed on vital sign flow sheet or in nurses' notes (per agency policy). Record any signs of BP alterations in nurses' notes. Report abnormal findings to nurse in charge, or physician, or health care provider.

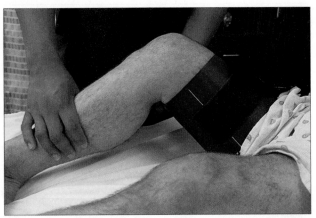

FIGURE **12-11** Lower extremity blood pressure cuff positioned above popliteal artery at midthigh with knee flexed.

stand the importance of this routine screening to detect children who are at risk for hypertension. The measurement of BP in infants and children is difficult for several reasons.

1. Different arm size requires careful and appropriate cuff size selection.
2. Readings are difficult to obtain in restless or anxious infants and children.
3. Placing stethoscope too firmly on the antecubital fossa causes errors in auscultation sounds.
4. Korotkoff sounds are difficult to hear in children because of low frequency and amplitude; a pediatric stethoscope bell is helpful.

The same auscultation method used with adults is appropriate for children. An infant or child younger than 5 years of age lies supine with the arm supported at heart level. Older children sit. It is important for the child to be relaxed and calm. A delay of at least 15 minutes before taking a reading is recommended to allow the child to recover from recent activity or apprehension. Use these 15 minutes for other quiet nursing activities. It helps to have a parent nearby. You prepare the child for the BP cuff's unusual sensation during inflation. Most children understand the analogy of a "tight hug on your arm" and will be more cooperative. Do not choose a cuff based on the name of the cuff. Average width of cuff bladder for an infant is $2\frac{1}{2}$ to $3\frac{1}{4}$ inches; average width of cuff bladder for a child is $4\frac{3}{4}$ to $5\frac{1}{2}$ inches.

## Respiration

Respiration is the mechanism the body uses to exchange gases between the atmosphere and the blood and the cells. Respiration involves three processes: **ventilation** (the mechanical movement of gases into and out of the lungs), **diffusion** (the movement of oxygen [$O_2$] and carbon dioxide

[$CO_2$] between the alveoli and the red blood cells), and **perfusion** (the distribution of red blood cells to and from the pulmonary capillaries). Analyzing respiratory efficiency requires integrating assessment data from all three processes. You assess ventilation by determining respiratory rate, respiratory depth, and respiratory rhythm, and you assess diffusion and perfusion by determining oxygen saturation.

### Assessment of Ventilation

Adults normally breathe in a smooth, uninterrupted pattern of 12 to 16 breaths per minute. Levels of $CO_2$ in the arterial blood normally regulate ventilation. The normal rate and depth of ventilation, **eupnea,** is interrupted by sighing. The sigh, a prolonged deeper breath, is a protective physiological mechanism for expanding small airways and alveoli not ventilated during a normal breath.

You first learn to recognize normal thoracic and abdominal movements to assess ventilation. During quiet breathing, the chest wall gently rises and falls. When breathing requires greater effort, the intercostal and accessory muscles work actively to move air in and out. The shoulders sometimes rise and fall, and the accessory muscles of ventilation in the neck visibly contract. Diaphragmatic movement becomes less noticeable as costal breathing increases.

### Measurement of Respiration

Accurate measurement of respiration requires observation and palpation of chest wall movement. A sudden change in the character of respirations is an important assessment finding. For example, a reduction in respirations occurring in a patient after head trauma signifies injury to the brain stem.

When assessing respiration, keep in mind the patient's usual ventilatory rate and pattern and the influence any disease or illness has on respiratory function. Also consider the relationship between respiratory and cardiovascular function and the influence of therapies on respiration. Box 12-14 summarizes factors influencing respiration. The objective measurement of respiration includes the rate and depth of breathing and the rhythm of ventilatory movements (Skill 12-4).

**RESPIRATORY RATE.** Observe a full inspiration and expiration when counting ventilations or respiratory rate. The respiratory rate varies with age (Table 12-10). A respiratory rate less than 12 per minute or lower than acceptable limits is **bradypnea,** whereas a rate over 16 or greater than the acceptable limits is **tachypnea. Apnea** is the lack of respiratory movements. A respiratory monitoring device that helps assess respiratory rate is the apnea monitor. This noninvasive device uses leads attached to the patient's chest wall to sense movement. An absence of chest wall movement triggers the apnea alarm. Apnea monitoring is used frequently with infants in the hospital and at home to observe for prolonged apneic events.

**VENTILATORY DEPTH.** You assess the depth of respirations by observing the degree of movement in the chest wall. You describe ventilatory movements as deep, normal, or shallow. A deep respiration involves a full expansion of

## BOX 12-14　Factors Influencing Character of Respirations

**Exercise**

Exercise increases respiration rate and depth to meet the body's need for additional oxygen and to rid the body of $CO_2$.

**Acute Pain**

Pain alters rate and rhythm of respirations; breathing becomes shallow.

Patient inhibits or splints chest wall movement when pain is in area of chest or abdomen.

**Anxiety**

Anxiety increases respiration rate and depth as a result of sympathetic stimulation.

**Smoking**

Chronic smoking changes pulmonary airways, resulting in increased respiratory rate at rest when not smoking.

**Body Position**

A straight, erect posture promotes full chest expansion.

A stooped or slumped position impairs ventilatory movement.

Lying flat prevents full chest expansion.

**Medications**

Narcotic analgesics, general anesthetics, and sedative hypnotics depress respiration rate and depth.

Amphetamines and cocaine increase rate and depth.

Bronchodilators slow rate by causing airway dilation.

**Neurological Injury**

Injury to the brain stem impairs the respiratory center and inhibits respiratory rate and rhythm.

**Hemoglobin Function**

Decreased hemoglobin levels (anemia) reduce oxygen-carrying capacity of the blood, which increases respiratory rate.

Increased altitude lowers the amount of saturated hemoglobin, which increases respiratory rate and depth.

Abnormal blood cell function (e.g., sickle cell disease) reduces ability of hemoglobin to carry oxygen, which increases respiratory rate and depth.

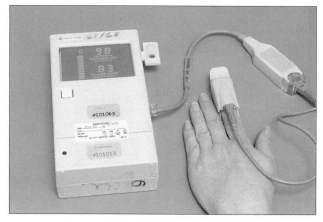

FIGURE **12-12** Pulse oximeter connected to finger sensor.

| TABLE 12-10 | Acceptable Range of Respiratory Rates for Age | |
|---|---|---|
| **Age** | | **Rate (breaths/min)** |
| Newborn | | 35-40 |
| Infant (6 months) | | 30-50 |
| Toddler (2 years) | | 25-32 |
| Child | | 20-30 |
| Adolescent | | 16-19 |
| Adult | | 12-16 |

the lungs with full exhalation. Respirations are shallow when only a small quantity of air passes through the lungs and ventilatory movement is difficult to see. You will need to use more objective techniques if you observe that chest excursion is unusually shallow (see Chapter 13).

**VENTILATORY RHYTHM.** Respiratory rhythm or breathing pattern is either regular or irregular. While assessing respiration, observe the interval between each respiratory cycle. With normal breathing, a regular interval occurs between each respiratory cycle. If you observe an irregular ventilatory rhythm, such as periods of apnea with shallow or deep breathing, you need a more detailed physical assess-

ment (see Chapter 28). Infants tend to breathe less regularly. The young child sometimes breathes slowly for a few seconds and then suddenly breathes more rapidly.

### Measurement of Arterial Oxygen Saturation

A pulse oximeter permits the indirect measurement of **oxygen saturation** for the patient's vital sign database (Skill 12-5). The pulse oximeter is a probe with a light-emitting diode (LED) and photosensor connected to an oximeter (Figure 12-12). Oxygenated and deoxygenated hemoglobin molecules absorb and then reflect light waves emitted by the LED. The photosensor detects the light-absorbing differences between each type of hemoglobin molecule, and the oximeter calculates pulse saturation ($SpO_2$). $SpO_2$ is a reliable estimate of $SaO_2$ (Grap, 2002). In adults the oximeter probe is applied to the earlobe, finger, toe, or bridge of the nose. The probe requires a highly vascular area to detect the degree of change in the transmitted light.

The measurement of $SpO_2$ is affected by factors that affect light transmission or peripheral arterial pulsations. An awareness of these factors will allow you to interpret abnormal $SpO_2$ measurements accurately (Box 12-15, p. 268). You can measure $SpO_2$ intermittently or continuously. You will use continuous $SpO_2$ monitoring to assess ongoing therapies. You can program alarm limits to alert you if the patient's $SpO_2$ drops to an unacceptable level.

*Text continued on p. 268*

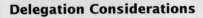

# SKILL 12-4 | Assessing Respiration

## Delegation Considerations

You can delegate the skill of respiration measurement to assistive personnel. Before delegation, instruct the assistive personnel about:

- Frequency of respiration measurement for select patient
- Usual values for the patient

- Patient history or risk for increased or decreased respiratory rate or irregular respiration
- Need to report any abnormalities that you will confirm

## Equipment

- Wristwatch with second hand or digital display
- Pen, pencil, vital sign flow sheet or record form

| STEP | RATIONALE |
| --- | --- |

### ASSESSMENT

1. Determine need to assess patient's respiration:
   a. Note risk factors for respiratory alterations.

   Conditions that place patient at risk for ventilatory alterations detected by changes in respiratory rate, depth, and rhythm include fever, pain, anxiety, diseases of chest wall or muscles, constrictive chest or abdominal dressings, presence of abdominal incisions, gastric distention, chronic pulmonary disease (emphysema, bronchitis, asthma), traumatic injury to chest wall, presence of a chest tube, respiratory infection (pneumonia, acute bronchitis), pulmonary edema and emboli, head injury with damage to brain stem, and anemia.

   b. Assess for signs and symptoms of respiratory alterations, such as bluish or cyanotic appearance of nail beds, lips, mucous membranes, and skin; restlessness, irritability, confusion, reduced level of consciousness; pain during inspiration; labored or difficult breathing; orthopnea; use of accessory muscles; adventitious breath sounds (see Chapter 13), inability to breathe spontaneously; thick, frothy, blood-tinged, or large amounts of sputum produced on coughing.

   Physical signs and symptoms sometimes indicate alterations in respiratory status related to ventilation.

2. Assess pertinent laboratory values:
   a. Arterial blood gases (ABGs) (values vary slightly within institutions):
      pH 7.35 to 7.45
      $PaCO_2$ 35 to 45 mm Hg
      Hg $PaO_2$ 80 to 100 mm Hg
      $SaO_2$ 94% to 98%

   Arterial blood gases measure arterial blood pH, partial pressure of $O_2$ and $CO_2$, and arterial $O_2$ saturation, which reflect patient's oxygenation status.

   b. Pulse oximetry ($SpO_2$): normal $SpO_2$ 90% to 100%; 85% to 89% is acceptable for certain chronic disease conditions; less than 85% is abnormal.

   $SpO_2$ less than 85% is often accompanied by changes in respiratory rate, depth, and rhythm.

   c. Complete blood count (CBC): normal CBC for adults (values may vary within institutions): hemoglobin: 14 to 18 g/100 ml, males; 12 to 16 g/100 ml, females; hematocrit: 40% to 54%, males; 38% to 47%, females; red blood cell count: 4.6 to 6.2 million/$mm^3$, males; 4.2 to 5.4 million/$mm^3$, females.

   Complete blood count measures red blood cell count, volume of red blood cells, and concentration of hemoglobin, which reflects patient's blood capacity to carry $O_2$.

3. Determine previous baseline respiratory rate (if available) from patient's record.

   Allows you to assess for change in condition. Provides comparison with future respiratory measurements.

4. Assess respirations after pulse measurement in adult.

   Inconspicuous assessment of respirations immediately after pulse assessment prevent patient from consciously or unintentionally altering rate and depth of breathing.

| STEP | RATIONALE |
|------|-----------|

## PLANNING

1. Be sure patient is in comfortable position, preferably sitting or lying with the head of the bed elevated 45 to 60 degrees. If patient has been active, wait about 5 to 10 minutes before assessing respirations.

Sitting erect promotes full ventilatory movement. Position of discomfort causes patient to breathe more rapidly. Exercise increases respiratory rate and depth. Assessing respirations while patient rests allows for objective comparison of values.

• *Critical Decision Point:* Assess patients with difficulty breathing (dyspnea), such as those with congestive heart failure or abdominal ascites or in late stages of pregnancy, in the position of greatest comfort. Repositioning will increase the work of breathing, which will increase respiratory rate.

## IMPLEMENTATION

1. Draw curtain around bed, and/or close door. Perform hand hygiene.

Maintains privacy. Prevents transmission of microorganisms.

2. Be sure patient's chest is visible. If necessary, move bed linen or gown.

Ensures clear view of chest wall and abdominal movements.

3. Place patient's arm in relaxed position across the abdomen or lower chest, or place your hand directly over patient's upper abdomen (see illustration).

A similar position used during pulse assessment allows you to assess respiratory rate subtly. Patient's hand or your hand rises and falls during respiratory cycle.

4. Observe complete respiratory cycle (one inspiration and one expiration).

You determine an accurate rate only after viewing the entire respiratory cycle.

5. After you observe a cycle, look at watch's second hand and begin to count rate: when sweep hand hits number on dial, begin time frame, counting one with first full respiratory cycle.

Timing begins with count of one. Respirations occur more slowly than pulse; thus timing does not begin with zero.

6. If rhythm is regular, count number of respirations in 30 seconds and multiply by 2. If rhythm is irregular, less than 12, or greater than 20, count for 1 full minute.

Respiratory rate is equivalent to number of respirations per minute. Suspected irregularities require assessment for at least 1 minute.

7. Note depth of respirations, subjectively assessed by observing degree of chest wall movement while counting rate. You also objectively assess depth by palpating chest wall excursion or auscultating the posterior thorax (see Chapter 13) after rate has been counted. Depth is shallow, normal, or deep.

Character of ventilatory movement reveals specific disease state restricting volume of air from moving into and out of the lungs.

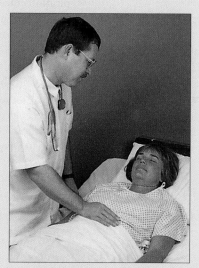

STEP 3 Nurse's hand over patient's abdomen to check respiratory rate.

---

SKILL 12-4 | Assessing Respiration—cont'd

| STEP | RATIONALE |
|---|---|
| **8.** Note rhythm of ventilatory cycle. Normal breathing is regular and uninterrupted. Do not confuse sighing with abnormal rhythm. Periodically people unconsciously take single deep breaths or sighs to expand small airways prone to collapse. | Character of ventilations reveals specific types of alterations. |

- *Critical Decision Point:* An irregular respiratory pattern or periods of apnea (the cessation of respiration for several seconds) are a symptom of underlying disease in the adult and must be reported to the physician or health care provider or nurse in charge. The patient may require further assessment (see Chapter 28) and need immediate intervention. An irregular respiratory rate and short apneic spells are normal for newborns.

| | |
|---|---|
| **9.** Replace bed linen and patient's gown. | Restores comfort and promotes sense of well-being. |
| **10.** Perform hand hygiene. | Reduces transmission of microorganisms. |

## EVALUATION

| | |
|---|---|
| **1.** Discuss findings with patient as needed. | Promotes participation in care and understanding of health status. |
| **2.** If you are assessing respiration for the first time, establish rate, rhythm, and depth as baseline if within normal range. | Used to compare future respiratory assessment. |
| **3.** Compare respiration with patient's previous baseline and normal rate, rhythm, and depth. | Allows you to assess for changes in patient's condition and for presence of respiratory alterations. |
| **4.** Correlate respiratory rate, depth, and rhythm with data obtained from pulse oximetry and arterial blood gas measurements if available. | Evaluation of ventilation, perfusion, and diffusion are interrelated. |

## RECORDING AND REPORTING

- Record respiratory rate and character in nurses' notes or vital sign flow sheet.
- Record abnormal depth and rhythm in narrative form in nurses' notes.
- Indicate type and amount of oxygen therapy if used by patient during assessment.
- Document measurement of respiratory rate after administration of specific therapies in narrative form in nurses' notes.
- Report abnormal findings to nurse in charge, physician, or health care provider.

## UNEXPECTED OUTCOMES AND RELATED INTERVENTIONS

- Respiratory rate is below 12 (bradypnea) or above 16 (tachypnea). Breathing pattern is irregular. Depth of respirations increase or decrease; patient complains of feeling short of breath.
  - Observe for related factors, including obstructed airway, noisy respirations, cyanosis, restlessness, irritability, confusion, productive cough, use of accessory muscles, and abnormal breath sounds.
  - Assist patient to supported sitting position (semi- or high-Fowler's) unless contraindicated, which improves ventilation.
  - Provide oxygen as ordered.
  - Assess for environmental factors that influence patient's respiratory rate such as secondhand smoke, poor ventilation, or gas fumes.

## SKILL 12-5 | Measuring Oxygen Saturation (Pulse Oximetry)

### Delegation Considerations

You can delegate the skill of oxygen saturation measurement to assistive personnel. Before delegation, instruct the assistive personnel about:

- Frequency of oxygen saturation measurements
- Appropriate sensor site, probe, and patient position for measurement of oxygen saturation
- Need to notify you immediately of any reading lower than 90%
- Factors that interfere with $SpO_2$ readings (see Box 12-15)

- Not using pulse oximetry as an assessment of heart rate because the oximeter will not detect an irregular rhythm

### Equipment

- Oximeter
- Oximeter probe appropriate for patient and recommended by oximeter manufacturer
- Acetone or nail polish remover if needed
- Pen, vital sign flow sheet or record form

| STEP | RATIONALE |
|---|---|

### ASSESSMENT

1. Determine need to measure patient's oxygen saturation:
   a. Note risk factors for alteration of oxygen saturation.

Certain conditions place patients at risk for decreased oxygen saturation: acute or chronic compromised respiratory function, recovery from general anesthesia or conscious sedation, traumatic injury to chest wall with or without collapse of underlying lung tissue, ventilator dependence, and changes in supplemental oxygen therapy or activity intolerance (Grap, 2002).

   b. Assess for signs and symptoms of alterations in oxygen saturation such as altered respiratory rate, depth, or rhythm; adventitious breath sounds (see Chapter 13); cyanotic appearance of nail beds, lips, mucous membranes, skin; restlessness, irritability, confusion; reduced level of consciousness; labored or difficult breathing.

Physical signs and symptoms indicate abnormal oxygen saturation.

2. Assess for factors that normally influence measurement of $SpO_2$ such as oxygen therapy, hemoglobin level, body temperature, and medications such as bronchodilators.

Allows you to accurately assess oxygen saturation variations. Peripheral hypothermia interferes with $SpO_2$ determination.

3. Review patient's medical record for physician's or health care provider's order, or consult agency policy or procedure manual for standard of care for measurement of $SpO_2$.

Medical order is sometimes required to assess oxygen saturation.

4. Determine most appropriate patient-specific site (e.g., finger, earlobe, bridge of nose) for sensor probe placement by measuring capillary refill (see Chapter 13). If capillary refill is less than 3 seconds, select alternative site.
   a. Site needs to have adequate local circulation and be free of moisture.
   b. Artificial nails and certain nail polish colors will alter readings (Grap, 2002); place probe on finger free of polish or artificial nail.
   c. If patient has tremors or is likely to move, use ear lobe.
   d. If patient is obese, clip-on probe may not fit properly. Obtain a single-use (tape-on) probe.

Sensor requires pulsating vascular bed to identify hemoglobin molecules that absorb emitted light. Changes in $SpO_2$ are reflected in the circulation of finger capillary bed within 30 seconds and the capillary bed of ear lobe within 5 to 10 seconds. Moisture prevents the sensor from detecting $SpO_2$ levels. Motion artifact is the most common cause of inaccurate readings.

### PLANNING

1. Determine previous baseline $SpO_2$ (if available) from patient's record.

Baseline information provides basis for comparison and assists in assessment of current status and evaluation of interventions.

## SKILL 12-5 Measuring Oxygen Saturation (Pulse Oximetry)—cont'd

| STEP | RATIONALE |
|---|---|
| 2. Obtain oximeter and appropriate probe for patient, and place at bedside. | Mixing probes from different manufacturers will result in burn injury to patient. If patient has latex sensitivity or a latex allergy, avoid adhesive sensors that contain latex. |
| 3. Explain purpose of procedure to patient and how you will measure oxygen saturation. Instruct patient to breathe normally. | Promotes patient cooperation and increases compliance. Prevents large fluctuations in minute ventilation and possible error in $SpO_2$ readings. |

### IMPLEMENTATION

| | |
|---|---|
| 1. Perform hand hygiene. | Reduces transmission of microorganisms. |
| 2. Position patient comfortably. If finger is the monitoring site, support lower arm. | Ensures probe positioning and decreases motion artifact that interferes with $SpO_2$ determination. |
| 3. If using the finger, remove fingernail polish with acetone if present. Acrylic nails without polish do not interfere with $SpO_2$ determination. | Opaque coatings decrease light transmission: nail polish containing blue pigment absorbs light emissions and falsely alters saturation (Grap, 2002). |
| 4. Attach sensor probe to monitoring site (see illustration). Instruct patient that clip-on probe will feel like a clothespin on the finger and will not hurt. | Patient may not expect pressure of sensor probe's spring tension on finger or earlobe. Select sensor site based on peripheral circulation and extremity temperature. Peripheral vasoconstriction alters $SpO_2$. |

• *Critical Decision Point:* Do not attach probe to finger, ear, or bridge of nose if area is edematous or skin integrity is compromised. Do not attach probe to fingers that are hypothermic. Select ear or bridge of nose if adult patient has a history of peripheral vascular disease. Do not use disposable adhesive sensors if patient is allergic to latex. Do not place sensor on same extremity as electronic BP cuff because blood flow to finger will be temporarily interrupted when cuff inflates and causes inaccurate readings that trigger alarms. Do not use earlobe and bridge of nose sensors for infants and toddlers because their skin is fragile.

| | |
|---|---|
| 5. Once sensor is in place, turn on oximeter by activating power. Observe pulse waveform/intensity display and audible beep. Correlate oximeter pulse rate with patient's radial pulse. | Pulse waveform/intensity display enables detection of valid pulse or presence of interfering signal. Pitch of audible beep is proportional to $SpO_2$ value. Double-checking pulse rate ensures oximeter accuracy. Oximeter pulse rate, patient's radial pulse, and apical pulse rate are normally the same. |
| 6. Inform patient that oximeter will sound if sensor falls off or if patient moves sensor. | |

• **Critical Decision Point:** If oximeter pulse rate, patient's radial pulse, and apical pulse are different, reevaluate oximeter probe placement and reassess pulse rates.

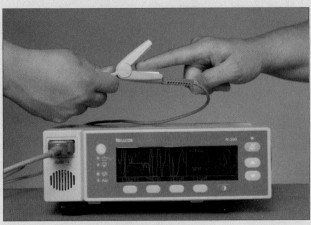

STEP 4 Attaching sensor probe to monitoring site.

| STEP | RATIONALE |
|---|---|
| 7. Leave probe in place until oximeter readout reaches constant value and pulse display reaches full strength during each cardiac cycle. Read SpO₂ on digital display. | Readings take 10 to 30 seconds depending on site selected. |
| 8. If you plan continuous SpO₂ monitoring, verify SpO₂ alarm limits and alarm volume, which are preset by the manufacturer at a low of 85% and a high of 100%. You determine the limits for SpO₂ and pulse rate alarms based on each patient's condition. Verify that alarms are on. Assess skin integrity every 2 hours under sensor probe. Relocate sensor probe at least every 24 hours or more frequently if skin integrity is altered or tissue perfusion compromised. | Ensures alarms are set at appropriate limits and volumes to avoid frightening patients and visitors. Spring tension of sensor probe or sensitivity to disposable sensor probe adhesive causes skin irritation and leads to disruption of skin integrity. |
| 9. Discuss findings with patient as needed. | Promotes participation in care and understanding of health status. |
| 10. If intermittent or spot-checking SpO₂ measurements are planned, remove probe and turn oximeter power off. Store probe in appropriate location. | Batteries will drain if oximeter is left on. Sensor probes are expensive and vulnerable to damage. |
| 11. Assist patient in returning to comfortable position. | Restores comfort and promotes sense of well-being. |
| 12. Perform hand hygiene. | Reduces transmission of microorganisms. |

## EVALUATION

| | |
|---|---|
| 1. Compare SpO₂ readings with patient baseline and acceptable values. | Comparison reveals presence of abnormality. |
| 2. Compare SpO₂ with SaO₂ obtained from ABG measurements (see Chapter 28) if available. | Documents reliability of noninvasive assessment. Pulse oximetry only warns of dangerous low levels of oxygen saturation. Values are not accurate under 80%. |
| 3. Correlate SpO₂ reading with data obtained from respiratory rate, depth, and rhythm assessment (see Skill 12-4). | Measurements assessing ventilation, perfusion, and diffusion are interrelated. |
| 4. During continuous monitoring, assess skin integrity underneath probe at least every 2 hours, based on patient's peripheral circulation. | Prevents tissue ischemia. |

## RECORDING AND REPORTING

- Record SpO₂ value on nurses' notes or vital sign flow sheet.
- Record type and amount of oxygen therapy used by patient during assessment.
- Record any signs and symptoms of reduced oxygen saturation in narrative form in nurses' notes.
- Document measurement of SpO₂ after administration of specific therapies in narrative form in nurses' notes.
- Report abnormal findings to nurse in charge, physician, or health care provider.
- Record in nurses' notes patient's use of continuous or intermittent pulse oximetry. Documents use of equipment for third-party payers.

## UNEXPECTED OUTCOMES AND RELATED INTERVENTIONS

- SpO₂ is less than 90%.
  - Verify that oximeter probe is intact and not influenced by outside light transmission.
  - Observe for signs and symptoms of decreased oxygenation: cyanosis, restlessness, and tachycardia.
  - Compare SpO₂ with SaO₂ from ABG to confirm low saturation.
  - Observe for and minimize factors that decrease SpO₂ such as lung secretions, increased activity, and hyperthermia.
  - Assist patient to a position that maximizes ventilatory effort; for example, place an obese patient in a high-Fowler's position.

---

**BOX 12-15** | **Factors Affecting Determination of Pulse Oxygen Saturation**

**Interference With Light Transmission**

Outside light sources interfere with the oximeter's ability to process reflected light.

Carbon monoxide (caused by smoke inhalation or poisoning) artificially elevates $SpO_2$ by absorbing light similar to oxygen.

Patient motion interferes with the oximeter's ability to process reflected light.

Jaundice interferes with the oximeter's ability to process reflected light.

Intravascular dyes (methylene blue) absorb light similar to deoxyhemoglobin and artificially lower saturation reading.

Dark skin pigment sometimes results in signal loss or overestimation of saturation.

**Interference With Arterial Pulsations**

Peripheral vascular disease (e.g., atherosclerosis) reduces pulse volume.

Hypothermia at assessment site decreases peripheral blood flow.

Pharmacological vasoconstrictors (e.g., epinephrine) decrease peripheral pulse volume.

Low cardiac output and hypotension decrease blood flow to peripheral arteries.

Peripheral edema obscures arterial pulsation.

Tight probe will record venous pulsations in the finger that compete with arterial pulsations.

---

**BOX 12-16** | PATIENT TEACHING

**Temperature**

- Identify patient's ability to initiate preventive health measures and recognize alteration in body temperature. Educate patients and family members about measures to prevent body temperature alterations.
- Teach patients risk factors for hypothermia and frostbite: fatigue; malnutrition; cold, wet clothing; alcohol intoxication.
- Teach patients risk factors for heat stroke: strenuous exercise in hot, humid weather; tight-fitting clothing in hot environments; exercising in poorly ventilated areas; sudden exposure to hot climates; poor fluid intake before, during, and after exercise.
- Teach patients the importance of taking and continuing antibiotics as directed until course of treatment is completed.

**Pulse Rate**

- Patients taking certain prescribed cardiac medications need to learn to assess their own pulse rates to detect side effects of medications. Patients undergoing cardiac rehabilitation need to learn to assess their own pulse rates to determine their response to exercise.

**Blood Pressure**

- Teach patient risk factors for hypertension. Persons with family history of hypertension are at significant risk. Obesity, cigarette smoking, heavy alcohol consumption, high blood cholesterol and triglyceride levels, and continued exposure to stress are factors linked to hypertension.

- Patients with hypertension need to learn about their blood pressure values, long-term follow-up care and therapy, the usual lack of symptoms, therapy's ability to control but not cure, and benefits of a consistently followed treatment plan.
- Instruct patients on the importance of appropriate-size blood pressure cuff for home use.
- Instruct primary caregiver to take blood pressure reading at same time each day and after patient has had a brief rest. Instruct caregivers to take measurements while patient is sitting or lying down and to use same position and arm each time they take blood pressure.
- Instruct primary caregiver that if it is difficult to hear the pressure, it is possible that the cuff is too loose, not big enough, or too narrow; the stethoscope is not over arterial pulse; cuff was deflated too quickly or too slowly; or cuff was not pumped high enough for systolic readings.

**Respiration**

- Patients who demonstrate decreased ventilation will benefit from being taught deep breathing and coughing exercises (see Chapter 28).
- Instruct family member to contact home care nurse, physician, or health care provider if unusual fluctuations in respiratory rate or rhythm occur.
- Teach patient signs and symptoms of hypoxemia: headache, somnolence, confusion, dusky color, shortness of breath, dyspnea.
- Teach patient effect of high-risk behaviors such as cigarette smoking on oxygen saturation.

---

## Patient Teaching and Vital Sign Measurement

The emphasis on health promotion and health maintenance, as well as early discharge from hospital settings, has resulted in an increase in the need for patients and their families to monitor vital signs in the home. Teaching considerations affect all vital sign measurements, and you will need to incorporate this into the patient's plan of care (Box 12-16). When considering how to teach patients and their families about vital sign measurement, the patient's age is an important factor. With the increasing older adult population, there is an increased need for caregivers to be aware of changes from normal vital sign values that are unique to older adults. Box 12-17 identifies some of these variations.

## BOX 12-17 CARE OF THE OLDER ADULT

### Temperature

- The temperature of older adults is at the lower end of the normal temperature range, 36° C (96.8° F). Therefore temperatures considered within normal range sometimes reflect a fever in an older adult.
- Older adults are very sensitive to slight changes in environment temperature because their thermoregulatory systems are not as efficient (Ebersole and others, 2004).
- A decrease in sweat gland reactivity in the older adult results in a higher threshold for sweating at high temperatures, which leads to hyperthermia and heatstroke.
- With aging, loss of subcutaneous fat reduces the insulating capacity of the skin; older men are at especially high risk for hypothermia.

### Pulse Rate

- It is often difficult to palpate the pulse of an older adult. A Doppler device will provide a more accurate reading.
- The older adult has a decreased heart rate at rest (Ebersole and others, 2004).
- It takes longer for the heart rate to rise in the older adult to meet sudden increased demands that result from stress, illness, or excitement. Once elevated, the pulse rate of an older adult takes longer to return to normal resting rate (Ebersole and others, 2004).
- When assessing the apical rate of an older woman, the breast tissue is gently lifted and the stethoscope placed at the fifth intercostal space (ICS) or the lower edge of the breast.
- Heart sounds are sometimes muffled or difficult to hear in older adults because of an increase in air space in the lungs.

### Blood Pressure

- The normal range for blood pressure is the same for older adults and younger people (NHBPEP, 2003).
- Older adults often have decreased upper arm mass, which requires special attention to selection of blood pressure cuff size.
- Older adults sometimes have an increase in systolic pressure related to decreased vessel elasticity while the diastolic pressure remains the same, resulting in a wider pulse pressure.
- Older adults are instructed to change positions slowly and wait after each change to avoid postural hypotension and prevent injuries.

### Respiration

- Aging causes ossification of costal cartilage and downward slant of ribs, resulting in a more rigid rib cage, which reduces chest wall expansion. Kyphosis and scoliosis that occur in older adults also restrict chest expansion and decrease tidal volume.
- Older adults depend more on accessory abdominal muscles during respiration than on weaker thoracic muscles.
- The respiratory system matures by the time a person reaches 20 years of age and begins to decline in healthy people after the age of 25. Despite this decline, older adults are able to breathe effortlessly as long as they are healthy. However, sudden events that require an increased demand for oxygen (e.g., exercise, stress, illness) can create shortness of breath in the older adult (Ebersole and others, 2004).
- Identifying an acceptable pulse oximeter probe site is difficult with older adults because of the likelihood of peripheral vascular disease, decreased cardiac output, cold-induced vasoconstriction, and anemia.

## Recording Vital Signs

Specific graphic flow sheets exist for recording vital signs (see Chapter 8). Identify and use the agency's policy for recording vital signs. In a community-based setting, you record vital signs on the progress notes for that particular clinic or home visit. In acute care and some restorative care settings you use a graphic flow sheet.

When you use a critical path, patients have their vital signs listed as outcomes. When a vital sign is above or below the expected value, you write a note in the patient's chart regarding the finding and related interventions.

## KEY CONCEPTS

- Vital sign measurement includes the physiological measurement of temperature, pulse, blood pressure, respiration, and oxygen saturation.
- You measure vital signs as part of a complete physical examination or in a review of a patient's condition.
- You evaluate vital sign changes with other physical assessment findings using clinical judgment to determine measurement frequency.
- Knowledge of the factors influencing vital signs assists in determining and evaluating abnormal values.
- Vital signs provide a basis for evaluating response to nursing interventions.
- Measure vital signs when the patient is inactive and the environment is controlled for comfort.
- Help the patient maintain body temperature by initiating interventions that promote heat loss, production, or conservation.
- A fever is one of the body's normal defense mechanisms.
- Measurement of temperature using the temporal artery is the least invasive, most accurate method of obtaining core temperature.
- To assess cardiac function, it is easy to measure pulse rate and rhythm using the radial or apical pulses.
- Respiratory assessment includes determining the effectiveness of ventilation, perfusion, and diffusion.

- Assessment of respiration involves observing ventilatory movements throughout the respiratory cycle.
- Variables affecting ventilation, perfusion, and diffusion influence oxygen saturation.
- Several hemodynamic variables contribute to blood pressure determination.

- Hypertension is diagnosed only after an average of readings made during two or more subsequent visits reveals an elevated blood pressure.
- Selecting and applying the blood pressure measurement cuff improperly will result in errors in blood pressure measurement.
- Changes in one vital sign often influence characteristics of the other vital signs.

## CRITICAL THINKING IN PRACTICE

*Mrs. Postemski, an 80-year-old widow, is a Polish-speaking immigrant. She has just been admitted to your unit following an abdominal hysterectomy. You learn during report that she has a history of hypertension. She understands some English but does not speak the language very well. This is her first hospitalization, and she has no children. She has an IV in the right antecubital fossa and an indwelling urinary catheter. She was transported from the recovery room using 2 L of oxygen via nasal cannula.*

1. a. List the vital signs you will obtain in order of priority.
   b. Which vital signs do you delegate to the nursing assistant?
   c. How often do you ask the nursing assistant to obtain vital signs?
2. After 30 minutes the nursing assistant informs you that Mrs. Postemski's blood pressure is 92/54 mm Hg and her heart rate is 110 beats per minute.
   a. What is your priority action?
   b. Which vital sign do you evaluate first?
   c. What directions do you give the nursing assistant related to vital sign measurement?
3. After 4 hours on your unit, the nursing assistant reports Mrs. Postemski's vitals signs as BP 130/64 mm Hg, heart rate 86 beats per minute, respiratory rate 16 breaths per minute, $SpO_2$ 90%, temporal temperature 100.0° F.
   a. What is your priority action?
   b. Which vital signs do you evaluate first?
   c. What directions do you give the nursing assistant related to vital sign measurement?
4. You are caring for Mrs. Postemski on her second postoperative day. As you are assisting her with walking in the hall, she says she is feeling a little light-headed and short of breath. You notice she is diaphoretic.
   a. What is your priority action?
   b. What is the priority vital sign you need to obtain?
   c. What directions do you give the nursing assistant related to vital sign measurement?

## NCLEX® REVIEW

1. A 68-year-old woman whose husband died last year walks into the wellness clinic of the assisted living facility. She reports that she feels depressed and tired all the time. She provides you with a list of medications, one of which her health care provider altered in the last 3 weeks, atenolol, a beta-adrenergic blocker. Which vital signs can you delegate to the clinic's medical assistant?
   1. Blood pressure and heart rate
   2. Temperature and respiratory rate
   3. Oxygen saturation and blood pressure
   4. Respiratory rate and heart rate
2. A patient's blood pressure is 102/58 mm Hg in the right arm. On his last visit, the blood pressure was 142/60 mm Hg in the left arm. What is your priority nursing action?
   1. Repeat the blood pressure in the right arm.
   2. Obtain the blood pressure in the left arm.
   3. Allow the patient to relax for 15 minutes.
   4. Notify the physician or health care provider.
3. A 53-year-old male patient has just returned from the postanesthesia care unit (PACU) following a small bowel resection. He has smoked two packs per day since he was 18 years old. His admission vital signs obtained by the nursing assistant are heart rate 114 beats per

minute, BP 118/72 mm Hg, tympanic temperature 97.8° F, respiratory rate 8 breaths per minute, and $SpO_2$ 94% using 3 L of oxygen via nasal cannula. How do you describe his vital signs?
   1. Bradycardia with apnea
   2. Tachycardia with hypoxia
   3. Bradycardia and bradypnea
   4. Tachycardia and bradypnea
4. Thirty minutes after returning from the PACU your patient's pulse oximeter alarms, and you note the $SpO_2$ is 89%. While she was sleeping, the oxygen cannula was dislodged. What is your priority nursing action?
   1. Reposition the oximeter probe.
   2. Reposition the nasal cannula.
   3. Obtain the patient's respiratory rate while asleep.
   4. Shake the patient to see if he wakes.
5. Poor oxygenation of the blood ordinarily will affect the pulse rate and cause it to become:
   1. Bounding
   2. Irregular
   3. Tachycardic
   4. Bradycardic

6. Six hours after surgery you dangle your patient on the side of the bed. The nursing assistant obtains a blood pressure of 92/58 mm Hg while he is sitting. The difference between his postoperative BP of 118/58 mm Hg and the sitting blood pressure is described as:
   1. Hypotensive response to surgery
   2. Normal response to repositioning
   3. Orthostatic hypotension
   4. Side effect of fluid shift

7. One day after surgery for a bowel obstruction, you help your patient get out of bed. He complains of dizziness and nausea. Your immediate action is to:
   1. Assist him to a supine position
   2. Assess blood pressure
   3. Report findings to the nurse in charge
   4. Question the patient about palpitations

8. Following surgery, your patient's systolic blood pressure drops 25 mm Hg when you are helping him out of bed. What is the likely cause for Mr. Meyer's change in blood pressure?
   1. Pain due to movement
   2. Fluid volume deficit
   3. Increase in heart rate due to stress
   4. Movement too soon after surgery

9. You have assigned the routine vital signs to a new nursing assistant recently hired by your clinic manager. You notice that the nursing assistant's last three patients have had unusually low blood pressures and heart rates that you have had to reconfirm. What is the most likely reason for the low blood pressures that the nursing assistant is obtaining?
   1. BP cuff too wide for arm circumference
   2. Bladder was inflated and deflated too slowly
   3. Patient's arm was not supported during measurement
   4. BP cuff not wrapped evenly around arm

10. An experienced nursing assistant complains about the vital signs that a newly hired nursing assistant has obtained. The experienced nursing assistant has been asked to retake a BP that the newly hired nursing assistant has taken 3 times this week. What action do you take?
    1. Do not delegate vital signs to the newly hired nursing assistant.
    2. Delegate only temperature and respiratory rate to the newly hired nursing assistant.
    3. Report the newly hired nursing assistant to your supervisor.
    4. Observe the newly hired nursing assistant as she obtains a blood pressure and pulse on a patient.

## REFERENCES

Anwar YA, White WB: Ambulatory monitoring of the blood pressure: device, analysis and clinical utility. In White WB, editor: *Blood pressure monitoring in cardiovascular medicines and therapeutics,* Totowa, NJ, 2001, Humana Press.

Armstrong RS: Nurses' knowledge of error in blood pressure measurement technique, *Int J Nurs Pract* 8:118, 2002.

Brashers VL: *Clinical application of pathophysiology,* St. Louis, 1998, Mosby.

Dochterman JM, Bulechek GM, editors: *Nursing interventions classification (NIC),* ed 4, St. Louis, 2004, Mosby.

Ebersole P and others: *Toward healthy aging: human needs and nursing response,* ed 6, St. Louis, 2004, Mosby.

Grap MJ: Pulse oximetry, *Crit Care Nurse* 22(3):69, 2002.

Hockenberry MJ and others: *Wong's nursing care of infants and children,* ed 7, St. Louis, 2003, Mosby.

Holtzclaw BJ: *Use of thermoregulatory principles in patient care: fever management,.* Glendale, Calif, 2003, CINAHL Information Systems, http://www.cinahl.com/cgi-bin/ojcishowdoc.cgi?vol05.htm.

The sixth report of the Joint National Committee on Detection, Evaluation, and Treatment of High Blood Pressure, *Arch Intern Med* 157:2413, 1997.

Jones DW and others: Measuring blood pressure accurately, *JAMA* 289(8):1027, 2003.

Maxton, FJ, Justin L, Gilles D: Estimating core temperature in infants and children after cardiac surgery: a comparison of six methods, *J Adv Nurs* 45(2):214, 2004.

Moorhead S, Johnson M, Mass M: *Nursing outcomes classification (NOC),* ed 3, St. Louis, 2004, Mosby.

National High Blood Pressure Education Program (NHBPEP); National Heart, Lung, and Blood Institute; National Institutes of Health: The seventh report of the Joint National Committee on Detection, Evaluation, and Treatment of High Blood Pressure, *JAMA* 289(19)2560, 2003.

Netea RT and others: Both body and arm position significantly influence blood pressure measurement, *J Hum Hypertens* 17(7):459, 2003.

Potter P and others: Evaluation of chemical dot thermometers for measuring body temperature of orally intubated patients, *Am J Crit Care* 12(5):403, 2003.

Sidberry GK and others. Comparison of temple temperatures with rectal temperatures in children under two years of age, *Clin Pediatr* 41:405, 2002.

Thibodeau GA, Patton, KT: *Anatomy & physiology,* ed 5, St. Louis, 2003, Mosby.

Thomas SA, DeKeyser F: Blood pressure, *Annu Rev Nurs* 14:3, 1996.

Thomas SA and others: A review of nursing research on blood pressure, *J Nurs Scholarsh* 34(4):313, 2002.

United States Environmental Protection Agency: *What should I do if I have a mercury spill?* 2005, http://www.epa.gov/epaoswer/hazwaste/mercury/spills.htm.

Whaley LF, Wong DL: *Nursing care of infants and children,* ed 6, St. Louis, 1999, Mosby.

Yarrows SA and others: Rapid oscillometric blood pressure measurement compared to conventional oscillometric measurement, *Blood Press Monit* 6(2):145, 2001.

# CHAPTER 13

# Health Assessment and Physical Examination

## MEDIA RESOURCES

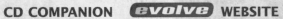

CD COMPANION  *evolve*  WEBSITE

http://evolve.elsevier.com/Potter/basic

- NCLEX® Review
- Audio Glossary
- English/Spanish Audio Glossary

## OBJECTIVES

- Discuss the purposes of physical examination.
- Describe the techniques used with each physical assessment skill.
- Discuss how cultural diversity influences health assessment.
- Describe proper patient positions for a physical examination.
- List techniques used to prepare a patient physically and psychologically before and during an examination.
- Describe interview techniques used to enhance communication during history taking.
- Make environmental preparations before an examination.

- Identify data to collect from the nursing history before an examination.
- Discuss normal physical findings in a young and middle-age adult compared with an older adult.
- Discuss ways to incorporate health promotion and health teaching into the examination.
- Use physical assessment skills during routine nursing care.
- Describe physical measurements made in assessing each body system.
- Identify self-screening examinations commonly performed by patients.

## KEY TERMS

acromegaly, p. 290
adventitious sounds, p. 302
alopecia, p. 287
aneurysm, p. 320
aphasia, p. 330
arcus senilis, p. 292
atherosclerosis, p. 308
atrophied, p. 321
auscultation, p. 275
basal cell carcinoma, p. 284
benign (fibrocystic) breast disease, p. 317
borborygmi, p. 319
bruit, p. 308
cerumen, p. 293
chancres, p. 321
clubbing, p. 311
conjunctivitis, p. 291
crackles, p. 302
cyanosis, p. 284
dysmenorrhea, p. 320
dyspnea, p. 300
dysrhythmia, p. 307
ectropion, p. 291
edema, p. 283
entropion, p. 291
erythema, p. 285
excoriation, p. 295
exostosis, p. 297

gingivae, p. 296
hematemesis, p. 318
hemorrhoids, p. 325
hernia, p. 324
hydrocephalus, p. 290
hypertonicity, p. 327
hypotonicity, p. 327
induration, p. 286
inspection, p. 274
jaundice, p. 284
kyphosis, p. 326
leukoplakia, p. 296
lordosis, p. 326
melanoma, p. 283
melena, p. 318
metastasize, p. 315
murmurs, p. 306
ophthalmoscope, p. 292
orthopnea, p. 300
osteoporosis, p. 326
otoscope, p. 293
ototoxicity, p. 294
pallor, p. 284
palpation, p. 274
palpitations, p. 305
Papanicolaou (Pap) smear, p. 322
paralytic ileus, p. 319
percussion, p. 275
peristalsis, p. 319
peritonitis, p. 319
PERRLA, p. 292

petechiae, p. 286
phlebitis, p. 312
pleural friction rub, p. 302
point of maximal impulse (PMI), p. 305
ptosis, p. 291
rhonchi, p. 302
scoliosis, p. 326

stenosis, p. 307
striae, p. 318
syncope, p. 307
thrill, p. 308
tinnitus, p. 292
turgor, p. 286
vertigo, p. 292
wheezes, p. 302

As a nurse, you will work in many settings, seeking information about patients' health status. You will possibly conduct health assessments at health fairs, clinics, in physicians' or health care providers' offices, in a patient's home, or in hospitals. Health screenings focus on a specific physical problem. For example, blood pressure screenings detect the risk for high blood pressure. If a screening determines that a patient has a risk for a disease, you refer the patient for a more complete physical examination. A complete health assessment involves a health history and behavioral and physical examination. The health history involves a lengthy patient interview to gather subjective data about the patient's condition. A physical examination is a head-to-toe review of body systems that offers objective information about the patient.

You will use physical assessment skills during an examination to make clinical judgments. The patient's condition and response affect the extent of your examination. The accuracy of your assessment will influence the choice of therapies a patient receives and the evaluation of response to those thera-

1. Do not stereotype aging patients. Most are able to adapt to change and to learn about their health. Similarly, they are reliable historians.
2. Recognize that sensory or physical limitations affect how quickly you are able to interview older adults and conduct examinations. Plan for more than one examination session. Sometimes it helps to give patients an initial health questionnaire before they come to a clinic or office (Ebersole and others, 2004).
3. Perform the examination with adequate space; this is especially important for patients with mobility aids such as a cane or walker.
4. During the examination use patience, allow for pauses, and observe for details. Recognize normalities of later life.
5. Certain types of health information are stressful for older patients to give. Illness is seen as a threat to independence and a step toward institutionalization.
6. Perform the examination near bathroom facilities if the patient has an urgent need to eliminate.
7. Be alert to signs that your patient is tiring, such as sighing, grimacing, irritability, leaning against objects for support, and drooping of head and shoulders.

## Physical Examination

Individual assessments for each body system constitute the physical examination. Patients with specific symptoms or needs require only portions of an examination. A complete health assessment follows the format of the health history (see Chapter 7). Obtain information from the history to focus attention on specific parts of the examination. For example, if the history shows that the patient experiences difficulty in breathing, conduct an examination of the thorax and lungs more carefully. The examination supplements information from the history to confirm or refute the data.

Be systematic and well organized about the examination so important assessments are not missed. A head-to-toe approach includes all body systems and helps you anticipate each step. In an adult begin by assessing the head and neck, progressing methodically down the body to include all body systems. Inspect both sides of the body, and compare for symmetry. If a patient is seriously ill, examine the body system most at risk for being abnormal. If a patient becomes fatigued, provide rest periods. Perform any painful procedures near the end of the examination. Record assessments in specific terms on a physical assessment form or in the nurses' notes. The use of common and accepted medical abbreviations helps to keep notes brief and concise.

### General Survey

Assessment begins when you first meet the patient. Determine the patient's reasons and expectations for seeking health care. Initial data from the general survey begins with a review of the patient's primary health problems. Make mental notes of the patient's behavior and appearance. Begin the examination with the general survey. The survey provides information about characteristics of an illness, a patient's hygiene and body image, emotional state, recent changes in weight, and the patient's developmental status. If you find any abnormalities or problems, closely assess the affected body system later.

**GENERAL APPEARANCE AND BEHAVIOR.** Assess appearance and behavior while you prepare the patient for the physical examination. The review of appearance and behavior includes the following:

1. *Gender and race.* A person's gender affects the type of examination performed and the manner in which you make assessments. Different physical features are related to gender and race. Certain illnesses are more likely to affect a specific gender or race; for example, skin cancer is more common in white patients and prostate cancer is higher in African-Americans. (American Cancer Society [ACS], 2005).
2. *Age.* Age influences normal physical characteristics and a person's ability to participate in some parts of the examination.
3. *Signs of distress.* There may be obvious signs or symptoms indicating pain (grimacing, splinting painful area) or difficulty in breathing (shortness of breath, sternal retraction) or anxiety. These signs help to establish priorities regarding what to examine first.
4. *Body type.* Observe if a patient appears trim and muscular, obese, or excessively thin. Body type reflects level of health, age, and lifestyle.
5. *Posture.* Normal standing posture is an upright stance with parallel alignment of hips and shoulders. Normal sitting involves some degree of rounding of the shoulders. Observe whether the patient has a slumped, erect, or bent posture. Posture often reflects mood or pain. Many older adults have a stooped, forward-bent posture, with hips and knees somewhat flexed and arms bent at the elbows, raising the level of the arms.
6. *Gait.* Observe the patient walk into the room or along the bedside (if ambulatory). Note if movements are coordinated or uncoordinated. A person normally walks with arms swinging freely at the sides, with the head and face leading the body.
7. *Body movements.* Observe whether movements are purposeful. Note any tremors involving the extremities. Determine if any body parts are immobile.
8. *Hygiene and grooming.* Note the patient's level of cleanliness by observing the appearance of the hair, skin, and fingernails. Note if the patient's clothes are clean. Grooming depends on the activities being performed just before the examination and the patient's occupation. Also note amount and type of cosmetics used.
9. *Dress.* Culture, lifestyle, socioeconomic level, and personal preference affect the type of clothes worn. Note if the type of clothing worn is appropriate for temperature

and weather conditions. Depressed or mentally ill persons may be unable to choose proper clothing. An older adult tends to wear extra clothing because of sensitivity to cold.

10. *Body odor.* An unpleasant body odor results from physical exercise, poor hygiene, or certain disease conditions.

11. *Affect and mood.* Affect is a person's feelings as they appear to others. Patients express mood or emotional state verbally and nonverbally. Note if verbal expressions match nonverbal behavior. Observe if mood is appropriate for the situation. Observe facial expressions while asking questions.

12. *Speech.* Normal speech is understandable and moderately paced. It shows an association with the person's thoughts. Note if the patient talks rapidly or slowly. An abnormal pace may be caused by emotions or neurological impairment. Observe if the patient speaks in a normal tone with clear inflection of words.

13. *Patient abuse.* Abuse of children, women, and older adults is a growing health problem. Obvious physical injury or neglect (e.g., evidence of malnutrition or presence of bruising on the extremities or trunk) are signs of possible abuse. Assess for the patient's fear of the spouse or partner, caregiver, parent, or adult child. Note if the partner or caregiver has a history of violence, alcoholism, or drug abuse. Is the person unemployed, ill, or frustrated in caring for the patient? Most states mandate a report to a social service center if you suspect abuse or neglect. When you suspect abuse, interview the patient in private. It is difficult to detect abuse because victims often will not complain or report that they are in an abusive situation (Kovach, 2004). Patients are more likely to reveal any problems to you when the suspected abuser is absent from the room (Kovach, 2004). Table 13-3 summarizes clinical indicators of abuse.

14. *Substance abuse.* Health care providers' recognition of patients who abuse alcohol, prescribed medications, or illegal drugs is typically poor. Substance abuse affects all socioeconomic groups. A single visit to a clinic does not always reveal the problem. Several visits often reveal behaviors that you can confirm with a well-focused history and physical examination. Approach the patient in a caring and nonjudgmental way because substance abuse involves both emotional and lifestyle issues. Patients to suspect for substance abuse include those listed in Box 13-3. When you suspect abuse, ask the following CAGE questions: Have you ever felt the need to CUT DOWN on your drinking or drug use? Have people ANNOYED you by criticizing your drinking or drug use? Have you ever felt bad or GUILTY about your drinking or drug use? Have you ever used or had a drink first thing in the morning as an EYE-OPENER to steady your nerves or feel normal? If two or more of the CAGE questions are positive, strongly suspect abuse and consider how to motivate the patient to seek treatment (Stuart and Laraia, 2005; Widlitz and Marin, 2002).

**VITAL SIGNS.** Generally you will measure vital signs (see Chapter 12) before the physical examination. Positioning or moving the patient can interfere with obtaining accurate values. You can also measure specific vital signs during individual body system assessments.

**HEIGHT AND WEIGHT.** Height and weight reflect a person's general level of health. Weight is a routine measure during health screenings and visits to physicians' or health care providers' offices or clinics. Weight is also an important indicator of fluid balance because trends in weight can reflect fluid loss or retention. Both height and weight are routine assessments during admission to a health care setting. Measuring an infant's or child's height and weight assesses their growth and development. In older adults, height and weight coupled with a nutritional assessment are important in determining cause and treatment for chronic disease and in assessing the older adult who has difficulty with feeding and other functional activities. Be sure to look for overall trends in height and weight changes.

A patient's weight normally will vary daily because of fluid loss or retention. Assessments screen for abnormal weight changes. First, ask the patient his or her current height and weight. Also assess weight gains or losses. A weight gain of 5 lb or 2.2 kg in a day indicates fluid-retention problems. If a change exists, assess the amount and the period over which the change occurred. Also assess changes in diet habits, appetite, prescription or over-the-counter drugs, or physical symptoms. Question whether the patient has a concern with the weight change or the body shape.

Weigh patients at the same time of day, on the same scale, and in the same clothes. This allows for an objective comparison of subsequent weights. Accuracy of weight measurement is important because health care providers will base medical and nursing decisions on changes. Patients capable of bearing their own weight use a standing scale. Calibrate a standard platform scale by moving the large and small weights to zero. Make the balance beam level and steady by adjusting the calibrating knob. The patient stands on the scale platform and remains still. Move the largest weight to the 50-lb or 22.5-kg increment under the patient's weight. Then adjust the smaller weight to balance the scale at the nearest $\frac{1}{4}$ lb or 0.1 kg (Seidel and others, 2003). Electronic scales are automatically calibrated each time they are used. Electronic scales automatically display weight within seconds.

Stretcher and chair scales are available for patients unable to bear weight. After being transferred to the scale, a hydraulic device lifts the patient above the bed and a balance beam or digital display measures the weight. Use caution when transferring patients to and from the scales.

Always weigh infants in baskets or on platform scales. Remove the infant's clothing and weigh the infant in dry, disposable diapers. Adjust the measurement later for the weight of the diaper, ensuring an accurate reading. Keep the room warm to prevent chills. A light cloth or paper placed on the scale's surface prevents cross infection from urine or feces. When placing infants in baskets or on platforms, hold

## TABLE 13-3 Clinical Indicators of Abuse

| Physical Findings | Behavioral Findings |
|---|---|
| **Child Sexual Abuse** | |
| Vaginal or penile discharge | Problem in sleeping or eating |
| Blood on underclothing | Fear of certain people or places |
| Pain or itching in genital area | Play activities recreate the abuse situation |
| Genital injuries | Regressed behavior |
| Difficulty sitting or walking | Sexual acting out |
| Pain while urinating; recurrent urinary tract infections | Knowledge of explicit sexual matters |
| Foreign bodies in rectum, urethra, or vagina | Preoccupation with other's or own genitals |
| Sexually transmitted diseases | Profound and rapid personality changes |
| Pregnancy in young adolescent | Rapidly declining school performance |
| | Poor relationship with peers |
| **Domestic Abuse** | |
| Injuries and trauma are inconsistent with reported cause | Attempted suicide |
| Multiple injuries involving head, face, neck, breasts, abdomen, and genitalia (black eyes, orbital fractures, broken nose, fractured skull, lip lacerations, broken teeth, strangulation marks) | Eating or sleeping disorders |
| | Anxiety |
| | Panic attacks |
| X-ray films show old and new fractures in different stages of healing | Pattern of substance abuse (follows physical abuse) |
| Abrasions, lacerations, bruises, welts | Low self-esteem |
| Burns | Depression |
| Human bites | Sense of helplessness |
| | Guilt |
| | Increased forgetfulness |
| | Stress-related complaints (headache, anxiety) |
| **Older Adult Abuse** | |
| Injuries and trauma are inconsistent with reported cause (e.g., cigarette burn, scratch, bruise, bite) | Dependent on caregiver |
| | Physically and/or cognitively impaired |
| Hematomas | Combative |
| Bruises at various stages of resolution | Wandering |
| Bruises, chafing, excoriation on wrist or legs (restraints) | Verbally belligerent |
| Burns | Minimal social support |
| Fractures inconsistent with cause described | Prolonged interval between injury and medical treatment |
| Dried blood | |

Data from Kovach K: Intimate partner violence, *RN* 67(8):38, 2004; Quinn, MJ: Undue influence and elder abuse: recognition and intervention strategies, *Geriatr Nurs* 23(1):11, 2002; Fulmer T: Elder abuse and neglect assessment, *J Gerontol Nurs* 29(1):8, 2003; and Hockenberry MJ and others: *Wong's essentials of pediatric nursing*, ed 7, St. Louis, 2005, Elsevier Mosby.

## BOX 13-3 Red Flags for Suspicion of Substance Abuse

Patients who frequently miss appointments

Patients who frequently request written excuses for work

Patients who have chief complaints of insomnia, "bad nerves," or pain that does not fit a particular pattern

Patients who often report lost prescriptions (e.g., tranquilizers, pain medications) or ask for frequent refills

Patients who make frequent emergency department visits

Patients who have a history of changing physicians or health care providers or who bring in medication bottles prescribed by several different providers

Patients with histories of gastrointestinal bleeds, peptic ulcers, pancreatitis, cellulitis, or frequent pulmonary infections

Patients with frequent sexually transmitted diseases, complicated pregnancies, multiple abortions, or sexual dysfunction

Patients who complain of chest pains or palpitations or who have histories of admissions to rule out myocardial infarctions

Patients who give histories of activities that place them at risk for human immunodeficiency virus (HIV) infections (multiple partners, multiple rapes)

Patients with family history of addiction; history of childhood sexual, physical, or emotional abuse; or social and financial or marital problems

Modified from Master S, Terpstra J: Recognition and diagnosis. In Schnoll SH and others: *Prescribing drugs with abuse liability*, Richmond, Va, 1992, DSAM, MCV-VCU; Friedman L and others: *Source book of substance abuse and addiction*, Baltimore, 1996, Williams & Wilkins; and Widlitz M, Marin D: Substance abuse in older adults: an overview: *Geriatrics* 57(12):29, 2002.

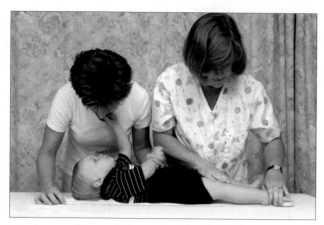

FIGURE 13-3 Measuring infant length.

a hand lightly above to prevent accidental falls. Measure weight in ounces and grams.

To measure the height of a weight-bearing patient have the patient remove his or her shoes. Place a paper towel on the scale platform so the feet remain clean. Have the patient stand erect. The platform scale has a metal rod attached to the back of the scale; this swings out and over the crown of the patient's head. Measure the patient's height in inches or centimeters.

Position a non–weight-bearing patient (such as an infant) supine on a firm surface (Figure 13-3). Portable devices are available that provide a reliable means to measure height. Place the infant on the device, having the parent hold the infant's head against the headboard. With the infant's legs straight at the knees, place the footboard against the bottom of the infant's feet. Record the infant's length to the nearest 0.5 cm or $\frac{1}{4}$ inch.

## Integument

The integument consists of the skin, nails, hair, and scalp. First inspect all skin surfaces or assess the skin gradually as you examine other body systems. Use the assessment skills of inspection, palpation, and olfaction to assess the function and integrity of the integument.

### Skin

Assessment of the skin reveals changes in oxygenation, circulation, nutrition, local tissue damage, and hydration. In a hospital setting the majority of patients are older adults, debilitated patients, or young but seriously ill patients. There are significant risks for skin lesions resulting from trauma to the skin while administering care, from exposure to pressure during immobilization, or from reaction to medications used in treatment. Patients most at risk are the neurologically impaired, chronically ill, and orthopedic patients. Others at risk are patients with diminished mental status, poor tissue oxygenation, low cardiac output, and in-

adequate nutrition. In nursing homes and extended care facilities, patients are often at risk for many of the same problems, depending on their level of mobility and presence of chronic illness. Routinely assess the skin to look for primary or initial lesions that develop. Without proper care, primary lesions quickly worsen to become secondary lesions that require more extensive nursing care.

The incidence of **melanoma,** an aggressive form of skin cancer, occurs primarily in light-pigmented people (ACS, 2005). To understand the nurse's role in detection of skin cancer, see Box 13-4. Over 1 million cases of the highly curable basal cell and squamous cell cancers occur yearly (ACS, 2005). Cutaneous malignancies are the most common neoplasms seen in patients. Incorporate a thorough skin assessment for all patients and educate them about self-examination (Box 13-4).

The condition of the patient's skin reveals the need for nursing intervention. Use your assessment findings to determine abnormalities and the type of hygiene measures required to maintain integrity of the integument (see Chapter 27). To treat excessively dry skin, tell the patient to avoid hot water, harsh soaps, and drying agents such as alcohol. Use a superfatted soap (e.g., Dove), and pat rather than rub the skin after bathing. Apply skin moisturizers regularly to reduce itching and drying, and wear cotton clothing (Hardy, 1996). Adequate nutrition and hydration become goals of therapy if you identify an alteration in the status of the integument.

You will need adequate illumination of the skin for accurate observations. The recommended choice is natural or halogen lighting. For detecting skin changes in the dark-skinned patient, sunlight is the best choice (Talbot and Curtis, 1996). Room temperature also affects skin assessment. A room that is too warm causes superficial vasodilation, resulting in an increased redness of the skin. A cool environment causes the sensitive patient to develop cyanosis (bluish color) around the lips and nail beds (Talbot and Curtis, 1996).

Use disposable gloves for palpation if open, moist, or draining skin lesions are present. Because you will inspect all skin surfaces, the patient will assume several positions. The examination includes inspecting the skin's color, moisture, temperature, texture, and turgor. Also note vascular changes, **edema,** and lesions. Carefully palpate abnormalities, and document your findings. Skin odors are usually noted in skinfolds, such as the axillae or under the female patient's breasts.

**HEALTH HISTORY.** Before assessing the skin, ask the patient about the presence of lesions, rashes, or bruises and determine whether the alterations are linked to heat, cold, and stress, exposure to toxic material or the sun, or new skin care products. Also determine if there has been a recent change in skin color or trauma to the skin. If a patient has been out in the sun, it is useful to know if the patient wore sunscreen. If not, the patient will require education on ways to safeguard the skin. Also assess for history of allergies, use of topical medications, and a family history of serious skin disorders.

| BOX 13-4 | USING EVIDENCE IN PRACTICE |
|---|---|

**Research Summary**

What is cancer? More specifically, what is skin cancer? Cancer by definition is an "uncontrolled growth and spread of abnormal cells" (ACS, 2005). Therefore skin cancer is characterized by abnormal skin cells, which can spread and invade other tissues. More importantly, what can we do about skin cancer? As nurses, it becomes our responsibility to assess for and educate our patients about all types of skin cancers, especially for the most serious form called melanoma. Melanoma was estimated to cause approximately 7,700 deaths in 2005; other skin cancer-related deaths were to reach around 2,800 (ACS, 2005). There are several risk factors for melanoma: major factors are positive family history of melanoma, a prior melanoma, and multiple or unusual moles. Other factors include fair complexion/skin that is sensitive to the sun; excessive exposure to the sun (especially before age 18), and the use of tanning beds/booths.

Research has indicated that skin cancer, when detected early and treated properly, is highly curable. Overall survival rates for melanoma at the 5-year mark is 91%, with 98% for localized melanoma; when it is grouped in regional and distant stages, the survival rates dramatically decrease (ACS, 2005). Therefore early intervention is of utmost importance.

**Application to Nursing Practice**

The results from the research studies have made it a nursing responsibility to screen and intervene for our patients' best interest. It is a necessity that we promote self-screening for all patients and their family members. We must also educate the general public.

Instruct your patients to conduct a complete monthly self-examination of the skin and scalp, noting moles, blemishes, and birthmarks. They can perform the examination after a bath or shower, including a head-to-toe check. Use a well-lit room and mirrors to examine all skin surfaces. If necessary, have the patient ask a family member/significant other to aid in the investigation. The ACS (2005) outlines the warning signs of skin cancer using the ABCD mnemonic: A is for **A**symmetry—look for uneven shape; B is for **B**order irregularity—look for edges that are blurred, notched, or ragged; C is for **C**olor—pigmentation is not uniform; blue, black, brown variegated and areas of pink, white, gray, blue, or red are abnormal (Hayes, 2003); and D is for **D**iameter, greater than the size of a typical pencil eraser. Also, teach your patients to contact their physician or health care provider if a skin lesion or mole starts to bleed or ooze or feels different (swollen, hard, lumpy, itchy, or tender to the touch). Especially instruct older adults, who tend to have delayed wound healing. Inform your patients of ways to prevent skin cancer by avoiding overexposure to the sun:

- Wear wide-brimmed hats and long sleeves.
- Apply broad-spectrum sunscreens with SPF of 15 or greater to protect against ultraviolet B (UVB) and ultraviolet A (UVA) rays approximately 15 minutes before going into the sun and after swimming or perspiring.
- Avoid tanning under the direct sun at midday (10 AM to 4 PM).
- Do not use indoor sunlamps, tanning parlors, or tanning pills.

Also, inform patients who are on medications that make the skin more sensitive to the sun (e.g., oral contraceptives, antiinflammatories, antihypertensives) to take extra precautions when spending time in the sun. Inform patients to protect their children from the sun. Severe sunburns in childhood greatly increase melanoma risk later in life (ACS, 2005). These interventions will provide the patient with self-screening measures to detect, prevent, and seek early treatment for skin cancer.

Data from American Cancer Society: *Cancer facts and figures 2005*, New York, 2005, The Society; and Hayes JL: Are you assessing for melanoma? *RN* 66(2):36, 2003.

**COLOR.** Skin color varies from body part to body part and from person to person. Despite individual variations, skin color is usually uniform over the body. Table 13-4 lists common variations. Normal skin pigmentation ranges from ivory or light pink to ruddy pink in white skin and from light to deep brown or black in dark skin. Sun-darkened or darker skin is common around knees and elbows.

**Basal cell carcinoma** is most common in sun-exposed areas and frequently occurs in a background of sun-damaged skin. In older adults pigmentation increases unevenly, causing discolored skin. While inspecting the skin, be aware that cosmetics or tanning agents sometimes mask color.

The assessment of color first involves areas of the skin not exposed to the sun, such as the palms of the hands. Note if the skin is unusually pale or dark. It is more difficult to note changes such as pallor or cyanosis in patients with dark skin. Usually color hues are best seen in the palms, soles of the feet, lips, tongue, and nail beds. Areas of increased color (hyperpigmentation) and decreased color (hypopigmentation) are common. Skin creases and folds are darker than the rest of the body in the dark-skinned patient.

Inspect sites where you can more easily identify abnormalities. For example, you can see **pallor** more easily in the face, buccal mucosa (mouth), conjunctivae, and nail beds. You observe **cyanosis** best in the lips, nail beds, palpebral conjunctivae, and palms.

In recognizing pallor in the dark-skinned patient, you observe that normal brown skin appears to be yellow-brown and normal black skin appears to be ashen gray. Also assess the lips, nail beds, and mucous membranes for generalized pallor. If pallor is present, the mucous membranes will be ashen gray. Assessment of cyanosis in the dark-skinned patient requires that you observe areas where pigmentation occurs the least (conjunctivae, sclera, buccal mucosa, tongue, lips, nail beds, and palms and soles). In addition, verify these findings with clinical manifestations (Talbot and Curtis, 1996).

The best site to inspect for **jaundice** (yellow-orange discoloration) is the patient's sclera. You see normal reactive hy-

| TABLE 13-4 | Skin Color Variations | | |
| --- | --- | --- | --- |
| **Color** | **Condition** | **Causes** | **Assessment Locations** |
| Bluish (cyanosis) | Increased amount of deoxygenated hemoglobin (associated with hypoxia) | Heart or lung disease, cold environment | Nail beds, lips, base of tongue, skin (severe cases) |
| Pallor (decrease in color) | Reduced amount of oxyhemoglobin | Anemia | Face, conjunctivae, nail beds, palms of hands |
| | Reduced visibility of oxyhemoglobin resulting from decreased blood flow | Shock | Skin, nail beds, conjunctivae, lips |
| Loss of pigmentation | Vitiligo | Congenital or autoimmune condition causing lack of pigment | Patchy areas on skin over face, hands, arms |
| Yellow-orange (jaundice) | Increased deposit of bilirubin in tissues | Liver disease, destruction of red blood cells | Sclera, mucous membranes, skin |
| Red (erythema) | Increased visibility of oxyhemoglobin caused by dilation or increased blood flow | Fever, direct trauma, blushing, alcohol intake | Face, area of trauma, sacrum, shoulders, other common sites for pressure ulcers |
| Tan-brown | Increased amount of melanin | Suntan, pregnancy | Areas exposed to sun: face, arms, areolae, nipples |

| TABLE 13-5 | Physical Findings of the Skin Indicative of Substance Abuse |
| --- | --- |
| **Physical Finding** | **Commonly Associated Drug** |
| Diaphoresis | Sedative hypnotic (including alcohol) |
| Spider angiomas | Alcohol, stimulants |
| Burns (especially fingers) | Alcohol |
| Needle marks | Opioids |
| Contusions, abrasions, cuts, scars | Alcohol, other sedative hypnotics |
| "Homemade" tattoos | Cocaine, IV opioids (prevents detection of injection sites) |
| Increased vascularity of face | Alcohol |
| Red, dry skin | Phencyclidine (PCP) |

Modified from Caulker-Burnett I: Primary care screening for substance abuse, *Nurse Pract* 19(6):42, 1994; and Friedman L and others: *Source book of substance abuse and addiction*, Baltimore, 1996, Williams & Wilkins.

peremia, or redness, most often in regions exposed to pressure such as the sacrum, heels, and greater trochanter (see Chapter 35).

Inspect for any patches or areas of skin color variation. Localized skin changes, such as pallor or **erythema** (red discoloration), often indicate circulatory changes. For example, localized vasodilation resulting from sunburn or fever is a cause for an area of erythema. In the dark-skinned patient, erythema is not easy to observe, so palpate the area for heat and warmth to note the presence of skin inflammation (Talbot and Curtis, 1996). An area of an extremity that appears unusually pale may result from an arterial occlusion or edema. It is important to ask if the patient has noticed any changes in skin coloring.

A pattern of findings that is becoming more common is that associated with patients who are chemically dependent and are intravenous (IV) drug abusers. It is sometimes difficult to recognize signs and symptoms after one examination. A patient who takes repeated IV injections has edematous, reddened, and warm areas along the arms and legs. This pattern suggests recent injections. Evidence of old injection sites appears as hyperpigmented and shiny or scarred areas. Table 13-5 summarizes additional physical findings associated with substance abuse.

**MOISTURE.** The hydration of skin and mucous membranes helps to reveal body fluid imbalances, changes in the skin's environment, and regulation of body temperature. Moisture refers to wetness and oiliness. The skin is normally smooth and dry. Skinfolds such as the axillae are normally moist. Minimal perspiration or oiliness is present in normal skin (Seidel and others, 2003). Increased perspiration is associated with activity, warm environments, obesity, anxiety, or excitement. Use ungloved fingertips to palpate skin surfaces and observe for dullness, dryness, crusting, and flaking. Flaking is the appearance of dandrufflike flakes when you lightly rub the skin surface. Scaling involves fishlike scales that are easily rubbed off the skin's surface. Both flaking and scaling are believed to indicate abnormally dry skin (Hardy, 1996). Excessively dry skin is common in older adults and persons who use excessive amounts of soap during bathing. Other factors causing dry skin include lack of humidity, exposure to sun, smoking, stress, excessive perspiration, and dehydration (Hardy, 1996). Excessive dryness worsens existing skin conditions.

**TEMPERATURE.** The temperature of the skin depends on the amount of blood circulating through the dermis. Increased or decreased skin temperature reflects an increase or decrease in blood flow. Localized erythema or redness of the skin is often accompanied by an increase in skin temper-

**Hair and Scalp Assessment**
- Instruct about basic hygiene measures including shampooing and combing of the hair (see Chapter 27).
- Instruct patients who have head lice to shampoo thoroughly with pediculicide (shampoo available at drug stores) in cold water, comb thoroughly with fine-tooth comb (following product directions), and discard comb. Caution against use of products containing lindane, a toxic ingredient known to cause adverse reactions. Repeat shampoo treatment 12 to 24 hours later.
- After combing, remove any remaining nits or nit cases with tweezers or between the fingernails. A dilute solution of vinegar and water helps loosen nits.
- Instruct patients and parents about ways to reduce transmission of lice:
  - Do not share personal care items with others.
  - Vacuum all rugs, car seats, pillows, furniture, and flooring thoroughly and discard vacuum bag.
  - Seal nonwashable items in plastic bags for 14 days if parents are unable to afford dry cleaning and do not have a vacuum.
  - Use thorough hand hygiene practices.
  - Launder all clothing, linen, and bedding in hot soap and water, and dry in a hot dryer for at least 20 minutes. Dry-clean nonwashable items.
  - Do not use insecticide.
- Instruct the patient to notify his or her partner if lice were sexually transmitted.
- Avoid physical contact with infested individuals and their belongings, especially clothing and bedding.
- Soak combs, brushes, and hair accessories in lice-killing products for 1 hour or in boiling water for 10 minutes.

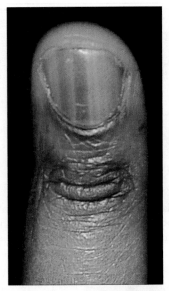

FIGURE **13-5** Pigmented bands in nail of patient with dark skin. (From Seidel HM and others: *Mosby's guide to physical examination,* ed 5, St. Louis, 2003, Mosby.)

even coloration. By carefully separating strands of hair, thoroughly examine the scalp for lesions. Note the characteristics of any scalp lesions. If lumps or bruises are found, ask if the patient has experienced recent head trauma. Moles on the scalp are common. You should warn the patient that combing or brushing sometimes causes a mole to bleed. Scaliness or dryness of the scalp is frequently caused by dandruff or psoriasis.

Careful inspection of hair follicles on the scalp and pubic areas may reveal lice or other parasites. Lice attach their eggs to hair. The head and body lice are tiny and have grayish white bodies. Crab lice have red legs. Lice eggs look like oval particles of dandruff. The lice themselves are difficult to see. Observe for bites or pustular eruptions in the follicles and in areas where skin surfaces meet, such as behind the ears and in the groin. The discovery of lice requires immediate treatment (Box 13-6).

## Nails

The condition of the nails reflects general health, state of nutrition, a person's occupation, and level of self-care. The most visible portion of the nails is the nail plate, the trans-

parent layer of epithelial cells covering the nail bed. The vascularity of the nail bed creates the nail's underlying color. The semilunar, whitish area at the base of the nail bed from which the nail plate develops is the lunula.

**HEALTH HISTORY.** Before assessing the nails ask if the patient has had any recent trauma. A blow to the nail changes the shape and growth of the nail, as well as loss of all or part of the nail plate. Have the patient also describe nail care practices. Improper care damages nails and cuticles. It is also important to find out if patients have acrylic nails or silk wraps, because these are areas for fungal growth. Question whether the patient has noticed changes in nail appearance or growth. Alterations occur slowly over time. Knowing if the patient has risks for nail or foot problems (e.g., diabetes, peripheral vascular disease, or older adulthood) will influence the level of hygienic care recommended.

**INSPECTION AND PALPATION.** Inspect the nail bed color, the thickness and shape of the nail, the texture of the nail, and the condition of tissue around the nail. The nails are normally transparent, smooth, and convex, with surrounding cuticles smooth, intact, and without inflammation. In whites, nail beds are pink with translucent white tips. In dark-skinned patients, nail beds are darkly pigmented with a blue or reddish hue. A brown or black pigmentation is normal with longitudinal streaks (Figure 13-5). Trauma, cirrhosis, diabetes mellitus, and hypertension cause splinter hemorrhages. Vitamin, protein, and electrolyte changes cause various lines or bands to form on nail beds.

Nails normally grow at a constant rate, but direct injury or generalized disease slows growth. With aging, the nails of

## BOX 13-7 Abnormalities of the Nail Bed

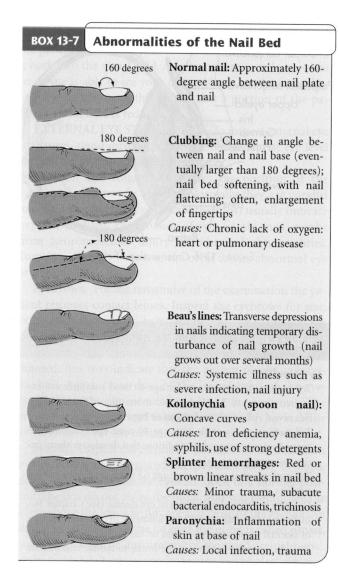

**160 degrees**

**Normal nail:** Approximately 160-degree angle between nail plate and nail

**180 degrees**

**Clubbing:** Change in angle between nail and nail base (eventually larger than 180 degrees); nail bed softening, with nail flattening; often, enlargement of fingertips
*Causes:* Chronic lack of oxygen: heart or pulmonary disease

**180 degrees**

**Beau's lines:** Transverse depressions in nails indicating temporary disturbance of nail growth (nail grows out over several months)
*Causes:* Systemic illness such as severe infection, nail injury

**Koilonychia (spoon nail):** Concave curves
*Causes:* Iron deficiency anemia, syphilis, use of strong detergents

**Splinter hemorrhages:** Red or brown linear streaks in nail bed
*Causes:* Minor trauma, subacute bacterial endocarditis, trichinosis

**Paronychia:** Inflammation of skin at base of nail
*Causes:* Local infection, trauma

## BOX 13-8 PATIENT TEACHING

### Nail Care

- Instruct the patient to cut nails only after soaking them about 10 minutes in warm water. (Exception: Diabetic patients are warned against soaking nails.)
- Instruct the patient to avoid using over-the-counter preparations to treat corns, calluses, or ingrown toenails.
- Tell the patient to cut nails straight across and even with the tops of the fingers or toes. If the patient has diabetes, tell the patient to file rather than cut the nails.
- Instruct the patient to shape nails with a file or emery board.
- If patient is diabetic:
  ○ Wash feet daily in warm water. Inspect feet each day in good light, looking for dry places and cracks in the skin. Soften dry feet by applying a cream or lotion such as Nivea, Eucerin, or Alpha Keri.
  ○ Do not put lotion between the toes.
  ○ Caution patient against using sharp objects to poke or dig under toenail or around the cuticle.
  ○ Have patient see a podiatrist for treatment of ingrown toenails and nails that are thick or tend to split.

Calluses and corns often occur on the toes or fingers. A callus is flat and painless, resulting from thickening of the epidermis. Friction and pressure from shoes causes corns, usually over bony prominences. During the examination instruct the patient in proper nail care (Box 13-8.)

## Head and Neck

An examination of the head and neck includes the head, eyes, ears, nose, mouth, pharynx, and neck (lymph nodes, carotid arteries, thyroid gland, and trachea). During the assessment of peripheral arteries, also assess the carotid arteries. You need to understand each anatomical area and its normal function. Assessment of the head and neck uses inspection, palpation, and auscultation.

### Head

**HEALTH HISTORY.** The history allows you to screen for possible intracranial injury if necessary. Ask whether the patient experienced recent trauma to the head or if neurological symptoms such as headache (note onset, duration, character, pattern, and associated symptoms), dizziness, seizures, poor vision, or loss of consciousness have occurred. The history also includes a review of the patient's occupation, focusing on those patients who wear safety helmets. In addition, ask if the patient participates in contact sports, cycling, roller blading, or skateboarding.

**INSPECTION AND PALPATION.** Inspect the patient's head, noting the position, size, shape, and contour. The head is normally held upright and midline to the trunk. A hori-

the fingers and toes become harder and thicker. Longitudinal striations develop, and the rate of nail growth slows. Nails become more brittle, dull, and opaque and turn yellow in older adults because of insufficient calcium. Also with age the cuticle becomes less thick and wide.

Inspection of the angle between the nail and nail bed normally reveals an angle of 160 degrees (Box 13-7). A larger angle and softening of the nail bed indicate chronic oxygenation problems. Palpate the nail base to determine firmness and condition of circulation. The nail base is normally firm. To palpate, gently grasp the patient's finger and observe the color of the nail bed. Next, apply gentle, firm, quick pressure with the thumb to the nail bed and release. As you apply pressure, the nail bed appears white or blanched; however, the pink color should return immediately on release of pressure. Failure of the pinkness to return promptly indicates circulatory insufficiency. An ongoing bluish or purplish cast to the nail bed occurs with cyanosis. A white cast or pallor results from anemia.

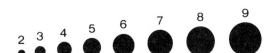

FIGURE **13-8** Chart depicting pupillary size in millimeters.

ularity in the surface indicates an abrasion or tear that requires further examination by a physician or health care provider. Both conditions are quite painful. Note the color and details of the underlying iris. In an older adult the iris becomes faded. A thin, white ring along the margin of the iris, called an **arcus senilis,** is common with aging but is abnormal in anyone under age 40. To test for the corneal blink reflex, see Table 13-12, p. 333, in the cranial nerve function section of this chapter.

**Pupils and Irises.** Observe the pupils for size, shape, equality, accommodation, and reaction to light. The pupils are normally black, round, regular, and equal in size (3 to 7 mm in diameter) (Figure 13-8). Cloudy pupils indicate cataracts. Dilated or constricted pupils result from neurological disorders or the effect of ophthalmic or certain systemic drugs. Pinpoint pupils are a common sign of opioid intoxication. When you shine a beam of light through the pupil and onto the retina, you stimulate the third cranial nerve and cause the muscles of the iris to constrict. Any abnormality along the nerve pathways from the retina to the iris alters the ability of the pupils to react to light. Changes in intracranial pressure, lesions along the nerve pathways, locally applied eye drugs, and direct trauma to the eye alter pupillary reaction.

Test pupillary reflexes (to light and accommodation) in a dimly lit room. While the patient looks straight ahead, bring a penlight from the side of the patient's face, directing the light onto the pupil (Figure 13-9). If the patient looks at the light, there will be a false reaction to accommodation. A directly illuminated pupil constricts, and the opposite pupil constricts consensually. Observe the quickness and equality of the reflex. Repeat the examination for the opposite eye.

To test accommodation, ask the patient to gaze at a distant object (the far wall) and then at a test object (finger or pencil) held by you approximately 10 cm (4 inches) from the bridge of the patient's nose. The pupils normally converge and accommodate by constricting when looking at close objects. The pupil responses are equal. If assessment of pupillary reaction is normal in all tests, record the abbreviation **PERRLA** (pupils equal, round, reactive to light and accommodation).

**INTERNAL EYE STRUCTURES.** The examination of internal eye structures through the use of an **ophthalmoscope** is beyond the scope of a new graduate nurse's practice. Patients in greatest need of the examination are those with diabetes, hypertension, and intracranial disorders.

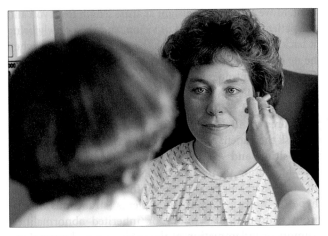
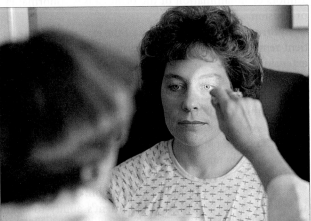

FIGURE **13-9 A,** To check pupil reflexes, first hold penlight to side of patient's face. **B,** Illumination of pupil causes pupillary constriction.

# Ears

The ear assessment determines the integrity of ear structures and hearing acuity. You will inspect and palpate external ear structures, inspect middle ear structures with the otoscope, and test the inner ear by measuring the patient's hearing acuity. Assessment of patients with hearing impairment provides useful data for you in planning effective communication techniques.

**HEALTH HISTORY.** The patient's health history includes a review of risks for hearing problems (e.g., hypoxia at birth, meningitis, intake of aspirin, ototoxic drugs, and exposure to noise), a history of ear surgery or trauma, and the patient's current exposure to high noise levels. Determine if the patient has ear pain, itching, discharge, **tinnitus** (ringing in ears), **vertigo** (loss of equilibrium), or change in hearing. Note behaviors indicative of hearing loss, such as failure to respond when spoken to, requests to repeat comments, leaning forward to hear, and a child's inattentiveness. If the patient has had a recent hearing problem, determine the onset, contributing factors, and effect on ADLs. Also assess if the patient wears a hearing aid and how the patient normally cleans the ears.

**AURICLES.** With the patient sitting, inspect the position, color, size, shape, and symmetry of the auricle. Be sure to examine lateral and medial surfaces and surrounding tissue. The auricles are normally of equal size and level with each other. The upper point of attachment to the head is normally in a straight line with the outer canthus, or corner of the eye. Ears that are low set or at an unusual angle are a sign of chromosome abnormality (e.g., Down syndrome). The color is the same as the face without moles, cysts, deformities, or nodules. Redness is a sign of inflammation or fever. Extreme pallor indicates frostbite. Palpate the auricles for texture, tenderness, swelling, and skin lesions. Auricles are normally smooth, firm, mobile, and without lesions. If the patient complains of pain, gently pull the auricle and press on the tragus and palpate behind the ear over the mastoid process. If palpating the external ear increases the pain, an external ear infection is likely. If palpation of the auricle and tragus does not influence the pain, the patient may have a middle ear infection. Tenderness in the mastoid area indicates mastoiditis.

Inspect the opening of the ear canal for size and presence of discharge. If discharge is present, wear gloves during the examination. A swollen or occluded meatus is not normal. A yellow, waxy substance called **cerumen** is common. Yellow or green foul-smelling discharge indicates infection or a foreign body.

**EAR CANALS AND EARDRUMS.** Observe the deeper structures of the external and middle ear with the use of an **otoscope.** A special ear speculum attaches to the battery tube of the ophthalmoscope. For best visualization select the largest speculum that fits comfortably in the patient's ear. Before inserting the speculum, check for foreign bodies in the opening of the auditory canal.

Make sure the patient avoids moving the head during the examination to avoid damage to the canal and tympanic membrane. Infants and young children often need to be restrained. Lie infants supine with their heads turned to one side and their arms held securely at their sides. Have young children sit on their parents' laps with their legs held between the parents' knees.

Turn on the otoscope by rotating the dial at the top of the battery tube. To insert the speculum properly, ask the patient to tip the head slightly to the opposite shoulder. Hold the handle of the otoscope in the space between the thumb and index finger, supported on your middle finger. This leaves the ulnar side of your hand to rest against the patient's head, stabilizing the otoscope as it is inserted into the canal (Seidel and others, 2003). There are two types of grips for the otoscope. In one, you hold the battery tube along the patient's neck with your fingers against the neck. In the other grip, lightly brace the inverted otoscope against the side of the patient's head or cheek. Insert the scope while pulling the auricle upward and backward in the adult and older child (Figure 13-10). This maneuver straightens the ear canal. In infants pull the auricle back and down. Insert the speculum slightly down and forward, 1.0 or 1.5 cm (½ inch) into the ear canal.

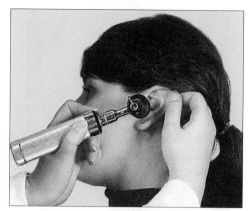

FIGURE **13-10** Otoscopic examination. (From Seidel HM and others: *Mosby's guide to physical examination,* ed 5, St. Louis, 2003, Mosby.)

---

| **BOX 13-10** | **PATIENT TEACHING** |
| --- | --- |

**Ear and Hearing Health**
- Instruct the patient in the proper way to clean the outer ear (see Chapter 27), avoiding use of cotton-tipped applicators and sharp objects such as hairpins, which may cause impaction of cerumen deep in ear canal.
- Tell the patient to avoid inserting pointed objects into the ear canal.
- Encourage patients over age 65 to have regular hearing checks. Explain that a reduction in hearing is a normal part of aging (see Chapter 36).
- Instruct family members of patients with hearing losses to avoid shouting and instead speak in low tones and to be sure the patient sees the speaker's face.

---

Take care not to scrape the sensitive lining of the ear canal, which is painful. The ear canal normally has little cerumen and is uniformly pink with tiny hairs in the outer third of the canal. Observe for color, discharge, scaling, lesions, foreign bodies, and cerumen. Normally cerumen is dry (light brown to gray and flaky) or moist (dark yellow or brown) and sticky. Dry cerumen occurs in Asians and Native Americans about 85% of the time (Seidel and others, 2003). A reddened canal with discharge is a sign of inflammation or infection. In older adults, accumulated cerumen is a common problem. Buildup of cerumen creates a mild hearing loss. During the examination ask the patient how he or she normally cleans the ear canal (Box 13-10). Caution the patient on the danger of inserting pointed objects into the canal. Avoid the use of cotton-tipped applicators to clean the ears because this causes impaction of cerumen deep in the ear canal.

The light from the otoscope allows visualization of the eardrum (tympanic membrane). Know the common anatomical landmarks and their appearance (Figure 13-11). Move the

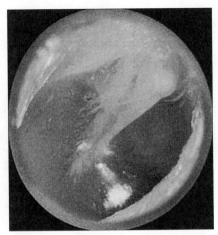

Figure **13-11** Normal tympanic membrane. (Courtesy Dr. Richard A. Buckingham, Abraham Lincoln School of Medicine, University of Illinois, Chicago.)

auricle to see the entire drum and its periphery. Because the eardrum is angled away from the ear canal, the light from the otoscope appears as a cone shape rather than a circle. The umbo is near the center of the drum, behind which is the attachment of the malleus. The underlying short process of the malleus creates a knoblike structure at the top of the drum. Check carefully to be sure there are no tears or breaks in the membrane of the eardrum. The normal eardrum is translucent, shiny, and pearly gray. It is free from tears or breaks. A pink or red bulging membrane indicates inflammation. A white color reveals pus behind it. The membrane is taut, except for the small triangular pars flaccida near the top. If cerumen is blocking the tympanic membrane, warm water irrigation will safely remove the wax.

**HEARING ACUITY.** You can often tell if the patient has a hearing loss from a response to conversation. The three types of hearing loss are conduction, sensorineural, and mixed. A conduction loss involves an interruption of sound waves as they travel from the outer ear to the cochlea of the inner ear because they are not transmitted through the outer and middle ear structures. A sensorineural loss involves the inner ear, the auditory nerve, or the hearing center of the brain. Sound is conducted through the outer and middle ear structures, but the continued transmission of sound becomes interrupted at some point beyond the bony ossicles. A mixed loss involves a combination of conduction and sensorineural loss.

Patients working or living around loud noises are at risk for hearing loss. Older adults experience an inability to hear high-frequency sounds and consonants (e.g., *s*, *z*, *t*, and *g*). Deterioration of the cochlea and thickening of the tympanic membrane causes older adults to gradually lose hearing acuity. They are especially at risk for hearing loss caused by **ototoxicity** (injury to the auditory nerve) resulting from high maintenance doses of antibiotics (e.g., aminoglycosides).

To conduct a hearing assessment, have the patient remove the hearing aid if worn. Note the patient's response to questions. Normally the patient responds without excess requests to have you repeat questions. If you suspect a hearing loss, check the patient's response to the whispered voice. Test one ear at a time while the patient occludes the other ear with a finger. Ask the patient to gently move the finger up and down during the test. While standing 30 cm (1 foot) from the ear you are testing, cover your mouth so the patient is unable to read lips. After exhaling fully, whisper softly toward the unoccluded ear, reciting random numbers with equally accented syllables such as "nine-four-ten." If necessary, gradually increase voice intensity until the patient correctly repeats the numbers. Then test the other ear for comparison. Seidel and others (2003) report that patients normally hear numbers clearly when whispered. You may use a ticking watch to test hearing acuity, but using the spoken word allows for more accuracy and control in testing.

If a hearing loss is present, there are tests that experienced practitioners perform using a tuning fork or audiometry.

### Nose and Sinuses

Assess the integrity of the nose and sinuses by inspection and palpation. The patient sits during the examination. A penlight allows for gross examination of each naris. A more detailed examination requires using a nasal speculum to inspect deeper nasal turbinates. Do not use a speculum unless a qualified practitioner is present.

**HEALTH HISTORY.** It is useful to know whether the patient's health history indicates exposure to dust or pollutants, allergies, nasal obstruction, recent trauma, discharge, frequent infections, headaches, or postnasal drip. An assessment for a history of nosebleed (epistaxis) includes review of frequency, amount of bleeding, treatment, and difficulty stopping bleeding. Also determine whether the patient has a history of using nasal spray or drops, including the amount, frequency, and duration of use (Box 13-11). Ask patients if they have been told that they snore or if they have difficulty breathing.

**NOSE.** When inspecting the external nose, observe the shape, size, skin color, and presence of deformity or inflammation. The nose is normally smooth and symmetrical, with the same color as the face. Recent trauma causes edema and discoloration. If swelling or deformities exist, gently palpate the ridge and soft tissue of the nose by placing one finger on each side of the nasal arch and gently moving fingers from the nasal bridge to the tip. Note any tenderness, masses, and underlying deviations. Nasal structures are usually firm and stable.

Air normally passes freely through the nose when a person breathes. To assess patency of the nares, place a finger on the side of the patient's nose and occlude one naris. Ask the patient to breathe with the mouth closed. Repeat the procedure for the other naris.

As you illuminate the anterior nares, inspect the mucosa for color, lesions, discharge, swelling, and evidence of bleeding. If discharge is present, apply gloves. Normal mucosa is pink and moist without lesions. Pale mucosa with clear discharge indicates allergy. A mucoid discharge indicates rhinitis. A sinus infection results in yellowish or greenish discharge. Habitual use of intranasal cocaine and opioids causes puffiness and increased vascularity of the nasal mucosa. For the patient with a nasogastric tube, check for local **excoriation** of the naris, characterized by redness and skin sloughing.

To view the septum and turbinates, have the patient tip the head back slightly to give you a clearer view. Illuminate the septum and look for alignment, perforation, or bleeding. Normally the septum is close to the midline and thicker anteriorly than posteriorly. Normal mucosa is pink and moist, without lesions. A deviated septum obstructs breathing and interferes with passage of a nasogastric tube. Perforation of the septum often occurs after repeated use of intranasal cocaine. Note any polyps (tumorlike growths) or purulent drainage. Advanced, experienced clinicians use a nasal speculum for this procedure.

**SINUSES.** The examination of the sinuses is limited to palpation. In cases of allergies or infection, the interior of the sinuses becomes inflamed and swollen. The most effective way to assess for tenderness is by externally palpating the frontal and maxillary facial areas (Figure 13-12). Palpate the frontal sinus by exerting pressure with the thumb up and under the patient's eyebrow. Gentle upward pressure elicits tenderness easily if sinus irritation is present. Do not apply pressure to the eyes. If tenderness of sinuses is present, the sinuses may be transilluminated. This procedure, however, requires advanced experience.

## Mouth and Pharynx

Assess the mouth and pharynx to detect signs of overall health, determine oral hygiene needs, and develop therapies for patients with dehydration, restricted intake, oral trauma, or oral airway obstruction. To assess the oral cavity use a

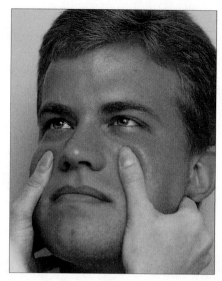

FIGURE **13-12** Palpation of maxillary sinuses.

penlight and tongue depressor or single gauze square. Wear gloves when contacting mucous membranes. Have the patient sit or lie during the examination. You are also able to assess the oral cavity while administering oral hygiene.

**HISTORY.** Determine if the patient wears dentures or retainers and if they fit comfortably. An assessment of a recent change in appetite or weight often points to a problem with chewing or swallowing. Assess the patient's dental hygiene practices and when the patient last visited a dentist. To rule out risks for mouth and throat cancer, ask if the patient smokes, chews tobacco, or smokes a pipe and consumes alcohol. Also assess for a history of pain or lesions of the mouth and pain with chewing. It helps to know if a tonsillectomy or adenoidectomy has been performed.

**LIPS.** Inspect the lips for color, texture, hydration, contour, and lesions. With the patient's mouth closed, view the lips from end to end. Normally they are pink, moist, symmetrical, smooth, and without lesions. Lip color in the dark-skinned patient varies from pink to plum. Have female patients remove their lipstick before the examination. Anemia causes pallor of the lips, with cyanosis caused by respiratory or cardiovascular problems. Any lesions such as nodules or ulcerations can be related to infection, irritation, or skin cancer.

**MUCOSA.** To view the inner oral mucosa, have the patient open the mouth slightly and gently pull the lower lip away from the teeth (Figure 13-13, A). Repeat this process for the upper lip. Inspect the mucosa for color, hydration, texture, and lesions such as ulcers, abrasions, or cysts. Normally the mucosa is a glistening pink. Varying shades of hyperpigmentation are normal in 10% of whites after age 50 and up to 90% of blacks by the same age. Palpate any lesions with a gloved hand for tenderness, size, and consistency.

To inspect the buccal mucosa, ask the patient to open the mouth and then gently retract the cheeks with a

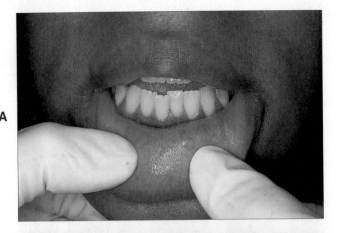

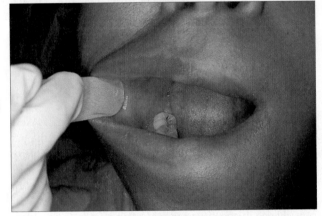

FIGURE **13-13 A,** Inspection of inner oral mucosa of lower lip. **B,** Retraction allows for clear view of buccal mucosa.

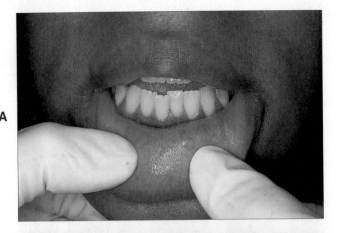

<table>
<tr><td>BOX 13-12</td><td>PATIENT TEACHING</td></tr>
</table>

**Mouth and Pharynx Health**

• Discuss proper techniques for oral hygiene, including brushing and flossing.
• Explain the early warning signs of oral cancer, including a sore that bleeds easily and does not heel, a lump or thickening, and red or white patch on the mucosa that persists (ACS, 2005). Difficulty chewing or swallowing is a late symptom.
• Encourage regular dental examinations every 6 months for children, adults, and older adults.
• Identify older patients who have difficulty in chewing and changes in the teeth. Teach patients to eat soft foods and to cut food into small pieces.

tongue depressor or gloved finger covered with gauze (Figure 13-13, *B*). A penlight illuminates the posterior mucosa. View the surface of the mucosa from right to left and top to bottom. Normal mucosa is glistening, pink, soft, moist, and smooth. For patients with normal pigmentation the buccal mucosa is a good site to inspect for jaundice and pallor. In older adults, the mucosa is normally dry because of reduced salivation. Thick white patches (**leukoplakia**) are often a precancerous lesion seen in heavy smokers and alcoholics. Palpate for any buccal lesions by placing the index finger within the buccal cavity and the thumb on the outer surface of the cheek.

**GUMS AND TEETH.** Examine the gums or **gingivae** for color, edema, retraction, bleeding, and lesions. If a patient wears dentures, irregularity or lesions of the gums creates discomfort and significantly impairs the ability to chew. Ask the patient to remove dentures for a complete assessment. Healthy gums are pink, moist, smooth, and tightly fit around each tooth. Dark-skinned patients may have patchy pigmentation. In older adults the gums are usually pale. Using gloves, palpate the gums to assess for lesions, thickening, or masses. Normally, there is no tenderness. Spongy gums that bleed easily indicate periodontal disease or vitamin C deficiency.

Ask the patient to clench the teeth and smile to observe teeth occlusion. The upper molars normally rest directly on the lower molars, and the upper incisors slightly override the lower incisors. Note the position and alignment of teeth. Probe each tooth gently with a tongue blade when the patient complains of any localized discomfort. The teeth are normally firmly set.

Determine the quality of a patient's dental hygiene by inspecting the teeth (Box 13-12). To examine the posterior surface of the teeth, have the patient open the mouth with lips relaxed. You will need a tongue depressor to retract the lips and cheeks, especially when viewing the molars. Note the color of teeth and the presence of dental caries, tartar, and extraction sites. Normal healthy teeth are smooth, white, and shiny. A chalky white discoloration of the enamel is an early indication that caries are forming. Brown or black discolorations indicate formation of caries. A stained yellow color is from tobacco use, whereas coffee, tea, and colas cause a brown stain. In the older adult, loose or missing teeth are common because bone resorption increases. An older adult's teeth often feel rough when tooth enamel calcifies. Yellow and darkened teeth are also common in the older adult because of general wear and tear that exposes the darker underlying dentin.

**TONGUE AND FLOOR OF MOUTH.** Carefully inspect the tongue on all sides and the floor of the mouth. The patient first relaxes the mouth and sticks the tongue out halfway. If the patient protrudes the tongue too far, sometimes you elicit the gag reflex. Using the penlight, examine the tongue for color, size, position, texture, movement, and coating or lesions. A normal tongue appears medium or dull red in color, moist, slightly rough on the top surface, and smooth along the lateral margins. The tongue remains at midline. Ask the patient to raise the tongue and move it from side to side. The tongue should move freely.

The undersurface of the tongue and floor of the mouth are highly vascular. Take extra care to inspect this area, a common site of origin for oral cancer lesions. The patient

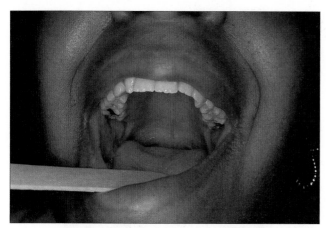

FIGURE **13-14** Tongue depressor allows view of pharynx and posterior soft palate.

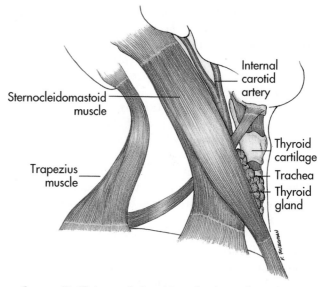

FIGURE **13-15** Anatomical position of major neck structures.

lifts the tongue by placing its tip on the palate behind the upper incisors. Inspect for color, swelling, and lesions such as cysts. The ventral surface of the tongue is pink and smooth with large veins between the frenulum folds.

**PALATE.** Have the patient extend the head backward, holding the mouth open to allow you to inspect the hard and soft palates. The hard palate, or roof of the mouth, is located anteriorly. The whitish hard palate is dome shaped. The soft palate extends posteriorly toward the pharynx. It is normally light pink and smooth. Observe the palates for color, shape, texture, and extra bony prominences or defects. A bony growth, or **exostosis,** between the two palates is common.

**PHARYNX.** Perform an examination of the pharyngeal structures to rule out infection, inflammation, or lesions. Have the patient tip the head back slightly, open the mouth wide, and say "Ah" while you place the tip of a tongue depressor on the middle third of the tongue. Take care not to press the lower lip against the teeth (Figure 13-14). If you place the tongue depressor too far anteriorly, the posterior part of the tongue mounds up, obstructing the view. Placing the tongue depressor on the posterior tongue elicits the gag reflex.

With a penlight, first inspect the uvula and soft palate. Both structures, which are innervated by the tenth cranial nerve (vagus), rise centrally as the patient says "Ah." Examine the anterior and posterior tonsillar pillars, and note the presence or absence of tonsillar tissue. The posterior pharynx is behind the pillars. Normally pharyngeal structures are smooth, pink, and well hydrated. Small irregular spots of lymphatic tissue and small blood vessels are normal. Note edema, petechiae (small hemorrhages), lesions, or exudate. Patients with chronic sinus problems frequently exhibit a clear exudate that drains along the wall of the posterior pharynx. Yellow or green exudate indicates infection. A patient with a typical sore throat has a reddened and edematous uvula and tonsillar pillars with possible presence of yellow exudate.

## Neck

Assessment of the neck includes assessing the neck muscles, lymph nodes of the head, carotid arteries, jugular veins, thyroid gland, and trachea (Figure 13-15). Postpone an examination of the carotid arteries and jugular veins until you assess the vascular system (p. 307). Inspect the neck to determine the integrity of neck structures and to examine the lymphatic system. An abnormality of superficial lymph nodes sometimes reveals the presence of infection or malignancy. Examination of the thyroid gland and trachea also aids in ruling out malignancies. Perform this examination with the patient sitting.

**HEALTH HISTORY.** Determine if the patient has had a recent cold or infection or feels weak or fatigued. Screening for hypothyroidism and hyperthyroidism and risk factors for human immunodeficiency virus (HIV) infection is necessary. Also assess if the patient has been exposed to radiation, toxic chemicals, or infection. Ask the patient to describe any history of thyroid problems, head or neck injury, or pain of head and neck structures. Finally, ask if the patient is taking thyroid medication or has a family history of thyroid disease.

**NECK MUSCLES.** With the patient sitting and facing you, inspect the gross neck structures. Observe for symmetry of neck muscles, alignment of the trachea, and any subtle fullness at the neck. Any distention or prominence of jugular veins and carotid arteries is abnormal. Ask the patient to flex the neck with the chin to the chest, hyperextend the neck backward, and move the head laterally to each side and then sideways with the ear moving toward the shoulder. This tests the sternocleidomastoid and trapezius muscles. The neck normally moves freely without discomfort.

**LYMPH NODES.** An extensive system of lymph nodes collects lymph from the head, ears, nose, cheeks, and lips

(Figure 13-16). With the patient's chin raised and head tilted slightly back, first inspect the area where lymph nodes are distributed and compare both sides. This position stretches the skin slightly over any possible enlarged nodes. Inspect visible nodes for edema, erythema, or red streaks. Nodes are not normally visible.

Use a methodical approach to palpate the lymph nodes to avoid overlooking any single node or chain. The patient relaxes muscles and tissues by keeping the neck flexed slightly forward and, if needed, toward you. Palpate both sides of the neck for comparison. During palpation either face or stand to the side of the patient for easy access to all nodes. Using the pads of the middle three fingers of each hand, gently palpate in a rotary motion over the nodes. Check each node methodically in the following sequence: occipital nodes at the base of the skull, postauricular nodes over the mastoid, preauricular nodes just in front of the ear, retropharyngeal nodes at the angle of the mandible, submandibular nodes, and submental nodes in the midline behind the mandibular tip. Try to detect enlargement, and note the location, size, shape, surface characteristics, consistency, mobility, tenderness, and warmth of the nodes. If the skin is mobile, move the skin over the area of the nodes (Figure 13-17) (Seidel and others, 2003). It is important to press underlying tissue in each area and not simply move the fingers over the skin. However, if you apply excessive pressure, you will miss small nodes and destroy palpable nodes.

To palpate supraclavicular nodes ask the patient to bend the head forward and relax the shoulders. You may have to hook the index and third finger over the clavicle, lateral to the sternocleidomastoid muscle, to palpate these nodes. Palpate the deep cervical nodes only with your fingers hooked around the sternocleidomastoid muscle.

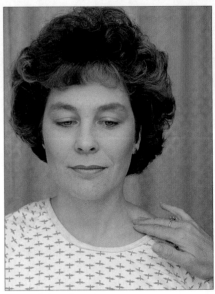

FIGURE **13-17** Supraclavicular lymph node palpation.

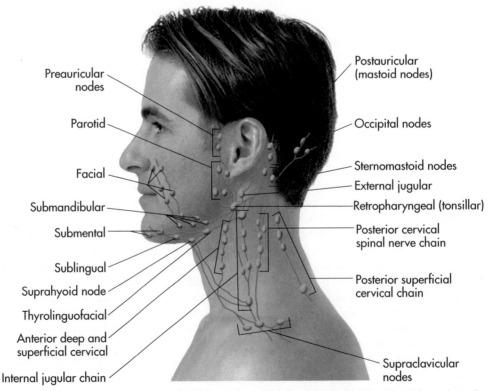

FIGURE **13-16** Lymphatic drainage system of the head and neck. (From Seidel HM and others: *Mosby's guide to physical examination*, ed 5, St. Louis, 2003, Mosby.)

Normally lymph nodes are not easily palpable. Lymph nodes that are large, fixed, inflamed, or tender indicate a problem such as local infection, systemic disease, or neoplasm (Seidel and others, 2003). Tenderness almost always indicates inflammation (Box 13-13). A problem involving a lymph node of the head and neck may mean an abnormality in the mouth, throat, abdomen, breasts, thorax, or arms. These are the areas drained by the head and neck nodes.

**THYROID GLAND.** The thyroid gland lies in the anterior lower neck, in front of and to both sides of the trachea. The gland is fixed to the trachea with the isthmus overlying the trachea and connecting the two irregular, cone-shaped lobes (Figure 13-18). Inspect the lower neck over the thyroid gland for obvious masses and symmetry. Offer the patient a glass of water, and, while observing the neck, have the patient swallow. This maneuver helps to visualize an abnormally enlarged thyroid gland. More-experienced nurses examine the thyroid by palpating for more subtle masses; this technique will not be discussed here.

**TRACHEA.** The trachea is a part of the upper airway that you directly palpate. It is normally located in the midline above the suprasternal notch. Masses in the neck or mediastinum and pulmonary abnormalities cause displacement laterally. Have the patient sit or lie down during palpation. Determine the position of the trachea by palpating at the suprasternal notch, slipping the thumb and index fingers to each side. Note if your finger and thumb shift laterally. Do not apply forceful pressure to the trachea because this elicits coughing.

## Thorax and Lungs

Examination of the thorax and lungs includes an in-depth look at ventilatory and respiratory functions of the lungs. If the lungs are affected by disease, other body systems are also affected. For example, reduced oxygenation causes changes in mental alertness because of the brain's sensitivity to lowered oxygen levels. This data is used from all body systems to determine the nature of pulmonary alterations.

Before assessing the thorax and lungs, be familiar with the landmarks of the chest (Figure 13-19). These landmarks help you locate findings and use assessment skills correctly. The patient's nipples, angle of Louis, suprasternal notch, costal angle, clavicles, and vertebrae are key landmarks that provide a series of imaginary lines for sign identification. You should keep a mental image of the location of the lobes of the lung and the position of each rib (Figure 13-20). The proper orientation to anatomical structures ensures a thorough assessment of the anterior, lateral, and posterior thorax.

Locating the position of each rib is critical to visualizing the lobe of the lung being assessed. The angle of Louis, at the junction between the manubrium and the body of the sternum, is the starting point for locating the ribs anteriorly. Knowing that the second rib extends from the angle makes it easy to locate and palpate the intercostal spaces (between the ribs) in succession. The spinous process of the third thoracic vertebra and the fourth, fifth, and sixth ribs serve to locate the lobes of the lung laterally (Figure 13-21). The lower lobes project laterally and anteriorly.

Posteriorly the tip or inferior margin of the scapula lies approximately at the level of the seventh rib. After you identify the seventh rib, count upward to locate the third thoracic vertebra and align it with the inner borders of the scapula to locate the posterior lobes (Figure 13-22).

The examination requires the patient to be undressed to the waist, with good lighting. The examination begins with the patient sitting for assessment of the posterior and lateral chest. Have the patient sit or lie for assessment of the anterior chest.

### Health History

A complete health history includes determining if the patient has a history of tobacco or marijuana use. Record the number of years the patient smoked, age started, number of

**BOX 13-13** PATIENT TEACHING

**Neck Assessment**
- Stress the importance of regular compliance with medication schedule to patients with thyroid disease.
- Instruct patients about lymph nodes and how infection commonly causes node tenderness.
- Instruct patients to call the physician or health care provider when they notice a lump or mass in the neck.
- Teach patients risk factors for HIV and other sexually transmitted diseases.

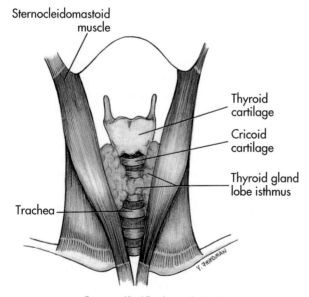

FIGURE **13-18** Thyroid gland.

Sternocleidomastoid muscle

Thyroid cartilage

Cricoid cartilage

Thyroid gland lobe isthmus

Trachea

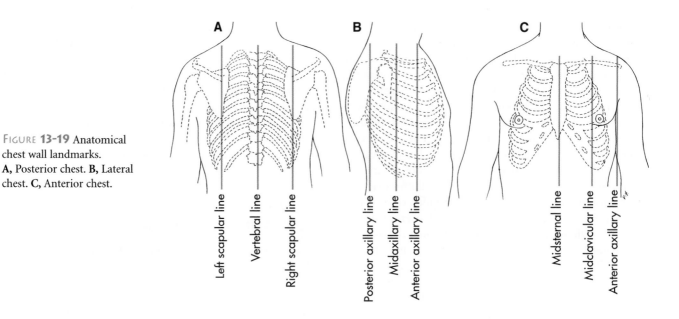

FIGURE **13-19** Anatomical chest wall landmarks. **A,** Posterior chest. **B,** Lateral chest. **C,** Anterior chest.

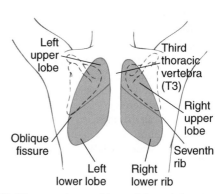

FIGURE **13-20** Anterior position of lung lobes in relation to anatomical landmarks.

FIGURE **13-22** Posterior position of lung lobes in relation to anatomical landmarks.

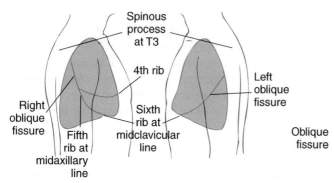

FIGURE **13-21** Lateral position of lung lobes in relation to anatomical landmarks.

cigarettes or cigars daily, and length of time since smoking stopped. To screen for warning signals of lung cancer, ask if the patient has a persistent cough, sputum production, chest pain, or recurrent attacks of pneumonia or bronchitis. Ask the patient about symptoms of **orthopnea** (difficulty in breathing; must be in upright position to breathe), shortness of breath, **dyspnea** (breathlessness) during exertion or at rest, and poor activity tolerance. This reveals cardiopulmonary problems. Review the presence of pollutants in the work environment or at home to assess a patient's risk for having lung disease. Also, review the patient's family history for cancer, tuberculosis, allergies, or chronic obstructive pulmonary disease.

Tuberculosis (TB) is on the decrease in the United States (Frakes and Evans, 2004); however, be alert for patients at risk. Those at risk are persons with HIV infection, substance abusers, residents and employees of nursing homes and shelters, homeless individuals, prison inmates, family members of TB patients, and immigrants to the United States from a country where TB is prevalent (Frakes and Evans, 2004). Evaluate at-risk patients and those who exhibit symptoms of persistent cough, hemoptysis, unexplained weight loss, fatigue, anorexia, night sweats, and fever for tuberculosis and/or HIV infection.

The history also includes assessment of allergies to airborne irritants, foods, drugs, or chemical substances. It is important to learn if a patient has had pneumonia or influenza vaccine and a TB test. The very young, the very old, and those with chronic respiratory problems or with immunosuppressive diseases are at increased risk for respiratory disease. If the patient has not been vaccinated, educate the individual on the need for vaccination to protect against illnesses.

## Posterior Thorax

Begin examination of the posterior thorax by observing for any signs or symptoms in other body systems that indicate pulmonary problems. Reduced mental alertness, nasal flaring, somnolence, and cyanosis are examples of signs assessed during other portions of the examination that indicate oxygenation problems. Inspect the posterior thorax by observing the shape and symmetry of the chest from the patient's back and front. Note the anteroposterior diameter. Body shape or posture significantly impairs ventilatory movement. Normally the chest contour is symmetrical, with the anteroposterior diameter one third to one half the size of the transverse or side-to-side diameter. A barrel-shaped chest (anteroposterior diameter equals transverse) characterizes aging and chronic lung disease. Infants have an almost round shape. Congenital and postural alterations cause abnormal contours. A patient may lean over a table or splint the side of the chest because of a breathing problem. Splinting or holding the chest wall because of pain causes a patient to bend toward the affected side. Such a posture impairs ventilatory movement.

Standing at a midline position behind the patient, look for deformities, position of the spine, slope of the ribs, retraction of the intercostal spaces during inspiration, and bulging of the intercostal spaces during expiration. The spine is normally straight without lateral deviation. The scapulae normally are symmetrical and closely attached to the chest wall. Posteriorly, the ribs tend to slope across and down. The ribs and intercostal spaces are easier to see in a thin person. Normally no bulging or active movement occurs within the intercostal spaces during breathing. Bulging indicates that the patient is using great effort to breathe.

You also assess the rate and rhythm of breathing at this time (see Chapter 12). Observe the thorax as a whole. The thorax normally expands and relaxes with equality of movement bilaterally. In healthy adults the normal respiratory rate varies from 12 to 20 respirations per minute.

Palpation of the posterior thorax assesses further characteristics. Palpate the thoracic muscles and skeleton for

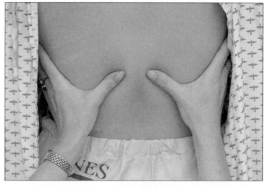

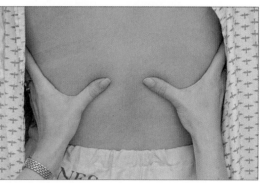

FIGURE **13-23 A,** Position of hands for palpation of posterior thorax excursion. **B,** When the patient inhales, the movement of chest excursion separates the thumbs.

lumps, masses, pulsations, and unusual movement. If pain or tenderness is noted, avoid deep palpation. Fractured rib fragments could be displaced against vital organs. Normally the chest wall is not tender. If you detect a suspicious mass or swollen area, lightly palpate it for size, shape, and typical qualities of a lesion.

To measure chest excursion or depth of breathing, stand behind the patient and place the thumbs along the spinal processes at the tenth rib, with the palms lightly contacting the posterolateral surfaces. Place your thumbs about 5 cm (2 inches) apart, pointing toward the spine and fingers pointing laterally (Figure 13-23, A). Press the hands toward the spine so that a small skinfold appears between the thumbs. Do not slide the hands over the skin. Instruct the patient to take a deep breath after exhaling. Note movement of the thumbs (Figure 13-23, B). Chest excursion is symmetrical, separating the thumbs 3 to 5 cm (1¼ to 2 inches). Reduced chest excursion is caused by pain, postural deformity, or fatigue. In older adults, chest excursion normally declines because of costal cartilage calcification and respiratory muscle atrophy.

Auscultation assesses the movement of air through the tracheobronchial tree and detects mucus or obstructed airways. Normally air flows through the airways in an unobstructed pattern. Recognizing the sounds created by normal air flow allows for detection of sounds caused by airway obstruction.

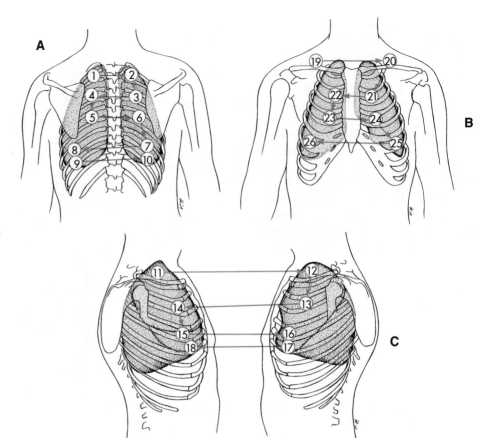

FIGURE **13-24** **A to C,** A systematic pattern (posterior-lateral-anterior) is followed for auscultation.

Place the diaphragm of the stethoscope over the posterior chest wall between the ribs. The patient folds the arms in front of the chest and keeps the head bent forward while taking slow, deep breaths with the mouth slightly open. Listen to an entire inspiration and expiration at each position of the stethoscope (Figure 13-24, *A*). If sounds are faint, as with an obese patient, ask the patient to breathe harder and faster temporarily. Breath sounds are much louder in children because of their thin chest walls. In children the bell works best because of a child's small chest. Use a systematic pattern comparing the sounds in one region on one side of the body with sounds in the same region on the opposite side.

Auscultate for normal breath sounds and abnormal sounds (**adventitious sounds**). Normal breath sounds differ in character, depending on the area being auscultated. Sounds normally heard over the posterior thorax include bronchovesicular and vesicular sounds. Bronchovesicular sounds are medium-pitched blowing sounds normally heard posteriorly between the scapulae. The sounds have equal inspiratory and expiratory phases. The character of bronchovesicular sounds is related to the larger underlying airways. You hear vesicular sounds over the periphery of the lungs. Air moving through the smaller airways creates these sounds. Vesicular sounds are soft, breezy, and low pitched, and the inspiratory phase is about three times longer than the expiratory phase.

Abnormal sounds result from air passing through moisture, mucus, or narrowed airways. They also result from alveoli suddenly reinflating or from an inflammation between the pleural linings of the lung. Adventitious sounds often occur superimposed over normal sounds. The four types of adventitious sounds are **crackles, rhonchi, wheezes,** and **pleural friction rub.** Each sound is caused by a specific entity and is characterized by typical auditory features (Table 13-6). During auscultation note the location and characteristics of the sounds, and listen for the absence of breath sounds (found in patients with collapsed or surgically removed lobes).

### Lateral Thorax

Usually you extend the assessment of the posterior thorax to the lateral sides of the chest (Figure 13-24, *B*). The patient sits during the lateral chest examination. Also have the patient raise the arms to improve access to lateral thoracic structures. Use inspection, palpation, and auscultation skills. You cannot assess excursion laterally. Normally the breath sounds heard are vesicular.

### Anterior Thorax

Inspect the anterior thorax for the same features as the posterior thorax. The patient sits or lies down with the head elevated. Observe the accessory muscles of breathing: sternocleidomastoid, trapezius, and abdominal muscles. The

| TABLE 13-6 | Adventitious Sounds | | |
|---|---|---|---|
| **Sound** | **Site Auscultated** | **Cause** | **Character** |
| Crackles | Are most commonly heard in dependent lobes: right and left lung bases | Random, sudden reinflation of groups of alveoli; disruptive passage of air | Fine crackles are high-pitched fine, short, interrupted crackling sounds heard during end of inspiration, usually not cleared with coughing. Moist crackles are lower, more moist sounds heard during middle of inspiration; not cleared with coughing. Coarse crackles are loud, bubbly sounds heard during inspiration, not cleared with coughing |
| Rhonchi (sonorous wheeze) | Are primarily heard over trachea and bronchi; if loud enough, can be heard over most lung fields | Muscular spasm, fluid, or mucus in larger airways, cause turbulence | Are loud, low-pitched, rumbling coarse sounds heard most often during inspiration or expiration; may be cleared by coughing |
| Wheezes (sibilant wheeze) | Can be heard over all lung fields | High-velocity airflow through severely narrowed bronchus | Are high-pitched, continuous musical sounds like a squeak heard continuously during inspiration or expiration; usually louder on expiration. |
| Pleural friction rub | Is heard over anterior lateral lung field (if patient is sitting upright) | Inflamed pleura, parietal pleura rubbing against visceral pleura | Has dry, grating quality heard best during inspiration; does not clear with coughing; heard loudest over lower lateral anterior surface |

Data from Seidel HM and others: *Mosby's guide to physical examination,* ed 5, St. Louis, 2003, Mosby.

accessory muscles move little with normal passive breathing. When a patient requires effort to breathe as a result of strenuous exercise or disease (Box 13-14), the accessory muscles and abdominal muscles contract. Some patients produce a grunting sound.

Observe the width of the costal angle. It is usually larger than 90 degrees between the two costal margins. You will more often assess respiratory rate and rhythm anteriorly (see Chapter 12). The male patient's respirations are usually diaphragmatic, whereas the female's are more costal.

Palpate the anterior thoracic muscles and skeleton for lumps, masses, tenderness, or unusual movement. The sternum and xiphoid are relatively inflexible. To measure chest excursion anteriorly, place your thumbs parallel along the costal margin 6 cm (2½ inches) apart with the palms touching the anterolateral chest. Push the thumbs toward the midline to create a skinfold. As the patient inhales deeply, the thumbs normally separate approximately 3 to 5 cm (1¼ to 2 inches), with each side expanding equally.

Auscultation of the anterior thorax also follows a systematic pattern (Figure 13-24, *C*). Have the patient sit, if possible, to maximize chest expansion. Give special attention to the lower lobes, where mucous secretions commonly gather. You will hear bronchovesicular and vesicular sounds above and below the clavicles and along the lung periphery. You can hear an additional normal breath sound, a bronchial sound, over the trachea. Bronchial sounds are loud, high pitched, and hollow sounding, with expiration lasting longer than inspiration (3:2 ratio).

PATIENT TEACHING

**Lung Health**

- Explain the risk factors for chronic lung disease and lung cancer, including cigarette smoking, history of smoking for over 20 years, exposure to environmental pollution, and radiation exposure from occupational, medical, and environmental sources. Residential radon exposure also increases risk, especially for cigarette smokers. Exposure to sidestream cigarette smoke increases risk for nonsmokers (ACS, 2005).
- Share brochures on lung cancer from the American Cancer Society with patient and family.
- Discuss the warning signs of lung cancer, such as a persistent cough, sputum streaked with blood, chest pains, and recurrent attacks of pneumonia or bronchitis.
- Counsel older adults on benefits of receiving influenza and pneumonia vaccinations because of a greater susceptibility to respiratory infection.
- Instruct patients with chronic obstructive pulmonary disease in coughing and pursed-lip–breathing exercises (see Chapter 28).
- Refer persons at risk for tuberculosis who visit clinics or health care centers for skin testing.

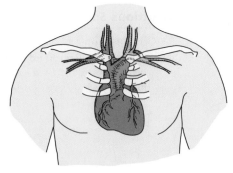

FIGURE **13-25** Anatomical position of the heart.

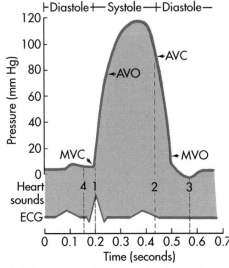

FIGURE **13-26** Cardiac cycle. *MVC,* Mitral valve closes; *AVO,* aortic valve opens; *AVC,* aortic valve closes, *MVO,* mitral valve opens.

## Heart

Compare your assessment of heart function with findings from the vascular examination. Alterations in either system sometimes manifest as changes in the other. A patient with signs and symptoms of heart problems may have a life-threatening condition requiring immediate attention. In this case, you quickly act and conduct only portions of the examination that are absolutely necessary. When a patient is more stable, you will conduct a more thorough examination.

Assess cardiac function through the anterior thorax. Form a mental image of the heart's exact location (Figure 13-25). In the adult the heart is located in the center of the chest (precordium) behind and to the left of the sternum, with a small section of the right atrium extending to the right of the sternum. The base of the heart is the upper portion, and the apex is the bottom tip. The surface of the right ventricle constitutes most of the heart's anterior surface. A section of the left ventricle shapes the left anterior side of the apex. The apex actually touches the anterior chest wall at approximately the fourth to fifth intercostal space along the midclavicular line. This is known as the apical impulse.

An infant's heart is positioned more horizontally. The apex of the heart is at the third or fourth intercostal space, just to the left of the midclavicular line. By the age of 7 years a child's apical impulse is in the same location as the adult's. In tall, slender persons the heart hangs more vertically and is positioned more centrally. With increased stockiness and shortness, the heart tends to lie more to the left and horizontally (Seidel and others, 2003).

To assess heart function, you need to understand the cardiac cycle and the physiological signs of each event (Figure 13-26). The heart normally pumps blood through its four chambers in a methodical, even sequence. Events on the left side occur just before those on the right. As the blood flows through each chamber, valves open and close, pressures within chambers rise and fall, and chambers contract. Each event creates a physiological sign. Both sides of the heart function in a coordinated fashion.

There are two phases to the cardiac cycle: systole and diastole. During systole the ventricles contract and eject blood from the left ventricle into the aorta and from the right ventricle into the pulmonary artery. During diastole the ventricles relax and the atria contract to move blood into the ventricles and fill the coronary arteries.

Heart sounds occur in relation to physiological events in the cardiac cycle. As systole begins, ventricular pressure rises and closes the mitral and tricuspid valves. Valve closure causes the first heart sound ($S_1$), often described as "lub." The ventricles then contract, and blood flows through the aorta and pulmonary circulation. After the ventricles empty, ventricular pressure falls below that in the aorta and pulmonary artery. This allows the aortic and pulmonary valves to close, causing the second heart sound ($S_2$), described as "dub." As ventricular pressure continues to fall, it drops below that of the atria. The mitral and tricuspid valves reopen to allow ventricular filling. Rapid ventricular filling may create a third heart sound ($S_3$). You hear this more often in children and young adults. You hear an $S_3$ as an abnormality in adults over 30 years of age. You hear a fourth heart sound ($S_4$) when the atria contract to enhance ventricular filling. You may hear the $S_4$ in healthy older adults, children, and athletes, but it is not normal in adults. Because $S_4$ also indicates an abnormal condition, report it to a physician or health care provider.

## Health History

The health history focuses on risk factors for cardiovascular disease (Box 13-15). Assess the patient's history of smoking, alcohol intake, caffeine intake, use of prescriptive and recreational drugs, exercise habits, and dietary patterns including fat and sodium intake. Does the patient have a stressful lifestyle? If so, what are the physical demands or emotional stresses? It is important to know if the patient takes medications for cardiovascular function (e.g., antidysrhythmics or antihypertensives). Also assess for signs and symptoms suggestive of heart disease, including chest pain or discomfort, **palpitations** (pounding or racing of heart), excess fatigue, cough, dyspnea, edema of the feet, cyanosis, fainting, or orthopnea. If the patient reports chest pain, determine if it is cardiac in nature; anginal pain is usually a deep pressure or ache that is substernal and diffuse, radiating to one or both arms, the neck, or the jaw. Determine whether the patient has preexisting diabetes, lung disease, obesity, or hypertension. Finally, assess the patient's personal and family history for heart disease.

## Inspection and Palpation

Use the skills of inspection and palpation simultaneously. The examination begins with the patient supine and the upper body elevated 45 degrees because patients with heart disease frequently suffer shortness of breath while lying flat. Stand at the patient's right side. Do not let the patient talk, especially when you auscultate heart sounds. Good lighting in the room is essential.

Direct your attention to the anatomical sites best suited for assessment of cardiac function. You feel the sternal angle or angle of Louis as a ridge in the sternum approximately 2 inches below the sternal notch. Slip your fingers along the angle on each side of the sternum to feel the adjacent ribs. The intercostal spaces are just below each rib. The second intercostal space allows for identification of each of the six anatomical landmarks (Figure 13-27). The second intercostal space on the right is the aortic area, and the left second intercostal space is the pulmonic area. You will need deeper palpation to feel the spaces in obese or heavily muscled patients. After locating the pulmonic area, move your fingers down the patient's left sternal border to the third intercostal space, called the second pulmonic area. The tricuspid area is located at the fourth left intercostal space along the sternum. To find the apical area or **point of maximal impulse (PMI)**, locate

---

| BOX 13-15 | PATIENT TEACHING |

**Heart Health**

- Explain the risk factors for heart disease, including high dietary intake of saturated fat or cholesterol, lack of regular aerobic exercise, smoking, excess weight, stressful lifestyle, hypertension, and family history of heart disease.
- Refer patients (if appropriate) to resources available for controlling or reducing risks (e.g., nutritional counseling, exercise class, stress reduction programs).
- Explain that research shows clinical benefit from reducing dietary intake of cholesterol and saturated fats. Tell patients that about 70 % to 75% of saturated fatty acids come from meats, poultry, fish, and dairy products. The American Heart Association recommends a diet that includes an intake of total fat less that 35% of calories, saturated fatty acids less than 10% of calories, and cholesterol less than 300 mg/100 ml (Moore, 2005).
- Encourage patients to have regular measurement of total blood cholesterol levels and triglycerides. Desirable levels are less than 200 mg/100 ml. You will need more than one cholesterol measurement to assess the blood cholesterol level accurately. Low-density lipoprotein (LDL) cholesterol is the major component of atherosclerotic plaques. Separate measurement of LDL cholesterol is wise in a patient with high total blood cholesterol levels. An LDL cholesterol level of 160 mg/100 ml or higher is high risk (Moore, 2005).
- Encourage patients to have a periodic C-reactive protein (CRP) level drawn upon advice of their physician or health care provider. CRP levels assess a patient's cardiovascular disease risk.
- Advise patients to avoid cigarette smoke because nicotine causes vasoconstriction.
- Advise patients to quite smoking because this lowers the risk for coronary heart disease and coronary vascular disease (ACS, 2005).
- Patients who have known angina benefit from taking a daily low dose of aspirin. Consult physician or health care provider before starting therapy.

---

the fifth intercostal space just to the left of the sternum and move your fingers laterally to the left midclavicular line. Locate the apical area with the palm of the hand or your fingertips. Normally the apical pulse is a light tap felt in an area 1 to 2 cm ($\frac{1}{2}$ to $\frac{3}{4}$ inch) in diameter at the apex. Another landmark is the epigastric area at the tip of the sternum. It is typically used to palpate for aortic abnormalities.

As you locate the six anatomical landmarks of the heart, inspect and palpate each area. Look for the appearance of pulsations, viewing each area over the chest at an angle to the side. Normally you will not see pulsations except perhaps at the apical impulse in thin patients or at the epigastric area as a result of abdominal aortic pulsation. You palpate for pulsations best using the proximal halves of the four fingers together and then alternating with the ball of the hand. Touch the areas gently to allow movements to lift the hand.

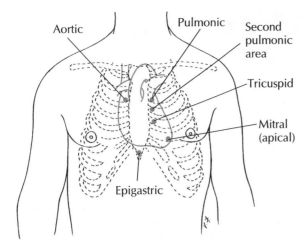

FIGURE **13-27** Anatomical sites for assessment of cardiac function.

Normally you do not feel any pulsations or vibrations in the second, third, or fourth intercostal spaces. Loud murmurs cause a vibration. If you palpate pulsations or vibrations, time their occurrence in relation to systole or diastole by auscultating heart sounds simultaneously.

The apical impulse or PMI should be felt easily. If not, have the patient turn onto the left side, moving the heart closer to the chest wall. Estimate the size of the heart by noting the diameter of the PMI and its position relative to the midclavicular line. In cases of serious heart disease, the cardiac muscle enlarges, with the PMI found to the left of the midclavicular line. The PMI is sometimes difficult to find in older adults because the chest deepens in its anteroposterior diameter. It is also difficult to find in muscular or overweight patients. An infant's PMI is usually at the third or fourth intercostal space. It is easy to palpate because of the child's thin chest wall.

## Auscultation

Auscultation of the heart detects normal heart sounds, extra heart sounds, and **murmurs** (blowing or humming sounds). You will need concentration to detect the low-intensity sounds caused by valve closure. To begin auscultation eliminate all sources of room noise and explain the procedure to relieve the patient's anxiety. Follow a systematic pattern beginning with the aortic area and inching the stethoscope along each of the six landmarks. Be sure you hear the complete cycle ("lub-dub") of heart sounds clearly at each location. Then repeat the sequence using the bell of the stethoscope. Sometimes you will ask the patient to assume three different positions during the examination (Figure 13-28):

- Sitting up and leaning forward (good for all areas and to hear high-pitched murmurs)
- Supine (good for all areas)
- Left lateral recumbent (good for all areas; best position to hear low-pitched sounds in diastole)

You must learn to identify the first ($S_1$) and second ($S_2$) heart sounds. At normal rates, $S_1$ occurs after the long diastolic

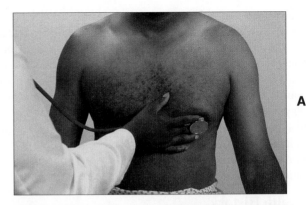

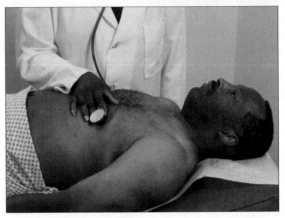

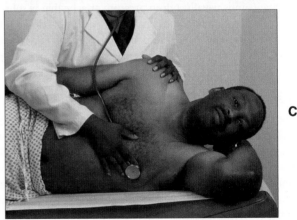

FIGURE **13-28** Sequence of patient positions for heart auscultation. **A,** Sitting. **B,** Supine. **C,** Left lateral recumbent. (From Seidel HM and others: *Mosby's guide to physical examination,* ed 5, St. Louis, 2003, Mosby.)

pause and preceding the short systolic pause. $S_1$ is high pitched, dull in quality, and heard best at the apex. If you have difficulty hearing $S_1$, time it in relation to the carotid pulse. It occurs just before the carotid pulsation. $S_2$ follows the short systolic phase and precedes the long diastolic phase. You hear it best at the aortic area.

Auscultate for rate and rhythm after you hear both sounds clearly. Each combination of $S_1$ and $S_2$ or "lub-dub" counts as one heartbeat. Count the rate for 1 minute, and listen for the interval between $S_1$ and $S_2$, and then the time between $S_2$ and the next $S_1$. A regular rhythm involves regular intervals of time between each sequence of beats. There is a distinct silent pause between $S_1$ and $S_2$. Failure of the heart to beat at regular successive intervals is a **dysrhythmia.** Some dysrhythmias are life threatening.

When the heart rhythm is irregular, compare apical and radial pulse rates to determine if a pulse deficit exists. Auscultate the apical pulse first, and then immediately assess the radial pulse (one-examiner technique). When two examiners are available, the apical and radial rates are assessed at the same time. Compare the two rates. When a patient has a pulse deficit, the radial pulse is slower than the apical because ineffective contractions fail to send pulse waves to the periphery. Report a difference in pulse rates to the physician or health care provider immediately.

Assess extra heart sounds and murmurs at each auscultatory site. Assess these low-pitched sounds (such as $S_3$ and $S_4$ gallops, clicks, or rubs) using the bell of the stethoscope. Presence of these sounds usually indicates a pathological condition. Report it immediately. Typically, advanced practice nurses perform this portion of the examination.

## Vascular System

Examination of the vascular system includes measuring the blood pressure (see Chapter 12) and assessing the integrity of the peripheral vascular system. Use the skills of inspection, palpation, and auscultation. You can perform portions of the vascular examination during other body system assessments.

### Health History

The history includes determining if the patient has leg cramps, numbness or tingling in the extremities, or the continual sensation of cold hands or feet. These signs and symptoms may indicate vascular disease. Also learn if the patient has noted swelling or cyanosis of the feet, ankles, or hand or pain in the feet or legs. If the patient has leg pain or cramps, ask if symptoms are aggravated by walking or standing for long periods or during sleep. This question helps to clarify if the problem is musculoskeletal or vascular in nature. For example, arterial occlusion creates muscle ischemia or claudication. This particular type of pain is a dull ache and cramping, usually appearing during sustained exercise and disappearing after a short rest. Musculoskeletal pain is not generally relieved when exercise ends. Also ask if patients wear tight-fitting garters or hosiery and sit or lie in bed with their legs crossed. These activities impair venous return. The history includes a review of the patient's medical history for heart disease, hypertension, phlebitis, diabetes, or varicose veins. Finally, risk factors assessed earlier for smoking, exercise, and nutritional problems are important when assessing the vascular system.

### Carotid Arteries

When the left ventricle pumps blood into the aorta, the arterial system transmits pressure waves. The carotid artery reflects heart function better than peripheral arteries, because

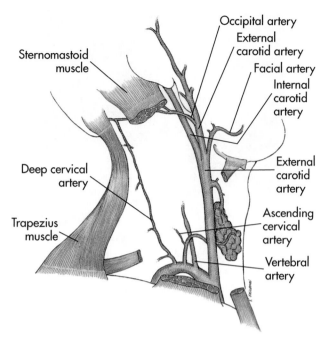

FIGURE **13-29** Anatomical position of carotid artery.

its pressure correlates with that of the aorta. The carotid artery supplies oxygenated blood to the head and neck (Figure 13-29). The overlying sternocleidomastoid muscle protects it.

To examine the carotid arteries, have the patient sit or lie supine with the head of the bed elevated 15 to 30 degrees. Examine one carotid artery at a time. If you occlude both arteries simultaneously during palpation, the patient will lose consciousness as a result of inadequate circulation to the brain. Do not palpate or massage the carotid arteries vigorously because the carotid sinus is in the upper third of the neck. The sinus sends impulses along the vagus nerve. Its stimulation causes a reflex drop in heart rate and blood pressure, which causes **syncope** (light-headedness) or circulatory arrest. This is a particular problem for older adults.

Begin inspection of the neck for obvious pulsation of the artery. Have the patient turn the head slightly away from the artery being examined. Sometimes you see the wave of the pulse. An absent pulse wave indicates arterial occlusion (blockage) or **stenosis** (narrowing).

To palpate the pulse, ask the patient to look straight ahead or turn the head slightly to the side being examined. Turning relaxes the sternocleidomastoid muscle. Slide the tips of your index and middle fingers around the medial edge of the sternocleidomastoid muscle. Gently palpate to avoid occlusion of circulation (Figure 13-30).

The normal carotid pulse is localized rather than diffuse. As a strong pulse, the carotid has a thrusting quality. As the patient breathes, no change occurs. Rotation of the neck or a shift from a sitting to a supine position does not change the carotid's quality. Both carotid arteries are normally equal in pulse rate, rhythm, and strength and are equally elastic. Diminished or unequal carotid pulsations indicate

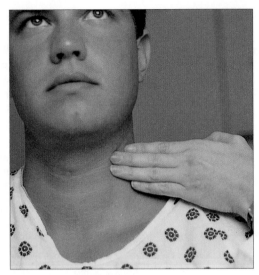

FIGURE **13-30** Palpation of the internal carotid artery.

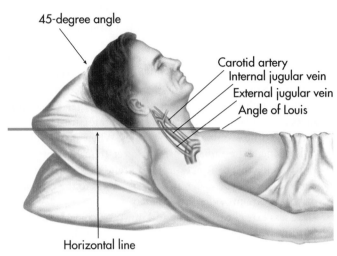

FIGURE **13-31** Position of patient to assess jugular vein distention. (From Thompson JM and others: *Mosby's clinical nursing*, ed 5, St. Louis, 2001, Mosby.)

**atherosclerosis** (plaque buildup in arteries) or other forms of arterial disease.

The carotid is the most commonly auscultated pulse. Auscultation is especially important for middle-age or older adults or patients suspected of having cerebrovascular disease. When the lumen of a blood vessel is narrowed, its blood flow is disturbed. As blood passes through the narrowed section, it creates a turbulence, causing a blowing or swishing sound. The blowing sound is called a **bruit** (pronounced "brew-ee"). Place the bell of the stethoscope over the carotid artery at the base of the neck, and move it gradually toward the jaw. Ask patients to hold their breath for a moment so that breath sounds do not obscure a bruit. Normally you will not hear any sound during carotid auscultation. If you hear a bruit, gently palpate the artery lightly for a **thrill** (palpable bruit).

## Jugular Veins

The most accessible veins for examination are the internal and external jugular veins in the neck. Both veins drain bilaterally from the head and neck into the superior vena cava. The external jugular lies superficially and you will see it just above the clavicle. The internal jugular lies deeper, along the carotid artery. Normally when a patient lies in the supine position, the external jugular distends and becomes easily visible. In contrast, the jugular veins normally flatten when the patient is in a sitting or standing position. A patient with heart disease, however, has distended jugular veins when sitting.

As an entry-level nurse you learn to assess for jugular venous distention. Inspect the patient's jugular veins in the supine position (normally veins protrude), when standing (normally veins are flat), and when sitting at a 45-degree angle (jugular veins distended only if patient has right-sided heart failure) (Figure 13-31). An advanced practitioner completes the specific measurement of jugular venous pressure.

## Peripheral Arteries

The most accurate assessment of peripheral arteries involves palpation over arteries that are close to the body surface and lie over bones. An arterial pulsation is a bounding wave of blood that diminishes in intensity with increasing distance from the heart (Seidel and others, 2003).

Assess the arterial pulses in the extremities to determine sufficiency of the entire arterial circulation. Factors such as coagulation disorders, local trauma or surgery, constricting casts or bandages, and systemic disease such as diabetes or arteriosclerosis impair circulation to the extremities. Discuss risk factors for circulatory problems with the patient (Box 13-16).

Examine each peripheral artery using the distal pads of your second and third fingers. The thumb helps anchor the brachial and femoral artery. Apply firm pressure, but avoid occluding a pulse. When a pulse is difficult to find, it helps to vary pressure and feel all around the pulse site. Be sure not to palpate your own pulse.

Routine vital signs usually include assessment of the rate and rhythm of the radial artery, because it is easily accessible (see Chapter 12). Count the pulse for either 30 seconds or a full minute, depending on the character of the pulse. Always count an irregular pulse for 60 seconds. With palpation you normally feel the pulse wave at regular intervals. When an interval is interrupted by an early, late, or missed beat, the pulse rhythm is irregular. In emergencies the carotid artery is chosen because it is accessible and closest to the heart and thus most useful in evaluating heart activity. To check local circulatory status of tissues, palpate the peripheral arteries long enough to note that a pulse is present.

Assess each peripheral artery for elasticity of vessel wall, strength, and equality. The arterial wall is normally elastic, making it easily palpable. After you depress the artery, it will spring back to shape when you release pressure. An abnormal artery is described as hard, inelastic, or calcified.

The strength of a pulse is a measurement of the force with which blood is ejected against the arterial wall. Some examiners use a rating from 0 (zero) to 4+ (Seidel and others, 2003):

0    Absent, not palpable
1+   Pulse is diminished, barely palpable
2+   Easily palpable, normal pulse
3+   Full, increased pulse
4+   Bounding, cannot be obliterated

Measure all peripheral pulses for equality and symmetry. Compare the left radial pulse with that of the right, the left brachial pulse with that of the left radial, and so on. Lack of symmetry indicates impaired circulation such as a localized obstruction or an abnormally positioned artery.

In the upper extremities the brachial artery channels blood to the radial and ulnar arteries of the forearm and hand. If circulation in this artery becomes blocked, the hands will not receive adequate blood flow. If circulation in the radial or ulnar arteries becomes impaired, the hand will still receive adequate perfusion. An interconnection between the radial and ulnar arteries guards against arterial occlusion (Figure 13-32).

To locate pulses in the arm, have the patient sit or lie down. You will find the radial pulse along the radial side of the forearm at the wrist. In a thin individual a groove is formed lateral to the flexor tendon of the wrist. You feel the radial pulse with light palpation in the groove (Figure 13-33). The ulnar pulse is on the opposite side of the wrist and feels less prominent (Figure 13-34). Palpate the ulnar pulse only when you expect arterial insufficiency to the hand.

To palpate the brachial pulse, find the groove between the biceps and triceps muscle above the elbow at the antecubital fossa (Figure 13-35). The artery runs along the medial side of the extended arm. Palpate the artery with the fingertips of your first three fingers in the muscle groove.

The femoral artery is the primary artery in the leg, delivering blood to the popliteal, posterior tibial, and dorsalis pedis arteries (Figure 13-36). An interconnection between the posterior tibial and dorsalis pedis arteries guards against local arterial occlusion. Find the femoral pulse with

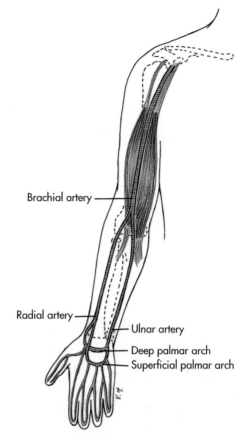

FIGURE **13-32** Anatomical positions of brachial, radial, and ulnar arteries.

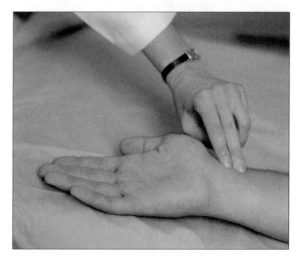

FIGURE **13-33** Palpation of radial pulse.

the patient lying down with the inguinal area exposed (Figure 13-37). The femoral artery runs below the inguinal ligament, midway between the symphysis pubis and the anterosuperior iliac spine. You sometimes need to use deep palpation to feel the pulse. Bimanual palpation is effective in obese patients. Place your fingertips of both hands on opposite sides of the pulse site. You will feel a

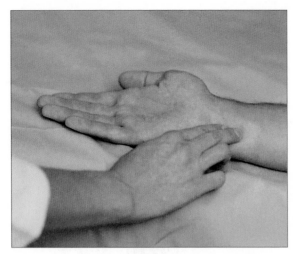

FIGURE **13-34** Palpation of ulnar pulse.

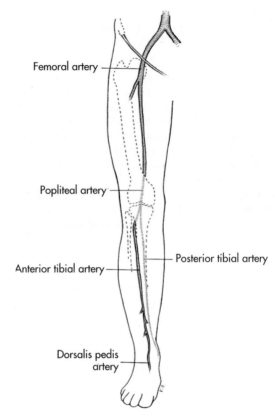

FIGURE **13-36** Anatomical position of femoral, popliteal, dorsalis pedis, and posterior tibial arteries.

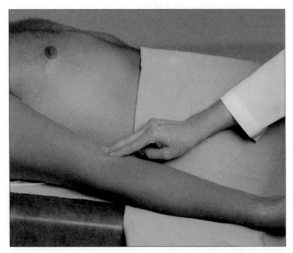

FIGURE **13-35** Palpation of brachial pulse.

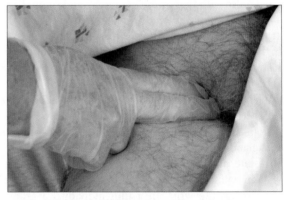

FIGURE **13-37** Palpation of femoral pulse.

pulsatile sensation when the arterial pulsation pushes your fingertips apart.

The popliteal pulse runs behind the knee (Figure 13-38). The patient should slightly flex the knee with the foot resting on the examination table. The patient also assumes a prone position with the knee slightly flexed. Instruct the patient to keep leg muscles relaxed. Palpate with the fingers of both hands deeply into the popliteal fossa, just lateral to the midline. The popliteal pulse is difficult to locate.

With the patient's foot relaxed locate the dorsalis pedis pulse. The artery runs along the top of the foot in a line with the groove between the extensor tendons of the great toe and first toe (Figure 13-39). You often find the pulse by placing your fingertips between the great and first toe and slowly inching up the foot. This pulse is sometimes congenitally absent. You find the posterior tibial pulse on the inner side of each ankle (Figure 13-40). Place your fingers behind and below the pa-

tient's medial malleolus (anklebone). You can easily locate the artery with the patient's foot relaxed and slightly extended.

**ULTRASOUND STETHOSCOPES.** If you have difficulty palpating a pulse, an ultrasound stethoscope is a useful tool that amplifies sounds of a pulse wave. Apply a thin layer of transmission gel to the patient's skin at the pulse site or directly onto the transducer tip of the probe. Turn on the volume control, and place the tip of the probe at a 45- to 90-degree angle on the skin. Move the probe until hearing a pulsating "whooshing" sound that indicates that arterial blood flow is present.

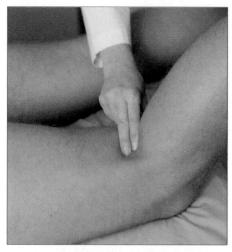

FIGURE **13-38** Palpation of popliteal pulse.

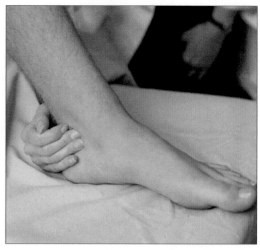

FIGURE **13-40** Palpation of posterior tibial pulse.

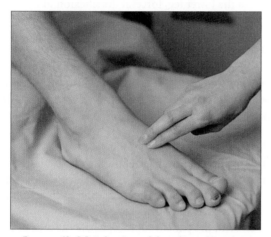

FIGURE **13-39** Palpation of dorsalis pedis pulse.

| TABLE 13-7 | **Signs of Venous and Arterial Insufficiency** | |
| --- | --- | --- |
| Assessment Criterion | Venous | Arterial |
| Color | Normal or cyanotic | Pale; worsened by elevation of extremity; dusky red when extremity lowered |
| Temperature | Normal | Cool (blood flow blocked to extremity) |
| Pulse | Normal | Decreased or absent |
| Edema | Often marked | Absent or mild |
| Skin changes | Brown pigmentation around ankles | Thin, shiny skin; decreased hair growth; thickened nails |

## Tissue Perfusion

The condition of the skin, mucosa, and nail beds offers useful data about the status of circulatory blood flow. Examine the face and upper extremities first, looking at the color of skin, mucosa, and nail beds. The presence of cyanosis requires special attention. Heart disease sometimes causes central cyanosis, which indicates poor arterial oxygenation. A bluish discoloration of the lips, mouth, and conjunctivae are characteristics of this. Blue lips, earlobes, and nail beds are signs of peripheral cyanosis, which indicates peripheral vasoconstriction. When cyanosis is present, consult with a physician or health care provider to have laboratory testing of oxygen saturation to determine severity of the problem. Examination of the nails involves inspection for **clubbing,** a bulging of the tissues at the nail base. Insufficient oxygenation at the periphery resulting from conditions such as congenital heart disease and chronic emphysema causes clubbing.

Inspect the lower extremities for changes in color, temperature, and condition of the skin indicating either arterial or venous alterations (Table 13-7). This is a good time to ask the patient about history of pain in the legs. If an arterial occlusion is present, the patient has signs resulting from absence of blood flow. Pain will be distal to the occlusion. The three *P*'s characterize an occlusion—*pain, pallor,* and *pulselessness.* Venous congestion causes tissue changes indicating inadequate circulatory flow back to the heart.

During examination of the lower extremities, you also inspect skin and nail texture; hair distribution on the lower legs, feet, and toes; venous pattern; and scars, pigmentation, or ulcers. The absence of hair growth over the legs indicates circulatory insufficiency. Remember, do not confuse an absence of hair on the legs with shaven legs. Also, many men have less hair around the calves because of tight-fitting dress socks or jeans. Chronic recurring ulcers of the feet or lower legs are a serious sign of circulatory insufficiency and require a physician or health care provider's intervention.

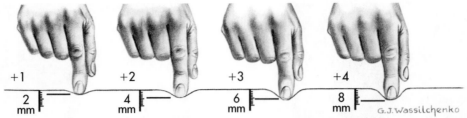

FIGURE **13-41** Assessing for pitting edema. (From Seidel HM and others: *Mosby's guide to physical examination*, ed 5, St. Louis, 2003. Mosby.)

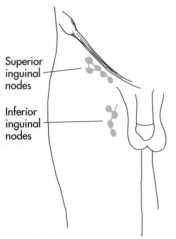

FIGURE **13-42** Inguinal lymph nodes.

## Peripheral Veins

Assess the status of the peripheral veins by asking the patient to assume sitting and standing positions. Assessment includes inspection and palpation for varicosities, peripheral edema, and phlebitis. Varicosities are superficial veins that become dilated, especially when legs are in a dependent position. They are common in older adults because the veins normally fibrose, dilate, and stretch. They are also common in people who stand for prolonged periods. Varicosities in the anterior or medial part of the thigh and the posterolateral part of the calf are abnormal.

Dependent edema around the feet and ankles is a sign of venous insufficiency or right-sided heart failure. Dependent edema is common in older adults and persons who spend a lot of time standing (e.g., nurses, waitresses, and security guards). To assess for pitting edema use your thumb to press firmly 1 to 2 seconds and then release over the medial malleolus or the shins. A depression left in the skin indicates edema. Grading +1 through +4 characterizes the severity of the edema (Figure 13-41).

**Phlebitis** is an inflammation of a vein that occurs commonly after trauma to the vessel wall, infection, immobilization, or prolonged insertion of IV catheters (see Chapter 15). Phlebitis promotes clot formation, a potentially dangerous situation because a clot within a deep vein of the leg can become dislodged and travel through the heart, causing a pulmonary embolus. To assess for phlebitis inspect the calves for localized redness, tenderness, and swelling over vein sites. Gentle palpation of calf muscles reveals warmth, tenderness and firmness of the muscle. Unilateral edema of the affected leg is one of the most reliable findings of phlebitis (Day, 2003). Also check for Homans' sign by supporting the leg while dorsiflexing the foot. If phlebitis is present in the lower leg, forceful dorsiflexion of the foot often causes pain in the calf. However, Homans' sign is not always a reliable indicator of phlebitis and is present in other conditions (Crowther and McCourt, 2004; Day, 2003). If there is a strong suspicion of phlebitis, testing for Homans' sign is contraindicated. If a clot is present, it may become dislodged from its original site during this test, resulting in a pulmonary embolism.

## Lymphatic System

Assess the lymphatic drainage of the lower extremities during examination of the vascular system or during the female or male genital examination. Superficial and deep lymph nodes drain the legs, but only two groups of superficial nodes are palpable. With the patient supine, palpate the area of the superior superficial nodes in the groin area (Figure 13-42). Then move your fingertips toward the inner thigh, feeling for any palpable inferior nodes. Use a firm but gentle pressure when palpating over each lymphatic chain. Multiple nodes are not normally palpable, although a few soft, nontender nodes are not unusual. Enlarged, hardened, tender nodes reveal potential sites of infection or metastatic disease.

## Breasts

It is important to examine the breasts of female and male patients. A small amount of glandular tissue, a potential site for the growth of cancer cells, is located in the male breast. In contrast, the majority of the female breast is glandular tissue.

### Female Breasts

New cases of breast cancer were expected to affect 211,240 women in the United States in 2005 (ACS, 2005). The disease is second to lung cancer as the leading cause of death in women with cancer. Early detection is the key to cure. A major responsibility for you is to teach patients health behaviors such as breast self-examination (BSE) (Box 13-17).

## BOX 13-17 FEMALE BREAST HEALTH

**Breast Self-Examination**

Tell patients to do a breast self-examination (BSE) once a month so that they become familiar with the usual appearance and feel of their breasts. Familiarity makes it easier to notice any changes in the breast from one month to another. Early discovery of a change from what is "normal" is the main idea behind BSE.

For patients who menstruate, the best time to do BSE is the last day of the menstrual cycle, when their breasts are least likely to be tender or swollen. For patients who no longer menstruate, pick a day, such as the first day of the month, to remind them it is time to do BSE.

Teach the following steps:

1. Stand before a mirror. Inspect both breasts for anything unusual, such as any discharge from the nipples, puckering, dimpling, or scaling of the skin.

   The next two steps are designed to emphasize any change in the shape or contour of your breasts. As you do them, you will be able to feel your chest muscles tighten.

2. Watching closely in the mirror, clasp your hands behind your head and press your hands forward.

3. Next, press your hands firmly on your hips and bow slightly toward your mirror as you pull your shoulders and elbows forward.

Some women do the next part of the examination in the shower. Fingers glide over soapy skin, making it easy to appreciate the texture underneath.

4. Raise your left arm over your head. Use three or four fingers of your right hand to explore your left breast firmly, carefully, and thoroughly. Beginning at the outer edge, press the flat part of your fingers in small circles, moving the circles slowly around the breast. Gradually work toward the nipple. Be sure to cover the entire breast. Pay special attention to the area between the breast and the armpit (upper outer quadrant), including the armpit itself. Feel for any unusual lump or mass under the skin.

5. Gently squeeze the nipple and look for a discharge. Repeat the examination on your right breast.

6. Repeat Steps 4 and 5 lying down. Lie flat on your back, with your left arm raised back, and hand behind your neck and a pillow or folded towel under your left shoulder. This position flattens the breast and makes it easier to examine. Use the same circular motion described earlier.

   Repeat on your right breast.

- Have the patient perform return demonstration of BSE, and offer the opportunity to ask questions.
- Explain recommended frequency of mammography and assessment by a health care provider.
- Discuss signs and symptoms of breast cancer.
- Discuss signs and symptoms of fibrocystic disease.
- Inform a woman who is obese or who has a family history of breast cancer that she is at higher risk for the disease (ACS, 2005). Encourage dietary changes, including limiting meat consumption to well-trimmed, lean beef, pork, or lamb; removing skin from cooked chicken before eating it; selecting tuna and salmon packed in water and not oil; and using low-fat dairy products.
- Encourage the patient to reduce intake of caffeine. Although controversial, decreasing caffeine intake is believed to reduce symptoms of benign (fibrocystic) breast disease.

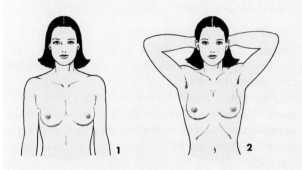

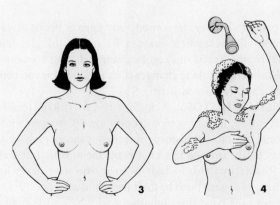

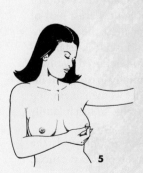

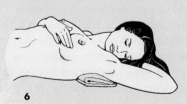

From Seidel HM and others: *Mosby's guide to physical examination,* ed 5, St. Louis, 2003, Mosby.

**BOX 13-18 Normal Changes in the Breast During a Woman's Life Span**

**Puberty (8 to 20 Years)***

Breasts mature in five stages. One breast may grow more rapidly than the other. The ages at which changes occur and rate of developmental progression vary.

**Stage 1 (Preadolescent)**

This stage involves elevation of the nipple only.

**Stage 2**

The breast and nipple elevate as a small mound, and the areolar diameters enlarge.

**Stage 3**

There is further enlargement and elevation of the breast and areola, with no separation of contour.

**Stage 4**

The areola and nipple project into the secondary mound above the level of the breast (does not occur in all girls).

**Stage 5 (Mature Breast)**

Only the nipple projects, and the areola recedes (varies in some women).

**Young Adulthood (20 to 30 Years)**

Breasts reach full (nonpregnant) size. Shape is generally symmetrical. Breasts are sometimes unequal in size.

**Pregnancy**

Breast size gradually enlarges to two to three times the previous size. Nipples enlarge and become erect. Areolae darken, and diameters increase. Superficial veins become prominent. The nipples expel a yellowish fluid (colostrum).

**Menopause**

Breasts shrink. Tissue becomes softer, sometimes flabby.

**Older Adulthood**

Breasts become elongated, pendulous, and flaccid as a result of glandular tissue atrophy. The skin of the breasts tends to wrinkle, appearing loose and flabby.

Nipples become smaller, flatter, and lose erectile ability.† Nipples invert because of shrinkage and fibrotic changes.‡

Data from:
*Hockenberry MJ and others: *Wong's essentials of pediatric nursing*, ed 7, St. Louis, 2005, Elsevier Mosby.
†Seidel HM and others: *Mosby's guide to physical examination*, ed 5, St. Louis, 2003, Mosby.
‡Ebersole P and others: *Toward healthy aging*, ed 6, St. Louis, 2004, Elsevier Mosby.

If the patient already performs self-examination, assess the method she uses and the time she does the examination in relation to her menstrual cycle. The best time for a self-examination is on the last day of the menstrual period, when the breast is no longer swollen or tender from hormone elevations. If the woman is postmenopausal, advise her to check her breasts on the same day each month. The pregnant woman should also check her breasts on a monthly basis.

Older women require special attention when reviewing the need for BSE. Fixed incomes limit many older women, and thus they fail to pursue regular clinical breast examination and mammography. Unfortunately, many older women ignore changes in their breasts, assuming they are a part of aging. In addition, physiological factors affect the ease with which older women can perform BSE. Musculoskeletal limitations, diminished peripheral sensation, reduced eyesight, and changes in joint range of motion limit palpation and inspection abilities. Find resources for older women, including free screening programs. Often you are able to teach family members to perform examinations.

The American Cancer Society (2005) recommends the following guidelines for the early detection of breast cancer:

1. Women 20 years of age and older need to perform BSE monthly.

2. Women need an examination by a physician or health care provider every 3 years from ages 20 to 40, and yearly for women over 40.
3. Women with a family history of breast cancer need a yearly examination by a physician or health care provider.
4. Asymptomatic women need a screening mammogram by age 40; women age 40 and over need a mammogram annually.
5. For women with a history of breast cancer, the ACS recommends a yearly examination.

The patient's history alerts you to any signs of breast disease and normal development changes. Because of this glandular structure, the breast undergoes changes during a woman's life. Knowledge of these changes (Box 13-18) helps you complete an accurate assessment.

**HEALTH HISTORY.** A history reveals risk factors for breast cancer, including women over age 40, women with a personal or family history of breast cancer, early-onset menarche (before age 13), or late-age menopause (after age 50). Risk factors also include women who have never had children, who gave birth to their first child after age 30, who have not breast-fed their infants, or who have diets high in fat. A history also determines whether a patient (both sexes) has signs and symptoms of breast cancer such as a lump,

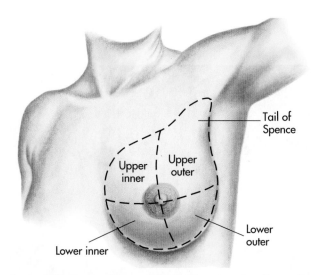

FIGURE **13-43** Quadrants of the left breast and axillary tail of Spence. (From Seidel HM and others: *Mosby's guide to physical examination,* ed 5, St. Louis, 2003, Mosby.)

thickening, pain, or tenderness of the breast; discharge, distortion, retraction, or scaling of the nipple; or change in breast size. Determine the patient's use of medications that create risk, such as oral contraceptives, digitalis, diuretics, steroids, or estrogen. Assess the patient's caffeine intake to review risk factors for fibrocystic disease. Ask if the patient performs monthly BSE. If so, determine the time of month she performs the examination in relation to her menstrual cycle. Have the patient describe or demonstrate the method used. If the patient reports a breast mass, perform a symptom analysis.

**INSPECTION.** Have the patient remove the top gown or drape to allow simultaneous visualization of both breasts. Have the patient stand or sit with her arms hanging loosely at her sides. If possible, place a mirror in front of the patient during inspection so she sees what to look for when performing self-examination. To recognize abnormalities, the patient needs to be familiar with the normal appearance of her breasts.

Describe observations or findings in relation to imaginary lines that divide the breast into four quadrants and a tail. The lines cross at the center of the nipple. Each tail extends outward from the upper outer quadrant (Figure 13-43).

Inspect the breasts for size and symmetry. Normally the breasts extend from the third to the sixth ribs, with the nipple at the level of the fourth intercostal space. It is common for one breast to be smaller. However, inflammation or a mass can cause a difference in size. As the woman becomes older, the ligaments supporting the breast tissue weaken, causing the breasts to sag and the nipples to lower.

Observe the contour or shape of the breasts, and note masses, flattening, retraction, or dimpling. Breasts vary in shape from convex to pendulous or conical. Retraction or dimpling results from invasion of underlying ligaments by tu-

mors. The ligaments fibrose and pull the overlying skin inward toward the tumor. Edema also changes the contour of the breasts. To bring out the presence of retraction or changes in the shape of the breasts, ask the patient to assume three positions: raise arms above the head, press hands against the hips, and extend arms straight ahead while sitting and leaning forward. Each maneuver causes a contraction of the pectoral muscles, which will accentuate the presence of any retraction.

Carefully inspect the skin for color; venous pattern; and presence of edema, lesions, or inflammation. Lift each breast when necessary to observe lower and lateral aspects for color and texture changes. The breasts are the color of neighboring skin, and venous patterns are the same bilaterally. You see venous patterns more easily in thin patients or pregnant women. Women with large breasts often have redness and excoriation of the undersurface caused by rubbing of skin surfaces.

Inspect the nipple and areola for size, color, shape, discharge, and the direction the nipples point. The normal areolae are round or oval and nearly equal bilaterally. Color ranges from pink to brown. In light-skinned women the areola turns brown during pregnancy and remains dark. In dark-skinned women the areola is brown before pregnancy (Seidel and others, 2003). Normally the nipples point in symmetrical directions, are everted, and have no drainage. If the nipples are inverted, ask if this has been a lifetime history. A recent inversion or inward turning of the nipple indicates an underlying growth. Rashes or ulcerations are not normal on the breast or nipples. Note any bleeding or discharge from the nipple. Clear yellow discharge 2 days after childbirth is common. While inspecting the breasts, explain the characteristics seen. Teach the patient the significance of abnormal signs or symptoms.

**PALPATION.** Palpation allows you to determine the condition of underlying breast tissue and lymph nodes. Breast tissue consists of glandular tissue, fibrous supportive ligaments, and fat. Glandular tissue is organized into lobes that end in ducts opening onto the nipple's surface. The largest portion of glandular tissue is in the upper outer quadrant and tail of each breast. Suspensory ligaments connect to skin and fascia underlying the breast to support the breast and maintain its upright position. Fatty tissue is located superficially and to the sides of the breast.

A large proportion of lymph from the breasts drains into axillary lymph nodes. If cancerous lesions **metastasize** or spread, the nodes commonly become involved. You need to learn the location of supraclavicular, infraclavicular, and axillary nodes (Figure 13-44). The axillary nodes drain lymph from the chest wall, breasts, arms, and hands. A tumor of one breast sometimes involves nodes on the opposite side, as well as those on the same side.

To palpate lymph nodes have the patient sit with arms at her sides and muscles relaxed. While facing the patient and standing on the side being examined, support the patient's arm in a flexed position and abduct the arm from the chest wall. Place

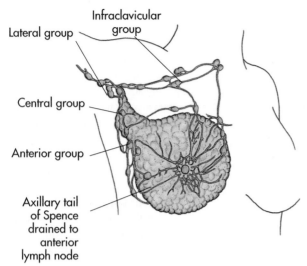

FIGURE **13-44** Anatomical position of axillary and clavicular lymph nodes.

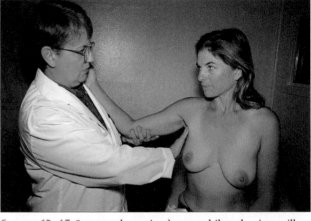

FIGURE **13-45** Support the patient's arm while palpating axillary lymph nodes.

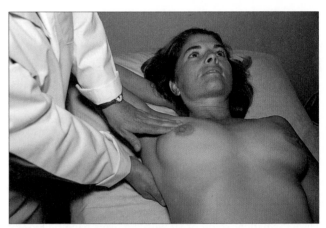

FIGURE **13-46** Patient lies flat with arm abducted and hand under head to help flatten breast tissue evenly over the chest wall. Palpate each breast in systematic fashion.

your free hand against the patient's chest wall and high in the axillary hollow (Figure 13-45). With your fingertips press gently down over the surface of the ribs and muscles. Palpate the axillary nodes with your fingertips gently rolling soft tissue. Palpate four areas of the axilla at the edge of the pectoralis major muscle along the anterior axillary line, the chest wall in the midaxillary area, the upper part of the humerus, and the anterior edge of the latissimus dorsi muscle along the posterior axillary line. Normally lymph nodes are not palpable. A palpable node feels like a small mass that is hard, tender, or immobile. Also palpate along the upper and lower clavicular ridges. Reverse the procedure for the patient's other side.

It is sometimes difficult for the patient to learn to palpate for lymph nodes. Lying down with the arm abducted makes the area more accessible. Instruct your patient to use her left hand for the right axillary and clavicular areas and vice versa. Take the patient's fingertips, and move them in the proper fashion.

You perform palpation of breast tissue best with the patient lying supine and one arm behind the head (alternating with each breast). The supine position allows the breast tissue to flatten evenly against the chest wall. The patient raises her hand and places it behind the neck to further stretch and position breast tissue evenly. Place a small pillow or towel under the patient's shoulder blade to further position breast tissue.

The consistency of normal breast tissue varies widely. The breasts of a young patient are firm and elastic. In an older patient the tissue may feel stringy and nodular. The patient's familiarity with the texture of her own breasts is most important. Patients gain familiarity through monthly BSE (see Box 13-17).

If the patient complains of a mass, examine the opposite breast first to ensure an objective comparison of normal and abnormal tissue. Use the pads of your first three fingers to compress breast tissue gently against the chest wall, noting tis-

sue consistency (Figure 13-46). Perform palpation systematically in one of three ways: *(A)* using a vertical technique with the fingers moving up and down each quadrant; *(B)* clockwise or counterclockwise, forming small circles with the fingers along each quadrant and the tail; or *(C)* palpating from center of the breast in a radial fashion, returning to the areola to begin each spoke (Figure 13-47). Whatever approach you use, be sure to cover the entire breast and tail, directing attention to any areas of tenderness. When palpating large, pendulous breasts, use a bimanual technique. Support the inferior portion of the breast in one hand while you use your other hand to palpate breast tissue against the supporting hand.

During palpation note the consistency of breast tissue. It normally feels dense, firm, and elastic. With menopause, breast tissue shrinks and becomes softer. The lobular feel of glandular tissue is normal. The lower edge of each breast feels firm and hard. This is the normal inframammary ridge

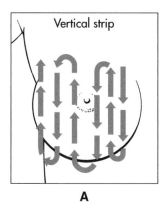
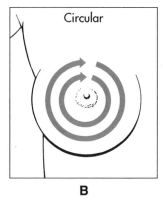
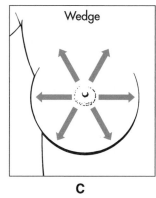

| **A** | **B** | **C** |

FIGURE **13-47** Various methods for breast palpation. **A,** Palpate from top to bottom in vertical strips. **B,** Palpate in concentric circles. **C,** Palpate out from the center in wedge sections. (From Seidel HM and others: *Mosby's guide to physical examination,* ed 5, St. Louis, 2003, Mosby.)

and is not a tumor. It helps to move the patient's hand so she feels normal tissue variations. Palpate abnormal masses to determine location in relation to quadrants, diameter in centimeters, shape (e.g., round or discoid), consistency (soft, firm, or hard), tenderness, mobility, and discreteness (clear or unclear borders). Cancerous lesions are hard, fixed, nontender, irregular in shape, and usually unilateral.

A common benign condition of the breast is **benign (fibrocystic) breast disease.** Bilateral lumpy, painful breasts and sometimes nipple discharge characterize this condition. Symptoms are more apparent during the menstrual period. When palpated, the cysts (lumps) are soft, well differentiated, and moveable. Deep cysts feel hard.

Give special attention to palpating the nipple and areola. Palpate the entire surface gently. Use your thumb and index finger to compress the nipple, and note any discharge. As you examine the nipple and areola, the nipple may become erect with wrinkling of the areola. These changes are normal.

After completing the examination, have the patient demonstrate self-palpation. Observe the patient's technique, and emphasize the importance of a systematic approach. Urge the patient to see her physician or health care provider if she discovers an abnormal mass during monthly self-examination.

## Male Breasts

Examination of the male breast is relatively easy. Inspect the nipple and areola for nodules, edema, and ulceration. An enlarged male breast results from obesity or glandular enlargement. Breast enlargement in young males results from steroid use. Fatty tissue feels soft, whereas glandular tissue is firm. Use the same techniques to palpate for masses used in examination of the female breast. Because male breast cancer is relatively rare, routine self-examinations are unnecessary.

## Abdomen

The abdominal examination is complex because of the number of organs located within and near the abdominal cavity. The organs are assessed anteriorly and posteriorly. A system of landmarks helps to map out the abdominal region. The

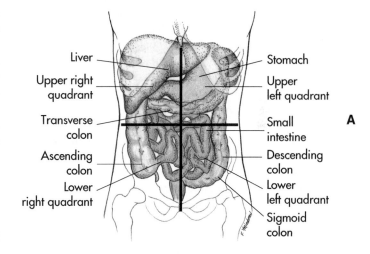

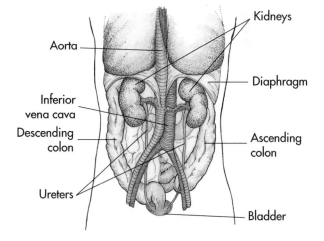

FIGURE **13-48 A,** Anterior view of abdomen divided by quadrants. **B,** Posterior view of abdominal sections.

xiphoid process (tip of the sternum) is the upper boundary of the anterior abdominal region. The symphysis pubis delineates the lower boundary. By dividing the abdomen into four imaginary quadrants (Figure 13-48, *A*), refer to assessment findings and record them in relation to each quadrant. Posteriorly, the lower ribs and heavy back muscles protect the kidneys, which are located from the T13 to L3 vertebrae (Figure 13-48, *B*). The costovertebral angle formed by the last rib and vertebral column is a landmark used during palpation of the kidney.

The examination includes an assessment of structures of the lower gastrointestinal (GI) tract in addition to the liver, stomach, kidneys, and bladder. Abdominal pain is one of the most common symptoms patients will report when seeking medical care. An accurate assessment requires matching patient history data with a careful assessment of the location of physical symptoms.

During the abdominal examination, the patient needs to be relaxed. A tightening of abdominal muscles hinders palpation. Ask the patient to void before beginning. Be sure the room is warm, and drape the patient's upper chest and legs. The patient lies supine or in a dorsal recumbent position with the arms at the sides and knees slightly bent. Place small pillows beneath the knees. If the patient places the arms under the head, the abdominal muscles tighten. Proceed calmly and slowly, being sure there is adequate lighting. Expose the abdomen from just above the xiphoid process down to the symphysis pubis. Warm hands and stethoscope further promote relaxation. Ask the patient to report pain and point out areas of tenderness. Assess tender areas last.

The order for an abdominal examination differs slightly from previous assessments. The nurse begins with inspection and then auscultation. By using auscultation before palpation, there is less chance of altering the frequency and character of bowel sounds. During the examination you need a tape measure and marking pen.

### Health History

Ask whether the patient has abdominal or low back pain, and assess the character of the pain in detail (see Chapter 30). Also review the patient's normal bowel habits and stool character. Ask if the patient uses laxatives. Determine if the patient has had abdominal surgery, trauma, or diagnostic tests of the GI tract. Signs and symptoms of belching, difficulty swallowing, flatulence, bloody emesis (**hematemesis**), black tarry stools (**melena**), heartburn, diarrhea, or constipation reveal a pattern of a problem. Also ask if the patient has had a recent weight change or intolerance to diet. If the patient takes antiinflammatory drugs (e.g., aspirin, ibuprofen, or steroids) and antibiotics, there is risk for GI upset or bleeding. Inquire about a family history of cancer, kidney disease, alcoholism, hypertension, or heart disease. Assess the patient's usual intake of alcohol. Also determine if the female patient is pregnant, and note her last menstrual period. Review the patient's history for risk factors of hepatitis B virus exposure. Finally, ask the patient to locate tender areas before beginning the examination.

### Inspection

Make it a habit to observe the patient during routine care activities. Note the patient's posture, and look for evidence of abdominal splinting, lying with the knees drawn up, or moving restlessly in bed. A patient free from abdominal pain will not stoop or splint the abdomen. To inspect the abdomen for abnormal movement or shadows, stand on the patient's right side and inspect the abdomen from above. By sitting down to look across the abdomen, you assess abdominal contour. Direct the examination light over the abdomen.

Inspect the skin over the abdomen for color, scars, venous patterns, lesions, and **striae** (stretch marks). The skin is subject to the same color variations as the rest of the body. Venous patterns are normally faint, except in thin patients. Artificial openings indicate drainage sites resulting from surgery or an ostomy. Scars reveal evidence of past trauma or surgery that created permanent changes in underlying organ anatomy. Bruising indicates accidental injury, physical abuse, or a type of bleeding disorder. Ask if the patient self-administers injections (e.g., insulin or low-molecular-weight heparin). Unexpected findings include generalized color changes such as jaundice or cyanosis. A glistening taut appearance indicates ascites.

Inspection continues with the umbilicus. Note the position; shape; color; and presence of inflammation, discharge, or protruding masses. A normal umbilicus is flat or concave with the color the same as surrounding skin. Inspect for contour, symmetry, and surface motion of the abdomen, noting any masses, bulging, or distention. A flat abdomen forms a horizontal plane from the xiphoid process to the symphysis pubis. A round abdomen protrudes in a convex sphere from a horizontal plane. A concave abdomen appears to sink into the muscular wall. Each of these findings is normal if the shape of the abdomen is symmetrical. In older adults there is often an overall increased distribution of adipose tissue.

The presence of masses on only one side, or asymmetry, indicates an underlying pathological condition. Observe the contour of the abdomen while asking the patient to take a deep breath and hold it. Normally the contour remains smooth and symmetrical. To evaluate abdominal musculature, have the patient raise the head. This position causes superficial abdominal wall masses, hernias, and muscle separations to become more apparent.

Intestinal gas, tumor, or fluid in the abdominal cavity causes distention (swelling). When distention is generalized, the entire abdomen protrudes. The skin often appears taut, as if it were stretched over. When gas causes distention, the flanks do not bulge. However, if fluid is the source of the problem, such as in ascites, the flanks bulge. Ask the patient to roll onto one side. A protuberance forms on the dependent side if fluid is the cause of the distention. Ask the patient if the abdomen feels unusually tight. Be careful not to confuse distention with obesity. In obesity the abdomen is large, rolls of adipose tissue are often present along the flanks, and the patient does not complain of tightness in the abdomen. If you expect abdominal distention, measure the girth of the abdomen by placing a tape measure around the abdomen at the level of the umbilicus. Consecutive measurements will show any increase or decrease in distention. Use a marking pen to indicate where you applied the tape measure.

Next inspect for movement. Normally men breathe abdominally and women breathe more costally. If the patient has severe pain, it diminishes respiratory movement and the pa-

PATIENT TEACHING

**Abdominal Health**
- Explain factors that promote normal bowel elimination, such as diet, regular exercise, limited use of over-the-counter drugs causing constipation, establishment of a regular elimination schedule, and a good fluid intake (see Chapter 33). Stress importance for older adults.
- Caution patients about dangers of excessive use of laxatives or enemas.
- Instruct patients to have acute abdominal pain evaluated by a health care provider.
- If the patient has chronic pain, explain measures used for pain relief (e.g., relaxation exercises, positioning) (see Chapter 30).
- Instruct the patient about warning signs of colon cancer, including bleeding from the rectum, pain, black or tarry stools, blood in the stool, and a change in bowel habits (constipation or diarrhea).
- If patient is a health care worker or has contact with blood or body fluids of affected persons, encourage patient to receive series of three hepatitis B vaccine doses.

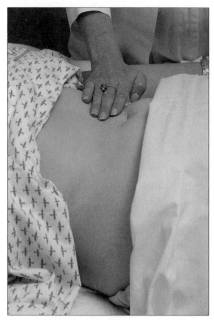

FIGURE **13-49** Light palpation of the abdomen.

tient tightens abdominal muscles to guard against the pain. Also observe for peristaltic movement or aortic pulsation by looking across the abdomen from the side. You see these movements in thin patients; otherwise no movement is present.

## Auscultation

Auscultate the abdomen to listen to the bowel sounds of normal intestinal contractions (**peristalsis**) and to detect vascular sounds. Patients with GI tubes connected to suction need them temporarily turned off before beginning the examination. Place the warmed diaphragm of the stethoscope lightly over each of the four quadrants. Ask the patient not to speak. Normally air and fluid move through the intestines, creating soft gurgling or clicking sounds that occur irregularly 5 to 35 times per minute (Seidel and others, 2003). Sounds may last 1½ seconds to several seconds. It normally takes 5 to 20 seconds to hear a bowel sound. However, it may take 5 minutes of continuous listening before determining bowel sounds are absent. Auscultate all four quadrants to be sure you do not miss any sounds. The best time to auscultate is between meals. Sounds are generally described as normal, audible, absent, hyperactive, or hypoactive.

Absent sounds indicate cessation of GI motility that results from late-stage bowel obstruction, **paralytic ileus** (decreased or absent peristalsis), or **peritonitis** (inflammation of the peritoneum). Hyperactive sounds are loud, "growling" sounds called **borborygmi,** which indicate increased GI motility. Inflammation of the bowel, anxiety, bleeding, excess ingestion of laxatives, and reaction of the intestines to certain foods cause increased motility (Box 13-19).

Bruits indicate narrowing of major blood vessels and disruption of blood flow. Presence of bruits in the abdominal area reveal aneurysms or stenotic vessels. Use the bell of the stethoscope to auscultate in the epigastric region and each of the four quadrants. Normally there are no vascular sounds over the aorta (midline through the abdomen) or femoral arteries (lower quadrants). Report a bruit immediately to a physician or health care provider.

## Palpation

Palpation primarily detects areas of abdominal tenderness, abnormal distention, or masses. As you become more skilled, you will learn to palpate for specific organs such as the liver. You will use light and deep palpation.

Perform light palpation over each abdominal quadrant. Initially avoid areas previously identified as problem spots. Lay the palm of your hand with fingers extended and approximated lightly on the abdomen. Explain the maneuver to the patient, and then with the palmar surface of your fingers depress 1.3 cm (½ inch) in a gentle dipping motion (Figure 13-49). Avoid quick jabs, and use smooth, coordinated movements. For ticklish patients, first place your hand under the patient's abdomen until they tolerate palpation. Feel for muscular resistance, tenderness, and superficial organs or masses. While palpating, observe the patient's face for signs of discomfort. The abdomen is normally smooth with consistent softness and nontender without masses. The older adult often lacks abdominal tone.

With experience you will perform deep palpation (Figure 13-50) to delineate abdominal organs and to detect less obvious masses. A qualified examiner will assist you until you become skilled in the technique. You will need to have short fingernails. It is important for the patient to be relaxed while your hands are depressed approximately 2.5 to 7.5 cm (1 to 3 inches) into the abdomen. Never use deep palpation over a surgical incision or over extremely tender organs. It is also unwise to use deep palpation on abnormal masses. Deep

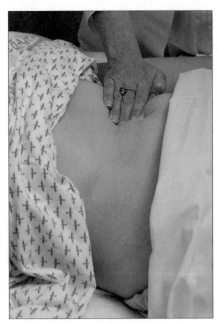

FIGURE **13-50** Deep palpation of the abdomen.

pressure causes tenderness in the healthy patient over the cecum, sigmoid colon, and aorta and in the midline near the xiphoid process (Seidel and others, 2003).

Survey each quadrant systematically. Palpate masses for size, location, shape, consistency, tenderness, pulsation, and mobility. If you note tenderness, check for rebound tenderness. Perform this test by pressing your hand slowly and deeply into the involved area and then let go quickly. If you elicit pain with the release of the hand, the test is positive. Rebound tenderness occurs in patients with peritoneal irritation such as in appendicitis; pancreatitis; or any peritoneal injury causing bile, blood, or enzymes to enter the peritoneal cavity.

To assess aortic pulsation, palpate with the thumb and forefinger of one hand deeply into the upper abdomen just left of the midline. Normally a pulsation is transmitted forward. If there is enlargement of the aorta from an **aneurysm** (localized dilation of a vessel wall), the pulsation expands laterally. Do not palpate a pulsating abdominal mass. In obese patients it is often necessary to palpate with both hands, one on each side of the aorta.

## Female Genitalia

Examination of the female genitalia, including external and internal sex organs, is embarrassing to the patient unless you use a calm, relaxed approach. The gynecological examination is one of the most difficult experiences for adolescents. Cultural background further adds to apprehension. For example, female Mexican-Americans have a strong social value that women do not expose their bodies to men or even to other women. Provide a thorough explanation as to the rea-

son for the procedures used in the examination. The lithotomy position assumed during the examination is an added source of embarrassment. You achieve comfort through correct positioning and draping. Be sure to explain each portion of the examination in advance so that patients anticipate your actions. Adolescents sometimes choose to have parents present in the examination room.

Sometimes a patient requires a complete examination, including assessing external genitalia and performing a vaginal examination. The nurse may examine external genitalia while performing routine hygiene measures or preparing to insert a urinary catheter. An examination is a part of each woman's preventive health care, because ovarian cancer causes more deaths than any other cancer of the female reproductive system (ACS, 2005).

Adolescents and young adults are examined because of the growing incidence of sexually transmitted diseases (STDs). The average age of menarche among young girls has declined, and the majority of male and female teenagers are sexually active by age 19 (Hockenberry and others, 2005). You can easily combine rectal and anal assessments with this examination because the patient assumes a lithotomy or dorsal recumbent position.

### Health History

The history reviews the patient's previous illnesses or surgeries involving reproductive organs, including STDs. A review of the menstrual history includes age at menarche, frequency and duration of cycle, character of flow, presence of **dysmenorrhea,** pelvic pain, dates of last two menstrual periods, and premenstrual symptoms. You also assess for signs of bleeding, vaginal discharge, or pain outside the normal menstrual period or after menopause. A review of the patient's obstetrical history is also valuable. Ask your patient if she has symptoms of genitourinary problems such as burning during urination, frequency, urgency, nocturia, hematuria, incontinence, or stress incontinence.

Ask the patient to describe her obstetrical history, including each pregnancy and history of abortions or miscarriages. Also question the patient about current and past contraceptive practices and problems encountered. It is important to determine if your patient uses safe sex practices. Discuss risks of STDs and HIV infection. Determine if the patient has signs and symptoms of vaginal discharge, painful or swollen perianal tissues, or genital lesions. Also review a patient's risk for developing cervical, endometrial, or ovarian cancer (Box 13-20).

### Preparing the Patient

As a beginning nurse, your responsibility will be assisting the patient's primary health care provider with the examination. You perform this examination best with the patient lying on an examination table or with the patient in bed with the legs supported with pillows or bath blankets. You will need the following equipment for a complete examination: examination table with stirrups; vaginal speculum of correct size; ad-

PATIENT TEACHING

**Female Genitalia Health**

- Instruct the patient about the purpose and recommended frequency of Papanicolaou (Pap) smears and gynecological examinations. Explain that the Pap smear is relatively painless and needed annually with a pelvic examination for women who are sexually active or who are over age 21. At age 30 or after, women who have three consecutive normal tests are screened every 2 to 3 years (ACS, 2005). Patients are screened more often if certain risk factors exist such as a weak immune system, multiple sex partners, smoking, and a history of infections (e.g., human papillomavirus [HPV]).
- Counsel patients with STDs about diagnosis and treatment.
- Instruct on genital self-examination: Using a mirror, position self to examine the area covered by the pubic hair. Spread the hair apart, looking for bumps, sores, or blisters, Also, look for any warts, which appear as small, bumpy spots and that enlarge to fleshy, cauliflower-like lesions. Next, spread the outer vaginal lips apart and look at the clitoris for bumps, blisters, sores, or warts. Also look at both sides of the inner vaginal lips. Inspect the area around the urinary and vaginal opening for bumps, blisters, sores, or warts.
- Explain warning signs of STDs: pain or burning on urination, pain during sex, pain in the pelvic area, bleeding between menstruation, an itchy rash around the vagina, and vaginal discharge (different from usual).
- Teach measures to prevent STDs (e.g., male partner's use of condoms, restricting number of sexual partners, avoidance of sex with persons who have several other partners, perineal hygiene measures).
- Tell patients with STDs to inform their sexual partner of the need for an examination.
- Reinforce the importance of perineal hygiene (as appropriate).

justable light source; sink; clean, disposable gloves; glass microscopic slides; plastic spatula and/or Cytobrush; and specimen bottles with fixative spray (hairspray).

Make sure equipment is ready before the examination begins. Ask the patient to empty her bladder so that she does not expel urine accidentally during the examination. Often it is necessary to collect a urine specimen. Assist the patient to the lithotomy position, in bed or on an examination table, for an external genitalia assessment. Assist the patient into stirrups for a speculum examination. Have the woman stabilize each foot in a stirrup, and then have her slide the buttocks down to the edge of the examining table. Place your hand at the edge of the table and instruct the patient to move until touching the hand. The patient's arms are at her sides or folded across the chest to prevent tightening of abdominal muscles.

A woman suffering from pain or deformity of the joints is sometimes unable to assume a lithotomy position. In this situation, it is necessary to have the patient abduct only one leg or to have another assist in separating the patient's thighs. Also, use the side-lying position with the patient on the left side and the right thigh and knee drawn up to her chest.

Give a square drape or sheet to the patient. She holds one corner over her sternum, the adjacent corners fall over each knee, and the fourth corner falls over the perineum. After the examination begins, lift the drape over the perineum. The male examiner always needs to have a female in attendance during the examination. A female examiner may prefer to work alone but should have a female attendant if the patient is particularly anxious or emotionally unstable.

## External Genitalia

Make sure the perineal area is well illuminated. Apply gloves on both hands. The perineum is extremely sensitive and tender; do not touch the area suddenly without warning the patient. It is best to touch the neighboring thigh first before advancing to the perineum.

While sitting at the end of the examination table or bed, inspect the quantity and distribution of hair growth. Preadolescents have no pubic hair. During adolescence hair grows along the labia, becoming darker, coarser, and curlier. In an adult, hair grows in a triangle over the female perineum and along the medial surface of the thighs. Hair is normally free of nits and lice.

Inspect surface characteristics of the labia majora. The skin of the perineum is smooth, clean, and slightly darker than other skin. The mucous membranes appear dark pink and moist. The labia majora are gaping or closed and appear dry or moist. They are usually symmetrical. After childbirth the labia majora separate, causing the labia minora to become more prominent. When a woman reaches menopause, the labia majora become thinned. With advancing age they become **atrophied** (decrease in size). The labia majora are normally without inflammation, edema, lesions, or lacerations.

To inspect the remaining external structures, use your nondominant hand and gently place the thumb and index finger inside the labia minora and retract the tissues outward (Figure 13-51). Be sure to have a firm hold to avoid repeated retraction against the sensitive tissues. Use your other hand to palpate the labia minora between the thumb and second finger. On inspection the labia minora are normally thinner than the labia majora, and one side may be larger. The tissue feels soft on palpation and without tenderness. The size of the clitoris is variable, but it normally does not exceed 2 cm in length and 0.5 cm in diameter. Look for atrophy, inflammation, or adhesions. If inflamed, the clitoris will be a bright cherry red. In young women it is a common site for syphilitic lesions or **chancres,** which appear as small open ulcers that drain serous material. Older women may have malignant changes that result in dry, scaly, nodular lesions.

Inspect the urethral orifice carefully for color and position. It is normally intact and without inflammation. The urethral meatus is anterior to the vaginal orifice and is pink. It appears as a small slit or pinhole opening just above the vaginal canal. Note any discharge, polyps, or fistulas.

Inspect the vaginal introitus next for inflammation, edema, discoloration, discharge, and lesions. Normally the

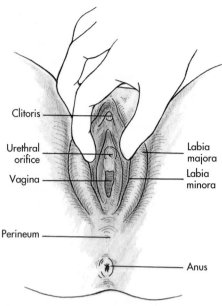

FIGURE **13-51** Female external genitalia.

introitus is a thin vertical slit or a large orifice. The tissue is moist. In women who have had several children, the opening to the vaginal canal may extend upward, blocking the view of the urethra. While inspecting the vaginal orifice or introitus, notice the condition of the hymen, which is just inside the introitus. In the virgin the hymen restricts the opening of the vagina. Only remnants of the hymen remain after sexual intercourse.

Inspect the anus looking for lesions and hemorrhoids (see rectal examination). After completion of the external examination, dispose of your gloves and offer your patient perineal hygiene.

Patients who are at risk for contracting STDs need to learn to perform a genital self-examination (see Box 13-21). The purpose of the examination is to detect any signs or symptoms of STDs. Many persons do not know they have an STD (e.g., chlamydia), and some STDs (e.g., syphilis) remain undetected for years.

### Speculum Examination of Internal Genitalia

An examination of internal genitalia requires much skill and practice. Advanced practice nurses and primary care providers will perform this examination. Beginning students will more than likely only observe the procedure or assist the examiner by helping the patient with positioning, handing off specimen supplies, and comforting the patient.

The examination involves use of a plastic or metal speculum, consisting of two blades and an adjustable thumbscrew. The examiner inserts the speculum into the vagina to assess the vaginal walls and cervix for cancerous lesions and other abnormalities. During the examination the examiner will collect a **Papanicolaou (Pap) smear** to test for cervical and vaginal cancer. This examination will not be discussed here.

## Male Genitalia

An examination of the male genitalia assesses the integrity of the external genitalia, inguinal ring, and canal. Because the incidence of STDs in adolescents and young adults is high, an assessment of the genitalia needs to be a routine part of any health maintenance examination for this age-group. Use a calm, gentle approach to lessen the patient's anxiety. The position and exposure obtained during the examination is embarrassing for some. It often helps to minimize the patient's anxiety by offering explanations of each step of the examination so the patient anticipates all actions. Manipulate the genitalia gently to avoid causing erection or discomfort. Examine the genitalia carefully and completely but also briskly.

### Health History

Assess the patient's normal urinary pattern, including frequency of voiding; character and volume of urine; daily fluid intake; and symptoms of burning, urgency and frequency, difficulty starting stream, and hematuria. The history also includes a review of previous surgery or illness involving urinary or reproductive organs, including STDs. The patient's sexual history and use of safe sex habits will alert you to any risks for HIV or other STDs. Patients at risk require extensive education (see Box 13-22). A number of disorders influence a patient's sexual performance; thus ask if the patient has difficulty achieving erection or ejaculation. Also review medications that influence sexual performance, including diuretics, sedatives, antihypertensives, and tranquilizers. Ask if the patient has noted penile pain or swelling, lesions of the genitalia, or urethral discharge (signs and symptoms of STDs). The patient's knowledge of testicular self-examination will guide you in health teaching (Box 13-21). Ask the patient if he has noticed heaviness or painless enlargement of a testis or irregular lumps (warning signs of testicular cancer). Finally, if the patient reports an enlargement in the inguinal area, assess if it is intermittent or constant; associated with straining or lifting; painful; and whether pain is affected by coughing, lifting, or straining at stool (signs and symptoms indicative of inguinal hernia).

### Sexual Maturity

The examination begins by having the patient void. Make sure the examination room is warm. Have the patient lie supine with the chest, abdomen, and lower legs draped or stand during the examination. Apply disposable gloves. First, note the sexual maturity of the patient by observing the size and shape of the penis and testes; the size, color, and texture of scrotal skin; and the character and distribution of pubic hair. The testes first increase in size in preadolescence. During this time there is no pubic hair. By the end of puberty, the testes and penis enlarge to adult size and shape and scrotal skin darkens and becomes wrinkled. With puberty, hair is coarse and abundant in the pubic area. The penis has no hair, and the scrotum has scant amounts. Also inspect the

| BOX 13-21 | MALE GENITALIA HEALTH |

**Male Genital Self-Examination**

All men 15 years and older need to perform this examination monthly using the following steps:

**Genital Examination**

Perform the examination after a warm bath or shower when the scrotal sac is relaxed.

Stand naked in front of a mirror, hold the penis in your hand, and examine the head. Pull back the foreskin if uncircumcised.

Inspect and palpate the entire head of the penis in a clockwise motion, looking carefully for any bumps, sores, blisters, or unusual discharge. Look also for any bumpy warts.

Look at the opening at the end of the penis for discharge.

Look along the entire shaft of the penis for the same signs.

Be sure to separate pubic hair at the base of the penis and carefully examine the skin underneath.

**Testicular Self-Examination**

Look for swelling or lumps in the skin of the scrotum while looking in the mirror.

Use both hands, placing the index and middle fingers under the testicles and the thumb on top (see the illustration).

Gently roll the testicle, feeling for lumps, thickening, or a change in consistency (hardening).

Find the epididymis (a cordlike structure on the top and back of the testicle; it is not a lump).

Feel for small, pea-size lumps on the front and side of the testicle. The lumps are usually painless and are abnormal.

Call your physician or health care provider if you find a lump.

**Prostate Health**

- Counsel patients with STDs about diagnosis and treatment.
- Explain warning signs of STDs:
  - Pain on urination and during sex
  - Penile discharge (different from usual)
  - Swollen lymph nodes
  - Rash or ulcer on skin or genitalia
- Teach measures to prevent STDs:
  - Use of condoms
  - Avoiding sex with infected partners
  - Restricting number of sexual partners
  - Avoiding sex with persons who have multiple partners
  - Using regular perineal hygiene
- Tell patients with STDs to inform sexual partners of the need to have an examination.
- Instruct patient to seek treatment as soon as possible if partner becomes infected with an STD.
- Instruct patients on how to perform genital self-examination.

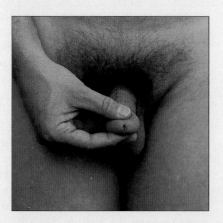 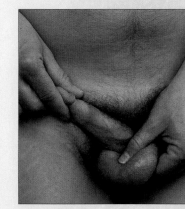

Illustrations from Seidel HM and others: *Mosby's guide to physical examination,* ed 5, St. Louis, 2003, Mosby.

skin covering the genitalia for lice, rashes, excoriations, or lesions. Normally the skin is clear, without lesions.

## Penis

To inspect penile surfaces thoroughly, manipulate the genitalia or have the patient assist. Inspect the corona, prepuce (foreskin), glans, urethral meatus, and shaft (Figure 13-52). In uncircumcised males retract the foreskin to reveal the glans and urethral meatus. The foreskin usually retracts easily. A bit of white, cheesy smegma sometimes collects under this foreskin. In the circumcised male, the glans is exposed; in either case, the glans should look smooth and pink along all surfaces.

Observe for discharge, lesions, edema, and inflammation. The urethral meatus is slitlike and normally positioned at the tip of the glans. In some congenital conditions the meatus is displaced along the penile shaft. The area between the foreskin and glans is a common site for venereal lesions.

Gentle compression of the glans between your thumb and index finger opens the meatus to allow inspection for discharge, lesions, and edema. (The patient may perform this maneuver.) Normally the opening is glistening and pink without discharge. Palpate any lesion gently to note tenderness, size, consistency, and shape. When you complete inspection of the glans, pull the foreskin down to its original

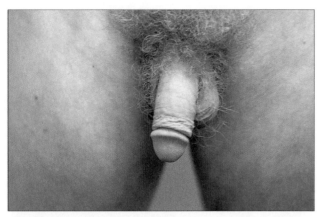

FIGURE **13-52** Normal male genitalia (circumcised). (From Seidel HM and others: *Mosby's guide to physical examination*, ed 5, St. Louis, 2003, Mosby.)

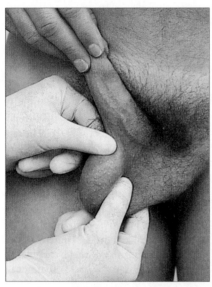

FIGURE **13-53** Palpating contents of scrotal sac. (From Seidel HM and others: *Mosby's guide to physical examination*, ed 5, St. Louis, 2003. Mosby.)

position. Continue by inspecting the entire shaft of the penis, including the undersurface, looking for any lesions, scars, or areas of edema. Palpate the shaft between the thumb and first two fingers to detect localized areas of hardness or tenderness. A patient who has lain in bed for a prolonged time may develop dependent edema in the penile shaft.

It is important for any male patient to learn to perform a genital self-examination to detect signs and symptoms of STDs. Many people who have an STD do not know it. Self-examination is a routine part of self-care (Box 13-23).

### Scrotum

Be especially cautious while inspecting and palpating the scrotum because the structures that lie within the scrotal sac are very sensitive. The scrotum is divided internally into halves. Each half contains a testicle, epididymis, and the vas deferens, which travels upward into the inguinal ring. The left testicle is normally lower than the right. Inspect the size, color, shape, and symmetry of the scrotum while observing for lesions or edema.

Gently lift the scrotum to view the posterior surface. The scrotal skin is usually loose, and the surface is coarse. The skin color is often more deeply pigmented than body skin. Tightening or loss of wrinkling reveals edema. The size of the scrotum normally changes with temperature variations because its dartos muscle contracts in cold and relaxes in warm temperature. Lumps in the scrotal skin are commonly sebaceous cysts.

Testicular cancer is a solid tumor commonly found in young men ages 18 to 34 years. Early detection is critical. Explain testicular self-examination while examining the patient. While the patient retracts the penis upward, gently palpate the testes and epididymis between the thumb and first two fingers (Figure 13-53).

Note the size, shape, and consistency of tissue, and ask if the patient feels any tenderness. The testes are normally sensitive but not tender. The underlying testicles are normally ovoid and approximately 2 by 4 cm ($\frac{4}{5}$ by $1\frac{3}{5}$ inches) in size. The testes feel smooth and rubbery and are free from nodules. The epididymis is resilient. In the older adult the testicles decrease in size and are less firm during palpation. The most common symptoms of testicular cancer are a painless enlargement of one testis and appearance of a palpable small, hard lump about the size of a pea on the front or side of the testicle.

Continue to palpate the vas deferens separately as it forms the spermatic cord toward the inguinal ring, noting nodules or swelling. It normally feels smooth and discrete.

### Inguinal Ring and Canal

The external inguinal ring provides the opening for the spermatic cord to pass into the inguinal canal. The canal forms a passage through the abdominal wall, a potential site for hernia formation. A **hernia** is a protrusion of a portion of intestine through the inguinal wall or canal. An intestinal loop may even enter the scrotum. The patient stands during this portion of the examination.

During inspection ask the patient to strain or bear down. The maneuver will help to make a hernia more visible. Look for obvious bulging in the inguinal area.

Complete the examination by palpating for inguinal lymph nodes. You will normally find small, nontender, mobile horizontal nodes. Any abnormality indicates local or systemic infection or malignant disease.

## Rectum and Anus

A good time to perform the rectal examination is after the genital examination. The procedure is uncomfortable, so explaining all steps helps the patient relax. Usually you will not perform the examination on young children or adolescents.

**PATIENT TEACHING**

### Colorectal and Anal Health

- Discuss the American Cancer Society's guidelines (2005) for early detection of colorectal cancer for both men and women. The American Cancer Society (2005) recommends the following examination schedule (consult your health care provider):

  Digital rectal examination yearly after age 50

  Fecal occult blood test (FOBT) or fecal immunochemical test (FIT) yearly after age 50

  Flexible sigmoidoscopy (FSIG): visual inspection of the rectum and lower colon with a hollow, lighted tube performed by a physician every 5 years after age 50 on advice of physician or health care provider

  Double-contrast barium enema every 5 years

  Colonoscopy every 10 years

- Individuals at increased risk need to discuss options with their physician or health care provider.
- Discuss warning signs of colorectal cancer.
- Discuss dietary planning to reduce fat and increase fiber content.
- Warn patients against problems caused by overuse of laxatives, cathartic medications, codeine, or enemas.
- Discuss with male patients the American Cancer Society's guidelines (2005) for early detection of prostatic cancer:

  Digital rectal examination should be performed annually after age 50.

  Men age 50 and over need an annual prostate-specific antigen (PSA) blood test.

  If either test is suspicious, health care providers perform a prostate ultrasonographic examination.

  African-American men or those with a first-degree relative diagnosed with prostate cancer begin testing at age 45.

  Discuss with male patients the warning signs of prostate cancer.

The examination detects colorectal cancer in its early stages. In men the rectal examination also detects prostatic tumors.

## Health History

The history includes review of the patient's personal history of colorectal cancer, polyps, or inflammatory bowel disease. If the patient is over age 40, ask if the patient has ever had a rectal examination or proctosigmoidoscopy. Ask the patient about symptoms of bleeding from the rectum, black or tarry stools (melena), rectal pain, or change in bowel habits, all of which indicate colorectal cancer. The patient's dietary habits, including intake of high-fat foods or deficient fiber content, are linked to colon cancer. To screen male patients for possible prostate cancer ask if your patient has experienced weak or interrupted urine flow; an inability to urinate; difficulty in starting or stopping the urinary stream; polyuria; nocturia; hematuria; dysuria; or continuing pain in the lower back, pelvis, or upper thighs. Also review the patient's use of laxatives, cathartics, codeine, or iron preparations, which can cause elimination problems (Box 13-22).

## Inspection

Female patients remain in the dorsal recumbent position following genitalia examination, or they assume a side-lying (Sims') position. The best way to examine men is to have the patient stand and bend over forward with the hips flexed and upper body resting across the examination table. Examine a nonambulatory patient in Sims' position. Use disposable gloves.

Using your nondominant hand, gently retract the buttocks to view the perianal and sacrococcygeal areas. Perianal skin is smooth and more pigmented and coarser than skin overlying the buttocks. Inspect anal tissue for skin characteristics, lesions, external **hemorrhoids** (dilated veins that appear as reddened skin protrusions), ulcers, inflammation, rashes, or excoriation. Anal tissues are moist and hairless, and the anus is held closed by the voluntary sphincter. Next, ask the patient to bear down as though having a bowel movement. Any internal hemorrhoids or fissures will appear at this time. Use clock referents (e.g., 12 o'clock or 5 o'clock) to describe the location of findings. There normally is no protrusion of tissue.

## Digital Palpation

You will use digital palpation to examine the anal canal and sphincters. In male patients, palpate the prostate gland to rule out enlargement. Usually advanced practitioners perform this portion of the examination.

# Musculoskeletal System

You will do the musculoskeletal assessment as a separate examination or integrated with other parts of the total physical examination. You can also assess this system while performing other nursing care measures such as bathing or positioning. The assessment of musculoskeletal integrity is especially important when the patient reports pain or loss of function in a joint or muscle. Frequently, muscular disorders are the result of neurological disease. For this reason health care providers often conduct a neurological assessment simultaneously.

While examining the patient's musculoskeletal function, you visualize the anatomy of bone and muscle placement and joint structure. Joints vary in their degree of mobility. Some, as in the knee, are freely moveable. The spinal vertebrae are examples of slightly moveable joints. For a complete examination expose the muscles and joints so that they are free to move. Depending on the muscle groups you are assessing, the patient assumes a sitting, supine, prone, or standing position.

## Health History

A history includes the patient's description of any problems in bone, muscle, or joint function, including history of recent falls, trauma, lifting heavy objects, fractures, and bone or joint disease. Ask the patient to point out locations of any alterations. It is useful to assess the patient's normal activity pattern, including the type of exercise routinely performed

**PATIENT TEACHING**

**Musculoskeletal Health**

- Instruct the patient about correct postural alignment. Consult with a physical therapist to provide the patient with exercises for improving posture.
- Recommend women age 65 and older be routinely screened for osteoporosis (U.S. Preventative Services Task Force, 2003). Recommend men for screening as well; they are equally at risk for development of osteoporosis as they age (Lewis, 2003).
- To reduce bone demineralization, instruct older adults about a proper exercise program (e.g., walking) to follow 3 or more times a week.
- Encourage intake of calcium to meet the recommended daily allowance. Increased vitamin D will aid calcium absorption.
- Recommendations for calcium supplements are 1200 mg/day, especially in older women (Moore, 2005).
- Explain to patients with low back pain that they will benefit from modification of worker risk factors (e.g., lifting heavy weights, use of protective equipment), regular aerobic exercise, exercises that strengthen the back and increase trunk flexibility, and learning how to lift properly.
- Instruct the patient in use of assistive devices (e.g., zippers on clothing instead of buttons, elevation of chairs to minimize bending of knees and hips) when he or she is unable to perform ADLs.
- Instruct older adults and those with osteoporosis in proper body mechanics and range of motion and moderate weight-bearing exercises (e.g., swimming, walking) to minimize trauma and subsequent bone fractures.
- Instruct older patients to pace activities to compensate for loss in muscle strength.

(Box 13-23). Also assess the nature and extent of pain or stiffness and determine if a musculoskeletal problem affects the patient's ability to perform ADLs and participate in social activities. Determine if the patient is involved in competitive sports (particularly involving collision and contact), fails to warm up adequately, is in poor physical condition, or had a rapid growth spurt (adolescents). Review the patient's history for osteoporosis risk factors, including heavy alcohol use; cigarette smoking; constant dieting; calcium intake less than 500 mg daily; thin and light body frame; nulliparous; menopause before age 45; postmenopause; family history of osteoporosis; or white, Asian, or Native American, or northern European ancestry. Also assess for excessive caffeine intake; advanced age; history of fractures/falls; chronic diseases (e.g., Cushing's disease, hyperthyroidism and hypothyroidism, malabsorption/malnutrition disorders, and neoplasms); and long-term use of corticosteroids, methotrexate, phenytoin, and aluminum-containing antacids (Peterson, 2001).

## General Inspection

Observe the patient's gait and posture when entering the examination room. When a patient is unaware of your observation, gait is more natural. Later a more formal test has the patient walk in a straight line away from you. Note how the patient walks, sits, and rises from a sitting position. Normally patients walk with arms swinging freely at the sides and the head leading the body. Older adults walk with smaller steps and a wider base of support. Note foot dragging, limping, shuffling, and the position of the trunk in relation to the legs.

Observe the patient from the side in a standing position. The normal standing posture is an upright stance with parallel alignment of the hips and shoulders (Figure 13-54). There should be an even contour of the shoulders, level scapulae and iliac crests, alignment of the head over the gluteal folds, and symmetry of extremities. Looking sideways at the patient, note the normal cervical, thoracic, and lumbar curves. Holding the head erect is normal. As the patient sits, some degree of rounding of the shoulders is normal. Older adults tend to assume a stooped, forward-bent posture, with hips and knees somewhat flexed and arms bent at the elbows, raising the level of the arms. Common postural abnormalities include kyphosis, lordosis, and scoliosis. **Kyphosis,** or hunchback, is an exaggeration of the posterior curvature of the thoracic spine. This postural abnormality is common in the older adult. **Lordosis,** or swayback, is an increased lumbar curvature. A lateral spinal curvature is called **scoliosis.**

Loss of height is frequently the first clinical sign of osteoporosis, in which height loss occurs in the trunk as a result of vertebral fracture and collapse. **Osteoporosis** is a metabolic bone disease that causes a decrease in quality and quantity of bone. Lewis (2003) reports that osteoporosis affects 28 million Americans, the majority of which are women. This disease now affects 2 million men, and it will affect another 3 million men (Lewis, 2003). Although you expect a small amount of height loss with aging, if the amount of loss is great, osteoporosis is likely. As men and women age, they are more likely to have osteoporotic fractures of the wrists, hips, and vertebrae (Pachucki-Hyde, 2001). Osteoporosis-related fractures occur in half of all postmenopausal women; of those, 25% will have vertebral deformities and 15% will suffer from hip fractures (U.S. Preventative Services Task Force, 2003).

During general inspection look at the extremities for overall size, gross deformity, bony enlargement, alignment, and symmetry. Normally there is bilateral symmetry in length, circumference, alignment, and position and numbering of skinfolds (Seidel and others, 2003). A general review pinpoints areas requiring specialized assessment.

## Palpation

Apply gentle palpation to all bones, joints, and surrounding muscles during a complete examination. In the case of a focused assessment, you only need to examine an involved area. Note any heat, tenderness, edema, or resistance to pressure. The patient should feel no discomfort when you apply palpation. Muscles should be firm.

## Range-of-Joint Motion

Ask the patient to put each major joint and its muscle groups through full range of motion (ROM) (Table 13-8). The examination includes comparison of both active and passive

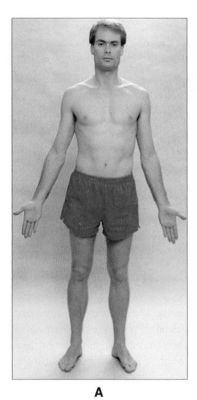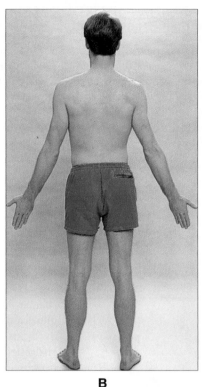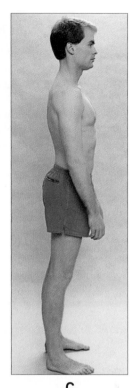

A    B    C

FIGURE 13-54 Inspection of overall body posture. **A,** Anterior view. **B,** Posterior view. **C,** Lateral view. (From Seidel HM and others: *Mosby's guide to physical examination,* ed 5, St. Louis, 2003, Mosby.)

ROM. To assess ROM passively, ask the patient to relax and then passively move the joints until you feel the end of range. Compare the same body parts for equality in movement. Do not force a joint into a painful position. Know the normal range of each joint and the extent to which the patient's joints can be moved. Ideally you assess the patient's normal range to determine a baseline for assessing later change. Joints are typically free from stiffness, instability, swelling, or inflammation. There should be no discomfort when you apply pressure to bones and joints. In older adults joints often become swollen and stiff, with reduced ROM resulting from cartilage erosion and fibrosis of synovial membranes. If a joint appears swollen and inflamed, palpate it for warmth.

## Muscle Tone and Strength

Assess muscle strength and tone during ROM measurement. Note muscle tone, the slight muscular resistance felt as you passively move the relaxed extremity through its ROM. Ask the patient to allow an extremity to relax or hang limp. This is often difficult, particularly if the patient feels pain in the extremity. Support the extremity and grasp each limb, moving it through the normal ROM (Figure 13-55). Normal tone causes a mild, even resistance to passive movement through the entire range.

If a muscle has increased tone, or **hypertonicity,** you will meet considerable resistance with sudden passive movement of a joint. Continued movement eventually causes the muscle to relax. A muscle that has little tone (**hypotonicity**) feels flabby. The involved extremity hangs loosely in a position determined by gravity.

For assessment of muscle strength the patient assumes a stable position. The patient performs maneuvers demonstrating strength of major muscle groups (Table 13-9). Compare symmetrical muscle pairs for strength, based on a grading scale of 0 to 5 (Table 13-10). The arm on the dominant side is normally stronger than the arm on the nondominant side. In the older adult a loss of muscle mass causes bilateral weakness, but muscle strength remains greater in the dominant arm or leg.

Examine each muscle group. Ask the patient first to flex the muscle to be examined and then to resist when you apply opposing force against that flexion. It is important to not allow the patient to move the joint. Gradually increase pressure to a muscle group (e.g., elbow extension). The patient resists the pressure you apply by attempting to move against resistance (e.g., elbow flexion). The patient resists until instructed to stop. As you vary the amount of pressure applied, the joint moves. If you identify a weakness, compare the size of the muscle with its opposite counterpart by measuring the circumference of the muscle body with a tape measure. A muscle that has atrophied (reduced in size) feels soft and baggy when palpated.

## Neurological System

An assessment of neurological function alone is quite time consuming. For efficiency, integrate neurological measurements with other parts of the physical examination. For example, test cranial nerve function during the survey of the

| TABLE 13-8 | Terminology for Normal Range-of-Motion Positions | |
|---|---|---|
| **Term** | **Range of Motion** | **Examples of Joints** |
| Flexion | Movement decreasing angle between two adjoining bones; bending of limb | Elbow, fingers, knee |
| Extension | Movement increasing angle between two adjoining bones | Elbow, knee, fingers |
| Hyperextension | Movement of body part beyond its normal resting extended position | Head |
| Pronation | Movement of body part so that front or ventral surface faces downward | Hand, forearm |
| Supination | Movement of body part so that front or ventral surface faces upward | Hand, forearm |
| Abduction | Movement of extremity away from midline of body | Leg, arm, fingers |
| Adduction | Movement of extremity toward midline of body | Leg, arm, fingers |
| Internal rotation | Rotation of joint inward | Knee, hip |
| External rotation | Rotation of joint outward | Knee, hip |
| Eversion | Turning of body part away from midline | Foot |
| Inversion | Turning of body part toward midline | Foot |
| Dorsiflexion | Flexion of toes and foot upward | Foot |
| Plantar flexion | Bending of toes and foot downward | Foot |

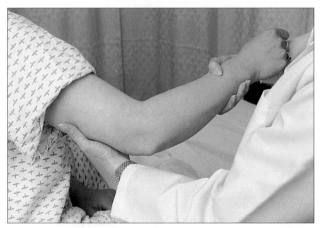

Figure **13-55** Assess muscle tone when moving the extremity passively.

head and neck. Observe mental and emotional status during the initial interview.

You will consider many variables when deciding the extent of the examination. A patient's level of consciousness influences the ability to follow directions. General physical status influences tolerance to assessment. The patient's chief complaint also helps to determine the need for a thorough neurological assessment. If the patient complains of headache or a recent loss of function in an extremity, the patient will need a complete neurological review. This requires special equipment, including reading material, vials of aromatic substances (e.g., vanilla extract and coffee), opposite tip of cotton swab or tongue blade broken in half, Snellen eye chart, penlight, vials of sugar or salt, tongue blade, two test tubes (one containing hot water, the other containing cold), cotton balls or cotton-tipped applicators, tuning fork, and reflex hammer.

## Health History

Gather a history that includes a screening for symptoms of headache, seizures, tremors, dizziness, vertigo, numbness or tingling of body parts, visual changes, weakness, pain, or changes in speech. The presence of any symptom then requires a more detailed review (e.g., onset, severity, precipitating factors, or sequence of events). Review the patient's use of analgesics, alcohol, sedatives, hypnotics, antipsychotics, antidepressants, nervous system stimulants, or recreational drugs. Also ask the patient's family if they have noticed any recent changes in the patient's behavior (e.g., increased irritability, mood swings, memory loss, or change in energy level). Ask about any noticeable changes in vision, hearing, smell, taste, and touch. A history of head or spinal cord trauma, meningitis, congenital anomalies, neurological disease, or psychiatric counseling will focus your assessment of select findings. If an older adult patient displays sudden acute confusion (delirium), review history for drug toxicity, serious infections, metabolic disturbances, heart failure, and severe anemia.

## Mental and Emotional Status

You can learn a great deal about mental capacities and emotional state by interacting with the patient. Ask questions during an examination to gather data and observe the appropriateness of emotions and thoughts. There are special assessment tools designed to assess a patient's mental status. The Mental Status Questionnaire (MSQ) developed by Kahn and others (1960) is a 10-item instrument and a widely used tool. The Mini–Mental State Examination (MMSE) is another assessment instrument developed by Folstein and others (1975) that measures patient's orientation and cognitive function. Box 13-24 offers examples of questions found on the MMSE. A maximum score on the MMSE is 30. Patients with scores of 21 or less generally reveal cognitive impairment requiring further evaluation.

To ensure an objective assessment consider the patient's cultural and educational background, values, beliefs, previous experiences, and current level of coping. Such factors influence response to questions. An alteration in mental or emotional status reflects a disturbance in cerebral functioning. The cerebral cortex controls and integrates intellectual and emotional functioning. Primary brain disorders, med-

| TABLE 13-9 | Maneuvers to Assess Muscle Strength |
| --- | --- |
| Muscle Group | Maneuver |
| Neck (sternocleido-mastoid) | Place hand firmly against patient's upper jaw. Ask patient to turn head laterally against resistance. |
| Shoulder (trapezius) | Place hand over midline of patient's shoulder, exerting firm pressure. Have patient raise shoulders against resistance. |
| Elbow | |
| Biceps | Pull down on forearm as patient attempts to flex arm. |
| Triceps | As patient flexes arm, apply pressure against forearm. Ask patient to straighten arm. |
| Hip | |
| Quadriceps | When patient is sitting, apply downward pressure to thigh. Ask patient to raise leg up from table. |
| Gastrocnemius | Patient sits, holding shin of flexed leg. Ask patient to straighten leg against resistance. |

| TABLE 13-10 | Muscle Strength | | | |
| --- | --- | --- | --- | --- |
| | | Scales | | |
| Muscle Function Level | Grade | % Normal | Lovett Scale |
| No evidence of contractility | 0 | 0 | 0 (zero) |
| Slight contractility, no movement | 1 | 10 | T (trace) |
| Full range of motion, gravity eliminated* | 2 | 25 | P (poor) |
| Full range of motion with gravity | 3 | 50 | F (fair) |
| Full range of motion against gravity, some resistance | 4 | 75 | G (good) |
| Full range of motion against gravity, full resistance | 5 | 100 | N (normal) |

From Barkauskas VH and others: *Health and physical assessment,* ed 2, St. Louis, 1998, Mosby.
*Passive movement.

ications, and metabolic changes are examples of factors that change cerebral function.

## Level of Consciousness

A person's level of consciousness exists along a continuum from being fully awake, alert, and cooperative to unresponsiveness to any form of external stimuli. Talk with the patient, asking questions about events involving the patient or concerns about any health problem. A fully conscious patient responds to questions quickly and expresses ideas logically. With a lowering of the patient's consciousness, you use the Glasgow Coma Scale (GCS) for an objective measurement of consciousness on a numerical scale (Table 13-11). The patient needs to be as alert as possible before testing. Use caution when using the scale if a patient has sensory losses (e.g., vision or hearing).

The GCS allows you to evaluate a patient's neurological status over time. The higher the score, the better the patient's neurological function. Ask short, simple questions, such as "What is your name?" or "Where are you?" Also ask the patient to follow simple commands, such as "Move your toes."

If the patient's consciousness is lowered to the point of being unable to follow commands, try to elicit a response by applying firm pressure with your thumb over the root of the

| BOX 13-24 | MMSE Sample Questions |
| --- | --- |

Orientation to time
  "What is the date?"
Registration
  "Listen carefully. I am going to say three words. You say them back after I stop.
  Ready? Here they are . . .
  HOUSE (pause), CAR (pause), LAKE (pause). Now repeat those words back to me."
  [Repeat up to 5 times, but score only the first trial.]
Naming
  "What is this?" [Point to a pencil or pen.]
Reading
  "Please read this and do what it says." [Show examinee the words on the stimulus form.]
  CLOSE YOUR EYES

| TABLE 13-11 | Glasgow Coma Scale | |
|---|---|---|
| **Action** | **Response** | **Score** |
| Eyes open | Spontaneously | 4 |
| | To speech | 3 |
| | To pain | 2 |
| | None | 1 |
| Best verbal response | Oriented | 5 |
| | Confused | 4 |
| | Inappropriate words | 3 |
| | Incomprehensible sounds | 2 |
| | None | 1 |
| Best motor response | Obeys commands | 6 |
| | Localized pain | 5 |
| | Flexion withdrawal | 4 |
| | Abnormal flexion | 3 |
| | Abnormal extension | 2 |
| | Flaccid | 1 |
| | TOTAL SCORE  15 | |

patient's fingernail. The normal response to painful stimuli is withdrawal of the body part from the stimulus.

## Behavior and Appearance

Behaviors, moods, hygiene, grooming, and choice of dress reveal pertinent information about mental status. Remain perceptive of the patient's mannerisms and actions during the entire physical assessment. Note both nonverbal and verbal behaviors. Does the patient respond appropriately to directions? Does the patient's mood vary with no apparent cause? Does the patient show concern about appearance? Is the patient's hair clean and neatly groomed, and are the nails trim and clean? The patient should behave in a manner expressing concern and interest in the examination. The patient should make eye contact with you and express appropriate feelings that correspond to the situation. Normally the patient's appearance will show some degree of personal hygiene.

Choice and fit of clothing reflects socioeconomic background or personal taste rather than deficiency in self-concept or self-care. Avoid being judgmental, and focus assessments on the appropriateness of clothing for the weather. Older adults sometimes neglect their appearance because of a lack of energy, finances, or reduced vision.

## Language

Normal cerebral function allows a person to understand spoken or written words and to express the self through written words or gestures. Observe the patient's voice inflection, tone, and manner of speech. Normally the patient's voice has inflections, is clear and strong, and increases in volume appropriately. Speech is fluent. When communication is clearly ineffective (e.g., omission or addition of letters and words, misuse of words, or hesitations), assess for **aphasia.** Injury to the cerebral cortex results in aphasia.

The two types of aphasia are sensory (or receptive) and motor (or expressive). With receptive aphasia a person cannot understand written or verbal speech. With expressive aphasia a person understands written and verbal speech but cannot write or speak appropriately when attempting to communicate. A patient sometimes suffers from a combination of receptive and expressive aphasia. Assessment requires that you ask the patient to name familiar objects when pointing at them. You also ask the patient to respond to simple verbal commands, such as "Stand up." Finally, you ask the patient to read a simple sentence out loud. Normally a patient names objects correctly, follows commands, and reads sentences correctly.

## Intellectual Function

Intellectual function includes memory, knowledge, abstract thinking, and judgment. Testing each aspect of function involves a specific technique. However, because cultural and educational background influences the ability to respond to test questions, do not ask questions related to concepts or ideas with which the patient is unfamiliar.

**MEMORY.** Assess immediate recall and recent and remote memory. Immediate recall is reflected in the ability of the patient to repeat a series of numbers in the order they are presented or in reverse order. Patients normally recall five to eight digits forward or four to six digits backward.

Ask if you can test the patient's memory. Then state clearly and slowly the name of three unrelated objects. After you say all three, ask the patient to repeat each. Continue until the patient is successful. Then, later in the assessment, ask the patient to repeat the three words again. The patient should be able to identify the three words. Another test for recent memory involves asking the patient to recall events occurring during the same day (e.g., what was eaten for breakfast). Validate information with a family member.

To assess past memory, you ask the patient to recall the maiden name of the patient's mother, a birthday, or a special date in history. It is best to ask open-ended questions rather than simple yes-or-no questions. A patient usually has immediate recall of such information. With older adults do not interpret a hearing loss as confusion. Good communication techniques are necessary throughout the examination to ensure the patient clearly understands all the directions and testing.

**KNOWLEDGE.** You assess the patient's knowledge by asking how much he or she knows about the illness or the reason for hospitalization. By assessing a patient's knowledge, you determine the patient's ability to learn or understand. If there is an opportunity to teach information, test the patient's mental status by asking for feedback during a follow-up visit.

**ABSTRACT THINKING.** Interpreting abstract ideas or concepts reflects the capacity for abstract thinking. For an individual to explain common sayings, such as "A stitch in time saves nine" or "Don't count your chickens before they're hatched," requires a higher level of intellectual functioning. Note whether the patient's explanations are relevant and concrete. The patient with an altered mental state will probably interpret the phrase literally or will merely rephrase the words.

**JUDGMENT.** Judgment requires a comparison and evaluation of facts and ideas to understand their relationships and to form appropriate conclusions. Attempt to measure

| TABLE 13-12 | Cranial Nerve Function and Assessment | | | |
|---|---|---|---|---|
| Number | Name | Type | Function | Method |
| I | Olfactory | Sensory | Sense of smell | Ask patient to identify different nonirritating aromas such as coffee and vanilla. |
| II | Optic | Sensory | Visual acuity | Use Snellen chart or ask patient to read printed material while wearing glasses. |
| III | Oculomotor | Motor | Extraocular eye movement | Assess directions of gaze. |
| | | | Pupil constriction and dilation | Measure pupil reaction to light reflex and accommodation. |
| IV | Trochlear | Motor | Upward and downward | Assess directions of gaze. |
| | | | movement of eyeball | |
| V | Trigeminal | Sensory and motor | Sensory nerve to skin of face | Lightly touch cornea with wisp of cotton. |
| | | | Motor nerve to muscles of jaw | Assess corneal reflex. Measure sensation of light pain and touch across skin of face. Palpate temples as patient clenches teeth. |
| VI | Abducens | Motor | Lateral movement of eyeballs | Assess directions of gaze. |
| VII | Facial | Sensory and motor | Facial expression | As patient smiles, frowns, puffs out cheeks, and raises and lowers eyebrows, look for asymmetry. |
| | | | Taste | Have patient identify salty or sweet taste on front of tongue. |
| VIII | Auditory | Sensory | Hearing | Assess ability to hear spoken word. |
| | | | Taste | |
| IX | Glossopharyngeal | Sensory and motor | Ability to swallow | Ask patient to identify sour or sweet taste on back of tongue. Use tongue blade to elicit gag reflex. |
| X | Vagus | Sensory and motor | Sensation of pharynx | Ask patient to say "Ah." Observe palate and pharynx movement. |
| | | | Movement of vocal cords | Assess speech for hoarseness. |
| XI | Spinal accessory | Motor | Movement of head and shoulders | Ask patient to shrug shoulders and turn head against passive resistance. |
| XII | Hypoglossal | Motor | Position of tongue | Ask patient to stick out tongue to midline and move it from side to side. |

the patient's ability to make logical decisions with questions such as "Why did you decide to seek health care?" or "What would you do if you suddenly became ill at home?" Normally a patient makes logical decisions.

## Cranial Nerve Function

You will assess all 12 cranial nerves or a single nerve or related group of nerves. A dysfunction in one nerve reflects an alteration at some point along the distribution of the cranial nerve. Measurements used to assess the integrity of organs within the head and neck also assess cranial nerve function. A complete assessment involves testing the 12 cranial nerves in order of their number. To remember the order of the nerves, use this simple phrase: "On old Olympus' towering tops a Finn and German viewed some hops." The first letter of each word in the phrase is the same as the first letter of the names of the cranial nerves listed in order (Table 13-12).

## Sensory Function

The sensory pathways of the central nervous system conduct the sensations of pain, temperature, position, vibration, and crude and finely localized touch. Different nerve pathways relay the various types of sensations. Most patients require only a quick screening of sensory function, unless there are symptoms of reduced sensation, motor impairment, or paralysis.

Normally a patient has sensory responses to all stimuli tested. A patient feels sensations equally on both sides of the body in all areas. Perform all sensory testing with the patient's eyes closed so that the patient is unable to see when or where a stimulus strikes the skin (Table 13-13). Then apply stimuli in a random, unpredictable order to maintain the patient's attention and to prevent detection of a predictable pattern. The patient will tell you when, what, and where he or she felt each stimulus. You compare symmetrical areas of the body while applying stimuli to the arms, trunk, and legs.

## Motor Function

An assessment of motor function includes measurements made during the musculoskeletal examination. In addition, you determine cerebellar function. The cerebellum coordinates muscular activity, maintains balance and equilibrium, and helps to control posture. Patients with any degree of motor dysfunction are at risk for injury (Box 13-25, p. 332).

**BALANCE.** Assess balance by asking the patient to stand with the feet together and arms at the sides, with eyes open and

| TABLE 13-13 | Assessment of Sensory Nerve Function | | |
|---|---|---|---|
| **Function** | **Equipment** | **Method** | **Precautions** |
| Pain | End of paper clip or end of cotton applicator | Ask patient to voice when dull or sharp sensation is felt. Alternately apply sharp and blunt ends of paper clip to skin's surface. Note areas of numbness or increased sensitivity. | Remember that areas where skin is thickened, such as heel or sole of foot, are less sensitive to pain. |
| Temperature | Two test tubes, one filled with hot water and the other with cold | Touch skin with tube. Ask patient to identify hot or cold sensation. | Omit test if pain sensation is normal. |
| Light touch | Cotton ball or cotton-tipped applicator | Apply light wisp of cotton to different points along skin's surface. Ask patient to voice when the sensation is felt. | Apply at areas where skin is thin or more sensitive (e.g., face, neck, inner aspect of arms, top of feet and hands). |
| Vibration | Tuning fork | Apply stem of vibrating fork to distal interphalangeal joint of fingers and interphalangeal joint of great toe, elbow, and wrist. Have patient voice when and where the vibration is felt. | Be sure patient feels vibration and not merely pressure. |
| Position | | Grasp finger or toe, holding it by its sides with thumb and index finger. Alternate moving finger or toe up and down. Ask patient to state when finger is up or down. Repeat with toes. | Avoid rubbing adjacent appendages as finger or toe is moved. Do not move joint laterally; return to neutral position before moving again. |
| Two-point discrimination | Two ends of paper clip | Lightly apply one or both ends of paper clip simultaneously to skin's surface. Ask patient if one or two pricks are felt. Find the distance at which patient no longer distinguishes two points. | Apply paper clip tips to same anatomical site (e.g., fingertips, palm of hand, upper arms). Minimum distance at which patient discriminates two points varies (2 to 8 mm on fingertips). |

| BOX 13-25 | PATIENT TEACHING |
|---|---|

**Neurological Health**

- Explain to family or friends the implications of any behavioral or mental impairment shown by the patient.
- If the patient has sensory or motor impairments, explain measures to ensure safety (e.g., use of ambulation aids, use of safety bars in bathrooms or on stairways).
- Teach older adults to plan enough time to complete tasks because their reaction time is slower.
- Teach older adults to observe skin surface for areas of trauma because their perception of pain is reduced.

closed. Standing close to the patient prevents an accidental fall. Expect slight swaying of the body in the Romberg's test. A loss of balance (positive Romberg) causes a patient to fall to the side.

**COORDINATION.** To avoid confusion, demonstrate each coordination assessment maneuver and then have the patient repeat it while you observe for smoothness and balance in the patient's movement. In older adults normally slow reaction time causes movements to be less rhythmical.

To assess fine motor function, have the patient extend the arms out to the sides and touch each forefinger alternately to the nose (first with eyes open, then with eyes closed). Normally the patient alternately touches the nose smoothly. Performing rapid, rhythmical, alternating movements demonstrates coordination in the upper extremities. While sitting, the patient begins by patting the knees with both hands. Then the patient alternately turns up the palm and back of the hands while continuously patting. Patients should do the maneuver smoothly and regularly with increasing speed.

Test lower extremity coordination with the patient lying supine, legs extended. Place your hand at the ball of the patient's foot. The patient taps your hand with the foot as quickly as possible. Test each foot for speed and smoothness. The feet do not normally move as rapidly or evenly as the hands.

## After the Examination

Record findings from the physical assessment during the examination or at the end. Special forms are available to record data. Review all findings before assisting the patient with dressing in case of a need to recheck any information or gather additional data. Integrate physical assessment findings into the plan of care.

After completing the assessment, give the patient time to dress. The hospitalized patient sometimes needs help with hygiene and returning to bed. When the patient is comfortable, it helps to share a summary of the assessment findings. If the findings have revealed serious abnormalities such as a highly irregular heart rate, consult the patient's physician or health care provider before revealing any findings. It is the physician's or health care provider's responsibility to make definitive medical diagnoses. Explain the type of abnormality found and the need for the physician or health care provider to conduct an additional examination.

Sometimes you delegate support staff to clean the examination area. Use infection control practices in removing materials or instruments soiled with potentially infectious wastes. If the patient's bedside was the site for the examination, clear away soiled items from the bedside table and makes sure the bed linen is dry and clean. The patient will appreciate a clean gown and the opportunity to wash the face and hands. Afterward, be sure to perform hand hygiene.

Be sure to record a complete assessment. If you delayed entering any items into the assessment form, enter them at this time to avoid forgetting important information. If you made entries periodically during the examination, review them for accuracy and thoroughness. Communicate significant findings to appropriate medical and nursing personnel, either verbally or in the patient's written care plan.

The patient often needs a number of ancillary examinations such as x-ray film examinations, laboratory tests, or ultrasonography after a physical examination. The tests provide additional screening information to rule out and to help diagnose specific abnormalities found during the examination. Explain the purpose of these tests and the sensations that the patient will experience.

## KEY CONCEPTS

- Baseline assessment findings reflect the patient's functional abilities when you first assess the patient and serve as the basis for comparison with subsequent assessment findings.
- Physical assessment of a child or infant requires that you apply principles of physical growth and development.
- You should recognize that the normal process of aging affects physical findings collected from an older adult.
- Integrate patient teaching throughout the examination to help patients learn about health promotion and disease prevention.
- Inspection requires good lighting, full exposure of the body part, and a careful comparison of the part with its counterpart on the opposite side of the body.
- Palpation involves the use of parts of the hand to detect different types of physical characteristics.
- Use auscultation to assess the character of sounds created in various body organs.
- Perform a physical examination only after proper preparation of the environment and equipment and after preparing the patient physically and psychologically.
- Throughout the examination keep the patient warm, comfortable, and informed of each step of the assessment process.
- A competent examiner learns to be systematic while combining assessments of different body systems simultaneously.

- Information from the history helps you to focus on body systems likely to be affected.
- When assessing a seriously ill patient, concentrate on the body systems most likely to be affected.
- Creating a mental image of internal organs in relation to external anatomical landmarks enhances accuracy in assessing the thorax, heart, and abdomen.
- When assessing heart sounds, imagine events occurring during the cardiac cycle.
- Never palpate the carotid arteries simultaneously.
- When examining a woman's breasts, explain the techniques for breast self-examination.
- The abdominal assessment differs from other portions of the examination in that auscultation follows inspection.
- During assessment of the genitalia, explain the technique for genital self-examination.
- Conduct an assessment of musculoskeletal function when observing the patient ambulate or participate in other active movements.
- Assess mental and emotional status by interacting with the patient throughout the examination.
- At the end of the examination provide for the patient's comfort, and then document a detailed summary of physical assessment findings.

## CRITICAL THINKING IN PRACTICE

*You are caring for Mr. Neal, 76, a resident of a long-term care facility. He had a colon resection for cancer 2 days ago. The morning shift has just started, and the night nurse reported that he had an "uneventful" night. Your patient is NPO, has an IV line for parenteral fluids, a nasogastric (NG) tube to low intermittent suction, an abdominal dressing, and a urethral (Foley) catheter to gravity.*

1. a. What focused systems assessments do you complete?
   b. Describe the key elements in these assessments.
2. Upon entrance into Mr. Neal's room, you observe that he appears agitated and confused. How do you further evaluate his mental status?
3. After reorienting Mr. Neal, you receive his cooperation to continue with your assessment. Upon auscultation of the lateral and posterior lung fields, you hear a crackling noise upon inspiration. What does this noise indicate?
4. You next assess his cardiac status. The apical heart rate is 84 beats per minute, rhythm regular. You know that this is considered:
   a. Abnormal
   b. Bradycardia
   c. Normal
   d. Tachycardia

5. Mr. Neal complains of abdominal incisional pain. After evaluation of his pain status, you administer pain relief medication. Following completion of this task, you inspect and then auscultate his abdomen. Prior to auscultation you would first (1) _____.
   After completion of the above task (1), you listen for 30 seconds at a site below and to the left of the umbilicus. You are unable to hear bowel sounds. The best assessment of this situation is that:
   a. You are not listening in the correct place
   b. You need to listen longer
   c. Your patient has a partial bowel obstruction
   d. Your patient has peritonitis
6. When you are examining Mr. Neal's lower extremities, he tells you that his left calf is tender to your touch; you note unilateral leg swelling, and the area is reddened and warm to the touch. Your assessment of this situation is:
   a. Your patient has developed a phlebitis
   b. Your patient has muscle fatigue
   c. Your patient should not be concerned—all patients have these symptoms after major surgery
   d. Your patient should have a Homans' sign test performed as soon as possible.

## NCLEX® REVIEW

1. The first technique you employ when conducting a patient's physical examination is:
   1. Palpation
   2. Inspection
   3. Percussion
   4. Auscultation
2. To assess the patient's posterior tibial pulse, you palpate:
   1. Behind the knee
   2. Over the lateral malleolus
   3. In the groove behind the medial malleolus
   4. Lateral to the extensor tendon of the great toe
3. The main reason you auscultate before palpation of the patient's abdomen is to:
   1. Prevent distortion of vascular sounds
   2. Prevent distortion of the bowel sounds
   3. Determine any areas of tenderness or pain
   4. Allow the patient to relax and be comfortable
4. To correctly palpate the patient's skin for temperature, you will use the:
   1. Base of your hands
   2. Fingertips of your hands
   3. Dorsal surface of your hands
   4. Palmar surface of your hands
5. To assess a patient's superficial lymph nodes, you:
   1. Deeply palpate using entire hand
   2. Deeply palpate using a bimanual technique
   3. Lightly palpate using a bimanual technique
   4. Gently palpate using the pads of your index and middle fingers

6. To spread the breast tissue evenly over the chest wall during an examination, you ask the patient to lie supine with:
   1. Hands clasped just above the umbilicus
   2. Both arms overhead with palms upward
   3. The dominant arm straight alongside the body
   4. The ipsilateral arm overhead with a small pillow under the shoulder
7. In performing a breast assessment on a female patient, you teach the patient that it is especially important to palpate the upper outer quadrant of breast tissue because this area is:
   1. The largest area of the breast
   2. More prone to calcifications
   3. Where breast tumors are often located
   4. Where most lymph nodes are located
8. You need to teach the patient to inspect all skin surfaces and to report pigmented skin lesions that:
   1. Are symmetrical
   2. Have irregular borders
   3. Are uniform in color
   4. Are less than 5 mm in diameter
9. You are assessing the patient for range-of-joint movement. You ask the patient to move the arm away from the body, evaluating the movement of:
   1. Flexion
   2. Extension
   3. Abduction
   4. Adduction

10. The patient's respiratory assessment reveals bilateral high pitches, continuous musical sounds heard loudest upon expiration. The nurse interprets these sounds as:
    1. Normal
    2. Crackles
    3. Rhonchi
    4. Wheezes

11. When auscultating the adult patient's thorax, you:
    1. Instruct the patient to take deep, rapid breaths
    2. Instruct the patient to breathe in and out through the nose
    3. Use the bell of the stethoscope held lightly against the chest
    4. Use the diaphragm of the stethoscope held firmly against the chest

12. You are auscultating the patient's lung fields. The systematic pattern you use for comparison is:
    1. Side to side
    2. Top to bottom
    3. Anterior to posterior
    4. Interspace to interspace

13. You are teaching a patient how to perform a testicular self-examination. You tell the patient:
    1. "Contact your physician or health care provider if you feel a painless pea-sized nodule."
    2. "The testes are normally round, moveable, and have a lumpy consistency."

3. "The best time to do a testicular self-examination is before your bath or shower."
4. "Perform a testicular self-examination every week to detect signs of testicular cancer."

14. When testing sensory pathways, you:
    1. Use a predictable order
    2. Perform each test quickly
    3. Compare symmetrical areas
    4. Ensure that the patient's eyes remain open

15. You ask the patient to smile, frown, and raise and lower the eyebrows; these actions test cranial nerve number:
    1. VII—facial
    2. V—trigeminal
    3. III—oculomotor
    4. XII—hypoglossal

16. To examine for hernias, ask the patient to:
    1. Jump in place
    2. Lift a heavy object
    3. Strain or bear down
    4. Assume the prone position

17. While auscultating heart sounds, you document that $S_1$ is heard best at the apex. This sound correlates with closure of the:
    1. Aortic and mitral valves
    2. Mitral and tricuspid valves
    3. Aortic and pulmonic valves
    4. Tricuspid and pulmonic valves

## REFERENCES

American Cancer Society: *Cancer facts and figures 2005,* New York, 2005, The Society.

Barkauskas VH and others: *Health and physical assessment,* ed 2, St. Louis, 1998, Mosby.

Caulker-Burnett I: Primary care screening for substance abuse, *Nurse Pract* 19(6):42, 1994.

Crowther M, McCourt K: Get the edge on deep vein thrombosis, *Nurs Manage* 35(1):22, 2004.

Day MW: Recognizing and management: DVT—deep vein thrombosis, *Nursing 2003* 33(5):36. 2003.

Ebersole P and others: *Toward healthy aging,* ed 6, St. Louis, 2004, Elsevier Mosby.

Folstein MF and others: Mini-Mental State: a practical method for grading the cognitive state of patients for the clinician, *J Psychiatr Res* 13:189, 1975.

Frakes MA, Evans T: TB—your vigilance is vital, *RN* 67(11):30, 2004.

Friedman L and others: *Source book of substance abuse and addiction,* Baltimore, 1996, Williams & Wilkins.

Fulmer T: Elder abuse and neglect assessment, *J Gerontol Nurs* 29(1):8, 2003

Hardy M: What can you do about your patient's dry skin? *J Gerontol Nurs* 22(5):10, 1996.

Hayes JL: Are you assessing for melanoma? *RN* 66(2):36, 2003.

Hockenberry MJ and others: *Wong's essentials of pediatric nursing,* ed 7, 2005, Elsevier Mosby

Kahn RL and others: Brief objective measures for the determination of mental status in the aged, *Am J Psychiatry* 117:326, 1960.

Kovach K: Intimate partner violence, *RN* 67(8):38, 2004.

Lewis C: Osteoporosis: a man's issue, *Prepared Foods* 172(1):99, 2003.

Master S, Terpstra J: Recognition and diagnosis. In Schnoll SH and others: *Prescribing drugs with abuse liability,* Richmond, Va, 1992, DSAM, MCV-VCU.

Meiner SE, Lueckenotte A: *Gerontologic nursing,* ed 3, St. Louis, 2006, Mosby.

Moore MC: *Pocket guide to nutritional care,* ed 5, St. Louis, 2005, Elsevier Mosby.

Pachuki-Hyde L: Assessment of risk factors for treatment and prevention of osteoporosis, *Nurs Clin North Am* 36(3):401, 2001.

Peterson JA: Osteoporosis overview, *Geriatr Nurs* 22(1):17, 2001.

Quinn MJ: Undue influence and elder abuse: recognition and intervention strategies, *Geriatr Nurs* 23(1):11, 2002.

Seidel HM and others: *Mosby's guide to physical examination,* ed 5, St. Louis, 2003, Mosby.

Stuart G, Laraia M: *Principles and practice of psychiatric nursing,* ed 8, St. Louis, 2005, Elsevier Mosby.

Talbot L, Curtis L: The challenges of assessing skin indicators in people of color, *Home Healthc Nurse* 14(3):167, 1996.

Thompson JM and others: *Mosby's clinical nursing,* ed 5, St. Louis, 2001, Mosby.

U.S. Preventative Services Task Force: Screening for osteoporosis in postmenopausal women: recommendations and rationale, *Am J Nurs* 103(1):73, 2003.

Widlitz M, Marin D: Substance abuse in older adults: an overview, *Geriatrics* 57(12):29, 2002.

# CHAPTER 14

# Administering Medications

## MEDIA RESOURCES

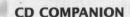 CD COMPANION 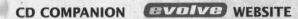 WEBSITE

http://evolve.elsevier.com/Potter/basic

- **NCLEX® Review**
- **Audio Glossary**
- **English/Spanish Audio Glossary**
- **Video Clips**

## OBJECTIVES

- Discuss the nurse's legal responsibilities in medication prescription and administration.
- Describe the physiological mechanisms of medication action.
- Differentiate toxic, idiosyncratic, allergic, and side effects of medications.
- Discuss developmental factors that influence pharmacokinetics.
- Discuss factors that influence medication actions.
- Discuss methods used to teach a patient about prescribed medications.
- Describe the roles of the pharmacist, physician or health care provider, and nurse in medication administration.

- Describe factors to consider when choosing routes of medication administration.
- Correctly calculate a prescribed medication dosage.
- Discuss factors to include in assessing a patient's needs for and response to medication therapy.
- List the six rights of medication administration.
- Correctly prepare and administer subcutaneous, intramuscular, and intradermal injections; intravenous medications; oral and topical skin preparations; eye, ear, and nose drops; vaginal instillations; rectal suppositories; and inhalants.

## KEY TERMS

absorption, p. 341
adverse effects, p. 343
allergic reactions, p. 343
anaphylactic reactions, p. 343
apothecary system, p. 347
biotransformation, p. 342
buccal, p. 346
concentration, p. 344
detoxify, p. 342
idiosyncratic reaction, p. 343
infusions, p. 347
inhalation, p. 347
injections, p. 347
instillation, p. 346
intradermal (ID), p. 346
intramuscular (IM), p. 346
intraocular, p. 347
intravenous (IV), p. 346
irrigations, p. 347
medication abuse, p. 340
medication allergy, p. 343
medication dependence, p. 340

medication error, p. 352
medication interaction, p. 344
metered-dose inhalers (MDIs), p. 381
metric system, p. 347
ophthalmic, p. 371
opioids, p. 352
parenteral administration, p. 346
pharmacokinetics, p. 341
polypharmacy, p. 361
prescriptions, p. 347
serum half-life, p. 344
side effect, p. 343
solution, p. 347
subcutaneous (Sub-Q), p. 346
sublingual, p. 346
synergistic effect, p. 344
therapeutic effect, p. 342
toxic effects, p. 343
transdermal disk, p. 346
Z-track injection, p. 404

Patients with acute or chronic health changes use a variety of medications. A medication is a substance used in the diagnosis, treatment, relief, or prevention of health alterations. No matter where patients receive their health care, you as the nurse will play an essential role in medication administration and teaching. You will also evaluate the effectiveness of medications in restoring or maintaining health. Your role in medication administration will differ based on which healthcare setting you to choose to practice.

In the primary care setting, the patient often self-administers medications. In this setting you are responsible for evaluating the effects of the medications on the patient's health status and teaching the patient about medications and their side effects. You are also responsible for ensuring patient adherence to medication regimens and evaluating the patient's medication administration technique. In the acute care setting, nurses spend much time administering medications to patients. Before discharge you make sure that patients are adequately prepared to administer their medications when they return to the community. In the home, patients usually administer their own medications. When patients cannot administer their own medications, family caregivers are sometimes responsible for medication administration. In this setting as the nurse, you assess the effects the patient's medications have on restoring or maintaining health and provide continued education to the patient, family, or caregiver in all aspects of medication administration.

## Scientific Knowledge Base

Because medication administration is essential to nursing practice, you need to be knowledgeable about the actions and effects of the medications you give to patients. To safely and accurately administer medications, you need to have an understanding of pharmacokinetics (the movement of drugs in the human body), growth and development, nutrition, and mathematics.

## Application of Pharmacology in Nursing Practice

**NAMES.** A medication sometimes has as many as three different names. A medication's chemical name provides an exact description of the medication's composition and molecular structure. In clinical practice, health care workers rarely use chemical names. An example of a chemical name is *N*-acetyl-*para*-aminophenol, which is commonly known as Tylenol. The manufacturer who first develops the medication gives the generic or nonproprietary name, with United States Adopted Name Council (USANC) approval. Acetaminophen is an example of a generic name. It is the generic name for Tylenol. The generic name becomes the official name that is listed in publications such as the *United States Pharmacopeia* (USP). The trade or brand name (e.g., Tylenol) is the name under which a manufacturer markets a medication. The trade name has the symbol ® at the upper right of the name, indicating that the manufacturer has copyrighted the medication's name. You will find medications under a variety of different names. Some medications often have similar spellings and may sound similar (e.g., ephedrine and epinephrine). These types of medications are called look-alike drugs. Medication errors often occur with look-alike drugs. Therefore the Joint Commission of Accreditation of Healthcare Organizations (JCAHO) now requires hospitals and other health care organizations to implement effective safety plans to prevent errors associated with look-alike medications (Institute of Safe Medication Practices [ISMP], 2004c). One JCAHO safety requirement plan states that health care organizations need to develop a list of at least 10 look-alike/sound-alike medications commonly used and set specific safety strategies for these medications (JCAHO, 2004b). Box 14-1 lists examples of strategies that help prevent medication errors caused by look-alike drugs.

**CLASSIFICATION.** Medications with similar characteristics are grouped into classifications. Medication classification indicates the effect of the medication on a body system, the symptoms the medication relieves, or the medication's desired effect. Usually each class contains more than one medication that physicians or health care providers can prescribe for a type of health problem. For example, patients who have type 2 diabetes often take oral medications to lower their blood sugar. This class of medication is called *oral hypoglycemic agents*. There are five different types of hypoglycemic agents and more than 20 different oral hypoglycemic agents (American Diabetes Association [ADA], 2005a). The physical and chemical compositions of medications within a class are sometimes slightly different. A physician or health care provider chooses a particular oral hypoglycemic medication based on patient characteristics, cost, efficacy, dosing frequency, or experience with the medication. A medication may also be part of more than one class.

| BOX 14-1 | **Ways to Prevent Medication Errors Associated With Look-Alike Drugs** |

- Order medication by generic name (e.g., when brand names look alike/sound alike).
- Include diagnosis on prescription.
- Repeat verbal orders back to the prescriber and spell the name of the drug.
- Discuss with patients the name of the drug, indication, and instructions for use.
- Reinforce the prescriber's instructions at the time of patient counseling—a critical step in identifying errors.
- Advise patients to check the labels on their medications before taking them.
- Before administering the medication, review the name and indication with the patient if possible, and check that the patient's diagnosis matches the drug's indication.
- Have patients report any changes in medication appearance (e.g., size, color, smell) to their nurse, pharmacist, prescriber, and/or health care professional.
- Stock similar named products by generic name if products are stored via brand name and vice versa (e.g., separate the look-alike products).
- Place stickers with "Tall Man" letters near the similar named products (e.g., HydrALAzine Hydrochloride and HydrOXYzine Hydrochloride).
- Alert all staff to the potential for error and any actual errors that have occurred.

From: United States Pharmacopeia: *Similar drug names continue to be reported*, 2003, http://www.usp.org/patientSafety/newsletters/practitionerReportingNews/prn1082003-10-23.html.

For example, aspirin is an analgesic, an antipyretic, and an antiinflammatory medication.

**MEDICATION FORMS.** Medications are available in a variety of forms or preparations. The form of the medication determines its route of administration. Manufacturers make many medications in several forms, such as tablets, capsules, elixirs, and suppositories. When administering a medication, be certain to use the proper form (Table 14-1).

## Medication Legislation and Standards

**GOVERNMENTAL REGULATION OF MEDICATIONS.** The role of the U.S. government in regulation of the pharmaceutical industry is to protect the health of the people by ensuring that medications are safe and effective. The first U.S. law to regulate medications was the Pure Food and Drug Act. This law simply requires all medications to be free of impure products. Subsequent legislation has set standards related to safety, potency, and effectiveness. Enforcement of medication laws rests with the Food and Drug Administration (FDA). The FDA ensures that all medications on the market undergo vigorous review before allowing manufacturers to distribute them to the public. State and local medication laws must comply with federal laws. Some individual states have stricter controls than the federal government.

| TABLE 14-1 | Forms of Medication by Route of Administration |
|---|---|

**Medication Forms Commonly Prepared for Administration by Oral Route**

**Solid Forms**

| | |
|---|---|
| Caplet | Solid dosage form for oral use; shaped like a capsule and coated for ease of swallowing. |
| Capsule | Medication encased in a gelatin shell. |
| Tablet | Powdered medication compressed into hard disk or cylinder. |
| Enteric coated | Tablet that is coated so that it does not dissolve in stomach; meant for intestinal absorption. |

**Liquid Forms**

| | |
|---|---|
| Elixir | Clear fluid containing water and alcohol; designed for oral use; usually has sweetener added. |
| Extract | Concentrated medication form made by removing the active portion of medication from its other components. |
| Glycerite | Solution of medication combined with glycerin for external use. |
| Solution | Liquid preparation that may be used orally, parenterally, or externally; can also be instilled into body organ or cavity (e.g., bladder irrigation); must be sterile for parenteral use. |
| Suspension | Finely dissolved particles in a liquid medium; when left standing, particles settle to bottom of container; not used intravenously. |
| Syrup | Medication dissolved in a concentrated sugar solution. |

**Other Oral Forms and Terms Associated With Oral Preparations**

| | |
|---|---|
| Troche (lozenge) | Flat, round dosage form containing medication that dissolves in mouth; not meant for ingestion. |
| Aerosol | Aqueous medication sprayed and absorbed in the mouth and upper airway; not meant for ingestion. |
| Sustained release | Tablet or capsule that contains small particles of a medication coated with material that requires a varying amount of time to dissolve. |

**Medication Forms Commonly Prepared for Administration by Topical Route**

| | |
|---|---|
| Ointment (salve or cream) | Semisolid, externally applied preparation, usually containing one or more medications. |
| Liniment | Oily liquid. |
| Lotion | Emollient liquid that can be clear solution, suspension, or emulsion. |
| Paste | Medication preparation that is thicker than ointment; absorbed through the skin more slowly than ointment. |
| Transdermal patch | Disk or patch embedded with a medication that is absorbed through the skin over a designated period of time. |

**Medication Forms Commonly Prepared for Administration by Parenteral Route**

| | |
|---|---|
| Solution | Preparation that contains water with one or more dissolved compounds. The solution must be sterile. |
| Powder | Particles of medication that are reconstituted with water, dissolved, and administered parenterally. The solution must be sterile. |

**Medication Forms Commonly Prepared for Instillation Into Body Cavities**

| | |
|---|---|
| Suppository | Solid dosage form mixed with gelatin and shaped in the form of a pellet for insertion into a body cavity (rectum or vagina). The suppository melts when it reaches body temperature and is then absorbed. |
| Intraocular disk | Disk (similar to a contact lens) embedded with a medication that is inserted into the client's eye. The medication is absorbed over a designated period of time. |

In 1993 the FDA instituted the MedWatch program. The voluntary program encourages nurses and other health care professionals to report when a medication, product, or medical event causes serious harm to a patient. Mandatory reporting is required for medication manufacturers, distributors, and packers. MedWatch forms are available to report such events (FDA, 2005).

**HEALTH CARE INSTITUTIONS AND MEDICATION LAWS.** Health care institutions establish individual policies to meet federal, state, and local regulations. The size of an institution, the types of services it provides, and the types of professional personnel it employs influence these policies.

Institutional policies are often more restrictive than governmental controls. An institution is concerned primarily with preventing health problems resulting from medication use. A common institutional policy is the automatic discontinuation of narcotic analgesics after a set number of days. Although a prescriber may reorder the medication, this policy helps to control unnecessarily prolonged medication therapy.

**MEDICATION REGULATIONS AND NURSING PRACTICE.** State Nurse Practice Acts have the most influence over nursing practice by defining the scope of a nurse's professional functions and responsibilities. In general, most practice acts are purposefully broad so as not to limit the professional re-

| BOX 14-2 | Guidelines for Safe Opioid Administration and Control |
| --- | --- |

- Keep all opioids in a locked, secure place (e.g., cabinet or computerized medication cart).
- During an institution's change of shift, a nurse going off duty counts all opioids and controlled substances with a nurse coming on duty. Both nurses sign the opioid record, indicating the count is correct.
- Report discrepancies in counts immediately.
- Keep a record each time someone dispenses an opioid. The record includes the patient's name, date, time of drug administration, name of drug, and dosage. If the facility keeps a paper record, the nurse dispensing the drug signs the record. If the facility uses a computerized system, the computer records the nurse's name.
- Keep an ongoing record of opioids used and opioids remaining in the facility.
- If you have to waste part of a controlled substance, a second nurse must witness the disposal of the unused portion. Both nurses record their names on the controlled substance record.

| BOX 14-3 | Nursing Interventions to Improve Compliance With Medications |
| --- | --- |

Establish a therapeutic nurse-patient relationship.

Involve the patient in deciding dosage schedule and regimen for drug preparation.

Simplify the medication regimen as much as possible.

Explain medication instructions in simple, easy-to-understand words.

Educate patients so they make informed decisions about medications.

Educate patients about expected side effects of medications and how to reduce, eliminate, or manage the side effects.

Review the patient's medications regularly, and consult with the prescriber if unnecessary or duplicate medications are prescribed or if discrepancies exist between what the patient should be taking and what the patient is actually taking.

Evaluate the effectiveness of communication between you and the patient and the effectiveness of medication education.

Call patients who miss appointments with their health care providers to keep the patients involved with their care.

Data from Ebersole P and others: *Toward healthy aging: human needs and nursing response,* ed 6, St. Louis, 2004, Mosby; and Haynes RB and others: Interventions for helping patients to follow prescriptions for medications, *Cochrane Database Syst Review* 4:2004.

sponsibilities of the nurse. Institutions and agencies interpret specific actions allowed under the acts, but they are not able to modify, expand, or restrict the act's intent. The primary intent of state Nurse Practice Acts is to protect the public from unskilled, undereducated, and unlicensed nurses.

You are responsible for following legal provisions when administering controlled substances or opioids, which are controlled through federal and state guidelines. Nurses who violate the Controlled Substances Act can face fines, imprisonment, and loss of nurse licensure. Hospitals and other health care institutions have policies for the proper storage and distribution of narcotics (Box 14-2).

**NONTHERAPEUTIC MEDICATION USE.** Misuse includes overuse, underuse, erratic use, and contraindicated use of medications. Patients of all ages misuse medications. However, there is a greater risk of this with older adults. Some people use medications for purposes other than their intended effect. Factors such as peer pressure, curiosity, and the pursuit of pleasure are some motivators for nontherapeutic medication use. Problems with medication use are not limited to heroin, cocaine, and other street drugs. The incidence of prescription and over-the-counter (OTC) drug misuse and abuse is also on the rise. The most commonly abused prescription medications include opioids, stimulants, tranquilizers, and sedatives. Common OTC medications patients misuse or abuse include aspirin and cough syrup (U.S. Department of Health and Human Services Substance Abuse and Mental Health Services Administration [USDHHS SAMHSA], 2004).

You have ethical and legal responsibilities to understand the problems of persons using medications improperly. When caring for patients with suspected **medication abuse** or **medication dependence,** be aware of your values and attitudes about the willful use of potentially harmful substances. You develop therapeutic relationships with patients when your personal values do not interfere with the acceptance or understanding of their needs. Knowing the physical, psychological, and social changes resulting from medication abuse allows you to identify patients with medication problems.

Health professionals also misuse medications. Stress in the workplace, personal problems, and the strong desire to perform well are some factors that cause nurses to misuse medications. Recognize and understand the problems of colleagues who abuse medications. Many programs are available to assist these nurses toward recovery. These programs are offered through the institution's employees' assistance program (EAP), the State Board of Nursing, or community agencies.

**Nonadherence.** Ethically, you need to understand why patients are nonadherent with their medications. Nonadherence is the failure of a patient to take a medication as it is prescribed. Research shows that approximately 50% of patients do not take their medications as prescribed (Haynes and others, 2004). Poor patient education or a patient's perception that a medication is not needed cause nonadherence. Nonadherence with medications is one of the biggest issues that affect the health and safety of all patients. For example, between 20% and 70% of older adults who live in the community do not adhere to their medication schedules (Ebersole and others, 2004). Many factors cause nonadherence in older adult populations, such as depression, a dislike for the side effects, a busy and active lifestyle, and an inability to afford medications. Carefully assess the medications your patient takes and compare them with what was prescribed. If you suspect nonadherence, investigate contributing factors and work with the patient to develop a medication regimen the patient will follow. Box 14-3 provides interventions that help promote

**BOX 14-4** USING EVIDENCE IN PRACTICE

**Research Summary**

Nonadherence in patients who have congestive heart failure often results in frequent hospitalizations and increased morbidity and mortality rates. Studies have shown that 47% of patients who are 70 years of age or older and who have congestive heart failure are rehospitalized within 90 days of discharge. Many times the reason for readmission is related to noncompliance with recommended medications and other treatments. The researchers in this study compared the compliance of patients who were 65 years old or older with the compliance of patients who were less than 65 years old. The researchers also asked the older patients why they had difficulty following health care recommendations and evaluated the relationship between the difficulty levels of the recommended therapies with how well the older patients complied with their treatments.

The researchers found that both the older and younger groups of patients were more compliant with keeping their medical appointments, taking their medications, and not smoking or drinking alcohol. Although both groups had difficulty following the recommended diet and exercise guidelines, the older group had more difficulties than the younger group. One fourth of the older patients reported difficulty going to medical appointments and taking their prescribed medications. When asked why they were having problems following their heart failure management plans, the older patients stated that the following contributed to their nonadherence: lack of transportation, costs of medications, forgetfulness, unpleasant side effects of medications, lack of motivation and self-control, and lack of energy.

**Application to Nursing Practice**

The results from this study provide helpful insights into why patients have difficulty complying with their medical treatment regimens. To help patients become more compliant, nurses need to investigate reasons for noncompliance and implement nursing interventions that will help patients overcome barriers to health care. Keeping medication schedules and treatment plans simple will improve patient compliance. Providing individualized teaching and counseling that addresses the specific concerns of the patient give patients, especially those who are older, the support and knowledge needed to manage their illness successfully.

From Evangelista LS and others: Compliance behaviors of elderly patients with advanced heart failure, *J Cardiovasc Nurs* 18(3):197, 2003.

medication compliance. Because of the negative outcomes associated with nonadherence, determining how to better help patients to comply with medication schedules and other associated therapies has recently been a major focus of nursing research (Box 14-4).

## Pharmacokinetics as the Basis of Medication Actions

For a medication to be therapeutically useful, it is taken into a patient's body; is absorbed and distributed to cells, tissues, or a specific organ; and alters physiological functions. **Pharmacokinetics** is the study of how medications enter the body, reach their site of action, metabolize, and exit the body (McKenry and Salerno, 2003). You will use your knowledge of pharmacokinetics to time medication administration, select the route of administration, judge the patient's risk for alterations in medication action, and evaluate the patient's response to the medication.

ABSORPTION. **Absorption** refers to passage of medication molecules into the blood from the site of administration. Factors that influence medication absorption are the route of administration, ability of the medication to dissolve, blood flow to the site of administration, body surface area, and lipid solubility of the medication.

**Route of Administration.** You will administer medications by various routes. Each route has a different rate of absorption. When you place medications on the skin, absorption is slow because of the physical makeup of the skin. The body sometimes absorbs oral medications at a slow rate because they first pass through the gastrointestinal (GI) tract to be absorbed. The body absorbs medications placed on the mucous membranes and in respiratory airways quickly, because these tissues contain many blood vessels. Intravenous (IV) injection produces the most rapid absorption, because this route provides immediate access to the systemic circulation.

**Ability of the Medication to Dissolve.** The ability of an oral medication to dissolve depends largely on its form of preparation. Solutions and suspensions are already in a liquid state and are easier for the body to absorb than tablets or capsules. Acidic medications pass through the gastric mucosa rapidly, whereas medications that are alkaline are not absorbed before reaching the small intestine.

**Blood Flow to the Area of Absorption.** The blood supply to the site of administration determines how quickly the body absorbs a drug. Sites with rich blood supplies absorb medications more quickly. For example, a medication administered in the muscle (intramuscular [IM] route) is absorbed faster than a medication administered in the subcutaneous tissue (subcutaneous route) because the blood supply to muscle is richer than the blood supply to subcutaneous tissue.

**Body Surface Area.** The size of the surface the medication comes in contact with affects how quickly the body absorbs the medication. If the surface area is large, the medication will be absorbed more quickly; thus the medication's effects will occur more quickly. This explains why many medications are absorbed more quickly and take effect faster when they absorbed in the small intestine rather than the stomach (McKenry and Salerno, 2003).

**Lipid Solubility of the Medication.** Medications that are highly lipid soluble are easier for the body to absorb because they readily cross the cell membrane, which is made of a lipid layer. Another factor that affects absorption of a medication is the presence of food in the stomach. Some oral medications are absorbed more quickly on an empty stomach, whereas other medications are unaffected by gastric contents. In addition, some medications interfere with the absorption of each other if given at the same time. Know the factors that alter or impair absorption of the medications that have been prescribed for your patients. This knowledge ensures that you administer all prescribed medications at the correct time to allow for correct absorption of the drug.

**DISTRIBUTION.** After a medication is absorbed, it is distributed within the body to tissues and organs and ultimately to its specific site of action. The rate and extent of distribution depend on the physical and chemical properties of medications and the physiology of the person taking the medication.

**Circulation.** Once a medication enters the bloodstream, the blood carries it throughout the tissue and organs of the body. How fast it gets there depends on the vascularity of the various tissues and organs. When conditions that limit blood flow exist or intended sites of action have a poor blood supply, this inhibits the distribution of a medication. For example, solid tumors have poor blood supply and sometimes do not respond to therapy intended to destroy them.

**Membrane Permeability.** To be distributed to an organ, a medication needs to pass through all the biological membranes of that organ. Some membranes serve as barriers to the passage of medications. For example, the blood-brain barrier allows only fat-soluble medications to pass into the brain and cerebrospinal fluid. Therefore central nervous system (CNS) infections require treatment with antibiotics injected directly into the subarachnoid space in the spinal cord. Older patients often experience adverse effects (e.g., confusion) as a result of the change in the permeability of the blood-brain barrier, with easier passage of fat-soluble medications. The placental membrane is a nonselective barrier to medications. Fat-soluble and non–fat-soluble agents cross the placenta and produce fetal deformities and respiratory depression. If the mother abuses narcotics, the fetus will suffer withdrawal symptoms when it is born.

**Protein Binding.** The degree to which medications bind to serum proteins, such as albumin, affects medication distribution. Most medications bind to protein to some extent. When medications bind to albumin, they do not exert any pharmacological activity. The unbound, or "free," medication is the active form of the medication. Older adults or patients with liver disease or malnutrition have decreased albumin in the bloodstream. Because more medication is unbound in these patients, they are at risk for an increase in medication activity, toxicity, or both.

**METABOLISM.** After a medication reaches its site of action, it becomes metabolized. **Biotransformation** occurs under the influence of enzymes that **detoxify**, degrade (break down), and remove biologically active chemicals. Most biotransformation occurs within the liver, although the lungs, kidneys, blood, and intestines also metabolize medications. The liver is especially important because its specialized structure oxidizes and transforms many toxic substances. The liver

degrades many harmful chemicals before they become distributed to the tissues. If a decrease in liver function occurs, such as with aging or liver disease, the body eliminates a medication more slowly, resulting in a buildup of the medication. When organs that metabolize medications do not function correctly, patients are at risk for medication toxicity.

**EXCRETION.** After medications are metabolized, they exit the body through the kidneys, liver, bowel, lungs, and exocrine glands. The chemical makeup of a medication determines which organ excretes the medication.

The kidneys are the main organs that excrete medications. Some medications escape extensive metabolism and exit unchanged in the urine. Other medications undergo biotransformation in the liver before the kidney excretes them. If renal function declines, a patient is at risk for medication toxicity. If the kidney cannot adequately excrete a medication, it is necessary to reduce the dose. Maintenance of an adequate fluid intake (50 ml/kg/day) promotes proper elimination of medications for the average adult.

Gaseous and volatile compounds, such as nitrous oxide and alcohol, exit through the lungs. Deep breathing and coughing (see Chapter 37) help the postoperative patient to eliminate anesthetic gases more quickly. The exocrine glands excrete lipid-soluble medications. When medications exit through sweat glands, the skin sometimes becomes irritated. The nurse assists the patient in good hygiene practices (see Chapter 27) to promote cleanliness and skin integrity.

The GI tract is another route for medication excretion. Many medications enter the hepatic circulation to be broken down by the liver and excreted into the bile. After chemicals enter the intestines through the biliary tract, the intestines reabsorb them. Factors that increase peristalsis (e.g., laxatives, enemas) accelerate medication excretion through the feces, whereas factors that slow peristalsis (e.g., inactivity, improper diet) prolong a medication's effects.

Medications are often excreted through the mammary glands. In these cases there is a risk that a nursing infant will ingest the chemicals. Have mothers check on the safety of any medication used while breast-feeding.

## Types of Medication Action

Medications vary considerably in the way they act and their types of action. Factors other than characteristics of the medication also influence medication actions. A patient does not always respond in the same way to each successive dose of a medication, or the same medication dosage sometimes causes very different responses in different patients. Box 14-5 lists important variables that influence medication action.

**THERAPEUTIC EFFECTS.** The **therapeutic effect** is the intended or desired physiological response of a medication. Each medication has a desired therapeutic effect. For example, you administer nitroglycerin to reduce cardiac workload and increase myocardial oxygen supply, thus decreasing or eliminating chest pain. Sometimes a single medication has many therapeutic effects. For example, aspirin is an analgesic, antipyretic, and antiinflammatory, and it reduces platelet aggregation (clumping of blood platelets). It is

---

## BOX 14-5 Factors Influencing Drug Actions

### Genetic Differences

- A person's genetic makeup influences drug metabolism. Members of a family sometimes share sensitivity to a medication.

### Physiological Variables

- Gender, age, body weight, nutritional status, and disease states all affect drug actions.
- Hormonal differences between men and women affect drug metabolism.
- Children usually require lower drug doses than adults. However, sometimes they need larger doses depending on the medication. The changes accompanying aging alter the influence of drugs.
- There is a direct relationship between the concentration of the medication administered and how quickly the medication is absorbed by body tissues.
- Diseases that impair the function of an organ responsible for normal pharmacokinetics also impair drug action (e.g., if a patient has liver failure, the metabolism of medications will be slower).

### Environmental Conditions

- Stress and the exposure to heat and cold affect drug actions. For example, patients receiving vasodilators require lower drug dosages in warm weather.
- The setting in which a person takes a drug influences a patient's reaction. When patients are alone or isolated, they may need more pain medication than if they were in a room with other patients or if their families frequently visit them.

### Psychological Factors

- A patient's attitude, reaction to the meaning of a drug, and the nurse's behavior affect drug actions. If a patient understands and accepts the need for a drug and if you administer it with supportive behavior, this enhances the drug's effect.

### Diet

- Drug and nutrient interactions alter a drug's action or the effect of a nutrient. For example, mineral oil decreases the absorption of fat-soluble vitamins.
- Proper drug metabolism relies on good nutrition.

---

important to know the expected therapeutic effect for each medication your patients receive. This will allow you to properly teach the patient about the medication's intended effect and to evaluate the effectiveness of the medication.

**SIDE EFFECTS/ADVERSE REACTIONS.** Medications can react in the body to produce unpredictable and sometimes unexplainable response (McKenry and Salerno, 2004). A **side effect** is a predictable and often unavoidable secondary effect produced at a usual therapeutic dose. For example, some antihypertensive medications and antidepressants often cause impotence in male patients. Some side effects are harmless, and some cause injury. If the side effects are serious enough to cancel the beneficial effects of a medication's therapeutic action, physicians or health care providers usually discontinue the medication. Patients often stop taking medications because of side effects. The most common are anorexia, nausea, vomiting, constipation, and diarrhea.

**Adverse effects** are undesired, unintended, and often unpredictable responses to medication. For example, a patient becomes comatose after taking a drug. When adverse responses to medications occur, the prescriber immediately discontinues the medication. Some adverse effects are unexpected effects that researchers did not discover during drug testing. When this situation occurs, health care providers are obligated to report the adverse effect to the FDA. Be alert to assess any unusual individual responses to drugs, especially with newly released medications. There is a continuum of adverse drug effects ranging from mild to severe. Clients most at risk for adverse medication reactions include the very young and elderly, women, clients taking multiple medications, clients extremely underweight or overweight, and clients with renal or liver disease.

**Toxic Effects. Toxic effects** develop after prolonged intake of a medication or when a medication accumulates in the blood because of impaired metabolism or excretion.

Excess amounts of a medication within the body have lethal effects, depending on the medication's action. Sometimes antidotes are available to treat specific types of medication toxicity. For example, a patient experiencing toxic effects of morphine has severe respiratory depression. In this case you give Narcan to reverse the toxic effects of the morphine.

**Idiosyncratic Reactions.** Some medications cause unpredictable effects, such as an **idiosyncratic reaction** in which a patient overreacts or underreacts to a medication or has a reaction different from what is expected. For example, a child receiving an antihistamine (e.g., Benadryl) becomes extremely agitated or excited instead of drowsy.

**Allergic Reactions. Allergic reactions** are also unpredictable responses to a medication. Some patients become immunologically sensitized to a medication after taking the first dose. With repeated administration, the patient develops an allergic response to the medication, its chemical preservatives, or a metabolite. The medication or chemical acts as an antigen, triggering the release of the body's antibodies. A patient's **medication allergy** may be mild or severe. Allergic symptoms vary, depending on the individual and the medication. Table 14-2 summarizes common, mild allergy symptoms. Sudden constriction of bronchiolar muscles, edema of the pharynx and larynx, and severe wheezing and shortness of breath all characterize severe or **anaphylactic reactions.** Antihistamines, epinephrine, and bronchodilators are used to treat anaphylactic reactions.

In anaphylaxis a patient also becomes severely hypotensive, necessitating emergency resuscitation measures. A patient with a known history of an allergy to a medication should avoid reexposure and wear an identification bracelet or medal (Figure 14-1) that alerts health care providers to the allergy if the patient is unconscious when receiving medical care.

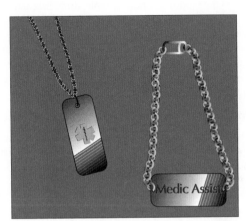

FIGURE **14-1** Identification bracelet and medal.

| TABLE 14-3 | Common Dosage Administration Schedules |
|---|---|
| Abbreviation | Meaning |
| AC, ac | Before meals |
| ad lib | As desired |
| BID, bid | Twice each day |
| daily | Every day |
| PC, pc | After meals |
| prn | Whenever there is a need |
| qAM | Every morning, every AM |
| h, hr | Hour |
| qh | Every hour |
| q2h | Every 2 hours |
| q4h | Every 4 hours |
| q6h | Every 6 hours |
| q8h | Every 8 hours |
| QID, qid | 4 times per day |
| stat | Give immediately |
| TID, tid | 3 times per day |

| TABLE 14-2 | Mild Allergic Reactions |
|---|---|
| Symptom | Description |
| Urticaria (hives) | Raised, irregularly shaped skin eruptions with varying sizes and shapes; have reddened margins and pale centers. |
| Eczema (rash) | Small, raised vesicles that are usually reddened; often distributed over entire body |
| Pruritus | Itching of skin; accompanies most rashes |
| Rhinitis | Inflammation of mucous membranes lining nose; causes swelling and clear, watery discharge |
| Wheezing | Constriction of smooth muscles that surround bronchioles; occurs mainly on inspiration and can lead to airway obstruction |
| Angioedema | Short-term subcutaneous or submucosal swellings of the face, neck, lips, larynx, hands, feet, genitalia, or viscera |

| TABLE 14-4 | Terms Associated With Medication Actions |
|---|---|
| Term | Meaning |
| Onset | Time it takes after you administer a drug for it to produce a response |
| Peak | Time it takes for a drug to reach its highest effective concentration |
| Trough | Minimum blood serum concentration of a drug reached just before the next scheduled dose |
| Duration | Time during which the drug is present in a concentration great enough to produce a response |
| Plateau | Blood serum concentration of a drug reached and maintained after repeated fixed doses |

**MEDICATION INTERACTIONS.** When one medication modifies the action of another medication, a **medication interaction** occurs. A medication sometimes enhances or diminishes the action of other medications and alters the way in which the body absorbs, metabolizes, or eliminates another medication. When two medications have a **synergistic effect,** the effect of the two medications combined is greater than the effects of the medications when given separately. For example, alcohol is a CNS depressant that has a synergistic effect on antihistamines, antidepressants, barbiturates, and narcotic analgesics.

Sometimes, a medication interaction is desirable. Often a physician or health care provider orders combination medication therapy to create a medication interaction for the patient's benefit. For example, a patient with moderate hypertension typically receives several medications, such as diuretics and vasodilators, that act together to control blood pressure.

**MEDICATION DOSE RESPONSES.** A medication undergoes absorption, distribution, metabolism, and excretion after it enters the body. Except when administered intravenously, medications take time to enter the bloodstream.

All medications have a **serum half-life,** which is the time it takes for excretion to lower the serum medication **concentration** by half. To maintain a therapeutic plateau, the patient receives regular fixed doses. For example, research has shown that pain medications are most effective when they are given "around the clock" rather than when the patient intermittently complains of pain. This results in a constant serum level of pain medication. After an initial medication dose, the patient receives each successive dose when the previous dose reaches its half-life.

You and the patient will follow prescribed doses and dosage intervals. Table 14-3 lists common dosage schedules

| TABLE 14-5 | Factors Influencing Choice of Administration Routes |
| --- | --- |

| Advantages by Route | Disadvantages/Contraindications |
| --- | --- |
| **Oral, Buccal, Sublingual Routes** | |
| Routes are convenient and comfortable for patient. Routes are economical. Medications sometimes produce local or systemic effects. Routes rarely cause anxiety for patient. | Avoid these routes when patient has alterations in GI function (e.g., nausea, vomiting), reduced GI motility (after general anesthesia or bowel inflammation), gastric suction, surgical resection of portion of GI tract, and reduced ability to swallow. Oral medications sometimes irritate lining of GI tract, discolor teeth, or have unpleasant tastes. |
| **Parenteral (Sub-Q, IM, IV, ID, Epidural)** | |
| Routes provide means of administration when oral drugs are contraindicated. More rapid absorption occurs than with topical or oral routes. IV infusion provides drug delivery when patient is critically ill. If peripheral perfusion is poor, IV route is preferred over injections. Epidural provides excellent pain control. | There is risk of introducing infection, drugs are expensive, and you need to avoid these routes in patients with bleeding tendencies. There is risk of tissue damage with these routes. IM and IV routes are dangerous because of rapid absorption. These routes cause considerable anxiety in many patients, especially children. Limits mobility during medication administration. Risk of infection. |
| **Topical** | |
| Skin applications primarily provide local effect. Route is painless. Limited side effects occur. | Extensive applications are bulky and often impair physical mobility. Do not apply if skin abrasions are present. |
| **Transdermal** | |
| Transdermal applications provide prolonged systemic effects, with limited side effects. | Application leaves oily or pasty substance on skin and soils clothing. |
| **Eyes, Ears, Nose, Vaginal, Rectal, Buccal, and Sublingual\*** | |
| Local application to involved sites provides therapeutic effects. Aqueous solutions are readily absorbed and capable of causing systemic effects. Mucous membranes provide route of administration when oral drugs are contraindicated. | Mucous membranes are highly sensitive to some drug concentrations. Insertion of rectal and vaginal medication often causes embarrassment. Patient with ruptured eardrum cannot receive irrigations. Rectal suppositories are contraindicated if patient has had rectal surgery or if active rectal bleeding is present. |
| **Inhalation** | |
| Inhalation provides rapid relief for local respiratory problems. Route provides easy access for introduction of general anesthetic gases. | Some local agents cause serious systemic effects. |
| **Intraocular Disk** | |
| Route is advantageous in that it does not require frequent administration like eye drops. | Local reactions can occur. Patient must be taught how to insert and remove disk. Expensive. Contraindicated with eye infections. |

\*Includes eyes, ears, nose, vagina, rectum, buccal, and sublingual routes.

used in acute care settings. When you teach patients about dosage schedules, use language that is familiar to the patient. For example, when teaching a patient about twice-daily medication dosing, instruct the patient to take the medication in the morning and again in the evening. Knowledge of the time intervals of medication action will help you anticipate a medication's effect. With this knowledge, instruct the patient when to expect a response. Table 14-4 lists common terms associated with medication actions.

## Routes of Administration

The route prescribed for administering a medication depends on the medication's properties and its desired effect. The route also depends on the patient's physical and mental condition (Table 14-5). Collaborate with the prescriber in determining the best route for a patient's medication. For example, you are caring for a patient who has 650 mg of acetaminophen ordered by mouth every 4 hours as needed for a temperature greater than 38.0° C (100.4° F).

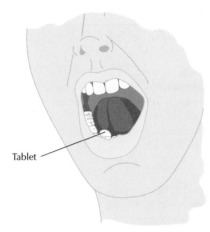

FIGURE **14-2** Sublingual administration of a tablet.

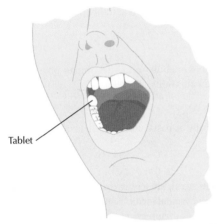

FIGURE **14-3** Buccal administration of a tablet.

Your patient has a temperature of 38.5°C (101.2° F), is vomiting, and is unable to tolerate oral fluids. Knowing your patient cannot tolerate oral medications at this time, you consult with the prescriber and have the medication changed to a rectal suppository.

**ORAL ROUTES.** The oral route is the easiest and the most commonly used. Medications are given by mouth and swallowed with fluid. Oral medications have a slower onset of action and a more prolonged effect than parenteral medications. Patients generally prefer the oral route.

**Sublingual Administration.** Some medications are designed to be readily absorbed after being placed under the tongue to dissolve (Figure 14-2). A medication given by the **sublingual** route should not be swallowed or chewed, or the desired effect will not be achieved. Nitroglycerin is commonly given by the sublingual route. Do not have the patient take a drink, eat, or chew gum until the medication is completely dissolved.

**Buccal Administration.** Administration of a medication by the **buccal** route involves placing the solid medication in the mouth and against the mucous membranes of the cheek until the medication dissolves (Figure 14-3). Teach patients to alternate cheeks with each dose to avoid mucosal irritation. Also teach patients not to chew or swallow the medication or to take any liquids with it. A buccal medication acts locally on the mucosa or systemically as it is swallowed in a person's saliva.

**PARENTERAL ROUTES. Parenteral administration** involves injecting a medication into body tissues. The four major parenteral routes are as follows:

1. **Subcutaneous (Sub-Q):** injection into tissues just below the dermis of the skin
2. **Intramuscular (IM):** injection into a muscle
3. **Intravenous (IV):** injection into a vein
4. **Intradermal (ID):** injection into the dermis just under the epidermis

You administer some medications into body cavities through other routes, including epidural, intraperitoneal, intrathecal or intraspinal, intracardiac, intrapleural, intra-arterial, intraosseous, and intra-articular routes. Nurses with advanced education or in advanced practice administer medications by these routes. Medication routes such as intracardiac or intra-articular are usually limited to physician administration. Regardless of who actually administers the medication by these routes, you are responsible for monitoring the integrity of the system of medication delivery, understanding the therapeutic value of the medication, and evaluating the patient's response to the therapy.

**TOPICAL ADMINISTRATION.** Medications applied to the skin and mucous and respiratory membranes generally have local effects. Topical medication is applied to the skin by painting or spreading it over an area, applying moist dressings, soaking body parts in a solution, or giving medicated baths. Systemic effects occur if a patient's skin is thin, if the medication concentration is high, or if contact with the skin is prolonged.

Some medications (e.g., nitroglycerin, Catapres, estrogens) have systemic effects because you apply them topically by a **transdermal disk** or patch. The disk firmly holds the medicated ointment to the skin. You apply these topical applications for as little as 12 hours or as long as 7 days.

You can apply medications to mucous membranes in a variety of ways, including the following:

1. By directly applying a liquid or ointment (e.g., eye drops, gargling, swabbing the throat)
2. By inserting a medication into a body cavity (e.g., placing a suppository in rectum or vagina, inserting medicated packing into vagina)
3. By instilling fluid into a body part or cavity (e.g., ear drops, nose drops, bladder or rectal **instillation** [fluid is retained])
4. By irrigating a body cavity (e.g., flushing eye, ear, vagina, bladder, or rectum with medicated fluid [fluid is not retained])
5. By spraying a medication into a body cavity (e.g., instillation into nose and throat)

**Inhalation Route.** The deeper passages of the respiratory tract provide a large surface area for medication absorption. You can administer medications through the nasal passages, oral passage, or tubes placed into the patient's mouth to the trachea. Medications that are administered by the **inhalation** route are readily absorbed and work quickly because of the rich vascular alveolar-capillary network in the pulmonary tissue. Inhaled medications sometimes have local or systemic effects.

**Intraocular Route. Intraocular** medication delivery involves administering medication into the eye. One kind of intraocular route involves inserting a medication similar to a contact lens into the patient's eye. The eye medication disk has two soft outer layers that have medication enclosed in them. You insert the disk into the patient's eye, much like a contact lens. The disk remains in the patient's eye for up to 1 week, if prescribed. Pilocarpine, a medication used to treat glaucoma, is the most common medication disk used.

## Systems of Medication Measurement

The proper administration of a medication requires the ability to compute medication doses accurately and measure medications correctly. A careless mistake in placing a decimal point or adding a zero to a dose can lead to a fatal error. Check the dose carefully before giving a medication.

The health care industry uses the metric, apothecary, and household systems of measurement for medication therapy. Most nations, including Canada, use the metric system as their standard of measurement. Although the U.S. Congress has not officially adopted the metric system, most health professionals in the United States use it. Physicians usually write **prescriptions** that are to be self-administered at home by patients in household measures. Use of the **apothecary system** is rare.

**METRIC SYSTEM.** As a decimal system, the **metric system** is the most logically organized. Metric units are easy to convert and calculate using simple multiplication and division. Each basic unit of measurement is organized into units of 10. In multiplication the decimal point moves to the right; in division the decimal moves to the left. For example:

$$10.0 \text{ mg} \times 10 = 100.0 \text{ mg}$$
$$10.0 \text{ mg} \div 10 = 1.0 \text{ mg}$$

The basic units of measurement in the metric system are the meter (length), liter (volume), and gram (weight). For medication calculations you use only the volume and weight units. In the metric system you use lower-case or upper-case letters to designate units:

$$\text{Gram} = \text{g or Gm}$$
$$\text{Liter} = \text{l or L}$$
$$\text{Milligram} = \text{mg}$$
$$\text{Milliliter} = \text{ml}$$

A system of Latin prefixes designates subdivision of the basic units: deci- ($\frac{1}{10}$ or 0.1), centi- ($\frac{1}{100}$ or 0.01), and milli-

| TABLE 14-6 | Equivalents of Measurement | |
|---|---|---|
| **Metric** | **Apothecary** | **Household** |
| 1 ml | 15-16 minims (m) | 15 drops (gtt) |
| 4-5 ml | 1 fluidram (f3) | 1 teaspoon (tsp) |
| 16 ml | 4 fluidrams (f3) | 1 tablespoon (tbsp) |
| 30 ml | 1 fluid ounce (f3) | 2 tablespoons (tbsp) |
| 240 ml | 8 fluid ounces (f3) | 1 cup (c) |
| 480 ml (approximately 500 ml) | 1 pint (pt) | 1 pint (pt) |
| 960 ml (approximately 1 L) | 1 quart (qt) | 1 quart (qt) |
| 3840 ml (approximately 5 L) | 1 gallon (gal) | 1 gallon (gal) |

($\frac{1}{1000}$ or 0.001). Greek prefixes designate multiples of the basic units: deka- (10), hecto- (100), and kilo- (1000). When writing medication doses in metric units, you use fractions or multiples of a unit. Always give fractions in decimal form:

$$500 \text{ mg or } 0.5 \text{ g, not } \frac{1}{2} \text{ g}$$
$$10 \text{ ml or } 0.01 \text{ L, not } \frac{1}{100} \text{ L}$$

Many actual and potential medication errors occur with the use of fractions. Therefore practice standards are used when medications are ordered in fractions to prevent medication errors. To make the decimal point more visible, a leading zero is always placed in front of a decimal (e.g., use 0.5, not .5). However, the use of a zero after a decimal point, also called a trailing zero, is not recommended because if a health care worker does not see the decimal point, the patient may end up receiving 10 times more medication than what is prescribed (e.g., use 5 not 5.0) (National Coordinating Council for Medication Error Reporting and Prevention [NCCMERP], 2001).

**HOUSEHOLD MEASUREMENTS.** Household units of measure are familiar to most people. The disadvantage with household measures is their inaccuracy. Household utensils, such as teaspoons and cups, often vary in size. Scales to measure pints or quarts are often not well calibrated. Household measures include drops, teaspoons, tablespoons, and cups for volume and pints and quarts for weight. Although pints and quarts are considered household measures, they are also used in the apothecary system.

The advantages of household measurements are their convenience and familiarity. When the accuracy of a medication dose is not critical, it is safe to use household measures. For example, you can safely measure many OTC medications by this method. Table 14-6 gives common equivalents from each measurement unit.

**SOLUTIONS.** Solutions of various concentrations are used for **injections, irrigations,** and **infusions.** A **solution** is a given mass of solid substance dissolved in a known volume of fluid or a given volume of liquid dissolved in a known volume of another fluid. When a solid is dissolved in a fluid, the concentration is in units of mass per units of volume (e.g., g/ml, g/L, or mg/ml). You also express a concentration of a solution as a percentage. For example, a 10% solution is 10 g of solid dissolved in 100 ml of solution. A proportion also expresses concentrations. A $\frac{1}{1000}$ solution represents a solution containing 1 g of solid in 1000 ml of liquid or 1 ml of liquid mixed with 1000 ml of another liquid.

## Clinical Calculations

To administer medications safely, you need to understand basic math to calculate medication dosages, to mix solutions, and to perform a variety of other activities. This is important because you will not always dispense medications in the unit of measure in which they are ordered. Medication companies package and bottle certain standard equivalents. For example, the physician or health care provider orders 250 mg of a medication that is available only in grams. You are responsible for converting available units of volume and weight to the desired doses. Therefore be aware of approximate equivalents in all major measurement systems.

**CONVERSIONS WITHIN ONE SYSTEM.** Converting measurements within one system is relatively easy. In the metric system you will use division or multiplication. For example, to change milligrams to grams, divide by 1000 or move the decimal three points to the left:

$$1000 \text{ mg} = 1 \text{ g}$$
$$350 \text{ mg} = 0.35 \text{ g}$$

To convert liters to milliliters, multiply by 1000 or move the decimal three points to the right:

$$1 \text{ L} = 1000 \text{ ml}$$
$$0.25 \text{ L} = 250 \text{ ml}$$

To convert units of measurement within the apothecary or household system, you need to know the equivalent. For example, when converting fluid ounces to quarts, you know that 32 ounces is the equivalent of 1 quart. To convert 8 ounces to a quart measurement, divide 8 by 32 to get the equivalent, $\frac{1}{4}$ or 0.25 quart.

**CONVERSION BETWEEN SYSTEMS.** Frequently you will determine the correct dose of a medication by converting weights or volumes from one system of measurement to another. For example, metric units are converted to equivalent household measures to ease medication administration at home. To convert from one measurement system to another, it is necessary to use equivalent measurements. Tables of equivalent measurements are available in all health care institutions. If a table is not available, the pharmacist is also a good resource for this information.

Before making a conversion, you compare the measurement system available with what was ordered. For example, a health care provider orders 30 ml of Robitussin for your patient. To provide proper instruction to the patient, you will convert "ml" to a common household measurement. By referring to a table, such as Table 14-6, you determine that 30 ml = 2 tablespoons. Therefore you instruct the patient to take 2 tablespoons of Robitussin.

**DOSAGE CALCULATIONS.** You can use many formulas to calculate medication dosages. Apply the following basic formula when preparing solid or liquid forms:

$$\frac{\text{Dose ordered}}{\text{Dose on hand}} \times \text{Amount on hand} = \text{Amount to administer}$$

The dose ordered is the amount of medication prescribed. The dose on hand is the weight or volume of medication available in units supplied by the pharmacy. It is expressed on the medication label as the contents of a tablet or capsule or as the amount of medication dissolved per unit volume of liquid. The amount on hand is the basic unit or quantity of the medication that contains the dose on hand. For solid medications, the amount on hand may be one capsule. The amount of liquid on hand may be 1 ml or 1 L. The amount to administer is the actual amount of available medication you will administer. The amount to administer is always expressed in the same unit as the amount on hand.

**Example 1.** Your patient needs to receive Demerol, 50 mg IM (dose ordered). The medication is available only in ampules containing 100 mg (dose on hand) in 1 ml (amount on hand). You apply the formula as follows:

$$\frac{50 \text{ mg}}{100 \text{ mg}} \times 1 \text{ ml} = 0.5 \text{ ml (amount to administer)}$$

After working the equation, you know to prepare 0.5 ml in a syringe.

**Example 2.** The physician or health care provider orders 0.125 mg orally (PO) of digoxin. The medication is available in tablets containing 0.25 mg. You apply the formula as follows:

$$\frac{0.125 \text{ mg}}{0.25 \text{ mg}} \times 1 \text{ tablet} = 0.5 \text{ tablets (amount to administer)}$$

Therefore you administer $\frac{1}{2}$ tablet.

**Example 3.** The order states, "Erythromycin suspension 250 mg PO." The pharmacy delivers 100-ml bottles with the labels stating, "5 ml contains 125 mg of erythromycin." You apply the formula as follows:

$$\frac{250 \text{ mg}}{125 \text{ mg}} \times 5 \text{ ml} = 10 \text{ ml (amount to administer)}$$

Therefore you prepare 10 ml in a medication cup to administer to the patient.

**PEDIATRIC DOSAGES.** Calculating children's medication dosages requires caution (Hockenberry and others, 2003). A child's age, weight, and maturity of body systems affect the ability to metabolize and excrete medications. For example, premature infants have livers and kidneys that are not matured. Therefore they are especially susceptible to the harmful effects of medications. As children develop out of the newborn period, they metabolize drugs more quickly. This results in a need to give medications more frequently to achieve the desired effect of the medication. You will some-

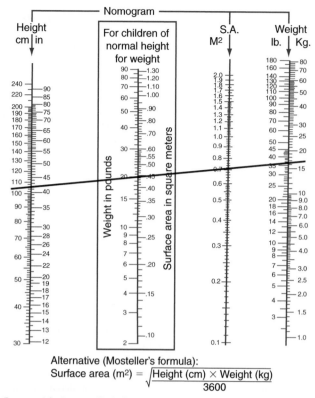

Alternative (Mosteller's formula):

Surface area (m2) = $\sqrt{\dfrac{\text{Height (cm)} \times \text{Weight (kg)}}{3600}}$

FIGURE **14-4** Mosteller's formula and West nomogram for estimation of surface areas in children. A straight line is drawn on West nomogram between height and weight. The point where the line crosses the surface area column is the estimated body surface area. (From Behrman RE and others: *Nelson textbook of pediatrics,* ed 17, Philadelphia, 2004, WB Saunders; modified from data of Boyd E, by West CD.)

times have difficulty evaluating the child's response to the medication, especially when the child cannot communicate with you verbally. For example, a side effect of Vancomycin, an antibiotic, is ototoxicity. If a child who cannot talk yet is taking Vancomycin, assessing for ototoxicity is challenging.

There are different formulas used to calculate drug dosages in children. The most accurate method of calculating pediatric dosages is based on a child's body surface area (BSA). You estimate body surface area by the child's height and weight. Use Mosteller's formula or the standard nomogram (e.g., the West nomogram) for estimation of a child's body surface area (Figure 14-4).

To calculate a pediatric dose, a formula that reflects the ratio of the child's body surface area compared with the body surface area of an average adult (1.7 square meters [$m^2$]) is used:

$$\text{Child's dose} = \frac{\text{Surface area of child}}{1.7\ m^2} \times \text{Normal adult dose}$$

For example, the prescriber orders ampicillin for a child weighing 12 kg. The normal adult dose for ampicillin is 250 mg. The West nomogram shows that a child weighing 12 kg has a

body surface area of 0.54 $m^2$. Using this information, you calculate the appropriate child's dose:

$$\frac{0.54\ m^2}{1.7\ m^2} \times 250\ mg = 79.4\ mg\ of\ ampicillin$$

JCAHO (2004a) has established medication safety standards that address the specific needs of children. Some medications cause significant harm to the patient if you do not give them correctly. These medications are called high alert medications. Many high alert medications are given in emergency situations and are ordered in different concentrations based on the age or weight of the child. Individualized concentrations of high alert medications have been associated with fatal medication errors and higher infection rates. Therefore high alert medications are provided only in standard concentrations. The medication order states the actual drug dose, not the volume. The order also contains the dose calculation, including the patient's weight, dose per unit weight, and rate of administration. This allows the pharmacist and the nurse the ability to verify the medication calculation to ensure a safe dose is administered to the child.

To increase the safety associated with medications administered to children in emergency situations, many institutions use color-coded tapes, such as the Braslow Tape. To use this system, measure the child from the head to the heel with the tape. The color the child fits into on the tape matches color-coded drawers, bins, or bags that provide safe drug doses, as well as other emergency equipment, such as nasogastric tubes, endotracheal tubes, and Foley catheters in sizes that are appropriate for the child.

## Administering Medications

You do not have sole responsibility for medication administration. The prescriber (e.g., physician or advanced practice nurse) and pharmacist also help to ensure the right medication gets to the right patient. However, you are accountable for knowing what medications are prescribed and their therapeutic and nontherapeutic effects and for knowing the patient's needs and abilities related to medication administration. You also are responsible for evaluating the desired effects of the patient's medications.

**PRESCRIBER'S ROLE.** The physician or health care provider prescribes the patient's medications. The prescriber writes an order on a form in the patient's medical record, in an order book, on a legal prescription pad, or through a computer terminal. Telephone or verbal orders are given when written or electronic communication between the prescriber and the nurse is not possible.

When a written or telephone order is received, the nurse who took the order writes the name of the prescriber ordering the medication followed by the nurse's signature. The prescriber will countersign the order at a later time, usually within 24 hours after making the order. Box 14-6 provides guidelines for taking verbal or telephone orders for medications safely. Institutional policies vary regarding who can take verbal or telephone orders. Generally, nursing students

| BOX 14-6 | Recommendations to Reduce Medication Errors Associated With Verbal Medication Orders and Prescriptions (NCCMERP, 2001) |

**Preamble**

In these recommendations, verbal orders are prescriptions or medication orders that are communicated as oral, spoken communications between senders and receivers face to face, by telephone, or by other auditory device.

**Recommendations**

1. Verbal communication of prescription or medication orders should be limited to urgent situations where immediate written or electronic communication is not feasible.
2. Health care organizations* should establish policies and procedures that:
   - Describe limitations or prohibitions on use of verbal orders
   - Provide a process to ensure validity/authenticity of the prescriber
   - List the elements required for inclusion in a complete verbal order
   - Describe situations in which verbal orders may be used
   - List and define the individuals who may send and receive verbal orders
   - Provide guidelines for clear and effective communication of verbal orders
3. Leaders of health care organizations should promote a culture in which it is acceptable, and strongly encouraged, for staff to question prescribers when there are any questions or disagreements about verbal orders. Questions about verbal orders should be resolved prior to the preparation, or dispensing, or administration of the medication.
4. Verbal orders for antineoplastic agents should **NOT** be permitted under any circumstances. These medications are not administered in emergency or urgent situations, and they have a narrow margin of safety.

5. Elements that should be included in a verbal order include:
   - Name of patient
   - Age and weight of patient, when appropriate
   - Drug name
   - Dosage form (e.g., tablets, capsules, inhalants)
   - Exact strength or concentration
   - Dose, frequency, and route
   - Quantity and/or duration
   - Purpose or indication (unless disclosure is considered inappropriate by the prescriber)
   - Specific instructions for use
   - Name of prescriber, and telephone number when appropriate
   - Name of individual transmitting the order, if different from the prescriber.
6. The content of verbal orders should be clearly communicated:
   - The name of the drug should be confirmed by any of the following:
     ○ Spelling
     ○ Providing both the brand and generic drug names
     ○ Providing the indication for use
   - In order to avoid confusion with spoken numbers, a dose such as 50 mg should be communicated as "fifty milligrams . . . five zero milligrams" to distinguish from "fifteen milligrams . . . one five milligrams."
   - Instructions for use should be provided without abbreviations. For example, "1 tab tid" should be communicated as "Take/give one tablet three times daily."
7. The entire verbal order should be repeated back to the prescriber, or the individual transmitting the order, using the principles outlined in these recommendations.
8. All verbal orders should be reduced immediately to writing and signed by the individual receiving the order.
9. Verbal orders should be documented in the patient's medical record by the prescriber as soon as possible.

*Health care organizations include community pharmacies, physicians' offices, hospitals, nursing homes, home care agencies, etc.

cannot take medication orders. You cannot give any medication without an order.

Common abbreviations are often used when writing orders. The abbreviations indicate dosage frequencies or times, routes of administration, and special information for giving the medication (see Table 14-3). However, the National Coordinating Council for Medication Error Reporting and Prevention (NCCMERP, 2005) recommends not using abbreviations when writing medication orders because of the high number of medication errors that occur related to the use of abbreviations. Table 14-7 lists abbreviations that are associated with a high incidence of medication errors. These abbreviations should not be used; rather, they should be writ-

ten out. In addition, JCAHO (2005) developed an official "do not use" list of abbreviations in 2004. This list was updated in 2005, and more abbreviations will probably be added to this list over time (Table 14-8). Do not use these abbreviations when documenting medication orders or when documenting other information about medications.

**TYPES OF ORDERS IN ACUTE CARE AGENCIES.** Five common types of medication orders are based on the frequency and/or urgency of medication administration.

**Standing Orders.** You carry out a standing order until the physician or health care provider cancels it by another order or until a prescribed number of days elapse. A standing order sometimes indicates a final date or number of

| TABLE 14-7 | **Dangerous Abbreviations** | |
|---|---|---|
| Abbreviation | Intended Meaning | Common Error |
| U | Units | Mistaken as a zero or a four (4) resulting in overdose. Also mistaken for "cc" (cubic centimeters) when poorly written. |
| μg | Micrograms | Mistaken for "mg" (milligrams) resulting in a tenfold overdose. |
| Q.D. | Latin abbreviation for every day | The period after the "Q" has sometimes been mistaken for an "I," and the drug has been given "QID" (four times daily) rather than daily. |
| QOD | Latin abbreviation for every other day | Misinterpreted as "QD" (daily) or "QID" (four times daily). If the "O" is poorly written, it looks like a period or "I." |
| SC or SQ | Subcutaneous | Mistaken as "SL" (sublingual) when poorly written. |
| TIW | Three times a week | Misinterpreted as "three times a day" or "twice a week." |
| D/C | Discharge; also discontinue | Patient's medications have been prematurely discontinued when D/C (intended to mean "discharge") was misinterpreted as "discontinue," because it was followed by a list of drugs. |
| HS | Half strength | Misinterpreted as the Latin abbreviation "HS" (hour of sleep). |
| cc | Cubic centimeters | Mistaken as "U" (units) when poorly written. |
| AU, AS, AD | Latin abbreviation for both ears; left ear; right ear | Misinterpreted as the Latin abbreviation "OU" (both eyes); "OS" (left eye); "OD" (right eye). |
| IU | International Unit | Mistaken as IV (intravenous) or 10 (ten) |
| MS, $MSO_4$, $MgSO_4$ | Confused for one another | Can mean morphine sulfate or magnesium sulfate |

Prescribers should not use vague instructions such as "Take as directed" or "Take/Use as needed" as the sole direction for use. Specific directions to the patient are useful to help reinforce proper medication use, particularly if therapy is to be interrupted for a time. Clear directions are a necessity for the dispenser to (1) check the proper dose for the patient and (2) enable effective patient counseling.

In summary, the council recommends:

Don't Wait . . . Automate!
When In Doubt, Write It Out!
When In Doubt, Check It Out!
Lead, Don't Trail!

dosages. Many institutions have policies for automatically discontinuing standing orders. The following are examples of standing orders:

Tetracycline, 500 mg PO q6h, and Decadron,

10 mg PO daily × 5 days

**prn Orders.** The physician or health care provider sometimes orders a medication to be given only when a patient requires it. This is a prn order. You use objective and subjective assessment and nursing discretion to determine whether the patient needs the medication. Often the physician or health care provider sets minimum intervals for the time of administration. This means you cannot give the medication any more frequently than what is prescribed. Examples of prn orders include the following:

Morphine sulfate, 10 mg IM q3-4h prn for incisional pain, and Maalox, 30 ml prn for heartburn

When you administer prn medications, document the assessment data you used to decide to give the medication and the time of medication administration. Frequently evaluate the effectiveness of the medication, and record findings in the appropriate record.

**Single (One-Time) Orders.** A prescriber will often order a medication to be given only once at a specified time. This is common for preoperative medications or medications given before diagnostic examinations. For example:

Versed, 25 mg IM on call to OR

**Stat Orders.** A stat order means that you give a single dose of a medication immediately and only once. Health care providers usually write stat orders for emergencies when the patient's condition changes suddenly. For example:

Give Apresoline, 10 mg IM stat

**Now Orders.** A now order is more specific than a one-time order and is used when a patient needs a medication quickly but not right away, as in a stat order. When you receive a now order, you have up to 90 minutes to administer the medication. Only administer medications ordered now one time. For example:

Give Vancomycin 1 gram IV piggyback now

| TABLE 14-8 | Abbreviations Prohibited by JCAHO |
|---|---|

**Prohibited and Error-Prone Abbreviations***

| Abbreviation | Preferred Term |
|---|---|
| U (unit) | Write "unit" |
| IU (International Unit) | Write "International Unit" |
| Q.D., QD, q.d., qd (daily) | Write "daily" |
| Q.O.D., QOD, q.o.d., qod (every other day) | Write "every other day" |
| Trailing zero (X.0 mg)† | Write "X mg" |
| Lack of a leading zero (.X mg) | Write "0.X mg" |
| MS, MSO₄ (morphine sulfate) | Write "morphine sulfate" |
| MgSO₄ (magnesium sulfate) | Write "magnesium sulfate" |
| HS (half strength) | Write out half strength |
| SC or SQ (subcutaneous) | Write out Sub-Q or SubQ |
| D/C (discharge) | Write out discharge |
| cc (cubic centimeter) | Write ml |

**Additional Abbreviations, Acronyms, and Symbols**
(Will possibly be included in a future "Do Not Use" List)

| | |
|---|---|
| > (greater than) | Write "greater than" |
| < (less than) | Write "less than" |
| Abbreviations for drug names | Write drug names in full |
| Apothecary units | Use metric units |
| @ | Write "at" |
| μg | Write "mcg" or "micrograms" |

Adapted from Joint Commission on Accreditation of Healthcare Organizations, http://www.jointcommission.org/PateintSafety/DoNotUseList, accessed on March 21, 2006. Institute for Safe Medication Practices, List of Error-Prone Abbreviations, Symbols, and Dose Designations, http://www.ismp.org/tools/errorproneabbreviations.pdf, accessed on May 7, 2006.
*Applies to all orders and all medication-related documentation that is handwritten (including free-text computer entry) or on preprinted forms.
†Exception: A "trailing zero" is used only when needed to show precision of a reported value (e.g., laboratory test results), studies that report the size of lesions, or catheter and tube sizes. A "trailing zero" cannot be used in medication orders or medication-related documentation.

Some conditions change the status of a patient's medication orders. For example, surgery automatically cancels all the patient's preoperative medications (see Chapter 37). A transfer from a general medical unit to an intensive care unit also cancels all the patient's medication orders. Because the patient's condition changes after surgery or after transferring to an intensive care unit, the prescriber writes new orders. When a patient is transferred to another health care agency or to a different unit within a hospital or is discharged, the prescriber reviews the medications and writes new orders as indicated.

**PRESCRIPTIONS.** Prescriptions are written for patients who are to take medications outside the hospital. The prescription includes more detailed information than a regular order because the patient needs to understand how to take the medication and when to refill the prescription if necessary. The parts of a prescription are included in Figure 14-5.

**PHARMACIST'S ROLE.** The pharmacist prepares and distributes prescribed medications. Pharmacists also assess the medication plan and evaluate the patient's medication-related needs. The pharmacist is responsible for filling prescriptions accurately and for being sure that prescriptions are valid.

**DISTRIBUTION SYSTEMS.** Systems for storing and distributing medications vary. Pharmacists provide the medications, but nurses distribute medications to patients. Institutions providing nursing care have special areas for stocking and dispensing medications, such as special medication rooms, portable locked carts, computerized medication cabinets, and individual storage units in patients' rooms. Medication storage areas need to be locked when unattended.

**Unit Dose.** The unit-dose system uses portable carts containing a drawer with a 24-hour supply of medications for each patient. The unit dose is the ordered dose of medication the patient receives at one time. Each tablet or capsule is wrapped separately. At a designated time each day, the pharmacist refills the drawers in the cart with a fresh supply. The cart also contains limited amounts of prn and stock medications for special situations. The unit-dose system is designed to reduce the number of medication errors and saves steps in dispensing medications.

**Computer-Controlled Dispensing Systems.** Computer-controlled dispensing systems are used successfully throughout the United States (Figure 14-6). They are especially useful for the delivery and control of **opioids.** Each nurse has a security code, allowing access to the system. In these systems you select the patient's name and the desired medication, dosage, and route. The system dispenses the medication to the nurse, records it, and charges it to the patient. Most systems do not document medication administration.

**Nurse's Role.** The administration of medications to patients requires knowledge and a set of skills that are unique to nursing. Responsibilities of medication administration include assessing the patient's ability to self-administer medications and determining whether a patient should receive a medication at a given time. You as the nurse are also responsible for administering medications correctly and monitoring the effects of prescribed medications. Patient and family education about proper medication administration and monitoring is an integral part of the nurse's role. Never delegate this to assistive personnel.

## Medication Errors

A **medication error** may cause or lead to inappropriate medication use or client harm while the medication is in the control of a health care professional. Medication errors include inaccurate prescribing, administration of the wrong medication, route, and time interval, as well as administering extra doses or failing to administer a medication. Medication errors can be related to professional practice, health care product design, or procedures and systems such as product labeling and distribution. When an error occurs, the client's safety and well-being become the top priority. As the nurse, assess and examine the client's condition and notify the physician or prescriber of the incident as soon as possible.

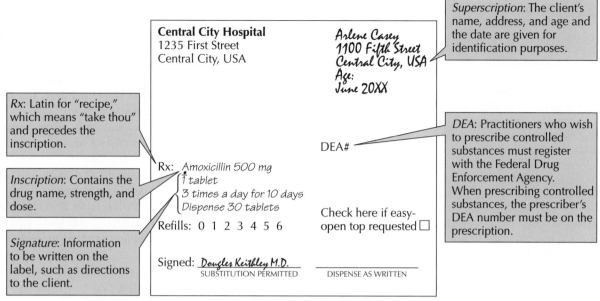

**Superscription:** The client's name, address, and age and the date are given for identification purposes.

**Central City Hospital**
1235 First Street
Central City, USA

Arlene Casey
1100 Fifth Street
Central City, USA
Age:
June 20XX

*Rx:* Latin for "recipe," which means "take thou" and precedes the inscription.

*Inscription:* Contains the drug name, strength, and dose.

DEA#

**DEA:** Practitioners who wish to prescribe controlled substances must register with the Federal Drug Enforcement Agency. When prescribing controlled substances, the prescriber's DEA number must be on the prescription.

Rx: Amoxicillin 500 mg
1 tablet
3 times a day for 10 days
Dispense 30 tablets

Refills: 0 1 2 3 4 5 6

Check here if easy-open top requested ☐

*Signature:* Information to be written on the label, such as directions to the client.

Signed: *Douglas Keithley M.D.*
SUBSTITUTION PERMITTED        DISPENSE AS WRITTEN

FIGURE **14-5** Example of a medication prescription.

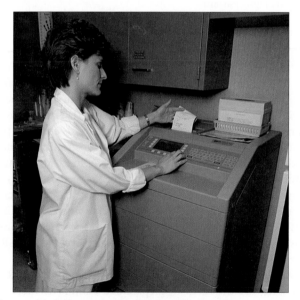

FIGURE **14-6** Computer-controlled medication dispensing system.

Once the client is stable, report the incident to the appropriate person in the institution (e.g., manager or supervisor).

You are also responsible for preparing a written incident report that usually must be filed within 24 hours of the incident. The report includes client identification information; the location and time of the incident; an accurate, factual description of what occurred and what was done; and the signature of the nurse involved. The incident report is not a permanent part of the medical record and should not be referred to in the record. This is to legally protect the health care professional and institution. Institutions use incident reports to track incident patterns and to initiate quality improvement programs as needed.

It is good risk management to report all medication errors, including mistakes that do not cause obvious or immediate harm or near misses. A nurse should feel comfortable in reporting an error and not fear repercussions from managerial staff. Even when a client suffers no harm from a medication error, the institution can still learn why the mistake occurred and what can be done to avoid similar errors in the future. Prevention is the key. Box 14-7 lists steps to take in preventing medication errors.

## Critical Thinking

### Synthesis

Critical thinking is extremely important in the administration of medications. The growing number of medications readily available to patients, the acute and complex nature of patient problems, higher acuity levels in acute care settings, and reductions in nursing and pharmacy staff contribute to the need for critical thinking. The skill of medication administration requires the synthesis of all factors that influence a patient's reaction to prescribed medications. This requires more than the knowledge of the medication's classification, desired effect, and common side effects. You will synthesize knowledge, experience, attitudes, and standards in order to apply the nursing process appropriately when administering medications.

**KNOWLEDGE.** You will use knowledge from many disciplines when administering medications. Knowledge of physiology and pathophysiology helps you understand why a particular medication has been prescribed for a patient and

| BOX 14-7 | **Steps to Take in Preventing Medication Errors** |
|---|---|

- Follow the six rights of medication administration.
- Be sure to read labels at least 3 times (comparing MAR with label): before, during, and after administering the medication.
- Use at least two patient identifiers (e.g., name band, client pronouncing name) whenever administering a medication.
- Do not allow any other activity to interrupt your administration of medication to a client.
- Double-check all calculations, and verify with another nurse.
- Do not interpret illegible hand writing; clarify with prescriber.
- Question unusually large or small doses.
- Document all medications as soon as they are given.
- When you have made an error, reflect on what went wrong; ask how you could have prevented the error.
- Evaluate the context or situation in which a medication error occurred. This helps to determine if nurses have the necessary resources for safe medication administration.
- When repeated medication errors occur within a work area, identify and analyze the factors that may have caused the errors, and take corrective action.
- Attend in-service programs that focus on the medications you commonly administer.

how this medication will alter the patient's physiology as it exerts its therapeutic effect. Knowledge about growth and development principles is also useful in medication administration. For example, knowledge about child development indicates that children often perceive medication administration as a negative experience. You use principles from child development to ensure that the child cooperates with medication administration.

**EXPERIENCE.** As a nursing student, you have limited experience with medication administration as it applies to professional practice. However, clinical experience provides you with the opportunity to apply the nursing process to medication administration. As you gain experience in medication administration, psychomotor skills (e.g., the preparation and actual administration of a medication) become more refined. As you acquire experience in observing patients' responses to medications, you will become more able to anticipate and evaluate the effects of medications.

**ATTITUDES.** To administer medications safely to patients, several critical thinking attitudes are essential. For example, you show discipline when you take adequate time to prepare and administer medications. You take the time to read your patient's history and physical, review your patient's orders, look up medications you do not know in a medication reference book, and determine why your patient is taking each of his or her prescribed medications. Every step of safe medication administration requires a disciplined attitude and a comprehensive, systematic approach.

Responsibility and accountability are other critical thinking attitudes that are essential to medication administration. When you administer a medication to a patient, you accept the responsibility that the medication or the nursing actions

in administering it will not harm the patient in any way. You are responsible for knowing that the medication that is ordered for the patient is the correct medication and the correct dose. You are accountable for administering an ordered medication that is obviously inappropriate for the patient. Therefore be familiar with the therapeutic effect, usual dosage, anticipated changes in laboratory data, and side effects of all medications that you administer.

**STANDARDS.** Professional standards guide medication administration. The American Nurses Association's (ANA's) *Standards of Nursing Practice* (see Chapter 2), based on the nursing process, apply to the activity of medication administration. Other professional nursing standards also apply. For example, the Association of Perioperative Registered Nurses (AORN) has developed a guidance statement that helps maintain safe medication nursing practices in perioperative settings (AORN, 2002).

To ensure safe medication administration, be aware of the six rights of medication administration:

1. The right medication
2. The right dose
3. The right patient
4. The right route
5. The right time
6. The right documentation

**Right Medication.** A medication order is required for any medication that you administer. Sometimes prescribers write orders by hand in the patient's chart. Alternatively, some agencies use computerized physician order entry (CPOE). CPOE allows the prescriber to electronically enter ordered medications. This eliminates the need for written orders. Regardless of how the order for the medication is received, you compare the physician's or health care provider's written orders with the medication administration record (MAR) when health care providers first order medications. Also, verify medication information whenever new MARs are written or distributed (ISMP, 2004b).

Once you determine that the information on the MAR is accurate, use the MAR to prepare and administer medications. When preparing medications in bottles or containers, compare the label of the medication container with the medication administration order three times: (1) before removing the container from the drawer or shelf, (2) as you remove the amount of medication ordered from the container, and (3) before returning the container to storage. Never prepare medications from unmarked containers or containers with illegible labels. With unit-dose packaged medications, you check the medication's label and dosage when you take it out of the medication dispensing system. Finally, you verify all medications at the patient's bedside with the patient's MAR using at least two patient identifiers before giving the patient any medications (ISMP, 2004a).

Because the nurse who administers the medication is responsible for any errors related to that medication, you only administer medications you prepare. If a patient questions a medication, it is important not to ignore these concerns. An alert patient will know whether a medication is different from those received before. In most cases the patient's medication order has been changed; however, the patient's questions often reveal an error. Withhold the medication until you recheck it against the prescriber's orders. If a patient refuses a medication, discard it rather than returning it to the original container. You can save unit-dose medications if they are not opened.

At home, have patients keep medications in their original labeled containers. It helps to have patients use a written schedule to remember which medications they need to take.

**Right Dose.** The unit-dose system is designed to minimize errors. When you prepare a medication from a larger volume or strength than needed or when the prescriber orders a system of measurement different from what the pharmacist supplies, the chance of error increases. Have another qualified nurse check the calculated doses when performing medication calculations or conversions.

After calculating dosages, prepare the medication using standard measurement devices. Use graduated cups, syringes, and scaled droppers to measure medications accurately. At home, have patients use kitchen measuring spoons rather than teaspoons and tablespoons, which vary in volume.

Only break tablets that are scored by the manufacturer. When it is necessary to break a scored tablet, make sure the break is even. Cut a tablet in half by using a knife edge or by using a cutting device. Discard tablets that do not break evenly. Some agencies allow you to save the part of the medication tablet that remains for the next dose if the remaining medication is repackaged and labeled. Verify agency policy before administering a tablet that has been opened, cut, and repackaged.

Sometimes you crush a tablet so you can mix it in food. Make sure the crushing device is completely cleaned before crushing the tablet. Remnants of previously crushed medications increase a medication's concentration or result in the patient receiving a portion of an unprescribed medication. Mix crushed medications with very small amounts of food or liquid. Do not use the patient's favorite foods or liquids because medications alter their taste and decrease the patient's desire for them. This is especially a concern with pediatric patients.

You cannot crush all medications. Some medications, such as time-released or extended-release capsules, have special coatings to keep the medication from being absorbed too quickly. Refer to a medication reference to ensure that you can safely crush the medication.

**Right Patient.** An important step in administering medications safely is being sure you give the medication to the right patient. It is difficult to remember every patient's name and face. Therefore, before giving a medication to a patient, you need to use at least two patient identifiers whenever administering medications (JCAHO, 2004a). Acceptable patient identifiers include the patient's name, an identification number assigned by a health care agency, or a telephone number. Do not use the patient's room number as an identifier. To identify a patient correctly in an acute care setting,

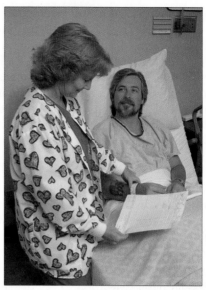

FIGURE **14-7** Before administering any medications, check the patient's identification and allergy bracelets. (From deWit S: *Fundamental concepts and skills for nursing,* ed 2, Philadelphia, 2005, WB Saunders.)

compare the patient identifiers on the MAR with the patient's identification bracelet at the patient's bedside (Figure 14-7). If an identification bracelet becomes illegible or is missing, get a new one for the patient. In health care settings that are not acute care settings, JCAHO does not require the use of armbands for identification. However, you still need to use a system that verifies the patient's identification with at least two identifiers before administering medications.

JCAHO does not require that patients state their names and other identifiers when administering medications (JCAHO, 2004a). The required identification process mandates collecting patient identifiers reliably when the patient is admitted to a health care agency. Once the identifiers are assigned to the patient (e.g., putting identifiers on an armband and placing the armband on the patient), you use the identifiers to match the patient with the MAR, which lists the correct medications. Asking patients to state their full names and identification information provides you with a third way to verify that you are giving medications to the right person.

In addition to using two identifiers, some agencies use a wireless bar code scanner to help identify the right patient. This system requires you to scan a personal bar code that is commonly placed on your name tag first. Then, you scan a bar code on the single-dose medication package. Finally, you scan the patient's armband. This information is then stored in a computer for documentation purposes. This system helps eliminate medication errors because it provides another step to ensure that the right patient receives the right medication.

**Right Route.** Always consult the prescriber when an order does not specify a route of administration. Likewise, if the specified route is not the recommended route or is not an appropriate route, alert the prescriber immediately.

When you administer injections, precautions are necessary to ensure that you give the medications correctly. It is also important to prepare injections only from preparations designed for parenteral use. The injection of a liquid designed for oral use produces local complications, such as sterile abscess or fatal systemic effects. Medication companies label parenteral medications "for injectable use only."

**Right Time.** Know why a medication is ordered for certain times of the day and whether you can alter the time schedule. For example, two medications are ordered, one q8h (every 8 hours) and the other tid (3 times per day). You will give both medications 3 times within a 24-hour period. The prescriber intends for you to give the q8h medication every 8 hours around the clock to maintain therapeutic blood levels of the medication. In contrast, you give the tid medication 3 times a day during the waking hours. Each agency has a recommended time schedule for medications ordered at frequent intervals.

The prescriber often gives specific instructions about when to administer a medication. A preoperative medication to be given "on call" to surgery means that you will give the medication when the operating room staff members tell you they are coming to get the patient for surgery. You give a medication ordered PC (after meals) within 30 minutes after a meal when the patient has a full stomach. You give a stat medication immediately.

Give priority to medications that must act at certain times. For example, you need to administer insulin at a precise interval before a meal. Give antibiotics on time around the clock to maintain therapeutic blood levels. Give all routinely ordered medications within 60 minutes of the time ordered (30 minutes before or after the prescribed time) (Centers for Medicare and Medicaid Services [CMS], 2003).

Some medications require your clinical judgment when determining the proper time for administration. Administer a prn sleeping medication when the patient is prepared for bed. Also, use nursing judgment when giving prn analgesics. For example, you sometimes need to obtain a stat order from the prescriber if the patient requires a medication before the prn interval has elapsed. Document whenever you call the patient's health care provider to obtain a change in a medication's order.

At home some patients have to take many medications throughout the day. Help plan schedules based on recommended medication intervals and the patient's daily schedule. For patients who have difficulty remembering when to take medications, make a chart that lists the times when to take each medication or prepare a special container that organizes and stores medications according to when the patient needs to take them (Figure 14-8).

**Right Documentation.** Several authors added this right to the traditional five rights of medication administration to improve medication safety (Aschenbrenner and others, 2002). Nurses and other health care providers use accurate documentation to communicate with each other. Many medication errors result from inaccurate documentation.

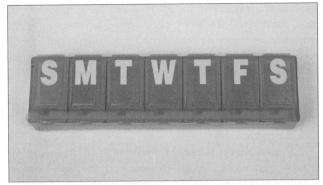

FIGURE **14-8** Medication organization container to help patients remember to take medications.

Therefore ensure that accurate and appropriate documentation exists before and after giving medications.

Before you administer medications, documentation indicates the patient's full name, the name of the ordered medications written out in full (no medication name abbreviations), the time the medication is to be administered, and the medication's dose, route, and frequency. If any of this information is missing or if dangerous drug abbreviations are used, contact the prescriber immediately to verify the order.

After you administer medications, indicate which medications you gave on your patient's MAR per agency policy to show that you gave the medications as ordered. Inaccurate documentation of medications, such as failing to document giving a medication or documenting an incorrect dose, leads to errors in subsequent decisions about your patient's care. For example, errors in documentation about insulin often result in negative patient outcomes. Consider the following situation: A patient receives insulin before breakfast but the insulin dose is not documented. The nurse caring for the patient goes home, and the patient has a new nurse for the day. The new nurse notices that the insulin is not documented and assumes that the previous nurse did not give the insulin. Therefore the new nurse gives the patient another dose of insulin. About 2 hours later, the patient experiences a low blood sugar, which causes the patient to have seizures. Accurate documentation would have prevented this situation from happening.

There are many nursing actions you take to ensure the right documentation. First, make sure that the information on your patient's MAR corresponds exactly with the prescriber's order and with the label on the medication's container. Do not administer medications that have illegible or incomplete orders. Verify inaccurate documentation before giving medications. It is better to give the correct medication at a later time than to give your patient the wrong medication. Record the administration of each medication on the MAR as soon as you give the medication. Never document that you have given a medication until you have actually given it. The name of the medication, the dose, the time of administration, and the route need to be documented on the MAR. Also document the site of any injections you give. Document the patient's responses to medications, either positive or negative, in the nursing notes. Notify the patient's physician or health care provider of any negative responses to medications and document the time, date, and name of the physician or health care provider you notified in the patient's chart. The efforts you make in ensuring the right documentation will help you to provide safe care to your patients.

**MAINTAINING PATIENTS' RIGHTS.** In accordance with *The Patient Care Partnership* (American Hospital Association [AHA], 2003) and because of the potential risks related to medication administration, a patient has the right to:

1. Be informed of medication name, purpose, action, and potential undesired effects
2. Refuse a medication regardless of the consequences
3. Have qualified nurses or physicians or health care providers assess a medication history, including allergies and use of herbals
4. Be properly advised of the experimental nature of medication therapy and to give written consent for its use
5. Receive labeled medications safely without discomfort in accordance with the six rights of medication administration (see section on medication delivery)
6. Receive appropriate supportive therapy in relation to medication therapy
7. Not receive unnecessary medications
8. Be informed if prescribed medications are a part of a research study

## Nursing Process

### Assessment

You will assess many factors to determine a patient's need for and potential response to medication therapy. You perform a thorough assessment on all your patients to help ensure safe medication administration.

**HISTORY.** Before administering medications, obtain or review the patient's medical history. A patient's medical history will provide any indications or contraindications for medication therapy. Disease or illness places patients at risk for adverse medication effects. For example, if a patient has a gastric ulcer, compounds containing aspirin will increase the likelihood of bleeding. Long-term health problems require specific medications. This knowledge will help you anticipate the medications your patient requires. A patient's surgical history indicates use of medications. For example, after a thyroidectomy a patient requires thyroid hormone replacement.

**History of Allergies.** All members of the health care team need to know the patient's history of allergies to medications and foods. Many medications have ingredients found in food sources. For example, if your patient is allergic to shellfish, the patient may be sensitive to any product containing iodine, such as Betadine or dyes used in radiological testing. In an acute care setting, patients sometimes wear identification bands that list medication allergies. All allergies and the types of reactions are noted on the patient's admission notes, medication records, and history and physical.

**Medication History.** When taking a medication history, you assess what medications the patient takes, including prescription and nonprescription drugs and herbal supplements. You also assess the length of time the patient has taken each drug, current dosage schedule, and whether the patient has experienced any adverse effects to any of the medications. In addition, you review information about the medications, including action, purpose, normal dosages, routes, side effects, and nursing implications for administration and monitoring. Be sure that a safe dose is ordered, especially when caring for older adults or children. Also, be aware of medication interactions and special nursing interventions needed for medication administration. Often, you need to consult several references to gather needed information. Pharmacology textbooks and handbooks; electronic medication manuals available on a desktop, laptop or handheld computer; nursing journals; the *Physician's Desk Reference* (PDR); medication package inserts; and pharmacists are valuable resources. You are responsible for knowing as much as possible about each medication your patients receive.

**Diet History.** An effective dosage schedule is planned around normal eating patterns and food preferences. Some medications interact with food. Teach patients who take these medications to avoid those foods that interact with medications.

**PATIENT'S PERCEPTUAL OR COORDINATION PROBLEMS.** For a patient with perceptual or coordination limitations, self-administration is sometimes difficult. Assess the patient's ability to prepare doses (e.g., open containers or fill syringes) and take medications (e.g., perform self-injection or instill eye drops) correctly. If the patient is unable to self-administer medications, you will need to assess whether family or friends will be available to assist.

**PATIENT'S CURRENT CONDITION.** The ongoing physical or mental status of a patient affects whether you give a medication and how you administer it. Assess a patient carefully before giving any medication. For example, check the patient's blood pressure before giving an antihypertensive. If the blood pressure is unusually low (e.g., systolic pressure below 100 mm Hg), hold the medication and notify the prescriber. Assessment findings serve as a baseline in evaluating the effects of medication therapy.

**PATIENT'S ATTITUDE ABOUT MEDICATION USE.** The patient's attitudes about medications reveal a level of medication dependence or drug avoidance. Patients do not usually express their feelings about taking a particular medication, particularly if dependence is a problem. Observe the patient's behavior for evidence of medication dependence or avoidance. Also assess the patient's cultural and personal beliefs about Western medicine to determine if the patient's beliefs interfere with medication compliance (see Box 14-8 and Chapter 17).

| BOX 14-8 | CULTURAL FOCUS |
| --- | --- |

The Hispanic population is one of the fastest growing ethnic populations in the United States. It is estimated that 12% of the current U.S. population is Hispanic. The Hispanic population has many health risks. For example, people who are Hispanic have a 40% greater chance of becoming infected with the hepatitis C virus when compared to the general American population. Currently, liver disease is the seventh highest cause of death among Hispanic people from the age of 25 to 44 and the third highest cause of death in Hispanics between 45 and 64 years of age (Stevenson and others, 2004).

The Hispanic community faces cultural, socioeconomic, and education barriers that are especially challenging in the diagnosis and treatment of chronic hepatitis C. Hepatitis C is primarily spread by contact with blood and blood products. Usually, people who have chronic hepatitis C do not experience any symptoms of the disease. Therefore screen people who report risk factors for hepatitis C, whether they feel sick or not. Once someone is diagnosed with hepatitis C, there are many medications available to treat it. These medications are expensive and have many adverse effects. The adverse effects to medications prescribed for hepatitis C include flulike symptoms (e.g., fever, chills, headache, nausea, and fatigue), anemia, neutropenia, and injection site reactions.

In the Hispanic culture, people who feel well are considered to be healthy. Therefore it is sometimes difficult to convince a Hispanic patient to be screened for hepatitis C if the patient does not feel sick. Also, the Hispanic population frequently uses folk medicines or remedies to treat illnesses and their symptoms. This can make your Hispanic patient reluctant to accept medical treatments, including medications.

Once you understand how Hispanic people view health, illness, and medical treatment, you apply the following principles when caring for Hispanic-Americans who are susceptible to becoming infected with hepatitis C:

- Determine your patient's perception of hepatitis C.
- Include the patient's significant other when making decisions about screening for hepatitis C and medical treatment, including medications.
- Be nonjudgmental, and use words that your patient understands and accepts.
- If your patient is diagnosed with hepatitis C, provide patient education materials about medications when possible. Consider providing information printed in both English and Spanish.
- If your patient does not understand English, and you cannot speak Spanish, find an interpreter to help you explain prescribed medication therapy to your patient.
- When using an interpreter for medication teaching, face and talk to the patient and watch the patient's nonverbal cues. Use short, simple sentences, and speak clearly.
- Explore financial resources if your patient cannot afford the prescribed medications.

Data from Stevenson L and others: Chronic hepatitis C virus and the Hispanic community: cultural factors impacting care, *Gastroenterol Nurs* 27(5):230, 2004.

**Patient's Knowledge and Understanding of Medication Therapy.** The patient's knowledge and understanding of medication therapy influence the willingness or ability to follow a medication regimen. Unless a patient understands a medication's purpose, the importance of regular dosage schedules and proper administration methods, and the possible side effects, compliance is unlikely. Questions used to assess the patient's knowledge of a medication include the following: What is it for? How is it taken? When is it taken? What side effects have there been? Have you ever stopped taking doses? Is there anything else you do not understand and would like to know about the medication? If the patient cannot afford medications, discuss financial resources.

**PATIENT'S LEARNING NEEDS.** During assessment, you will discover that some patients do not understand their medications. When this happens, you need to explain to patients the action and purpose of medications, expected side effects, correct administration techniques, and ways to help patients remember their medication schedule. In addition, you need to teach patients ways to change medication schedules to fit into their lifestyles. If a patient has been placed on a newly prescribed medication, the patient may need more involved instruction (Box 14-9).

 **Nursing Diagnosis**

Assessment provides data about the patient's condition, ability to self-administer medications, and medication compliance, which you will use to determine actual or potential problems with medication therapy. When you cluster certain data together, there are defining characteristics that reveal nursing diagnoses. For example, if a patient admits to missing a medication dose, this data often indicates the diagnosis of *noncompliance* regarding a medication regimen. Once you select the diagnosis, you need to identify the appropriate related factor. The related factors of inadequate resources versus lack of knowledge require different interventions. If the patient's noncompliance is related to inadequate finances, you collaborate with family members, social workers, or community agencies to help a patient receive necessary medications. If the related factor is lack of knowledge, you implement a teaching plan with follow-up. The following is a list of nursing diagnoses that you will use when administering medications to patients:

- Anxiety
- Ineffective health maintenance
- Health-seeking behaviors

<table>
<tr><td>

| BOX 14-9 | PATIENT TEACHING |

You are a home care nurse assigned to care for Esther, an 85-year-old woman who is taking a lot of medications for several health reasons. You have found that Esther needs education on how to self-administer her medications safely. You develop the following teaching plan for Esther:

**Outcome**

At the end of the teaching session, Esther will self-administer her medications safely and correctly.

**Teaching Strategies**

- Sit with Esther at her kitchen table when you provide medication teaching.
- Ensure that the room is well lit, and limit distractions (e.g., television off).
- Include Esther's spouse and any other family caregivers in your educational sessions.
- Have Esther bring all of her medications to the table, and remind her to keep each drug in its original labeled container. Throw away outdated medications.
- Review information about medications, including desired effect, dose, frequency, and adverse effects with Esther.
- Provide patient teaching materials about prescribed medications. Ensure that the print on the teaching sheets is large enough for Esther to see.

**Evaluation Strategies**

- Ask Esther questions about her medications (e.g., Why are you taking these medications? When do you take your medications?).
- Ask Esther to write out a medication schedule that includes how much of each medication she should take and when she should take them.
- On a return visit, ask Esther to show you where she stores her medication, and review which medications she has.
- Have Esther verbalize symptoms related to adverse effects of medications that she will report to her physician or health care provider.
- Have Esther set up her medications for the whole day while you are visiting her.

</td></tr>
</table>

- Deficient knowledge (medications)
- Noncompliance (medications)
- Effective therapeutic regimen management
- Ineffective family therapeutic regimen management

## Planning

Organize nursing activities to ensure the safe administration of medications. Hurrying to give patients medications or getting interrupted while you prepare and administer medications will lead to errors. Therefore give all your attention to what you are doing. Give yourself adequate time, and avoid interruptions and distractions when you prepare and administer medications. Another way to avoid medication errors is to have all the equipment you need available when you prepare medications. Diligent planning and following a safe routine every time you prepare and administer medications ensures safe medication administration.

Plan to teach patients about their medications while you are administering medications. Family members usually reinforce the importance of medication regimens. Therefore collaborate with the patient's family or friends when you provide instruction. When patients are hospitalized, do not postpone instruction until the day of discharge.

In the community, ensure that the patient knows where and how to obtain medications and that the patient is able to read medication labels. Whether a patient attempts self-administration or you assume responsibility for administering medications, you set goals and related outcomes to use time wisely during medication administration. For example, if you are caring for a patient with newly diagnosed hypertension, you establish the following goal and related outcomes:

*Goal:* The patient will safely administer all medications before discharge.
*Outcomes:*
1. The patient will verbalize understanding of desired effects and adverse effects of medications.
2. The patient will state signs, symptoms, and treatment of hypertension.
3. The patient will establish a daily routine that will promote compliance with ordered medications.

## Implementation

**HEALTH PROMOTION ACTIVITIES.** In promoting or maintaining the patient's health, remember that health beliefs, personal motivation, socioeconomic factors, and habits (e.g., excessive alcohol intake) influence the patient's compliance with the medication regimen. Several nursing interventions promote adherence to a medication regimen. These include teaching patients and their families about the benefit of a medication and why they need to take it correctly, integrating the patient's health beliefs and cultural practices into the treatment plan, and making referrals to community resources if the patient is unable to afford or cannot arrange transportation to obtain necessary medications.

**Patient and Family Teaching.** If you do not inform patients properly about medications, it is possible that they will take their medications incorrectly, or they will not take their medications at all. Provide information about the purpose of medications and their actions and effects. Many health care institutions offer easy-to-read patient education sheets on specific types of medications. A patient needs to know how to take a medication properly and what will happen if he or she fails to do so. For example, after receiving a prescription for an antibiotic, a patient needs to understand the importance of taking the full prescription. Failure to do this leads to a worsening of the condition, as well as the development of bacteria resistant to the medication.

When your patients depend on daily injections, they need to learn to prepare and administer an injection correctly using aseptic technique. Teach family members or friends to give injections in case the patient becomes ill or physically unable to handle a syringe. Provide specially designed equipment such as syringes with enlarged calibrated scales for easier reading or braille-labeled medication vials for patients with visual alterations.

Patients need to be aware of the symptoms of medication side effects or toxicity. Inform family members of medication side effects, such as changes in behavior, because they are often the first persons to recognize these effects. Your patients are better able to cope with problems caused by medications if they understand how and when to act. All patients need to learn the basic guidelines for medication safety. These guidelines ensure the proper use and storage of medications in the home.

**ACUTE CARE ACTIVITIES.** In the acute care setting, expert nursing observation and documentation of responses to medications are essential. Several nursing interventions are critical to provide safe and effective medication administration when receiving a medication order.

**Receiving Medication Orders.** A medication order is required for you to administer any medication to a patient. The medication order needs to contain all the elements in Box 14-10. If the medication order is incomplete, contact the prescriber to verify the order. Medication orders can only be given verbally or by telephone by the prescriber to the nurse when immediate written or electronic communication is not possible (NCCMERP, 2001). A verbal order is a medication or treatment order received in the presence of the prescriber. You enter verbal orders into the patient's medical record and transcribe them the same way as if the prescriber wrote the orders himself or herself. Telephone orders are medication or treatment orders the prescriber gives to the nurse over the phone, generally after the prescriber has been updated about a change in the patient's condition. JCAHO (2004a) requires that the nurse who takes a verbal or telephone order read back the complete order after entering it into the patient's chart. Health care workers must follow institutional policies regarding the receiving, recording, and transcription of verbal and telephone orders. Generally the provider has to sign verbal or telephone orders within 24 hours. When the prescriber is present, policies discourage the use of verbal orders and instead prefer written ones. As a student you are prohibited from receiving verbal and telephone orders.

**Correct Transcription and Communication of Orders.** Once you receive and process a medication, place the physician's or health care provider's complete order on the appropriate medication form, the MAR. The MAR includes the patient's name, room, and bed number, as well as the names, dosages, frequencies, and routes of administration for each medication. As a nurse you complete or update the MAR. Sometimes a computer system generates the MAR. When you use a computer printout, it lists all currently ordered medications with dosage information (Figure 14-9). You can use the same printout to record medications given. Each time you prepare a medication dosage, refer to the MAR. When transcribing orders, ensure the names of medications,

---

**BOX 14-10** | **Components of Medication Orders**

A medication order needs to have the following:

*Patient's full name.* The patient's full name distinguishes the patient from other persons with the same last name.

*Date and time that the order is written.* Include the day, month, year, and time. Designating the time that an order is written clarifies when certain orders are to stop automatically. If an incident occurs involving a medication error, it is easier to document what happened when this information is available.

*Drug name.* The physician or advanced practice nurse will order a generic or trade-name drug. Correct spelling is essential in preventing confusion with drugs with similar spellings.

*Dosage.* Include the amount or strength of the medication.

*Route of administration.* Drug route is important because you administer some drugs by more than one route. Be sure to clarify unsafe or illegible abbreviations with the prescriber to avoid medication errors.

*Time and frequency of administration.* You need to know when to initiate drug therapy. Orders for multiple doses establish a routine schedule for drug administration.

*Signature of prescriber.* The signature makes the order a legal request.

---

dosages, routes, and times are legible. Clarify and rewrite any illegible transcriptions, and, whether the MAR is handwritten or computer generated, carefully verify that all information on the MAR is complete and accurate.

The nurse checks all medication orders for accuracy and thoroughness. When orders are transcribed, the same information needs to be checked again by the nurse. It is essential that you verify the accuracy of every medication you give to the patient with the patient's orders. The process of verification of medications varies among health care agencies. However, if an order seems incorrect or inappropriate or if there is a discrepancy between the written order and what is on the MAR, you consult the prescriber. When you give the wrong medication or an incorrect dose, **you** are legally responsible for the error.

**Accurate Dosage Calculation and Measurement.** You calculate each dose when preparing medications. To avoid calculation errors, pay close attention to the process of calculation, and avoid interruptions from other people or nursing activities. If you are in doubt about the accuracy of your calculation or if you are calculating a new or unusual dose, ask another nurse to double-check your calculations against the prescriber's order. If you are administering a liquid medication, be sure to use a standard measuring container.

**Correct Administration.** Before administering a medication to a patient, verify the patient's identity by using at least two patient identifiers (JCAHO, 2004a). In the acute care setting, the most frequently used patient identifiers are the patient's name and an identification number, such as the patient's birth date. These identifiers are usually on a patient's armband. You compare the two identifiers with the MAR to ensure that you are giving the medications to the correct patient. You also ask the patient to state his or her name as a third identifier. Use aseptic technique and proper procedures when handling and giving medications. Some medications require an assessment before administration (e.g., assessing heart rate before giving a cardiac glycoside).

**Recording Medication Administration.** After administering a medication, you record it immediately on the appropriate record form (see Figure 14-9). Never chart a medication before administering it. Recording immediately after administration prevents errors.

The recording of a medication includes the name of the medication, dosage, route, and exact time of administration. Some agency policies also require that you record the location of an injection.

If a patient refuses a medication or is undergoing tests or procedures that result in a missed dose, explain why you did not give the medication in the nurses' notes. Some agencies require that you circle the prescribed administration time on the medication record when a patient misses a dose. Be sure to follow all agency policies when documenting medication administration.

**RESTORATIVE CARE ACTIVITIES.** Because of the numerous types of restorative care settings, medication administration activities vary. You may need to administer all medications to patients with functional limitations. However, in the home care and rehabilitation settings, your patient usually administers his or her own medications. Regardless of the type of medication activity, you remain responsible for medication instruction. You are also responsible for monitoring compliance with medications and determining the effectiveness of medications that have been prescribed.

**SPECIAL CONSIDERATIONS FOR ADMINISTERING MEDICATIONS TO SPECIFIC AGE-GROUPS.** A patient's developmental level affects how you administer medications. Knowledge of your patient's developmental needs helps you anticipate responses to medication therapy.

**Infants and Children.** Children vary in age; weight; surface area; and the ability to absorb, metabolize, and excrete medications. Children's medication dosages are usually lower than those of adults, but with some medications, children require higher dosages than adults. Therefore take special caution when preparing medications for children. Medications are usually not prepared and packaged in standardized dose ranges for children. Preparing an ordered dosage from an available amount requires careful calculation.

A child's parents often are valuable resources for determining the best way to give the child medications. Sometimes it is less traumatic for the child if a parent gives the medication while you supervise. Tips for administering medications to children are in Box 14-11.

**Older Adults.** Older adults also require special consideration during medication administration (Box 14-12). In addition to physiological changes of aging (Figure 14-10), behavioral and economic factors influence an older person's use of medications.

*Polypharmacy.* Polypharmacy happens when a patient uses two or more medications to treat the same illness, when a patient takes two or more medications from the same chemical class, or when the patient uses two or more medications with the same or similar actions to treat different illnesses (Brager and Sloland, 2005; Ebersole and others, 2004). Polypharmacy also occurs when your patient mixes nutritional supplements or herbal products with medications. Because many older adults suffer chronic health problems, polypharmacy is common in older adults. However, it is also becoming more common in children. When the patient experiences polypharmacy, there is a high risk of medication interactions with other medications and with foods that the patient eats. There is also an increased risk of the patient's having an adverse reaction to the medications.

Rational polypharmacy happens when polypharmacy is needed to treat the patient's illnesses. Rational polypharmacy is commonly found in older adults. For example, many older adults need to take multiple medications to lower their blood pressure. Irrational polypharmacy happens when the patient takes more medications than needed. Irrational polypharmacy has many causes. For example, older patients often visit several health care providers to treat different illnesses. If an accurate medication history is not taken and if the health care providers do not communicate with each other, the patients will end up taking many different medications, which increases the risk of polypharmacy (Brager and Sloland, 2005).

To decrease the risks associated with polypharmacy in older adults or to help an older adult experiencing polypharmacy, start with taking a detailed medication history. Because older adults may have a hard time remembering all their medications, ask them if they take specific medications. For example, ask what pills, eye drops, ointments, suppositories, herbal supplements, and OTC medications they take. Then notify all the patient's health care providers of what medications the patient takes. Work with your patient's prescribers to make sure that the best and fewest medications are ordered to treat your patient's health problems (Brager and Sloland, 2005).

*Self-Prescribing of Medications.* Older adults experience a variety of symptoms (e.g., pain, constipation, insomnia, and indigestion). All of these symptoms are amenable to OTC medications. Many of these OTC preparations have ingredients that, when used inappropriately, cause undesirable side effects or adverse reactions or are contraindicated in the patient's condition. Self-prescription of medications contributes to polypharmacy. Therefore, in addition to using the same interventions you use when the patient has polypharmacy, educate the patient on the dangers of self-prescribing of medications and tell the patient to take medications only if prescribed by his or her health care provider.

## Evaluation

Evaluate your patient's response to medications on an ongoing basis. This requires that you know the desired effect, side effects, and nursing implications of each medication. A change in your patient's condition can be related to a change in health status or may result from medications or both. The goal of safe and effective medication administration involves a careful evaluation of the patient's response to therapy and ability to assume responsibility for self-care.

Room: 3700-03

Patient: PDM, Pharmacy
Birth: 11/30/79   Admit: 01/01/00
MRN: 2000403   Acct: 900015
A Doctor: Jim Smith

Age: 20 y   Ht: 5 ft 2 in     Wt: 125.2 lbs
Metric:     Ht: 1 m 57 cm   Wt: 56.79 kg

### Saint Francis Medical Center

**MEDICATION ADMINISTRATION RECORD**

**Date:** 01/18/00 – 01/19/00

**ADEs/Nondrug allergies:** Latex – Zosyn – Amoxicillin – Insulins – Darvocet – Lugols soln. – Antihi +

| Medication | 0800 | 0900 | 1000 | 1100 | 1200 | 1300 | 1400 | 1500 | 1600 | 1700 | 1800 | 1900 | 2000 | 2100 | 2200 | 2300 | 2400 | 0100 | 0200 | 0300 | 0400 | 0500 | 0600 | 0700 |
|---|---|---|---|---|---|---|---|---|---|---|---|---|---|---|---|---|---|---|---|---|---|---|---|---|
| P00014 Bacitracin ointment<br>AKA: Bacitracin ointment<br>Dose: Apply   STRGH: 30 gm/tube<br>TID   Topical: Right lower leg<br>For external use only<br>Testing | | | RL 10 | | | | | | | | | | | | | | | | | | | | | |
| P00029 Insulin/human regular<br>AKA: Humulin R   Dose: 15 units<br>Strgh: 1 ml = 100 units AC SQ | RL 0730 | | | | | | | | | | | | | | | | | | | | | | | |
| P00030 Fexofenadine 60 mg/psuedo 120 mg<br>AKA: Allegra–D Sr Tab<br>Dose: 1 tab   STRGH: 60/120/tab<br>BID   Oral<br>Auto Sub: 1 Allegra–D Tab bid<br>For Claritin–D 12 hr and 24 hr<br>Per P&T Comm | | | RL 10 | | | | | | | | | | | | | | | | | | | | | |
| P00036 Aspirin<br>AKA: Aspirin 325 mg Tab<br>Dose: 2 tab 650 mg   STRGH: 325 mg/tab<br>Q3–4h   Oral<br>Testing | | | | | | | RL 1315 | | | | | | | | | | | | | | | | | |
| P00039 Haloperidol tablet<br>AKA: Haldol 0.5 mg tab<br>Dose: 1 mg   STRGH: 1 mg/tab<br>QHS   Oral | | | | | | | | | | | | | | | | | | | | | | | | |
| P00035 Zolpidem<br>AKA: Ambien 5 mg tab<br>Dose: 5 mg   STRGH: 5/tab<br>QHS PRN   Oral<br>MR × 1<br>Testing | | | | | | | | | | | | | | | | | | | | | | | | |

**Circle = Dose not given**
**Initials = Dose given**   Page: 01 (continued)
**Deltoid = R.D., L.D.**
**Vastus Lateralis = R.V.L., L.V.L.**
**Lower Abdominal = R.L.A., L.L.A.**
**Anterior Gluteal = R.A.G., L.A.G.**
**Posterior Gluteal = R.P.G., L.P.G.**

| Initials and signature | Initials and signature | Initials and signature |
|---|---|---|
| Rita Lassater RL | | |
| Initials and signature | Initials and signature | Initials and signature |
| | | |
| Initials and signature | Initials and signature | Initials and signature |

FIGURE **14-9** Example of medication administration record (MAR). (Courtesy OSF Saint Francis Medical Center, Peoria, Ill.)

## BOX 14-11  Tips for Administering Medications to Children

### Oral Medications

- Liquids are safer to swallow to avoid aspiration.
- Offer juice, a soft drink, or a frozen juice bar after child swallows a drug.
- A carbonated beverage poured over finely crushed ice reduces nausea.
- When mixing drugs with palatable flavorings, such as syrup or honey, use only a small amount. Children sometimes refuse to take all of a larger mixture.
- Avoid mixing medications in foods or liquids the child enjoys because the child may then refuse them.
- A plastic disposable syringe is the most accurate device for preparing liquid dosages. Cups, teaspoons, and droppers are inaccurate.
- When administering liquid medications, a spoon, plastic cup, or syringe without a needle is useful.

### Injections

- Be very careful when selecting IM injection sites. Infants and small children have underdeveloped muscles.
- Children can be unpredictable and uncooperative. Have someone available to hold a child if needed.
- Always awaken a sleeping child before giving an injection.
- Distracting the child with conversation or a toy reduces pain perception.
- Give the injection quickly, and do not fight with the child.
- Apply a lidocaine ointment to an injection site before the injection to reduce the pain perception during the injection.

## BOX 14-12  CARE OF THE OLDER ADULT

- Space medication times so they do not interfere with meal times.
- Have patient take medications in a comfortable setting that is free from distractions.
- Include a family member or caregiver when providing education about medications.
- If the patient has difficulty swallowing a large capsule or tablet, ask the physician or health care provider to substitute a liquid medication if possible. However, remember that cutting the tablet in half or crushing it and placing it in applesauce or fruit juice will distort the action of some medications, reduce the dose, or cause choking or aspiration of particles of medication or applesauce.
- Provide memory aids in print large enough for the patient to see.
- Watch the patient remove the caps from pill bottles and prepare medications to ensure that they are preparing and taking medications accurately.
- Teach alternatives to medications if approved by the prescriber, such as proper diet instead of vitamins, exercise instead of laxatives, bedtime snacks instead of hypnotics, weight reduction, and limited salt or fats in diet instead of antihypertensive agents.

Modified from Ebersole P and others: *Toward healthy aging: human needs and nursing response,* ed 6, St. Louis, 2004, Mosby.

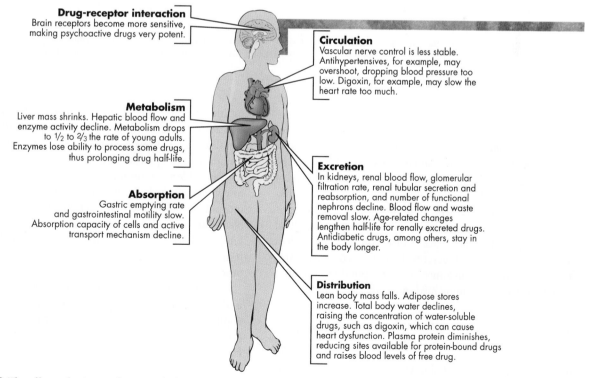

FIGURE **14-10** The effects of aging on drug metabolism. (From Lewis SM and others: *Medical-surgical nursing,* ed 5, St. Louis, 2000, Mosby.)

---

| TABLE 14-9 | Example Evaluations for Patient Goals |
|---|---|

| Goal | Expected Outcomes | Evaluative Measure With Example |
|---|---|---|
| Patient and family understand drug therapy. | Patient and family describe information about drug, dosage, schedule, purpose, and adverse effects. | Written measurement: Have patient write out medication schedule for a 24-hour period. |
| | | Oral questioning: Ask patient to describe purpose, dosage, and adverse effects of each prescribed medication. |
| | Patient and family identify situations that require medical intervention. | Oral questioning: Have family describe what to do when a patient has adverse effects from a medication. |
| | Patient and family demonstrate appropriate administration technique. | Direct observation: Have patient demonstrate filling of an insulin syringe and self-injection. |
| Patient safely self-administers medications. | Patient follows prescribed treatment regimen. | Anecdotal notes: Have family keep log of patient's compliance with therapy for 1 week. |
| | Patient performs techniques correctly. | Direct observation: Observe patient instill eye drops. |
| | Patient identifies available resources for obtaining necessary medication. | Oral questioning: Ask family to identify how to contact local pharmacy or community clinic for necessary medications. |

---

| BOX 14-13 | Interventions to Prevent Aspiration of Medications in Patients With Dysphagia |
|---|---|

Allow the patient to self-administer medications if possible.

Position the patient in an upright, seated position with feet flat on the floor, hips and knees at 90 degrees, the head midline, and back erect if possible.

When the patient puts the medication in the mouth, make sure the chin is tucked or tilted down slightly. When the patient swallows, the chin can be lifted and the head tilted back to help the medication get into the stomach.

If the patient has unilateral weakness, place the medication in the stronger side of the mouth. Turning the head toward the weaker side helps the medication move down the stronger side of the esophagus.

Administer medications one at a time, ensuring that the patient swallows each medication before introducing the next one.

Thicker liquids are often easier to tolerate. Thicken regular liquids or offer fruit nectars to enhance swallowing.

You can crush some medications and place them into pureed foods if necessary.

Straws decrease the amount of control the patient has over the amount of fluid taken into the mouth. Therefore do not have the patient use a straw.

Time medications to coincide with meals if appropriate.

Give medications at times when the patient is well rested and awake.

Minimize distractions during medication administration times.

If dysphagia is severe, explore alternative routes of administration.

Modified from Dahlin C: Oral complications at the end of life: although dysphagia and stomatitis can have devastating effects on the quality of a patient's life, there are many ways to manage them, *Am J Nurs* 104(7):40, 2004; and West JF: Feeding the adult with neurogenic disorders, *Topics in Geriatric Rehabilitation* 20(2):131, 2004.

---

You will use many different measures to evaluate patient responses to medications: direct observation of behavior or response, rating scales (e.g., pain scale) and checklists, and verbal questioning. The type of measurements used varies with the action being evaluated, the reading skill and knowledge level of the patient, and the patient's cognitive and psychomotor ability. One type of measurement commonly used is a physiological measure. Examples of physiological measures are blood pressure, heart rate, and visual acuity. You also use patient statements as evaluative measures. Table 14-9 contains examples of goals, expected outcomes, and corresponding evaluative measures when determining medication therapy results.

## Oral Administration

The easiest and most desirable way to administer medications is by mouth (Skill 14-1). Patients usually are able to ingest or self-administer oral medications with a minimum of problems. Most tablets and capsules need to be swallowed and administered with approximately 60 to 100 ml of fluid (as allowed). However, there are some situations that contraindicate the patient's ability to receive medications by mouth. Table 14-5 summarizes the primary contraindications to giving oral medications. There are many medications that interact with food and herbal supplements. You are responsible for knowing about these interactions. Understanding how food and herbals affect medication absorption helps you determine the best time to give oral medications (Jordan and others, 2003).

An important precaution to take when administering any oral preparation is to protect patients from aspiration. Aspiration occurs when food, fluid, or medication intended for GI administration goes into the respiratory tract. Evaluate your patient's ability to swallow before administering oral medications. When there is a risk of aspiration, you will use certain interventions (Box 14-13). Properly positioning the patient is essential in preventing aspiration.

*Text continued on p. 370*

## SKILL 14-1 Administering Oral Medications

### Delegation Considerations

Do not delegate this skill.
Instruct assistive personnel about:

- Potential side effects of medications and to report their occurrence

### Equipment

- Disposable medication cups
- Glass of water, juice, or preferred liquid
- Drinking straw
- Pill-crushing or pillating device (optional)
- MAR or computer printout

| STEP | RATIONALE |
|------|-----------|

### ASSESSMENT

1. Check accuracy and completeness of each MAR or computer printout with prescriber's original medication order. Check patient's name, drug name and dosage, route of administration, and time for administration. Recopy or re-print any portion of MAR that is difficult to read.

The prescriber's order is the most reliable source and only legal record of drugs patient is to receive. Ensures patient receives the right medications. Illegible MARs are a source of medication errors.

2. Assess for any contraindications to patient receiving oral medication: Is patient able to swallow? Is patient able to have food and drink by mouth? Is patient suffering from nausea and vomiting? Was patient diagnosed as having bowel inflammation or reduced peristalsis? Has patient had recent GI surgery? Does patient have gastric suction?

Alterations in GI function interfere with drug absorption, distribution, and excretion. Patients with GI suction will not receive benefit from the medication because it may be suctioned from the GI tract before it can be absorbed. Giving medications to patients who cannot swallow increases the risk of aspiration.

3. Assess risk for aspiration (see Chapter 32). Is patient able to swallow? Assess patient's swallow, cough, and gag reflexes.

Aspiration occurs when blood, fluid, or medication inadvertently enters the respiratory tract. Patients with impaired swallowing are at higher risk for aspiration.

4. Assess patient's medical history, history of allergies, medication history, and diet history. Make sure patient's food and drug allergies are listed on each page of the MAR and prominently displayed on the patient's medical record per agency policy.

Identifies potential food and drug interaction. Reflects patient's need for medications. Effective communication of allergies is essential for all health care providers to provide safe, effective care.

5. Gather and review assessment and laboratory data that influences drug administration, such as medication history, vital signs, and renal and liver function laboratory findings.

Physical examination or laboratory data sometimes contraindicate drug administration. Alterations in liver and kidney function affect metabolism and excretion of medications (McKenry and Salerno, 2003).

---

• **Critical Decision Point:** If there are any contraindications to patient's receiving oral medications, or if in doubt about patient's ability to swallow oral medications, temporarily withhold medication and notify prescriber.

---

6. Assess patient's knowledge regarding health and medication usage.

Determines patient's need for medication education and assists in identifying patient's adherence to drug therapy at home. Assessments reveal drug use problems, such as drug tolerance, abuse, addiction, or dependency.

7. Assess patient's preferences for fluids. Maintain ordered fluid restriction (when applicable). Can medication be given with preferred fluid?

Fluids ease swallowing and facilitate absorption from the GI tract. It is necessary to maintain fluid restrictions. Some fluids may interfere with drug absorption.

┌ ─ ─ ─ ─ ─ ─ ┐
**SKILL 14-1** | **Administering Oral Medications—cont'd**
└ ─ ─ ─ ─ ─ ─ ─ ─ ─ ─ ─ ─ ─ ─ ─ ─ ─ ─ ─ ─ ─ ─ ─ ─ ─ ─ ─ ─ ┘

| STEP | RATIONALE |
|---|---|

## PLANNING

1. Expected outcomes following completion of procedure:
   - Patient experiences desired medication effect within time of medication onset.

     *Medication has exerted its therapeutic action.*
   - Patient denies adverse effects of medications.

     *Avoidance of adverse effects improves compliance with drug therapy (Ebersole and others, 2004).*
   - Patient explains purpose of medications and dosage schedule.

     *Demonstrates understanding of medication therapy.*

---

- *Critical Decision Point:* Clarify incomplete or unclear orders or orders using dangerous abbreviations with prescriber before giving patient medications.

---

## IMPLEMENTATION

1. Prepare medications:
   a. Perform hand hygiene.

      *Reduces transfer of microorganisms.*
   b. Arrange medication tray in medication preparation room or move medication cart outside patient's room.

      *Organization of equipment saves time and reduces error.*
   c. Unlock medicine drawer or cart, or log onto computerized medication dispensing system.

      *Medications are safeguarded when locked in cabinet, cart, or computerized medication dispensing system.*
   d. Prepare medications for one patient at a time. Keep all pages of MARs or computer printouts for one patient together.

      *Prevents preparation errors.*
   e. Select correct drug from stock supply or unit-dose drawer by comparing label of medication with MAR or computer printout (see illustration).

      *Reading label and comparing it with transcribed order reduce errors.*
   f. Check expiration date on all medications.

      *Medications used past their expiration date are sometimes inactive, less effective, or harmful to patient.*
   g. Calculate drug dose as necessary. Double-check calculation.

      *Double checking reduces risk of error.*
   h. When preparing controlled substance, check record for previous drug count and compare with supply available.

      *Controlled substance laws require careful monitoring of dispensed narcotics.*
   i. Prepare solid forms of oral medications:
      (1) To prepare tablets or capsules from a floor stock bottle, pour required number into bottle cap and transfer medication to medication cup. Do not touch medication with fingers. Return extra tablets or capsules to bottle. Break medications that need to be broken to administer half the dosage using a gloved hand, or cut with a pillating device (see illustration). Make sure these tablets are prescored. Identify prescored tablets by a manufactured line that traverses the center of the tablet.

         *Maintains clean technique required of medication administration. Tablets that are prescored can be split to ensure giving the patient an accurate dose.*
      (2) To prepare unit-dose tablets or capsules, place packaged tablet or capsule directly into medicine cup. (Do not remove wrapper; see illustration.)

         *Wrapper maintains cleanliness of medications and identifies drug name and dosage.*

| STEP | RATIONALE |
|---|---|

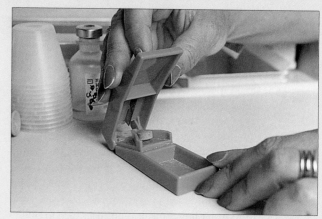

STEP **1e** Check the label of the medication with the patient's MAR.

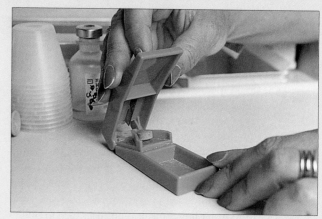

STEP **1i(1)** Place tablet in pillating device, and cut in half.

(3) Place all tablets or capsules to be given to patient at same time in one medicine cup. Place medications requiring preadministration assessments (e.g., pulse rate, blood pressure) in separate cups.

Keeping medications that require preadministration assessments separate from others makes it easier for you to remember to make special assessments and withhold drugs as necessary.

(4) If patient has difficulty swallowing and liquid medications are not an option, use a pill-crushing device, such as a mortar and pestle, to grind pills. If a pill-crushing device is not available, place tablet between two medication cups and grind with a blunt instrument. Mix ground tablet in small amount of soft food (e.g., custard, applesauce).

Large tablets are difficult to swallow. Ground tablet mixed with palatable soft food is usually easier to swallow.

---

• *Critical Decision Point:* Not all drugs can be crushed (e.g., capsules, enteric-coated drugs). Consult pharmacist when in doubt.

---

j. Prepare liquids:

(1) Gently shake container. Remove bottle cap from container and place cap upside down, or open the unit-dose container. If unit-dose container has correct amount to administer, no further preparation is necessary.

Shaking container ensures medication is mixed before administration. Placing cap of bottle upside down prevents contamination of inside of cap.

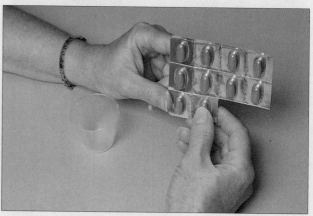

STEP **1i(2)** Place tablet into medicine cup without removing wrapper.

---

# SKILL 14-1 Administering Oral Medications—cont'd

| STEP | RATIONALE |
|---|---|
| (2) Hold bottle with label against palm of hand while pouring. | Spilled liquid will not soil or fade label. |
| (3) Hold medication cup at eye level, and fill to desired level (see illustration A). Make sure scale is even with fluid level at its surface or base of meniscus, not edges. For small doses of liquid medications, draw liquid into a calibrated 10-ml syringe without needle (see illustration B). | Ensures accuracy of measurement. Use of syringe is more accurate for measuring small doses of liquid medications. |
| (4) Discard any excess liquid into sink. Wipe lip and neck of bottle with paper towel. | Prevents contamination of bottle's contents and prevents bottle cap from sticking. |
| (5) Administer liquid medications packaged in single-dose cups directly from the single-dose cup. Do not pour them into medicine cups. | Avoids unnecessary manipulation of dose. |
| k. Compare MAR with prepared drug and container. | Reading label second time reduces error. |
| l. Return stock containers or unused unit-dose medications to shelf or drawer, and read label again. | Checking label of medications in multiple-dose containers for a third time reduces administration errors. |
| m. Do not leave drugs unattended. | Nurse is responsible for safekeeping of drugs. |
| 2. Administer medications: | |
| a. Take medications to patient at correct time, and perform hand hygiene. | Administer medications within 30 minutes before or after prescribed time to ensure intended therapeutic effect. Give stat or single-order medications at the time ordered. Hand hygiene decreases transfer of microorganisms. |
| b. Verify patient's identity by using at least two patient identifiers. Compare patient's name and one other identifier, such as hospital identification number on identification bracelet, with MAR. Ask patient to state name if possible for a third identifier (see Figure 14-7). | Complies with JCAHO requirements and improves medication safety. In most acute care settings, patient's name and identification number on armband and MAR are used to identify patients. Identification bracelets are made at time of patient's admission and are most reliable source of identification. Patient's room number is **not** an acceptable identifier (JCAHO, 2004a). |

• *Critical Decision Point:* Replace patient identification bracelets that are missing, illegible, or faded.

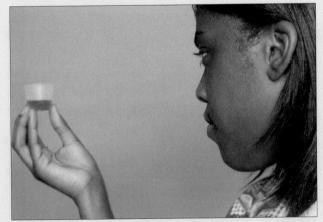

A

STEP **1j(3)A** Pour the desired volume of liquid so that base of meniscus is level with line on scale.

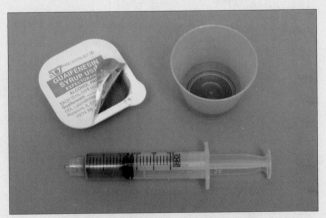

B

STEP **1j(3)B** Use needleless syringe to draw up volumes under 10 ml.

| STEP | RATIONALE |
|---|---|
| c. Compare label of medications with MAR at patient's bedside. | Final check of medication label against MAR at patient's bedside reduces medication administration errors. |
| d. Explain purpose of each medication and its action to patient. Allow patient to ask any questions about drugs. | Patient has right to be informed about medication therapy. Questions indicate need for education or noncompliance with therapy. |
| e. Assist patient to sitting or Fowler's position. Use side-lying position if sitting is contraindicated. | Sitting position prevents aspiration during swallowing (Dahlin, 2004). Remaining seated for 30 minutes helps medications move through the stomach (Jordan and others, 2003). |
| f. Administer medication: | |
| (1) **For tablets:** Patients sometimes wish to hold solid medications in hand or cup before placing in mouth. | Patient will become familiar with medications by seeing each drug. |
| (2) Offer water or juice to help patient swallow medications. Give cold carbonated water if available and not contraindicated. | Choice of fluid promotes patient's comfort and will improve fluid intake. Taking tablets and capsules with a full glass of water or other liquid helps medications enter stomach (Jordan and others, 2003). |
| (3) **For sublingual medications:** Have patient place medication under tongue and allow it to dissolve completely. Caution patient against swallowing tablet whole (see Figure 14-2). | Drug is absorbed through blood vessels of undersurface of tongue. If swallowed, gastric juices will destroy the drug or the liver will rapidly detoxify it so that the patient will not attain therapeutic blood levels. |
| (4) **For buccal medications:** Have patient place medication in mouth against mucous membranes of the cheek until it dissolves (see Figure 14-3). Avoid administering liquids until buccal medication has dissolved. | Buccal medications act locally on mucosa or systemically as the patient swallows them in saliva. |
| (5) Caution patient against chewing or swallowing lozenges. | Drug acts through slow absorption through oral mucosa, not gastric mucosa. |
| (6) **For powdered medications:** Mix with liquids at bedside, and give to patient to drink. | When prepared in advance, powdered drugs thicken and even harden, making swallowing difficult. |
| (7) Give effervescent powders and tablets immediately after dissolving. | Effervescence improves unpleasant taste of drug and often relieves GI problems. |
| g. If patient is unable to hold medications, place medication cup to the lips and gently introduce each drug into the mouth, one at a time. Do not rush. | Administering single tablet or capsule eases swallowing and decreases risk of aspiration. |
| h. If tablet or capsule falls to the floor, discard it and repeat preparation. | Drug is contaminated when it touches floor. |
| i. Stay until patient has completely swallowed each medication. Ask patient to open mouth if uncertain whether patient has swallowed medication. | You are responsible for ensuring that patient receives ordered dosage. If left unattended, patient may not take dose or may save drugs, causing risk to health. |
| j. For highly acidic medications (e.g., aspirin), offer patient nonfat snack (e.g., crackers) if not contraindicated by patient's condition. | Reduces gastric irritation. |
| k. Assist patient in returning to comfortable position. | Maintains patient's comfort. |
| l. Dispose of soiled supplies, and perform hand hygiene. | Reduces transmission of microorganisms. |
| m. Replenish stock, such as cups and straws, return cart to medicine room, and clean work area. | Clean working space assists other staff in completing duties efficiently. |

## SKILL 14-1 Administering Oral Medications—cont'd

| STEP | RATIONALE |
| --- | --- |

### EVALUATION

1. Evaluate patient's response to medications at times that correlate with the medication's onset, peak, and duration. Evaluate patient for both desired effect and adverse effects.

Evaluates drug's therapeutic benefit and detects onset of side effects or allergic reactions.

2. Ask patient or family member to identify drug name and explain purpose, action, dose schedule, and potential side effects of medication.

Determines patient's or family member's understanding of medication.

### RECORDING AND REPORTING

■ Record administration of oral medications on computerized or paper copy of MAR immediately after administering medication. If using paper copy of MAR, include your initials or signature.

■ If you withheld any medication, record the reason and follow agency's policy to record withheld medication on MAR.

■ Report adverse effects to prescriber.

■ Report evaluation of medication effect to prescriber if required.

### UNEXPECTED OUTCOMES AND RELATED INTERVENTIONS

■ Patient exhibits side or adverse effects.
  • Assess for symptoms such as urticaria, rash, **pruritus**, rhinitis, and wheezing that indicate allergic reaction.

  • Always notify prescriber and pharmacy when the patient exhibits adverse effects.
  • Withhold further doses.
  • Add allergy information to patient's chart.
■ Patient refuses medication.
  • Explore reasons why patient does not want medication.
  • Educate if misunderstandings of medication therapy are apparent.
  • Do not force patient to take medication.
  • Remember that patients have the right to refuse treatment.
  • If patient continues to refuse medication despite education, record why the drug was withheld on patient's chart and notify prescriber.

When possible, place the patient in a seated or Fowler's position. You also place the patient in the side-lying position when your patient's swallow, gag, and cough reflexes are intact. If your patient has difficulty swallowing, consult appropriate personnel (e.g., speech therapist) for a swallow evaluation before administering oral medications and use other routes of medication administration (e.g., intravenous or subcutaneous). Sometimes, you will give medications through the nasogastric or feeding tube when the patient cannot swallow. Box 14-14 summarizes guidelines for administering medications through gastric tubes.

## Topical Medication Applications

Topical medications are medications applied locally, most often to intact skin. They come in the form of lotions, pastes, or ointments (see Table 14-1). They are also applied to mucous membranes.

### Skin Applications

Because many locally applied medications, such as lotions, pastes, and ointments, create systemic and local effects, wear gloves and use applicators when administering them. Use sterile technique if the patient has an open wound. Skin encrustation and dead tissues harbor microorganisms and block contact of medications with the tissues to be treated. Therefore clean the skin thoroughly before applying topical medications.

Spread the medication evenly over the involved surface when applying ointments or pastes. In some cases you apply a gauze dressing over the medication to prevent soiling of clothes and wiping away of the medication. Apply each type of medication according to directions to ensure proper penetration and absorption. Spread lotions and creams lightly onto the skin's surface, because rubbing causes irritation. Apply a liniment by rubbing it gently but firmly into the skin. You dust a powder lightly to cover the affected area with a thin layer. Before and during any application, assess the

| BOX 14-14 | PROCEDURAL GUIDELINES FOR |
| --- | --- |

## Administering Medications Through a Nasogastric Tube, G-Tube, J-Tube, or Small-Bore Feeding Tube

**Delegation Considerations:** Do not delegate this skill. Instruct assistive personnel about the potential side effects of medications and the need to report their occurrence.

**Equipment:** 60-ml syringe (catheter tip for large-bore tubes; Luer-Lok tip for small-bore tubes), gastric pH test tape (scale of 0.0 to 11.0 or 14.0 preferred), graduated container, water, medication to be administered, pill crusher if medication in tablet form, medication administration record, disposable gloves

1. Check accuracy and completeness of each MAR or computer printout with prescriber's written medication order. Check patient's name, drug name and dosage, route of administration, and time for administration.
2. Investigate and use alternative routes of medication administration if possible (e.g., transdermal, rectal).
3. Avoid complicated medication regimens that frequently interrupt enteral feedings.
4. Prepare medication (see Skill 14-1, Implementation steps 1a-m). Check label of medication with MAR two times.
5. Be sure the medication is compatible with the enteral feeding before administering medications. If the medication is incompatible with the feeding, stop the feeding 1 to 2 hours before giving the medication, and restart the feeding 1 to 2 hours after giving the medication. Never add medications directly to the tube feeding.
6. Administer medications in a liquid form (suspension, elixir, solution) when possible to prevent obstruction of the tube.
7. Before crushing medications, be sure they should be crushed. Do not crush buccal, sublingual, enteric-coated, or sustained-release medications.
8. Take medications to patient at correct time, and perform hand hygiene.
9. Verify patient's identity by using at least two patient identifiers. Compare patient's name and one other identifier, such as hospital identification number on identification bracelet, with MAR. Ask patient to state name if possible for a third identifier.
10. Compare label of medications against MAR one more time at patient's bedside.
11. Explain procedure to patient, and educate patient about medications.
12. Dissolve crushed tablets, gelatin capsules, and powders in 15 to 30 ml of warm water.
13. Do not give whole or undissolved medications through the feeding tube.
14. Put on clean, disposable gloves.
15. Verify placement of any tube that enters the mouth or nose using pH testing (see Chapter 31).
16. Assess gastric residual (see Chapter 31).
17. Flush tube with 30 ml warm water.
18. Draw up medication in syringe. Do **not** mix medications together.
19. Connect syringe with medication to nasogastric tube, G-tube, J-tube, or small-bore feeding tube.
20. Administer medication by either pushing the medication through the tube with the syringe or by allowing medication to flow into body freely by using gravity. Administer each medication separately
21. Flush tube with 15 to 30 ml of water between each medication. Unless contraindicated, the total amount of liquid volume administered to the patient for each medication is approximately 60 ml.
22. Once you have given all medications, flush tube once more with 30 to 60 ml warm water.
23. Clean area, and put supplies away.
24. Remove gloves, and perform hand hygiene.
25. Document administration of medications on MAR.
26. Continually evaluate the patient's response to medication therapy. If the patient does not achieve the desired effect, a different medication or route of administration may be indicated because of problems with drug bioavailability when given by the enteral route.

Modified from Jordan and others: Administration of medicines. II. Pharmacology, *Nurs Stand* 18(3):45, 2003.

skin thoroughly. Note the area applied and condition of skin in the patient's chart, and document the name and administration of the medication on the MAR.

## Nasal Instillation

Patients with nasal sinus alterations often receive medications by spray, drops, or tampons (Box 14-15). The most commonly administered form of nasal instillation is decongestant spray or drops, used to relieve symptoms of sinus congestion and colds. Caution your patient to avoid abuse of nose drops and sprays, because overuse leads to rebound nasal congestion. In addition, when patients swallow excess decongestant solution, serious systemic effects develop, especially in children. Saline drops are safer as a decongestant

for children than nasal preparations that contain sympathomimetics (e.g., Afrin, Neo-Synephrine).

It is easier to have the patient self-administer sprays, because the patient can control the spray and inhale as it enters the nasal passages. If patients use nasal sprays repeatedly, observe the nares for irritation. You usually treat severe nosebleeds with packing or nasal tampons, which are treated with epinephrine, to reduce blood flow. Usually a physician or health care provider places nasal tampons.

## Eye Instillation

Common medications used by patients are eye drops and ointments, including OTC preparations (e.g., Visine or Murine). Many patients receive prescribed **ophthalmic**

**BOX 14-15** PROCEDURAL GUIDELINES FOR

## Administering Nasal Instillations

**Delegation Considerations:** Do not delegate this skill. Instruct assistive personnel about the potential side effects of medications and the need to report their occurrence

**Equipment:** prepared medication with clean dropper or spray container, facial tissue, small pillow (optional), washcloth (optional), gloves (if patient has extensive nasal drainage), medication administration record or computer printout

1. Check accuracy and completeness of each MAR or computer printout with prescriber's original medication order. Check patient's name, drug name and dosage, route of administration, and time for administration.
2. Determine which sinus is affected by referring to medical record if giving nasal drops.
3. Assess patient's medical history (e.g., history of hypertension, heart disease, diabetes mellitus, and hyperthyroidism) and allergies to medications and foods. Make sure patient's drug and food allergies are listed on the MAR and are prominently displayed on the patient's medical record per agency policy.
4. Using a penlight, inspect condition of nose and sinuses. Palpate sinuses for tenderness.
5. Assess patient's knowledge regarding use of nasal instillations and technique for instillation and willingness to learn self-administration.
6. Prepare medication: See Skill 14-1, Implementation steps 1a-h, k-m. Be sure to compare label of medication against MAR at least two times while preparing medication.
7. Take medications to patient at correct time, and perform hand hygiene.
8. Verify patient's identity by using at least two patient identifiers. Compare patient's name and one other identifier, such as hospital identification number on identification bracelet, with MAR. Ask patient to state name if possible for a third identifier.
9. Compare MAR with medication labels at patient's bedside.
10. Explain procedure to patient regarding positioning and sensations to expect, such as burning or stinging of mucosa or choking sensation as medication trickles into throat.

11. Arrange supplies and medications at bedside. Apply gloves if patient has nasal drainage.
12. Gently roll or shake container.
13. Instruct patient to clear or blow nose gently unless contraindicated (e.g., risk of increased intracranial pressure or nosebleeds).
14. Administer nasal drops:
    a. Assist patient to supine position, and position head properly:
       (1) For access to posterior pharynx, tilt patient's head backward.
       (2) For access to ethmoid or sphenoid sinus, tilt head back over edge of bed or place small pillow under patient's shoulder and tilt head back (see illustration).
       (3) For access to frontal or maxillary sinus, tilt head back over edge of bed or pillow with head turned toward side to be treated (see illustration).
    b. Support patient's head with nondominant hand.
    c. Instruct patient to breathe through mouth.
    d. Hold dropper 1 cm (½ inch) above nares, and instill prescribed number of drops toward midline of ethmoid bone.
    e. Have patient remain in supine position 5 minutes.
    f. Offer facial tissue to blot runny nose, but caution patient against blowing nose for several minutes.
15. Assist patient to a comfortable position after drug is absorbed.
16. Dispose of soiled supplies in proper container, and perform hand hygiene.
17. Document adminstration of medication on MAR.
18. Observe patient for onset of side effects 15 to 30 minutes after administration. Ask if patient is able to breathe through nose after decongestant administration. May be necessary to have patient occlude one nostril at a time and breathe deeply.
19. Evaluate patient's response to medications at times that correlate with the medication's onset, peak, and duration. Evaluate patient for both desired effect and adverse effects.

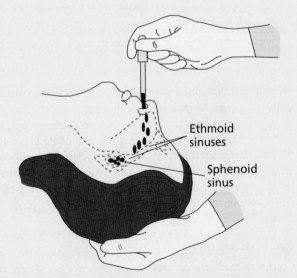

STEP **14a(2)** Position for instilling nose drops into ethmoid or sphenoid sinus.

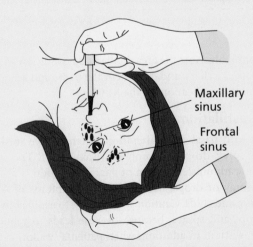

STEP **14a(3)** Position for instilling nose drops into frontal and maxillary sinus.

medications for eye conditions such as glaucoma or after cataract extraction. Many patients who receive eye medications are older adults. Age-related problems, including poor vision, hand tremors, and difficulty grasping or manipulating small containers, affect the ability of older adults to self-administer eye medications. Educate your patients and their family members about the proper techniques for administering eye medications (Skill 14-2). Evaluate the patient's and family's ability to self-administer through a return demonstration of the procedure. Showing patients each step of the procedure for instilling eye drops will improve their compliance. Apply the following principles when administering eye medications:

1. Avoid instilling any form of eye medication directly onto the cornea. The cornea of the eye is richly supplied with pain fibers and thus very sensitive to anything applied to it.
2. Avoid touching the eyelids or other eye structures with eye droppers or ointment tubes. The risk of transmitting infection from one eye to the other is high.
3. Use eye medication only for the patient's affected eye.
4. Never allow a patient to use another patient's eye medications.

You will administer some medications using an intraocular disk (see Skill 14-2). Intraocular medicated disks resemble a contact lens. The medication is placed onto the conjunctival sac, where it remains in place for up to 1 week. Teach your patient receiving medications in this way to monitor for adverse reactions to the disk as well as methods of insertion and removal.

*Text continued on p. 377*

---

## SKILL 14-2 ▕ Administering Eye Medications

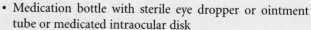

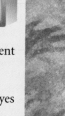

### Delegation Considerations

Do not delegate this skill.
Instruct assistive personnel about:
• Potential side effects of medications and to report their occurrence
• Potential for patients to become impaired after administration of eye medications

### Equipment

• Medication bottle with sterile eye dropper or ointment tube or medicated intraocular disk
• Cotton ball or tissue
• Washbasin filled with warm water and washcloth if eyes have crust or drainage
• Eye patch and tape (optional)
• Clean gloves
• MAR or computer printout

| STEP | RATIONALE |
|---|---|
| **ASSESSMENT** | |
| 1. Check accuracy and completeness of each MAR or computer printout with prescriber's original medication order. Check patient's name, drug name and dosage (e.g., number of drops [if a liquid] and eye [right = O.D.; left = O.S.; both = O.U.]), route of administration, and time for administration. | The prescriber's order is the most reliable source and only legal record of drugs patient is to receive. Ensures patient receives the right medications. |
| 2. Recopy or re-print any portion of the MAR that is difficult to read. | Illegible MARs are a source of medication errors. |
| 3. Assess condition of external eye structures. (You may also do this just before drug instillation.) | Provides baseline to later determine if local response to medications occurs. Also indicates need to clean eye before drug application. |
| 4. Determine whether patient has any known allergies to eye medications. Also ask if patient has allergy to latex. | Protects patient from risk of allergic drug response. If patient has a latex allergy, use nonlatex gloves. |
| 5. Determine whether patient has any symptoms of visual alterations. | Certain eye medications act to either lessen or increase these symptoms. Ensures that you are able to recognize change in patient's condition. |
| 6. Assess patient's level of consciousness and ability to follow directions. | If patient becomes restless or combative during procedure, a greater risk of accidental eye injury exists. |

| STEP | RATIONALE |
|---|---|
| 7. Assess patient's knowledge regarding drug therapy and desire to self-administer medication. | Patient's level of understanding indicates need for health teaching. Motivation influences teaching approach. |
| 8. Assess patient's ability to manipulate and hold equipment necessary for eye medication (e.g., dropper, tube of ointment, intraocular disk). | Reflects patient's ability to self-administer drug. |

## PLANNING

| | |
|---|---|
| 1. Expected outcomes following completion of procedure:<br>• Patient experiences desired effect of medication. | Medication is administered correctly without injury to patient and has exerted its therapeutic action. |
| • Patient denies discomfort or other adverse effects of medication. | Absence of adverse effects improves compliance with drug therapy (Ebersole and others, 2004). |
| • Patient is able to discuss information about medication. | Demonstrates understanding of medication therapy. |
| • Patient is able to self-administer medication correctly. | Demonstrates learning. |

## IMPLEMENTATION

| | |
|---|---|
| 1. Prepare medication: See Skill 14-1, Implementation steps 1a-h, k-m. Be sure to check the label two times while preparing medication. | Following the same routine when preparing medications, eliminating distractions, and checking the label of the medication with transcribed order reduces error. |
| 2. Take medications to patient at correct time, and perform hand hygiene. | Administer medications within 30 minutes before or after prescribed time to ensure intended therapeutic effect. Give stat or single-order medications at the time ordered. Hand hygiene decreases transfer of microorganisms. |
| 3. Verify patient's identity by using at least two patient identifiers. Compare patient's name and one other identifier, such as hospital identification number on identification bracelet, with MAR. Ask patient to state name if possible for a third identifier. | Complies with JCAHO requirements and improves medication safety. In most acute care settings, patient's name and identification number on armband and MAR are used to identify patients. Identification bracelets are made at time of patient's admission and are most reliable source of identification. Patient's room number is **not** an acceptable identifier (JCAHO, 2004a). |
| 4. Compare label of medication against MAR for third time. | Final check of medication against MAR decreases risk of medication errors. |
| 5. Explain procedure to patient regarding positioning and sensations to expect, such as burning or stinging of mucosa or choking sensation as medication trickles into throat. | Relieves anxiety about medication being instilled into eye. |
| 6. Arrange supplies at bedside; apply clean gloves. If eye drops are stored in refrigerator, allow eye drops to come to room temperature before giving eye drops. | Reduces transmission of microorganisms and follows Centers for Disease Control and Administration (CDC) recommendations to prevent accidental exposure to body fluids (OSHA, 2001). Warming eye drops reduces irritation to eye. |
| 7. Gently roll container. | Ensures medication is mixed before administration. Shaking container creates bubbles, which makes medication administration difficult. |
| 8. Ask patient to lie supine or sit back in chair with head slightly hyperextended. | Position provides easy access to eye for medication instillation and minimizes drainage of medication through tear duct. |

• *Critical Decision Point:* If the patient has a cervical spine injury, do not hyperextend the neck.

| STEP | RATIONALE |
|---|---|

9. If crusts or drainage is present along eyelid margins or inner canthus, gently wash away. Apply damp washcloth or cotton ball over eye for a few minutes to soak crusts that are dried and difficult to remove. Always wipe clean from inner to outer canthus.

Crusts or drainage harbors microorganisms. Soaking allows easy removal and prevents pressure from being applied directly over eye. Cleansing from inner to outer canthus avoids entrance of microorganisms into lacrimal duct.

10. Hold cotton ball or clean tissue in nondominant hand on patient's cheekbone just below lower eyelid.

Cotton or tissue absorbs medication that escapes eye.

11. With tissue or cotton resting below lower lid, gently press downward with thumb or forefinger against bony orbit.

Technique exposes lower conjunctival sac. Retraction against bony orbit prevents pressure and trauma to eyeball and prevents fingers from touching eye.

12. Ask patient to look at ceiling.

Action retracts sensitive cornea up and away from conjunctival sac and reduces stimulation of blink reflex.

13. Administer ophthalmic medication.
    a. To instill eye drops:
       (1) With dominant hand resting on patient's forehead, hold filled medication eye dropper or ophthalmic solution approximately 1 to 2 cm ($\frac{1}{2}$ to $\frac{3}{4}$ inch) above conjunctival sac (see illustration).

Helps prevent accidental contact of eye dropper with eye structures, thus reducing risk of injury to eye and transfer of infection to dropper. Ophthalmic medications are sterile.

       (2) Drop prescribed number of medication drops into conjunctival sac.

Conjunctival sac normally holds 1 or 2 drops. Provides even distribution of medication across eye.

       (3) If patient blinks or closes eye or if drops land on outer lid margins, repeat procedure.

Therapeutic effect of drug is obtained only when drops enter conjunctival sac.

       (4) After instilling drops, ask patient to close eye gently.

Helps to distribute medication. Squinting or squeezing of eyelids forces medication out of conjunctival sac (VisionRx, 2004).

       (5) When administering drugs that cause systemic effects, apply gentle pressure with your finger and clean tissue on the patient's nasolacrimal duct for 30 to 60 seconds.

Prevents overflow of medication into nasal and pharyngeal passages. Prevents absorption into systemic circulation.

    b. To instill eye ointment:
       (1) Ask patient to look at ceiling.

Action retracts sensitive cornea up and away from conjunctival sac and reduces stimulation of blink reflex.

       (2) Holding ointment applicator above lower lid margin, apply thin stream of ointment evenly along inner edge of lower eyelid on conjunctiva (see illustration) from the inner canthus to outer canthus.

Distributes medication evenly across eye and lid margin.

       (3) Have patient close eye and roll eye behind closed eyelid.

Further distributes medication without traumatizing eye.

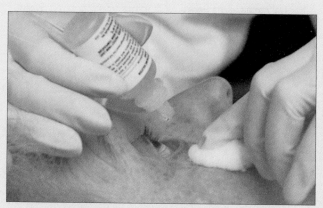

STEP **13a(1)** Hold eye dropper above conjunctival sac.

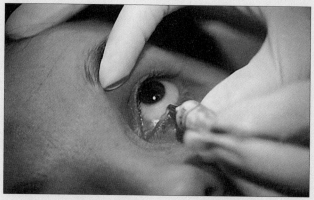

STEP **13b(2)** Apply ointment along lower eyelid.

## SKILL 14-2 ¦ Administering Eye Medications—cont'd

| STEP | RATIONALE |
|---|---|

c. To administer intraocular disk:

  (1) Application:

    (a) Open package containing the disk. Apply gloves. Gently press your fingertip against the disk so that it adheres to your finger. Position the convex side of the disk on your fingertip (see illustration).

*Allows you to inspect disk for damage or deformity.*

    (b) With your other hand, gently pull the patient's lower eyelid away from the eye. Ask patient to look up.

*Prepares conjunctival sac for receiving medicated disk.*

    (c) Place the disk in the conjunctival sac so that it floats on the sclera between the iris and lower eyelid (see illustration).

*Ensures delivery of medication.*

    (d) Pull the patient's lower eyelid out and over the disk (see illustration).

*Ensures accurate medication delivery.*

---

• *Critical Decision Point:* You should not be able to see the disk at this time. Repeat step (d) if you can see the disk.

---

  (2) Removal:

    (a) Perform hand hygiene, and put on gloves.

*Prevents transfer of microorganisms and follows CDC recommendations to prevent accidental exposure to body fluids (OSHA 2001).*

    (b) Explain procedure to patient.

*Relieves anxiety about manipulation of disk in eye.*

    (c) Gently pull down on the patient's lower eyelid.

*Exposes intraocular disk.*

    (d) Using your forefinger and thumb of your opposite hand, pinch the disk and lift it out of the patient's eye (see illustration).

14. If excess medication is on eyelid, gently wipe it from inner to outer canthus.

*Promotes comfort and prevents trauma to eye (VisionRx, 2004).*

15. If patient had eye patch, apply clean one by placing it over affected eye so entire eye is covered. Tape securely without applying pressure to eye.

*Clean eye patch reduces chance of infection.*

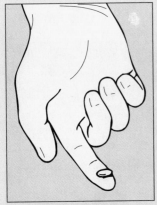

STEP **13c(1)(a)** Gently position the convex side of the disk against your fingertip.

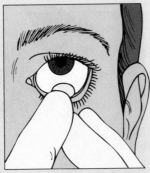

STEP **13c(1)(c)** Place disk in the conjunctival sac between the iris and lower eyelid.

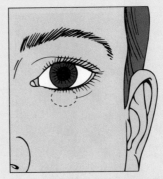

STEP **13c(1)(d)** Gently pull lower eyelid over the disk.

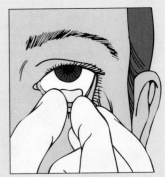

STEP **13c(2)(d)** Carefully pinch the disk to remove it from patient's eye.

| STEP | RATIONALE |
|---|---|
| 16. If patient receives more than one eye medication to the same eye at the same time, wait at least 5 minutes before administering the next medication. | Allows medication to absorb and avoids interaction between medications (VisionRx, 2004). |
| 17. If patient receives eye medication to both eyes at the same time, use a different tissue or cotton ball with each eye. | Prevents cross contamination between eyes. |
| 18. Remove gloves, dispose of soiled supplies in proper receptacle, and perform hand hygiene. | Maintains neat environment at bedside and reduces transmission of microorganisms. |

## EVALUATION

| | |
|---|---|
| 1. Note patient's response to instillation; ask if he or she felt any discomfort. | Determines if you performed procedure correctly and safely and if patient is experiencing adverse effects of medication. |
| 2. Observe response to medication by assessing visual changes and noting any side effects. | Evaluates effects of medication. |
| 3. Ask patient to discuss drug's purpose, action, side effects, and technique of administration. | Determines patient's level of understanding. |
| 4. Have patient demonstrate self-administration of next dose. | Provides feedback regarding competency with skill. |

## RECORDING AND REPORTING

■ Record drug, concentration, number of drops, time of administration, and eye (left, right, or both) that received medication on electronic or printed MAR.

■ Record appearance of eye in nurses' notes.

## UNEXPECTED OUTCOMES AND RELATED INTERVENTIONS

■ Patient cannot instill drops without supervision.
- Reinforce teaching, and allow patient to self-administer drops as much as possible to enhance confidence.
- If patient cannot self-administer drops, teach others, such as family members, to instill drops into the patient's eye.

■ Patient displays signs of allergic reaction (e.g., tearing, reddened sclera) or systemic response (e.g., bradycardia) to medication.
- Hold medication, and speak with prescriber.
- Follow institutional policy or guidelines for reporting of adverse or allergic reaction to medications.
- Add information about allergy to medical record per agency policy.

## Ear Instillation

Internal ear structures are very sensitive to temperature extremes. Failure to instill ear drops or irrigating fluid at room temperature causes vertigo (severe dizziness) or nausea. Although the structures of the outer ear are not sterile, you use sterile drops and solutions in case the eardrum is ruptured. The entrance of nonsterile solutions into middle ear structures will result in infection. If the patient has ear drainage, check with the physician or health care provider to be sure the patient does not have a ruptured eardrum before instilling ear drops. Never occlude the ear canal with the dropper or irrigating syringe. Forcing medication into an occluded ear canal creates pressure that will injure the eardrum. When administering medications into the ear, you straighten the ear canal properly to allow medications to reach the deeper, external ear structures. Box 14-16 provides guidelines for administering ear drops and ear irrigations and describes how to straighten the ear canal for children and for adults.

## Vaginal Instillation

Vaginal medications are available as suppositories, foams, jellies, or creams. Suppositories come individually packaged and are stored in a refrigerator to prevent them from melting. After inserting a suppository into the vaginal cavity, body temperature causes it to melt and be distributed and absorbed. You administer foams, jellies, and creams with an applicator or inserter. You give a suppository with a gloved hand in accordance with standard precautions. Patients often prefer administering their own vaginal medications. Give the patient privacy to do this. After instillation of the med-

| BOX 14-16 | PROCEDURAL GUIDELINES FOR |
|---|---|

## Administering Ear Medications

**Delegation Considerations:** Do not delegate this skill. Instruct assistive personnel about the potential side effects of medications and the need to report their occurrence.

**Equipment:** *drops:* medication bottle with dropper, cotton-tipped applicator, cotton ball (optional), clean gloves if patient has drainage from ear; *irrigation:* irrigating syringe, kidney basin, towel; MAR.

1. Check accuracy and completeness of each MAR or computer printout with prescriber's written medication order. Check patient's name, drug name and dosage, route of administration, and time for administration.
2. Prepare medication (see Skill 14-1, Implementation steps 1a-h, k-m). Be sure to compare the label of the medication with the MAR at least two times during medication preparation.
3. Take medication to patient at correct time, and perform hand hygiene.
4. Verify patient's identity by using at least two patient identifiers. Compare patient's name and one other identifier, such as hospital identification number on identification bracelet, with MAR. Ask patient to state name if possible for a third identifier.
5. Compare the label of the medication with the MAR one more time at the patient's bedside.
6. Explain procedure to patient regarding positioning and sensations to expect, such as hearing bubbling or feeling of water in ear as medication trickles into ear.
7. Teach patient about medication.
8. *Administer ear drops:*
   a. Place patient in side-lying position if not contraindicated by patient's condition, with ear to be treated facing up. The patient may also sit in a chair or at the bedside.
   b. Straighten ear canal by pulling auricle down and back for children or upward and outward for adults.
   c. Instill prescribed drops holding dropper 1 cm (½ inch) above ear canal (see illustration).
   d. Ask patient to remain in side-lying position for 2 to 3 minutes. Apply gentle massage or pressure to tragus of ear with finger.
   e. If you place a cotton ball into the outermost part of ear canal, do not press cotton ball into the canal. Remove cotton after 15 minutes.
9. *Administer ear irrigations:*
   a. Assess the tympanic membrane, or review medical record

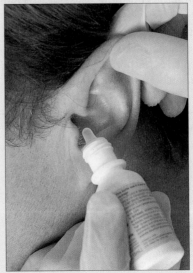

STEP **8c** Instill prescribed drops holding dropper above ear canal.

   for history of eardrum perforation, which contraindicates ear irrigation.
   b. Assist patient into sitting or lying position with head tilted or turned toward affected ear. Place towel under patient's head and shoulder, and have patient hold basin under affected ear.
   c. Fill irrigating syringe with solution (approximately 50 ml) at room temperature.
   d. Gently grasp auricle, and straighten ear by pulling it down and back for children or upward and outward for adults.
   e. Slowly instill irrigating solution by holding tip of syringe 1 cm (½ inch) above opening of ear canal. Allow fluid to drain out during instillation. Continue until you cleanse the canal or use all solution.
10. Clean area, and put supplies away.
11. Remove gloves, and perform hand hygiene.
12. Document medication administration on MAR.
13. Evaluate patient's response to the medication.

---

ication, some patients wish to wear a perineal pad to collect drainage. Because you will often give vaginal medications to treat infection, discharge is usually foul-smelling. Follow aseptic techniques, and offer your patient frequent opportunities to maintain perineal hygiene (see Chapter 27). Box 14-17 describes the steps to take when administering vaginal medications.

## Rectal Instillation

Rectal suppositories are thinner and more bullet-shaped than vaginal suppositories. The rounded end prevents anal trauma during insertion. Rectal suppositories contain medications that exert local effects, such as promoting defecation, or systemic effects, such as reducing nausea. Rectal suppositories are stored in the refrigerator until administered.

## BOX 14-17 PROCEDURAL GUIDELINES FOR

## Administering Vaginal Medications

**Delegation Considerations:** Do not delegate this skill. Instruct assistive personnel about the potential side effects of medications and the need to report their occurrence.

**Equipment:** vaginal cream, foam, jelly, or suppository or irrigating solution with applicator (if required); clean gloves; towels and/or washcloth; perineal pad; drape or sheet; water-soluble lubricating jelly; MAR

1. Check accuracy and completeness of each MAR or computer printout with prescriber's written medication order. Check patient's name, drug name and dosage, route of administration, and time for administration.
2. Prepare medication (see Skill 14-1, Implementation steps 1a-h, k-m). Compare the label of the medication with the MAR two times while preparing the medication.
3. Take medication to patient at the correct time, and perform hand hygiene.
4. Verify patient's identity by using at least two patient identifiers. Compare patient's name and one other identifier, such as hospital identification number on identification bracelet, with MAR. Ask patient to state name if possible for a third identifier.
5. Compare label of medication against the MAR one more time at the patient's bedside.
6. Explain procedure to patient regarding positioning and sensations to expect, such as feelings of moisture or wetness in the vaginal area. Be sure patient understands the procedure if she plans to self-administer medication. Teach patient about the medication.
7. Close room door or pull curtain to provide privacy.
8. Put on clean gloves.
9. Be sure there is adequate lighting to visualize vaginal opening. Assess vaginal area, noting the appearance of any discharge and the condition of the external genitalia. Cleanse area with towel or washcloth if needed.

10. *Administer vaginal suppository:*
    a. Remove suppository from wrapper, and apply liberal amount of sterile water-based lubricating jelly to smooth or rounded end. Lubricate gloved index finger of dominant hand.
    b. With nondominant gloved hand, gently separate and hold labial folds.
    c. With dominant gloved hand, gently insert rounded end of suppository along posterior wall of vaginal canal entire length of finger (7.5 to 10 cm or 3 to 4 inches) (see illustration).
    d. Withdraw finger, and wipe away remaining lubricant from around vaginal opening and labia.
11. *Administer cream or foam:*
    a. Fill cream or foam applicator following package directions.
    b. With nondominant gloved hand, gently separate and hold labial folds.
    c. With dominant gloved hand, gently insert applicator about 5 to 7.5 cm (2 to 3 inches). Push applicator plunger to deposit medication into vagina (see illustration).
    d. Withdraw applicator, and place on paper towel. Wipe off residual cream from labia or vaginal opening.
12. Dispose of supplies, remove gloves, and perform hand hygiene.
13. Instruct patient to remain on back for at least 10 minutes.
14. Document medication administration on MAR.
15. If applicator is used, wearing gloves, wash with soap and warm water, rinse, and store for future use.
16. Offer perineal pad to patient when she begins to ambulate.
17. Evaluate patient's response to medication.

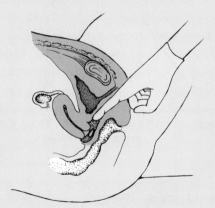

STEP **10c** Insertion of a suppository into the vaginal canal.

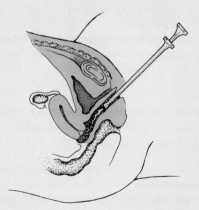

STEP **11c** Instillation of medication in vaginal canal.

During administration, place the unwrapped suppository past the internal anal sphincter and against the rectal mucosa. Otherwise, the patient will expel the suppository before it dissolves and is absorbed into the mucosa. You will feel the sphincter relaxing around the finger when you administer the suppository. Do not force suppositories into a mass of fecal material. You will need to clear the rectum with a small cleansing enema before inserting a suppository. Box 14-18 describes the steps to use when administering rectal medications.

---

## BOX 14-18    PROCEDURAL GUIDELINES FOR

### Administering Rectal Suppositories

**Delegation Considerations:** Do not delegate this skill. Instruct assistive personnel about the potential side effects of medications and the need to report their occurrence.

**Equipment:** rectal suppository, clean gloves, drape or sheet, water-soluble lubricating jelly, tissue, MAR

1. Check accuracy and completeness of each MAR or computer printout with prescriber's written medication order. Check patient's name, drug name and dosage, route of administration, and time for administration.
2. Prepare medication (see Skill 14-1, Implementation steps 1a-h, k-m). Be sure to compare the label of the medication with the MAR two times during medication preparation.
3. Take medication to patient at the correct time, and perform hand hygiene.
4. Verify patient's identity by using at least two patient identifiers. Compare patient's name and one other identifier, such as hospital identification number on identification bracelet, with MAR. Ask patient to state name if possible for a third identifier.
5. Compare the label of the medication with the MAR one more time at the patient's bedside.
6. Explain procedure to patient regarding positioning and sensations to expect, such as feelings of needing to defecate. Be sure patient understands the procedure if he or she plans to self-administer medication. Teach patient about the medication.
7. Close room door or pull curtain to provide privacy.
8. Put on clean gloves.
9. Assist patient to the Sims' position. Keep patient draped with only anal area exposed.
10. Be sure there is adequate lighting to visualize anus. Assess external condition of anus, and palpate rectal walls as needed (see Chapter 33). Dispose of gloves in proper receptacle if soiled.
11. Apply disposable gloves if gloves were thrown away in previous step.
12. Remove suppository from wrapper and lubricate rounded end with sterile water-soluble lubricating jelly (see illustration). Lubricate index finger of dominant hand with water-soluble jelly.
13. Ask patient to take slow deep breath through mouth and relax anal sphincter.
14. Retract buttocks with nondominant hand. Using dominant hand, insert suppository gently through anus, past internal sphincter and against rectal wall, 10 cm (4 inches) in adults, or 5 cm (2 inches) in children and infants (see illustration). You may need to apply gentle pressure to hold buttocks together momentarily.
15. Withdraw finger, and wipe anal area with tissue.

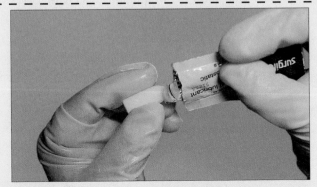

STEP **12** Lubricate tip of rectal suppository with water-soluble jelly.

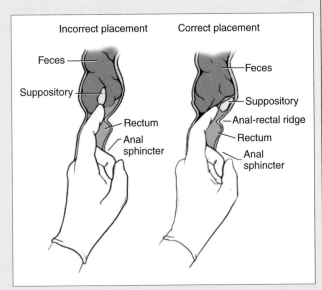

STEP **14** Inserting a rectal suppository. (From deWit S: *Fundamental concepts and skills for nursing,* ed 2, Philadelphia, 2005, WB Saunders.)

16. Dispose of supplies, remove gloves, and perform hand hygiene.
17. Instruct patient to remain on side for at least 5 minutes.
18. If suppository is a laxative or stool softener, place call light within reach of the patient.
19. Document medication administration on MAR.
20. Evaluate patient's response to medication.

## Administering Medications by Inhalation

Medications administered with handheld inhalers are dispersed through an aerosol spray, mist, or powder that penetrates lung airways. The alveolar-capillary network absorbs medications rapidly. **Metered-dose inhalers (MDIs)** and dry powder inhalers (DPIs) are usually designed to produce local effects, such as bronchodilation. However, some medications create serious systemic side effects. MDIs use a chemical propellant to push the medicine out of the inhaler, whereas DPIs use energy created by the patient during inhalation to push the medication out of the inhaler (MayoClinic.com, 2003a).

Patients who receive medications by inhalation frequently have a chronic respiratory disease, such as chronic asthma, emphysema, or bronchitis. Medications given by inhalation provide these patients with control of airway obstruction. Proper use of MDIs improves patient outcomes and decreases mortality associated with chronic airway diseases (Pereira and others, 2002). Therefore patients who need to take these medications need to learn how to administer them correctly (Skill 14-3).

To use an MDI a patient must use 5 to 10 lb of pressure to activate the aerosol. Assess if your patient has sufficient strength to correctly use the MDI by having the patient manipulate the device. Many patients who use MDIs are children or older adults. Because these two populations have diminished hand strength, it is especially important to assess if patients in these age-groups have enough strength to use the MDI. Your patient can use a spacer with the MDI. A spacer is a 4- to 8-inch–long tube that attaches to the MDI and allows the particles of medication to slow down and break into smaller pieces. This helps the medication get deeper into the lungs and enhances absorption (MayoClinic.com, 2003b). Spacers are helpful when the patient has difficulty coordinating the steps involved in self-administering inhaled medications.

DPIs hold dry, powdered medication and create an aerosol when the patient inhales through a reservoir to deliver the medication. DPIs require less manual dexterity. Because the patient activates the DPI when breathing, there is no need to coordinate puffs with inhalation, as when using an MDI. DPIs do not require a spacer. However, if the patient is in a humid climate, the medication sometimes clumps. The patient must be able to inhale fast enough to administer the entire dose of the medication.

*Text continued on p. 385*

## SKILL 14-3 ┃ Using Metered-Dose or Dry Powder Inhalers

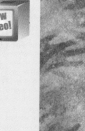

### Delegation Considerations

Do not delegate this skill.
Instruct assistive personnel about:
- Potential side effects of medications and to report their occurrence
- The need to report to the nurse any change in respiratory status, increased coughing or breathing difficulties

### Equipment

- MDI or DPI
- Spacer (optional with MDI)
- Facial tissues (optional)
- Wash basin or sink with warm water
- Paper towel
- MAR or computer printout

| STEP | RATIONALE |
|---|---|
| **ASSESSMENT** | |
| 1. Check accuracy and completeness of each MAR or computer printout with prescriber's written medication order. Check patient's name, drug name and dosage, route of administration, and time for administration. Recopy or re-print any portion of MAR that is difficult to read. | The order sheet is the most reliable source and only legal record of drugs patient is to receive. Ensures patient receives the right medications. Illegible MARs are a source of medication errors. |
| 2. Assess respiratory pattern and auscultate breath sounds. | Establishes baseline or airway status for comparison during and after treatment. |
| 3. If previously instructed in self-administration of inhaled medicine, assess patient's technique in using an inhaler. | Nurse's instruction sometimes only requires simple reinforcement, depending on patient's level of dexterity. |
| 4. Assess patient's ability to hold, manipulate, and depress canister and inhaler. | Any impairment of grasp or coordination impairs patient's ability to use MDI or DPI correctly. |
| 5. Assess patient's readiness to learn: patient asks questions about medication, disease, or complications; requests education in use of inhaler; is mentally alert; participates in own care. | Influences patient's motivation to understand explanations and actively participate in teaching process. |

## SKILL 14-3 | Using Metered-Dose or Dry Powder Inhalers—cont'd

| STEP | RATIONALE |
|---|---|
| 6. Assess patient's ability to learn: make sure patient is not fatigued, in pain, or in respiratory distress; assess level of understanding of technical vocabulary terms. | Mental or physical limitations affect patient's ability to learn and methods nurse uses for instruction. |
| 7. Assess patient's knowledge and understanding of disease and purpose and action of prescribed medications. | Knowledge of disease and medications is essential for patient to realistically understand use of inhaler. |
| 8. Determine drug schedule and number of inhalations prescribed for each dose. | Influences explanations nurse provides for use of inhaler. |

## PLANNING

| | |
|---|---|
| 1. Expected outcomes following completion of procedure:<br>  • Patient's breathing pattern improves, and airways become clear. | Desired effect of medication achieved. |
|   • Patient has adequate gas exchange. | Medication administered properly and therapeutic effect achieved. |
|   • Patient describes need for medication, dose, frequency, and how to use inhaler. | Demonstrates learning. |
|   • Patient correctly self-administers inhaler. | Patient is able to administer medication correctly. |
| 2. Provide adequate time for teaching session. | Prevents interruptions and enhances learning. |

## IMPLEMENTATION

| | |
|---|---|
| 1. Prepare medication: See Skill 14-1, Implementation steps 1a-h, k-m. Be sure to compare the label of the medication with the MAR two times while preparing the medication. | Following the same routine when preparing medication, eliminating distractions, and comparing the medication label with the MAR decreases risk of medication administration errors. |
| 2. Verify patient's identity by using at least two patient identifiers. Compare patient's name and one other identifier, such as hospital identification number on identification bracelet, with MAR. Ask patient to state name if possible for a third identifier. | Complies with JCAHO requirements and improves medication safety. In most acute care settings, patient's name and identification number on armband and MAR are used to identify patients. Identification bracelets are made at time of patient's admission and are most reliable source of identification. Patient's room number is **not** an acceptable identifier (JCAHO, 2004a). |
| 3. Compare the label of the medication with the MAR one more time at the patient's bedside. | Final comparison of medication label with the MAR decreases risk of medication administration errors. |
| 4. Help patient get into a comfortable position, such as sitting in chair in hospital room or sitting at kitchen table in home. | Patient will be more likely to remain receptive of nurse's explanations. |
| 5. Have patient manipulate inhaler, canister, and spacer device. Explain and demonstrate how canister fits into inhaler. | Patient needs to be familiar with how to use equipment. |

• *Critical Decision Point:* If patient is using an MDI and the inhaler is new or has not been used for several days, push a "test spray" into the air. You do not need to do this for a DPI.

| | |
|---|---|
| 6. Explain what metered dose is, and warn patient about overuse of inhaler and medication side effects. | Makes sure patient does not administer excessive inhalations because of risk of serious side effects. Side effects are minimized if patients take medication as ordered. |
| 7. Explain steps for administering inhaled dose of MDI (demonstrate steps when possible):<br>  a. Insert MDI canister into the holder.<br>  b. Remove mouthpiece cover from inhaler. | Use of simple, step-by-step explanations allows patient to ask questions during procedure. |

| STEP | RATIONALE |
|---|---|

---

• *Critical Decision Point:* If dirt or foreign objects are in mouthpiece, clean before using inhaler to avoid inhalation of unwanted material.

---

| STEP | RATIONALE |
|---|---|
| c. Shake inhaler strongly five or six times | Aerosolizes fine particles. |
| d. Tell patient to sit up straight or stand and take a deep breath and exhale. | Empties lungs and prepares the patient's airway to receive the medication. |
| e. Teach patient to position the inhaler in one of two ways: | Proper positioning of inhaler is essential to administering medication correctly. |
| (1) Close mouth around MDI with opening toward back of throat (see illustration). | |
| (2) Position MDI 2 to 4 cm (1 to 2 inches) in front of the mouth (see illustration). | |
| f. With the inhaler positioned correctly, have patient hold inhaler with thumb at the mouthpiece and the index finger and middle finger at the top. This is called a three-point or lateral hand position. | MDIs work best when patients use a three-point or lateral hand position to activate canisters. |
| g. Instruct patient to tilt head back slightly and inhale slowly and deeply through mouth for 3 to 5 seconds while fully pressing down on canister. | Medication is distributed to airways during inhalation. Inhalation through mouth rather than nose draws medication into airways better. |
| h. Have patient hold breath for as long as comfortable, up to 10 seconds. | Allows the medication to settle into the patient's airway (MayoClinic.com, 2003b). |
| i. Remove MDI from mouth and exhale slowly through pursed lips. | Keeps small airways open during exhalation. |
| 8. Explain steps to administer MDI using a spacer, such as an Aerochamber (demonstrate steps when possible): | Use of simple, step-by-step explanations allows patient to ask questions at any point during procedure. |
| a. Remove mouthpiece cover from inhaler and spacer. Inspect spacer for foreign objects, and if the spacer has a valve, make sure it is intact. | Inhaler fits into end of spacer. |
| b. Insert MDI into end of spacer. | Spacer breaks up and slows down the medication particles, increasing the absorption of medication into the airway (MayoClinic.com, 2003b). |
| c. Shake inhaler strongly five to six times. | Ensures fine particles are aerosolized. |
| d. Have patient take a deep breath and exhale completely before closing mouth around spacer's mouthpiece. Tell patient to avoid covering small exhalation slots with the lips (see illustration). | Empties the lungs and prepares the patient's airway to receive the medication. |
| e. Have patient press medication canister one time, spraying one puff into spacer. | MDI releases spray that allows finer particles to be inhaled. Large droplets are kept in spacer. |

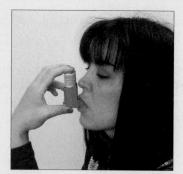

STEP **7e(1)** One technique for use of the inhaler. The patient opens lips and places inhaler in mouth with opening toward back of throat.

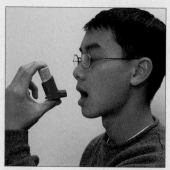

STEP **7e(2)** One technique for use of the inhaler. The patient positions the mouthpiece 1 to 2 inches from the mouth. This is considered the best way to deliver the medication.

SKILL 14-3 | Using Metered-Dose or Dry Powder Inhalers—cont'd

| STEP | RATIONALE |
| --- | --- |

STEP **8d** Have patient place mouthpiece in mouth and close lips, being careful to keep exhalation slots exposed.

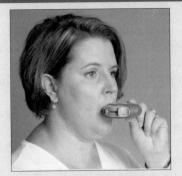

STEP **9d** Have patient place mouthpiece of DPI between lips.

| STEP | RATIONALE |
| --- | --- |
| f. Instruct patient to inhale slowly and deeply through mouth for 3 to 5 seconds. | Maximizes amount of medication that enters the lungs. |
| g. Hold breath for approximately 10 seconds. | Allows distribution of all medication. |
| h. Remove MDI and spacer before exhaling. | Allows patient to exhale normally. |
| 9. Explain steps to administer DPI (demonstrate when possible): | Use of simple step-by-step explanations allows patient to ask questions at any point during the procedure. |
| a. Remove mouthpiece cover. Do not shake DPI. | |
| b. Hold inhaler upright, and turn wheel to the right and then to the left until you hear a click. | Primes inhaler, which allows medication to be delivered to the patient. |
| c. Exhale away from the inhaler. | Prevents loss of powder. |
| d. Position mouthpiece between lips (see illustration). | Keeps medication from escaping through mouth. |
| e. Inhale deeply and forcefully through the mouth. | Creates aerosol. |
| f. Hold full breath for 5 to 10 seconds. | Allows distribution of medication. |
| 10. Instruct patient to wait at least 1 minute between inhalations of all devices or as ordered by prescriber. | Patients need to inhale medications slowly. First inhalation opens airways and reduces inflammation. Second or third inhalation penetrates deeper airways. |

• **Critical Decision Point:** If patient uses a corticosteroid, have patient rinse mouth with water or salt water or brush teeth after inhalation to reduce risk of fungal infection. Also teach patient to inspect oral cavity daily for redness, sores, or white patches. Report abnormal assessment findings to the patient's health care provider (MayoClinic.com, 2003b).

| STEP | RATIONALE |
| --- | --- |
| 11. Tell patient not to repeat inhaler doses until next scheduled dose. | Health care providers prescribe medications at intervals during the day to provide constant drug levels and minimize side effects. |
| 12. Explain that patient may feel gagging sensation in throat caused by droplets of medication on pharynx or tongue. | Results when inhalant is sprayed and inhaled incorrectly. |
| 13. Instruct patient in how to clean inhaler: | |
| a. Once a day, rinse inhaler and cap in warm running water. Make sure inhaler is completely dry before using. | Accumulation of spray around mouthpiece interferes with proper distribution during use (MayoClinic.com, 2003b). |
| b. Twice a week, wash the L-shaped plastic mouthpiece with antibacterial soap and warm water. Rinse and air dry well before putting canister back into mouthpiece (National Heart, Lung and Blood Institute, 1995). | Removes residual medication and decreases transfer of microorganisms. |

| STEP | RATIONALE |
|------|-----------|

## EVALUATION

1. Ask if patient has any questions.
2. Have patient explain and demonstrate steps in use of inhaler.
3. Ask patient to explain medication schedule, side effects, and when to call health care provider.
4. Ask patient to calculate how many days the inhaler will last.
5. After medication has been taken, assess patient's respiratory status, including ease of respirations, auscultation of lungs, and use of pulse oximetry to assess patient's oxygenation status.

Clarifies information.

Return demonstration provides feedback for measuring patient's learning.

Understanding of schedule and medication improves likelihood of compliance with therapy.

Helps patient determine when to reorder prescription.

Determines status of breathing pattern and adequacy of ventilation.

## RECORDING AND REPORTING

■ Document in the nurses' notes the skills you taught and patient's ability to perform skills.
■ Record medication, time of administration, and the amount of puffs on the MAR.
■ Report any undesirable effects from medication.

## UNEXPECTED OUTCOMES AND RELATED INTERVENTIONS

■ Patient needs a bronchodilator more than every 4 hours.
  • Indicates respiratory problems; reassess type of medication and delivery methods needed; consult with prescriber.

■ Patient experiences cardiac dysrhythmias, especially if receiving beta-adrenergics.
  • If patient experiences symptoms with the dysrhythmias (e.g., light-headedness, syncope), withhold all further doses of medication. Discuss with prescriber.
■ Patient is not able to self-administer medication properly.
  • Explore alternative delivery routes or methods.
■ Patient experiences paroxysms of coughing.
  • Aerosolized particles irritate posterior pharynx. Notify prescriber; need to reassess type of medication or delivery method.

Help your patients determine when the MDI and DPI are empty and need to be replaced. Do not float the MDI in water to determine how much medication is left because extra propellant in the MDI will allow the container to float even if it is empty. Some DPIs have an indicator that shows how many doses are left. However, these are not always accurate. Therefore the best way to calculate how long medication in an MDI or DPI will last requires you to divide the number of doses in the container by the number of doses your patient takes per day. For example, your patient is to take albuterol, a beta-adrenergic agonist bronchodilator. The ordered dose is 2 puffs 4 times a day (qid). The canister has a total of 200 puffs. You complete the following calculations to determine how long the MDI will last:

$$2 \text{ puffs} \times 4 \text{ times a day} = 8 \text{ puffs per day}$$
$$200 \text{ puffs} \times 8 \text{ puffs per day} = 25 \text{ days}$$

Therefore the canister will last 25 days. To ensure that the patient does not run out of medication, teach your patient to refill the medication at least 7 to 10 days before it runs out (MayoClinic.com, 2003b).

## Administering Medications By Irrigation

Some medications irrigate or wash out a body cavity and are delivered through a stream of solution. Sterile water, saline, or antiseptic solution irrigations of the eye, ear, throat, vagina, and urinary tract are common. If there is a break in the skin or mucosa, you use the aseptic technique. When the cavity to be irrigated is not sterile, as is the case with the ear canal (see Box 14-16) or vagina (see Box 14-17), clean technique is acceptable. Irrigations cleanse an area, instill a medication, or apply hot or cold to injured tissue.

## Parenteral Administration of Medications

Parenteral administration of medications is the administration of medications by injection. When you administer medications this way, it is an invasive procedure that you per-

| BOX 14-19 | Preventing Infection During an Injection |

- To prevent contamination of solution in an ampule, quickly draw the medication into the syringe. Do not allow the ampule to stand open.
- Do not allow the needle to touch a contaminated surface (e.g., outer edges of ampule or vial, outer surface of needle cap, your hands, the countertop).
- Avoid touching the length of the plunger or inner part of the barrel. Keep tip of syringe covered with cap or needle.
- Wash skin soiled with dirt, drainage, or feces with soap and water. Use friction and a circular motion while cleaning with an antiseptic swab. Swab from center of site, and move outward in a 2-inch radius.

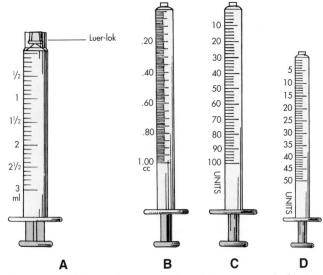

**A**     **B**     **C**     **D**

FIGURE **14-11** Types of syringes. **A,** Luer-Lok syringe marked in 0.1 (tenths). **B,** Tuberculin syringe marked in 0.01 (hundredths) for doses less than 1 ml. **C,** Insulin syringe marked in units (100). **D,** Insulin syringe marked in units (50).

form using aseptic techniques (Box 14-19). After a needle pierces the skin, there is risk of infection. Each type of injection requires certain skills to ensure that the medication reaches the proper location. The effects of a parenterally administered medication develop rapidly, depending on the rate of medication absorption. Therefore closely observe the patient's response to the medication.

## Equipment

A variety of syringes and needles are available, each designed to deliver a certain volume of a medication to a specific type of tissue. Use nursing judgment when determining the syringe or needle that will be most appropriate.

**SYRINGES.** Syringes have a cylindrical barrel with a close-fitting plunger and a tip designed to fit the hub of a hypodermic needle. Syringes in general are classified as being Luer-Lok or non–Luer-Lok. This name is based on the design on the syringe's tip. Luer-Lok syringes (Figure 14-12, *A*) require special needles, which are twisted onto the tip and lock themselves in place. This design prevents the inadvertent removal of the needle. Non–Luer-Lok syringes (Figure 14-12, *B* to *D*) require needles that slip onto the tip.

To fill a syringe, pull the plunger outward while the needle tip remains immersed in the prepared solution. To maintain sterility, touch the outside of the syringe barrel and the handle of the plunger, but do not touch the tip or inside of the barrel, the hub, the shaft of the plunger, and the needle (Figure 14-13).

Syringes come in a number of sizes, ranging from 0.5 to 60 ml. It is unusual to use a syringe larger than 5 ml for an injection. A 1- to 3-ml syringe is usually adequate for IM and Sub-Q injections. You use large syringes to administer certain IV medications, add medications to IV solutions, and irrigate wounds or drainage tubes. Some syringes come prepackaged with a needle attached. However, sometimes you need to change the needle based on the route of administration and the size of the patient.

The tuberculin syringe (see Figure 14-11, *B*) has a long, thin barrel with a preattached thin needle. The syringe is calibrated in sixteenths of a minim and hundredths of a milli-

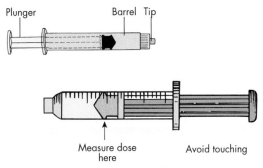

FIGURE **14-12** Parts of a syringe.

liter and has a capacity of 1 ml. You use tuberculin syringes to prepare small amounts of medications. You also use them for ID and Sub-Q injections.

Insulin syringes (see Figure 14-11, *C* and *D*) hold 0.3 to 1 ml and are calibrated in units. Most insulin syringes are U-100s, designed for use with U-100 strength insulin. Each milliliter of solution contains 100 units of insulin.

**NEEDLES.** Sometimes needles come attached to syringes. Other needles come packaged individually to allow flexibility in selecting the right needle for a patient. Needles are disposable, with most made of stainless steel.

The needle has three parts: the hub, which fits onto the tip of a syringe; the shaft, which connects to the hub; and the bevel, or slanted tip (see Figure 14-12). The tip of a needle, or the bevel, is always slanted. When injected into tissue, the bevel creates a narrow slit that quickly closes when you remove the needle. This prevents leakage of medication, blood, or serum. Long beveled tips are sharp and narrow, which

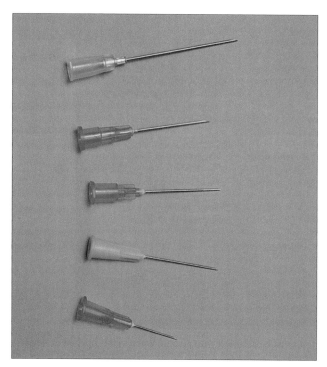

FIGURE **14-13** Hypodermic needles *(top to bottom):* 19 gauge, 1½-inch length; 20 gauge, 1-inch length; 21 gauge, 1-inch length; 23 gauge, 1-inch length; and 25 gauge, ⅝-inch length.

minimizes discomfort when entering tissue used for Sub-Q or IM injections.

Needles vary in length from ¼ to 3 inches (Figure 14-13). The needle length you choose depends on the patient's size and weight and the route of administration. A child or slender adult generally requires a shorter needle. Use longer needles (1 to 1½ inches) for IM injections and shorter needles (⅜ to ⅝ inch) for Sub-Q injections. As the needle gauge gets smaller, the needle diameter becomes larger (see Figure 14-13). The selection of a gauge depends on the viscosity of fluid you will inject or infuse. The rationale for needle selection is included in each skill.

**DISPOSABLE INJECTION UNITS.** Disposable, single-dose, prefilled syringes are available for some medications. With these syringes you do not have to prepare medication dosages, except perhaps to expel portions of unneeded medications.

The Carpuject Syringe System includes reusable plastic syringe holders and disposable, prefilled, sterile, glass cartridge units (Figure 14-14). When using this system, you load the cartridge Luer tip first into the plastic syringe holder, and then you secure it (following package directions) and check for air bubbles in the syringe. You advance the plunger to expel air and excess medication, as with a regular syringe. You can use the glass cartridge with needleless systems or safety needles. After giving the medication, you dispose of the glass cartridge easily and safely in a puncture-proof and leakproof receptacle. This design reduces the risk of needle-stick injury.

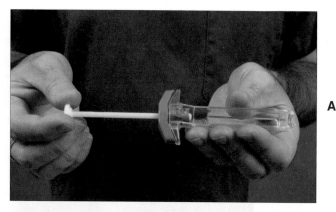

A

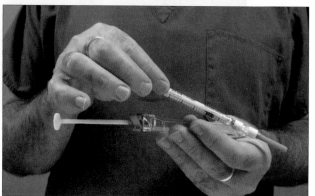

B

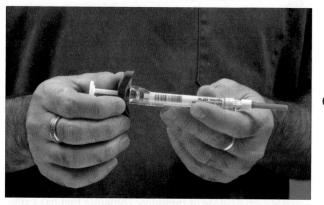

C

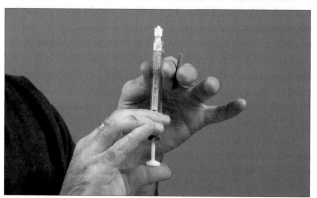

D

FIGURE **14-14** **A,** Carpuject syringe and prefilled sterile cartridge with needle. **B,** Assembling the Carpuject. **C,** The cartridge slides into the syringe barrel, turns, and locks at the needle end. The plunger then screws into the cartridge end. **D,** Expel excess medication to obtain accurate dose.

---
**SKILL 14-4** | Preparing Injections—cont'd
---

| STEP | RATIONALE |
|------|-----------|

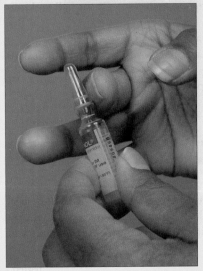

STEP **2A(1)** Tapping ampule moves fluid down neck.

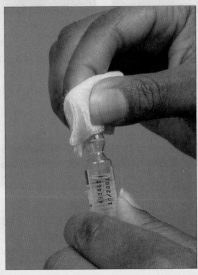

STEP **2A(2)** Gauze pad placed around neck of ampule.

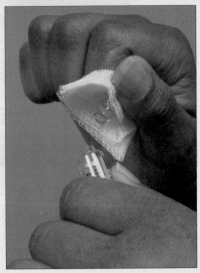

STEP **2A(3)** Snapping neck away from hands.

(4) Draw up medication quickly, using a filter needle long enough to reach bottom of ampule.

System is open to airborne contaminants. Makes sure needle is long enough to access medication for preparation. Filter needles are used to filter out any fragments of glass (Nicoll and Hesby, 2002).

(5) Hold ampule upside down, or set it on a flat surface. Insert filter needle into center of ampule opening. Do not allow needle tip or shaft to touch rim of ampule.

Broken rim of ampule is considered contaminated. When ampule is inverted, solution dribbles out if needle tip or shaft touches rim of ampule.

(6) Aspirate medication into syringe by gently pulling back on plunger (see illustrations).

Withdrawal of plunger creates negative pressure within syringe barrel, which pulls fluid into syringe.

(7) Keep needle tip under surface of liquid. Tip ampule to bring all fluid within reach of the needle.

Prevents aspiration of air bubbles.

(8) If you aspirate air bubbles, do not expel air into ampule.

Air pressure forces fluid out of ampule, and medication will be lost.

(9) To expel excess air bubbles, remove needle from ampule. Hold syringe with needle pointing up. Tap side of syringe to cause bubbles to rise toward needle. Draw back slightly on plunger, and then push plunger upward to eject air. Do not eject fluid.

Withdrawing plunger too far will remove it from barrel. Holding syringe vertically allows fluid to settle in bottom of barrel. Pulling back on plunger allows fluid within needle to enter barrel so you do not expel fluid. You then expel air at top of barrel and within needle.

(10) If syringe contains excess fluid, use sink for disposal. Hold syringe vertically with needle tip up and slanted slightly toward sink. Slowly eject excess fluid into sink. Recheck fluid level in syringe by holding it vertically.

Safely disperses medication into sink. Position of needle allows you to expel medication without it flowing down needle shaft. Rechecking fluid level ensures proper dose.

(11) Cover needle with its safety sheath or cap. Replace filter needle with regular needle.

Minimizes needle sticks. Do not use filter needles for injection.

| STEP | RATIONALE |
|---|---|

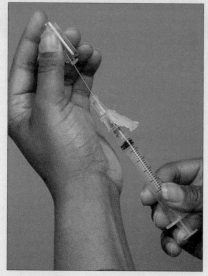 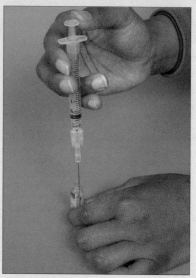

STEP **2A(6)** **A,** Medication aspirated with ampule inverted. **B,** Medication aspirated with ampule on flat surface.

### B. Vial Containing a Solution:

(1) Remove cap covering top of unused vial to expose sterile rubber seal. If a multidose vial has been used before, cap is already removed. Firmly and briskly wipe surface of rubber seal with alcohol swab, and allow it to dry.

(2) Pick up syringe, and remove needle cap or cap covering needleless vial access device (see illustration). Pull back on plunger to draw amount of air into syringe equivalent to volume of medication to be aspirated from vial.

(3) With vial on flat surface, insert tip of needle or needleless vial access device through center of rubber seal (see illustration). Apply pressure to tip of needle during insertion.

Vial comes packaged with cap that cannot be replaced after seal removal. Not all drug manufacturers guarantee that caps of unused vials are sterile. Therefore swab caps with alcohol before preparing medication. Allowing alcohol to dry prevents it from coating needle and mixing with medication. Injecting air into vial prevents buildup of negative pressure in vial when aspirating medication.

Center of seal is thinner and easier to penetrate. Using firm pressure prevents coring of rubber seal, which could enter vial or needle.

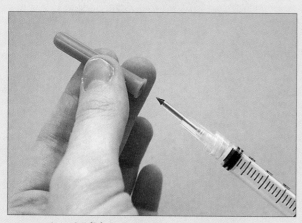

STEP **2B(2)** Syringe with needleless adapter.

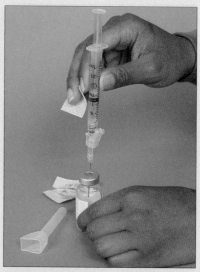

STEP **2B(3)** Insert safety needle through center of vial diaphragm (with vial flat on table).

SKILL 14-4 Preparing Injections—cont'd

| STEP | RATIONALE |
|---|---|
| (4) Inject air into the vial's air space, holding on to plunger. Hold plunger with firm pressure; plunger sometimes is forced backward by air pressure within the vial. | You need to inject air before aspirating fluid to create vacuum needed to get medication to flow into syringe. Injecting into vial's air space prevents formation of bubbles and inaccuracy in dosage. |
| (5) Invert vial while keeping firm hold on syringe and plunger (see illustration). Hold vial between thumb and middle fingers of nondominant hand. Grasp end of syringe barrel and plunger with thumb and forefinger of dominant hand to counteract pressure in vial. | Inverting vial allows fluid to settle in lower half of container. Position of hands prevents forceful movement of plunger and permits easy manipulation of syringe. |
| (6) Keep tip of needle below fluid level. | Prevents aspiration of air. |
| (7) Allow air pressure from the vial to fill syringe gradually with medication. If necessary, pull back slightly on plunger to obtain correct amount of solution. | Positive pressure within vial forces fluid into syringe. |
| (8) When you obtain desired volume, position needle into vial's air space; tap side of syringe barrel carefully to dislodge any air bubbles. Eject any air remaining at top of syringe into vial. | Forcefully striking barrel while needle is inserted in vial may bend needle. Accumulation of air displaces medication and causes dosage errors. |
| (9) Remove needle or needleless vial access device from vial by pulling back on barrel of syringe. | Pulling plunger rather than barrel causes plunger to separate from barrel, resulting in loss of medication. |
| (10) Hold syringe at eye level, at 90-degree angle, to ensure correct volume and absence of air bubbles. Remove any remaining air by tapping barrel to dislodge any air bubbles (see illustration). Draw back slightly on plunger; then push plunger upward to eject air. Do not eject fluid. | Holding syringe vertically allows fluid to settle in bottom of barrel. Pulling back on plunger allows fluid within needle to enter barrel so you do not expel fluid. You then expel air at top of barrel and within needle. |
| (11) If you need to inject medication into patient's tissue, change needle to appropriate gauge and length according to route of medication administration. | Inserting needle through a rubber stopper dulls beveled tip. New needle is sharper. Because no fluid is along shaft, needle will not track medication through tissues. You cannot inject needleless access device into the body. |

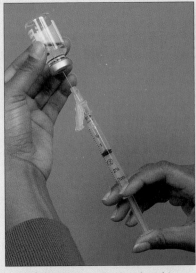

STEP 2B(5) Withdraw fluid with vial inverted.

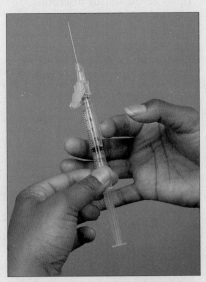

STEP 2B(10) Hold syringe upright, tap barrel to dislodge air bubbles.

| STEP | RATIONALE |
|---|---|
| (12) For multidose vial, make label that includes date of opening vial and your initials. | Ensures that nurses will prepare future doses correctly. You discard some drugs after certain number of days after opening a vial. |
| **C. Vial Containing a Powder (Reconstituting Medications):** | |
| (1) Remove cap covering vial of powdered medication and cap covering vial of proper diluent. Firmly swab both caps with alcohol swab, and allow to dry. | Not all drug manufacturers guarantee that caps of unused vials are sterile. Allowing alcohol to dry prevents it from coating needle and mixing with medication. |
| (2) Draw up diluent into syringe following steps 2B(2) through 2B(10). | Prepares diluent for injection into vial containing powdered medication. |
| (3) Insert tip of needle or needleless access device through center of rubber seal of vial of powdered medication. Inject diluent into vial. Remove needle. | Diluent begins to dissolve and reconstitute medication. |
| (4) Mix medication thoroughly. Roll in palms. Do not shake. | Ensures proper dispersal of medication throughout solution. |
| (5) Reconstituted medication in vial is ready for you to draw into new syringe. Read label, and compare with the MAR carefully to determine dose after reconstitution. | Once you add diluent, concentration of medication (mg/ml) determines dose you give. Comparing label of medication with the MAR decreases administration errors. |
| (6) Draw up reconstituted medication in syringe following steps 2B(2) through 2B(12). | Prepares medication for administration. |

---

· *Critical Decision Point:* Some institutions require that you verify medications prepared for parenteral administration for accuracy by another nurse. Check institutional guidelines before administering medication.

---

| | |
|---|---|
| 3. Dispose of soiled supplies. Place broken ampule and/or used vials and used needle or needleless access device in puncture-proof and leakproof container. Clean work area, and perform hand hygiene. | Proper disposal of glass and needle prevents accidental injury to staff. Controls transmission of infection. |

## EVALUATION

| | |
|---|---|
| 1. Compare dose in syringe with desired dose. | Determines dose is accurate. |

## UNEXPECTED OUTCOMES AND RELATED INTERVENTIONS

■ Air bubbles remain in syringe.
  · Expel air from syringe, and add medication to syringe until you prepare the correct dose.

■ You prepared incorrect dose.
  · Discard prepared dose.
  · Prepare corrected new dose.

SKILL 14-5 | Administering Injections—cont'd

| STEP | RATIONALE |
|------|-----------|
| **B. Intramuscular:** | |
| (1) Position nondominant hand just below site and pull skin approximately 2.5 to 3.5 cm down or laterally with ulnar side of hand to administer in a Z-track. Hold position until medication is injected. With dominant hand, inject needle quickly at 90-degree angle into muscle. | Z-track creates zigzag path through tissues that seals needle track to avoid tracking of medication. A quick, dartlike injection reduces discomfort. Z-track injections are used for all IM injections (Nicoll and Hesby, 2002). |
| (2) *Option:* If patient's muscle mass is small, grasp body of muscle between thumb and fingers. | Ensures that medication reaches muscle mass (Hockenberry and others, 2003). |
| (3) After needle pierces skin, grasp lower end of syringe barrel with nondominant hand to stabilize syringe. Continue to pull skin tightly with nondominant hand. Move dominant hand to end of plunger. Do not move syringe. | Smooth manipulation of syringe reduces discomfort from needle movement. Skin remains pulled until after you inject drug to ensure Z-track administration. |
| (4) Pull back on plunger 5 to 10 seconds. If no blood appears, inject medication slowly at a rate of 1 ml/10 sec. | Aspiration of blood into syringe indicates IV placement of needle. Slow injection reduces pain and tissue trauma (Nicoll and Hesby, 2002). |

---

• ***Critical Decision Point:*** If blood appears in syringe, remove needle, dispose of medication and syringe properly, and prepare another dose of medication for injection.

---

| STEP | RATIONALE |
|------|-----------|
| (5) Wait 10 seconds, then smoothly and steadily withdraw needle and release skin. | Allows time for medication to absorb into muscle before removing syringe. |
| **C. Intradermal:** | |
| (1) With nondominant hand, stretch skin over site with forefinger or thumb. | Needle pierces tight skin more easily. |
| (2) With needle almost against patient's skin, insert it slowly at a 5- to 15-degree angle until resistance is felt. Then advance needle through epidermis to approximately 3 mm (⅛ inch) below skin surface. You will see needle tip through skin. | Ensures that needle tip is in dermis. You will obtain inaccurate results if you do not inject needle at correct angle and depth (CDC, 2004). |
| (3) Inject medication slowly. Normally you feel resistance. If not, needle is too deep; remove and begin again. | Slow injection minimizes discomfort at site. Dermal layer is tight and does not expand easily when you inject solution. |
| (4) While injecting medication, note that small bleb (approximately 6 mm [½ inch]) resembling mosquito bite appears on skin surface (see illustration). | Bleb indicates you deposited medication in dermis. |

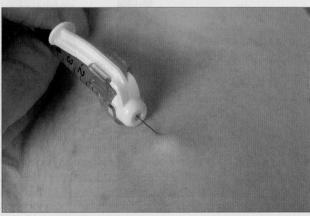

STEP **14C(4)** Injection creates a small bleb.

| STEP | RATIONALE |
|---|---|
| 17. After withdrawing needle apply alcohol swab or gauze gently over site. | Support of tissue around injection site minimizes discomfort during needle withdrawal. Dry gauze minimizes discomfort associated with alcohol on nonintact skin. |
| 18. Apply gentle pressure. Do not massage site. Apply bandage if needed. | Massage damages underlying tissue. Massage of ID site disperses medication into underlying tissue layers and alters test results. |
| 19. Assist patient to comfortable position. | Gives patient sense of well-being. |
| 20. Discard uncapped needle or needle enclosed in safety shield and attached syringe into puncture-proof and leakproof receptacle. | Prevents injury to patient and health care personnel. Recapping needles increases risk of needle-stick injury (OSHA, 2001). |
| 21. Remove disposable gloves, and perform hand hygiene. | Reduces transmission of microorganisms. |
| 22. Stay with patient, and observe for any allergic reactions. | Dyspnea, wheezing, and circulatory collapse are signs of severe anaphylactic reaction. |

## EVALUATION

| | |
|---|---|
| 1. Return to room, and ask if patient feels any acute pain, burning, numbness, or tingling at injection site. | Continued discomfort indicates injury to underlying bones or nerves. |
| 2. Inspect site, noting any bruising or induration. | Bruising or induration indicates complication associated with injection. Document findings, and notify health care provider. Provide warm compress to site. |
| 3. Observe patient's response to medication at times that correlate with the medication's onset, peak, and duration. | The body rapidly absorbs IM medications. Adverse effects of parenteral medications develop rapidly. Evaluate effect of medication based on the medication's onset, peak, and duration of action. |

• *Critical Decision Point:* Read tuberculin (TB) test at 48 to 72 hours. Induration (hard, dense, raised area) of skin around injection site indicates positive TB reaction of:
  ◦ 15 mm or more in patients with no known risk factors for TB
  ◦ 10 mm or more in patients who are recent immigrants; injection drug users; residents and employees of high-risk settings; patients with certain chronic illnesses; children less than 4 years of age; and infants, children, and adolescents exposed to high-risk adults
  ◦ 5 mm or more in patients who are human immunodeficiency virus (HIV) positive, immunocompromised patients, or patients recently exposed to TB (CDC, 2004)

| | |
|---|---|
| 4. Ask patient to explain purpose and effects of medication. | Evaluates patient's understanding of information taught. |
| 5. *For ID injections,* use skin pencil and draw circle around perimeter of injection site. Read site within appropriate amount of time, designated by type of medication or skin test you give. | Pencil mark makes site easy to find. You determine the results of skin testing at various times, based on the type of medication used or the type of skin testing completed. Refer to the manufacturer's directions to determine when to read the test's results. |

## RECORDING AND REPORTING

■ Document medication dose, route, site, time, and date given on MAR.
■ Report any undesirable effects from medication to prescriber.
■ Record patient's response to medications in nurses' notes.

## UNEXPECTED OUTCOMES AND RELATED INTERVENTIONS

■ Raised, reddened, or hard zone (induration) forms around ID test site.
  • Notify patient's health care provider.
  • Document sensitivity to injected allergen or positive test if tuberculin skin testing was completed.
■ Hypertrophy of skin develops from repeated Sub-Q injections.

┌─────────────┐
│ SKILL 14-5  │ Administering Injections—cont'd
└─────────────┘

- Do not use this site for future injections.
- Instruct patient not to use site for 6 months.
■ Patient develops signs and symptoms of allergy or side effects.
  - Follow institutional policy or guidelines for appropriate response to adverse drug reactions.
  - Notify patient's health care provider immediately.
  - Enter allergy information into patient's medical record.
■ Patient complains of localized pain, numbness, or tingling or burning at injection site.

- Severe pain related to medication administration is not normal.
- Sometimes potential injury to nerve or tissues has occurred.
- Assess injection site.
- Document findings.
- Notify patient's health care provider.

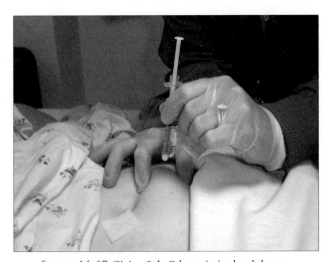

FIGURE **14-18** Giving Sub-Q heparin in the abdomen.

for heparin injections is the abdomen (Figure 14-18). The site used for low-molecular-weight (LMW) heparin (e.g., enoxaparin) is on the right or left side of the abdomen at least 2 inches from the umbilicus. This area is often called the patient's "love handles" (Aventis, 2003). Sub-Q sites for other medications include the scapular areas of the upper back and the upper ventral or dorsal gluteal areas. Choose an injection site that is free of skin lesions, bony prominences, and large underlying muscles or nerves.

When you give U-100 insulin, use U-100 insulin syringes with preattached 26- to 31-gauge needles (ADA, 2005b). Use 1-ml tuberculin syringes when you give U-500 insulin (Cohen, 2002). Recommended Sub-Q insulin injections sites include the upper arm, anterior and lateral portions of the thigh, buttocks, and abdomen. Rotating injections within the same body part for a sequence of injections provides more consistency in the absorption of insulin. For example, if you inject the morning insulin into the patient's arm, then you give the next injection in a different place of the same

arm. The rate of absorption is another factor in site selection for insulin administration. The abdomen has the quickest absorption rate, followed by the arms, thighs, and buttocks (ADA, 2004).

Give only small doses (0.5 to 1 ml) of water-soluble medications subcutaneously because the tissue is sensitive to irritating solutions and large volumes of medications. Collection of medications within the tissues causes sterile abscesses, which appear as hardened, painful lumps under the skin.

A patient's body weight indicates the depth of the Sub-Q layer. Therefore base the needle length and angle of insertion on the patient's weight. Generally a 25-gauge ⅝-inch needle inserted at a 45-degree angle (Figure 14-19) or a ½-inch needle inserted at a 90-degree angle deposits medications into the Sub-Q tissue of a normal-size patient. A child usually requires only a ½-inch needle. If the patient is obese, pinch the tissue and use a needle long enough to insert through fatty tissue at the base of the skinfold. Thin patients sometimes have insufficient tissue for Sub-Q injections. Therefore the upper abdomen is the best site for injection with this type of patient. To ensure a Sub-Q medication reaches the subcutaneous tissue, you use the following rule to determine the appropriate angle of injection: if you are able to grasp 2 inches (5 cm) of tissue, insert the needle at a 90-degree angle; if you are able to grasp 1 inch (2.5 cm), insert the needle at a 45-degree angle (Rushing, 2004).

**INTRAMUSCULAR INJECTIONS.** The IM route provides faster medication absorption than the Sub-Q route because of a muscle's greater vascularity. There is less danger of causing tissue damage when medications enter deep muscle, but the risk of inadvertently injecting medications directly into blood vessels exists. You use a longer and heavier-gauge needle to pass through Sub-Q tissue and penetrate deep muscle tissue (see Skill 14-6). Weight and the amount of adipose tissue influence needle size selection. An obese patient requires a needle 3 inches long, whereas a thin patient only requires a ½- to 1-inch needle (Nicoll and Hesby, 2002).

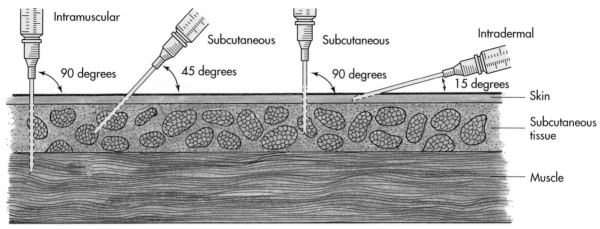

FIGURE **14-19** Comparison of angles of insertion for IM (90 degrees), Sub-Q (45 and 90 degrees), and ID (15 degrees) injections.

Administer intramuscular injections so that the needle is perpendicular to the patient's body and as close to a 90-degree angle as possible (Nicoll and Hesby, 2002) (see Figure 14-19). Muscle is less sensitive to irritating and viscous drugs. A normal, well-developed patient tolerates as much as 3 ml of medication in a larger muscle without much pain (Nicoll and Hesby, 2002). However, the body does not absorb larger medication volumes well. Children, older adults, and thin patients tolerate only 2 ml of an IM injection. Small children and infants (e.g., under the age of 2 years) receive no more than 1 ml of medication in one injection (Hockenberry and others, 2003).

Assess the muscle before giving an injection. Make sure the muscle is free of tenderness. Repeated injections in the same muscle cause severe discomfort. With the patient relaxed, palpate the muscle to rule out any hardened lesions. Help the patient assume a comfortable position to minimize discomfort during an injection.

**Sites.** When selecting an IM site, consider the following: Is the area free of infection or necrosis? Are there local areas of bruising or abrasions? What is the location of underlying bones, nerves, and major blood vessels? What volume of medication will you administer? Each site has certain advantages and disadvantages (Box 14-22).

***Ventrogluteal.*** The ventrogluteal muscle involves the gluteus medius and minimus and is a safe site for all patients. Research has shown that injuries such as fibrosis, nerve damage, abscess, tissue necrosis, muscle contraction, gangrene, and pain have been associated with all the common IM sites except the ventrogluteal site. The only published case study of a complication at the ventrogluteal site reported a local reaction to the medication, which is not a complication associated with the site itself (Nicoll and Hesby, 2002). The ventrogluteal site is the preferred injection site for adults. This site is also appropriate for children over 7 months old who are receiving irritating or viscous solutions (Hockenberry and others, 2003; Nicoll and Hesby, 2002).

To locate the ventrogluteal muscle, place the heel of your hand over the greater trochanter of the patient's hip with the

---

**BOX 14-22    Characteristics of Intramuscular Sites**

**Vastus Lateralis**

- Lacks major nerves and blood vessels
- Rapid drug absorption
- Preferred site for infants (less than 12 months) receiving immunizations
- Also used in toddlers and older children receiving immunizations

**Ventrogluteal**

- A deep site, situated away from major nerves and blood vessels
- Less chance of contamination in incontinent patients or infants
- Easily identified by prominent bony landmarks
- Preferred site for medications (e.g., antibiotics) that are larger in volume, more viscous, and irritating for adults, children, and infants over 7 months of age

**Deltoid**

- Easily accessible but muscle not well developed in most patients
- Used for small amounts of drugs
- Not used in infants or children with underdeveloped muscles
- Potential for injury to radial and ulnar nerves or brachial artery
- Used for immunizations for toddlers, older children, and adults
- Recommended site for hepatitis B vaccine and rabies injections

---

wrist perpendicular to the femur. Use the right hand for the left hip and the left hand for the right hip. Point your thumb toward the patient's groin with your index finger pointed to the anterosuperior iliac spine. Point your middle finger back along the iliac crest toward the buttock. Your index finger, the middle finger, and the iliac crest form a V-shaped triangle. The injection site is the center of the triangle (Figure 14-20). The patient lies on the side or back. Flexing of the knee and hip helps the patient relax this muscle.

***Vastus Lateralis.*** The vastus lateralis muscle is another injection site used in adults and children. The muscle is thick and well developed and is located on the anterior lateral aspect of the thigh. It extends in an adult from a handbreadth above

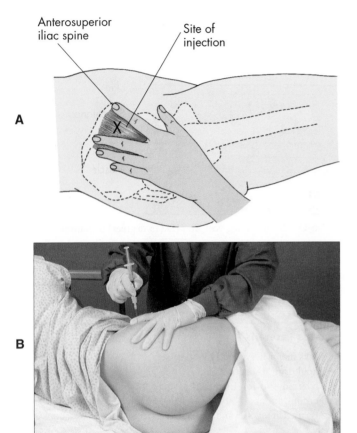

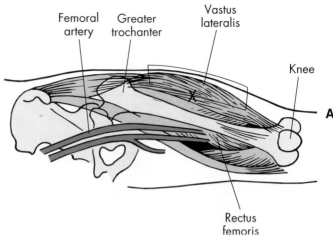

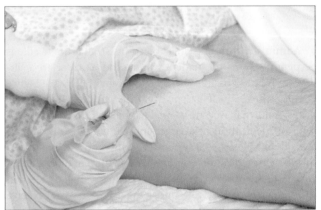

FIGURE **14-20 A,** Landmarks for ventrogluteal site. **B,** Giving IM injection in ventrogluteal site.

FIGURE **14-21 A,** Landmarks for vastus lateralis site. **B,** Giving IM injection in vastus lateralis muscle.

the knee to a handbreadth below the greater trochanter of the femur (Figure 14-21). Use the middle third of the muscle for injection. The width of the muscle usually extends from the midline of the thigh and the midline of the thigh's outer side. With young children or cachectic patients, grasp the body of the muscle during injection to be sure that you deposit the medication in muscle tissue. To help relax the muscle, have the patient lie flat with the knee slightly flexed or assume a sitting position. The vastus lateralis site is preferable for infants, toddlers, and children receiving biologicals (e.g., immune globulins, vaccines, or toxoids) (Nicoll and Hesby, 2002).

***Dorsogluteal.*** In the past, nurses used the dorsogluteal muscle for IM injections. However, the exact location of the sciatic nerve varies from one person to another. If a needle hits the sciatic nerve, the patient experiences adverse outcomes, including permanent or partial paralysis of the involved leg. Therefore this site is **not** used for IM injections any more (Nicoll and Hesby, 2002).

***Deltoid.*** Because the radial and ulnar nerves and brachial artery lie within the upper arm along the humerus (Figure 14-22, *A*), use this site only for small medication volumes or when other sites are inaccessible because of dressings or casts. Locate the deltoid muscle by fully exposing the patient's upper arm and shoulder and having the patient relax the arm at

the side and flex the elbow. Do not roll up a tight-fitting sleeve. Have the patient sit, stand, or lie down (Figure 14-22, *B*). Palpate the lower edge of the acromion process, which forms the base of a triangle in line with the midpoint of the lateral aspect of the upper arm. The injection site is in the center of the triangle, about 2.5 to 5 cm (1 to 2 inches) below the acromion process (see Figure 14-22, *A*). You also can locate the site by placing four fingers across the deltoid muscle, with the top finger along the acromion process. The injection site is then three finger widths below the acromion process.

**Technique in Intramuscular Injections**

***Z-Track Method.*** It is recommended that you use the **Z-track injection** method when giving IM injections to minimize irritation by sealing the medication in muscle tissue (Nicoll and Hesby, 2002). To use the Z-track method, apply a new needle to the syringe after preparing the medication so that no solution remains on the outside needle shaft. Then choose an IM site, preferably in a larger, deeper muscle such as the ventrogluteal muscle. Pull the overlying skin and Sub-Q tissues approximately 2.5 to 3.5 cm (1 to 1½ inches) laterally to the side with the ulnar side of the nondominant hand. Hold the skin in this position until you administer the injection. After preparing the site with an antiseptic swab, inject the needle deep into the muscle. Slowly inject the

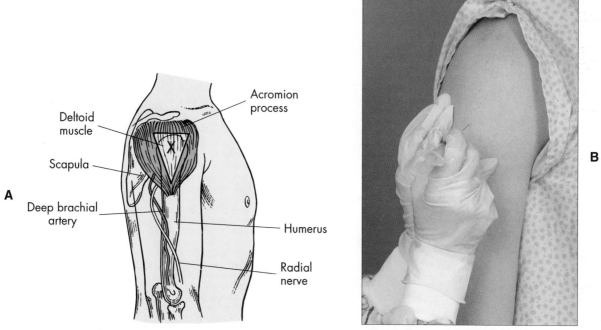

FIGURE **14-22 A,** Landmarks for deltoid site. **B,** Giving IM injection in deltoid muscle.

medication if there is no blood return on aspiration. Keep the needle inserted for 10 seconds to allow the medication to disperse evenly. Then release the skin after withdrawing the needle. This leaves a zigzag path that seals the needle track where tissue planes slide across each other (Figure 14-23). The medication cannot escape from the muscle tissue.

**INTRADERMAL INJECTIONS.** ID injections are usually used for skin testing (e.g., tuberculin screening or allergy tests). Because these medications are potent, you inject them into the dermis, where blood supply is reduced and medication absorption occurs slowly. A patient will possibly have a severe anaphylactic reaction if the medications enter the circulation too rapidly.

You need to assess the injection site for changes in color and tissue integrity. Therefore choose an ID site that is lightly pigmented, free of lesions, and relatively hairless. The inner forearm and upper back are ideal locations.

To administer an injection intradermally, use a tuberculin or small syringe with a short ($\frac{1}{4}$ to $\frac{1}{2}$ inch), fine-gauge (26 or 27) needle. The angle of insertion for an ID injection is 5 to 15 degrees (see Figure 14-19). As you inject the medication, a small bleb resembling a mosquito bite will appear on the skin's surface (see Skill 14-6). If a bleb does not appear or if the site bleeds after needle withdrawal, there is a good chance the medication entered Sub-Q tissues. In this case, test results will not be valid.

### SAFETY IN ADMINISTERING MEDICATIONS BY INJECTION

**Needleless Devices.** The most frequent route of exposure to blood-borne disease is from needle-stick injuries (American Nurses Association, 2002; Perry and others, 2003). These injuries commonly occur when health care workers recap nee-

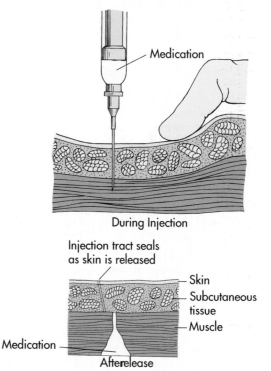

FIGURE **14-23** Z-Track method of injection prevents deposit of medication into sensitive tissues.

dles, mishandle IV lines and needles, or leave stray needles at a patient's bedside. Exposure to blood-borne pathogens is one of the deadliest hazards nurses are exposed to on a daily basis. However, over 80% of needle-stick injuries are preventable with the implementation of safe needle devices (American Nurses Association, 2002). The Needlestick Safety and

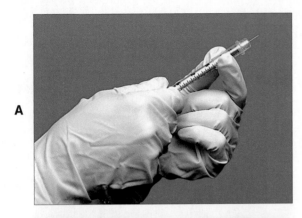

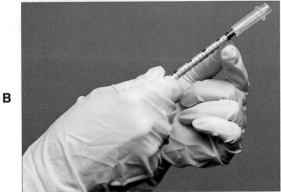

FIGURE **14-24** Needle with plastic guard to prevent needle sticks. **A,** Position of guard before injection. **B,** After injection, the nurse locks the guard in place, covering the needle.

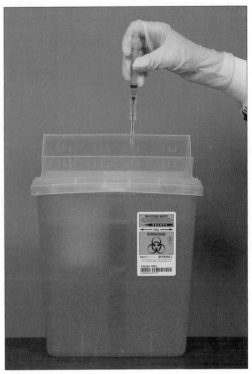

FIGURE **14-25** Sharps disposal using only one hand.

Prevention Act is a federal law that became effective in April 2001. This federal law mandates health care facilities to use safe needle devices to reduce the frequency of needle-stick injury.

Special syringes are designed with a sheath or guard that covers the needle after it is withdrawn from the skin (Figure 14-24). The guard immediately covers the needle, eliminating the chance for a needle-stick injury. You dispose of the syringe and sheath together in a receptacle. Use "needleless" devices whenever possible to reduce the risk of needle-stick injuries (OSHA, 2001).

Always dispose of needles and other instruments considered "sharps" into clearly marked, appropriate containers (Figure 14-25). The proper containers are puncture-proof and leakproof. Never force a needle into a full needle disposal receptacle, and never place used needles and syringes in a wastebasket, in your pocket, on a patient's meal tray, or at the patient's bedside. Box 14-23 summarizes recommendations for the prevention of needle-stick injuries.

## Intravenous Administration

You administer medications intravenously by the following methods:

1. As mixtures within large volumes of IV fluids
2. By injection of a bolus, or small volume, of medication through an existing IV infusion line or intermittent venous access (heparin or saline lock)

---

| BOX 14-23 | **Recommendations for the Prevention of Needle-Stick Injuries** |
|---|---|

- Avoid using needles when effective needleless systems or Sharps with Engineered Sharps Injury Protections (SESIP) safety devices are available.
- Do not recap any needle.
- Plan safe handling and disposal of needles before beginning the procedure.
- Immediately dispose of needles, needleless systems, and SESIP into puncture-proof and leak-proof sharps disposal containers.
- Maintain a sharps injury log that includes:
  ○ Type and brand of device involved in the incident
  ○ Location of the incident (e.g., department or work area)
  ○ Description of the incident
  ○ Procedure to maintain privacy of the employees who have had sharps injuries

From Occupational Safety and Health Administration: Occupational exposure to bloodborne pathogens: needlestick and other sharps injuries—final rule, *Federal Register,* CFR 29, part 1910 (*Federal Register* #66:5317-5325), January 18, 2001. http://www.osha.gov/pls/oshaweb/owadisp.show_document?p-table=STANDARDS&p_id=10051.

3. By piggyback infusion of a solution containing the prescribed medication and a small volume of IV fluid through an existing IV line

In all three methods the patient has either an existing IV infusion line or an IV site that is accessed intermittently for infusions (sometimes called a heparin or saline lock). In most institutions, policies and procedures identify the medications that nurses are allowed to administer intravenously. These policies are based on the medication, capability and availability of staff, and type of monitoring equipment available.

Chapter 15 describes the technique for performing venipuncture and establishing continuous IV fluid infusions. Medication administration is only one reason for supplying IV fluids. You use IV fluid therapy primarily for fluid replacement in patients unable to take oral fluids and as a means of supplying electrolytes and nutrients.

When using any method of IV medication administration, observe patients closely for symptoms of adverse reactions. After a medication enters the bloodstream, it begins to act immediately and there is no way to stop its action. Therefore, avoid errors in dose calculation and preparation. Follow the six rights of safe medication administration, understand the desired action and side effects of the medication, and document the medication according to agency policy. If the medication has an antidote, have it available during administration. When administering potent medications, assess vital signs before, during, and after the infusion.

Administering medications by the IV route has advantages. Often you use the IV route in emergencies when you need to deliver a fast-acting medication quickly. The IV route is also best when it is necessary to establish constant therapeutic blood levels. Some medications are highly alkaline and irritating to muscle and Sub-Q tissue. These medications cause less discomfort when given intravenously.

**LARGE-VOLUME INFUSIONS.** Of the three methods of administering IV medications, mixing medications in large volumes of fluids is the safest and easiest. You dilute medications in large volumes (500 ml or 1000 ml) of compatible IV fluids, such as normal saline or lactated Ringer's solution (Skill 14-6). In most institutions to ensure asepsis, the IV fluids come premixed from the manufacturer, or the pharmacist adds medications to the primary container of IV solution. Because the medication is not in a concentrated form, the risk of side effects or fatal reactions is lessened when infused over the prescribed time frame. Vitamins and potassium chloride are two types of medications commonly added to IV fluids. However, there is a danger with continuous infusion. If the IV fluid is infused too rapidly, the patient suffers circulatory fluid overload.

*Text continued on p. 411*

---

## SKILL 14-6 | Adding Medications to Intravenous Fluid Containers

### Delegation Considerations

Do not delegate this skill. Only registered professional nurses perform this skill. However, in some institutions the pharmacist adds drugs to primary containers of IV solutions to ensure asepsis and enhance medication safety.
Instruct assistive personnel about:
- Potential side effects of medications and to report their occurrence

### Equipment

- Vial or ampule of prescribed medication
- Syringe of appropriate size (1 to 20 ml)

- Sterile needle (1 to 1½ inch, 19 to 21 gauge) with special filters if indicated
- Correct diluent if indicated (e.g., sterile water, normal saline)
- Sterile IV fluid container (bag or bottle, 25 to 1000 ml in volume)
- Alcohol or antiseptic swab
- Label to attach to IV bag or bottle
- MAR or computer printout

| STEP | RATIONALE |
|------|-----------|

### ASSESSMENT

1. Check accuracy and completeness of each MAR or computer printout with prescriber's written medication order. Check patient's name, drug name and dosage, route of administration, and time for administration. Recopy or re-print any portion of MAR that is difficult to read.
2. Assess patient's medical history.
3. Collect information necessary to administer drug safely, including action, purpose, side effects, normal dose, time of peak onset, and nursing implications.

The order sheet is the most reliable source and only legal record of drugs patient is to receive. Ensures patient receives the right medications. Illegible MARs are a source of medication errors.

Identifies need for medication.
Allows you to give drug safely and to monitor patient's response to therapy.

Adding Medications to Intravenous Fluid Containers—cont'd

| STEP | RATIONALE |
|---|---|
| 4. When you add more than one medication to IV solution, assess for compatibility of medications. | Drugs often are incompatible when mixed together. Chemical reactions that occur result in clouding or crystallization of IV fluids. Check institutional policy for drug compatibility list. |
| 5. Assess patient's systemic fluid balance, as reflected by skin hydration and turgor, body weight, pulse, and blood pressure. | In continuous IV infusions there is a danger that fluids will infuse too rapidly, causing circulatory overload, especially in older adults or children (Ebersole and others, 2004; Hockenberry and others, 2003). |
| 6. Assess patient's history of drug allergies. | IV administration of drugs causes rapid effects. Allergic response is immediate. |
| 7. Perform hand hygiene. Assess IV insertion site for signs of infiltration or phlebitis (see Chapter 15). Assess patency of existing IV infusion line. | An intact, properly functioning site and infusion ensures that you give medication safely. |
| 8. Assess patient's understanding of purpose of drug therapy. | Reveals any need for education. |

## PLANNING

| | |
|---|---|
| 1. Expected outcomes following completion of this procedure: | |
| • Patient experiences no medication side effects or adverse reactions. | Medication administered safely with desired therapeutic effect achieved. |
| • Patient develops no signs or symptoms of fluid volume overload. | Intravenous rate is correctly maintained. |
| • Intravenous site is free of swelling or inflammation. | IV fluid delivered without infusion site complications. |
| • Patient explains purpose and side effects of medication. | Demonstrates learning. |

## IMPLEMENTATION

| | |
|---|---|
| 1. Prepare medication: See Skill 14-4, using aseptic technique. Check label of medication carefully with MAR two times while preparing medication. | Ensures medication is sterile; preparation techniques differ for ampules and vial. Ensures right medication is given to patient. |
| 2. Perform hand hygiene. | Reduces transfer of microorganisms. |
| 3. Compare labels of medication and IV fluid bag with the MAR. | Ensures right medication is injected into right IV fluid. |
| 4. Add medication to new container (usually done in medication room or at medication cart): | |
| a. *Solutions in a bag:* Locate medication injection port on plastic IV solution bag. Port has small rubber stopper at end. Do not select port for the IV tubing insertion or air vent. | Medication injection port seals itself to prevent introduction of microorganisms after repeated use. |
| b. *Solutions in bottles:* Locate injection site on IV solution bottle. Often a metal or plastic cap covers it. | Accidental injection of medication through main tubing port or air vent alters pressure within bottle and causes fluid leaks through air vent. Cap seals bottle to maintain its sterility. |
| c. Wipe off port or injection site with alcohol or antiseptic swab (see illustration). | Reduces risk of introducing microorganisms into bag during needle insertion. |
| d. Remove needle cap or sheath from syringe, and insert needle of syringe through center of injection port or site; inject medication (see illustration). | Insertion of needle into sides of port sometimes produces leak and leads to fluid contamination. |
| e. Withdraw syringe from bag or bottle. | Withdrawal automatically self-seals the injection port, preventing introduction of microorganisms. |

| STEP | RATIONALE |
|---|---|
| f. Mix medication and IV solution by holding bag or bottle and turning it gently end to end. | Allows even distribution of medication. |
| g. Complete medication label with name and dose of medication, date, time, and your initials. Stick it on bottle or bag. *Optional (check institution's policy): Apply a flow strip that identifies the time you hung the solution and intervals indicating fluid levels (see illustration).* | Label is easily read during infusion of solution and informs other nurses and physician or health care providers of contents of bag or bottle. Do not use felt-tip markers on plastic surfaces. The ink will penetrate the plastic and leach into the IV solution. |
| h. If new tubing is required, spike bag or bottle with IV tubing, prime IV tubing. | Prepares container for infusion. |
| 5. Bring assembled items to patient's bedside at right time, and perform hand hygiene. | Organization reduces errors. Hand hygiene reduces transfer of microorganisms. |
| 6. Verify patient's identity by using at least two patient identifiers. Ask patient to state name if possible for a third identifier. | Complies with JCAHO requirements and improves medication safety. In most acute care settings, you use patient's name and identification number on armband and MAR to identify patients. Identification bracelets are made at time of patient's admission and are most reliable source of identification. Patient's room number is **not** an acceptable identifier (JCAHO, 2004a). |
| 7. Compare label on IV bag with the MAR a final time. | Final comparison of medication label with the MAR decreases risk of medication administration errors. |
| 8. Prepare patient by explaining that you will give medication through an existing IV line or that you will start a new IV line. Explain that patient will feel no discomfort during drug infusion. Encourage patient to report symptoms of discomfort. | Most IV medications do not cause discomfort when diluted. However, potassium chloride is sometimes irritating. Pain at insertion site is possible early indication of infiltration. |

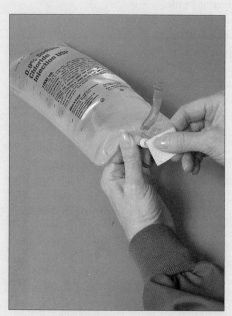

STEP **3c** Cleanse injection port with antiseptic swab.

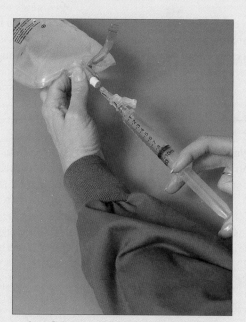

STEP **3d** Inject medication through port.

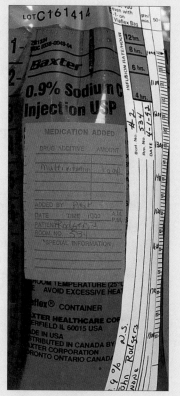

STEP **3g** Affix label to IV bag.

## SKILL 14-6  Adding Medications to Intravenous Fluid Containers—cont'd

| STEP | RATIONALE |
|---|---|
| 9. Connect new infusion tubing or spike container with existing tubing. Regulate infusion at ordered rate (see Chapter 15). | Prevents rapid infusion of fluid. |

• *Critical Decision Point:* Some medications (e.g., potassium chloride) cause serious adverse reactions, including fatal cardiac dysrhythmias. Infuse these medications on an IV pump. Check institutional guidelines or policies indicating which IV medications require administration on an IV pump.

| | |
|---|---|
| 10. Add medication to existing container:<br> a. Check volume of solution remaining in bottle or bag. | You need proper minimal volume (see drug insert) to dilute medication adequately. |

• *Critical Decision Point:* Because there is no way to know exactly how much IV fluid is in an existing hanging IV container, there is no way to determine the exact concentration of the medication in the IV solution. Therefore it is recommended that you add medications to new IV fluid containers whenever possible.

| | |
|---|---|
| b. Close off IV infusion clamp. | Prevents medication from directly entering circulation as you inject it into bag or bottle. |
| c. Wipe off medication injection port with an alcohol or antiseptic swab. | Mechanically removes microorganisms that enter container during needle insertion. |
| d. Remove needle cap or sheath from syringe, insert syringe needle through injection port, and inject medication. | Injection port seals itself and prevents fluid leaks. |
| e. Withdraw syringe from bag or bottle. | Self-seals medication port. |
| f. Lower bag or bottle from IV pole, and gently mix. Rehang bag. | Ensures even distribution of medication. |
| g. Complete medication label, and stick it to bag or bottle. | Informs other nurses and physicians or health care providers of contents of bag or bottle. |
| h. Regulate infusion at ordered rate (see Chapter 15). | Prevents rapid infusion of fluid. |
| 11. Properly dispose of equipment and supplies. Do not cap needle of syringe. Discard specially sheathed needles as a unit with needle covered. | Proper disposal of needle prevents injury to nurse and patient. Capping of needles increases risk of needle-stick injuries. |
| 12. Perform hand hygiene. | Reduces transmission of microorganisms. |

## EVALUATION

| | |
|---|---|
| 1. Observe patient for signs or symptoms of drug reaction. | IV medications cause rapid effects. |
| 2. Observe for signs and symptoms of fluid volume excess. | Rapid uncontrolled infusion causes circulatory overload. |
| 3. Periodically return to patient's room to assess IV insertion site and rate of infusion. | Over time IV sites sometimes become infiltrated or needles move and are not positioned correctly. Flow rate changes according to patient's position or volume left in container. |
| 4. Observe for signs or symptoms of IV infiltration. | Infiltrated drugs injure tissue. |
| 5. Ask patient to explain purpose and effects of medication therapy. | Demonstrates learning. |

## RECORDING AND REPORTING

■ Record solution and medication added to parenteral fluid on appropriate form.

■ Report any adverse effects to patient's health care provider, and document adverse effects according to institutional policy.

## UNEXPECTED OUTCOMES AND RELATED INTERVENTIONS

■ Patient has adverse or allergic reaction to medication.
  • Follow institutional policy or guidelines for appropriate response to and reporting of adverse drug reactions.
  • Notify patient's health care provider immediately.

■ Patient develops signs of fluid volume overload (e.g., abnormal breath sounds, shortness of breath, intake greater than output).
  • Assess patient for compromised circulatory regulation.
  • Stop IV infusion.
  • Notify patient's health care provider immediately.

■ IV site becomes swollen, warm, reddened, and tender to touch (see Chapter 15).
  • Indicates phlebitis.
  • Stop IV infusion.
  • Discontinue IV infusion.
  • Treat IV site as indicated by institutional policy.
  • Insert new IV site if continuing IV therapy.

■ IV site becomes cool, pale, and swollen (see Chapter 15).
  • Indicates signs of infiltration.
  • Determine how harmful IV medication is to subcutaneous tissue by referring to a medication reference or consulting with a pharmacist.
  • Provide IV extravasation care (e.g., inject phentolamine [Regitine] around the IV infiltration site) as indicated by institutional policy, or use a medication reference or manual, or consult a pharmacist to determine appropriate follow-up care.

**INTRAVENOUS BOLUS.** An IV bolus involves introducing a concentrated dose of a medication directly into the systemic circulation (Skill 14-7). Because a bolus requires only a small amount of fluid to deliver the medication, it is an advantage when the amount of fluid the patient takes is restricted. The IV bolus is the most dangerous method for administering medications because the body absorbs the medication as soon as you administer it, so there is no time to correct errors. In addition, a bolus sometimes causes direct irritation to the lining of blood vessels. Before administering a bolus, confirm placement of the IV line. Never give an IV medication if the insertion site appears puffy or edematous or the IV fluid does not flow at the proper rate. Accidental injection of a medication into the tissues around a vein causes pain, sloughing of tissues, and abscesses.

You usually determine the rate of administration of an IV bolus medication by the amount of medication that the IV will give each minute. Look up each medication to determine the recommended concentration and rate of administration. Consider the purpose for which a medication is prescribed and any potential adverse effects related to the rate or route of administration when giving a medication by IV push.

**VOLUME-CONTROLLED INFUSIONS.** Another way of administering IV medications is through small amounts (25 to 100 ml) of compatible IV fluids. The fluid is in a secondary fluid container separate from the primary fluid bag. The container connects directly to the primary IV line or to separate tubing that inserts into the primary line. Different types of containers used include volume-control administration sets (e.g., Volutrol, Pediatrol), piggyback sets, and mini-infusers. Using volume-controlled infusions has the following advantages:

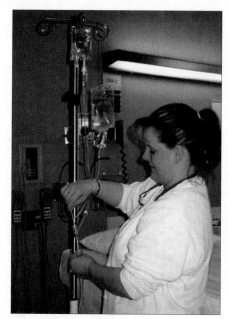

FIGURE **14-26** Piggyback setup.

1. Volume-controlled infusions dilute and infuse medications over longer time intervals (e.g., 30 to 60 minutes), reducing risks to the patient associated with IV push.
2. You can administer medications (e.g., antibiotics) that are stable for a limited time in solution.
3. This way of administration controls IV fluid intake.

**Piggyback.** A piggyback is a small (25 to 250 ml) IV bag or bottle connected to a short tubing line that connects to the *upper* Y-port of a primary infusion line (Figure 14-26) or

*Text continued on p. 417*

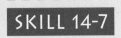

---

SKILL 14-7 | ## Administering Medications by Intravenous Bolus

### Delegation Considerations

Do not delegate this skill. Only registered professional nurses perform this skill.

Instruct assistive personnel about:

- Potential side effects of medications and the need to report their occurrence
- The need to report discomfort at infusion site as soon as possible
- Obtaining any required vital signs and reporting these findings

### Equipment

- Watch with second hand
- MAR or computer printout

- Disposable gloves
- Antiseptic swab
- Medication in vial or ampule
- Syringe
- Needleless device or sterile needle (21 to 25 gauge)
- Intravenous lock: vial of appropriate flush solution (saline most common, but heparin may also be used; if heparin is used, most common concentration is 10 to 100 units; check agency policy)

| STEP | RATIONALE |
|---|---|

### ASSESSMENT

1. Check accuracy and completeness of each MAR or computer printout with prescriber's written medication order. Check patient's name, drug name and dosage, route of administration, and time for administration. Recopy or re-print any portion of MAR that is difficult to read.

The order sheet is the most reliable source and only legal record of drugs patient is to receive. Ensures patient receives the right medications. Illegible MARs are a source of medication errors.

---

- *Critical Decision Point:* Some IV medications can be pushed safely only when the patient is continuously monitored for dysrhythmias, blood pressure changes, or other adverse effects. Therefore you can push some medications only in specific areas within a health care agency. Confirm institutional guidelines regarding requirements for special monitoring before giving these medications (Zurlinden, 2002).

---

2. Collect drug reference information necessary to administer drug safely, including action, purpose, side effects, normal dose, time of peak onset, how slowly to give the medication, and nursing implications, such as the need to dilute the medication or administer it through a filter.

Allows you to give drug safely and to monitor patient's response to therapy.

3. If you will give drug through existing IV line, determine compatibility of medication with IV fluids and any additives within IV solution.

Intravenous medication is sometimes not compatible with IV solution and/or additives.

4. Perform hand hygiene. Assess condition of IV needle insertion site for signs of infiltration or phlebitis.

Do not administer medication if site is edematous or inflamed.

5. Check patient's medical history and drug allergies.

Intravenous bolus delivers drug rapidly. Allergic reaction could prove fatal.

6. Check date of expiration for medication vial or ampule.

Drug potency sometimes increases or decreases when medications are outdated.

7. Assess patient's understanding of purpose of drug therapy.

May reveal need for education.

### PLANNING

1. Expected outcomes following completion of procedure:
   - Patient experiences no medication side effects or adverse reactions.
   - Intravenous site remains clear, without swelling.
   - Patient explains purpose and side effects of medication.

Medication administered safely with desired therapeutic effect achieved.
Medication infuses without complications to IV site.
Demonstrates learning.

| STEP | RATIONALE |
|---|---|

• *Critical Decision Point:* Some IV medications require dilution before administration. Verify with agency policy. If a small amount of medication is given (e.g., less than 1 ml), dilute medication in 5 to 10 ml of normal saline or sterile water so that the medication does not collect in the "dead spaces" (e.g., Y-site injection port, IV cap) of the IV delivery system.

## IMPLEMENTATION

1. Prepare medication dose from ampule or vial (See Skill 14-4, using aseptic techniques). Check label of medication carefully with MAR two times.

Ensures that medication is sterile. Preparation techniques differ for ampule and vial. Ensures correct medication is administered to patient.

2. Take medication to patient at right time, and perform hand hygiene.

Ensures patient experiences effect of medication at correct time and reduces transmission of microorganisms.

3. Verify patient's identity by using at least two patient identifiers. Ask patient to state name if possible for a third identifier.

Complies with JCAHO requirements and improves medication safety. In most acute care settings, you use patient's name and identification number on armband and MAR to identify patients. Identification bracelets are made at time of patient's admission and are most reliable source of identification. Patient's room number is **not** an acceptable identifier (JCAHO, 2004a).

4. Compare the label of the medication with the MAR one more time at the patient's bedside.

Final comparison of medication label with the MAR decreases risk of medication administration errors.

5. Explain procedure to patient. Encourage patient to report symptoms of discomfort at IV site.

Informs patient of planned therapies, keeps patient involved in care, and helps identify possible infiltration early.

6. Put on disposable gloves.

Follows Centers for Disease Control and Prevention recommendations to prevent accidental exposure to blood and body fluids (OSHA, 2001).

7. **Intravenous push (existing line):**
   a. Select injection port of IV tubing closest to patient. Whenever possible, use a stopcock or other needleless injection port.

Follows provisions of The Needle Safety and Prevention Act of 2001 (OSHA, 2001).

   b. Clean port with antiseptic swab.

Prevents transfer of microorganisms during needle insertion.

   c. Connect syringe to IV line: Insert needleless tip of syringe or small-gauge needle containing drug through center of port (see illustration).

Prevents damage to port diaphragm.

   d. Occlude IV line by pinching tubing just above injection port (see illustration). Pull back gently on syringe's plunger to aspirate for blood return.

Final check ensures that medication is delivered into bloodstream.

• *Critical Decision Point:* In some cases, especially with a smaller gauge IV needle, blood return sometimes is not aspirated, even if IV is patent. If IV site does not show signs of infiltration and IV fluid is infusing without difficulty, proceed with IV push.

   e. Release tubing, and inject medication within amount of time recommended by institutional policy, pharmacist, or medication reference manual. Use a watch to time administrations. You can pinch the intravenous line while pushing medication and release it when not pushing medication (see illustration). Allow IV fluids to infuse when not pushing medication.

Ensures safe drug infusion. Rapid injection of IV drug can be fatal. Allowing IV fluids to infuse while pushing IV drug enables medication to be delivered to patient at prescribed rate.

Administering Medications by Intravenous
Bolus—cont'd

| STEP | RATIONALE |
|------|-----------|

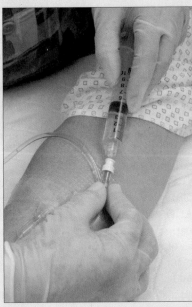

STEP **7c** Connecting syringe to IV line with blunt needleless cannula tip.

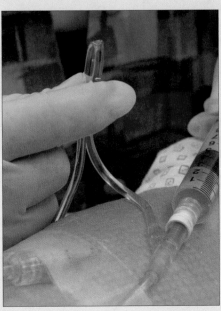

STEP **7d** Intravenous line pinched above injection port for medication infusion.

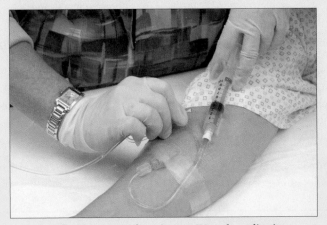

STEP **7e** Using a watch to time an IV push medication.

• **Critical Decision Point:** If IV medication is incompatible with IV fluids, stop the IV fluids, clamp the IV line, flush with 10 ml of normal saline or sterile water, give the IV bolus over the appropriate amount of time, flush with another 10 ml of normal saline or sterile water at the same rate as the medication was administered, and then restart the IV fluids at the prescribed rate. This allows you to give IV push medication through the existing line without creating potential risks associated with IV incompatibilities. If IV that is currently hanging is a medication (e.g., ranitidine), disconnect IV and administer IV push medication as outlined in step 6 to avoid giving a sudden bolus of the medication in the existing IV line to the patient. Verify institutional policy regarding the stopping of IV fluids or continuous IV medications. If unable to stop IV infusion, start a new IV site (see Chapter 15) and administer medication using the IV push (IV lock) method.

| STEP | RATIONALE |
|---|---|
| f. After injecting medication, withdraw syringe, and recheck fluid infusion rate. | Injection of bolus often alters rate of fluid infusion. Rapid fluid infusion causes circulatory fluid overload. |

**8. Intravenous push (intravenous lock):**

a. Prepare flush solutions according to hospital policy.

   (1) *Saline flush method (preferred method):* Prepare two syringes filled with 2 to 3 ml of normal saline (0.9%).

Normal saline is effective in keeping IV locks patent and is compatible with a wide range of medications.

   (2) *Heparin flush method (traditional method):*

     (a) Prepare one syringe with ordered amount of heparin flush solution.

     (b) Prepare two syringes with 2 to 3 ml of normal saline (0.9%).

b. Administer medication:

   (1) Clean lock's injection port with antiseptic swab.

Prevents transfer of microorganisms during needle insertion.

   (2) Insert syringe with normal saline 0.9% through injection port of IV lock (see illustrations).

   (3) Pull back gently on syringe plunger, and check for blood return.

Indicates if needle or catheter is in vein.

---

• *Critical Decision Point:* In some cases, especially with a smaller gauge IV needle, blood return is usually not aspirated, even if IV is patent. If IV site does not show signs of infiltration, and IV flushes without difficulty, proceed with IV push.

---

   (4) Flush IV site with normal saline by pushing slowly on plunger.

Cleans needle and reservoir of blood. Flushing without difficulty indicates patent IV.

---

• *Critical Decision Point:* Carefully observe the area of skin above the IV catheter. Note any puffiness or swelling as you flush the IV. Swelling indicates infiltration into the vein and requires removal of catheter.

---

   (5) Remove saline-filled syringe.

   (6) Clean lock's injection port with antiseptic swab.

Prevents transmission of infection.

   (7) Insert syringe containing prepared medication through injection port of IV lock.

Allows administration of medication.

   (8) Inject medication within amount of time recommended by institutional policy, pharmacist, or medication reference manual. Use a watch to time administration.

Many medication errors are associated with IV pushes being administered too quickly. Following guidelines for IV push rates promotes patient safety (Karch and Karch, 2003).

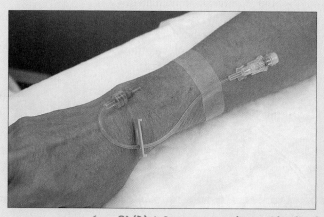 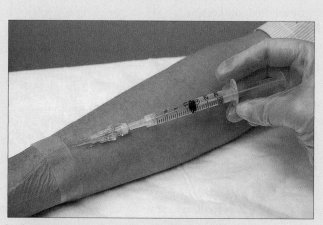

STEP **8b(2) A,** Intravenous catheter with saline lock adapter. **B,** Syringe inserted into injection port.

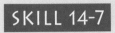

SKILL 14-7 | Administering Medications by Intravenous Bolus—cont'd

| STEP | RATIONALE |
|---|---|
| (9) After administering bolus, withdraw syringe. | |
| (10) Clean lock's injection site with antiseptic swab. | Prevents transmission of infection. |
| (11) Flush injection port. | |
| (a) Attach syringe with normal saline, and inject normal saline flush at the same rate the medication was delivered. | Flushing IV line with saline prevents occlusion of IV access device and ensures all medication delivered. Flushing IV site at same rate as medication ensures that any medication remaining within IV needle is delivered at the correct rate. |
| (b) *Heparin flush option:* After instilling saline, attach syringe containing heparin flush. Inject heparin slowly, and then remove syringe. | Maintains patency of IV needle by inhibiting clot formation. SASH method: *S*aline, *A*dministration of medication, *S*aline, *H*eparin. |
| 9. Dispose of uncapped needles and syringes in puncture-proof and leakproof container. | Prevents accidental needle-stick injuries and follows CDC guidelines for disposal of sharps (OSHA, 2001). |
| 10. Remove gloves, and perform hand hygiene. | Reduces transfer of microorganisms. |

## EVALUATION

| | |
|---|---|
| 1. Observe patient closely for adverse reactions during administration and for several minutes thereafter. | Intravenous medications act rapidly. |
| 2. Observe IV site during injection for sudden swelling. | Swelling indicates infiltration into tissues surrounding vein. |
| 3. Assess patient's status after giving medication to evaluate the effectiveness of the medication. | Some IV bolus medications cause rapid changes in the patient's physiological status. Some drugs require careful monitoring and assessment and possibly future laboratory testing (e.g., vasopressors and antiarrhythmics require blood pressure and heart rate monitoring, whereas heparin requires laboratory studies after administration to determine if it is in a therapeutic level). |
| 4. Ask patient to explain drug's purpose and side effects. | Evaluates learning. |

## RECORDING AND REPORTING

■ Record medication administration, including drug name, dose, route, and time of administration.
■ Report any adverse reactions to patient's health care provider. Patient's response may indicate need for additional medical therapy.
■ Record patient's response to medication in nurses' notes.

## UNEXPECTED OUTCOMES AND RELATED INTERVENTIONS

■ Patient develops adverse reaction to medication.
• Stop delivering medication immediately, and follow institutional policy or guidelines for appropriate response and reporting of adverse drug reactions.
• Notify patient's health care provider of adverse effects immediately.

• Add allergy information to patient's medical record per agency policy.
■ Intravenous site becomes cool, pale, and swollen (see Chapter 15), indicating signs of infiltration.
• Stop IV infusion immediately.
• Provide extravasation care as indicated by institutional policy or prescriber.
• See other related interventions for infiltration in Skill 14-6.
■ Patient is unable to explain medication information.
• Patient requires reinstruction or is unable to learn at this time.

to an intermittent venous access. The piggyback tubing is a microdrip or macrodrip system (see Chapter 15). The set is called a piggyback because the small bag or bottle is set higher than the primary infusion bag or bottle. In the piggyback setup, the main line does not infuse when the piggybacked medication is infusing. The port of the primary IV line contains a back-check valve that automatically stops flow of the primary infusion once the piggyback infusion flows. After the piggyback solution infuses and the solution within the tubing falls below the level of the primary infusion drip chamber, the back-check valve opens and the primary infusion begins to flow again.

**Volume-Control Administration.** Volume-control administration sets (e.g., Volutrol, Buretrol, Pediatrol) are small (50 to 150 ml) containers that attach just below the primary infusion bag or bottle. The set is attached and filled in a manner similar to that used with a regular IV infusion. However, the priming filling of the set is different, depending on the type of filter (floating valve or membrane) within the set. Follow package directions for priming sets (Skill 14-8).

**Mini-infusion Pump.** The mini-infusion pump is battery operated and delivers medications in very small amounts of fluid (5 to 60 ml) within controlled infusion times. It uses standard syringes (see Skill 14-8).

**INTERMITTENT VENOUS ACCESS.** An intermittent venous access (commonly called a heparin lock or saline lock) is an IV catheter with a small "well" or chamber covered by a rubber cap. You insert special rubber-seal injection caps into most IV catheters (see Chapter 15). Advantages to intermittent venous access include the following:

1. Cost savings resulting from the omission of continuous IV therapy
2. Saving nurses' time by eliminating constant monitoring of IV flow rates
3. Increased mobility, safety, and comfort for patient by eliminating the need for a continuous IV line

After you administer an IV bolus or piggyback medication through an intermittent venous access, flush with a solution to keep it patent. Generally, saline is effective as a flush solution. Some institutions require the use of heparin. Be sure to check and follow institutional policies regarding the care and maintenance of the IV site.

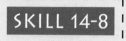

### Administering Intravenous Medications by Piggyback, Intermittent Intravenous Infusion Sets, and Mini-infusion Pumps

#### Delegation Considerations

Do not delegate this skill. Usually only registered professional nurses perform this skill. Refer to your nurse practice act; some states certify licensed practical nurses (LPNs) to administer some IV piggyback medications.
Instruct assistive personnel about:
• Potential side effects of medications and to report their occurrence

#### Equipment

• Adhesive tape (optional)
• Antiseptic swab
• IV pole or rack
• MAR or computer printout

*Piggyback or Mini-infusion Pump*
• Medication prepared in 5- to 250-ml labeled infusion bag or syringe
• Short microdrip or macrodrip IV tubing set (may have needleless system attachment)
• Needleless device or stopcocks if available
• Needles (21 or 23 gauge, only if stopcocks or other needleless methods are not available)
• Mini-infusion pump if indicated
*Volume-Control Administration Set*
• Volutrol or Buretrol
• Infusion tubing (may have needleless system attachment)
• Syringe (1 to 20 ml)
• Vial or ampule of ordered medication

| STEP | RATIONALE |
|---|---|
| **ASSESSMENT** | |
| 1. Check accuracy and completeness of each MAR or computer printout with prescriber's written medication order to determine type of IV solution you will use, type of medication, dose, route, and time of administration. Recopy or re-print any portion of MAR that is difficult to read. Also check patient's name. | The order sheet is the most reliable source and only legal record of drugs patient is to receive. Ensures patient receives the right medications. Illegible MARs are a source of medication errors. |

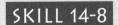

**SKILL 14-8** Administering Intravenous Medications by Piggyback, Intermittent Intravenous Infusion Sets, and Mini-infusion Pumps—cont'd

| STEP | RATIONALE |
|---|---|
| 2. Determine patient's medical history. | Patient's overall physical condition dictates type of IV solution used. Ensures safe and accurate drug administration. |
| 3. Collect information necessary to administer drug safely, including action, purpose, side effects, normal dose, time of peak onset, and nursing implications. | Allows you to give drug safely and to monitor patient's response to therapy. |
| 4. Assess compatibility of drug with existing IV solution. | Drugs that are incompatible with IV solutions result in clouding or crystallization of solution in IV tubing, which will harm the patient. |

• *Critical Decision Point:* Never administer IV medications through tubing that is infusing blood, blood products, or parenteral nutrition solutions.

| STEP | RATIONALE |
|---|---|
| 5. Assess patency of patient's existing IV infusion line (see Chapter 15). | In order for medication to reach venous circulation effectively, IV line needs to be patent and fluids should infuse easily. |

• *Critical Decision Point:* If the patient's IV site is saline locked, cleanse the port with alcohol and assess the patency of the IV line by flushing the IV line with 2 to 3 ml of sterile normal saline. Attach appropriate IV tubing to the saline lock, and administer the medication via piggyback, mini-infusion, or volume-control administration set. When the infusion is completed, disconnect the tubing, cleanse the port with alcohol, and flush the IV line with 2 to 3 ml sterile normal saline. Maintain sterility of IV tubing between intermittent infusions.

| STEP | RATIONALE |
|---|---|
| 6. Perform hand hygiene. Assess IV insertion site for signs of infiltration or phlebitis: redness, pallor, swelling, or tenderness on palpation. | Confirmation of placement of IV needle or catheter and integrity of surrounding tissues ensures you administer medication safely. |
| 7. Assess patient's history of drug allergies. | Effects of medications develop rapidly after IV infusion. Be aware of patients at risk. |
| 8. Assess patient's understanding of purpose of drug therapy. | Reveals any need for education. |

## PLANNING

| 1. Expected outcomes following completion of procedure: | |
|---|---|
| • Medication infuses without adverse reactions. | Gave drug safely with desired therapeutic effect. |
| • Medication infuses within desired time frame. | Intravenous line remains patent. |
| • Intravenous site remains intact without signs of swelling or inflammation or symptoms of tenderness at site. | Fluid infuses into vein, not tissues. |
| • Patient is able to explain drug purposes, action, side effects, and dosage. | Demonstrates learning. |

## IMPLEMENTATION

| 1. Assemble medication and supplies at bedside. | Drug preparation usually is not required. |
|---|---|
| 2. Compare the label of the medication with the MAR at least two times while preparing supplies. | Following the same routine when preparing medication, eliminating distractions, and comparing the medication label with the MAR decreases risk of medication administration errors. |

| STEP | RATIONALE |
|---|---|
| **3.** Give medication to patient at right time, and perform hand hygiene. | Ensures patient will experience effect of medication at right time and reduces transmission of microorganisms. |
| **4.** Verify patient's identity by using at least two patient identifiers. Ask patient to state name if possible for a third identifier. | Complies with JCAHO requirements and improves medication safety. In most acute care settings, you use patient's name and identification number on armband and MAR to identify patients. Identification bracelets are made at time of patient's admission and are most reliable source of identification. Patient's room number is **not** an acceptable identifier (JCAHO, 2004a). |
| **5.** Explain purpose of medication and side effects to patient, and explain that you will give medication through existing IV line. Encourage patient to report symptoms of discomfort at site. | Keeps patient informed of planned therapies, minimizing anxiety. Patients who verbalize pain at the IV site help detect IV infiltrations early, lessening damage to surrounding tissues. |
| **6.** Compare the label of the medication with the MAR one more time. | Final comparison of medication label with the MAR decreases risk of medication administration errors. |
| **7.** Administer infusion: | |
| **A. Piggyback Infusion:** | |
| (1) Connect infusion tubing to medication bag (see Chapter 15). Allow solution to fill tubing by opening regulator flow clamp. Once tubing is full, close clamp and cap end of tubing. | Filling of infusion tubing with solution and freeing of air bubbles prevent air embolus. |
| (2) Hang piggyback medication bag above level of primary fluid bag (see Figure 14-29). (Use hook to lower main bag.) | Height of fluid bag affects rate of flow to patient. |
| (3) Connect tubing of piggyback infusion to appropriate connector on primary infusion line: | |
| (a) *Needleless system:* Wipe off needleless port of main IV line, and insert tip of piggyback infusion tubing (see illustration). | The CDC strongly recommends needleless connections to prevent accidental needle-stick injuries (OSHA, 2001). Allows IV medication to enter main IV line. |
| (b) *Stopcock:* Wipe off stopcock port with alcohol swab, and connect tubing. Turn stopcock to open position. | Stopcock eliminates need for needle. |
| (c) *Tubing port:* Connect sterile needle to end of piggyback infusion tubing, remove cap, cleanse injection port on main IV line, and insert needle through center of port. Secure by taping connection. | Prevents introduction of microorganisms during needle insertion. |
| (4) Regulate flow rate of medication solution by adjusting regulator clamp or IV pump infusion rate (see Chapter 15). (Infusion times vary. Refer to medication reference or institutional policy for safe flow rate.) | Provides slow, safe infusion of medication and maintains therapeutic blood levels. |
| (5) After medication has infused, check flow rate on primary infusion. The primary infusion automatically begins to flow after the piggyback solution is empty. If stopcock is used, turn stopcock to off position. | Back-check valve on piggyback stops flow of the primary infusion until medication infuses. Checking flow rate ensures proper administration of IV fluids. |
| (6) Regulate main infusion line to ordered rate if necessary. | Infusion of piggyback sometimes interferes with the main line infusion rate. |
| (7) Leave IV piggyback bag and tubing in place for future drug administration, or discard in appropriate containers. | Establishment of secondary line produces route for microorganisms to enter main line. Repeated changes in tubing increase risk of infection transmission (check institutional policy). |

SKILL 14-8 | Administering Intravenous Medications by Piggyback, Intermittent Intravenous Infusion Sets, and Mini-infusion Pumps—cont'd

| STEP | RATIONALE |
| --- | --- |

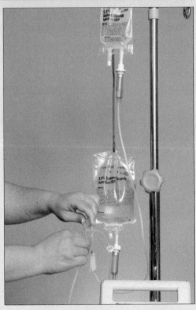

STEP **7A(3)(a)** For the needleless system, insert tip of piggyback infusion tubing into port.

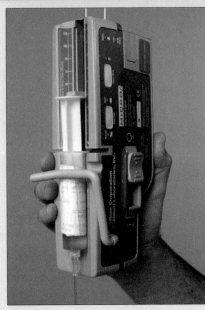

STEP **7B(3)** Ensure syringe is secure after placing it into mini-infusion pump.

**B. Mini-infusion Administration:**

(1) Connect prefilled syringe to mini-infusion tubing.

Special tubing designed to fit syringe delivers medication to main IV line.

(2) Carefully apply pressure to syringe plunger, allowing tubing to fill with medication.

Ensures tubing is free of air bubbles to prevent air embolus.

(3) Place syringe into mini-infusion pump (follow product directions). Be sure syringe is secured (see illustration).

Correct placement is necessary for proper infusion.

(4) Connect mini-infusion tubing to main IV line.

    (a) *Needleless system:* Wipe off needleless port of IV tubing, and insert tip of the mini-infusion tubing.

OSHA recommends needleless system to reduce risk of needle-stick injuries (2001).

    (b) *Stopcock:* Wipe off stopcock port with alcohol swab, and connect tubing. Turn stopcock to open position.

Stopcock reduces risk of needle-stick injuries.

    (c) *Needle system:* Connect sterile needle to mini-infusion tubing, remove cap, cleanse injection port on main IV line or saline lock, and insert needle through center of port. Consider placing tape where IV tubing enters port to keep connection secured.

Cleansing reduces transmission of microorganisms.

(5) Hang infusion pump with syringe on IV pole alongside main IV bag. Set pump to deliver medication within time recommended by institutional policy, a pharmacist, or a medication reference manual. Press button on pump to begin infusion.

Pump automatically delivers medication at safe, constant rate based on volume in syringe.

| STEP | RATIONALE |
|---|---|

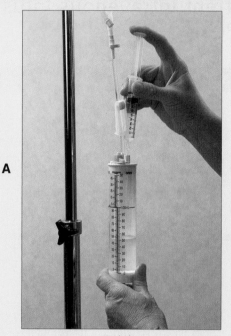 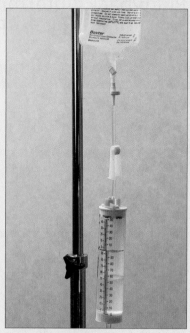

STEP **5C(4)** **A,** Inject medication into device. **B,** Prepared dose.

|   |   |
|---|---|
| (6) After medication has infused, check flow rate on primary infusion. The infusion automatically begins to flow once the pump stops. Regulate main infusion line to desired rate as needed. (NOTE: If using a stopcock, turn off mini-infusion line.) | Maintains patency of primary IV line. |

**C. Volume-Control Administration Set (e.g., Volutrol):**

|   |   |
|---|---|
| (1) Fill Volutrol with desired amount of fluid (50 to 100 ml) by opening clamp between Volutrol and main IV bag. | Small volume of fluid dilutes IV medication and reduces risk of fluid infusing too rapidly. |
| (2) Close clamp, and check to be sure clamp on air vent of Volutrol chamber is open. | Prevents additional leakage of fluid into Volutrol. Air vent allows fluid in Volutrol to exit at regulated rate. |
| (3) Clean injection port on top of Volutrol with antiseptic swab. | Prevents introduction of microorganisms during needle insertion. |
| (4) Remove needle cap or sheath, and insert syringe needle through port, then inject medication (see illustrations). Gently rotate Volutrol between hands. | Rotating mixes medication with solution in Volutrol to ensure equal distribution. |
| (5) Regulate IV infusion rate to allow medication to infuse in time recommended by institutional policy, a pharmacist, or a medication reference manual. | For optimal therapeutic effect, drug needs to infuse in prescribed time interval. |
| (6) Label Volutrol with name of drug, dosage, total volume including diluent, and time of administration. | Alerts nurses to drug being infused. Prevents other medications from being added to Volutrol. |
| (7) Dispose of uncapped needle or needle enclosed in safety shield and syringe in proper container. | Prevents accidental needle sticks. |
| (8) Discard supplies in appropriate container. Perform hand hygiene. | Reduces transmission of microorganisms. |

| SKILL 14-8 | Administering Intravenous Medications by Piggyback, Intermittent Intravenous Infusion Sets, and Mini-infusion Pumps—cont'd |

| STEP | RATIONALE |
| --- | --- |

## EVALUATION

1. Observe patient for signs of adverse reactions.

IV medications act rapidly.

2. During infusion, periodically check infusion rate and condition of IV site.

IV needs to remain patent for proper drug administration. Development of infiltration necessitates discontinuing infusion.

3. Ask patient to explain purpose and side effects of medication.

Evaluates patient's understanding of instruction.

## RECORDING AND REPORTING

■ Record drug, dose, route, and time administered on MAR or computer printout.

■ Record volume of fluid in medication bag or Volutrol on intake and output form.

■ Report any adverse reactions to patient's health care provider.

## UNEXPECTED OUTCOMES AND RELATED INTERVENTIONS

■ Patient develops adverse drug reaction.
  • Stop medication infusion immediately.
  • Follow institutional policy or guidelines for appropriate response and reporting of adverse drug reactions.
  • Notify patient's health care provider of adverse effects immediately.
  • Add allergy information to patient's medical record per agency policy.
■ Medication does not infuse over desired period.
  • Determine reason (e.g., improper calculation of flow rate, poor positioning of IV needle at insertion site, infiltration)
  • Take corrective action as indicated.

■ IV site becomes swollen, warm, reddened, and tender to touch (see Chapter 15). Indicates phlebitis.
  • Stop IV infusion.
  • Discontinue IV infusion.
  • Treat IV site as indicated by institutional policy.
  • Insert new IV site if continuing IV therapy.
■ IV site becomes cool, pale, and swollen (see Chapter 15). Indicates signs of infiltration.
  • Determine how harmful IV medication will be to Sub-Q tissue by referring to a medication reference or consulting with a pharmacist.
  • Provide IV extravasation care (e.g., injecting phentolamine [Regitine] around IV infiltration site) as indicated by institutional policy, or use a medication reference or consult a pharmacist to determine appropriate follow-up care.

## KEY CONCEPTS

• Learning medication classifications helps you better understand nursing implications for administering medications with similar characteristics.
• You handle all controlled substances according to strict procedures that account for each medication.
• You apply understanding of the physiology of medication action when timing administration, selecting routes, initiating actions to promote the potency of the medication, and observing responses to medications.

• The older adult's body undergoes structural and functional changes that alter medication actions and influence the manner in which nurses provide medication therapy.
• You compute children's medication doses on the basis of body surface area or weight.
• The body absorbs medications given parenterally more quickly than medications administered by other routes.
• Each medication order includes the patient's name; the time and date the order was written; the medication name;

dosage, route, and time and frequency of administration; and the prescriber's signature.
- You need to clarify medication orders that are illegible or that contain dangerous abbreviations.
- A medication history reveals allergies, medications a patient is taking, and the patient's compliance with therapy.
- The six rights of medication administration ensure accurate preparation and administration of medication doses.
- Only administer medications you prepare, and never leave medications unattended.
- Document medications immediately after administration.
- Use clinical nursing judgment when determining the best time to administer prn medications.

- Report medication errors immediately.
- When preparing medications, check the medication container label against the MAR or computer printout three times.
- When administering medication to patients, you verify your patients' identity by using at least two patient identifiers. Ask your patients to state their name if possible for a third identifier.
- The Z-track method for IM injections protects Sub-Q tissues from irritating parenteral fluids.
- Failure to select injection sites by anatomical landmarks leads to tissue, bone, or nerve damage.

## CRITICAL THINKING IN PRACTICE

*You are caring for Jennifer Bloom, a 58-year-old woman who recently had a hemorrhagic stroke. As a result of her stroke, Jennifer is unable to swallow, so her physician has inserted a gastrostomy tube (G-tube). Jennifer is receiving tube feedings at 80 ml per hour. Jennifer started having seizures early this morning. Therefore her physician has ordered Dilantin (phenytoin) 300 mg IV push tid today and then Dilantin 300 mg liquid suspension down the G-tube daily at bedtime.*

1. What information do you need to know about the Dilantin before you start the IV dose today?
2. Five 2-ml vials of Dilantin arrive from the pharmacy. The label on the vials says, "50 mg Dilantin/ml." How much Dilantin will you prepare in the syringe for the first IV dose?
3. Jennifer has a saline lock in her right wrist. After you have verified that the medication is correct, performed hand hygiene, prepared the medication, and verified Jennifer's identity, what will you do next in administering the IV push medication?
   a. Push the medication in slowly.
   b. Flush the IV site with heparin.
   c. Observe for adverse reactions.
   d. Assess the IV insertion site for signs of infiltration or phlebitis.
4. While you are flushing Jennifer's saline lock with saline before administering the IV Dilantin, you assess swelling, warmth, redness, and tenderness at the IV site. Which of the following interventions do you implement? (Mark all that apply.)
   a. Stop flushing the IV with normal saline.
   b. Infuse the medication slowly.
   c. Reposition the IV cannula.
   d. Discontinue the saline lock.
   e. Insert a new saline lock at a different site.

5. The next day has come, and it is now 1800. Jennifer is scheduled to receive her Dilantin through her G-tube tonight before she goes to bed. Your agency's policy states that you give medications ordered for bedtime at 2100. After looking up Dilantin in your medication reference manual, it states that you are supposed to hold tube feedings 1 hour before giving Dilantin and for 2 hours after giving Dilantin. This is because Dilantin can bind to tube feedings. What time will you stop Jennifer's feedings, what time will you give the Dilantin, and what time will you restart Jennifer's tube feedings?
6. The pharmacy has sent Dilantin suspension up to your floor. The label on the bottle says, "Dilantin 125 mg/5 ml." How much Dilantin will you give down the G-tube?
7. Listed below are different steps you will take to administer the Dilantin through Jennifer's G-tube. Place the steps in order.
   a. Draw up the Dilantin in a syringe.
   b. Evaluate Jennifer's response to the medication.
   c. Flush tube with 30 ml warm tap water before capping G-tube.
   d. Flush tube with 30 ml warm tap water before giving medication.
   e. Push Dilantin into the G-tube.
   f. Assess gastric residual.
8. Jennifer is going to be discharged home soon. Her oldest daughter and her husband will be caring for Jennifer. They have never administered medications in a G-tube before. They are asking you questions about how they will do this at home. What is the appropriate nursing diagnosis at this time? Provide an outcome, and list interventions necessary to help Jennifer's caregivers become more familiar with administering medications down a G-tube. What evaluation methods do you use to determine if the caregivers are able to administer G-tube medications at home?

## NCLEX® REVIEW

1. A patient receiving an antihypertensive medication is complaining of postural hypotension. This is an example of:
   1. A side effect
   2. A toxic effect
   3. An allergic reaction
   4. An idiosyncratic reaction

2. Immediately after administering an intradermal injection, the nurse should:
   1. Apply an alcohol swab or small gauze pad gently to the site
   2. Massage the site to decrease pain
   3. Perform hand hygiene
   4. Recap the needle

3. A patient is being discharged with nitroglycerin sublingually as needed for angina. The nurse knows the patient understands medication teaching about the sublingual route when the patient states:
   1. "It will take a long time for this medication to work."
   2. "I should put the tablet under my tongue and not swallow it."
   3. "I should drink 8 ounces of water whenever I take this medication."
   4. "I should alternate cheeks when I take multiple doses of this medication."

4. A patient is to receive an IM injection of morphine sulfate. The patient is 5 feet, 10 inches tall and weighs 185 lb. The nurse plans to administer the injection in the ventrogluteal muscle. The most appropriate needle size to use for this injection is:
   1. 20 gauge, 1 inch
   2. 23 gauge, $\frac{5}{8}$ inch
   3. 25 gauge, $\frac{1}{2}$ inch
   4. 22 gauge, $1\frac{1}{2}$ inch

5. The patient has an order for 2 tablespoons of milk of magnesia. The nurse, converting this to the metric system, would give the patient:
   1. 2 ml
   2. 5 ml
   3. 16 ml
   4. 32 ml

6. A physician's order for a medication states: "Insulin 5u reg and 10 u L BID." The physician is very busy and does not like to be bothered. The nurse should:
   1. Consult a pharmacist to interpret the order
   2. Call the physician and have the order verified
   3. Administer 5 units of regular insulin and 10 units of Lente insulin Sub-Q 2 times a day
   4. Talk to the unit secretary on the floor who is good at reading the physician's handwriting

7. A patient is to receive cephalexin (Keflex), 500 mg PO. The pharmacy has sent 250-mg tablets. The nurse should give:
   1. $\frac{1}{2}$ tablet
   2. 1 tablet
   3. $1\frac{1}{2}$ tablets
   4. 2 tablets

8. You have to give the following medications to the following patients. Which patient should you give medications to first?
   1. A patient who is to receive 325 mg aspirin who has a history of coronary artery disease
   2. A patient who needs 2 tablets of Vicodin (acetaminophen/hydrocodone) who is rating his incisional pain at a 10 on a 0 to 10 pain scale
   3. A patient who is to get Capoten (Captopril) 25 mg for a history of hypertension whose current blood pressure is 125/72 mm Hg
   4. A patient who is receiving Bactrim DS (trimethoprim/sulfamethoxazole) for a urinary tract infection

9. Which of the following assessment findings indicates a positive TB reaction in a patient with no known risk factors for TB?
   1. A large area of redness and swelling at the injection site
   2. An induration of 18 mm
   3. Frequent, productive cough and fever
   4. Sudden onset of shortness of breath and wheezing

10. Which statement, when made by a patient with diabetes who is taking insulin 2 times a day, indicates that he needs further instruction?
    1. "I need to carry some hard candy in my pocket whenever I go out of the house."
    2. "I need to check my blood sugars at least 2 times a day."
    3. "When I prepare my insulin, I put the NPH in the syringe before the regular insulin."
    4. "I keep my insulin in the refrigerator when I am not using it."

## REFERENCES

American Diabetes Association: Insulin administration: position statement, *Diabetes Care* 27(1S): S106, 2004.

American Diabetes Association: Class action, *Diabetes Forecast* 58(1):RG6, 2005a.

American Diabetes Association: Insulin delivery, *Diabetes Forecast* 58(1):RG16, 2005b.

American Hospital Association: *The patient care partnership*, 2003, http://www.hospitalconnect.com/aha/ptcommunication/partnership/index.html.

American Nurses Association: *American Nurses Association needlestick prevention guide: safe needles save lives*, 2002, http://www. nursingworld.org/needlestick/needleguide.pdf.

Aschenbrenner DS and others: *Drug therapy in nursing*, Philadelphia, 2002, Lippincott.

Association of Perioperative Registered Nurses: AORN guidance statement: safe medication practices in perioperative practice settings, *AORN J* 75(5):1008, 2002.

Aventis: *Lovenox: enoxaparin sodium injection*, 2003, http://www. lovenox.com.

Behrman RE and others: *Nelson textbook of pediatrics*, ed 17, Philadelphia, 2004, WB Saunders.

Brager R, Sloan E: The spectrum of polypharmacy, *Nurse Pract* 30(6):44, 2005.

Centers for Disease Control and Prevention: *Mantoux tuberculin skin test facilitator guide*, 2004, http://www.cdc.gov/nchstp/tb/pubs /Mantoux/ images/Mantoux.pdf.

Centers for Medicare and Medicaid Services: Clarifying policies related to the responsibilities of Medicare-partner hospitals in the treatment of individuals with emergency conditions, update 10/2003, CMS-1063-F, USH HHS Baltimore, Md, http://www.cms.hhs.gov.

Cohen MR: Drop that insulin syringe, *Nursing* 32(1):18, 2002.

Dahlin C: Oral complications at the end of life: although dysphagia and stomatitis can have devastating effects on the quality of a patient's life, there are many ways to manage them, *Am J Nurs* 104(7):40, 2004.

deWit S: *Fundamental concepts and skills for nursing*, ed 2, Philadelphia, 2005, WB Saunders.

Ebersole P and others: *Toward healthy aging: human needs and nursing response*, ed 6, St. Louis, 2004, Mosby.

Evangelista LS and others: Compliance behaviors of elderly patients with advanced heart failure, *J Cardiovasc Nurs* 18(3):197, 2003.

FDA: *MedWatch Reporting Forms*, 2005, http://www.fda.gov/medwatch/index.html.

Haynes RB and others: Interventions for helping patients to follow prescriptions for medications, *Cochrane Database Syst Review* 4:2004.

Hockenberry MJ and others: *Wong's nursing care of infants and children*, ed 7, St. Louis, 2003, Mosby.

Institute of Safe Medication Practices: *Oops, sorry, wrong patient! Applying the JCAHO "two-identifier" rule beyond the patient's room*, 2004a, http://www.ismp.org/MSAarticles/OOpsPrint.htm.

Institute of Safe Medication Practices: *Root causes: a roadmap to action*, 2004b, http://www.ismp.org/MSAarticles/RootPrint.htm.

Institute of Safe Medication Practices: What's up with tall man letters? *Nurse Advise-ERR* 2(9):2, 2004c.

Joint Commission on Accreditation of Healthcare Organizations: *2004 national patient safety goals FAQs*, 2004a, http://www. jcaho.org/accredited+organizations/patient+safety/04+npsg/ 04_npsgs_final2.pdf.

Joint Commission on Accreditation of Healthcare Organizations: *2005 national patient safety goals FAQs*, 2004b, http://www.jcaho. org/accredited+organizations/patient+safety/05+npsg/lasa.pdf.

Joint Commission on Accreditation of Healthcare Organizations: The official "do not use" list, 2005, http://www.jcaho.org/accredited+organizations/patient+safety/dnu.htm.

Jordan and others: Administration of medicines. II. Pharmacology, *Nurs Stand* 18(3):45, 2003.

Karch AM, Karch FE: Not so fast! *Am J Nurs* 103(8):71, 2003.

Lewis SM and others: *Medical-surgical nursing*, ed 5, St. Louis, 2000, Mosby.

MayoClinic.com: *Asthma inhalers: how they work*, 2003a, http://www.mayoclinic.com/printinvoker.cfm?objectid=87D67A 9F-B323-4C73-B42F99D100BE8D13.

MayoClinic.com: *Metered dose inhalers: how to use them properly*, 2003b, http://www.mayoclinic.com/printinvoker.cfm?objectid= 2C653B70-E5AF-4805-A15DF80E565409CB.

McKenry LM, Salerno E: *Mosby's pharmacology in nursing*, ed 21, St. Louis, 2003, Mosby.

National Coordinating Council for Medication Error Reporting and Prevention: *Recommendations to reduce medication errors associated with verbal medication orders and prescriptions*, 2001, http://www. nccmerp.org/council/council2001-02-20.html? USP_Print=true.

National Coordinating Council for Medication Error Reporting and Prevention: *Recommendations to enhance accuracy of prescription writing*, 2005, http://www.nccmerp.org/council/council1996-09-04.html.

Nicoll LH, Hesby A: Intramuscular injection: an integrative research review and guideline for evidence-based practice, *Appl Nurs Res* 16(2):149, 2002

Occupational Safety and Health Administration: Occupational exposure to bloodborne pathogens: needlestick and other sharp injuries—final rule, *Federal Register*, CFR 29, part 1910(66:5317-5325), January 18, 2001, http://www.osha.gov/pls/oshaweb/ owadisp.show_document?p_table=STANDARDS&p_id=10051.

Pereira LMP and others: Understanding and use of inhaler medication by asthmatics in specialty care in Trinidad, *Chest* 121(6): 1833, 2002.

Perry J and others: Nurses and needlesticks, then and now, *Nursing* 33(4):22, 2003.

Pope BB: How to administer subcutaneous and intramuscular injections, *Nursing* 32(1):50, 2002.

Rushing J: How to administer a subcutaneous injection, *Nursing* 34(6):32, 2004.

Stevenson L and others: Chronic hepatitis C virus and the Hispanic community: cultural factors impacting care, *Gastroenterol Nurs* 27(5):230, 2004.

United States Department of Health and Human Services Substance Abuse and Mental Health Services Administration: *The DSAIS report: characteristics of primary prescription and OTC treatment admissions: 2002*, 2004, http://www.oas.samhsa.gov/2k4/prescriptionTX/ prescription.htm.

United States Pharmacopeia: *Similar drug names continue to be reported*, 2003, http://www.usp.org/patientSafety/newsletters/ practitionerReportingNews/prn1082003-10-23.html

VisionRx: *Encyclopedia: eye drops*, 2004, http://www.visionrx.com/ library/enc/enc_eyedrops.asp.

West, JF: Feeding the adult with neurogenic disorders, *Topics in Geriatric Rehabilitation* 20(2):131, 2004.

Zurlinden J: Double check IV push, *Nurs Spectr* 15(25IL):16, 2002.

# Fluid, Electrolyte, and Acid-Base Balance

## MEDIA RESOURCES

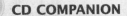 **CD COMPANION** 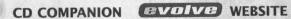 **WEBSITE**

http://evolve.elsevier.com/Potter/basic

- **NCLEX® Review**
- **Audio Glossary**
- **English/Spanish Audio Glossary**
- **Video Clips**
- **Butterfield's Fluids and Electrolytes Program**

## OBJECTIVES

- Describe the basic physiological mechanism responsible for maintaining fluid and electrolyte balance.
- Describe the processes involved in acid-base balance.
- Discuss common disturbances in fluid, electrolyte, and acid-base balances.
- Discuss variables that affect fluid, electrolyte, and acid-base balances.
- Discuss clinical assessments for fluid, electrolyte, and acid-base imbalances.
- List and discuss appropriate nursing interventions for patients with fluid, electrolyte, and acid-base imbalances.

- Describe procedures for initiating and maintaining fluid balance.
- Discuss complications of intravenous therapy.
- Discuss complications of total parenteral nutrition.
- Describe the procedure for initiating a blood transfusion and the complications of blood therapy.
- Identify appropriate nursing interventions for nurses to delegate.

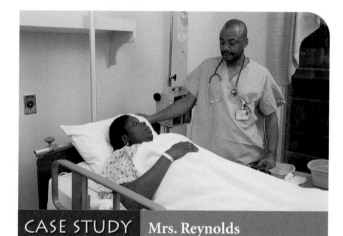

## CASE STUDY  Mrs. Reynolds

Susan Reynolds, a 42-year-old African-American married accountant, has just been admitted to the medical-surgical unit with a history of nausea, loss of appetite for 3 days, and vomiting and diarrhea for 2 days. She feels her symptoms are related to "bad food" she had on her recent business trip. Past medical history includes hypertension controlled by Lasix 40 mg once a day and a no-salt-added diet. After obtaining a blood sample for electrolytes, complete blood count, and an electrocardiogram (ECG), the physician has admitted her for observation. He has ordered that she have nothing by mouth (NPO) and have an intravenous (IV) infusion of 0.45% normal saline at 125 ml/hr inserted. He has also ordered for her to be on intake and output (I&O) recordings and vital signs every 4 hours, with daily weights.

Robert is a junior nursing student assigned to Mrs. Reynolds. He is 35 years old, married with three young children, and a former paramedic. Although this is somewhat of a career change for him, after two semesters of medical-surgical nursing he has enjoyed each rotation and he is sure a career in nursing is for him.

## KEY TERMS

active transport, p. 429
aldosterone, p. 430
angiotensin, p. 430
anion gap, p. 434
anions, p. 428
antidiuretic hormone (ADH), p. 430
autologous transfusion, p. 474
buffer, p. 431
cations, p. 428
colloid osmotic pressure, p. 429
concentration gradient, p. 428
dehydration, p. 430
diffusion, p. 428
electrolyte, p. 428
electronic infusion device, p. 446
extracellular fluid (ECF), p. 428
filtration, p. 429
fluid volume deficit (FVD), p. 436
fluid volume excess (FVE), p. 445
hemolysis, p. 474
homeostasis, p. 429
hydrostatic pressure, p. 429
hypertonic, p. 429
hypotonic, p. 429

hypovolemia, p. 429
infiltration, p. 466
infusion pump, p. 460
insensible water loss, p. 430
interstitial fluid, p. 428
intracellular fluid (ICF), p. 428
intravascular fluid, p. 428
isotonic, p. 429
metabolic acidosis, p. 434
metabolic alkalosis, p. 434
milliequivalents per liter (mEq/L), p. 428
oncotic pressure, p. 429
osmolality, p. 429
osmolarity, p. 429
osmoreceptors, p. 429
osmosis, p. 428
osmotic pressure, p. 428
parenteral nutrition (PN), p. 445
peripherally inserted central catheter (PICC), p. 447
phlebitis, p. 466

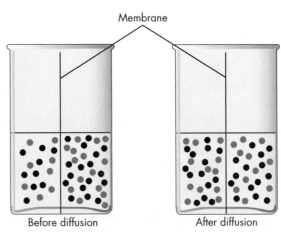

FIGURE **15-1** Diffusion across a semipermeable membrane. (From Lewis SM and others: *Medical-surgical nursing: assessment and management of clinical problems,* ed 4, St. Louis, 2002, Mosby.)

Fluid, electrolyte, and acid-base balances within the body are necessary to maintain health and function in all body systems. Intake and output of water and electrolytes, their distribution in the body, and the regulation of renal and pulmonary function contribute to maintain homeostasis. Imbalances result from many factors, including illnesses, altered fluid intake, or prolonged episodes of vomiting or diarrhea. Acid-base balance is necessary for many physiological processes. Imbalances alter respiration, metabolism, cardiovascular and renal function, and the functioning of the central nervous system.

## Scientific Knowledge Base

Water is the largest single component of the body; 60% of the average 30-year-old adult male and 50% of the average female weight is fluid. A healthy, mobile, well-oriented adult is usually capable of maintaining normal fluid, electrolyte, and acid-base balances because of the body's adaptive physiological mechanisms.

### Distribution of Body Fluids

Body fluids are distributed in two distinct compartments, one containing **intracellular fluid (ICF)** and the other **extracellular fluid (ECF)**. ICF comprises all fluid within body cells. This fluid contains dissolved solutes essential to fluid and electrolyte balance and metabolism. In adults approximately 40% of body weight is ICF (Huether and McCance, 2004).

ECF is all fluid outside a cell, which is divided into two smaller compartments: **interstitial** and **intravascular fluids.** Interstitial fluid is the fluid between cells and outside the blood vessels. Intravascular fluid is blood plasma. Other extravascular fluids are the lymph, transcellular, and organ fluids (Huether and McCance, 2004). ECF makes up about 20% of the total body weight.

### Composition of Body Fluids

Body fluid contains substances that are sometimes called minerals or salts but are technically known as electrolytes. An **electrolyte** is an element or compound that, when dissolved in water or another **solvent,** separates into ions and is able to carry an electric current. Positively charged electrolytes are **cations.** Negatively charged electrolytes are **anions.** Although the accumulation of electrolytes differs in ECF and ICF, the total number of anions and cations in each fluid compartment is usually the same. You measure electrolytes in **milliequivalents per liter (mEq/L).**

### Movement of Body Fluids

Fluids and electrolytes constantly shift from compartment to compartment to meet a variety of metabolic needs. The movement of fluids depends on cell membrane permeability.

**Diffusion** (Figure 15-1) is a process in which a **solute** (gas or substance) in a **solution** moves from an area of higher concentration to an area of lower concentration, evenly distributing the solute in the solution. For example, when you pour a small amount of cream into a cup of black coffee, the cream mixes or diffuses through the whole cup of coffee. The difference in the two concentrations is known as a **concentration gradient.** Fluids and electrolytes diffuse across cellular membranes. For a substance to cross the membrane, the membrane must be permeable to it.

**Osmosis** is the movement of water across a semipermeable membrane from an area of lower concentration to one that has a higher concentration (Figure 15-2). Osmosis equalizes the concentration of molecules (ions) on each side of the membrane. Boiling a hot dog is an example of osmosis. The concentration of molecules inside the hot dog is greater than in water. The water passes through the hot dog skin, which is a semipermeable membrane, in an attempt to equalize the number of molecules on both sides of the membrane. Finally, when the hot dog is unable to hold more water, the skin, or semipermeable membrane, ruptures.

When you have a more concentrated solution on one side of a selectively permeable membrane and a less concentrated solution on the other side, there is a pull called **osmotic pressure** that draws the water through the membrane to the

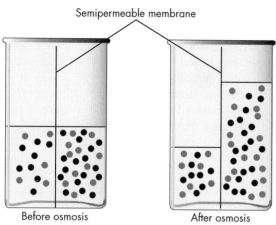

FIGURE **15-2** Osmosis through a semipermeable membrane. (From Lewis SM and others: *Medical-surgical nursing: assessment and management of clinical problems,* ed 4, St. Louis, 2002, Mosby.)

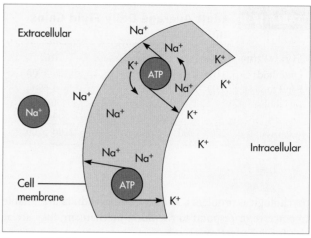

FIGURE **15-3** The sodium-potassium pump. (From Lewis SM and others: *Medical-surgical nursing: assessment and management of clinical problems,* ed 4, St. Louis, 2002, Mosby.)

more concentrated side. When the solutions on both sides of the semipermeable membrane have established equilibrium, or are equal in concentration, they are isotonic. The measure of a solution's ability to create osmotic pressure and thus affect the movement of water is **osmolality.** Changes in extracellular osmolality sometimes results in changes in both ECF and ICF volume.

**Osmolarity,** another term used to describe the concentration of solutions, reflects the number of molecules in a liter of solution and is measured in milliosmoles per liter (mOsm/L). Solutions are classified as **hypertonic, isotonic,** or **hypotonic.** Hypertonic (a solution of higher osmotic pressure) solutions pull fluid from cells; isotonic (a solution of same osmotic pressure) solutions expand the body's fluid volume without causing a fluid shift from one compartment to another; and hypotonic (a solution of lower osmotic pressure) solutions move into the cells, causing them to enlarge. Each of these actions occurs through osmosis.

Diffusion and osmosis are passive processes that do not require energy from the body's cells. **Active transport** is the movement of molecules or ions "uphill" against osmotic pressures to areas of higher concentration. An example of active transport found in the body is the sodium-potassium-ATPase pump, which moves sodium to the outside of the cell and then returns potassium to the inside of the cell (Figure 15-3).

**Hydrostatic pressure** is the force of the fluid pressing outward against a surface. When there is a difference in the hydrostatic pressure on two sides of a membrane, water and diffusible solutes move out of the solution that has the higher hydrostatic pressure. This process is called **filtration.** At the arterial end of the capillary, the hydrostatic pressure is greater than the **colloid osmotic pressure** (oncotic pressure), causing fluid and diffusible solutes to move out of the capillary into the interstitial space. At the venous end, the colloid osmotic pressure (**oncotic pressure**), or pull, is

greater than the hydrostatic pressure, and fluids and some solutes move into the capillary from the interstitial space. The lymph channels return excess fluid and solutes in the interstitial space to the intravascular compartment. The pressure at the capillary bed is called colloid osmotic pressure. The body does not allow blood plasma proteins to pass freely because the capillary membrane is impermeable to proteins (colloids). Forcing the blood proteins to stay within the capillary enhances the osmotic pressure.

### Regulation of Body Fluids

Body fluids maintain balance through the process of **homeostasis.** Fluid intake, hormonal controls, and fluid output regulate body fluids. In health, the body readily responds to disturbances in fluids and electrolytes to prevent or repair damage.

**FLUID INTAKE.** The thirst mechanism, a major factor influencing fluid intake, primarily regulates fluid intake. The thirst-control center is in the hypothalamus. The **osmoreceptors** continually monitor the serum osmotic pressure, and when osmolality increases, the hypothalamus stimulates thirst. Eating salty foods increases the osmotic pressure of the body fluids and stimulates the thirst mechanism. Increased plasma osmolality occurs with any condition that interferes with the oral ingestion of fluids, or it occurs with the intake of hypertonic fluids. The hypothalamus also is stimulated when excess fluid is lost, and **hypovolemia** occurs, as in excessive vomiting and hemorrhage.

The average adult's fluid intake (Table 15-1) is about 2200 to 2700 ml per day; oral intake accounts for 1100 to 1400 ml, solid foods about 800 to 1000 ml, and oxidative metabolism 300 ml daily (Heitz and Horne, 2005). Water oxidation (oxidative metabolism) is the by-product of cellular metabolism of ingested solid foods. Fluid intake requires an alert state. Infants, patients with neurological or

| TABLE 15-1 | Adult Average Daily Fluid Gains and Losses | | |
|---|---|---|---|
| **Fluid Gains** | **(ml)** | **Fluid Losses** | **(ml)** |
| Oral fluids | 1100-1400 | Kidneys | 1200-1500 |
| Solid foods | 800-1000 | Skin | 500-600 |
| Metabolism | 300 | Lungs | 400 |
| | | Gastrointestinal | 100-200 |
| TOTAL GAINS | 2200-2700 | TOTAL LOSSES | 2200-2700 |

psychological problems, and some older adults are unable to perceive or respond to the thirst mechanism; they are at risk for **dehydration.**

**HORMONAL REGULATION. Antidiuretic hormone (ADH)** stored in the posterior pituitary gland is released in response to changes in the blood osmolarity. ADH prevents diuresis, thus causing the body to save water. When there is an increase in the osmolarity, stimulation of the osmoreceptors in the hypothalamus causes a release of ADH. The ADH works directly on the renal tubules and collecting ducts to make them more permeable to water. This in turn causes water to return to the systemic circulation, diluting the blood and decreasing its osmolarity. The patient will experience a decrease in urinary output as the body tries to compensate. When the blood has been sufficiently diluted, the osmoreceptors stop the release of ADH.

The adrenal cortex releases **aldosterone** in response to increased plasma potassium levels or as a part of the renin-angiotensin-aldosterone mechanism to counteract hypovolemia. It acts on the distal portion of the renal tubule to increase the reabsorption (saving) of sodium and the secretion and excretion of potassium and hydrogen. Because sodium retention leads to water retention, the release of aldosterone acts as a volume regulator (Heitz and Horne, 2005).

**Renin,** an enzyme, responds to decreased renal perfusion secondary to a decrease in extracellular volume. Renin acts to produce angiotensin I, which causes some vasoconstriction. However, **angiotensin** I almost immediately becomes reduced by an enzyme that converts angiotension I into angiotensin II. Angiotensin II then causes massive selective vasoconstriction of many blood vessels and relocates and increases the blood flow to the kidney, improving renal perfusion. In addition, angiotensin II also stimulates the release of aldosterone.

**FLUID OUTPUT REGULATION.** Fluid output (see Table 15-1) occurs through four organs of water loss: the kidneys, skin, lungs, and gastrointestinal (GI) tract. The kidneys are the major regulatory organs of fluid balance. They receive approximately 180 L of plasma to filter each day and produce 1200 to 1500 ml of urine. The sympathetic nervous system regulates water loss from the skin by activating sweat glands. Water loss from the skin is either a sensible or insensible loss. The human body loses an average of 500 to 600 ml of sensible and insensible fluid via the skin each day (Heitz

and Horne, 2005). **Insensible water loss** is continuous and nonperceptual. **Sensible water loss** occurs through excess perspiration that the patient or the nurse assesses through inspection. The amount of sensible perspiration is directly related to the stimulation of the sweat glands.

The lungs expire about 400 ml of water daily. This insensible water loss sometimes increases in response to changes in respiratory rate and depth. In addition, devices for giving oxygen increase insensible water loss from the lungs.

Under normal conditions, the GI tract accounts for only 100 to 200 ml of fluid loss each day, yet it plays a vital role in fluid regulation because it is the site of nearly all intake of fluid. In disease, however, the GI tract sometimes becomes a site of major fluid loss because approximately 3 to 6 L of isotonic fluid is secreted into and reabsorbed out of the GI tract daily.

## Regulation of Electrolytes

**CATIONS.** Major cations within the body fluids include sodium ($Na^+$), potassium ($K^+$), calcium ($Ca^{++}$), and magnesium ($Mg^{++}$). Cations interchange when one cation leaves the cell and another one replaces it. This occurs because cells tend to maintain electrical neutrality.

**Sodium Regulation.** Sodium is the most abundant cation (90%) in ECF. Sodium ions are the major contributors to maintaining water balance through their effect on serum osmolality, nerve impulse transmission, regulation of acid-base balance, and participation in cellular chemical reactions (Huether and McCance, 2004). Dietary intake and aldosterone secretion regulate sodium. The normal extracellular sodium concentration is 135 to 145 mEq/L.

**Potassium Regulation.** Potassium is the predominant intracellular cation; only 2% is in ECF. It regulates many metabolic activities and is necessary for glycogen deposits in the liver and skeletal muscle, transmission and conduction of nerve impulses, normal cardiac rhythms, and skeletal and smooth muscle contraction (Huether and McCance, 2004). The normal range for serum potassium concentrations is 3.5 to 5 mEq/L. Dietary intake and renal excretion regulate potassium. The body does not conserve potassium well, so any condition that increases urine output will result in decreased serum potassium.

**Calcium Regulation.** Bone, plasma, and body cells store calcium. Ninety-nine percent of calcium is in the bones, and only 1% is in ECF. Approximately 50% of calcium in the plasma is bound to protein, primarily albumin, and 40% is free ionized calcium. Normal serum ionized calcium ranges from 4 to 5 mEq/L. Normal total calcium is 8.5 to 10.5 mg/dl. Bone and teeth formation, blood clotting, hormone secretion, cell membrane integrity, cardiac conduction, transmission of nerve impulses, and muscle contraction require calcium.

**Magnesium Regulation.** Magnesium is essential for enzyme activities, neurochemical activities, and cardiac and skeletal muscle excitability. Plasma concentrations of magnesium range from 1.5 to 2.5 mEq/L. Dietary intake, renal mechanisms, and actions of parathyroid hormone (PTH) regulate serum magnesium.

**ANIONS.** The three major anions of body fluids are chloride ($Cl^-$), bicarbonate ($HCO_3$), and phosphate ($PO_4^{-3}$) ions.

**Chloride Regulation.** Chloride is the major anion in ECF. The transport of chloride follows sodium. Normal concentrations of chloride range from 95 to 108 mEq/L. Dietary intake and the kidneys regulate serum chloride. A person with normal renal function who has a high chloride intake will excrete a higher amount of urine chloride.

**Bicarbonate Regulation.** Bicarbonate is the major chemical base buffer within the body. The bicarbonate ion is in ECF and ICF. The bicarbonate ion is an essential component of the carbonic acid-bicarbonate buffering system essential to acid-base balance. The kidneys regulate bicarbonate. Normal arterial bicarbonate levels range between 22 and 26 mEq/L; venous bicarbonate is measured as carbon dioxide content, and the normal value is 24 to 30 mEq/L.

**Phosphorus-Phosphate Regulation.** Nearly all the phosphorus in the body exists in the form of phosphate ($PO^{-}_4$), which assists in the regulation of acid-base regulation. Phosphate and calcium help to develop and maintain bones and teeth. Generally calcium and phosphate are inversely proportional; if one rises, the other falls. Phosphate also promotes normal neuromuscular action and participates in carbohydrate metabolism. The body normally absorbs phosphate through the GI tract. Dietary intake, renal excretion, intestinal absorption, and PTH regulate phosphate. The normal serum level is 2.5 to 4.5 mg/dl.

## Regulation of Acid-Base Balance

Metabolic processes maintain a steady balance between acids and bases for optimal functioning of cells. Arterial pH is an indirect measurement of hydrogen ion ($H^+$) concentration. For example, the greater the concentration of $H^+$ ions, the more acidic the solution and the lower the pH; the lower the concentration of $H^+$ ions, the more alkaline the solution and the higher the pH. pH is also a reflection of the balance between carbon dioxide ($CO_2$), which the lungs regulate, and bicarbonate ($HCO_3$), a base, which the kidneys regulate. Acid-base balance exists when the net rate at which the body produces acids or bases equals the rate at which the body excretes acids or bases. This balance results in a stable concentration of hydrogen ions ($H^+$) in body fluids, expressed as the pH value. Normal hydrogen ion level is necessary to maintain cell membrane integrity and the speed of cellular enzymatic reactions. A pH value of 7 is neutral; below 7 is acid, and above 7 is alkaline. Normal values in arterial blood range from 7.35 to 7.45.

The three general types of acid-base regulators within the body are chemical (the carbonic acid-bicarbonate buffer system), biological (the absorption and release of hydrogen ions by cells), and physiological buffering systems (the lungs and the kidneys). A **buffer** is a substance or a group of substances that absorb or release $H^+$ to correct an acid-base imbalance.

## Disturbances in Electrolyte, Fluid, and Acid-Base Balance

Disturbances in electrolyte, fluid, or acid-base balances seldom occur alone and disrupt normal body processes (Table 15-2). When there is a loss of body fluids because of burns, illnesses, or trauma, the patient is also at risk for electrolyte imbalances. In addition, some untreated electrolyte imbalances (e.g., potassium loss) result in acid-base disturbances.

### ELECTROLYTE IMBALANCES

**Sodium Imbalances.** Hyponatremia is a lower-than-normal concentration of sodium in the blood (serum), which occurs with a net sodium loss or net water excess (see Table 15-2). Clinical treatment depends on the cause and whether the EDF volume is normal, decreased, or increased. The usual situation is a loss of sodium without a loss of fluid, and this results in a decrease in the osmolality of ECF. The initial body adaptation is the reduction of water excretion and thus sodium excretion to maintain serum osmolality at near-normal levels. As the sodium loss continues, the body preserves the blood and interstitial (tissue) volume. As a result, the sodium in ECF becomes diluted.

Hypernatremia is a greater-than-normal concentration of sodium in ECF. Excess water loss or overall sodium excess is often the cause of this (see Table 15-2). When the cause of hypernatremia is increased aldosterone secretion, the body retains sodium and excretes potassium. When hypernatremia occurs, the body attempts to conserve as much water as possible through renal reabsorption.

**Potassium Imbalances.** Hypokalemia is one of the most common electrolyte imbalances in which an inadequate amount of potassium circulates in ECF (see Table 15-2). When severe, hypokalemia affects cardiac conduction and function. Because the normal amount of serum potassium is so small, there is little tolerance for fluctuations. The most common cause is the use of potassium-wasting diuretics, such as thiazide and loop diuretics.

Hyperkalemia is a greater-than-normal amount of potassium in the blood. Severe hyperkalemia produces marked cardiac conduction abnormalities. The primary cause of hyperkalemia is renal failure because any decrease in renal function diminishes the amount of potassium the kidney is able to excrete.

**Calcium Imbalances.** Hypocalcemia represents a drop in serum and/or ionized calcium. It results from several illnesses, some of which directly affect the thyroid and parathyroid glands (see Table 15-2). Another cause is renal insufficiency (kidneys unable to excrete phosphorus, causing the phosphorus level to rise and the calcium level to decline). Signs and symptoms are related to the physiological role of serum calcium in neuromuscular function.

Hypercalcemia is an increase in the total serum concentration of calcium and/or ionized calcium. Hypercalcemia is frequently a symptom of an underlying disease resulting in excess bone resorption with release of calcium.

## TABLE 15-2  Electrolyte Imbalances

| Causes | Signs and Symptoms |
|---|---|
| **Hyponatremia** | |
| Kidney disease resulting in salt wasting<br>Adrenal insufficiency<br>GI losses<br>Increased sweating<br>Use of diuretics, especially when combined with low-sodium diet<br>Psychogenic polydipsia<br>Syndrome of inappropriate ADH (SIADH) | *Physical examination:* apprehension, personality change, confusion, postural hypotension, postural dizziness, abdominal cramping, nausea and vomiting, diarrhea, tachycardia, convulsions, coma, and fingerprints remaining on sternum after palpation<br>*Laboratory findings:* serum sodium level <135 mEq/L, serum osmolality <280 mOsm/kg, and urine specific gravity <1.010 (if not caused by SIADH) |
| **Hypernatremia** | |
| Ingestion of large amounts of concentrated salt solutions<br>Iatrogenic administration of hypertonic saline solution parenterally<br>Excess aldosterone secretion<br>Diabetes insipidus<br>Increased sensible and insensible water loss<br>Water deprivation | *Physical examination:* thirst, dry and flushed skin, dry and sticky tongue and mucous membranes, fever, agitation, convulsions, restlessness, and irritability<br>*Laboratory findings:* serum sodium levels >145 mEq/L, serum osmolality >295 mOsm/kg, and urine specific gravity >1.030 (if not caused by diabetes insipidus) |
| **Hypokalemia** | |
| Use of potassium-wasting diuretics<br>Diarrhea, vomiting, or other GI losses<br>Alkalosis<br>Excess aldosterone secretion<br>Polyuria<br>Extreme sweating<br>Excessive use of potassium-free IV solutions<br>Treatment of diabetic ketoacidosis with insulin | *Physical examination:* weakness and fatigue, decreased muscle tone, intestinal distention, decreased bowel sounds, ventricular dysrhythmias, paresthesias, and weak, irregular pulse<br>*Laboratory findings:* serum potassium level <3.5 mEq/L and ECG abnormalities (e.g., ventricular dysrhythmias)* |
| **Hyperkalemia** | |
| Renal failure<br>Fluid volume deficit<br>Massive cellular damage such as from burns and trauma<br>Iatrogenic administration of large amounts of potassium intravenously<br>Adrenal insufficiency<br>Acidosis, especially diabetic ketoacidosis<br>Rapid infusion of stored blood<br>Use of potassium-sparing diuretics | *Physical examination:* anxiety, dysrhythmias, paresthesias, weakness, abdominal cramps, and diarrhea<br>*Laboratory findings:* serum potassium level >5.3 mEq/L and ECG abnormalities (bradycardia, heart block, dysrhythmias); eventually QRS pattern widens and cardiac arrest occurs* |

**Magnesium Imbalances.** Table 15-2 summarizes disturbances in magnesium levels. Symptoms are the result of changes in neuromuscular excitability.

**Chloride Imbalances.** Hypochloremia occurs when the serum chloride level falls below normal. Vomiting or prolonged and excessive nasogastric or fistula drainage sometimes results in hypochloremia because of the loss of hydrochloric acid. The use of loop and thiazide diuretics also increases chloride excretion as sodium is excreted. When serum chloride levels fall, metabolic alkalosis occurs. The body adapts by increasing reabsorption of the bicarbonate ion to maintain electrical neutrality.

Hyperchloremia occurs when the serum chloride level rises above normal, which usually occurs when the serum bicarbonate value falls or sodium level rises. Hypochloremia and hyperchloremia rarely occur as single disease processes but are commonly associated with acid-base imbalance. There is no single set of symptoms associated with these two alterations.

**FLUID DISTURBANCES.** The basic types of fluid imbalances are isotonic and osmolar. Isotonic deficit and excess exist when water and electrolytes are either gained or lost in equal proportions. In contrast, osmolar imbalances are losses or excesses of only water, affecting the concentration (osmolality) of the serum. Table 15-3 lists the causes and symptoms of common fluid disturbances.

**ACID-BASE IMBALANCES.** Arterial blood gas (ABG) analysis is the best way of evaluating acid-base balance. When we measure ABG levels, we look at six components:

| **TABLE 15-2** | **Electrolyte Imbalances—cont'd** |
|---|---|
| **Causes** | **Signs and Symptoms** |

| **Causes** | **Signs and Symptoms** |
|---|---|
| **Hypocalcemia** | |
| Rapid administration of blood transfusions containing citrate<br>Hypoalbuminemia<br>Hypoparathyroidism<br>Vitamin D deficiency<br>Pancreatitis<br>Alkalosis | *Physical examination:* numbness and tingling of fingers and circumoral region, hyperactive reflexes, positive Trousseau's sign (carpopedal spasm with hypoxia), positive Chvostek's sign (contraction of facial muscles when facial nerve is tapped), tetany, muscle cramps, and pathological fractures (chronic hypocalcemia)<br>*Laboratory findings:* serum calcium level <4.0 mEq/L or 8.5 mg/100 ml and ECG abnormalities |
| **Hypercalcemia** | |
| Hyperparathyroidism<br>Malignant neoplastic disease<br>Paget's disease<br>Osteoporosis<br>Prolonged immobilization<br>Acidosis | *Physical examination:* anorexia, nausea and vomiting, constipation, weakness, lethargy, low back pain (from kidney stones), decreased level of consciousness, personality changes, and cardiac arrest<br>*Laboratory findings:* serum calcium level >5 mEq/L or 10.5 mg/100 ml; x-ray examination showing generalized osteoporosis, widespread bone cavitation, radiopaque urinary stones; elevated blood urea nitrogen (BUN) level >25 mg/100 ml and elevated creatinine level >1.5 mg/100 ml caused by fluid volume deficit (FVD) or renal damage caused by urolithiasis; and ECG abnormalities |
| **Hypomagnesemia** | |
| Inadequate intake: malnutrition and alcoholism<br>Inadequate absorption: diarrhea, vomiting, nasogastric drainage, fistulas; diseases of small intestine<br>Excessive loss resulting from thiazide diuretics<br>Aldosterone excess<br>Polyuria | *Physical examination:* muscular tremors, hyperactive deep tendon reflexes, confusion and disorientation, dysrhythmias, and positive Chvostek's sign and Trousseau's sign<br>*Laboratory findings:* serum magnesium level <1.5 mEq/L |
| **Hypermagnesemia** | |
| Renal failure<br>Excess oral or parenteral intake of magnesium | *Physical examination:* physical findings that are more frequent in acute elevations in magnesium levels: hypoactive deep tendon reflexes, decreased depth and rate of respirations, hypotension, and flushing<br>*Laboratory findings:* serum magnesium level >2.5 mEq/L |

*Data from Heitz U, Horne MM: *Mosby's pocket guide series: fluid, electrolyte, and acid-base balance,* ed 5, St. Louis, 2005, Mosby.

pH, $PaCO_2$, $PaO_2$, oxygen saturation, base excess, and $HCO_3^-$. Deviation from a normal value indicates that the patient is experiencing an acid-base imbalance.

**pH.** pH measures $H^+$ ion concentration in body fluids. Even a slight change is potentially life threatening. An increase in concentration of hydrogen ions ($H^+$) makes a solution more acidic; a decrease makes the solution more alkaline. The normal arterial blood pH value is 7.35 to 7.45 (acidic is less than 7.35, and alkalotic is more than 7.45).

**$PaCO_2$.** $PaCO_2$ is the partial pressure of carbon dioxide in arterial blood and is a reflection of the depth of pulmonary ventilation. Normal range is 35 to 45 mm Hg. A $PaCO_2$ of less than 35 mm Hg indicates that hyperventilation has occurred. As rate and depth of respiration increase,

the patient exhales more carbon dioxide and the carbon dioxide concentration decreases. A $PaCO_2$ of more than 45 mm Hg indicates hypoventilation. As rate and depth of respiration decrease, the patient exhales less carbon dioxide, retaining more carbon dioxide, which increases the concentration of carbon dioxide.

**$PaO_2$.** $PaO_2$ is the partial pressure of oxygen in arterial blood. It has no primary role in acid-base regulation if it is within normal limits. A $PaO_2$ less than 60 mm Hg leads to anaerobic metabolism, resulting in lactic acid production and metabolic acidosis. There is a normal decline in $PaO_2$ in older adults. Hypoxemia sometimes causes hyperventilation, resulting in respiratory alkalosis. Normal range is 80 to 100 mm Hg.

## FOCUSED PATIENT ASSESSMENT

TABLE 15-6

| Factors to Assess | Questions and Approaches | Physical Assessment Strategies |
|---|---|---|
| Vital signs | Ask patient about experiencing dizziness when changing positions. | When patient gets out of bed, monitor patient's blood pressure for decrease consistent with orthostatic hypotension. Observe patient for other signs of orthostatic hypotension (e.g., dizziness, light-headedness). |
| | Ask if patient feels a "racing heart rate." | Palpate patient's pulse, or auscultate heart rate. |
| Intake and output | Ask patient about usual I&O patterns. | Monitor patient's 24- and/or 36-hour I&O amount. |
| | Ask patient to specify if there has been a significant increase or decrease in I&O. | Inspect patient's urine and vomitus or diarrhea, if applicable. |
| | Determine cause of the I&O change. | |
| Skin turgor | Ask patient about skin dryness, or swelling. | Obtain a baseline weight, and monitor weight daily. Inspect patient's skin, palpate for turgor and edema. |
| | Determine if patient has experienced any itching or changes in the skin, and have patient explain. | Inspect for any skin changes. |

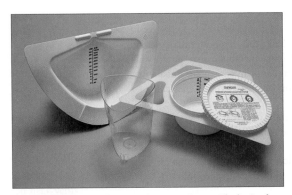

FIGURE **15-4** Graduated measuring containers. *Clockwise from top left:* "hat" receptacle, specimen, and measurement container.

electrolytes to determine the hydration status, the electrolyte concentration of the blood plasma, and acid-base balance. The frequency with which you measure these electrolytes depends on the severity of the patient's illness. You routinely perform serum electrolyte tests on any patient entering a hospital to screen for alterations and to serve as a baseline for future comparisons.

The complete blood count (CBC) is a measure of the number and type of red and white blood cells per cubic millimeter of blood. As long as a patient is not anemic, the hematocrit is an indication of the hydration status of the patient. The hematocrit will increase (become more concentrated) in situations where fluid is lost, whereas it will decrease in situations in which fluid is excessively retained in the vascular space.

Blood creatinine levels measure kidney function. Creatinine is a normal by-product of muscle metabolism, and the kidneys excrete it at fairly constant levels, regardless of factors such as fluid intake, diet, or exercise. Therefore it provides a measure of renal function that is relatively independent of the hydration status of the patient or the patient's dietary intake. BUN is the amount of nitrogenous substance present in the blood as urea. It is a rough indicator of kidney function.

Serum osmolality measures the concentration of the plasma. The osmolality decreases with hypoosmolar fluid imbalance (water excess) or hyponatremia. Decreased serum osmolality results in osmosis, which moves fluid into body cells (cellular edema). Osmolality increases with hyperosmolar fluid imbalance (water deficit) or hypernatremia or other gains of solutes such as glucose. Fluid moves out of body cells and into the interstitial space (cellular shrinkage). Both cellular edema and shrinkage disrupt normal cell processes.

The urine specific gravity test measures the urine's degree of concentration and evaluates the kidney's ability to conserve or excrete water. The specific gravity normally ranges between 1.010 and 1.025.

ABG analysis provides information on the status of acid-base balance and the effectiveness of ventilatory function in providing normal oxygen-carbon dioxide exchange (Table 15-7). You need to understand that you evaluate an ABG result in a systematic approach.

First, examine the pH; a value less than 7.35 is acidic and a value greater than 7.45 is alkalotic. Next, check the $PaCO_2$; the pH and $PaCO_2$ normally move in opposite directions. For example, as pH increases, the $PaCO_2$ normally decreases. Then you examine the $HCO_3^-$ (bicarbonate), and it is important to remember that the pH and $HCO_3^-$ move in the same direction. If the $PaCO_2$ and the $HCO_3^-$ are both abnormal, then you examine the value that corresponds more closely to the pH. The value that more closely corresponds to the pH and deviates more from the norm usually points to the primary disturbance responsible for altering the pH.

## SYNTHESIS IN PRACTICE

Robert reviews Mrs. Reynolds' clinical condition. The nursing history found in the medical record reveals that Mrs. Reynolds's loss of appetite, episodes of diarrhea, and continued use of Lasix (a non–potassium-sparing diuretic) for hypertension have placed her at risk for a fluid and electrolyte imbalance. The cause of her GI symptoms is unclear, although the physician or health care provider plans further diagnostic tests. Robert reviews the physiology of potassium as an electrolyte and studies the pathological findings of potassium excess and deficiency. He also reads recommendations in his pharmacology text on how to minimize the risk of hypokalemia when taking diuretics. Robert anticipates the need to perform a focused physical assessment of this patient tomorrow and to manage and monitor her IV therapy. He knows that patient education will eventually be important for this patient because her therapy for hypertension will likely continue.

Just a few weeks ago, Robert cared for a patient with ulcerative colitis. Although Mrs. Reynolds' condition is different, both patients had diarrhea. Robert knows that Mrs. Reynolds will require careful monitoring of I&O, as well as stabilization of GI function. The lessons learned from his previous patient will help Robert to be more alert if Mrs. Reynolds' clinical condition changes under his care.

Robert knows the importance of being accountable in completing an examination, assessing and documenting I&O, assessing vital signs, and administering medications in a timely manner. A well-organized approach to Mrs. Reynolds' care will minimize the chance of making errors.

Robert checks the policy and procedure manual at his institution for an IV therapy protocol. He reviews the new standards for dressing changes and is familiar with the procedure.

**PATIENT EXPECTATIONS.** Fluid and electrolyte or acid-base disturbances are either insidious or acute. If a patient is alert enough to discuss care with you, a review of expectations will sometimes reveal short-term needs, such as provision of comfort from nausea or IV placement, or long-term needs, such as understanding how to prevent alterations from occurring in the future. It is imperative that the patient understands the implications of fluid and electrolyte or acid-base changes in order to express expectations of care. Your competent response to sudden changes in patients' conditions and through communication with patients and/or family members will strengthen your patients' trust in you. Keeping your patients abreast of the changes and the interventions will allow them to be active participants in their care.

## Nursing Diagnosis

When caring for patients with suspected fluid, electrolyte, and acid-base imbalances, your skill in critical thinking is primary in formulating nursing diagnoses. The following is

### BOX 15-2 Laboratory Data for Fluid, Electrolyte, and Acid-Base Imbalances

**Fluid and Electrolytes**

Altered concentrations of sodium, potassium, magnesium, calcium, phosphates, chloride, and bicarbonate (venous $CO_2$ concentrations)

Increase in hematocrit, BUN, sodium, and osmolality in serum (related to loss of ECF fluid or gain of solutes)

Decrease in hematocrit, BUN, sodium, and osmolality in serum (related to gain of ECF fluid or loss of solutes)

Concentrated urine demonstrated by urine specific gravity >1.030

Dilute urine demonstrated by a specific gravity <1.012

**Metabolic Alkalosis**

pH >7.45
$PaCO_2$ normal or >45 mm Hg if lungs are compensating
$PaO_2$ normal
$O_2$ saturation ($SaO_2$) normal
$HCO_3^-$ >26 mEq/L
$K^+$ <3.5 mEq/L

**Metabolic Acidosis**

pH <7.35
$PaCO_2$ normal or <35 mm Hg if lungs are compensating
$PaO_2$ normal
$SaO_2$ normal
$HCO_3^-$ <22 mEq/L
$K^+$ >5.3 mEq/L
$K^+$ <3.5 mEq/L

**Respiratory Alkalosis**

pH >7.45
$PaCO_2$ <35 mm Hg
$PaO_2$ normal
$SaO_2$ normal
$HCO_3^-$ normal
$K^+$ <3.5 mEq/L

**Respiratory Acidosis**

pH <7.35
$PaCO_2$ >45 mm Hg
$PaO_2$ normal or <80 mm Hg, depending on cause of acidosis
$SaO_2$ normal or <95%, depending on cause of acidosis
$HCO_3^-$ normal if early respiratory acidosis or >26 mEq/L if kidneys are compensating
$K^+$ >5.3 mEq/L

an example of the multiple nursing diagnoses that you may identify from your patients' assessment data.

- Ineffective breathing pattern
- Decreased cardiac output
- Deficient fluid volume

SKILL 15-1 | Initiating a Peripheral Intravenous Infusion—cont'd

| STEP | RATIONALE |
|------|-----------|

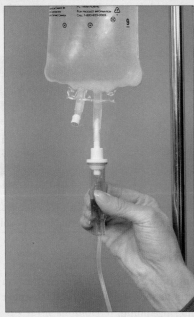

STEP **5f** Squeezing drip chamber to fill with fluid.

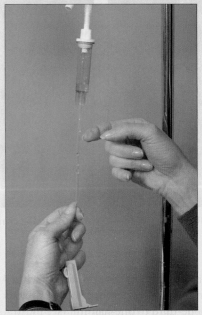

STEP **5h** Remove air bubbles from tubing.

---

• *Critical Decision Point:* You are able to add an extension tubing to IV tubing to allow for more length, which will enable patient to move more freely while still keeping IV line stable.

---

6. *Option:* Prepare heparin or normal saline lock for infusion:
   a. If a loop or short extension tubing is needed because of an awkward VAD site placement, use sterile technique to connect the IV plug (adapter) to the loop of short extension tubing. Inject 1 to 3 ml through the plug and through the loop or short extension tubing.

   Removes air to prevent introduction into the vein.

---

• *Critical Decision Point:* Gloves are not absolutely required to assess veins, but you need to apply them before insertion.

---

7. Identify accessible vein for placement of VAD. Apply tourniquet around arm above antecubital fossa (see illustration) or 4 to 6 inches (10 to 15 cm) above proposed insertion site. Do not apply tourniquet too tightly to avoid injury or bruising to skin. Check for presence of radial pulse. Tourniquet may be applied on top of a thin layer of clothing such as a gown sleeve. It will become necessary to remove tourniquet and move lower down arm. Optional: Apply blood pressure cuff instead of tourniquet. Inflate to a level just below the patient's normal diastolic pressure. Maintain inflation until venipuncture is completed.

   Tourniquet impedes venous return but should not occlude arterial flow. If vein cannot be found in antecubital fossa, move down along patient's arm to locate vessel in lower arm or hand.

   Use of blood pressure cuff reduces trauma to the underling skin and tissues.

| STEP | RATIONALE |
|------|-----------|
| 8. Select the vein for VAD insertion. The cephalic, basilic, and median cubital are preferred in adults (see Figure 15-5). | Venipuncture is performed distal to proximal, which increases the availability of other sites for future IV therapy. Hair impedes adherence of IV dressing. |
| a. Use the most distal site in the nondominant arm, if possible. Clip arm hair with scissors if necessary. | |

• *Critical Decision Point:* Do not shave area. Shaving may cause microabrasions and increase patient's risk for infection (INS, 2000).

| STEP | RATIONALE |
|------|-----------|
| b. Avoid areas that are painful to palpation. | May indicate inflammation. |
| c. Select a vein large enough for VAD. | Prevents interruption of venous flow while allowing adequate blood flow around the catheter. |
| d. Choose a site that will not interfere with patient's activities of daily living (ADLs) or planned procedures. | Keeps patient as mobile as possible. |
| e. Using your index finger, palpate the vein by pressing downward and noting the resilient, soft, bouncy feeling as you release pressure (see illustration). | Fingertip is more sensitive and is better to assess vein location and condition. |
| f. If possible, place extremity in dependent position from the heart. | Permits venous dilation and visibility. |
| g. Select well-dilated vein. Methods to foster venous distention include: | |
| (1) Stroking the extremity from distal to proximal below the proposed venipuncture site. | Promotes venous filling |
| (2) Applying warmth to the extremity for several minutes, for example, with a warm washcloth. | Increases blood supply and fosters venous dilation. |

• *Critical Decision Point:* Vigorous friction and multiple tapping of the veins, especially in older adults, will cause hematoma and/or venous constriction.

| STEP | RATIONALE |
|------|-----------|
| h. Avoid sites distal to previous venipuncture site, veins in antecubital fossa or inner wrist, sclerosed or hardened veins, infiltrate site or phlebotic vessels, bruised areas, and areas of venous valves. | Such sites cause infiltration of newly placed VAD and excessive vessel damage. Antecubital fossa is used for blood draws; also limits patient's mobility. |
| i. Avoid fragile dorsal veins in older adult patients and vessels in an extremity with compromised circulation (e.g., in cases of mastectomy, dialysis graft, or paralysis). | Venous alterations increase the risk of complications (e.g., infiltration and decreased catheter dwell time). |
| 9. Release tourniquet temporarily and carefully. | Restores blood flow while preparing for venipuncture. |

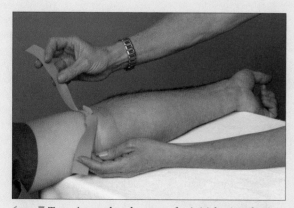

STEP **7** Tourniquet placed on arm for initial vein selection.

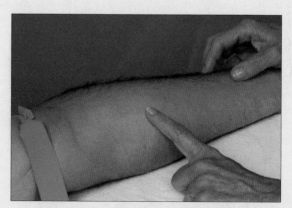

STEP **8e** Palpate vein for resilience.

| STEP | RATIONALE |
|---|---|
| 10. Apply disposable gloves. Wear eye protection and mask (see agency policy) if splash or spray of blood is possible. | Reduces transmission of microorganisms. Decreases exposure to HIV, hepatitis, and other blood-borne organisms (CDC, 2002) and prevents spraying of blood on nurse's mucous membranes. |
| 11. Place VAD adapter end of infusion set nearby on sterile gauze or sterile towel. | Permits smooth, quick connection of infusion to VAD once vein is accessed. |
| 12. If area of insertion appears to need cleansing, use soap and water first.) Use antiseptic swab agent to cleanse insertion site using friction in a horizontal plane, then a vertical plane followed with a circular motion (middle to outward); allow the agent to dry.<br><br>   Refrain from touching the cleansed site unless using sterile technique. | Mechanical friction in this pattern allows penetration of the antiseptic solution into the cracks and fissures of the epidermal layer of the skin (Crosby and Mares, 2001).<br>Antiseptic solutions should be allowed to air-dry completely to effectively reduce microbial counts (INS, 2000). If antiseptic solutions are used in combination, allow each to air-dry separately. Chlorhexidine 2% preparation is preferred (CDC, 2002).<br>Touching the cleansed area introduces organisms from your hand to the site. You would need to prepare the site again if you touch the clean area. |
| 13. Reapply tourniquet 10 to 12 cm (4 to 5 inches) above anticipated insertion site. Check presence of distal pulse. | Diminished arterial flow prevents venous filling. The pressure of the tourniquet causes the vein to dilate. |
| 14. Perform venipuncture. Anchor vein below site by placing thumb over vein and by stretching the skin against the direction of insertion 1½ to 2 inches (4 to 5 cm) distal to the site (see illustration). Warn patient of a sharp, quick stick. | Stabilizes vein for insertion. Places VAD parallel to vein. |
|   a. *Over-the-needle catheter (ONC) with safety device:* Insert with bevel up at 10- to 30-degree angle slightly distal to actual site of venipuncture in the direction of the vein. | Places needle at a 10- to 30-degree angle to the vein. When you puncture the vein, you reduce the risk of puncturing the posterior vein. Superficial veins require a smaller angle. Deeper veins require a greater angle. |
|   b. *IV catheter safety device:* Insert using same position as for ONC (see illustration). | IV safety devices should be available and used. |
|   c. *Winged cannula:* Hold needle at 10- to 30-degree angle with bevel up slightly distal to actual site of venipuncture. | |

• *Critical Decision Point:* Use each VAD only once for each insertion attempt.

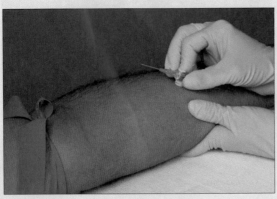

STEP **14** Stabilize vein below insertion site.

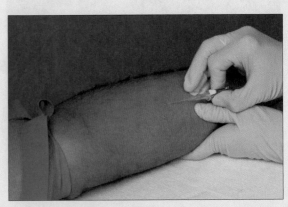

STEP **14b** Puncture skin with VAD at 10 to 30 degrees above vein.

| STEP | RATIONALE |
|---|---|
| **15.** Observe for blood return through flashback chamber of cannula or tubing of winged cannula, indicating that VAD has entered vein (see illustration). Lower catheter until almost flush with skin. Advance catheter approximately ¼ inch into vein and then loosen stylet if using ONC. Continue to hold skin taut and advance VAD into vein until hub rests at venipuncture site. *Do not reinsert the stylet once it is loosened.* Advance the safety device by using push-off tab to thread the catheter (see illustration). Advance winged cannula until hub rests at venipuncture site. | Increased venous pressure from tourniquet increases backflow of blood into catheter or tubing. Reinsertion of the stylet causes catheter breakage in the vein.<br>Allows for full penetration of the vein wall, placement of the cannula in the vein's inner lumen, and advancement of the cannula from the stylet. Reduces risk of introduction of microorganisms along cannula.<br>Reinsertion of stylet causes cannula shearing in vein. |

• *Critical Decision Point:* An individual nurse makes no more than two attempts at initiating the IV access.

| | |
|---|---|
| **16.** Stabilize cannula with one hand, and release tourniquet with other. Apply gentle but firm pressure with index finger of nondominant hand 1¼ inches (3 cm) above the insertion site (see illustration). Keep cannula stable. For the safety device, glide the catheter off the stylet while gliding the protective guard over the stylet. A click indicates the device is locked over the stylet. (NOTE: Techniques will vary with each IV device.) Remove the stylet of the ONC. If you can reach the sharps container, place the stylet directly into sharps container. If you cannot easily reach the sharps container, place the stylet on work area away from other supplies to prevent needlestick injury. | Permits venous flow, reduces backflow of blood, and allows connection with administration set with minimal blood loss. |

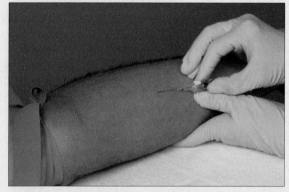 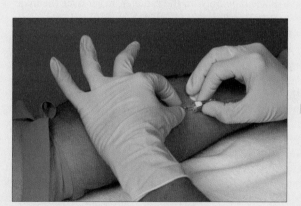

STEP **15 A,** Blood return in flashback chamber. **B,** Advance device into vein.

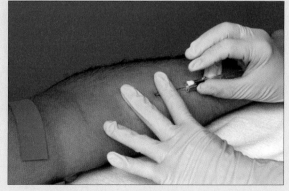 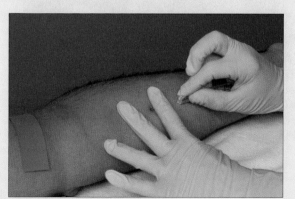

STEP **16 A,** Apply pressure above insertion site. **B,** Retract the stylet by pushing safety tab.

| STEP | RATIONALE |
|---|---|
| 17. Quickly connect end of the prepared saline lock (see illustration) or the infusion tubing set to end of catheter. Do not touch point of entry of connection. Secure connection. | Prompt connection of infusion set maintains patency of vein and prevents risk of exposure to blood. Maintains sterility. |
| 18. *Intermittent infusion:* Hold the sterile heparin/saline lock firmly with nondominant hand, cleaning with appropriate agent. Insert prefilled syringe containing flush solution into injection cap (see illustration). Flush slowly with flush solution. Withdraw the syringe while still flushing. | "Positive-pressure flushing" allows fluid to displace the removed needle, creates positive pressure in the catheter, and prevents reflux of blood during flushing. Stabilizing the cannula prevents accidental withdrawal or dislodgement. |
| 19. *Continuous infusion:* Begin infusion by slowly opening the slide clamp or adjusting the roller clamp of the IV tubing. | Initiates flow of fluid through IV catheter, preventing clotting of device. |

• *Critical Decision Point:* Be sure to calculate rate to regulate IV solution at prescribed rate.

| | |
|---|---|
| 20. Secure cannula (procedures can differ, follow agency policy). | |
|   a. *Transparent dressing:* Secure catheter with nondominant hand while preparing to apply dressing. | Prevents accidental dislodgement of catheter. |
|   b. *Sterile gauze dressing:* Place narrow piece (½ inch) of sterile tape under catheter hub with sticky side up, and cross tape over catheter hub (see illustrations). Place tape only on the catheter, never over the insertion site. Secure site to allow easy visual inspection. Avoid applying tape around the arm. | Prevents accidental removal of catheter from vein. Prevents back-and-forth motion, which irritates the vein and introduces bacteria on the skin into the vein. Adhesive tape is a potential source of bacteria. Use sterile tape close to IV site (CDC, 2002). |
| 21. Apply sterile dressing | |
|   **A. Transparent Dressing** | |
|     (1) Carefully remove adherent backing. Apply one edge of dressing, and then gently smooth remaining dressing over IV site, leaving connection between IV tubing and catheter hub uncovered (see illustration). Remove outer covering, and smooth dressing gently over site. | Occlusive dressing protects site from bacterial contamination. Connection between administration set and hub needs to remain uncovered to aid changing the tubing if necessary. The CDC (2002) does not recommend application of antimicrobial ointment to catheter site. |

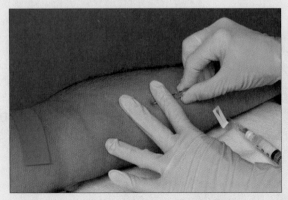

STEP **17** Connecting end of saline lock.

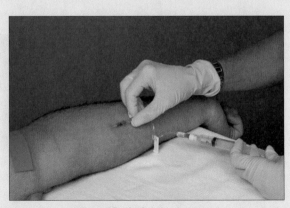

STEP **18** Flush injection cap.

| STEP | RATIONALE |
|---|---|

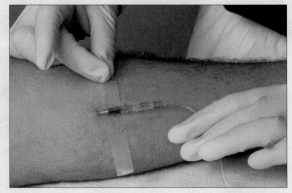
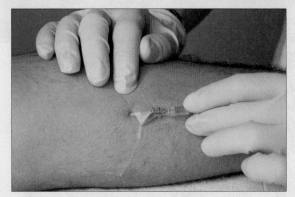

STEP **20B A,** Place tape under catheter hub. **B,** Chevron applied before gauze dressing.

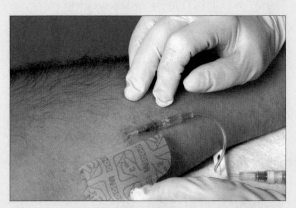
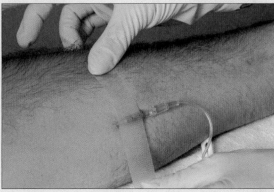

| STEP **21A(1)** Applying transparent dressing. | STEP **21A(2)** Place tape over transparent dressing. |
|---|---|

    (2) Take 1-inch piece of tape, and place it down from end of hub of catheter to insertion site, placing it over transparent dressing (see illustration).

    (3) Apply chevron, and place only over tape, not the transparent dressing.

**B. Sterile Gauze Dressing**

    (1) Fold a 2 × 2 gauze in half, and cover with a 1-inch-wide tape extending about an inch from each side. Place under the tubing/catheter hub junction (see illustration). Curl a loop of tubing alongside the arm, and place a second piece of tape directly over the tubing and padded 2 × 2, securing tubing in two places.

    (2) Place 2 × 2 gauze pad over insertion site and catheter hub. Secure all edges with tape. Do not cover connection between IV tubing and catheter hub.

22. Loop tubing alongside the arm, and place a second piece of tape directly over the tape covering the transparent dressing (see illustration) or over the padded 2 × 2.

23. For IV fluid administration, recheck flow rate to correct drops per minute (see Skill 15-2).

Tape on top of gauze makes it easier to access hub/tubing junction. Gauze pad elevates hub off skin to prevent pressure area. Securing loop of tubing reduces risk of dislodging catheter should the IV tubing get pulled (i.e., the loop would come apart before the catheter dislodges).

Secures IV tubing and reduces the risk of accidental dislodgement of IV catheter.

Manipulation of catheter during dressing application alters flow rate. Maintains correct rate of flow for IV solution. Flow fluctuates, so check it at intervals for accuracy.

| STEP | RATIONALE |
|---|---|

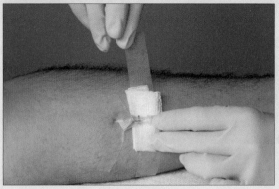

STEP **21B(1)** Place folded 2 × 2 gauze under cannula hub.

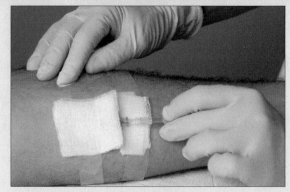

STEP **21B(2)** Apply 2 × 2 gauze dressing.

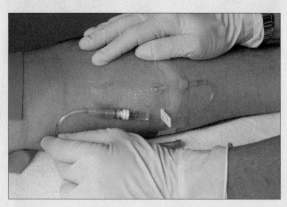

STEP **22** Loop and secure tubing.

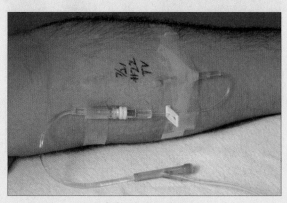

STEP **24** Label IV dressing.

24. Label dressing per agency policy. Information on label often includes date and time of IV insertion, VAD gauge size and length, and your initials (see illustration).

Provides immediate access to data as to when you inserted IV and when to make subsequent dressing changes.

25. Dispose of used stylet or other sharps in appropriate sharps container. Discard supplies. Remove gloves, and wash hands.

Reduces transmission of microorganisms and protects staff from infection and injury.

26. Instruct patient in how to move about in and out of bed without dislodging VAD.

## EVALUATION

1. Observe peripheral IV access. Peripheral IV access should be changed every 72 to 96 hours or per physician's or health care provider's orders or more frequently if complications occur (CDC, 2002).

Incidence of complications are higher when peripheral IV remains in a vein over 72 hours (CDC, 2002).

2. Observe patient every 1 to 2 hours:
   a. Check if correct amount of IV solution has infused by looking at time tape on IV container or by checking EID record.

Correct administration of fluid volume prevents fluid imbalance.

| STEP | RATIONALE |
|---|---|
| b. Count drip rate (if gravity drip) or check rate on EID. | Accurate monitoring of drip rate further ensures correct volume administration. |
| c. Check patency of VAD. | |
| d. Observe patient during palpation of vessel for signs of discomfort. | Tenderness is an early sign of phlebitis. |
| e. Inspect insertion site, noting color (e.g., redness or pallor). Inspect for presence of swelling, infiltration (see Table 15-9) and phlebitis (see Table 15-10). Palpate temperature of skin above dressing. | Redness, inflammation, tenderness, and warmth indicate vein inflammation or phlebitis. Swelling above insertion site and cool temperature indicate infiltration of fluid into tissues. |
| 3. Observe patient every 1 to 2 hours to determine response to therapy (e.g., I&O, weights, vital signs, postprocedure assessments). | IV fluids and additives are given to maintain or restore fluid and electrolyte balance. If I&O, weights, or vital signs change unexpectedly, fluid volume alterations will be serious. |

## RECORDING AND REPORTING

■ Record in nurses' notes number of attempts at insertion, insertion site by vessel, flow rate, size and type of catheter or other insertion device, type of solution and time you began infusion. Use an infusion therapy flow sheet if available.

■ If you are using an EID, document type and rate of infusion and identification number on the device.

■ Record patient's status, IV fluid, amount infused, and integrity and patency of system according to agency policy.

■ Report to oncoming nursing staff: type of fluid, flow rate, status of VAD site, amount of fluid remaining in present solution, expected time to hang subsequent IV container, and patient condition.

■ Report to physician or health care provider adverse reactions such as pulmonary congestion, shock, or thrombophlebitis.

## UNEXPECTED OUTCOMES AND RELATED INTERVENTIONS

■ Fluid volume deficit (FVD) as manifested by decreased urine output, dry mucous membranes, hypotension, tachycardia.
 • Notify physician or health care provider; infusion rate sometimes requires readjustment.

■ Fluid volume excess (FVE) as manifested by crackles in the lungs, shortness of breath, edema.
 • Reduce IV flow rate if symptoms appear, and notify physician or health care provider.

■ Electrolyte imbalances indicated by abnormal serum electrolyte levels, changes in mental status and neuromuscular function, changes in vital signs.
 • Notify physician or health care provider. Additives in IV or type of IV fluid sometimes need adjusting.

■ Infiltration as indicated by swelling and possible pitting edema, pallor, coolness, pain at insertion site, possible decrease in flow rate (Table 15-9).
 • Stop infusion, and discontinue IV.
 • Elevate affected extremity.
 • Restart new IV if continued therapy is necessary.

■ Phlebitis as indicated by pain, increased skin temperature, erythema along path of vein (Table 15-10).
 • Stop infusion, and discontinue IV. Restart new IV if continued therapy is necessary.
 • Place moist warm compress over area of phlebitis.

■ Bleeding occurs at venipuncture site.
 • Verify that the system is intact and change the dressing.
 • Restart new IV if bleeding from site does not stop or if IV is disloged.

| TABLE 15-9 | Infiltration Scale |
|---|---|
| Grade | Clinical Criteria |
| 0 | No symptoms |
| 1 | Skin blanched |
|  | Edema less than 1 inch in any direction |
|  | Cool to touch |
|  | With or without pain |
| 2 | Skin blanched |
|  | Edema 1 to 6 inches in any direction |
|  | Cool to touch |
|  | With or without pain |
| 3 | Skin blanched, translucent |
|  | Gross edema greater than 6 inches in any direction |
|  | Cool to touch |
|  | Mild to moderate pain |
|  | Possible numbness |
| 4 | Skin blanched, translucent |
|  | Skin tight, leaking |
|  | Skin discolored, bruised, swollen |
|  | Gross edema greater than 6 inches in any direction |
|  | Deep pitting tissue edema |
|  | Circulatory impairment |
|  | Moderate to severe pain |
|  | Infiltration of any amount of blood product, irritant, or vesicant |

From Intravenous Nurses Society (INS): 2000 infusion nursing standards of practice, *J Intraven Nurs* 23(6S):S51-S72, 2000.

| TABLE 15-10 | Phlebitis Scale |
|---|---|
| Grade | Clinical Criteria |
| 0 | No clinical symptoms |
| 1 | Erythema at access site with or without pain |
| 2 | Pain at access site with erythema and/or edema |
| 3 | Pain at access site with erythema and/or edema |
|  | Streak formation |
|  | Palpable venous cord |
| 4 | Pain at access site with erythema and/or edema |
|  | Streak formation |
|  | Palpable venous cord greater than 1 inch in length |
|  | Purulent drainage |

From Intravenous Nurses Society (INS): 2000 infusion nursing standards of practice, *J Intraven Nurs* 23(6S):S51-S72, 2000.

minimal rate used to keep a vein open and patent is about 10 to 15 ml/hr using a microdrip infusion set.

Infusion devices will assist you in maintaining a correct flow rate of IV fluids; many EIDs record the volume of the fluid infused. An electronic **infusion pump** is designed to deliver a measured amount of fluid over a period of time (e.g., 125 ml/hr) using positive pressure, whereas an electronic infusion controller is gravity dependent. EIDs have an electronic sensor and an alarm that will sound if it does not detect the appropriate rate. There are additional alarms to alert the nurse to increased system pressure that will occur from a variety of factors (e.g., obstruction in the IV tubing, infiltration of fluid into surrounding tissue, and occlusion by a clotting in the VAD).

Sometimes you will use other types of nonelectronic infusion devices, such as an IV controller (e.g., Dial-a-Flow) that delivers small amounts of fluid with the aid of gravity. The rate of infusion with an IV gravity controller depends on the height of the IV fluid container, IV tubing size, and fluid viscosity. The IV gravity controller is less precise than an EID in regulating IV fluids. With either device, the patient requires monitoring to verify the correct infusion of the IV solution and to detect the occurrence of any complication.

Patency of the VAD means that there are no clots at the tip of the cannula and that the cannula tip is not against the vein wall. An occluded or blocked cannula affects the infusion rate of the IV fluids. Infiltration, obstruction or kink in the tubing, height of the solution, and position of the patient's extremity also affect IV flow rates. Whenever a problem occurs with the infusion of the IV, perform an assessment of the IV system until you locate the problem. Start the assessment at the VAD site for signs and symptoms of infiltration and phlebitis. If the VAD site is without complication and fluid does not flow easily from the drip chamber when the roller clamp is opened, continue the assessment systematically until you reach the IV container. Other problems that sometimes contribute to the flow rate include the following:

- A tight, occluding VAD dressing impedes the flow.
- A clot occludes the cannula.
- The catheter tip is against the wall of the vein.

Inspect the tubing and area around the insertion site for anything blocking the flow of IV fluids. An obstruction or kink in the tubing will decrease the flow rate. Occasionally the cannula is kinked under a dressing, which will require you to remove the dressing for inspection. The flow rate frequently resumes after you relieve the tubing obstruction. Sometimes the patient also occludes the tubing by lying or sitting on it. The height of the IV container is sometimes too low. Raising the bag usually increases the rate because of increased hydrostatic pressure.

The position of the extremity, particularly at the wrist or elbow, decreases flow rates. Occasionally the use of an arm board helps to keep the joint extended and provides some protection to the site. Sometimes it is more comfortable for the patient to have an infusion started in a new location rather than dealing with a site that causes problems. However, before discontinuing the infusion hampered by an extremity position, start the infusion in another site to verify that the patient has other accessible veins.

An infiltration is often present when the insertion site is cool, clammy, swollen, and in some cases painful. An infiltration occurs when the needle or catheter has dislodged

*Text continued on p. 465*

## SKILL 15-2 Regulating Intravenous Flow Rate

### Delegation Considerations

The skill of regulating intravenous flow rate should not be delegated to assistive personnel. Delegation to LPNs varies by State Nurse Practice Acts.

Instruct assistive personnel about:

- The prescribed rate of flow and to report if the rate has slowed or increased
- Reporting if EID alarm sounds
- Reporting when patient complains about burning, swelling, bleeding, or coolness at the insertion site
- Reporting when the fluid container is almost complete

### Equipment

- Watch with second hand
- Paper or pencil
- Tape
- Label
- IV regulating device: electronic infusion device (EID) (optional), volume-control device (optional)

| STEP | RATIONALE |
|---|---|
| **ASSESSMENT** | |
| 1. Check patient's medical record for correct solution and additives. Follow six rights of medication administration (see Chapter 14). Usual order includes solution, additives or medications (if included) for 24 hours, usually divided into 2 or 3 L. Occasionally, IV order contains only 1 L to keep vein open (KVO). Record also shows time over which each liter is to infuse. | IV fluids are medications. Six rights prevent medication administration error. |
| 2. Perform hand hygiene. Observe patency of VAD and IV tubing. | For fluid to infuse at proper rate, make sure IV tubing and VAD are free of kinks, knots, and clots. |
| 3. Assess patient's knowledge of how positioning of IV site affects flow rate. | Fosters patient participation in maintaining most effective position of arm with IV equipment. The nurse or health care provider is responsible for positioning or setting control clamp or infusion device drip rate. |
| 4. Inspect IV site, and verify with patient how venipuncture site feels; for example, determine if there is pain or burning. Palpate site for tenderness. | Pain or burning is an early indication of phlebitis. Includes patient in decision making. |

### PLANNING

1. Collect and organize equipment.
2. Check patient's identification using two identifiers. Explain procedure.
3. Have paper and pencil or calculator to calculate flow rate.
4. Acquire calibration (drop factor) in drops per milliliter (gtt/ml) of infusion set:
   *Microdrip:* 60 gtt/ml
   *Macrodrip (depending on product manufacturer):*
   20 gtt/ml
   15 gtt/ml
   10 gtt/ml

| | |
|---|---|
| | Use mathematical calculations to determine correct IV flow rate. |
| | Microdrip tubing universally delivers 60 gtt/ml, and you use this when infusing small or very precise volumes. Microdrip tubing also prevents fluid overload with large-volume parenteral administration and is for patients who have cardiac and renal disorders. There are different commercial parenteral administration sets for macrodrip tubing. Use macrodrip tubing when large quantities or fast rates are necessary. |

## SKILL 15-2 | Regulating Intravenous Flow Rate—cont'd

| STEP | RATIONALE |
|------|-----------|

**5.** Determine ml/hr by dividing volume by hours.

$$\text{ml/hr} = \text{total infusion (ml)/hours of infusion}$$
$$1000 \text{ ml/8 hr} = 125 \text{ ml/hr}$$

Next, select one of the formulas to calculate flow rate.
(a) ml/hr/60 min = ml/min
   (1) Drop factor × ml/min = drops/min
*or*
(c) ml/hr × drop factor/60 min = drops/min

Once you determine hourly rate, these formulas give correct flow rate.

## IMPLEMENTATION

**1.** Read physician's or health care provider's orders, and follow six rights for correct solution and proper additives.

IV fluids are medications; following six rights decreases chance of medication error. Physician's/health care provider's order normally includes volume, solutions, additives, rate, and duration.

**2.** Obtain IV fluid/medication and appropriate tubing.

Use of correct tubing ensures accurate calculation for infusion delivery. Determines volume of fluid that infuses hourly.

---

• *Critical Decision Point:* It is common for physicians or health care providers to write an abbreviated IV order such as: "D₅W with 20 mEq KCl 125 ml/hr continuous." This order implies that you maintain the IV at this rate until order has been written for IV to be discontinued.

---

**3.** Confirm hourly infusion rate and place marked adhesive tape or commercial fluid indicator tape on IV container next to volume markings (see illustration)

Time taping IV container gives you visual cue as to whether fluids are being administered over the correct period of time. Use time tapes for all IV infusions, including those with EIDs.

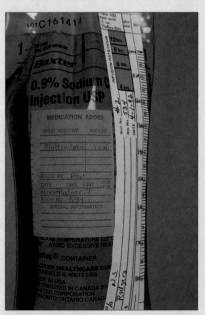

Step 3 IV fluid bag with time tape.

| STEP | RATIONALE |
|------|-----------|

• *Critical Decision Point:* Avoid drawing directly on IV containers made of polyvinyl chloride (PVC) with felt-tip pens or permanent markers because the ink is able to leak into the solution (Hadaway, 2003).

---

4. *For gravity transfusions:* Confirm hourly rate and minute rate calculated in planning. Microdrip infusion set has a drop factor of 60 gtt/ml. Regular drip or macrodrip infusion set used in this example has drop factor of 20 gtt/ml. Using formula (see Planning, step 5), calculate minute flow rates: Bottle 1:1000 ml with 20 mEq KCl over 8 hours.

*Microdrip:*
125 ml/hr × 60 gtt/ml = 7500 gtt/hr
7500 gtt ÷ 60 minutes = 125 gtt/min

*Macrodrip:*
125 ml/hr × 20 gtt/ml = 2500 gtt/hr
2500 gtt ÷ 60 minutes = 41 gtt/min

Allows nurse to calculate minute flow rate for regulation of infusion.

When using microdrip, milliliters per hour (ml/hr) always equals drops per minute (gtt/min).

Multiply volume by drop factor, and divide the product by time (in minutes).

5. Determine flow rate by counting drops in drip chamber for 1 minute by watch, then adjust roller clamp to increase or decrease rate of infusion (see illustration).

Adjusts flow to prescribed rate.

6. *For infusion using EID:* Follow manufacturer's guidelines for setup of EID.

EID sometimes regulates by positive pressure (pump) or gravity (controller).

   a. Consult manufacturer's directions for setup of the infusion. Place electronic eye over drip chamber (see illustration). If gravity controller is used, ensure that IV container is 36 inches above IV site.

IV controllers works by gravitational principle.

   b. Insert tubing into chamber of control mechanism, according to manufacturer's directions (see illustration).

Most electronic infusion devices use positive pressure to infuse.
Infusion pumps move fluid by compressing and milking IV tubing, thus propelling fluid through tubing.

   c. Required drops per minute or volume per hour are selected, door to control chamber is closed, power button is turned on, and start button is pressed (see illustrations).

---

• *Critical Decision Point:* Specific infusion tubing is required for most EIDs. Refer to manufacturer's specifications.

---

   d. Open regulator clamp completely while EID is in use.

Ensures that EID freely regulates infusion rate without obstruction.

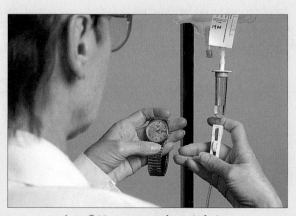

STEP **5** Nurse counts drops infusing.

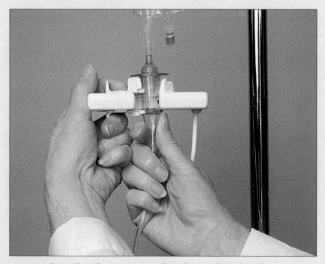

STEP **6a** Electronic eye placed over drip chamber.

SKILL 15-2 | Regulating Intravenous Flow Rate—cont'd

| STEP | RATIONALE |
|---|---|

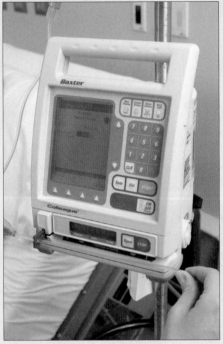

STEP **6b** Insert IV tubing into chamber of control mechanism.

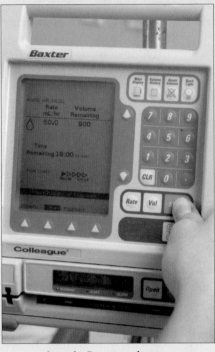

STEP **6c** Press start button.

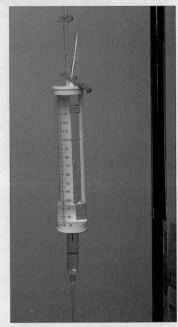

STEP **7a** Volume-metric device.

e. Monitor infusion rates and IV site for complications according to agency policy. Use watch to check rate of infusion, even when using EID.

f. Assess patency of system when alarm sounds.

EIDs are not perfect and do not replace frequent, accurate nursing assessment evaluation. Sometimes EIDs continue to infuse IV fluids after a complication has begun.

Alarm indicates that system flow is blocked. Empty solution bag or bottle, kink in tubing, closed clamp, infiltrated or clotted needle, and/or air in the tubing will all trigger the EID alarm.

7. For a volume-control device:

a. Place volume-metric device between IV container and insertion spike of infusion set (see illustration).

Allows infusion of small amount of fluid volume in incremental stages, but you must refill as volume becomes low. Reduces amount if sudden fluid infusion occurs.

b. Place 2 hours' allotment of fluid into device.

Promotes continuous fluid in tubing if you do not return in exactly 60 minutes to refill volume. In addition, if there is accidental increase in flow rate, patient receives at most only a 2-hour allotment of fluid.

c. Assess system at least hourly; add fluid to volume-control device. Regulate flow rate.

Maintains system patency and patient monitoring.

## EVALUATION

1. Monitor IV infusion at least every hour, noting volume of IV fluid infused and rate.

Ensures correct volume infuses over prescribed time period.

2. Observe patient for signs of overhydration or dehydration to determine response to therapy and restoration of fluid and electrolyte balance.

Signs and symptoms of dehydration or overhydration warrant changing rate of fluid infused.

3. Evaluate for signs of complications with IV flow rate: infiltration, inflammation at site, occluded VAD, or kink or obstruction in infusion tubing.

Complications cause decrease or cessation of flow rate.

## RECORDING AND REPORTING

■ Record rate of infusion, drops per minute or milliliters per hour in nurses' notes or parenteral fluid form according to agency policy.

■ Immediately record in nurses' notes any new IV fluid rates.

■ Document use of any electronic infusion device or controlling device and identification number on that device.

■ At change of shift or when leaving on break, report rate of and volume left in infusion to nurse in charge or next nurse assigned to care for patient.

## UNEXPECTED OUTCOMES AND RELATED INTERVENTIONS

■ Sudden infusion of large volume of solution occurs with patient having symptoms of dyspnea, crackles in the lung, and increased urine output, indicating fluid overload.

• Slow infusion to KVO rate.
• Place patient in high Fowler's position.
• Notify physician or health care provider immediately.
• Anticipate new IV orders.
• Administer diuretics if ordered.

■ IV fluid container becomes empty with subsequent loss of IV line patency.

• Restart new VAD.

■ The IV infuses more slowly than ordered rate.

• Check patient for positional change that affects rate, height of IV container, kinking of tubing or obstruction.
• Check condition of VAD site for complications.
• If volume infused is deficient, consult physician or health care provider for new order to provide necessary fluid volume.

---

from the vein and is in the subcutaneous space. When an infiltration occurs, you remove the VAD and insert a new one. Factors that alter IV flow rates occur with any patient at any time. When caring for a patient with an infusion, assess the site and the infusion rate at least every hour.

It is important for you to protect children, older adults, patients with severe head trauma, and patients susceptible to volume overload from sudden increases in infusion volumes. When certain IV controller devices are released, they allow a free flow of the IV fluid. An excessive amount of solution will inadvertently infuse until the tubing clamp is regulated. For example, a restless patient loosens the roller clamp with a sudden movement and increases the flow rate, or the flow rate is accidentally increased if the patient ambulates. A sudden increase in IV infusion rate causes a rapid increase in vascular volume, which will possibly make the patient critically ill or even cause death. Volume-control devices limit the amount of sudden excessive increases in the volume of IV solution infused by limiting the volume of fluid in the device. Safeguards are in place for EIDs to prevent free flow of infusion and sudden volume infusion when regulators are removed from the tubing housing.

***Maintaining the System.*** You need to maintain the system once the VAD is in place, the infusion is started, and the flow rate is regulated. In order to do this you: (1) keep the system sterile; (2) change solutions, tubing, and site dressings; and (3) assist the patient with self-care activities so he or she does not disrupt the system.

You will play an important role in maintaining the IV integrity to prevent the development of infection. Figure 15-7 demonstrates the potential sites for contamination of an intravascular device. The procedure for VAD insertion is designed to minimize the patient's microflora on the skin and

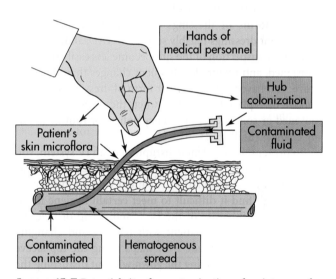

FIGURE **15-7** Potential sites for contamination of an intravascular device.

to reduce contamination during VAD insertion. You control the other factors through conscientious ongoing use of infection control principles. This begins with the use of thorough hand hygiene before and after you handle any part of the IV system.

You always maintain the integrity of the IV system. Never disconnect IV tubing because it becomes tangled or because it is more convenient in positioning or moving a patient. If a patient needs more room to maneuver, add extension tubing to an IV line. Stopcocks are available for connecting more than one IV solution to a single IV access site. Insert IV tubing into each port on a stopcock; otherwise, you attach a sterile cap to a nonused port. Do not allow a

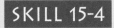

> ┌─────────────┐
> │ **SKILL 15-4** │ # Changing a Peripheral Intravenous
> └─────────────┘   Dressing—cont'd

| STEP | RATIONALE |
|---|---|
| 2. Remove tape, gauze, and/or transparent dressing from old dressing one layer at a time by pulling toward the insertion site (see illustration), leaving tape that secures VAD intact. Be cautious if IV tubing becomes tangled between two layers of dressing. When removing transparent dressing, hold cannula hub and tubing with non-dominant hand. | Prevents accidental displacement of VAD. |
| 3. Observe insertion site for signs and/or symptoms of infection: redness, swelling, and exudates. | Presence of infection indicates need to remove VAD at current site and insert a new VAD at another site. |
| 4. If complication exists or if ordered by physician or health care provider, discontinue the infusion. | Presence of infection indicates need to discontinue IV at current site. |
| 5. If IV is infusing properly, gently remove tape securing VAD. Stabilize VAD with one hand. Use adhesive remover to cleanse skin and remove adhesive residue, if needed. | Exposes venipuncture site. Stabilization prevents accidental displacement of VAD. Adhesive residue decreases ability of new tape to adhere tightly to skin. |

- *Critical Decision Point:* Keep one finger over cannula at all times until tape or dressing secures placement. It will help to have another staff member assist especially with restless patients or children.

| | |
|---|---|
| 6. Cleanse insertion site with antiseptic swab using friction. Use the first swab in a horizontal plane, cleansing the skin from side to side. Allow to dry. Apply the second swab on a vertical plane, up and down. Allow to dry. Apply the final swab in a circular pattern moving outward from the insertion site (see illustration). Allow to dry. | Mechanical friction in this pattern allows penetration of the antiseptic solution into the cracks and fissures of the epidermal layer of the skin (Crosby and Mares, 2001). Allowing antiseptic solutions to air-dry completely effectively reduces microbial counts (INS, 2000). When antiseptic solutions are used in combination, allow each one to dry. |
| 7. Apply skin protectant to the area where you will apply the tape or transparent dressing. Allow to dry. | Coats the skin with protective solution to maintain skin integrity, prevent irritation from the adhesive, and promote adhesion of the dressing. |
| 8. Apply dressing. See Skill 15-1, Implementation steps 21 to 22. | |
| 9. Reduce flow rate to correct drops per minute (see Skill 15-2). | Manipulation of catheter during dressing application can alter flow rate. |
| 10. Remove and discard gloves and mask. | Prevents transmission of microorganisms. |
| 11. Label dressing per agency policy. Information on label often includes date and time of IV insertion, VAD gauge size and length, and your initials. | Documents dressing change. |
| 12. Apply securement device (e.g., IV House Protective Device). | |
| 13. Discard equipment, and perform hand hygiene. | Reduces transmission of microorganisms. |

## EVALUATION

| | |
|---|---|
| 1. Regulate IV flow as ordered. | Validates that IV is patent and functioning correctly. |
| 2. Inspect condition of VAD site. Palpate for skin temperature, edema, and tenderness. | Complications such as phlebitis and infiltration require removal of VAD and insertion of new VAD at another site. |
| 3. Monitor patient's body temperature. | Elevated temperature indicates an infection that is sometimes associated with contamination of the venipuncture site. |

## RECORDING AND REPORTING

■ Record in nurses' notes time you changed IV dressing and type of dressing used. Include patency of system and description of venipuncture site.

■ Report to nurse in charge or oncoming nursing shift that you changed the dressing and any significant information about integrity of system.

■ Report to physician or health care provider any complications.

## UNEXPECTED OUTCOMES AND RELATED INTERVENTIONS

■ VAD is infiltrated, as evidenced by decreased flow rate or edema, pallor, or decreased temperature around insertion site.
  • Stop infusion, and remove VAD.
  • Restart new VAD in other extremity if continued therapy is necessary.
  • Elevate affected extremity.

■ Phlebitis is present, as evidenced by erythema and tenderness along vein pathway.
  • Stop infusion, and remove VAD.
  • Restart new VAD in other extremity if continued therapy is necessary.
  • Apply warm moist compress to area of phlebitis.

■ VAD is accidentally removed.
  • Restart VAD if continued therapy is needed.

■ Patient has an elevated temperature.
  • Notify physician or health care provider. You may remove and restart VAD. Patient will be evaluated for source of infection.

■ Insertion site is red and/or edematous and/or painful and/or has presence of exudate, indicating infection at venipuncture site.
  • Remove VAD. Antibiotic therapy is sometimes prescribed.
  • Apply warm, moist compress to area of inflammation.

---

removing the tape and dressing that is in place. Always stabilize the VAD when removing the dressing to minimize patient discomfort. Move the roller clamp to the "off" position to prevent spillage of IV fluid, and apply a sterile 2 × 2 gauze pad over the venipuncture site. Using the other hand, withdraw the cannula by pulling straight back away from the puncture site (Figure 15-8). Elevate the extremity and apply pressure to the site for 1 to 2 minutes to control bleeding and prevent hematoma formation. Patients who have received anticoagulants require longer pressure on the site because of the interference with blood-clotting mechanisms. If necessary, use alcohol or soap and water to remove dried blood or other drainage. You will need to apply a bandage over the venipuncture site if you believe a small amount of seepage will occur. You then record the amount of fluid infused and the time it was discontinued. Do not forget to go back and check the venipuncture site after you have discontinued the IV, especially if you had to apply a bandage over the wound.

**Blood Replacement.** Blood replacement or transfusion is the IV administration of whole blood or a component such as plasma, packed red blood cells (RBCs), or platelets. The objectives for blood transfusions include (1) to increase circulating blood volume after surgery, trauma, or hemorrhage; (2) to increase the number of RBCs and to maintain hemoglobin levels in patients with severe anemia; and (3) to provide selected cellular components as replacement therapy (e.g., clotting factors, platelets, or albumin).

***Blood Groups and Types.*** The most important grouping for transfusion purposes is the ABO system, which includes A, B, O, and AB blood types. The determination of blood

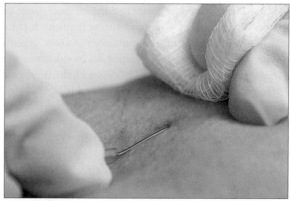

FIGURE **15-8** IV catheter is withdrawn slowly, keeping catheter parallel to vein.

groups is based on the presence or absence of A and B red cell antigens. Individuals with A antigens, B antigens, or no antigens belong to groups A, B, and O respectively. The person with A and B antigens has AB blood.

Individuals with type A blood naturally produce anti-B antibodies in their plasma. Similarly, type B individuals naturally produce anti-A antibodies. An individual with type O has neither type A nor type B antigen and thus is a universal donor. A type AB individual produces neither antibody, which is why type AB individuals are universal recipients and receive any type of blood. In the event blood that is mismatched with the patient's blood is transfused, a **transfusion reaction** occurs. The transfusion reaction is an antigen-antibody reaction and ranges from a mild response to severe anaphylactic shock and is potentially fatal.

Another consideration when matching for blood transfusions is the Rh factor, an antigenic substance in the erythrocytes of most people. A person with the factor is Rh positive, whereas a person without it is Rh negative.

*Autologous Transfusion.* **Autologous transfusion** (autotransfusion) is the collection and reinfusion of a patient's own blood. You obtain the blood for an autologous transfusion by having the patient make preoperative donation weeks before the scheduled procedure, depending on the type of surgery and the ability of the patient to maintain an acceptable hematocrit. The blood is tested for blood-borne transmissions, such as HIV and HBV. An autologous transfusion is also obtained during perioperative blood salvage (e.g., during vascular and orthopedic surgery, organ transplant surgery, and traumatic injuries) and reinfused during the surgery. Blood can also be salvaged postoperatively from mediastinal and chest-tube drains and after joint and spinal surgery. Autologous transfusions are safer for the patient because they decrease the risk of complications such as mismatched blood and exposure to blood-borne transmissions.

**Blood Transfusions.** Transfusing blood or blood components is a nursing procedure. It is your responsibility to assess the patient before, during, and after the transfusion and for regulation of the transfusion. If the patient has a VAD already in place, assess the site for signs of inflammation or infiltration and cannula patency. Determine the cannula gauge and recognize that a smaller gauge size affects the flow. It is necessary to insert a large gauge cannula such as 18 or larger if a rapid flow rate is required. The tubing for blood administration has an in-line filter (Figure 15-9). You fill the tubing with 0.9% normal saline to prevent **hemolysis** of RBCs.

Information obtained from the patient before the transfusion establishes whether the patient knows the reason for the blood transfusion and whether the patient has ever had a previous transfusion or transfusion reaction. A patient who has had a transfusion reaction is usually at no greater risk for a reaction with a subsequent transfusion. However, some patients are anxious about the transfusion, requiring nursing intervention. Before giving a transfusion, verify that the patient has signed an informed consent. Then explain the procedure to the patient and instruct him or her to report any side effects (e.g., chills, dizziness, or fever) once the transfusion begins.

Because of the danger of transfusion reactions, it is very important to use precautions in administering blood or blood products. Obtain the patient's baseline vital signs before the transfusion begins. This data will allow you to determine when changes in vital signs occur, which will indicate that a transfusion reaction is developing. To ensure that the right patient receives the correct type of blood or blood product, use a thorough procedure to check the identity of the blood products, the patient, and the compatibility of the blood and the patient. Although you are not involved in the blood labeling process, you are responsible for determining that the blood delivered to the patient corresponds to the patient's blood

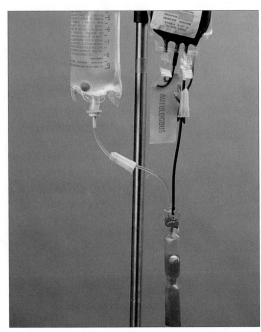

FIGURE **15-9** Tubing for blood administration has an in-line filter.

type listed in the medical record. Two registered nurses or one registered nurse and a licensed practical nurse (see agency policy) must simultaneously check the label on the blood product against the patient's identification number, blood group, and complete name. If even a minor discrepancy exists, the blood is withheld and the blood bank is notified immediately and the blood returned to the blood bank.

Initiation of a transfusion begins slowly to allow for the early detection of a transfusion reaction. Maintain the infusion rate, monitor for side effects, assess the patient's vital signs, and promptly record all findings. It is important that you stay with the patient during the first 15 minutes, the time when a reaction is most likely to occur. After that time you will need to continue to monitor the patient and obtain vital signs periodically during the transfusion as directed by agency policy. If you suspect a transfusion reaction, STOP the transfusion immediately, obtain vital signs, and notify the physician or health care provider.

The rate of transfusion is usually specified in the physician's or health care provider's orders. Ideally, a unit of whole blood or packed RBCs will transfuse in 2 hours. This time can be lengthened to 4 hours if the patient is at risk for FVE. Beyond 4 hours there is a risk of the blood becoming contaminated because of the rich medium for pathogen growth. If the patient cannot tolerate the volume of fluid within this time frame, the blood bank will divide the unit into smaller volumes.

When patients have a severe blood loss such as with hemorrhage, they receive rapid transfusions through a central venous catheter. A blood-warming device is often necessary, because the tip of the central venous pressure catheter lies in the superior vena cava, above the right atrium. Rapid administration of cold blood will result in cardiac dysrhythmia.

*Transfusion Reactions.* A transfusion reaction is a systemic response by the body to incompatible blood. Causes include red cell incompatibility or allergic sensitivity to the components of the transfused blood or to the potassium or citrate preservative in the blood. Blood transfusion can also result in the transmission of infectious disease. A second category of reactions includes diseases transmitted by infected blood donors who are asymptomatic. Diseases transmitted through transfusions are malaria, hepatitis, and HIV. Because all units of blood collected undergo serological testing and screening for HIV and HBV, the risk of acquiring blood-borne infections from blood transfusions is reduced.

Circulatory overload is a risk when a patient receives massive whole blood or packed RBC transfusions for massive hemorrhagic shock or when a patient with normal blood volume receives blood. Older adults and those with cardiopulmonary diseases are particularly at risk for circulatory overload. Blood transfusion reactions are life threatening, but prompt nursing intervention will maintain the patient's physiological stability (Box 15-5).

**Interventions for Acid-Base Imbalances.** Nursing interventions to promote acid-base balance support prescribed medical therapies and are aimed at reversing the acid-base imbalance that exists. Such imbalances are life threatening and require rapid correction. It is important that you maintain a functional IV line and frequently check the physician's or health care provider's orders for new medications or fluids. Give prescribed drugs, such as insulin or sodium bicarbonate, fluid and electrolyte replacement, and oxygen supportive therapy promptly.

In addition, you will need to monitor the patient closely for changes in acid-base balance. Any patient with acid-base disturbances usually needs repeated ABG analysis. This procedure involves obtaining arterial blood samples for analysis of hydrogen ion concentration.

*Arterial Blood Gases.* ABG determination requires the removal of a sample of blood from an artery to assess the patient's acid-base status and the adequacy of ventilation and oxygenation. You draw arterial blood from a peripheral artery (usually the radial) or from an arterial line inserted by a physician or health care provider. In some agencies, registered nurses are responsible for radial artery punctures. After obtaining the specimen, take care to prevent air from entering the syringe because this will affect the blood gas analysis. To reduce metabolism of cells, you submerge the syringe in crushed ice and have it transported immediately to the laboratory. It is necessary to apply pressure to the puncture site for at least 5 minutes to reduce the risk of a hematoma formation. You will need a longer period if the patient is on anticoagulant medications. You reassess the radial pulse after pressure has been removed.

**CONTINUING CARE.** After experiencing acute alterations in fluid and electrolyte or acid-base balance, patients often require ongoing maintenance to prevent a recurrence

| BOX 15-5 | **Nursing Interventions for Blood Transfusion Reaction** |

1. If you suspect a blood reaction, STOP the transfusion immediately.
2. Keep the IV line open. Disconnect the blood tubing at the hub of the VAD, and connect the primed tubing of 0.9% normal saline directly into the VAD. Place a sterile cap on the end of the blood tubing to maintain sterile system.
3. Do not turn off the blood and simply turn on the 0.9% normal saline that is connected to the Y-tubing infusion set. This causes blood remaining in the Y tubing to infuse into the patient. Even a small amount of mismatched blood is able to cause a major reaction.
4. If patient presents with anaphylactic shock, administer epinephrine within protocol guidelines.
5. Notify the physician or health care provider immediately.
6. Remain with the patient, observing signs and symptoms and monitoring vital signs as often as every 5 minutes.
7. Prepare to administer emergency drugs such as antihistamines, vasopressors, fluids, and steroids per physician's or health care provider's order.
8. Prepare to perform cardiopulmonary resuscitation.
9. Obtain a urine specimen, and send it to the laboratory.
10. If physician or health care provider orders discontinuation of transfusion, save the blood container, tubing, attached labels, and transfusion record, and return them to the laboratory.
11. Document the transfusion reaction, description, treatment, and outcome.

of health alterations. Older adults and the chronically ill require special considerations to prevent complications from developing.

**Home Intravenous Therapy.** IV therapy is often continued in the home setting for patients requiring long-term hydration, parenteral nutrition, or extended medication administration. A home IV therapy nurse will work closely with the patient to ensure that the patient maintains a sterile IV system and that the patient avoids complications or recognizes them promptly.

Box 15-6 summarizes patient education guidelines for home IV therapy.

**Nutritional Support.** Most patients who have had electrolyte disorders or metabolic acid-base disturbances require ongoing nutritional support. Depending on the type of disorder, you will encourage or restrict certain fluids or food. If patients are still responsible for preparing their own meals, make sure they learn to look at the lists of the nutrient content of foods and to read the labels of commercially prepared foods.

**Medication Safety.** Numerous drugs contain constituents or create potential side effects that alter fluid and electrolyte balance. Patients with chronic disease who are receiving multiple medications and those with renal or liver disorders are at significant risk for alterations to develop.

---

**BOX 15-6** PATIENT TEACHING

**Home Intravenous Therapy**

Although Robert knows that Mrs. Reynolds will not need home intravenous therapy, he knows that at some point in time he might have a patient who requires continued intravenous therapy in the home environment. As a result, he develops the following teaching plan:

**Outcome**

At the end of the teaching sessions a patient/caregiver will be able to safely monitor and maintain home IV therapy.

**Teaching Strategies**

- Explain to patient and caregiver the importance of IV therapy in maintaining hydration and access for medications delivery.
- Stress the importance of hand hygiene in infection control.
- Emphasize the risks involved when the IV system is not kept sterile.
- Show the patient and/or caregiver how to manipulate the required equipment, and provide opportunity to handle the equipment.
- Demonstrate to patient or caregiver how to change IV solutions, tubing, and dressing when they become soiled or dislodged. (NOTE: The home care nurse is sometimes able to visit frequently enough to perform scheduled tubing and dressing changes.)

- Instruct patient and caregiver about signs and symptoms of infiltration, phlebitis, and infection and to notify the home care nurse immediately.
- Instruct patient and caregiver to notify the home care nurse if the infusion slows or stops or if the patient sees blood in the tubing.
- Teach patient with caregiver's assistance how to ambulate, perform hygiene, and participate in other activities of daily living without dislodging or disconnecting VAD and tubing.
- Instruct patient and caregiver how to properly dispose of used infusion equipment.

**Evaluation Strategies**

- Observe patient's hydration status.
- Inspect VAD insertion site for signs of inflammation, phlebitis, infiltration.
- Observe patient and/or caregiver change IV solutions, tubing, dressings.
- Ask patient and caregiver to verbalize signs associated with infiltration, phlebitis, and infection.
- Ask patient and caregiver to describe how they are disposing of used equipment.

---

 OUTCOME EVALUATION | **TABLE 15-11**

| Nursing Action | Patient Response/Finding | Achievement of Outcome |
|---|---|---|
| Inspect oral mucous membranes. Assess skin turgor. | Mucous membranes are moist. Skin recoil is sluggish. | Fluid status improving; continue to support hydration. |
| Auscultate blood pressure (BP) with Mrs. Reynolds lying, sitting, and standing. | Mrs. Reynolds does not experience any changes in BP while changing positions. | Orthostatic hypotension has improved. Continue to encourage Mrs. Reynolds to get up slowly. |
| Measure urine output, and note color of urine with each void. | Mrs. Reynolds' urinary output is approximately equal to intake. Urine is dark amber. | I&O appears to have improved. Need to encourage fluid. Urine is still dark in color. |
| Monitor daily laboratory tests results. | Hematocrit and electrolyte levels are all within normal limits. | Laboratory results appear to indicate an improvement. Mrs. Reynolds will need encouragement to increase potassium in her diet. |

---

Patient and family education are essential to providing information regarding potential side effects or over-the-counter medications to avoid. Review all medications with patients, and encourage them to consult with their local pharmacist each time they try a new over-the-counter medication.

 **Evaluation**

**PATIENT CARE.** The evaluation of a patient's clinical status is especially important if an acute alteration in fluid and electrolyte or acid-base disturbance exists (Table 15-11). It is possible for the patient's condition to change very quickly, so

be able to recognize the signs and symptoms of impending problems by integrating the patient's presenting clinical status, the effects of the present treatment regimen, and the potential causative agent. The patient's assessment is ongoing, and you need to evaluate the therapies that are initiated for their effectiveness. For example, assessment of heart rate and rhythm, muscle tone, bowel sounds, and peripheral sensation will detect if a patient with hypokalemia is showing signs of improvement. The physical signs and symptoms of hypokalemia begin to disappear or lessen in intensity if your interventions are managing the hypokalemia.

## EVALUATION

Robert returns to the clinical area the next day and evaluates Mrs. Reynolds' progress. She remarks, "I feel much better. I have had no nausea since I saw you last and no diarrhea since yesterday morning." The IV of 0.45% normal saline is still in place, infusing at 125 ml/hr. However, the physician or health care provider has just visited and has ordered you to reduce the rate to 40 ml/hr. Mrs. Reynolds' 24-hour intake since yesterday is 2800 ml, and her output is 2200 ml. During examination Robert notices the oral mucosa is still slightly dry; skin turgor has returned to normal. Mrs. Reynolds' vital signs are blood pressure 126/78, pulse 88, and respirations 18. She is afebrile. The serum potassium level drawn at 6 AM was 4.0.

Robert tells Mrs. Reynolds he is pleased with her progress. He prepares her breakfast, during which she receives her first soft foods since entering the hospital. Robert plans time to discuss with Mrs. Reynolds the information she has learned from their discussion about food sources for potassium. Robert asks, "After discussing the importance of potassium in your diet, tell me what foods to select that include potassium." Mrs. Reynolds is again able to identify six different sources of potassium that she is able to routinely include in her diet.

### Documentation Note

"Denies nausea and reports feeling better. No diarrhea stool since yesterday morning. On inspection, oral mucosa remains dry, without lesions or inflammation. Skin turgor is normal. Bowel sounds are normal in all four quadrants, and abdomen is soft to palpation. IV of 0.45% normal saline is infusing in left cephalic vein in forearm at 125 ml/hr, without tenderness or inflammation at site. Is able to identify six food sources for potassium to include in her diet. Is resting comfortably, out of bed in a chair, family at the bedside. Will continue to monitor."

For patients with less acute alterations, evaluation likely occurs over a longer period of time. In this situation, you focus the evaluation more on behavioral changes (e.g., the patient's ability to follow dietary restrictions and medication schedules). The family's ability to anticipate alterations and prevent problems from recurring is also an important element to evaluate.

The patient's level of progress determines whether you need to continue or revise the plan of care. It is more than likely that you will need to communicate with the other members of the health care team about interventions that have and have not been successful. If you do not meet goals due to the failure to meet expected outcomes, there are several things you can do. You can increase the frequency of an intervention (e.g., provide more fluids to a dehydrated patient), introduce a new therapy (e.g., initiate insertion of an IV), or discontinue a therapy (e.g., consult with physician or health care provider in discontinuing a diuretic). Once you have met the outcomes, you are able to resolve the nursing diagnosis and focus on other priorities.

**PATIENT EXPECTATIONS.** Routinely review if you have met the patient's expectations of care. For example, ask the patient, "Tell me if I have helped you feel more comfortable." If the patient's concerns involve having a better understanding of a chronic problem, evaluate the patient's satisfaction with instruction. Often the patient's level of satisfaction with care also depends on your success in involving family and friends. If the patient has concerns about returning home or to a different care setting, it is important to evaluate if the patient feels prepared for the transition from acute care. Acknowledge these fears and concerns, and give honest and clear explanations.

Listening attentively to your patients and their families or significant others will assist you in planning and providing appropriate care. Often they are fearful of potential dangers that exist and are fearful of not knowing what to expect. Providing them with opportunities to ask questions and seek affirmation is part of the nursing care you will deliver.

## KEY CONCEPTS

- Body fluids are distributed in ECF and ICF compartments and contain electrolytes, cells, and water.
- Body fluids are regulated through fluid intake, output, and hormonal regulation.
- Volume disturbances include isotonic and osmolar deficits and excesses.
- Dietary intake and hormonal controls regulate electrolytes.
- Chronic and serious illnesses increase the risk of fluid, electrolyte, and acid-base imbalances.
- Patients who are very young or very old are at greater risk for fluid, electrolyte, and acid-base imbalances.
- Assessment for fluid, electrolyte, and acid-base alterations includes the nursing history; physical and behavioral assessment; measurements of I&O; daily weights; and specific laboratory data such as measurement of serum osmolality, serum electrolytes, BUN, urine specific gravity, and ABG levels.

- Enteral or parenteral administration of fluid will correct FVD and osmolar imbalances.
- Common complications of IV therapy include infiltration, phlebitis, infection, FVE, and bleeding at the infusion site.
- You give blood transfusions to replace fluid volume loss from hemorrhage, to treat anemia, or to replace coagulation factors.
- Administration of blood or blood products requires you to follow a specific procedure to identify transfusion reactions quickly.
- In addition to transfusion reactions, the risks of transfusion include hyperkalemia, hypocalcemia, FVE, and infection.
- Treatment for electrolyte disturbances includes dietary and pharmacological interventions.
- Acid-base balance depends on the hydrogen ion concentration in the blood.

- Chemical, biological, and physiological buffering systems shield the body from acid-base imbalances.
- The body's chemical buffering system responds first to acid-base abnormalities.
- Increased carbon dioxide and hydrogen ion concentrations characterize respiratory acidosis.
- Decreased carbon dioxide and hydrogen ion concentrations characterize respiratory alkalosis.

- A decrease in bicarbonate level and increase in hydrogen ion concentration characterize metabolic acidosis.
- An increase in bicarbonate level and decrease in hydrogen ion concentration characterize metabolic alkalosis.
- The goals of therapy for acid-base imbalances are to treat the underlying illness and to restore the arterial pH to normal.

## CRITICAL THINKING IN PRACTICE

*Mrs. Shuffield is a 73-year-old white woman admitted with abdominal pain. Her nursing history reveals that she has mid-epigastric abdominal pain and has been nauseated for 2 days with several episodes of vomiting and diarrhea. She tells the nurse that she has had little to eat and drink. The physician has ordered vital signs every 4 hours, nothing by mouth, intake and output, blood chemistry, IV of $D_5$ ½ NS at 125 ml/hr, analgesic, and abdominal x-ray films.*

1. What additional information should the nurse obtain from Mrs. Shuffield?
2. What considerations does the nurse include before she proceeds with starting the IV?

3. List nursing interventions for the nursing diagnosis *deficient fluid volume.*
4. Upon further assessment, Mrs. Shuffield presents with temperature of 100.9° F. How does this affect her condition?
5. What other indicators does the nurse expect with dehydration in Mrs. Shuffield?
6. What is the primary cause of Mrs. Shuffield's fluid imbalance?
7. What type of intravenous solution does Mrs. Shuffield's condition require?
   a. Hypotonic
   b. Hypertonic
   c. Isotonic

## NCLEX® REVIEW

1. The catheter tip of a PICC should be located in the:
   1. Aorta
   2. Cephalic vein
   3. Right atrium
   4. Superior vena cava
2. The most common cause of hypokalemia is:
   1. Dehydration
   2. Renal failure
   3. Thiazide and loop diuretics
   4. Too rapid blood transfusion
3. Which of the following IV solutions is isotonic?
   1. D2.5%W
   2. D5%W
   3. D10%W
   4. D50%W
4. The process of a solution moving from a higher concentration area to a lower concentration area is known as:
   1. Active transport
   2. Diffusion
   3. Homeostasis
   4. Osmosis
5. You just started a blood transfusion on your patient, and within 5 minutes he states that his throat feels like it is closing up. Which of the following nursing interventions should you do first?
   1. Give the patient some ice chips.
   2. Notify the physician or health care provider.

3. Stop the blood transfusion.
4. Take the patient's vital signs.
6. Your patient presents with arterial blood gas levels as follows: pH, 7.59; $HCO_3^-$, 39; $PaCO_2$, 48 mm Hg; base excess, positive. Which of the following acid-base imbalances does he have?
   1. Metabolic acidosis
   2. Metabolic alkalosis
   3. Respiratory acidosis
   4. Respiratory alkalosis
7. A patient admitted with acute renal failure has a 24-hour urine output of 75 ml. Which of the following is he most at risk of developing?
   1. Hypercalcemia
   2. Hyperkalemia
   3. Hypokalemia
   4. Metabolic alkalosis
8. The physician orders potassium chloride (KCl) 20 mEq/L to be given intravenously. Which of the following methods is the most appropriate?
   1. Direct IV push
   2. IV piggyback
   3. Added to the existing primary fluid
   4. Wait until the next primary fluid is due to be infused

## REFERENCES

Centers for Disease Control and Prevention: Guidelines for the prevention of intravascular catheter-related infections, *MMWR Morb Mortal Wkly Rep* 51 (No. RR-10):1, 2002.

Christensen BL, Kockrow EO: *Foundations of nursing,* ed 4, St. Louis, 2005, Mosby.

Crosby CT, Mares AK: Skin antisepsis: past, present, and future, *J Vasc Access Devices* 6(2):26, 2001.

Dochterman JM, Bulechek GM, editors: *Nursing interventions classification (NIC),* ed 4, St. Louis, 2004, Mosby.

Gorski LA, Czaplewski L: Peripherally inserted central catheters and midline catheters for the homecare nurse, *J Infus Nurs* 27(6):399, 2004.

Hankins J and others: *Infusion therapy in clinical practice,* Philadelphia, 2001, Saunders.

Heitz U, Horne MM: *Mosby's pocket guide series: fluid, electrolyte, and acid-base balance,* ed 5, St. Louis, 2005, Mosby.

Hockenberry MJ and others: *Wong's nursing care of infants and children,* ed 7, St. Louis, 2003, Mosby.

Huether SE, McCance KL: *Understanding pathophysiology,* ed 3, St. Louis, 2004, Mosby.

Ignatavicius DD, Workman ML: *Medical-surgical nursing: critical thinking for collaborative care,* ed 4, Philadelphia, 2002, WB Saunders.

Infusion Nurses Society (INS): 2000 infusion nursing standards of practice, *J Intraven Nurs* 23(6S):(5)S1-S72, 2000.

Lewis SM and others: *Medical-surgical nursing: assessment and management of clinical problems,* ed 4, St. Louis, 2002, Mosby.

McKenry LM, Salerno E: *Pharmacology in nursing,* ed 21 rev, St. Louis, 2003, Mosby.

Metheny N: *Fluid and electrolyte balance: nursing considerations,* ed 4, Philadelphia, 2000, Lippincott.

Millam AA, Hadaway LC: On the road to successful IV starts: expert clinicians share tips and insights based on 35 years' experience performing and teaching venipuncture techniques, *Nursing* 33(5):S1, 2003.

Moorhead S, Johnson M, Maas M, editors: *Nursing outcomes classification (NOC),* ed 3, St. Louis, 2004, Mosby.

Penney-Timmons E, Sevedge S: Outcome data for peripherally inserted central catheters used in an acute care setting, *J Infus Nurs* 27(6):431, 2004.

# CHAPTER 16

# Caring in Nursing Practice

## MEDIA RESOURCES

**CD COMPANION**  **evolve** **WEBSITE**

http://evolve.elsevier.com/Potter/basic

- **NCLEX® Review**
- **Audio Glossary**
- **English/Spanish Audio Glossary**

## OBJECTIVES

- Discuss the role that caring plays in building a nurse-patient relationship.
- Compare and contrast theories on the concept of caring.
- Discuss patients' perceptions of caring nurse behaviors
- Describe ways to convey caring through use of touch
- Describe how to provide presence when performing a nursing procedure.
- Describe the therapeutic benefit of listening to patients' stories.
- Explain the relationship between knowing a patient and clinical decision making.
- Discuss the importance of a nurse's ability to demonstrate caring toward families.

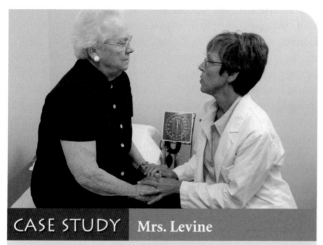

### CASE STUDY  Mrs. Levine

Mrs. Levine is an 82-year-old patient diagnosed 2 months ago with liver cancer. She has been having trouble with low back pain due to the spread of cancer to her spine. Mrs. Levine had been relatively independent before her diagnosis. She continued to go to her weekly bridge club and enjoyed going to lunch with friends from her church. Her son, Jim, lives only a few miles away and is a consistent resource when she needs transportation to the physician or repairs to her home. Mrs. Levine is to begin a new research protocol for chemotherapy treatments this week at the university oncology clinic.

Sue is a clinical nurse specialist who works in the oncology clinic. She has been an oncology nurse for over 10 years. She enters the examination room where Mrs. Levine is waiting, introduces herself, and sits down next to her patient. Sue states, "Mrs. Levine, I am here to understand your story. I am here to listen and learn how I can best support you." Sue uses eye contact during her explanation and leans toward Mrs. Levine to establish a physical presence. Mrs. Levine nods, smiles, and begins her story. "I have had such a good life, I guess it had to end." Sue replies, "Go on." Mrs. Levine explains, "The doctor tells me the cancer is serious. I worry about what is going to happen to me and how it will affect my son, Jim. I do not want to become so dependent on him." Sue responds in a calm, soothing tone, "Mrs. Levine, your concerns are not unusual. It is important for you to remain as independent as possible; let's talk about how we can do that."

### KEY TERMS

caring, p. 481
comforting, p. 486
nurturant, p. 482

presence, p. 485
transcultural, p. 482

In this clinical scenario Sue demonstrates an act of **caring** through her words and actions. Her calm presence, eye contact, and attention to the patient's concerns all convey a person-centered, comforting approach to care. Caring is central to nursing practice, but perhaps it has never been more important because of today's fast-paced health care environment. Pressure and time constraints on health care workers cause nurses, therapists, and others to be perceived as cold and indifferent to patients' needs. Technological advances and ever-increasing demands on caregivers often come first in health care, limiting the opportunity for interpersonal connections that are critical in therapeutic patient relationships. For many older adults, this is particularly difficult, because they can still remember what being in hospitals was like 25 to 30 years ago. At that time caregivers had more time to be attentive and to care for a patient over a course of several days. But today is different. Benner and Wrubel (1989) warn that technological advances are dangerous and inappropriate unless nurses practice with caring and compassion. It is time to value and embrace the caring practices and expert knowledge that are a part of nursing practice.

## Theoretical Views on Caring

Caring is universal. It affects the way we think, feel, and behave in relation to one another. Caring in nursing has been studied from a variety of philosophical and ethical perspectives since the time of Florence Nightingale. A number of nursing scholars have developed theories on caring because of its importance to the practice of nursing. This chapter does not cover all of the theories on caring, but it will help you as you begin your nursing career to understand that caring is at the heart of your ability to work with people in a respectful and therapeutic way.

## Caring Is Primary

After spending time studying the clinical stories of expert nurses, Patricia Benner (1984) describes caring as the essence of excellent nursing practice. Caring means that persons, events, projects, and things matter to people. It is a word that means being connected. Because caring determines what matters to a person, it describes a wide range of involvements, from parental love to friendship, from caring for one's work to caring for one's pet, to caring for and about one's patients. Benner and Wrubel (1989) note that "Caring creates possibility." In the case study example, Sue's concern for Mrs. Levine provides motivation and direction for Sue to better understand the meaning cancer has for Mrs. Levine and to provide the best approach in helping the patient cope with a serious illness.

Patients are not all the same. Each brings a different background of experiences, values, and cultural perspectives to a health care situation. Caring is always specific and relational for each nurse-patient meeting. Patients have different expectations of caring. For example, some patients will perceive caring as maintaining a silent presence in the room during an invasive procedure, while others perceive caring as your attempt to explain and console them. A nurse expresses caring differently for an older adult patient in pain versus a young mother who has had a miscarriage. As you acquire more nursing experience, you will learn that caring helps you to focus on the patient for whom you care. Caring improves your ability to know a patient, allowing you to recognize a patient's problems, to find solutions, and to implement those solutions (Benner and Wrubel, 1989).

In addition to their work in understanding caring, Benner and Wrubel (1989) describe the relationship between health, illness, and disease. Health is not the absence of illness, nor is illness identical with disease. Health is a state of being that people define in relation to their own values, personality, and lifestyle. Health exists along a continuum (see Chapter 1). Illness is the experience of loss or dysfunction, whereas disease is an abnormality at the cellular, tissue, or organ level. A patient may have a disease (e.g., arthritis or diabetes) but not have the sense of being ill. An individual does not usually seek health care until there is a disruption, loss, or concern. For example, a patient has had diabetes for a number of years but does not sense being ill until the disease begins to affect his vision, threatening the ability to work. Illness therefore takes on meaning within the context of the person's life. The patient begins to feel and experience symptoms as interruption to his normal way of life.

Benner and Wrubel (1989) argue that because illness is the human experience of loss or dysfunction, any treatment given without consideration of its meaning to the individual is likely to be worthless. Expert nurses understand the difference between health, illness, and disease. Through caring re-

lationships, nurses learn to listen to patients' stories about their illnesses so that they obtain an understanding of the meaning of illness for each patient. As Sue listened to Mrs. Levine's story about her concerns over cancer, Sue took the first steps providing therapeutic, patient-centered care.

## The Essence of Nursing and Health

Madeleine Leininger (1978) offers a **transcultural** perspective of caring. She describes the concept of care as the essence and dominant domain that sets nursing apart from other health disciplines. Care is an essential human need, necessary for the health and survival of all individuals. Care, unlike cure, assists an individual or group in improving a human condition. Acts of caring refer to the direct or indirect **nurturant** and skillful activities, processes, and decisions that assist people in ways that are empathetic, compassionate, and supportive. Caring acts are dependent on the needs, problems, and values of the individual you assist. Leininger's studies (1988) of numerous cultures around the world have found that care is essential for well-being, health, growth, survival, and facing handicaps or death. Care is vital to recovery from illness and to the maintenance of healthy life practices.

Leininger (1988) stresses the importance of nurses' understanding cultural caring behaviors. Even though human caring is a universal phenomenon, the expressions, processes, and patterns of caring vary among cultures. For example, the Papua New Guinean people of Melanesia value surveillance and protection as basic elements of care, whereas southern rural African-Americans in the United States value concern and support as care. Caring is personal, and thus its expression differs for each patient. For caring to affect cure, you as a nurse learn those culturally specific behaviors that define caring for patients in different cultures (see Chapter 17).

## Transpersonal Caring

Patients and their families expect a high quality of human interaction from nurses. Unfortunately, many of the conversations that occur between patients and their nurses are very brief and oftentimes disconnected. The demands that exist within today's health care settings often cause nurses to become more task oriented rather than person oriented. Dr. Jean Watson's transpersonal caring-healing theory (1979, 1988a, 1995) focuses on individuals and what is meaningful for them and their quality of life. The theory describes a conscious recognition that caring for a person involves sensitivity, respect, and a high moral and ethical commitment. Caring comes from the Greek word *Caritas,* which means to cherish, to appreciate, and to give special attention (Watson, 2003). The caring process is a deliberate one that involves choice and action (Watson, 1988b). Watson suggests that if nurses consciously hold thoughts that are caring, open, kind, and receptive in contrast to thoughts that are controlling or manipulative, their actions will be more beneficial to patients.

Watson's caring theory (1988a) rejects the disease orientation to health care and places care before cure. Caring be-

| TABLE 16-1 | Watson's 10 Carative Factors |
| --- | --- |
| **Carative Factor** | **Example in Practice** |
| Formation of humanistic-altruistic value system | As a nurse you practice loving-kindness through giving an extension of yourself when interacting with patients. You may use, for example, self-disclosure to foster a therapeutic alliance with the patient. |
| Instillation of faith-hope | You enable and sustain your own and the patient's deep belief system. You can provide a connectedness with the patient that offers purpose and direction when trying to find the meaning of illness. |
| Cultivation of sensitivity to one's self and to others | A caring nurse achieves what Maslow describes as self-actualization. You learn to accept yourself and others for their full potential in life. |
| Developing a helping-trusting, human caring relationship | You learn to develop and sustain a helping-trusting, authentic caring relationship through effective communication with patients. |
| Promoting and expressing positive and negative feelings | You support and accept patients' expression of positive and negative feelings as a connection with self and patients. You and the patient take risks in what you share with one another. |
| Use of creative problem-solving caring processes | You learn to apply the nursing process in systematic, scientific problem solving decision making in patient care. |
| Promotion of transpersonal teaching-learning | This carative factor separates care from cure. You educate the patient appropriately while the patient assumes responsibility for learning. |
| Provision for a supportive, protective, and/or corrective mental, physical, societal, and spiritual environment | You create a healing environment at all levels (physical and nonphysical; this promotes wholeness, beauty, comfort, dignity, and peace). |
| Assistance with gratification of human needs | You assist patients with basic needs, with an intentional caring and consciousness. |
| Allowance for existential-phenomenological-spiritual forces | A nurse allows spiritual forces to provide a better understanding of oneself. |

comes the ethical standard with which we measure nursing care. Caring preserves human dignity in a cure-dominated health care system. The emphasis of care is on the nurse-patient relationship. How a nurse chooses to be with a patient and family in any given moment influences the caring-healing relationship (Watson, 1999). Watson (2003) has identified 10 caring processes that when used by nurses foster therapeutic healing relationships and affect the one caring and the one being cared for (Table 16-1).

The 10 caring processes offer a framework for the nurse's approach to patient care (Bernick, 2004). A nurse acquires a high regard for the patient and an ability to be genuine in understanding each patient's situation. The carative factors become the nurse's tools in providing caring and humane nursing therapies.

## Swanson's Theory of Caring

In the development of her caring theory, Swanson (1991) conducted interviews with three different groups: women who had miscarried, parents and professionals in a newborn intensive care unit, and socially at-risk mothers who had received long-term, public health intervention. All groups were in a perinatal (before, during, or after the birth of a child) situation and had experienced the phenomenon of caring. Swanson asked each group how they experienced caring and how caregivers expressed caring in their situation. All three groups expressed common themes or principles. Swanson's theory of caring is a composite of these themes. The theory describes caring as consisting of five

processes (Table 16-2). Each process includes a number of different subdimensions, based on patients' perceptions. Swanson defines caring as a nurturing way of relating to a valued other toward whom one feels a personal sense of commitment and responsibility. The theory supports the claim that caring is a central nursing phenomenon but not necessarily unique to nursing practice.

Swanson's theory (1991) offers valuable direction for how to develop useful and effective caring strategies. Each of the caring processes has definitions and subdimensions that serve as the basis for nursing interventions. For example, the caring process of "being with" includes conveying ability. When a nurse prepares to perform a procedure (e.g., IV or urinary catheter insertion) for a patient, it is useful to explain, "I am going to make this as painless as possible. I have performed the procedure before. I will coach you as I go and explain how you can help me." A subdimension of "enabling" is generating alternatives. When a patient is preparing to go home, a nurse supports enabling though explaining the various options available in the community for the patient to obtain needed medical supplies.

## Summary of Theoretical Views

There are common themes in nursing caring theories. Caring is highly relational. The nurse and the patient enter into a relationship that is much more than one person simply "doing tasks for" another. There is a mutual give-and-take that develops as nurse and patient begin to know and care for one another.

| TABLE 16-2 | Swanson's Theory of Caring | |
|---|---|---|
| **Caring Process** | **Definitions** | **Subdimensions** |
| Knowing | Striving to understand an event as it has meaning in the life of the other | Avoiding assumptions<br>Centering on the one cared for<br>Assessing thoroughly<br>Seeking cues<br>Engaging the self or both |
| Being with | Being emotionally present to the other | Being there<br>Conveying ability<br>Sharing feelings<br>Not burdening |
| Doing for | Doing for the other as he or she would do for the self if it were at all possible | Comforting<br>Anticipating<br>Performing skillfully<br>Protecting<br>Preserving dignity |
| Enabling | Facilitating the other's passage through life transitions (e.g., birth, death) and unfamiliar events | Informing/explaining<br>Supporting/allowing<br>Focusing<br>Generating alternatives<br>Validating/giving feedback |
| Maintaining belief | Sustaining faith in the other's capacity to get through an event or transition and face a future with meaning | Believing in/holding in esteem<br>Maintaining a hope-filled attitude<br>Offering realistic optimism<br>"Going the distance" |

From Swanson K: Empirical development of a middle-range theory of caring, *Nurs Res* 40(3):161, 1991.

Caring seems highly invisible at times when you and a patient enter a relationship of respect, concern, and support. Your empathy and compassion become a natural part of every patient encounter. However, when caring is absent, it is very obvious. For example, if you show disinterest or choose to avoid a patient's request for assistance, your inaction will quickly convey an uncaring attitude. Patients are able to quickly tell when you fail to relate to them because of poor eye contact, inattention to a discussion, or changing topics of discussion. In contrast, when you practice caring, the patient senses a commitment on your part and is willing to enter into a relationship that allows you to gain an understanding of the patient and his or her experience of illness. In a study of oncology patients, one participant described a nurse's caring as "putting the heart in it" and "having an investment" that makes "patients feel that you are with them" (Radwin, 2000). Caring allows you to become a coach and partner rather than a detached provider of nursing care.

Understanding the context of the person's life and illness is another caring theme. It is difficult to care for other individuals without understanding who they are, their life experiences, and their perception of their illness. With experience you will appreciate the value of learning about the patient's situation: How did the patient first recognize the illness? How did the patient feel? How does the illness affect the patient's daily life practices? Knowing the context of a patient's illness helps you, as the nurse, to choose and individualize interventions that will actually help the patient. This approach is more successful than simply selecting interventions on the basis of the patient's symptoms or disease process.

## Patients' Perceptions of Caring

A number of researchers have studied caring from patients' perceptions (Table 16-3). The identification of those behaviors that patients perceive as caring emphasizes what patients expect from their caregivers. Patients have always valued nurses' effectiveness in performing tasks, but clearly patients also value the affective dimension of nursing care (Williams, 1997). Establishing a reassuring presence, recognizing an individual as unique, and keeping a close, attentive eye on the patient are recurrent caring behaviors that researchers have identified. All patients are unique; however, understanding common behaviors that patients associate with caring will help you learn to express caring in practice.

The study of patients' perceptions is important because health care organizations place great emphasis on patient satisfaction (see Chapter 2). What patients experience in their interactions with institutional services and health care professionals, and what they think of that experience, will determine how patients use the health care system and how they will benefit from it (Gerteis and others, 1993). When

| TABLE 16-3 | Nursing Care Behavior (as Perceived by Patients) | |
|---|---|---|
| **Parsons and others (1995)** **Perceptions of Surgical Outpatients** | **Attree (2001)** **Perceptions of General Medical Patients and Families** | **Radwin (2000)** **Perceptions of Cancer Patients** |
| Reassuring presence of the nurse | Checking up on patients | Expressing concern |
| Expressions of concern | Being compassionate and patient | Being nurturant |
| Attention to physical comfort | Demonstrating sensitivity and sympathy | Remembering the patient |
| Teamwork of nursing staff | Using a calm, gentle, and kind approach | Individualization or selecting therapies more |
| Provision of a relaxed and quiet environment | | likely to feel nurturing |
| Nurses' professional manner | | Being attentive |

patients sense that health care providers are interested in them as people, it is likely patients will be more willing to follow recommendations and therapeutic plans. Williams (1997) studied the relationship between patients' perceptions of caring and their satisfaction with nursing care. Patients indicated that they were most satisfied when they perceived nurses to be caring. Radwin (2000) found oncology patients described excellent nursing care as attentiveness, partnership, individualization, rapport, and caring. As institutions look for ways of improving patient satisfaction, creating an environment of caring is a necessary and worthwhile goal. Institutions create caring environments in the way they design and furnish patient rooms and waiting areas, provide nurses with the resources to meet individual needs of patients, and offer educational resources. Patients' satisfaction with nursing care is the most important factor in their decision to return to a hospital.

As you begin your clinical practice, it is important to observe and learn how patients perceive caring and how to implement caring practices daily as you provide care. The behaviors that researchers have associated with caring offer an excellent starting point. But remember that each patient has unique expectations. Researchers have learned that patients and nurses often differ in their perceptions of caring. For that reason, you build relationships that allow you to know what is important to patients. A patient who is fearful of having an intravenous (IV) catheter inserted may benefit more if you acquire assistance from a staff member who is able to quickly and skillfully insert the catheter than if you attempt to relieve anxiety through a lengthy description of the procedure. Knowing who patients are will help you to select those caring approaches that are most appropriate to the patients' needs.

## Caring in Nursing Practice

It is impossible to prescribe ways for you to become a caring nurse. Experts disagree as to whether caring is a teachable concept or not. Some believe it is fundamentally a way of being in the world. For those who find caring a normal part of their life, caring is a product of their culture, values, beliefs, experiences, and relationships with others. Persons who do not experience care in their lives often find it difficult to act in caring ways. As nurses deal with health and illness in their practice, they grow in their ability to care. Expert nurses understand the differences and relationships between health, illness, and disease. They become able to see patients in their own context, to interpret their needs, and to offer caring acts that improve patients' health. Caring is not a separate act that you perform. Caring is embedded within each encounter and each action that you share with a patient.

### Providing Presence

Watson's theory (1988a) of caring explains that a nurse is always present and open to exchanges with patients. Being present involves a conscious awareness of the relationship with one another (Bernick, 2004). Presence is more than mere physical presence, although the physical closeness is important. Presence also represents being "in tune" with each other. Nursing **presence** is a deep physical, psychological, spiritual, and energetic connection between the nurse and patient (Duis-Nittsche, 2002).

When you work on a busy nursing unit of a hospital it is difficult to find the moment needed to prepare for a patient encounter. However, the initial moments you spend with a patient affect how the nurse-patient relationship develops and evolves. Bernick (2004) explains that it is important when a nurse enters a patient's personal space to first pause and center. A centering act includes hand washing, the formal greeting made with a patient, the personal touch of eye contact or a handshake. Centering is an occasion to clear your energy and open up yourself to receive another person (Watson, 1999). When Sue first met Mrs. Levine, she introduced herself, sat down by Mrs. Levine, and made eye contact. These intentional acts created a focus to connect with Mrs. Levine and to convey a commitment to attend to her spoken words. The act of centering creates a shift from the intention to assess and recommend care measures to a genuine responsibility to begin to understand the complexity of a patient's situation (Bernick, 2004).

Eye contact, body language, voice tone, listening, and having a positive and encouraging attitude are all part of es-

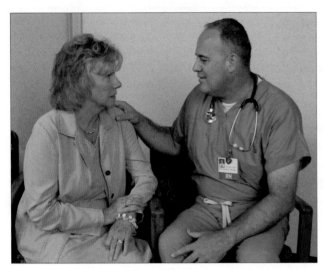

FIGURE **16-1** Nurse conveying presence to a patient.

tablishing an open presence (Figure 16-1). Openness and understanding convey the message that the patient's experience matters to you (Swanson, 1991). In the opening clinical scenario, Sue's gentle encouragement and willingness to listen conveyed a presence that allowed the patient to express her feelings. Being able to establish presence with a patient enhances your ability to learn from the patient. As a result, you strengthen your ability to provide adequate and appropriate nursing care each time you are with the patient.

It is especially important to establish presence when patients are experiencing stressful events or situations. Awaiting a physician's or health care provider's report of test results or preparing for an unfamiliar procedure are just two examples of events in the course of a person's illness that create unpredictability and dependency on care providers. Your presence helps to calm anxiety and fear related to stress. Giving reassurance and thorough explanations about a procedure, remaining at the patient's side, and coaching the patient through the experience all convey a presence that is invaluable to the patient's well-being.

## Comforting

**Comforting** is an approach that provides both physical and emotional calm. A nurse uses principles of comforting, patient privacy, and safety when delivering all nursing care interventions. For example, using the principles of hygiene and comfort described in Chapters 27 and 30 offers effective comforting strategies. Remember, it is not simply the "doing for" that is comforting; rather, it is a comforting approach that creates calm. For example, a patient who is undergoing chemotherapy often suffers from fatigue and has ulcerative lesions of the mouth. Anyone can provide mouth care as just another activity in the workday of a nurse. However, for the mouth care to be comforting, choose a time, outside of a routine, that best meets the patient's needs. Perhaps time the mouth care to coincide with 30 minutes after the patient has

had an analgesic. Provide gentle, cleansing mouth care, dim the room lights, reposition the patient, and offer some encouraging words to allow the patient to rest peacefully once the procedure is over.

## Touch

Patients face embarrassing, frightening, and painful situations. Nurses use touch as one comforting approach to reach out and communicate their support. Touch is a form of relating that involves contact and noncontact (Fredriksson, 1999). Contact touch involves obvious skin-to-skin contact, whereas noncontact touch refers to eye contact. Fredriksson (1999) describes both types of touch within three categories: task-oriented touch, caring touch, and protective touch.

Always use a task-oriented touch when performing nursing procedures. The skillful and gentle insertion of a catheter or the way you turn a patient conveys security and a sense of competence. Expert nurses learn that any procedure is more effective when it is done carefully and in consideration of any patient concern. For example, if a patient is anxious about having an IV started, you comfort the patient by explaining fully how you will perform the procedure and what the patient will feel. You also convey the sense that you will place the IV safely, skillfully, and successfully in the way you prepare supplies, position the patient, and gently manipulate the IV catheter. Talking quietly to a patient throughout a procedure offers reassurance and support. In contrast, when you perform a procedure efficiently in an automatic fashion, without attending to the patient's anxiety, the patient will perceive your competence as uncaring.

When you perform nursing procedures, always maintain eye contact with the patient as much as you can. Your ability to look at patients, especially when they ask questions or express emotions through groaning or sighing, shows you are interested in their well-being. Good eye contact reinforces to patients that you care and that what they say is important.

Caring touch is a form of nonverbal communication that successfully influences a patient's comfort and security and enhances self-esteem (Boyek and Watson, 1994). You convey caring touch in the way you hold a patient's hand, give a back rub, or participate in a conversation. Just holding a patient's hand for a few minutes is very calming when a patient is afraid, hurting, or confused. Sitting on the side of the bed as you hold a patient's hand, shows that you are not in a hurry and that the patient's needs are your main priority. Through caring touch you connect with the patient and show acceptance of the person.

Protective touch is a form of touch used to protect the nurse and/or patient (Fredriksson, 1999). Patients view protective touch both positively and negatively. The most obvious form of protective touch is when you use touch to prevent an accident. For example, you hold and brace a patient to avoid a fall. Protective touch also protects you as the nurse emotionally. You might push away or distance yourself from a patient when you need to escape from a stressful situation. In this example, protective touch can cause negative feelings in patients.

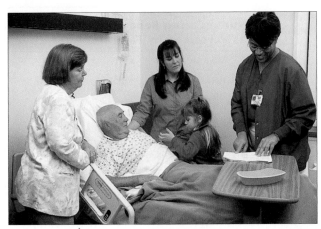

FIGURE **16-2** Nurse discusses patient's health care needs with family.

Because touch conveys many messages, use it with discretion. Patients usually accept task-oriented touch, because most individuals give nurses a license to enter their personal space to provide care. However, exceptions exist because of patients' cultural backgrounds (see Chapter 17). Always know if a patient accepts touch and how they will interpret your intentions.

## Listening

Caring involves an interpersonal interaction that is much more than two persons simply talking back and forth. In a caring relationship you establish trust, open lines of communication, and listen to what the patient has to say (Figure 16-2). Listening is key because it conveys your full attention and interest. It is not only "taking in" what a patient says, but also includes an interpretation and understanding of what is said and giving back that understanding to the person talking (Kemper, 1992). Listening to the meaning of what a patient says helps create a mutual relationship.

When individuals become ill, there usually is a story about the meaning of their illness. Any critical or chronic illness affects a patient's life choices and decisions. Being able to tell that story helps the patient break the distress of illness. Stories help you as the nurse to form a mental image that provides a better understanding of questions such as, What does it mean to be ill? What does it mean to feel comfortable? To tell a story a patient needs a listener. Frank (1998) described his own feelings during his experience with cancer, emphasizing his need to be able to express what he needed. The personal concerns that are part of a patient's illness story determine what is at stake for the patient. Caring for a patient enables you to participate in the patient's life. Give patients your undivided, full attention while they are telling their stories. Listening is not simply a task, but instead a gift; otherwise its efficacy, or power to effect, is lost (Frank, 1998).

When a patient chooses to tell his or her story, it involves reaching out to another human being. Telling the story implies a relationship that develops only if the clinician ex-

changes personal stories as well. Frank (1998) argues that professionals do not routinely take seriously their own need to be known as part of a clinical relationship. Yet, unless the professional acknowledges this need, there is no reciprocal relationship, only an interaction (Campo, 1997). You will feel pressure to know as much as possible about a patient without allowing a relationship to develop, but this isolates you from the patient. In contrast, in knowing and being known each supports the other (Frank, 1998). As a nurse you will hear and share a variety of stories from patients. To show that you are listening, tell parts of your own stories but do so in response to the ill person's story. For example, when a patient tells a story about how the patient's family is reacting to his or her illness, choose to share a personal family story that enforces a sense of hope as to how a family is able to cope with illness. To give the gift of listening is to appreciate receiving the gift of a patient's story and to then share a part of you.

Learning to listen is sometimes difficult. It is easy to become distracted by the tasks at hand and colleagues shouting instructions. However, the time you take to listen (and listen effectively) is worthwhile because you gain information and strengthen the nurse-patient relationship. When you take the time to listen to patients, the patients feel that you care about them and find what they need to express is important. Patients often share with their nurses things that they do not share with their physicians or health care providers and sometimes even their families. Listening involves paying attention to the patient's words and tone of voice and entering the patient's world. By observing the expressions and body language of the patient, you find cues to help assist the patient in exploring ways to make decisions, take action, or to do whatever a situation requires. Chapter 9 discusses additional listening techniques.

## Knowing the Patient

A concept important to a nurse's ability to care is "knowing the patient." Knowing is discussed by a number of different nurse researchers. Swanson (1991) describes knowing the patient as one of the five caring processes in her theory of caring. Through repeated experience in caring for patients with similar problems and needs, you begin to develop a level of knowing. For example, with experience you begin to know what a pressure ulcer looks like, how patients respond to analgesics, and how patients express fear. Through active listening and being present in a discussion, you begin to know patients in relation to what they believe are important to them (Bernick, 2004). To know a patient means to avoid assumptions, center on the patient, and engage in a caring relationship that reveals information and cues that promote critical thinking and clinical judgment. Knowing develops in the everyday practical work of patient care: getting a grasp of the patient, getting situated into what is occurring clinically, and understanding the patient's situation in context of the illness and the effects it has on the patient's life (Tanner and others, 1993). Knowing the patient is at the core of clinical decision making.

Expert nurses develop the ability to detect changes in patients' conditions almost effortlessly. A nurse learns to recognize particular responses and patterns: the effect of a slight change in an antihypertensive drug on a patient's blood pressure, the effect of physical turning on the patient's heart rate, and the avoidance of conversation as a patient's pain increases. Clinical decision making involves various aspects of knowing the patient. This includes responses to therapies, routines and habits, coping resources, physical capacities and endurance, and body typology and characteristics (Tanner and others, 1993). Additional factors that the experienced nurse knows about patients are their experiences, behaviors, feelings, and perceptions (Radwin, 1995). When you make clinical decisions accurately in the context of knowing a patient well, improved patient outcomes will result.

Knowing a patient is much more than simply gathering data about the patient's clinical signs and condition. Duis-Nittsche (2002) notes that hospitalized patients identify "knowing me" as part of the nurse's presence and ability to provide comforting and supportive care. Success in knowing a patient lies in the relationship that you establish. To know a patient is to enter into a caring, social process that sets the stage for the nurse-patient relationship to evolve into "working" and "changing" phases in which you help the patient to become involved in personal care and to accept help when needed.

## Healing Environments

The environment influences the caring-healing process (Watson, 1999). Often a health care setting is not one that creates a sense of calm or well-being. Factors that stimulate our senses such as noise, privacy, light levels, access to nature, space, and color affect the caring-healing process. Bernick explains that when you care for an older adult, small changes in the environment make a big difference (Box 16-1). It is important to create a caring environment that respects the older adult's dignity.

## Spiritual Caring

A person achieves spiritual health when he or she finds a balance between personal life values, goals, and belief systems and those of others. A person's beliefs and expectations affect the person's physical well-being. Establishing a caring relationship with a patient involves an interconnectedness between you and your patient. This is the reason why Watson (1999) describes the caring relationship in a spiritual sense.

Spirituality offers a sense of connectedness as well, intrapersonally (connected with oneself), interpersonally (connected with others and the environment), and transpersonally (connected with the unseen, God, or a higher power). In a caring relationship, a patient and nurse come to know one another and move toward a healing relationship by mobilizing hope for the patient and for the nurse. Both find an interpretation or understanding of illness, symptoms, or emotions that is acceptable to the patient. As a nurse you assist the patient in using social, emotional, or spiritual resources. Chapter 18 describes in detail the significance that spirituality plays in an individual's health.

## Family Care

People live their worlds in an involved way. Each individual experiences life through relationships with others. Caring for an individual therefore does not occur in isolation from that person's family. As a nurse, it is important for you to know the family almost as thoroughly as you know a patient. The patient's family is an important resource. Success with interventions often depends on the family's willingness to share information about the patient, their acceptance and understanding of therapies, whether the interventions fit with the family's daily practices, and whether the family is able to support and deliver the therapies recommended.

Caring for a family often begins with listening. When a family member has a concern about a patient, they want a caregiver to listen. Typically, family members want to know about the care and treatments that are being given to their relative. If you do not respond to them in a caring manner, they will be more likely to not trust you. A family member can become an invaluable partner when you care for a patient. Learn to know what family members expect from you. Also, be sensitive to any cultural factors that will affect the extent to which you should involve family members in patient care.

Mayer (1987) identified 10 nurse caring behaviors that families of patients with cancer perceived as most helpful (Box 16-2). Ensuring the patient's well-being and helping the family to become active participants are critical for family members. Although specific to families of patients with cancer, the behaviors offer useful guidelines for developing caring relationships with all families. Early in the nurse-patient relationship, ask who are members of the patient's family and what their roles are in the patient's life. Showing the family that you care about the patient creates an openness that enables a relationship to form with them. Caring for the family takes into consideration the context of the patient's illness and the stress it imposes on all members.

## The Challenge of Caring

Caring motivates people to become nurses, and it becomes the source of satisfaction when nurses know they have made a difference in their patients' lives. It is becoming more of a challenge to care in today's health care system. Being a part of the helping professions is difficult and demanding. Nurses are given less time to spend with patients, making it much harder to get to know the patient. Too often patients become just numbers, with their real needs either overlooked or ignored.

If health care is to make a positive difference in our patients' lives, we cannot treat human beings like machines or robots. Instead, health care must become more humanizing. As a professional you play an important role in making care an integral part of health care. This begins by making caring a part of the philosophy and environment in the workplace. Always conduct nursing rounds with an attentional focus and desire to create a presence that enables patients to tell their stories. Listen and learn; do not try to control or manipulate the interventions you choose. Instead, engage in a caring relationship that you shape using the patient's perspectives and what is important to him or her. Engage the patient in decisions about the best interventions to use. Always take time to get to know family members as well. Be committed to caring and be willing in your day-to-day practice to establish relationships with patients and families that afford personal, compassionate, and meaningful nursing care.

## KEY CONCEPTS

- According to Benner, *caring* is a word for being connected and is the essence of excellent nursing practice.
- Because illness is the human experience of loss or dysfunction, any treatment or intervention given without consideration of its meaning to the individual is likely to be worthless.
- Leininger stresses the importance of understanding that even though human caring is universal, the patterns and expressions of caring vary among cultures.
- Watson's transpersonal caring-healing theory explains that caring focuses on individuals and what is meaningful for them and their quality of life.
- Swanson's theory of caring includes five caring processes: knowing, being with, doing for, enabling, and maintaining belief.
- To care for another individual, understand the context of the person's life and illness.
- Patients and nurses often differ in their perceptions of caring.

- Patients tend to be more satisfied with nursing care when they perceive that nurses care.
- Presence involves a centering act that clears a nurse's energy and opens up the nurse's self to receive a patient.
- When you establish presence, eye contact, body language, voice tone, listening, and having a positive and encouraging attitude act together to create openness and understanding.
- The skillful and gentle performance of a nursing procedure conveys security and a sense of competence in a nurse.
- Listening involves paying attention to an individual's words and tone of voice and entering into his or her frame of reference.
- Knowing the patient is at the core of the process by which nurses make clinical decisions.
- You demonstrate caring by helping family members become active participants in a patient's care.

## CRITICAL THINKING IN PRACTICE

*Mrs. Levine has decided to receive chemotherapy treatments for her cancer. She comes to the outpatient surgery unit for the insertion of an implanted port. The port will allow the nursing staff to administer chemotherapeutic doses regularly. Sue begins preparation for the first dose of chemotherapy. She encourages Mrs. Levine to ask any questions about the procedure.*

1. As Sue prepares the supplies for administering chemotherapy, which of the following actions conveys a "caring touch"?
   a. Sue explains to Mrs. Levine that the chemotherapeutic drug will be instilled slowly.
   b. Sue plumps the pillows and assists Mrs. Levine with assuming a comfortable position in the recliner.

   c. Sue double-checks the label of the chemotherapeutic drug against the physician's or health care provider's order sheet.
   d. Sue places all the equipment she needs next to Mrs. Levine's recliner and methodically manipulates Mrs. Levine's port to prepare for the chemotherapy infusion.
2. Mrs. Levine says to Sue, "I am still worried about some of the side effects of this drug." Using Swanson's theory of caring, describe an intervention you use for each of the following:
   a. Maintaining belief
   b. Knowing

3. Mrs. Levine's son, Jim, comes to the clinic just as the chemotherapy begins. He asks to talk with Sue about his mother's treatment. Choose all of the following that are examples of centering used by Sue.
   a. Sue explains only the common risks of chemotherapy.
   b. Sue shakes Jim's hand as they begin their discussion.
   c. Sue asks Jim if his mother can be involved in the discussion.
   d. Sue invites Jim to sit down with her in the lounge; she leans forward and looks at Jim at eye level.

4. As Sue explains chemotherapy and its risks to Jim, she demonstrates behaviors that show she cares about Mrs. Levine. List three behaviors Sue uses to demonstrate to Jim that she cares for his mother.

## NCLEX® REVIEW

1. As part of your work in a teen pregnancy clinic you talk with a young teenage patient about her experience in relationships with young men. The teen needs to talk with her boyfriend about the use of a condom during intercourse. You respond to the teen, "From what you have told me, I think you know how to talk with your boyfriend. Tell me how you will explain the need for him to wear a condom." This is an example of:
   1. Knowing
   2. Enabling
   3. Doing for
   4. Maintaining belief

2. You enter a patient's room, greet the patient, and explain that you intend to check the IV medications infusing into the patient's arm. You increase the rate of the IV and wait a few minutes after checking vital signs to see if the patient's behavior changes in any way. Your combined actions are an example of:
   1. Knowing
   2. Presence
   3. Listening
   4. Doing for

3. When you change a patient's wound dressing, you drape the patient to expose only the wound and change the dressing without soiling the bed linen or pulling the skin unnecessarily. This series of actions exhibits:
   1. Enabling
   2. Being with
   3. Doing for
   4. Comforting

4. When you are able to demonstrate culturally specific behaviors that express caring, you are applying the theory of caring developed by:
   1. Benner
   2. Radwin
   3. Swanson
   4. Leininger

5. During the change-of-shift report, another nurse tells you that Mrs. Riza had a difficult night and was unable to sleep. She has had episodes of crying and called out frequently to the nurses. You have not cared for Mrs. Riza in the past. Upon first entering the patient's room you establish eye contact and offer to hold her hand, asking "Mrs. Riza, the nurses tell me you had a restless night; tell me what has been bothering you." This is an example of:
   1. Anticipating
   2. Being with
   3. Centering
   4. Knowing

6. Choose the action that best describes effective listening:
   1. Anticipating what the patient has to say
   2. Establishing initial eye contact
   3. Observing a patient's body language
   4. Choosing actions to control a patient's behavior

7. Jim, the nurse caring for Mr. Rosen, a 70-year-old patient who had a stroke, knew that food was central to Mr. Rosen's being. Mr. Rosen always enjoyed cooking his own meals and found great satisfaction in fresh, well-seasoned food. Jim's decision to attend to Mr. Rosen's dietary needs in a way that provided caring sustenance is addressed in which of the caring theories?
   1. Leininger
   2. Benner
   3. Swanson
   4. Watson

8. Howard has cared for Mr. Levin the last 2 days. Mr. Levin has terminal cancer and is probably in his last days of life. Howard checks on Mr. Levin frequently and stands at his bedside often to explain the comfort measures he provides. When Mr. Levin opens his eyes to see Howard, Howard responds, "I am here." This is an example of:
   1. Presence
   2. Centering
   3. Doing for
   4. Maintaining belief

## REFERENCES

Attree M: Patients' and relatives' experiences and perspectives of "good" and "not so good" quality care, *J Adv Nurs* 33(4):456, 2001.

Benner P: *From novice to expert,* Menlo Park, Calif, 1984, Addison-Wesley.

Benner P, Wrubel J: *The primacy of caring: stress and coping in health and illness,* Menlo Park, Calif, 1989, Addison-Wesley.

Bernick L: Caring for older adults: practice guided by Watson's caring-healing model, *Nurs Sci Q* 17(2):128, 2004.

Boyek K, Watson R: A touching story, *Elderly Care* 3:20, 1994.

Campo R: *The poetry of healing: a doctor's education in empathy, identification, and desire,* New York, 1997, WW Norton.

Duis-Nittsche ER: *A study of nursing presence,* unpublished doctoral dissertation, Galveston, Tex, 2002, University of Texas Medical Branch.

Frank AW: Just listening: narrative and deep illness, *Fam Syst Health* 16(3):197, 1998.

Fredriksson L: Modes of relating in a caring conversation: a research synthesis on presence, touch, and listening, *J Adv Nurs* 30(5):1167, 1999.

Gerteis M and others: What patients really want, *Health Manage Q* 15:2, 1993.

Kemper BJ: Therapeutic listening: developing the concept, *J Psychosoc Nurs* 7:21, 1992.

Leininger M: *Transcultural nursing: concepts, theories and practices,* New York, 1978, John Wiley & Sons.

Leininger M: *Care: the essence of nursing and health,* Detroit, 1988, Wayne State University Press.

Mayer DK: Cancer patients' and families' perceptions of nurse caring behaviors, *Top Clin Nurs* 8(2):63, 1986.

Mayer DK: Oncology nurses' versus cancer patients' perceptions of nurse caring behaviors: a replication study, *Oncol Nurs Forum* 14(3):48, 1987.

Parsons E and others: Perioperative nurse caring behaviors, *Adv Operating Room Nurs J* 57(5):1106, 1995.

Radwin L: Knowing the patient: a process model for individualized interventions, *Nurs Res* 44:364, 1995.

Radwin L: Oncology patients' perceptions of quality nursing care, *Res Nurs Health* 23:179, 2000.

Swanson KM: Empirical development of a middle-range theory of caring, *Nurs Res* 40(3):161, 1991.

Tanner C and others: The phenomenology of knowing the patient, *Image J Nurs Sch* 25:273, 1993.

Watson J: *Nursing: the philosophy and science of caring,* Boston, 1979, Little Brown.

Watson J: New dimensions of human caring theory, *Nurs Sci Q* 1:175, 1988a.

Watson J: *Nursing: human science and human care,* New York, 1988b, National League for Nursing.

Watson J: Nursing's caring-healing paradigm as exemplar for alternative medicine? *Altern Ther Health Med* 1(3):64, 1995.

Watson J: *Postmodern nursing and beyond,* Edinburgh, 1999, Churchill Livingstone.

Watson J: *Theory of human caring,* University of Colorado Health Sciences Center, School of Nursing, 2003, http://www2.uchsc.edu/son/caring, accessed Oct 15, 2004.

Williams SA: The relationship of patients' perceptions of holistic nurse caring to satisfaction with nursing care, *J Nurs Care Qual* 11(5):15, 1997.

# CHAPTER 17

# Cultural Diversity

## MEDIA RESOURCES

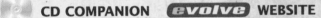

**CD COMPANION** *evolve* **WEBSITE**

http://evolve.elsevier.com/Potter/basic

- **NCLEX® Review**
- **Audio Glossary**
- **English/Spanish Audio Glossary**

## OBJECTIVES

- Identify the impact of demographic trends on health and nursing.
- Describe health disparities linked with racial and ethnic differences.
- Compare dominant and variant cultural contexts of health and illness.
- Analyze impact of culture in health, illness, and caring patterns.
- Describe steps toward developing cultural competence.
- Use cultural assessment to plan culturally competent care.
- Apply research findings in culturally competent care.

## KEY TERMS

acculturation, p. 499
assimilation, p. 499
*baridi,* p. 494
biases and prejudices, p. 494
bilineally, p. 499
botanica, p. 495
*confianza,* p. 501
cultural and linguistic competence, p. 496
cultural assessment, p. 497
cultural awareness, p. 495
cultural care accommodation or negotiation, p. 504
cultural care preservation or maintenance, p. 504
cultural care repatterning or restructuring, p. 504
cultural competence, p. 495
cultural encounters, p. 495
cultural imposition, p. 494
cultural knowledge, p. 495
cultural pain, p. 494
cultural skills, p. 495
culturally blind, p. 494
culturally congruent care, p. 495
culturally ignorant, p. 494
culture, p. 494

culture-bound syndromes, p. 494
culture care theory, p. 495
culturological nursing assessment, p. 497
discrimination, p. 494
disease, p. 494
dominant culture, p. 493
emic worldview, p. 495
ethnicity, p. 493
ethnocentrism, p. 494
ethnohistory, p. 499
etic worldview, p. 495
face-saving, p. 501
*fajita,* p. 503
*farmacia,* p. 495
fictive, p. 499
focused cultural assessment, p. 499
future orientation, p. 501
granny midwives, p. 503
*halal,* p. 500
*haram,* p. 500
*hilots,* p. 503
illness, p. 494
imam, p. 504
impression management, p. 498
karma, p. 495
*la curantena,* p. 503
*la dieta,* p. 503
*mal de ojo,* p. 502
matrilineal, p. 499

*parteras,* p. 502
patrilineal, p. 499
*personalismo,* p. 501
present time orientation, p. 501
race, p. 493
Ramadan, p. 501
*respeto,* p. 501
Sabbath, p. 500

*simpatia,* p. 501
stereotypes, p. 494
subcultures, p. 493
Sunrise Model, p. 495
transcultural nursing, p. 495
variant, p. 493
worldview, p. 494

The U.S. population is increasing in diversity. Nonwhite and Hispanic groups make up approximately 35% of the total population. In 2002, Hispanics have become the largest minority group, numbering 38.8 million (U.S. Bureau of the Census, 2003b). Asians have the highest growth rate (U.S. Bureau of the Census, 2003a). Within this context of increasing diversity, you need to recognize that in any society there is a **dominant culture** that exists along with other **variant** cultural patterns (Kluckhohn, 1976). These variant patterns are also called diverse cultures, subcultures, or minority cultures. Although subcultures have similarities with the dominant culture, they maintain their unique life patterns, values, and norms. In the United States, the dominant culture is Anglo-American with origins from Western Europe. **Subcultures** represent various ethnic, religious, and other groups with distinct characteristics from the dominant culture. **Ethnicity** refers to a shared identity related to social and cultural heritage such as values, language, geographical space, and racial characteristics. Members of an ethnic group feel a common sense of identity. For example, individuals declare their ethnic identity as Peruvian, Bosnian, or Korean. The term **race,** which is often wrongly interchanged with ethnicity, means the common biological characteristics shared by a group of people such as skin color (Leininger and McFarland, 2002; Spector, 2004). Some examples of racial classifications are African-Americans and Caucasians.

## Health Disparities

Health disparities are unequal burdens of disease morbidity and mortality rates experienced by racial and ethnic groups (Baldwin, 2003). Several studies have established the link between health and an individual's socioeconomic status, environment, ethnicity, and/or gender. For example, women of Vietnamese origin suffer from cervical cancer five times more than white women and death rates from heart disease for African-Americans are 40% higher than for whites (U.S. Department of Health and Human Services [USDHHS], 2000). Even when there is access to health services, researchers often find that racial and ethnic differences contribute to health care disparities. Racial and ethnic minorities experience a lower quality of health services and are less likely to receive even routine medical procedures than white Americans. Health provider bias, stereotyping, prejudice, clinical uncertainty (Smedley, Stith, and Nelson, 2002), and poor provider-patient communication contribute to racial and ethnic health disparities (Ashton and others, 2003; Van Ryn and Fu, 2003).

Although persons belonging to ethnic minority groups have increased health risks, most health care interventions and health care concepts have targeted middle-class, white populations. Health care practitioners often misinterpret the effect a person's culture has on health and are ill-prepared educationally and clinically to provide safe and effective care for culturally diverse populations (Kao, Hsu, and Clark, 2004). For example, a study of low-income African-American mothers and their children attending a clinic in transitional housing found that the women and children encountered barriers to access to care. The care these mothers and children received was fragmented and did not respond to their needs (Amen and Pacquiao, 2004).

## Cultural Conflicts

Culture has a significant influence on the patient and health care practitioners. Because culture is a cognitive system of meanings that provides the context for valuing, evaluating, and categorizing life experiences, members of a cultural group are predisposed to **ethnocentrism.** This is a tendency to hold one's own way of life as superior to others. It is also the source of **biases and prejudices** composed of beliefs and attitudes associating negative permanent characteristics to people who are perceived to be different from oneself. When a person acts with prejudice, **discrimination** occurs. Health care practitioners who are **culturally ignorant** or **culturally blind** about differences generally resort to **cultural imposition** and use their own values and customs as the absolute guide in dealing with patients and interpreting their behaviors. Although knowledge about particular cultures is important, avoid **stereotypes,** which result in a tendency to fit every person into a particular pattern without further as-

sessment. When practitioners disregard a patient's valued way of life, the patient experiences **cultural pain** (Leininger and McFarland, 2002).

## Culture in Health and Illness

Understanding the effect culture has on health is evident in the priorities for funding research by the National Institutes of Health and the initiative taken by the U.S. Department of Health and Human Services in eliminating health disparities. The Office of Minority Health (2000) defined **culture** as the "integrated patterns of human behavior that include the language, thoughts, communications, actions, customs, beliefs, values and institutions of racial, ethnic, religious or social groups." Culture is socially transmitted across generations and guides a particular group's thoughts, decisions, and actions (Leininger and McFarland, 2002; Purnell and Paulanka, 2003b). Culture provides the framework in which the meaning of illness is defined. **Illness** is the personal, interpersonal, and cultural reaction to disease, whereas **disease** is a malfunctioning or maladaptation of biological or psychological processes. People create their own interpretation and descriptions of biological and psychological malfunctions within their unique social and cultural context (Kleinman, 1980). **Culture-bound syndromes** are illnesses restricted to a particular culture or group because of its psychosocial characteristics (Andrews, 2003). The personal, social, and cultural explanations and reactions of a given society to perceived dysfunctions or abnormalities in its members make up these syndromes (Kleinman, 1980).

For example, among the Bena people of Tanzania, where communal values are the norm, the condition of **baridi** is attributed to disrespectful behavior within the family or transgression of cultural taboos. The person experiences physical symptoms (feeling cold, fatigue, restlessness, and loss of appetite and weight), psychological symptoms (mental disturbances, sexual disability), and social and economic losses (loss of job, property partner). Traditional healers detect the illness and treat it by having the ill person make a public admission and an apology, having the person make amends towards the family, or by using herbal remedies (Juntunen, 2005).

### Comparative Worldviews About Health and Illness

A **worldview** is a cognitive stance or perspective about phenomena characteristic of a particular cultural group. Note that professional worldviews about health and illness are often distinct from those of patients. Table 17-1 presents a comparison between distinct worldviews held by the dominant U.S. culture and those of variant groups. Health care professionals are educated in the dominant cultural norms of the society in which they practice. Consequently, they have a particular worldview that sometimes conflicts with that of other subcultures. In any intercultural encounter, there are two si-

| TABLE 17-1 | Comparative Cultural Worldviews About Health and Illness | |
| --- | --- | --- |
| | **Dominant United States** | **Variant Cultures** |
| Illness causation | Biomedical | Cosmological |
| | Scientific | Supernatural |
| | | Magico-religious |
| Treatment | Organ-specific | Holistic |
| | Specialty-driven | Mixed (magico-religious, supernatural, herbal, biomedical, etc.) |
| Practitioners/healers | Universal standards of practice | May be learned through apprenticeship |
| | Uniform qualifications for practice | Criteria for practice not uniform |
| | | Reputation established in community |
| Caring pattern | Self-care | Caring provided by others |
| | Self-determination | Group reliance and interdependence |

multaneous perspectives about the situation. There is an insider or native perspective (**emic worldview**) and an outsider's perspective (**etic worldview**).

For example, the Asian Indian belief in **karma** attributes mental illness to past deeds in one's previous life; hence the individual deserves suffering. Compounded by the cultural stigma attached to the illness, patients generally express their symptoms in somatic or physical symptoms and seek help only when the family is no longer able to manage the condition (Conrad and Pacquiao, 2005).

However, the dominant culture in the United States encourages self-care, which matches the societal value of self-reliance and individualism. The focus of care is the individual patient, who is responsible for changing his or her behavior to achieve health and well-being. In contrast, collectivistic cultures such as traditional Asians, Hispanics, and Africans rely on their family to care for the sick member. Members other than the patient will make decisions about care and perform the tasks of caring. Group caring often conflicts with health care institutional policies, such as limiting visitors at the bedside, informed consent, and confidentiality.

Table 17-2 presents folk healers or practitioners in specific cultural groups. These healers share the group's naturalistic, holistic, and supernatural worldview about causes of illness. Treatments are more holistic and not focused on one specific organ. The healers often use different methods, combining the spiritual, religious, and supernatural with natural means. Heat, massage, acupuncture, and herbs are common methods. Some folk healers learn their trade through apprenticeship, and some guard their trade with great secrecy such as in Santeria and voodoo. Hispanics seek folk healers and healing methods such as magic, religious, and herbal remedies from a **botanica** and obtain prescribed medications from a **farmacia**.

## Culturally Competent Care

Leininger's **culture care theory** emphasizes the central purpose of nursing, which is to provide **culturally congruent care**. This is care that fits personal valued life patterns and meanings generated by the individual, which are sometimes different from the professional's perspectives on the person's care. Leininger developed **transcultural nursing** as a distinct discipline focused on the comparative study of cultures to understand similarities (culture universal) and differences (culture-specific) among groups of people. Leininger's **Sunrise Model** (Figure 17-1) demonstrates how culturally congruent care comes from the cultural and social structure dimensions of a particular group that enables the health care practitioner to design care decisions and actions that correspond with those of the group. Leininger also describes folk care as a form of caring that is defined by the people. Folk care contrasts with health professionals' biomedical caring, which is based on scientific principles (Leininger and McFarland, 2002).

Campinha-Bacote (2003) defines **cultural competence** as a process in which the health care professional continually strives to achieve the ability and availability to work effectively with individuals, families, and communities. Cultural desire is the spiritual and pivotal energy source and motivation for one's journey into the process of developing the following:

**Cultural awareness**—gaining in-depth awareness of one's own background, stereotypes, biases, prejudices, and assumptions about other people

**Cultural knowledge**—obtaining knowledge of other cultures; gaining sensitivity to, respect for, and appreciation of differences

**Cultural skills**—developing cultural skills such as communication, cultural assessment, and culturally competent care

**Cultural encounters**—engaging in cross-cultural interactions, refining intercultural communication skills, gaining in-depth understanding of others and avoiding stereotypes, and cultural conflict management

Suh (2004) theorizes that cultural competence has four domains, attributes, and outcomes. The cognitive domain includes awareness of the need for cultural competence and gaining a foundation to understand other cultures. The affective domain involves cultural sensitivity and appreciation of

| TABLE 17-2 | Cultural Healers | |
|---|---|---|
| **Cultural Group** | **Healer** | **Nature of Practice** |
| Chinese and Southeast Asians | Herbalist | Combination of plant, animal, and mineral products in restoring balance based on yin/yang concepts |
| | Acupuncturist | Yin treatment using needles to restore balance and flow of *qi*; yang treatment using moxibustion or heat with acupuncture; may be indicated to restore yin/yang balance |
| | Fortune teller | Consultation to foretell outcomes of plans and seek spiritual advice to enhance good fortune and deal with misfortune |
| | Shaman | Combination of prayers, chanting, and herbs to treat illnesses caused by supernatural, psychological, and physical factors |
| Asian Indians | Ayurvedic practitioner | Combination of dietary, herbal, and other naturalistic therapies to prevent and treat illness |
| | Homeopath | Use of natural remedies in titrated doses |
| Native American | Shaman | Combination of prayers, chanting, and herbs to treat illnesses caused by supernatural, psychological, and physical factors |
| African-American | Old lady "granny midwife" | Consultation in diagnosing and treating common illnesses and care of women in childbirth and children |
| | Spiritualist | Spiritual advisement, counseling, and prayers to treat illness or cope with personal and psychosocial problems |
| | Voodoo practitioners *Hougan* (male) *Mambo* (female) | Combination of herbs, drumming, and symbolic offerings to cure illness, remove curses, and protect a person |
| Hispanic | *Curandero/a* | Combination of prayers, herbs, and other rituals to treat traditional illnesses, especially in children |
| | *Parteras* Lay midwives | Assistance for women in childbirth and newborn care |
| | *Yerbero* Herbalist | Consultation for herbal treatment of traditional illnesses |
| | *Sabador* Bonesetters | Massage and manipulation of bones and joints used to treat a variety of ailments, including musculoskeletal conditions |
| | *Espiritista* Spiritualist | Foretelling of future and interpretation of dreams; combination of prayers, herbs, potions, amulets, and prayers for curing illnesses, including witchcraft |
| | *Santeroa* | Combination of prayers, symbolic offerings, herbs, potions, and amulets against witchcraft and curses |

cultural differences. The behavioral domain includes skills in cultural assessment and intercultural communication. The environmental domain comprises encounters or situations that allow for cultural competence to develop. Attributes or characteristics of cultural competence are the ability to give care to diverse populations, openness to cultural differences, and flexibility or adaptability to different situations. Outcomes of cultural competence are evident in the patient (satisfaction with care and adherence to treatment), health care practitioner (personal growth and development), and health care outcomes (cost-effectiveness and quality of care).

Cultural competence is not limited to health practitioners; it also includes health care organizations. The Office of Minority Health (OMH) (2000) has defined **cultural and linguistic competence** as a "set of congruent behaviors, attitudes, and policies that come together in a system, agency, or among professionals that enables effective work in cross cultural situations. Competence implies having the capacity to function effectively as an individual and an organization

within the context of the cultural beliefs, behaviors, and needs presented by consumers and their communities." The OMH published 14 standards clustered into three sections: culturally competent care by health practitioners, provision of language access services, and organizational supports. Cultural competence is the ability to work with diverse social and cultural groups inclusive of race, ethnicity, religion, gender, sexual orientation, age, disability, socioeconomic status, English proficiency, literacy, and hearing function. For example, health care organizations have to provide support services such as interpreters and translators at no cost to patients who are not proficient in English. Organizations need to provide services accessible by culturally diverse patients through policy development and training of personnel.

Pacquiao (2003a) identifies three distinct levels of cultural competence at the practitioner, organizational, and societal levels. Culturally competent care is the ability of practitioners to bridge cultural gaps in caring, to work with cultural differences, and to enable patients and families to achieve meaning-

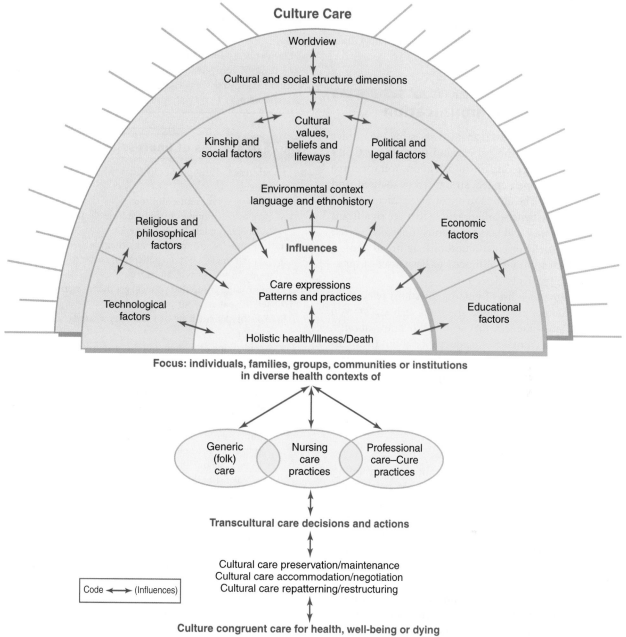

FIGURE **17-1** Leininger's culture care theory and Sunrise Model. (Reprinted with permission of the McGraw-Hill Companies.)

ful and supportive caring. Cultural competence is the synthesis of all three levels. Health care practitioners need system-wide support to implement culturally congruent care. Culturally competent communities and societies are knowledgeable and skilled in using health care services and articulating their rights and needs to practitioners and organizations. For example, members of the congregation of Jehovah's Witnesses approached local hospitals to provide surgery without transfusion of blood or blood products. Their demands for religious accommodation led to alternatives to blood transfusion in planned surgeries (bloodless surgery).

## Cultural Assessment

**Cultural assessment** or **culturological nursing assessment** (Andrews, 2003) is a systematic and comprehensive examination of the cultural care values, beliefs, and practices of individuals, families, and communities. The goal of cultural assessment is to generate from patients significant information and understanding that will enable the nurse to implement culturally congruent care (Leininger and McFarland, 2002). There are several models for cultural assessment, such as Purnell's Model for Cultural Competence (Purnell and

Paulanka, 2003a), Giger and Davidhizar's Transcultural Assessment Model (2004), Spector's HEALTH Traditions Model (2004), and Andrews and Boyle's Assessment Guide (Andrews, 2003).

## Intercultural Communication

The challenge in cultural assessment is assessing the insider or emic perspective of the patient and using the patient's own context for interpreting the information. You use three types of questions: open-ended, structured or focused, and contrast questions. The aim is to encourage patients to describe those values, beliefs, and practices that are significant to their care that they will take for granted unless otherwise uncovered. Culturally oriented questions are broad and require a lot of descriptions. You need to have a set of questions to elicit the patients' descriptions.

Box 17-1 provides a list of guiding questions relevant to nursing care. Do not ask a global question such as, "Do you have any cultural practices that we should know about?" Rather, ask patients more specific questions about their cultural practices, such as routines regarding mealtimes, praying, bathing, etc. Global questions require a higher level of understanding and expression in English and are especially difficult for patients who are not proficient in English or have a low level of literacy.

### Building Relationships

Cultural assessment tends to be intrusive and time consuming, and it requires a trusting relationship between participants. Establishing a trusting relationship with the patient and the family makes it easier to do this effectively. Miscommunication commonly occurs because of language and communication differences between and among participants, as well as different contextual frames for interpreting each other's behaviors. **Impression management** skills are essential for nurses. Impression management is based on one's ability to interpret the others' behaviors within their own context of meanings and behave in a culturally congruent way. In a sense it is managing the impression one makes on the other to achieve desired outcomes of communication (Pacquiao, 2000). Impression management requires linguistic skills, culturally congruent interpretation of behaviors of others, and listening and observation skills.

In cultural assessment the goal is to generate knowledge about the patients' values, beliefs, and practices about nursing and health care. If your behavior is offensive to the patient, he or she will not be likely to participate in the interaction. You communicate respect by not rushing the patient, being attentive to the patient, demonstrating genuine interest in the patient, and using appropriate group-centered approaches. Avoid judgmental comments about the patient's statements. Box 17-2 describes the general rules of impression management with specific recommendations when working with interpreters.

---

**BOX 17-1** **Questions Used in Cultural Care Assessment**

*Open-ended:* How would you like your bath done?
*Focused:* Whom would you like to help you with your bath?
*Contrast:* If your wife is not around, can one of the nurses give your bath?

---

**BOX 17-2** **Rules of Impression Management**

1. Address the group or individuals who are present with the patient.
2. Introduce your name and role.
3. Request each one to introduce himself or herself and how he or she is related to the patient.
4. Welcome the group, and thank them for coming to visit.
5. Request to talk with the patient, and offer to accompany the group to the waiting room.
6. Inform the group that you will get them when you are done.
7. Tell the patient your purpose.
8. Ask the patient if he or she wants a family member to be present.
9. Avoid asking the patient questions in front of family/spouse that can put him or her at risk with this group.
10. Ask the patient who is the person who needs to be consulted for major decisions and how to contact this person.
11. Observe nonverbal behavior, and match degree of distance exhibited by the patient.
12. If the patient needs an interpreter:
    • Introduce yourself to the interpreter.
    • Determine qualifications of interpreter.
      ○ Make sure that the interpreter can speak the dialect of the patient.
      ○ Ensure gender, age, and ethnic compatibility of interpreter with patient's preference and topic to be discussed.
      ○ Watch for differences in educational and socioeconomic status between the patient and the interpreter.
      ○ Orient the interpreter to your purpose and expectation.
    • Clarify your questions about the interpreter's training and compatibility between the patient's and interpreter's understanding of your expectations beforehand.
    • Introduce the interpreter to the patient.
    • Remember the distinct difference between interpretation and translation. Do not expect the interpreter to translate your statements word for word.
    • Pace your speech slowly, and allow time for the patient's response to be interpreted.
    • Direct your questions to the patient.
    • Request interpreter to ask the patient for feedback and clarification at regular intervals.
    • Observe the patient's nonverbal and verbal behaviors.
    • Thank both patient and interpreter.

---

You must determine a patient's spoken and written language(s) and need for an interpreter on admission to any health care facility. It is a federal mandate that patients have language access and interpreters at no cost. Working with interpreters and patients with little or no fluency in English requires skill development. Participate in educational programs and practice applications of principles of impression management before an intercultural encounter. It is not acceptable for family members to translate health care information, but they can assist with ongoing interaction during the patient's care.

## Selected Components of Cultural Assessment

You perform comprehensive **focused cultural assessments** by selecting components that are most relevant to the problem at hand. Background knowledge of the culture assists you with conducting a focused assessment when time is limited. Table 17-3 presents components of cultural assessment and specific areas for you to assess.

### Ethnic Heritage and Ethnohistory

**Ethnohistory** refers to significant historical experiences of a particular group. Knowledge of the country of origin, its history, and ecological contexts are significant to health care. For example, African cultures in the Caribbean colonized by Great Britain speak English, whereas those colonized by France speak French. Colonial influence is also apparent in their names.

People migrate to another country for various reasons and have different motivations for adapting to the new country. The process of adapting to and adopting a new culture is **acculturation** (Padilla, Wagatsuma, and Lindholm, 1984). Acculturation results in varying degrees of affiliation with the dominant culture. Refugees experience greater dislocation and deprivation compared with immigrants who enter the United States with specialized skills and education and have the option to return to their homeland. Age of immigration also determines the level of acculturation. Younger immigrants usually acculturate faster than older immigrants. Similarities shared by an immigrant group with the dominant culture in society are strong predictors that the group will change and integrate.

**Assimilation** results when an individual gives up his or her ethnic identity in favor of the dominant culture (Spector, 2004). White European immigrants experienced less difficulty in America and had greater motivation to assimilate than nonwhite immigrants. Although acculturation and length of residence in the new culture are related, other factors such as education, racial characteristics, and familiarity with the language and religion differentiate the outcomes. It is important to explore the patient's preimmigration and postimmigration status, available resources for medical coverage, health risks in the new environment, and availability of support systems.

### Biocultural History

Identify patients' health risks related to sociocultural and biological history during admission to a health care facility. Some distinct health risks are related to the ecological con-

text of a culture. For example, Hispanics living in the United States are almost twice as likely to die from diabetes than non-Hispanic whites. The rate of diabetes for Native Americans and Alaska natives is more than twice that for whites. The Pima of Arizona have one of the highest rates of diabetes in the world (USDHHS, 2000).

### Social Organization

Cultural groups consist of units of organization described by kinship, status hierarchy, and appropriate roles for members. In the dominant American society, the most common unit of social organization is the nuclear family, and married children and adults are expected to establish separate residences from their parents. In collective cultures, such as Hispanics and Filipinos, the family includes distant blood relatives across three generations and **fictive** or nonblood kin. Kinship is extended **bilineally** to both the father's and mother's side of the family or limited to the side of either father (**patrilineal**) or mother (**matrilineal**). Some Chinese and Hindu cultures have patrilineally extended families, where a woman moves into her husband's family after marriage and minimizes her kinship ties with her parents and siblings.

A patient's status within the social hierarchy is based on age and gender as well as achieved status such as education and position. The dominant culture in the United States emphasizes achievement as the determinant of status, whereas most collectivistic cultures give higher priority to age and gender. The eldest male is next to his father in terms of authority in many Arabic and African cultures.

Cultures based on age and gender define the roles of their members. Certain behaviors are acceptable in children, but not tolerated among adults. For example, in Muslim families, females perform the caretaking tasks whereas men make the major decisions about the care of family members. Make sure you determine the family social hierarchy as soon as possible to prevent offending your patients and their families. Working with established family hierarchy prevents delays and achieves timely outcomes in nursing care.

### Religious and Spiritual Beliefs

Religious and spiritual beliefs are major influences in the patient's worldview about health and illness, pain and suffering, and life and death. Unlike the United States, the distinction between religion and spirituality is blurred in other cultures. It is advisable to understand the emic perspective of the patient. Many cultures do not separate the two, whereas other cultures have a totally distinct concept of spirituality. For example, to an Igbo patient from Nigeria, spirits are those of dead ancestors or forces external to the person. To an Anglo-American, spirituality means an inner, personal relationship with God. Although discussion of religious and spiritual philosophies is difficult in a hospital setting, you are able to elicit this information from the patients' identified religion and practices (see Chapter 18).

Devout patients expect to continue their religious rituals in the hospital. Mormons who have gone through the sacra-

| TABLE 17-3 | Cultural Assessment Guide |
| --- | --- |
| **Categories** | **Questions** |
| Cultural identity/ancestry/heritage | Place of birth of patient and his or her parents/ancestors |
| | Reason for immigration |
| Ethnohistory | Length of time in the United States |
| | Age of immigration |
| | Degree of acculturation |
| Social organization | Living arrangements |
| | Family composition, definition and degree of contact with family members |
| | Position in family hierarchy and decision making |
| | Social support |
| | Family roles, expectations of each other, gender-appropriate roles |
| | Extent of family participation in care desired |
| Socioeconomic status | Occupation before and after immigration |
| | Educational attainment |
| | Type of residence |
| | Medical insurance |
| | Primary care provider, other care providers and specialists used |
| Biocultural ecology and health risks | Purpose of visit/consultation/hospitalization |
| | Perceived cause of problem |
| | Terms used to describe problem, feelings |
| | Preponderance of problem within family and community |
| | Folk treatment |
| | Effect of problem on self and family |
| | Expectations of care to be provided |
| | Presence of health risks |
| Language and communication | Languages spoken and written |
| | Preferred language when speaking and reading |
| | Preferred communication and manner of address |
| | Need and preference for an interpreter (gender, age, etc.) |
| | Literacy level and English proficiency |
| Religion/spirituality | Religion, spiritual leader, contact for religious/spiritual leader |
| | Religious/spiritual needs |
| | Religious rituals observed |
| | Dietary practices observed |
| Caring beliefs and practices | Measures to promote health |
| | Caring practices when sick |
| | Practices relevant to activities of daily living |
| | Folk and professional healers sought |
| | Healing modalities used for problem |
| | Expectations about care to be given |
| | Hygiene, dietary, and mobility considerations |
| | Age and gender considerations |
| | Beliefs and practices with regard to life transitions |
| Experience with professional health care | Evaluations of previous experiences |
| | Attributes of valued caregivers |

ments and are deemed worthy wear a white undergarment at all times except when taking a bath or shower. Devout Muslims pray five times daily and undergo an obligatory ritual cleansing of some parts of their body before praying. During **Sabbath** (sundown Friday to sundown Saturday) Orthodox Jewish patients refrain from using electrical appliances. This calls for creative accommodations by the nursing staff. In this case, you place articles of care near the patient so he or she does not need to use the call light or telephone to get assistance. You can also provide battery-operated candles during Sabbath.

Religious beliefs are evident in the patients' dietary practices. Devout Muslims eat **halal,** or foods permissible for Muslims to eat. These include meat, fish, fresh fruit, vegetables, eggs, milk, and cheese. Halal meat comes from animals that have been slaughtered during a prayer ritual. **Haram,** or prohibited foods, include nonhalal meat, animals with fangs, pork products, gelatin products, and alcohol (Akhtar, 2002).

During the 28 days of **Ramadan,** observed during the ninth lunar month, Muslims fast during the daylight hours. Although children and sick individuals are exempt from fasting, do not assume that these individuals will eat regular meals during Ramadan. Sometimes you will need to reschedule treatments and medications to prevent complications such as hypoglycemia. Observant Mormons avoid drugs, alcohol, and beverages containing stimulants such as coffee and cola.

The inability of Orthodox Jews to pray in groups at the bedside with the dying patient because of limitations in the number of visitors allowed will cause cultural pain in the patient and family. Always work with the family and their religious/spiritual leader to facilitate culturally congruent care (Pacquiao, 2003a).

## Communication Patterns

Different cultural groups have distinct linguistic and communication patterns. These patterns reflect the core cultural values of the society. The dominant American culture values assertive and direct communication. This communication pattern reflects the ideal of individual autonomy and self-determination. The individual is expected to say what he or she means and mean what he or she says. In collectivistic cultures the context of relationships among participants shapes communication. Promoting group harmony is a priority, so participants interact based on their expected positions and relationships within the social hierarchy. Differences in status and position, age, gender, and outsider versus insider determine the content and process of communication (Box 17-3).

Among Asian cultures, **face-saving** communication promotes harmony by indirect communication and avoiding conflict. Messages spoken sometimes have little to do with their meanings. For example, saying "no" to a superior or older person is not permitted in some cultures. A subordinate's affirmative response may only mean, "I heard you" rather than "Yes, I agree with you." This communication pattern is likely to happen when a physician or health care provider, who is perceived as an authority, speaks to some Asian, African, or Hispanic patients. Observing a patient's behavior and clarifying messages heard from a trusted insider will prevent misinterpretation.

In cultural groups with distinct linear hierarchy, negotiation of conflict occurs between persons within the same level of position or authority. Identifying and working with established family hierarchy will prevent miscommunication. In cultures with highly differentiated gender roles, some patients place more value on the advice of a male physician or health care provider than a female nurse. By recognizing and working within this cultural context, you will become more effective in achieving outcomes.

Culture also shapes nonverbal communication. Culture dictates the distance between participants in an interaction, the degree of eye contact, the extent of touching, and the degree to which individuals share private information. Individuals commonly use less distance when speaking to

| BOX 17-3 | CARE OF THE OLDER ADULT |
|---|---|

Henry Lee, who is 70 years old, is admitted for gastric discomfort and loss of appetite. The nurse is assigned to conduct his admission. His 50-year-old son and 30-year-old granddaughter accompany him. Mr. Lee immigrated to the United States from Taiwan at the age of 20 years. He supported himself through school and obtained a degree in chemistry. He retired from his job in a pharmaceutical company at age 65. When communicating with Mr. Lee:

- Address him formally unless otherwise directed by Mr. Lee.
- Demonstrate respect by using deferential tone of voice, listening, slower pacing, and sometimes avoidance of direct eye contact or touching.
- Provide privacy and a tranquil environment.
- Ask politely for Mr. Lee's consent before performing any procedure.
- Accommodate Mr. Lee's preference for gender-congruent care.
- Accommodate Mr. Lee's preference for family members to be present at the bedside to assist him with care.
- Accommodate Mr. Lee's food preferences.
- Expect that Mr. Lee will not verbally respond to all the questions.
- Observe nonverbal reactions.

trusted insiders and persons of the same age, gender, and position in the social hierarchy. Many ethnic groups tend to speak their own dialect with insiders for ease and privacy and as a marker of insider status. To minimize this distance when communicating with patients, you need to establish rapport and behave in a culturally congruent manner through impression management.

## Time Orientation

All cultures have past, present, and future time dimensions. Differences exist in the dimensions of time they emphasize and the manner of expressing time. Time orientation is reflected in communication patterns. **Future orientation** minimizes present time, so communication tends to be direct and focused on task achievement. Business time is separate and distinct from social time. This is the norm in the dominant American culture. In contrast, collectivistic cultures emphasize past and present times to preserve social hierarchy and promote group harmony. Communication is sometimes circular and indirect to avoid offending and disrespecting others. These cultures often emphasize social time and mix it with business time. Your patients will perceive rushed, hurried, and business-like communication as uncaring or disrespectful. This is true with Mexican-Americans who tend to trust (*confianza*) caregivers who interact with them in a personalistic (*personalismo*), warm, friendly (*simpatia*), and respectful (*respeto*) manner (Zoucha, 1998).

**Present time orientation** is in conflict with the dominant organizational norm in health care emphasizing punctuality and adherence to appointments. Expect conflicts, and make adjustments when dealing with other ethnic groups. Improve the accessibility of health services, so time schedules accommodate the cultural patterns of others. When making appointments and referrals, explore anticipated barriers to time adherence and manage them with the patient.

## Caring Beliefs and Practices

Care meanings, values, and beliefs are expressed in practices associated with life transitions. You need to determine how your patients and their families define meaningful and supportive caring. Caring expressions integrate the central values of the culture. In collectivistic cultures, caring means active involvement of the group, emphasizing mutual and reciprocal obligations of members to care for each other. This caring norm is different from the individualism and self-care ideology of the dominant American culture. As a nurse you will need to adopt a patient's caring ways and learn to work with patient's families, especially when providing patient education (Box 17-4).

Religious and spiritual beliefs are integrated in caring practices. For example, African-American churches play a critical role in caring for their community members. Gender-congruent care is a strong value among Muslims, Orthodox Jews, Hindus, and many other groups that emphasize female modesty. Whereas Americans value individual privacy, most Hispanics value group interdependence.

**CULTURAL PRACTICES DURING LIFE TRANSITIONS.** Life transitions are generally marked by rituals that symbolize cultural values and meanings attached to these transitions. Religious and spiritual beliefs are integrated in rituals associated with life transitions. Examining the practices surrounding these life events provides a glimpse of the cultural meanings and expressions relevant to these transitions.

**PREGNANCY.** Most cultures associate pregnancy with caring practices symbolic of its significance as a life transition in women. Some Asian, African, and Hispanic cultures believe that a mother's activities and predispositions also affect the fetus. Many cultures believe that if a pregnant woman's food craving is not met, negative consequences to the baby will occur.

Some cultures subscribe to the hot and cold theory of illness. For example, the Hindus view pregnancy as a hot state, so they encourage a pregnant woman to eat cold foods such as milk and milk products, yogurt, sour foods, and vegetables. They believe hot foods such as chilies, ginger, and animal products cause miscarriage and fetal abnormality. Although many cultures share the hot and cold theory, there is no agreement on what foods and beverages are classified as hot or cold. These classifications are associated with the ecological and ethnohistorical attributes of the culture.

Modesty is a strong value among Arab women (Kulwicki, 2003). Many avoid prenatal visits because of embarrassment, and sometimes they demand to be examined by a female practitioner. Religious beliefs sometimes interfere with prenatal testing, as in the case of a Filipino couple that refused

---

**BOX 17-4  PATIENT TEACHING**

Culture influences what a patient routinely eats. Type 2 diabetes is a chronic illness that requires diet education for successful disease management. The following shows how cultural care concepts are applied in an older adult Puerto Rican patient who has type 2 diabetes.

**Outcome**

At the end of the teaching session, the patient will verbalize dietary measures used to maintain stable blood glucose levels.

**Teaching Strategies**

- Assess cultural dietary preferences.
- Assess meanings of foods and meals.
- Refer patient to speak with a dietitian who is familiar with Hispanic diet.
- Provide brochures that describe healthy food choices that are related to the Hispanic diet.

**Evaluation Strategies**

- Ask patient to keep a food diary for 1 week and evaluate food choices.
- Ask patient to describe how commonly prescribed foods will be integrated into diabetes management plan.

---

amniocentesis because they believe that the outcome of pregnancy is God's will. Supernatural beliefs associated with pregnancy are evident among Hispanics who believe that baby showers early in pregnancy will bring bad luck or *mal de ojo* (evil eye) (Spector, 2004). Orthodox Jews avoid baby showers and do not announce the baby's name before the naming ceremony for the same reason.

**CHILDBIRTH.** Expressing pain and treating suffering vary cross culturally. Puerto Rican and Mexican women are verbally expressive of their pain during labor. *Parteras,* or lay midwives, commonly advise a screaming woman in labor to close her mouth because an open mouth will cause the uterus to rise (Juarbe, 2003). Middle Eastern mothers verbally express their labor pain by crying and screaming aloud. They often refuse pain medication.

Fear of drug addiction and belief that pain is a form of spiritual atonement for one's past deeds motivate most Filipino mothers to tolerate pain without much complaining or asking for medication (Pacquiao, 2001). Southeast Asian women believe that crying and screaming are shameful and expect to endure labor pains.

Some religious beliefs prohibit the presence of males, including husbands, from the delivery room. This is common among devout Muslims, Hindus, and Orthodox Jews. Husbands generally leave the room with the appearance of the bloody show. As soon as the child is born, a Muslim father or mother whispers the Islamic call to prayer in the newborn's ear, welcoming the baby into the life of the world where the responsibility to Allah's call is the greatest (Emerick, 2002).

Practitioners other than physicians or health care providers attend childbirth in some groups, such as *parteras* among Mexicans, **granny midwives** among Appalachian and southern African-Americans, and **hilots** among Filipinos (Pacquiao, 2003b). Known in their communities, these practitioners are affordable and accessible in remote areas. They use a combination of naturalistic, religious, and supernatural methods combining herbs, massage, and prayers.

**NEWBORN.** The age of the newborn varies in some cultures. Among traditional Vietnamese and Koreans, a newborn is a year old at birth. Once acculturated to Western culture, they assume a bicultural view and deduct 1 year from the age of the child when speaking to outsiders.

The name of the child reflects cultural values of the group. It is typical for a Hispanic baby to have several first names followed by the surnames of the father and mother (e.g., Maria Kristina Lourdes Lopez Vega). The bilineal tracing of descent from both the mother's and father's side in the Hispanic group is different from the patrilineal system, where the last name of the father precedes the child's first name. In the Chinese culture, descent is traced only from the paternal side. Hence the name Chen Lu means that Lu is the daughter of Mr. Chen.

Many societies consider newborns and young children vulnerable and use a variety of ways to prevent the evil eye, using amulets, religious medals, herbs, or spices. For example, some Catholic Filipinos keep newborns inside the home until after the baptism to ensure the baby's health and protection. The practice of using a cotton binder or *fajita* on the baby's abdomen to prevent gas and umbilical hernia is also evident among Filipinos and Hispanic groups (Pacquiao, 2003b). Filipinos sometimes rub warm oil on the baby's belly to prevent and relieve gas. Some traditional Iranians believe babies are vulnerable to cold and wind; hence they are not bathed for a number of days. They remain indoors with their mothers for a period of 30 to 40 days (Hafizi and Lipson, 2003).

Some cultures do not regard the colostrum (initial cloudy breast secretion following delivery) as healthy for the baby. For some Hindus and Muslims the colostrum is dirty and not fit for a newborn, so they postpone breast-feeding until regular milk appears. You will need to use alternative measures to promote lactation (Jambunathan, 2003).

**POSTPARTUM PERIOD.** In many non-Western cultures, people associate postpartum with vulnerability of the mother to cold. To restore balance, mothers sometimes refuse a shower and prefer a sponge bath. Cultural groups have preferences in terms of what types of foods are appropriate to restore balance in women after birth. Some Chinese mothers prefer soups, eggs, and tea, whereas rural Iranian families prefer pistachio nuts and eggs (Hafizi and Lipson, 2003; Wang, 2003). The length of the postpartum period is generally much longer (30 to 40 days) in non-Western cultures to provide much attention and support for the mother and her baby. This is one of the reasons given for the rarity of postpartum depression in these cultures when compared with the United States. Some Hispanic women go into a 40-day period of *la cuarantena,* when they follow a special diet *(la dieta)* and restrict physical activity. This cultural belief that the mother needs much rest and relaxation after delivery conflicts with the Western belief in early ambulation.

Some Filipinos, Mexicans, and Pacific Islanders use an abdominal binder to prevent air from entering the woman's uterus and to promote healing (Pacquiao, 2003b; Zoucha and Purnell, 2003). Orthodox Jewish, Islamic, and Hindu cultures associate bleeding with pollution. A woman has to go into a ritual bath after the bleeding stops before she is able to resume relations with her husband (Hafizi and Lipson, 2003; Selekman, 2003). In some African cultures in Ghana and Sierra Leone, women will not resume sexual relations with their husbands until after weaning the baby.

## Grief and Loss

Dying and death bring a resurgence of cultural traditions that have been meaningful to groups of people most of their lives (see Chapter 23). Societies assign different meanings to the death of a child, a young person, or an older adult. In Western cultures with strong future time orientation, a child is expected to survive his or her parent. The death of a young person is devastating. However, in cultures where infant mortality is high, the reality of the commonly observed risks of growing up temper the emotional distress over a child's death. Hence some cultures mourn the untimely death of an adult more deeply.

Societies that believe in the concept of reincarnation, such as devout Hindus and Buddhists, view death as a step toward rebirth. Care of the dying focuses on supporting the patient's preparation for a good death. The family prays and reads religious scriptures to the patient to improve his or her chances in the next cycle.

Culture strongly influences pain expression and the need for pain medication. Whereas a typical American believes in individual freedom and autonomy as synonymous with freedom from pain and suffering, other groups accept suffering. Do not assume that everyone values pain relief equally.

Advance directives, informed consent, and consent for hospice are examples of mandates that violate diverse values of people. Informed consent and advance directives (see Chapter 4) protect the right of the individual to know and make decisions ensuring continuity of these rights even when the individual is incapacitated. However, in some cultures, the group or family assumes decision making and is trusted to make the right decision for the individual. These cultures value group interdependence and view individual autonomy as an unnecessary burden for a loved one who is ill (Pacquiao, 2002, 2003a).

In the case of cultures that share the religious belief that events in their life are God's will, prognostication, or predicting the outcome of a disease, is not an acceptable human practice. Hence devout Muslims sometimes object to a diagnosis of terminal illness or cancer. This belief will hinder their ability to get into hospice programs unless organizational policies are flexibly applied to accommodate their values and beliefs (Pacquiao, 2002, 2003a).

Culture conditions rituals associated with dying and death. Orthodox Jews rally behind members of their congregation and provide care for the dying, as well as assistance to the family. They come in groups of about 10 and pray together with the patient and the family at the bedside. Orthodox Jews and Muslims call a special group knowledgeable in the religious rituals to perform postmortem care. They strictly observe gender-congruent care and provision of privacy as a show of respect for the dead person. They also generally schedule an immediate burial. Therefore always plan preparations with the family beforehand. Orthodox Jews generally bury the dead before sundown (Bonura and others, 2001). Some Buddhists refuse to move the dead body after death because of their belief that the spirit of the dead takes some time to leave the body. They define death as the absence of consciousness and loss of body warmth. Because of this belief, many other groups do not agree with using brain death as a criterion of death.

Religious beliefs also affect attitudes toward cremation, organ donation, or loss of a body part. Devout Muslims sometimes refuse an autopsy for fear of desecrating the dead and because of their belief that one has to be whole to appear in front of the creator. They prefer burial over cremation. In addition, some Muslim patients request a priest (**imam**) to bless the leg to be amputated before surgery (Pacquiao, 2003a).

## Experience With Professional Health Care

Understanding the patient's emic perspective of professional care is valuable in correcting misconceptions and preventing culturally offensive actions. Previous encounters with professional caregivers affect patients' decisions to seek health care. For example, southern African-Americans prefer their family members to make end-of-life decisions for them. Their reluctance to execute advance directives comes from their mistrust of the health care system and past experience with racism and discrimination by the white majority (Dupree, 2000). In order to elicit information about advance directives, there needs to be a trusting relationship between providers and patients.

Partnership between health care professionals and the community provides proactive and authentic feedback from culturally diverse patient groups. Such a dialogue clarifies the expectations cultural groups have of their health care providers.

## Culturally Competent Nursing Actions

After you have conducted a cultural care assessment, identify any area of potential conflicts between professional care and the patient's care values and practices. You do this by identifying similarities and differences between the dominant professional and organizational norms and the patient's cultural

---

| BOX 17-5 | **USING EVIDENCE IN PRACTICE** |

### Research Summary

Advance directives communicate the kind of care that people desire at the end of life. However, when compared to Caucasians, significantly fewer members of ethnic minority groups complete advance directives.

Forty-five Asian Indian immigrants recruited from a community center, a Midwestern university, and a mailing list of alumni from a university in India who were residing in the United States responded to the mailed survey. The survey, Hindu Voices on Care of the Dying, consisted of three parts: demographics, end-of-life, and Hindu religious beliefs and ritual scale. The study findings revealed only 9% of respondents had prepared a living will and none had a durable power of attorney. The stronger the religious beliefs and observance of Hinduism rituals, the less likely the respondent desired to complete advance directives.

### Application to Nursing Practice

Assessing the patient's religious and spiritual beliefs is important in predicting attitudes toward advance directives. Belief in karma creates acceptance of one's fate; hence advance directives are out of place. In addition, collectivistic cultures such as the Indian culture leave decisions about oneself to trusted family members. Examine relevance and meaning of policies and protocols in health care to patients. Use a more culturally congruent alternative to advance directives in collectivistic cultures. A durable power of attorney is suggested, because the patient is more likely to leave major decisions to family members. Thus designating a particular family member to make decisions follows organizational policy and allows the patient to maintain the Indian cultural values of caring by others and group reliance. Knowledge of the culture assists nurses in advocating for the patient and supports the patient's valued life patterns.

Data from Doorenbos AZ, Nies MA: The use of advance directives in a population of Asian Indian Hindus, *J Transcult Nurs* 14(1):6, 2003.

---

life patterns. Leininger and McFarland (2002) identified three nursing decision and action modes to achieve culturally congruent care. Use any or all of these action modes simultaneously. These actions require that you have the knowledge of the patient's culture and have the willingness, commitment, and skills to work with patients and their families in decision making.

**Cultural care preservation or maintenance**—Retain and/or preserve relevant care values so that patients are able to maintain their well-being, recover from illness, or face handicaps and/or death.

**Cultural care accommodation or negotiation**—Adapt or negotiate with the patient/family to achieve beneficial or satisfying health outcomes.

**Cultural care repatterning or restructuring**—Reorder, change, or greatly modify patient's/family's customs for new, different, and beneficial health care pattern.

In the following scenario, a nurse uses the action modes with a Pakistani patient. A male Pakistani patient is admitted for terminal pancreatic cancer. On admission he denies presence of pain. His main complaint is the inability to sleep. He admits to having "discomfort that goes away only when he is sleeping." Knowing the cultural background of the patient, being a South Asian male Muslim, the nurse understands his behavior is consistent with male behavioral norms of controlling his emotions. Stoicism is a valued trait and demonstrates a male's inner strength. Because of her cultural knowledge, the nurse interprets the patient's behavior in a culturally congruent manner.

The nurse then selects the nursing diagnosis: *disturbed sleep pattern related to discomfort.* She decides on the following plan of action: obtain an order for pain medication but present its purpose to the patient as an aid to promote sleep. She also communicates her plan to the other members of the team. She repatterns her own and her peers' thinking regarding the use of pain medication to promote sleep. She accommodates the patient's interpretation of his problem and does not try to convince him that his pain causes his difficulty sleeping. The nurse's decision is culturally congruent with the patient's life patterns and demonstrates the nurse's cultural competence. Nurses often use information from research studies to plan culturally competent care (Box 17-5).

## KEY CONCEPTS

- The central purpose of nursing is to provide culturally competent and congruent care.
- Even when there is access to health services, racial and ethnic differences contribute to health care disparities.
- Health care practitioners often misinterpret the impact of culture on health and are ill-prepared educationally and clinically to provide safe and effective care for culturally diverse populations.
- When practitioners disregard a patient's valued way of life, the patient experiences cultural pain.
- Collectivistic cultures rely on family to care for sick members.
- Attributes or characteristics of cultural competence are the ability to give care to diverse populations, openness to cultural differences, and flexibility or adaptability to different situations.

- Culturally competent communities and societies are knowledgeable and skilled in using health care services and articulating their rights and needs to practitioners and organizations.
- The goal of cultural assessment is to generate from patients significant information and understanding that will enable the nurse to implement culturally congruent care.
- In hospital settings it is a requirement to use a trained interpreter to communicate information about medical conditions to patients.
- Life transitions such as pregnancy, childbirth, and death are generally marked by rituals that symbolize cultural values and meanings attached to these transitions.
- Dying and death bring a resurgence of cultural traditions that have been meaningful to groups of people most of their lives.

## CRITICAL THINKING IN PRACTICE

*Afryea Vihma, a 60-year-old woman from Ghana with a history of hypercholesterolemia, moderate obesity, and hypertension is preparing for discharge. The nurse started to talk about Afryea's need to lose weight to improve her lipid profile and hypertension. It is obvious that the nurse, who is also Ghanaian, has a trusting relationship with the patient. In the middle of the nurse's presentation on foods to be avoided, Afryea chuckles and tells her, "Honey, I am leaving for Ghana next month. If I lose weight, my folks back there will think that my children in America abandoned me. Worse, people will think I have AIDS. Besides, I need to fit into my traditional outfits. As the village queen, I need to wear these outfits every day and they don't look good on me if I lose weight. Talk to me when I get back."*

- - - - - - - - - - - - - - - - - -

1. Africans tend to equate a more robust body with health.
   a. True
   b. False
2. The cultural conflict that exists between the nurse and Afryea stems from:
   a. Cultural imposition and stereotypes
   b. Cultural biases and prejudices

c. Contrasting worldviews of health and illness
   d. Discrimination and ethnocentrism
3. An appropriate short-term goal for Afryea is to:
   a. Send an appropriate menu for her to use during the trip
   b. Ask her daughter to make sure that the patient adheres to her diet
   c. Collaborate with Afryea in goal setting and planning care
   d. Remind Afryea of the dangers of uncontrolled hypertension and hypercholesterolemia
4. The nurse did not get upset or insist that Afryea follow her plan of action. She sat down with Afryea to determine her own priorities and decisions. The nurse's behavior is an example of:
   a. Unprofessional behavior
   b. Cultural self-repatterning
   c. Etic worldview
   d. Cultural awareness

# NCLEX® REVIEW

1. An older adult Filipino patient requested his wife to ask the nurse manager not to have the same nurse assigned to him. He refused to give any explanation to the nurse manager. His communication pattern demonstrates:
   1. Assertive communication
   2. Face-saving communication
   3. Direct communication
   4. Biased communication

2. An Iranian female patient refuses to have an abdominal examination done by a male care provider despite attempts to drape her. After several attempts, explaining the reason for the procedure, the care provider stepped out angrily and left the patient in tears. The behavior of the care provider is an example of:
   1. Cultural imposition
   2. Stereotypes
   3. Cultural accommodation
   4. Ethnocentrism

3. The behavior of the patient in question 2 is congruent with the Iranian cultural value of:
   1. Female modesty
   2. Short distance between unrelated males and females
   3. Female subservience to males
   4. Fatalism

4. Some cultures, such as Hindus and Orthodox Jews, avoid baby showers because of their belief that the practice will:
   1. Bring the evil eye to the newborn
   2. Expose the mother to bacterial infection
   3. Result in premature birth
   4. Transgress religious practices

5. A Mexican woman's refusal to take a shower during her entire postpartal stay in the hospital is a manifestation of:
   1. Poor hygiene
   2. Belief in hot and cold theory in illness
   3. Fear of bleeding
   4. Her need for attention

6. A *hilot* is a folk healer commonly used by traditional:
   1. Vietnamese
   2. Filipinos
   3. Chinese
   4. Koreans

7. Mrs. de la Cruz, an older adult Cuban matriarch, is hospitalized with congestive heart failure (CHF). The nurses are concerned that she is getting exhausted by the numerous visitors who stay at her bedside from early morning until late evening. She denies being exhausted by her visitors. Consistent presence of extended family members and fictive kin at the bedside of Mrs. de la Cruz is a manifestation of the Cuban cultural value of:
   1. Familism and close ties among extended kin
   2. Caring by others through presence and attention to the ill member
   3. Bilineal extension of kinship ties
   4. *Simpatia*

8. Cultural accommodation of the de la Cruzes is best done by:
   1. Collaborating with the family decision maker to schedule turns of limited number of visitors at her bedside
   2. Explaining repeatedly the visiting policy to Mrs. de la Cruz's visitors
   3. Informing the information desk not to allow all visitors to go up at the same time
   4. Requesting an early discharge for Mrs. de la Cruz

9. In some cultures, such as Asian, Hispanic, and Africans, food cravings of the pregnant woman are satisfied because:
   1. A mother's stressful condition creates stress in her baby
   2. The mother will be in danger of malnutrition
   3. It strengthens bonds between husband and wife
   4. It will result in twin births

10. Which of the following males is likely to respond on behalf of his wife?
    1. Orthodox Jew
    2. African-American
    3. Filipino
    4. White American

# REFERENCES

Akhtar S: Nursing with dignity. VIII. Islam, *Nurs Times* 98(16):40, 2002.

Amen M, Pacquiao DF: Contrasting experiences with child health care services by mothers and professional caregivers in a transitional housing, *J Transcult Nurs* 15(3):217, 2004.

Andrews M: Cultural competence in the health history and physical examination. In Andrews M, Boyle J: *Transcultural concepts in nursing care,* ed 4, Philadelphia, 2003, Lippincott Williams & Wilkins.

Ashton CM and others: Racial and ethnic differences in the use of health services: bias, preferences or poor communication? *J Gen Intern Med* 18(2):146, 2003.

Baldwin DM: Disparities in health and health care: focusing efforts to eliminate unequal burdens, *Online J Issues Nurs* 8(1):2, 2003.

Bonura D and others: Culturally-congruent end-of-life care for Jewish patients and their families, *J Transcult Nurs* 12(3):211, 2001.

Campinha-Bacote J: *The process of cultural competence in the delivery of healthcare services: a culturally competent model of care,* ed 4, Cincinnati, 2003, Transcultural C.A.R.E. Associates.

Conrad M, Pacquiao DF: Manifestation, attribution and coping with depression among Asian Indians from the perspective of healthcare practitioners, *J Transcult Nurs* 16(1):23, 2005.

Doorenbos AZ, Nies MA: The use of advance directives in a population of Asian Indian Hindus, *J Transcult Nurs* 14(1):6, 2003.

Dupree CY: The attitudes of black Americans toward advance directives, *J Transcult Nurs* 11(1):12, 2000.

Emerick Y: *The complete idiot's guide to understanding Islam,* Indianapolis, 2002, Pearson Education, Inc.

Giger J, Davidhizar R: *Transcultural nursing: assessment and intervention,* ed 4, St. Louis, 2004, Mosby.

Hafizi H, Lipson J: People of Iranian heritage. In Purnell LD, Paulanka BJ: *Transcultural health care: a culturally competent approach,* ed 2, Philadelphia, 2003, FA Davis.

Jambunathan J: People of Hindu heritage. Chapter on CD-ROM. In Purnell LD, Paulanka BJ: *Transcultural health care: a culturally competent approach,* ed 2, Philadelphia, 2003, FA Davis.

Juarbe J: People of Puerto Rican heritage. In Purnell LD, Paulanka BJ: *Transcultural health care: a culturally competent approach,* ed 2, Philadelphia, 2003, FA Davis.

Juntunen A: Baridi: a culture-bound syndrome among the Bena peoples in Tanzania, *J Transcult Nurs* 16(1):15, 2005.

Kao HF, Hsu MT, Clark L: Conceptualizing and critiquing culture in health research, *J Transcult Nurs* 15(4):269, 2004.

Kleinman A: *Patients and healers in the context of culture,* Berkeley, 1980, University of California Press.

Kluckhohn F: Dominant and variant value orientations. In Brink P, editor: *Transcultural nursing: a book of readings,* Upper Saddle River, NJ, 1976, Prentice Hall.

Kulwicki AD: People of Arab heritage. In Purnell LD, Paulanka BJ: *Transcultural health care: a culturally competent approach,* ed 2, Philadelphia, 2003, FA Davis.

Leininger MM, McFarland M: *Transcultural nursing concepts, theories, research and practice,* ed 3, New York, 2002, McGraw-Hill.

Office of Minority Health: National standards for culturally and linguistically appropriate services (CLAS) in health care, *Federal Register* 65(247), 80865, Washington, DC, 2000, Office of Minority Health.

Pacquiao DF: Impression management: an alternative to assertiveness in intercultural communication, *J Transcult Nurs* 11(1):5, 2000.

Pacquiao DF: Cultural incongruities of advance directives, *Bioethics Forum* 17(1):27, 2001.

Pacquiao DF: Ethics and cultural diversity: a framework for decision-making, *Bioethics Forum* 17(3-4):12, 2002.

Pacquiao DF: Cultural competence in ethical-decision-making. In Andrews M, Boyle J: *Transcultural concepts in nursing care,* ed 4, Philadelphia, 2003a, Lippincott Williams & Wilkins.

Pacquiao DF: People of Filipino heritage. In Purnell LD, Paulanka BJ: *Transcultural health care: a culturally competent approach,* ed 2, Philadelphia, 2003b, FA Davis.

Padilla AM, Wagatsuma Y, Lindholm KJ: Acculturation and personality as predictors of stress in Japanese and Japanese-Americans, *J Soc Psychol* 125(3):295, 1984.

Purnell LD, Paulanka BJ: The Purnell model for cultural competence. In Purnell LD, Paulanka BJ: *Transcultural health care: a culturally competent approach,* ed 2, Philadelphia, 2003a, FA Davis.

Purnell LD, Paulanka BJ: Transcultural diversity and healthcare. In Purnell LD, Paulanka BJ: *Transcultural health care: a culturally competent approach,* ed 2, Philadelphia, 2003b, FA Davis.

Selekman J: People of Jewish heritage. In Purnell LD, Paulanka BJ: *Transcultural health care: a culturally competent approach,* ed 2, Philadelphia, 2003, FA Davis.

Smedley BD, Stith AR, Nelson AR, editors: *Unequal treatment: confronting racial and ethnic disparities in health care—Institute of Medicine report,* Washington, DC, 2002, National Academies Press.

Spector R: *Cultural diversity in health and illness,* ed 6, Upper Saddle River, NJ, 2004, Prentice Hall.

Suh EE: The model for cultural competence through an evolutionary concept analysis, *J Transcult Nurs* 15(2):93, 2004.

U.S. Bureau of the Census: *Hispanic population reaches all-time high of 38.8 million, new census bureau estimates show,* 2003a, http://www.census.gov/Press-Release/www/releases/archives/hispanic_origin_population/001130.html.

U.S. Bureau of the Census: *U.S. Census 2000,* 2003b, http://www.cen2000.html.

U.S. Department of Health and Human Services: *Healthy people 2010: understanding and improving health,* Washington, DC, 2000, U.S. Government Printing Office.

Van Ryn M, Fu SS: Paved with good intentions: do public health and human service providers contribute to racial/ethnic disparities in health? *Am J Public Health* 93(2):248, 2003.

Wang Y: People of Chinese heritage. In Purnell LD, Paulanka BJ: *Transcultural health care: a culturally competent approach,* ed 2, Philadelphia, 2003, FA Davis.

Zoucha R: The experience of Mexican Americans receiving professional nursing care: an ethnonursing study, *J Transcult Nurs* 9(3):34, 1998.

Zoucha R, Purnell LD: People of Mexican heritage. In Purnell LD, Paulanka BJ: *Transcultural health care: a culturally competent approach,* ed 2, Philadelphia, 2003, FA Davis.

# CHAPTER 18

# Spiritual Health

## MEDIA RESOURCES

 **CD COMPANION** 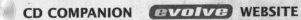 **WEBSITE**

http://evolve.elsevier.com/Potter/basic

- **NCLEX® Review**
- **Audio Glossary**
- **English/Spanish Audio Glossary**

# OBJECTIVES

- Describe the relationship between faith, hope, and spiritual well-being.
- Compare and contrast the concepts of religion and spirituality.
- Discuss the relationship of spirituality to an individual's total being.

- Perform an initial assessment of a patient's spirituality.
- Discuss nursing interventions designed to promote spiritual health.
- Establish presence with your patients.
- Evaluate how patients attain spiritual health.

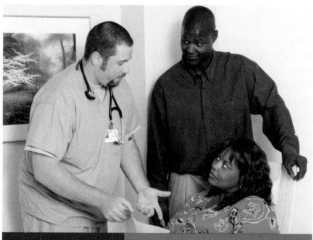

## CASE STUDY    Victoria Timms

Victoria Timms is a 48-year-old African-American college professor, diagnosed 3 months ago with breast cancer. She is married to Joe, an insurance salesman, and is the mother of two children: Valerie, who is 16 years old, and Peter, who is 12. Victoria describes her family as being very close and supportive.

Surgeons removed Victoria's cancerous tumor and two involved lymph nodes. Because of the lymphatic involvement, Victoria is at increased risk for the cancer to spread. Victoria has completed a course of radiation and now visits the local cancer clinic with her husband 3 times a week for chemotherapy treatments. She has received instruction from one of the clinic nurses about the side effects of chemotherapy. Both Victoria and Joe discuss their concern for their children. Valerie and Peter attend Sunday school weekly after going to church with their parents. Their Sunday school teacher informed Victoria and Joe that Valerie and Peter are very angry about their mother's illness and they are upset that Victoria has lost her hair as a result of her cancer therapy. Valerie's and Peter's classmates have been praying for Victoria's family during this difficult time.

Jeff is a 36-year-old, married student nurse assigned to the oncology clinic. One of the clinic case managers, who serves as Jeff's preceptor, assigns Jeff to follow Victoria during her clinic visits. Jeff is in his last semester at school and hopes to get a position in the clinic after graduation. Victoria's experience is significant for Jeff because he has children who are the same age as Victoria's, and he wonders how his children would react if his spouse became ill.

During one of their clinic visits, Victoria and Joe appear very calm and relaxed when discussing cancer therapy. Joe explains,

"We both have a lot of faith in God." Victoria responds, "Even though I know I have cancer, I hope to be able to continue to go to church with my family and my children. My family is very supportive, and together I know we will make it through this experience. But I am worried about my children. With God's help, I can help them cope with my illness better."

## KEY TERMS

agnostic, p. 510
atheist, p. 510
connectedness, p. 518
faith, p. 511
holistic, p. 509
hope, p. 511

self-transcendence, p. 511
spiritual distress, p. 512
spiritual well-being, p. 510
spirituality, p. 509

The word *spirituality* comes from the Latin word *spiritus*, which refers to breath or wind. The spirit gives life to a person. It signifies whatever is at the center of all aspects of a person's life (McEwan, 2004). **Spirituality** is an awareness of one's inner self and a sense of connection to a higher being, nature, or to some purpose greater than oneself (Mauk and Schmidt, 2004). A person's health depends on a balance of physical, psychological, sociological, cultural, developmental, and spiritual variables. This **holistic** view of health is the focus and heart of nursing practice. Spiritual care is often an overlooked part of nursing; however, the spiritual dimension does not exist in isolation from our physical and psychological being (Taylor, 2002). Spirituality is an important factor that helps to achieve the balance needed to maintain health and well-being and to cope with illness. Research on patients with chronic illness and survivors of abuse has shown that spirituality reduces a person's distress and even enhances personal growth and empowerment (Krebs, 2003; Musgrave, Allen, and Allen, 2002; Otis-Green and others, 2002).

Too often, nurses and other health care providers de-emphasize the spiritual dimension of human nature, either because it is not scientific enough or it is difficult to measure. In addition, there are health care providers who do not believe in God or an ultimate being (Friedemann, Mouch, and Racey, 2002). Frequently spirituality and religion are interchanged, but spirituality is a much broader and more unifying concept than religion. Florence Nightingale described spirituality as the sense of a presence higher than human, the divine intelligence that creates and sustains (Calabria and Macrae, 1994). The human spirit is powerful, and you are able to integrate it into your approach to care. Nursing care involves helping patients to use their spiritual resources as they identify and explore what is meaningful in their lives and to find ways to cope with illness and life's stressors (Krebs, 2003).

## Scientific Knowledge Base

Recently health care research has shown the association between spirituality and health. There are beneficial health outcomes when an individual is able to engage personal beliefs in a higher power and sense a source of strength or support. For example, Theis and others (2003) found that caregivers who cared for patients at home coped better with the stress of caregiving through prayer and social support from their church. Many people use prayer frequently as a method of coping because it is effective in minimizing physical stressors. Attending church often positively impacts health and the decision to participate in health promotion practices (Aaron, Levine, and Burstin, 2003). The increased interest in studying the effect of spirituality and health has greatly contributed to nursing science (Mauk and Schmidt, 2004).

Researchers do not fully understand the relationship between spirituality and healing. However, it is the individual's intrinsic spirit that seems to be the factor in healing. When you give patients a placebo (sugar pill) instead of a prescribed medication, often they improve, not because of the sugar pill but because of their belief in the effect of the treatment. The placebo phenomenon shows that healing often takes place because of believing.

Research shows a link between the mind, body, and spirit. An individual's beliefs and expectations have effects on the person's physical well-being (Taylor, 2002). Many of these effects are tied to hormonal and neurological function. Relaxation exercises and guided imagery, for example, improve individuals' immune function (Bakke, Purtzer, and Neton, 2002) and perceptions of pain and anxiety (Antall and Kresevic, 2004). Laughter raises pain thresholds, boosts antibodies, reduces stress hormones, relieves tension, and elevates mood (Hoare, 2004; MacDonald, 2004). In one study, researchers found that attending religious services was associated with decreasing the risk of heart disease in patients with diabetes (King, Mainous, and Pearson, 2002). A person's inner beliefs and convictions are powerful resources for healing. As a nurse you will be more successful in helping patients achieve desirable health outcomes after learning to support patients' and families' spiritually.

## Nursing Knowledge Base

### Concepts in Spiritual Health

It is important for you to understand the concepts that are at the foundation of spiritual health. The concepts of spirituality, faith, hope, spiritual well-being, and religion give direction in understanding the view each individual has of life and its value.

**SPIRITUALITY.**  Spirituality is unique for each of us. Our culture, development, life experiences, beliefs, and values about life all influence our definition of spirituality (Mauk and Schmidt, 2004). There are two important common characteristics of spirituality: (1) it is a unifying theme in people's lives and (2) it is a state of being. The definition of spirituality includes four themes: existential reality, transcendence, connectedness, and power/force/energy (Chiu and others, 2004). Existential reality is created when we find meaning, purpose, and hope in our lives. We become connected when we strengthen relationships with ourselves, others, a higher being, and nature. Spirituality transcends or goes beyond time and space, which allows us to develop new perspectives and have new experiences that go beyond ordinary physical boundaries. Power, force, and energy provide creative energy and motivation. They help us discover ourselves and help us grow.

Our spirituality enables us to love, to have faith and hope, to seek meaning in life, and to nurture relationships with others. Spirituality offers a sense of connectedness intrapersonally (connected with oneself), interpersonally (connected with others and the environment), and transpersonally (connected with God, the unseen, or a higher power). Through connectedness, patients are able to move beyond the stressors of everyday life and find comfort, faith, hope, peace, and empowerment (Tanyi, 2002). Elements of spirituality found in literature include **spiritual well-being,** spiritual needs, and spiritual awareness. Those who are spiritually healthy experience joy, are able to forgive themselves and others, accept hardship and mortality, report an enhanced quality of life, and have a positive sense of physical and emotional well-being (Fisch and others, 2003; Tanyi, 2002).

There are individuals who either do not believe in the existence of God (**atheist**) or who believe that any ultimate reality is unknown or unknowable (**agnostic**). This does not mean that spirituality is not an important concept for the atheist or agnostic (Taylor, 2002). Atheists search for meaning in life through their work and relationships with others. Because atheists feel they are alone, they sense a strong responsibility for themselves. They also tend to believe in a joint responsibility for others. In acting for themselves, they feel they also need to act for all of humankind. It is important for agnostics to discover meaning in what they do or how they live because they find no ultimate meaning for the way things are. They believe that we, as people, bring meaning to what we do.

Spirituality is an integrating theme in our lives. A person's concept of spirituality begins in childhood and continues to grow throughout adulthood (Narayanasamy and others,

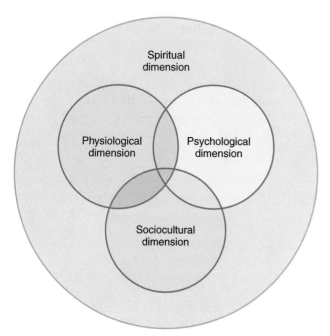

FIGURE **18-1** The spiritual dimension: the unifying approach. (With kind permission of Springer Science and Business Media.)

2004; Smith and McSherry, 2004). Spirituality represents the totality of one's being, serving as the overriding perspective that unifies the various aspects of an individual (Figure 18-1). Spirituality spreads throughout the physiological, psychological, and sociocultural dimensions of a person's life, whether or not the individual acknowledges or develops it.

**FAITH.** The concept of **faith** has two definitions. First, faith is defined as a cultural or institutional religion, such as Buddhism, Christianity, or Islam. Second, faith is a relationship with a divinity, higher power, authority, or spirit that incorporates a reasoning faith (belief) and a trusting faith (action) (Benner, 1985). Reasoning faith is a person's belief and confidence in something for which there is no proof. It is an acceptance of what our reasoning cannot reach. Sometimes it involves a belief in a higher power, spirit guide, God, or Allah (Mauk and Schmidt, 2004). However, faith also is the manner in which a person chooses to live life. Faith in this sense enables action. For example, a person believes that having a positive outlook on life is the best way to achieve life's goals. The belief that comes with faith involves **self-transcendence,** or an awareness of that which cannot be seen or known in ordinary physical ways (Davis, 2003; Perry, 2004). It gives purpose and meaning to an individual's life, allowing for action. For example, a patient living with cancer who has faith in a positive outlook on life decides to seek more knowledge about the disease and continues to pursue daily activities rather than resigning to the disease's symptoms. Self-transcendence allows nurses to provide unconditional care to all patients (Perry, 2004).

**RELIGION.** Religion is associated with the "state of doing," or a specific system of practices associated with a partic-

ular denomination, sect, or form of worship. Religion refers to the system of organized beliefs and worship that a person practices to outwardly express spirituality (Tanyi, 2002). Generally religion involves worshiping a supreme being. Many persons practice a faith or belief in the doctrines of a specific religion or sect, such as the Lutheran church within Christianity or Orthodox Judaism. People from different religions view spirituality differently (McSherry, Cash, and Ross, 2004). Religion influences how the person exercises a faith of belief and action. For example, a Buddhist believes in Four Noble Truths: life is suffering, suffering is caused by clinging, suffering can be eliminated by eliminating clinging, and to eliminate clinging and suffering, one follows an eight-fold path. The path includes the right understanding, intention, speech, action, livelihood, effort, mindfulness, and concentration. This path promotes wisdom, moral behavior, and meditation (Mauk and Schmidt, 2004). A Buddhist turns inward, valuing self-control, whereas a Christian looks to the love of God to provide enlightenment and direction in life.

When providing spiritual care to patients, you need to know the differences between religion and spirituality. Religious care helps patients maintain their faithfulness to their belief systems and worship practices. Spiritual care helps people maintain personal relationships and a relationship to a higher being or life force, in order to identify meaning and purpose in life.

**HOPE.** Spirituality and faith bring hope (Buckley and Herth, 2004; Chiu and others, 2004). When a person has the attitude of something to live for and look forward to, hope is present. **Hope** is a multidimensional concept that gives comfort while a person endures hardship and personal challenges (Buckley and Herth, 2004). It is a concept closely associated with faith. Hope is energizing, giving individuals a motivation to achieve and the resources to use toward that achievement. People express hope in all aspects of their lives as a force that helps them deal with life stressors. Hope is a valuable personal resource whenever someone faces a loss (see Chapter 23) or a challenge that seems difficult to achieve.

## Spiritual Health

People gain spiritual health by finding a balance between their life values, goals, and belief systems and their relationships within themselves and with others. Throughout life a person sometimes grows more spiritual, becoming increasingly aware of the meaning, purpose, and values of life. In times of stress, illness, loss, or recovery, a person often turns to previous ways of responding or adjusting to a situation. Often these coping styles lie within the person's spiritual beliefs.

Spiritual beliefs change as patients grow and develop (Table 18-1). Spirituality begins as children learn about themselves and their relationships with others. When you understand a child's spiritual beliefs, it is easier to care for and comfort the child (McEvoy, 2003). As children mature into adulthood, they experience spiritual growth by entering into lifelong relationships. An ability to care meaningfully for others and self is evidence of a healthy spirituality. Older

| TABLE 18-1 | Relationship Between Developmental Stage and Spiritual Beliefs |
|---|---|
| **Erickson's Developmental Stage** | **Spiritual Beliefs** |
| Trust vs mistrust<br>  Birth to 18 months | Spiritual well-being provided by parents<br>Trust provides a basis for hope<br>Love, affection, security, and a stimulating environment promote spirituality |
| Autonomy vs shame and doubt<br>  18-36 months | Fascination with magic and mystery<br>Often believes illness is related to bad behavior<br>Begins to learn the difference between right and wrong<br>Imitates parents' spiritual or religious actions, recites prayers and sings simple religious songs but does not understand their meanings<br>Interprets meanings literally |
| Initiative vs guilt<br>  3-6 years | Feels guilty when not acting responsibly<br>Influenced by spiritual and religious stories, examples, moods, and actions<br>Models moral behaviors of parents<br>Begins to ask about God or supreme beings |
| Industry vs inferiority<br>  6-12 years | Wants to learn about spirituality<br>Has a clear picture of God or supreme being, morality, and the difference between right and wrong<br>Sorts fantasy from fact<br>Demands proof of reality and believes literal meanings of spiritual stories |
| Identity vs identity confusion<br>  Adolescence | Reflects on inconsistencies in stories<br>Begins to question spiritual practices, forms own opinions, and occasionally discards parents' beliefs<br>Abstract reasoning leads to exploration of moral issues<br>Spirituality comes from connectedness with family, nature, and God or a supreme being |
| Intimacy vs isolation and loneliness<br>  Young adulthood | Establishes self-identity and world view<br>Forms independent beliefs, attitudes, and lifestyles<br>Uses principles to solve problems when individual's and society's rules conflict |
| Generativity vs stagnation<br>  Middle-age adulthood | Develops appreciation of past spiritual experiences<br>Embraces people from different faiths and religions<br>Reviews value system during crisis<br>Values others |
| Ego identity vs despair and disgust<br>  Older Adulthood | Values love and interactions with others<br>Focuses on overcoming oppression and violence<br>Beliefs vary based on many factors, such as gender, past experiences, religion, economic status, and ethnic background |

Data from Edelman CL, Mandle CL: *Health promotion throughout the lifespan*, ed 5, St. Louis, 2002, Mosby; Elkins M, Cavendish R: Developing a plan for pediatric spiritual care, *Holist Nurs Pract* 18(4):179, 2004; Smith J, McSherry W: Spirituality and child development: a concept analysis, *J Adv Nurs* 45(3):307, 2004; and Young C, Koopsen C: *Spirituality, health, and healing*, Thorofare, NJ, 2005, SLACK Inc.

adults often turn to important relationships and the giving of themselves to others as spiritual tasks.

## Spiritual Problems

When illness, loss, grief, or a major life change affects a person, spiritual resources help the person move to recovery. Without spiritual resources, concerns and doubts develop within an individual. **Spiritual distress** is a nursing diagnosis, defined as the disruption in the "life principle" that fills a person's entire being and that integrates and transcends one's biological and psychosocial nature (North American Nursing Diagnosis Association, 2003). For example, a catastrophic illness, like cancer, can upset a person's spiritual well-being enough to cause doubt and a loss of faith. Spiritual distress causes the person to feel alone or even abandoned by resources that at one time were very nurturing. Individuals question their spiritual values, raising questions about their whole way of life and purpose for living. Spiritual distress also occurs when there is conflict between a person's beliefs and prescribed health treatment plan or the inability to practice usual rituals.

**ACUTE ILLNESS.** Sudden, unexpected illness that threatens a patient's life, health, and/or well-being creates significant spiritual distress. For example, the 50-year-old man who has a heart attack and the 20-year-old who is injured in a motor vehicle accident both face crises that threaten their spiritual health. The illness or injury creates an unanticipated scramble to integrate and cope with new realities (e.g., disability). People look for ways to remain faithful to their beliefs and value systems through use of

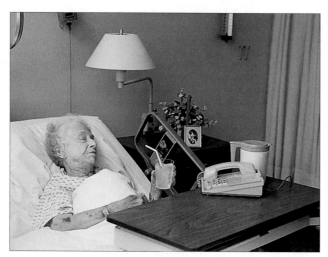

FIGURE **18-2** Spiritual distress often affects a person's adjustment to illness.

spiritual resources. Often conflicts develop around a person's beliefs and the meaning of life. Anger is common, and patients sometimes express it against God, their families, themselves, and their nurses or other health care providers. The strength of patients' spirituality influences their ability to cope with sudden illness and their ability to begin recovery. You play a key role in helping patients resolve feelings of spiritual distress. You create a healing environment and maximize recovery by enhancing your patients' spiritual well-being (Jackson, 2004).

**CHRONIC ILLNESS.** Persons with chronic illness often suffer debilitating symptoms that change their lifestyles. The uncertain and long-term nature of chronic illness, along with the potential for outcomes such as pain, changes in body image, and the need to confront death, all lead to spiritual distress. Patients struggle with questions about the meaning and purpose of their lives because their independence is threatened, causing fear, anxiety, and an overall dispiritedness. The nursing diagnosis *spiritual distress* is appropriate to use for patients who experience these symptoms (Figure 18-2). A person's spirituality is a significant factor in how he or she adapts to the changes resulting from chronic illness. Successfully adapting to those changes strengthens a person spiritually, but it sometimes takes a long-term plan to help the chronically ill patient achieve spiritual well-being. You, as the nurse, are in a unique position to help patients reevaluate their lives and achieve spiritual health (Mauk and Schmidt, 2004). Patients who have a sense of spiritual well-being have a much better chance to reestablish a self-identity and live to their potential.

**TERMINAL ILLNESS.** Terminal illness commonly causes fear of physical pain, isolation, the unknown, and dying. When patients feel uncertain about what death means, they are susceptible to spiritual distress. On the other hand, there are patients who have a spiritual sense of peace that enables them to face death without fear. Individuals experiencing a terminal illness often find themselves reviewing their

life and questioning its meaning. Common questions asked include, Why is this happening to me? or What have I done? Terminal illness affects family and friends just as much as the patient. It causes members of the family to ask important questions about life's meaning and how it will affect their relationship with the patient (see Chapter 23).

When the patient is terminally ill, make a referral to hospice. Hospice nurses work with an interdisciplinary health care team to assist patients and their families with having a peaceful death. Once the patient dies, hospice provides bereavement support to the family. While the patient and family receive hospice services, they often spend a lot of time in quiet, spiritual reflection. Spirituality helps patients and families find resolution and peace at the end of life (Mauk and Schmidt, 2004).

Wong and others (2004) investigated the health needs of patients who were dying at home. They found that except for trouble breathing, the patients' physical symptoms were generally well controlled. The patients and families were more concerned about the psychological aspects of dying. Family members, along with the patient, often experienced role changes during this time. For example, patients who were once caregivers became receivers of care. The patients expressed guilt, stress, fear, anger, anxiety, grief, and spiritual distress. However, these feelings decreased over time as the nurses provided soothing home care. Patients who had adequate social support and who viewed death as a part of life coped better with their illness. Dying is a holistic event that encompasses the patient's physical, social, psychological, and spiritual health.

**NEAR-DEATH EXPERIENCE.** You may care for a patient or have a family member who has had a near-death experience (NDE). An NDE is a psychological phenomenon of people who have either been close to clinical death or have recovered after being declared dead. It is not associated with a mental disorder. Instead, experts agree that NDE describes a powerfully close brush with physical, emotional, and spiritual death. Persons who experience an NDE after cardiopulmonary arrest, for example, often tell the same story of feeling themselves rising above their bodies and watching caregivers initiate lifesaving measures. Commonly, patients who experience an NDE describe feeling totally at peace, having an out-of-body experience, being pulled into a dark tunnel, being surrounded by bright light, and encountering people who preceded them in death. Instead of moving toward the light, they learn it is not time for them to die, and they return to life (James, 2004).

Patients who have an NDE are often reluctant to discuss it, thinking family or caregivers will not understand. Isolation and depression often occurs. However, individuals experiencing an NDE who discuss it openly with family or caregivers find acceptance and meaning from this powerful experience. They are often no longer afraid of death, and they have a decreased desire to achieve material wealth. They also report increased sensitivity to different chemicals, such as alcohol and medications. After patients have survived an NDE, you promote spiritual well-being by remaining open, giving patients a chance to explore what happened, and supporting patients as they share the experience with significant others (James, 2004).

# Critical Thinking

## Synthesis

The helping role is an important domain of nursing practice (Benner, 1984). Patients look to nurses for help that is different than the help they seek from other health care professionals. Your nursing expertise will allow you to anticipate the personal issues affecting patients' abilities to receive and seek help, including their spiritual well-being. Critical thinking, knowledge, and skills help you to enhance patients' spiritual well-being and health and to assist those in need of help and support in engaging their own spirituality for healing and recovery. While using the nursing process, you will apply knowledge, experience, attitudes, and standards in providing appropriate spiritual care.

**KNOWLEDGE.** Your knowledge about the concept of spirituality and a patient's faith and belief systems helps to provide appropriate spiritual care. Taking a faith history will reveal the individual's beliefs toward life, health, and a supreme being. Knowledge of a patient's culture will provide additional insight into a person's spiritual practices (Box 18-1). In addition, good communication principles (see Chapter 9) and caring (see Chapter 16) will help you to establish therapeutic trust with patients. An individual's spiritual beliefs are very personal and relational. When you are able to convey caring and openness to individuals, you will be more successful in promoting honest discussion about their spiritual beliefs.

When caring for patients with terminal illness, knowledge of loss and grief dynamics (see Chapter 23) is important. A person's reaction to loss is in part a function of the grief response, influenced by the person's spirituality. You also need to consider family dynamics while providing spiritual care (see Chapter 21). For many individuals, their spiritual health is often integrated with the relationships between family members. Therefore consider the family's beliefs when planning spiritual care for your patient.

Another area of knowledge for you to reflect on is your own spiritual beliefs and values. By fostering your own personal, emotional, and spiritual health, you become a resource for your patient (Jackson, 2004). You use your awareness of your own spirituality as a tool when caring for yourself and your patients. Differentiate your personal spirituality from that of the patient. This becomes important during the delivery of care, when you need to be able to engage a patient spiritually rather than try to exercise personal spiritual convictions. Your role is not to solve the spiritual problems of patients but to provide an environment where your patients are able to express their spirituality.

Finally, a sound understanding of ethics and values (see Chapter 5) is essential to providing spiritual care. A person's

---

**BOX 18-1** CULTURAL FOCUS

Through studying, Jeff found that one in every three American women diagnosed with cancer has breast cancer. Five-year survival rates for breast cancer have steadily improved. However, the survival rate for African-American women is lower than the survival rate for white women. Spiritual needs are often associated with cultural beliefs. Spiritual and cultural beliefs affect how women of different cultures experience health and illness. African-American women generally express Christian beliefs in their spirituality, which is associated with a deep relationship with God and strong moral and ethical values. Spirituality for African-Americans often provides a source of healing, coping, and peace. Jeff uses this understanding of breast cancer and spirituality among African-American women to develop a culturally competent plan of care for Victoria and her family.

### Implications for Practice

- Jeff encourages Victoria and her family to strengthen their spiritual health as they continue to cope with Victoria's breast cancer diagnosis and cancer treatment.
- Victoria's church has a parish nurse. Parish nurses care for the spiritual, emotional, and physical health of the members of a congregation. Because of their holistic approach to health, African-American people usually consider parish nurses to be helpful. Jeff talks with Victoria about the services her parish nurse provides. With Victoria's permission, he shares her health problems and concerns with the parish nurse. The parish nurse agrees to contact Victoria and arrange a time for them to meet.
- Many African-American women study the Bible and pray regularly. Jeff prays with Victoria and Joe during their visits to the oncology clinic and encourages them to continue to read the Bible together at home.
- African-American churches provide a great deal of social support and companionship, which is helpful to people who have cancer and their caregivers. Therefore Jeff encourages Joe to attend church even if Victoria is too ill to attend. He also contacts the Timms's pastor and arranges times for people from the church to come sit with Victoria for a few hours 2 days a week to allow Joe some time to take care of himself.

Data from Musgrave CF, Allen CE, Allen GJ: Spirituality and health for women of color, *Am J Public Health* 92(4):557, 2002; Newlin K, Knafl K, Melkus GD: African-American spirituality: a concept analysis, *ANS Adv Nurs Sci* 25(2):57, 2002; Phillips JS and others: African American women's experiences with breast cancer screening, *J Nurs Scholarsh* 33(2):135, 2001; Wallace DC and others: Client perceptions of parish nursing, *Public Health Nurs* 19(2):128, 2002.

---

values or beliefs about the worth of a given idea, attitude, or custom are linked to the individual's spiritual well-being. Application of ethical principles ensures respect for a patient's spiritual and religious convictions.

**EXPERIENCE.** Recognizing that spirituality is more than religion, you need to consider personal views and philosophies about life and reflect on whether your own spirituality is beneficial in assisting patients. If you sense a personal faith and hope regarding life, it is likely that you will be better able to help patients (Jackson, 2004). Previous personal and professional experiences with dying patients, patients with chronic disease, or patients who have experienced significant losses provide lessons in how to help patients face difficult challenges and how to offer support to family and friends (Wright, 2005).

**ATTITUDES.** Do not take a patient's reaction to illness or loss for granted. Humility becomes very important, particularly when caring for patients from diverse cultural and/or religious backgrounds. Recognize any limitations in your own knowledge about a patient's spiritual beliefs and religious practices, and be willing to pursue the knowledge needed to provide appropriate, individualized care. Show genuine concern for patients as you ask them about their beliefs and how spirituality influences their health (Mazanec and Tyler, 2004). Also exhibit integrity; realize the importance of refraining from expressing your opinions about religion or spirituality when they conflict with that of the patient. Finally, show confidence in dealing with spiritual issues as you build a caring relationship with the patient. Confidence works to build trust.

**STANDARDS.** A good critical thinker is thorough and ensures that information about a patient is significant and relevant when making decisions about patients' spiritual needs. The nature of a person's spirituality is complex and highly individualized. Therefore avoid making assumptions about the patient's religion and beliefs. Significance and relevance are standards of critical thinking that ensure you explore the issues that are most meaningful to patients and most likely to affect their spiritual well-being. Also, apply ethical standards of care when providing spiritual care.

The Joint Commission on Accreditation of Healthcare Organizations (JCAHO) sets standards for quality health care. JCAHO requires health care organizations to acknowledge patients' rights to spiritual care and provide for patients' spiritual needs through pastoral care or others who are certified, ordained, or lay individuals (LaPierre, 2003). The JCAHO requirements state that you need to assess the patient's denomination, beliefs, and spiritual practices (Mauk and Schmidt, 2004).

The Code of Ethics for Nurses (ANA, 2001) sets standards for quality nursing care. The Code requires you to practice nursing with compassion. You show compassion by accepting the dignity and worth of all your patients despite their socioeconomic status, personal characteristics or type of health problems. You promote an environment that respects your patients' values, customs, and spiritual beliefs.

## Nursing Process

Application of the nursing process from the perspective of a patient's spiritual needs is not simple. It goes beyond assessing a patient's religious practices. Understanding a patient's spirituality and then appropriately identifying the level of support and resources needed requires a new, broader perspective. Heliker (1992) described the importance of shared

community and compassion. *Compassion* comes from the Latin words *puti* and *cum,* meaning "to suffer with." *Community* comes from the Latin word meaning "fellowship." To be compassionate is to "enter into places of pain, to share in brokenness with other human beings" (Heliker, 1992). To practice compassion as a nurse requires awareness of the very human tie between patients and a healing community. Remove any personal biases or misconceptions from your assessment, and be willing to share and discover another person's meaning and purpose in life, sickness, and health. Learn to look beyond a personal view when establishing a patient relationship. This means identifying the common values that make us human and respecting the commitments and values that make humans unique.

Another important aspect of spiritual care is recognizing that a patient does not have to have a spiritual problem. Patients bring certain spiritual resources for you to use as resources to help them assume healthier lives, recover from illness, or face impending death. Supporting and recognizing the positive side of a patient's spirituality goes a long way in delivering effective, individualized nursing care.

## Assessment

Before you complete a spiritual assessment on your patient, you need to be aware of your own spiritual beliefs, values, and biases. Understanding your own spirit is essential when you provide spiritual care to your patients (Young and Koopsen, 2005). You also need to practice spiritual self-care. You practice spiritual self-care when you participate in religious practices, provide community service, and connect with your family and friends.

Your ability to gain a reliable picture of patients' spirituality will be limited if you have only periodic contact with patients (e.g., outpatient settings) or if you fail to build therapeutic relationships with them. But once you establish a trusting relationship with a patient, you and the patient will reach a point of learning together, and spiritual caring will occur (Taylor, 2003). Learn to consciously integrate an attitude of spiritual care into the nursing process. Make your assessment focus on aspects of spirituality most likely to be influenced by life experiences, events, and questions in the case of illness and hospitalization (Table 18-2). Conducting an assessment is therapeutic because it conveys a level of caring and support.

You assess a patient's spiritual health in several different ways. One way is to ask the patient direct questions. This approach requires you to feel comfortable asking others about their spirituality. The indicator-based method of spiritual assessment requires that you look for defining characteristics, such as anger or expressing concern about life, when you assess your patients. If your patient has these defining characteristics, then you make a nursing diagnosis. Finally, some institutions and researchers have created assessment tools to clarify values and assess spirituality (McSherry and Ross, 2002). For example, the B-E-L-I-E-F assessment tool

## FOCUSED PATIENT ASSESSMENT

TABLE 18-2

| Factors to Assess | Questions and Approaches | Physical Assessment Strategies |
| --- | --- | --- |
| Past experiences with loss | How would you describe the ways you cope spiritually when faced with difficult times? | Observe patient's facial expressions and mannerisms during the discussion. |
| Fear of the unknown resulting from a terminal illness | Describe the people who mean the most to you. In what way do you look to them for support? Do you consider yourself a spiritual person? If so, what gives you comfort? If not, what provides you a sense of peace? | Fear is associated with anxiety. Be alert for changes in vital signs. Observe the patient's mood, willingness to initiate conversation, and interest in surroundings. |

(McEvoy, 2003) helps pediatric nurses evaluate the child and family's spiritual and religious needs. The acronym stands for the following:

B—Belief system
E—Ethics or values
L—Lifestyle
I —Involvement in a spiritual community
E—Education
F—Future events

Assessment tools like the B-E-L-I-E-F scale help nurses remember important areas to assess and create a spiritual plan of care.

Nurse researchers developed the JAREL spiritual well-being scale to provide nurses and other health care professionals with a simple tool for assessing a patient's spiritual well-being (Hungelmann and others, 1996). The tool was developed for patients from Christian, non-Christian, and atheist belief systems. Items on the tool make up three key dimensions: the faith/belief dimension, life/self-responsibility, and life-satisfaction/self-actualization. The tool is simple to use and requires patients to rate their level of agreement with each item along a five-point scale (strongly agree to strongly disagree). If you use this tool with patients who have visual or literacy problems, you will need to read the items to the patient and record the patient's response. If the patient's score on any item, group of items, or a particular dimension is low, it indicates an area to explore further (Hungelmann and others, 1996). The tool helps you explore any perceptions or concerns a patient has. For example, if a patient disagrees about accepting life situations, you need to spend time learning how the patient accepts and manages his or her illness. Remember, when using any spiritual assessment tool, do not impose your personal value systems on the patient. This is particularly true when the patient's values and beliefs are similar to yours because it then becomes very easy to make false assumptions.

You will use any or all of these methods to perform a spiritual assessment. When you understand the overall approach to spiritual assessment, you are able to enter into thoughtful discussions with the patient, gain a greater awareness of the personal resources the patient brings to a situation, and incorporate the resources into an effective plan of care.

**FAITH/BELIEF.** Individuals have some source of authority and guidance in their lives that leads them to choose and act on their beliefs. The authority is sometimes a supreme being, a code of conduct, a religious leader, family or friends, oneself, or a combination of sources. Faith in an authority provides a sense of confidence that guides a person in exercising beliefs and experiencing growth. You assess a person's faith in an authority by asking, "Who do you look to for guidance in life?" The patient's response will likely open the door for a meaningful discussion. Listen carefully, and explore what is meaningful to the patient (Friedemann and others, 2002).

Determine if the patient has a religious source of guidance that conflicts with medical treatment plans. This seriously affects the treatment options nurses and other health care providers are able to offer patients. For example, if a patient is a Jehovah's Witness, blood products are not an acceptable form of treatment. Christian Scientists often refuse any medical intervention, believing that their faith will heal them.

It is also important to understand a patient's philosophy of life. Asking the patient, "Describe for me what is most important in your life" or "Tell me what gives your life meaning or purpose" helps to assess the basis of the patient's spiritual belief system (Taylor, 2003). This information reveals the patient's spiritual focus and will help to reflect the impact illness, loss, or disability has on the person's life. A patient's religious practices, views about health, and response to illness influence how you will provide support (Table 18-3).

**LIFE AND SELF-RESPONSIBILITY.** Spiritual well-being includes life and self-responsibility. Individuals who accept change in life, make decisions about their lives, and are able to forgive themselves and others in times of difficulty have a higher level of spiritual well-being. During illness, patients often are unable to accept limitations or know what to do to regain a functional and meaningful life. Their sense of helplessness reflects spiritual distress. However, if a patient is able to adapt to changes and seek solutions for how to deal with any limitations, spiritual well-being reflects an important coping resource. Assess the extent to which a patient understands any limitations or threats posed by an illness and the manner in which the patient chooses to adjust to them. Ask, "Tell me how you feel about the changes caused by your illness" and "How do these changes affect what you now need to do?"

| TABLE 18-3 | Religious Beliefs About Health | | |
|---|---|---|---|
| **Religious or Cultural Group** | **Health Care Beliefs** | **Response to Illness** | **Implications for Health and Nursing** |
| Hinduism | Accepts modern medical science. | Past sins cause illness. Prolonging life is discouraged. | Allow time for prayer and purity rituals. Allow use of amulets, rituals, and symbols. |
| Sikhism | Accepts modern medical science. | Females to be examined by females. Removing undergarments causes great distress. | Provide time for devotional prayer. Allow use of religious symbols. |
| Buddhism | Accepts modern medical science. | Sometimes refuses treatment on holy days. Nonhuman spirits invading the body cause illness. May want a Buddhist priest. May permit withdrawal of life support. Does not practice euthanasia. Often will not take time off from work or family responsibilities when sick. | Health is an important part of life. Good health is maintained by caring for yourself and others. Does not always accept medications because of belief that chemical substances in the body are harmful. |
| Islam | Must be able to practice the Five Pillars of Islam. Sometimes has a fatalistic view of health. | Uses faith healing. Family members are a comfort. Group prayer is strengthening. May permit withdrawal of life support. Does not practice euthanasia. Believes time of death is predetermined and cannot be changed. Maintains a sense of hope and often avoids discussions of death. | Women prefer female health care providers. During month of Ramadan, women cannot eat until after the sun goes down. Health and spirituality are connected. Family and friends visit during times of illness. Organ transplantation or donation and postmortem examinations are usually not considered. |
| Judaism | Believes in the sanctity of life. God and medicine have a balance. Observance of the Sabbath is important. Some refuse treatments on the Sabbath. | Visiting the sick is an obligation. Obligation to seek care, exercise, and sleep, eat well, and avoid drug and alcohol abuse. Euthanasia is forbidden. Life support is discouraged. | Believes it is important to keep yourself healthy. Expects nurses to provide competent health care. Allow patients to express their feelings. Allow family to stay with the dying patient. |
| Protestants and Catholics | Accept modern medical science. | Use prayer, faith healing. Appreciate visits from clergy. Some will use laying on of hands. Commonly take holy communion. Last rites given when individual near death (Catholic). | Are in favor of organ donation. Health is important to maintain. Allow time for patients to pray by themselves, with family or friends. |
| Navajos | Concepts of health have a fundamental place in their concept of humans and their place in the universe. | Blessingway is a practice that attempts to remove ill health by means of stories, songs, rituals, prayers, symbols, and sand paintings. | Prefer holistic approach to health care. Often are not on time for appointments. Promote physical, mental, spiritual, and social health of persons, families, and communities. Allow family members to visit. Provide teaching about wellness, not disease prevention, when possible. |
| Appalachians | Nature controls life and health. Accept folk healers. Good Christian members of community are called as servants to minister to disabled. | Dislike hospitals. Tend to not follow medical regimens but expect help when seeking episodic treatment. | Become anxious in unfamiliar settings. Encourage communication with family and friends when ill. |

of care (see care plan). Match the patient's needs with those interventions that are supported and recommended in the clinical and research literature. Focus on building a caring relationship with the patient so that you will enter into a healing relationship together.

**GOALS AND OUTCOMES.** A spiritual plan of care includes realistic and individualized goals along with relevant outcomes. This will require you to work closely with the patient in setting goals and outcomes and ultimately choosing nursing interventions. In cases where spiritual care requires helping patients adjust to loss or stressful situations, some goals are long term (e.g., regaining spiritual comfort or affirming a purpose in life). Short-term goals, such as renewing participation in religious practices, are helpful to allow a patient to move toward a more spiritually healthy situation. Outcomes need to relate to what you have learned about the patient. For example, if you know a patient once practiced regular prayer and meditation, you state an outcome for the goal of regaining spiritual comfort as "Patient will begin regular prayer and meditation daily."

**SETTING PRIORITIES.** Spiritual care is very personalized. Your relationship with the patient allows you to understand your patient's priorities. If you have developed a mutually agreed-on plan with the patient, he or she is able to relate what is most important. Spiritual priorities need not be sacrificed for physical care priorities. In the case of a terminally ill patient, for example, spiritual care is possibly the most important intervention you will provide.

**CONTINUITY OF CARE.** To ensure ongoing spiritual care, it sometimes becomes necessary to involve family members, significant others, and clergy to lend support. This means you learned from the assessment which individuals or groups have formed a fellowship with the patient. These individuals become involved in all levels of your plan. The patient's support network will assist in sharing quiet moments of prayer, reading scripture to the patient, and even giving physical care. In a hospital setting the pastoral care department is a valuable resource. These professionals provide insight about how and when to best support patients and families.

## Implementation

If a patient is in spiritual distress or has a health problem that requires the patient to use spiritual resources, a caring relationship between you and the patient is necessary. Both you and the patient must feel free to let go and discover together the meaning illness or loss poses for the patient and the impact it has on the meaning and purpose of life. When you achieve this level of understanding with a patient, it enables you to deliver care in a sensitive, creative, and appropriate manner.

**HEALTH PROMOTION.** Spiritual care needs to be a central theme in promoting an individual's overall well-being (Grant, 2004). Spirituality is one personal resource that affects the balance between health and illness. You will be able to use the interventions described here at any level of health care.

**Establishing Presence.** You contribute to a sense of well-being and provide hope for recovery when you spend time with your patients (Krebs, 2003). Behaviors that establish your presence include giving attention, answering questions, listening, and having a positive and encouraging (but realistic) attitude. Presence is part of the art of nursing. Benner (1984) explains that presence involves "being with" a patient versus "doing for" a patient. Presence is being able to offer a closeness with the patient: physically, psychologically, and spiritually. Presence helps to prevent emotional and environmental isolation (see Chapter 16).

When health promotion is the focus of care, your presence becomes important in instilling confidence in patients' abilities to take the steps necessary to remain healthy. You convey a caring presence by listening to patients' concerns, willingly involving family in discussions about the patient's health, and showing self-confidence when providing health instruction.

Trust is fundamental to any relationship. The attitude you convey when first interacting with a patient sets the tone for all conversations (see Chapter 9). Actively listening to the meaning of what a patient says is most important. It involves paying attention to the person's words, tone of voice, and entering his or her frame of reference. By observing the patient's expressions and body language, you will find cues to help the patient explore ways to achieve inner peace, take action, or manage pain (Otis-Green and others, 2002). Your role as a nurse is not to solve the spiritual problems of patients but to provide an environment where your patients can express spirituality (McEwan, 2004).

**Supporting a Healing Relationship.** When giving spiritual care, look beyond isolated patient problems and recognize the broader picture of a patient's holistic needs. For example, do not just look at a patient's back pain as a problem to solve with quick remedies but rather look at how the pain influences the patient's ability to function and achieve goals established in life. A holistic view enables you to assume a helping role. When you develop a helping role with your patients, you establish healing relationships (Benner, 1984). Three steps are evident when you establish healing relationships with your patients:

1. Mobilizing hope for you and for the patient
2. Finding an interpretation or understanding of the illness, pain, anxiety, or other stressful emotion that is acceptable to the patient
3. Assisting the patient in using social, emotional, or spiritual resources (Benner, 1984)

Mobilizing the patient's hope is central to a healing relationship. Hope motivates people to face challenges in life (Lohne and Severinsson, 2004). You will help patients find realistic things to hope for. A patient newly diagnosed with diabetes might hope to learn how to manage the disease so as to continue a productive and satisfying way of life. A terminally ill

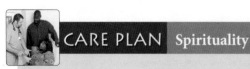

## CARE PLAN  Spirituality

### ASSESSMENT

Victoria has been told her prognosis is promising, although she will need treatment to prevent spread of her disease. Victoria expresses a **connectedness with her God,** "I do not feel alone; God is with me. I have a better appreciation of each day God gives me, and I believe God's strength will help me continue to be active in my church." Victoria and Joe **attend their church regularly and hope to continue** doing so even during the chemotherapy. Jeff learns that Joe encourages Victoria and has been trying to arrange work so that he is able to take her to the clinic. This means that he has less time in the evening to spend with the children. In the past, Joe and Victoria have always had discussions with the children during mealtime, but this has been difficult. **Members of their church have offered support** by taking Victoria to the clinic if Joe is unable.

Victoria worries about her children. During the last month she has spent less time with Valerie and Peter because of her cancer treatment and resultant fatigue. Peter is having some difficulty in school. Valerie has recently expressed concern about her mother dying. Both children reportedly have been acting angrily toward their parents. Before Victoria's illness the children were very **close to their parents and shared their faith in God.**

*Defining characteristics are shown in bold type.

---

**NURSING DIAGNOSIS** Readiness for enhanced spiritual well-being related to renewed appreciation of life after cancer diagnosis.

---

### PLANNING

| GOAL | EXPECTED OUTCOMES* |
|---|---|
| | ***Spiritual Health*** |
| • Victoria will restore connectedness with children (within 2 months). | • Victoria, Joe, and children will discuss patient's beliefs about the future and her hope of having the cancer cured (to be met in 2 weeks).<br>• Patient will report son and daughter's ability to discuss fears with mother (to be met in 4 weeks). |
| • Victoria will remain connected with herself, her husband, and God (within 1 month). | • Victoria will make time in her day to pray (to be met in 1 week).<br>• Victoria will report that she and her husband are able to discuss their feelings and fears on a daily basis (to be met in 3 weeks). |

*Outcomes classification label from Moorhead S, Johnson M, Maas M: *Nursing outcomes classification (NOC),* ed 3, St. Louis, 2004, Mosby.

---

| INTERVENTIONS† | RATIONALE |
|---|---|
| ***Spiritual Support*** | |
| • Use therapeutic communication (see Chapter 9) to establish presence and trust and to demonstrate empathy with Victoria and Joe. | Establishing rapport, active listening, and trust are necessary when caring for people with spiritual needs (Grant, 2004). |
| • Pray with Victoria and her family. | When people pray, they recognize the importance of their relationships with others and experience enhanced connectedness (O'Brien, 2003). |
| • Encourage Victoria and her husband to tell stories about positive past experiences that represented spiritual strength and mutual support with their children. | Storytelling about positive spiritual experiences helps the child and family feel they are not alone during times of crisis (Elkins and Cavendish, 2004). |
| ***Family Integrity Promotion*** | |
| • Identify typical family coping mechanisms during a conference scheduled late in afternoon at the cancer clinic when the children are able to attend. Provide discussion of their mother's progress. Establish a presence, and express a realistic hope of mother's prognosis. | Discussing coping mechanisms used in the past helps children cope with illness. Discussion of illness ensures children will have accurate perception of mother's clinical condition and treatment. Offering compassionate presence and support contributes to the patient's spiritual well-being (McEvoy, 2003). |
| • Encourage Victoria to identify tasks she needs assistance to complete at home, and help Joe and the children identify a plan to provide care to Victoria. | Virtues of sharing and concern of others contribute to the overall healthy development of children and their families (McEvoy, 2003). |
| • Encourage Victoria and Joe to maintain their positive relationship by spending time with each other every day to talk about feelings and fears. | Emotional support provided by husbands helps wives better cope with chronic illnesses and contributes to the health of a marriage (Kramer and Thompson, 2002). |

†Intervention classification labels from Dochterman JM, Bulechek GM, editors: *Nursing interventions classification (NIC),* ed 4, St. Louis, 2004, Mosby.

*Continued*

CARE PLAN Spirituality—cont'd

**EVALUATION**

- Ask Victoria about her daily routine. Determine if her routine includes time for prayer and communication with family.
- Have Victoria and Joe report on outcomes of discussions with children.

- Observe interactions between parents and children.
- Ask Victoria to describe feelings she has when communicating with husband and children about cancer.

patient may hope to attend a daughter's graduation and live each day to the fullest.

Hope has both short- and long-term implications. From a long-term perspective, hope gives individuals a determination to endure and carry on with life's responsibilities (Buckley and Herth, 2004). In the short-term view, hope provides an incentive for constructive coping with obstacles and for finding ways to realize the object of hope. Hope is future oriented and helps a patient work toward recovery. You help patients achieve hope by working with them to find explanations for their situations that are mutually acceptable. Then help each patient realistically exercise hope. This includes supporting a patient's positive attitude toward life or a desire to be informed and to make decisions.

To further support a healing relationship, remain aware of the patient's spiritual resources and needs. It is always important for patients to be able to express and exercise their beliefs and to find spiritual comfort. When illness or treatment creates confusion or uncertainty for the patient, recognize the possible effect this can have on a patient's well-being. How can spiritual resources be used and strengthened? Having a clear sense of what illness will be like for an individual helps the person to apply all resources toward recovery.

**ACUTE CARE.** Within an acute care setting, support and enhancement of a patient's spiritual well-being is a challenge when the focus of health care seems to be one of treatment and cure rather than care (McEwan, 2004). To overcome these challenges, display a soothing presence and supportive touch as you implement nursing interventions. Some patients are fearful of experiencing an illness that threatens their loss of control, and they look for someone to offer competent direction. Your artful use of hands, encouraging words of support, promotion of connectedness, and calm and decisive approach will establish a presence that builds trust. Work closely with patients to maximize resources that support their spirituality. For example, you build trust with your patients when you perform procedures competently. You promote connectedness and build trust by listening to the dying patient's concerns, providing reassurance and comfort, and helping the patient complete unfinished business (Narayanasamy and others, 2004).

**Support Systems.** Using support systems is important in any health care setting. Support systems serve as a human link connecting the patient, the nurse, and the patient's lifestyle before an illness. In today's society, support comes from many areas, including the family, friends, and support groups. Klemm and Wheeler (2005) found that an online support group for cancer caregivers helped caregivers express feelings such as hope, optimism, and pessimism. The members of the online support group formed a special bond with each other, even though many of them had never met in person. Part of the patient's caregiving environment is the regular presence of supportive family and friends. Families often influence how patients perceive their illness (Callahan, 2003). You enhance the patient's support network when you include the patient's family and friends in planning care. The patient's support system is a source of coping, faith, and hope that is a resource in religious rituals that are important for a patient (Callahan, 2003).

When a patient depends on family, friends, spiritual advisors, and members of the clergy for support, encourage them to visit the patient regularly. Make all the patient's visitors welcome on nursing units, and ensure privacy during visits to provide spiritual comfort. If possible, ask the pastoral care department to notify community clergy of their congregant's admission. Often illness and the hospital environment produce uncertainty that frightens family members and friends. Help the family to feel welcome, and use their support and presence to promote the patient's healing. For example, including family members in prayer is a thoughtful gesture if it is appropriate to the patient's religion and if family members are comfortable participating. Encouraging the family to bring meaningful religious symbols to the patient's bedside and facilitating the administration of sacraments, rites, and rituals offers significant spiritual support (Leininger and McFarland, 2002).

**Diet Therapies.** Food and nutrition are important aspects of nursing care. Food is also an important component of some religious observances. For example, some Hindu and Islamic sects are vegetarians. Muslims are not allowed to eat pork, and they fast during the month of Ramadan. Orthodox Jewish patients observe kosher dietary restrictions. Native Americans have food practices influenced by individual tribal beliefs. Like many aspects of a particular culture or religion, food and the rituals surrounding the preparation and serving of food are important to a patient's spirituality. When possible, you integrate the patient's dietary preferences into daily care and consult with the health care institution's dietitian when needed. In the event that a hospital or other health care agency cannot prepare food in the preferred way, ask the fam-

| BOX 18-2 | CARE OF THE OLDER ADULT |
|---|---|

- Religious activities, attitudes, and spiritual experiences are very common among older adults. Those who experience spiritual well-being have strong social support, better emotional health, and to some extent, improved physical health (Koenig, George, and Titus, 2004).
- Respecting privacy and dignity is an essential part of nursing care, especially when meeting spiritual needs of the older adult (Narayanasamy and others, 2004).
- Older adults use a variety of strategies such as exercise, physical therapy, and complementary medicine to cope with pain and chronic illness. Including religious activities positively enhances coping (Barry and others, 2004).
- Feelings of connectedness are important for the older adult. You enhance connectedness by helping the older patient find meaning and purpose in life, listening actively to concerns, and being present (Narayanasamy and others, 2004).
- Beliefs in the afterlife increase as adults grow older. Make visits from clergy, social workers, lawyers, and even financial advisors available so patients feel as though they have completed all unfinished business. Leaving a legacy to loved ones prepares the older adult to leave the world with a sense of meaning (Ebersole and Hess, 2004). Legacies include oral histories, works of art, publications, photographs, or other objects of significance.

| BOX 18-3 | PATIENT TEACHING |
|---|---|

At one of her clinic visits, Victoria tells Jeff, "My friend told me yesterday that when she had cancer, she used meditation to help her cope with the side effects of her chemotherapy. I was thinking that I might try meditating to see if it would help me. But, I don't know how to meditate. Can you help me?" Jeff develops the following teaching plan for Victoria:

### Outcome
Victoria will verbalize feelings of relaxation and self-transcendence after meditation.

### Teaching Strategies
- Provide a brief description of what will be taught.
- Give Victoria a patient teaching sheet that describes how to meditate.
- Help Victoria identify at least one quiet place in her home that has minimal interruptions.
- Tell her that soft background noise like a fan or soft music can be used during meditation to block out distractions.
- Teach Victoria the steps of meditation—sit in a comfortable position with the back straight; breathe slowly; and focus on a sound, a prayer, or an image.
- Encourage Victoria to meditate for 10 to 20 minutes 2 times a day.
- Answer any questions.
- Reinforce information as needed.

### Evaluation Strategies
- Ask Victoria to identify what she learned about herself and how she feels after meditating.

ily to bring meals that are appropriate for dietary restrictions posed by the patient's condition.

**Supporting Rituals.** You become active in your patients' spiritual care by supporting patients' participation in spiritual rituals and activities. This is especially important for older adults (Box 18-2). Plan care to allow time for religious readings, spiritual visitations, or even attendance at religious services. Some churches and synagogues offer audiotapes of religious services. Allow family members to plan a prayer session or an organized reading when appropriate. Taped meditations, religious music, and televised religious services provide other effective treatment options. Be respectful of icons, medals, prayer rugs, or crosses that patients bring to a health care setting, and make sure they are not accidentally lost or misplaced.

### RESTORATIVE AND CONTINUING CARE

**Prayer and Meditation.** The act of prayer gives an individual the opportunity to renew personal faith and belief in a higher being in a specific, focused way that is either highly ritualized and formal or quite spontaneous and informal. Prayer is an effective coping resource for physical and psychological symptoms (Wright, 2005). Patients pray in private or pursue opportunities for group prayer with family, friends, or clergy. Some patients pray while listening to music. Be supportive of prayer by giving the patient privacy if desired, by learning if the patient wishes to have you participate, and by suggesting prayer when it is known to be a coping resource for the patient. If prayer is not suitable for a patient, alterna-

tives include listening to calming music or reading a book, poetry, or inspirational texts selected by the patient.

Meditation is effective in creating a relaxation response that reduces daily stress. Patients who meditate often state they have an increased awareness of their spirituality and of the presence of God or a supreme being (Box 18-3). Meditation exercises give patients relief from chronic pain, insomnia, anxiety, and depression and help in coping with the side effects of uncomfortable therapy (Roberts, 2004). Meditation involves sitting quietly in a comfortable position with eyes closed and repeating a sound, phrase, or sacred word in rhythm with breathing, while disregarding intrusive thoughts. Individuals who meditate regularly (twice a day, for 10 or 20 minutes), experience decreased metabolism and heart rate, easier breathing, and slower brain waves. Chapter 30 addresses relaxation approaches.

### ✳ Evaluation

**PATIENT CARE.** Attainment of spiritual health is a lifelong goal. Patients will experience the need to clarify values (see Chapter 5), reshape philosophies, and live those experiences

## OUTCOME EVALUATION

**TABLE 18-4**

| Nursing Action | Patient Response/Finding | Achievement of Outcome |
|---|---|---|
| Ask Victoria to explain her daily routine. Does she include time for self-reflection and communication with Joe? | Victoria sits by herself in her garden daily and prays. Victoria meditates for 10-15 minutes a day. She and Joe spend time talking with each other nightly. | Outcome met. |
| Ask Victoria to describe how children reacted to discussion with her and Joe. Did children express concerns? | Children initially did not speak, only listened. With Joe's encouragement, daughter began to express her fears. | Outcome partially met. Recommend an additional session with children. |
| During next clinic visit observe manner in which Victoria and children interact. | Both children come to clinic with Victoria. They spontaneously ask questions of staff. Daughter stands close to mother and asks if chemotherapy infusion is uncomfortable. | Children showing closeness to mother and interest in her well-being. Recommend a final family conference after last round of chemotherapy. |

## EVALUATION

Victoria returns to the clinic the week after establishing a plan to enhance her spiritual health with Jeff. A member of her church accompanies Victoria because Joe is out of town on a business trip. Jeff wants to evaluate whether Victoria continues to feel connected with herself, Joe, her children, and God. Jeff asks, "Tell me, Mrs. Timms, have you had a chance yet to try any of the approaches we talked about last week to give yourself, Joe, and the kids a chance to talk about their feelings? If so, what were the results?" Victoria reports, "Yes, I spend at least 10 minutes every morning in prayer while I sit in my garden, and I have been meditating for 10 to 15 minutes every day. Joe and I set aside at least 15 minutes a day to talk in private after the kids go to bed. If he is not in town, we talk on the phone. Joe and I planned a family game night last Saturday evening with the kids. We shared lots of funny family stories and began to talk with them about my cancer treatment. The kids really seemed to enjoy being together as a family. They asked many questions, and we talked about chores they could help with around the house. They are looking forward to coming to the clinic Thursday. I hope this will help them settle down a bit and feel less frightened." Jeff also determines that Victoria has spoken with close friends from her church, and they plan to visit her this week. Victoria states she is going to see the physical therapist today.

In an effort to evaluate if the clinic has met Victoria's expectations, Jeff asks, "Do you believe we have helped you so far with your concerns about your family? Your faith is strong, and it is my hope you have felt comfortable in talking about your worries." Victoria replies, "The best thing you have done is listen and recognize how important my family is to me. Your suggestions have helped so far; I am encouraged by them."

**Documentation Note**

"The patient visited the clinic for her third week of chemotherapy. She denies nausea but is complaining of some soreness in the mouth and a loss of hair. She asks questions readily and has made an appointment with the physical therapist as recommended. She has enhanced her connectedness with herself and her family by taking time to pray and meditate, talking and listening with her family, and having fun with her children. She has expressed hope that her children will feel less frightened over the diagnosis. The children will be attending the next clinic visit."

that help to shape purpose in life. As you provide spiritual care, always evaluate whether the patient achieved planned outcomes and goals (Table 18-4). Compare the patient's level of spiritual health with the behaviors and perceptions noted in the nursing assessment (see case study). For example, if your assessment found the patient losing hope, the follow-up evaluation involves a discussion to determine if the patient has regained an attitude that life is worth living. Family and friends are a useful source of evaluative information. Successful outcomes reveal the patient developing an increased or restored sense of connectedness with family; maintaining, reviewing, or reforming a sense of purpose in life; and, for some, a confidence and trust in a supreme being or higher power.

For patients with a serious or terminal illness, evaluation focuses on the goal of helping the patient retain faith and hope or express openly the uncertainties life poses. Evaluate how well the patient is accepting the illness and whether hope has enabled the patient to recognize individual mortality and focus on living for each day. You cannot assume all patients have faith in a higher power. However, your support helps patients find meaning in life and death, accept their destiny, and be at peace (Wong and others, 2004).

**PATIENT EXPECTATIONS.** Evaluate whether you met patient expectations. When you evaluate spiritual care, determine if you respected the patient's spiritual practices and if the quality of the nurse-patient relationship was supportive. Both the patient and family should relate that opportunities were offered for religious rituals. With respect to the nurse-patient relationship, does the patient express trust and confidence in you? Is the patient able to discuss those things that are important spiritually? Taking time to ask the patient to reflect on the quality of the nurse-patient relationship is time well spent. Asking the patient, "Have you felt comfortable in saying what you feel is important to you spiritually?" will determine whether you developed an effective healing relationship.

## KEY CONCEPTS

- Attending to a patient's spirituality ensures a holistic focus to nursing practice.
- Frequently spirituality and religion are interchanged, but spirituality is a much broader and more unifying concept than religion.
- An individual's beliefs and spiritual well-being influence physical health status.
- Faith and hope are closely linked to a person's spiritual well-being, providing an inner strength for dealing with illness and disability.
- Religion is a system of organized beliefs that a person practices to outwardly express his or her spirituality.
- Being an atheist or agnostic does not eliminate spirituality as an important resource for a patient.
- Research suggests there is a link between a patient's spirituality and potential for healing.
- Acute and chronic illness, terminal illness, and near-death experiences pose spiritual problems for individuals.
- The provision of appropriate spiritual care requires you to critically apply knowledge from principles related to caring, cultural care, loss and grief, and therapeutic communication.

- Avoid biases when assessing and planning spiritual care.
- Learning to practice caring and compassion helps you to discover a patient's life values and meaning.
- Connectedness and fellowship with other persons are a source of hope for a patient.
- Patients often have spiritual strengths that you will use as resources to help them assume healthier lives.
- Interruptions or changes to customary religious practices affect the support that religion contributes to a person's well-being.
- Common religious rituals include private worship, prayer, singing, use of a rosary, and scripture reading.
- The personal nature of spirituality requires open communication and the establishment of trust between you and the patient.
- Establishing presence involves giving attention, answering questions, having an encouraging attitude, and conveying a sense of trust.
- Part of a patient's caregiving environment is the regular presence of family, friends, and spiritual advisors.

## CRITICAL THINKING IN PRACTICE

*Mr. Garcia is a 72-year-old man who is of Hispanic descent. He has been married for 50 years and has three grown children. He has macular degeneration and is going blind in both eyes. He is very independent and goes golfing in his free time. You are a nurse at the city health department. Mr. Garcia comes to the health department to have his blood pressure taken every other week. As you take him back to the examination room today, you notice he is having more trouble with his vision. When you ask him about his vision, Mr. Garcia replies, "Oh, it's nothing, really. God is just playing games with me these days." You decide you need to complete a spiritual assessment before you take Mr. Garcia's blood pressure.*

- - - - - - - - - - - - - - - - - -

1. List and describe three different methods you will use to perform a spiritual assessment. Which method is the most appropriate one in this case and why?
2. You pay close attention to what Mr. Garcia tells you during your assessment. You answer his questions about macular degeneration realistically and remain with Mr. Garcia until he tells you he needs to go home. These in-

terventions are examples of how nurses establish
_____.
3. During Mr. Garcia's spiritual assessment, you find out that he is Roman Catholic. Describe the difference between Mr. Garcia's spirituality and his religious beliefs.
4. Based on Mr. Garcia's assessment, you enter a nursing diagnosis of *spiritual distress related to negative feelings associated with visual loss.* Provide a goal, an outcome, and at least two nursing interventions for Mr. Garcia.
5. You decide that Mr. Garcia needs to regain his feelings of connectedness. Which of the following questions assess his feelings of connectedness? (Mark all that apply.)
   a. How happy or satisfied are you with your life?
   b. How do you feel after you pray?
   c. Who is the most important person in your life?
   d. How satisfied are you with your accomplishments in your life so far?
   e. Describe the relationship you have with your wife.
   f. When you have faced difficult times in the past, who has been your greatest resource?

## NCLEX® REVIEW

1. You enter the hospital room to discover that your patient is crying quietly in bed. You walk to the bedside, announce your entry, place your hand on the patient's shoulder, and softly ask, "Can you tell me what is bothering you?" In this example you are demonstrating:
   1. Coaching
   2. Presence
   3. Establishing hope
   4. Offering social resource

2. You are completing a spiritual assessment on a newly admitted 42-year-old man. When you ask him if he prays to God, he replies, "I don't pray because I do not believe in the existence of God." Based on his reply, this man most likely is an:
   1. Agnostic
   2. Atheist
   3. Anarchist
   4. Agenic

3. During your assessment of a patient at a neighborhood health clinic, you learn that the patient recently lost his job as a store manager. The patient states he has no health problems at this time. He continues to take his medication regularly for high blood pressure. The patient's wife is in the waiting room, and when the patient walked into the examination room, you observed the two arguing about what to tell the physician. The patient is likely experiencing the nursing diagnosis of:
   1. Spiritual distress
   2. Ineffective coping
   3. Risk for spiritual distress
   4. Ineffective health maintenance

4. You have been caring for a patient recently diagnosed with colon cancer. You enter the patient's room prepared to assess vital signs and to determine if the patient is having any discomfort. The patient interrupts you and says, "You know, I really am worried about how my family is going to take all of this." You stop placing the blood pressure cuff around the patient's arm and say, "Tell me what concerns you have." You are demonstrating an intellectual standard for critical thinking called:
   1. Humility
   2. Completeness

3. Significance
4. Risk taking

5. Your patient shows hope when she states:
   1. "I have had a great life and a good marriage."
   2. "My daughter is a major source of support for me."
   3. "My medicine is improving my health."
   4. "I will continue to find purpose in my life no matter what happens."

6. Which of the following nursing interventions support a healing relationship with a patient? (Mark all that apply.)
   1. Telling a patient that it is time to take a bath
   2. Helping a patient find meaning in a terminal illness
   3. Making a referral to the pastoral care department
   4. Calling dietary and ordering a hot fudge sundae for the patient
   5. Facilitating hopeful feelings despite the presence of chronic pain

7. Which of the following statements made by a patient who has experienced a miscarriage recently most requires follow-up by the nurse?
   1. "My husband sits with me when I cry."
   2. "I believe that my child is in heaven."
   3. "Sometimes it is hard to understand why bad things happen to good people."
   4. "I have not eaten lunch with my friends since my miscarriage."

8. A nurse is caring for a patient who had a near-death experience 2 months ago. He tells the nurse that he remembers seeing paramedics and physicians giving him CPR (cardiopulmonary resuscitation), and he is asking you questions about the event. The nurse's priority intervention is to:
   1. Ask the patient to describe what he remembers in greater detail
   2. Ask the patient's physician or health care provider to answer the patient's questions
   3. Inform the patient that it was probably just a dream
   4. Encourage him to share this experience with his wife immediately

## REFERENCES

Aaron KF, Levine D, Burstin H: African American church participation and health care practices, *J Gen Intern Med* 19(11):908, 2003.

American Nurses Association: *Code of ethics for nurses with interpretive statements,* 2001, http://www.nursingworld.org/ethics/code/protected_nwcoe303.htm.

Antall GF, Kresevic D: The use of guided imagery to manage pain in an elderly orthopaedic population, *Orthop Nurs* 23(5):335, 2004.

Bakke AC, Purtzer MZ, Neton P: The effect of hypnotic-guided imagery on psychological well-being and immune function in patients with breast cancer, *J Psychosom Res* 53(6):1131, 2002.

Barry LC and others: Identification strategies used to cope with chronic pain in older persons receiving primary care from a veterans affairs medical center, *J Am Geriatr Soc* 52(6):950, 2004.

Benner DG: *Baker encyclopedia of psychology,* Grand Rapids, Mich, 1985, Baker Book House.

Benner P: *From novice to expert,* Menlo Park, Calif, 1984, Addison-Wesley.

Buckley J, Herth K: Fostering hope in terminally ill patients, *Nurs Stand* 19(10):33, 2004.

Calabria M, Macrae J, editors: *Suggestions for thought by Florence Nightingale: selections and commentaries,* Philadelphia, 1994, University of Pennsylvania Press.

Callahan HE: Families dealing with advanced heart failure: a challenge and an opportunity, *Crit Care Nurs Q* 26(3):230, 2003.

Cavendish R and others: Nurses enhance performance through prayer, *Holist Nurs Pract* 18(1):26, 2004.

Chiu L and others: An integrative review of the concept of spirituality in the health sciences, *West J Nurs Res* 26(4):405, 2004.

Davis CM: Empathy and transcendence, *Geriatr Rehabil* 19(4):265, 2003.

Dochterman JM, Bulechek GM, editors: *Nursing interventions classification (NIC),* ed 4, St. Louis, 2004, Mosby.

Ebersole P, Hess P: *Toward healthy aging,* ed 6, St. Louis, 2004, Mosby.

Edelman CL, Mandle CL: *Health promotion throughout the lifespan,* ed 5, St. Louis, 2002, Mosby.

Elkins M, Cavendish R: Developing a plan for pediatric spiritual care, *Holist Nurs Pract* 18(4):179, 2004.

Farran CJ and others: Development of a model for spiritual assessment and intervention, *J Relig Health* 28(3):185, 1989.

Fisch MJ and others: Assessment of quality of life in outpatients with advanced cancer: the accuracy of clinician estimations and the relevance of spiritual well-being—a Hoosier Oncology Group study, *J Clin Oncol* 21(14):2754, 2003.

Friedemann ML, Mouch J, Racey T: Nursing the spirit: the framework of systemic organization, *J Adv Nurs* 39(4):325, 2002.

Grant D: Spiritual interventions: how, when, and why nurses use them, *Holist Nurs Pract* 18(1):36, 2004.

Heliker D: Reevaluation of a nursing diagnosis: spiritual distress, *Nurs Forum* 27(4):15, 1992.

Hoare J: The best medicine, *Nurs Stand* 19(14-16):18, 2004.

Hungelmann J and others: Focus on spiritual well-being: harmonious interconnectedness of mind-body-spirit—use of the JAREL spiritual well-being scale, *Geriatr Nurs* 18(6):262, 1996.

Jackson C: Healing ourselves, healing others: first in a series, *Holist Nurs Pract* 18(2):67, 2004.

James D: What emergency department staff need to know about near-death experiences: *Top Emerg Med* 26(1):29, 2004.

King D, Mainous AG, Pearson WS: C-reactive protein, diabetes, and attendance at religious services, *Diabetes Care* 25(7):1172, 2002.

Klemm P, Wheeler E: Cancer caregivers online: hope, emotional roller coaster, and physical/emotional/psychological responses, *Comput Inform Nurs* 23(1):38, 2005.

Koenig H, George LK, Titus P: Religion, spirituality, and heath in medically ill hospitalized older patients, *J Am Geriatr Soc* 52(4):554, 2004.

Kramer BJ, Thompson EH: *Men as caregivers: theory, research and service implications,* New York, 2002, Springer Publishing Co.

Krebs K: Complementary healthcare practices: the spiritual aspect of caring: an integral part of health and healing, *Gastroenterol Nurs* 26(5):212, 2003.

LaPierre LL: JCAHO safeguards spiritual care, *Holist Nurs Pract* 17(4):219, 2003.

Leininger M, McFarland MR: *Transcultural nursing: concepts, theories, research and practice,* ed 3, New York, 2002, McGraw-Hill.

Lohne V, Severinsson E: Hope during the first months after acute spinal cord injury, *J Adv Nurs* 47(3):279, 2004.

MacDonald CM: A chuckle a day keeps the doctor away: therapeutic humor and laughter, *J Psychosoc Nurs Ment Health Serv* 42(3):18, 2004.

Mauk KL, Schmidt NK: *Spiritual care in nursing practice,* Philadelphia, 2004, Lippincott Williams & Wilkins.

Mazanec P, Tyler MK: Cultural considerations in end-of-life care: how ethnicity, age, and spirituality affect decisions when death is imminent, *Home Healthc Nurse* 22(5):317, 2004.

McEvoy M: Culture and spirituality as an integrated concept in pediatric care, *MCN Am J Matern Child Nurs* 28(1):39, 2003.

McEwan W: Spirituality in nursing: what are the issues? *Orthop Nurs* 23(5):321, 2004.

McSherry W, Cash K, Ross L: Meaning of spirituality: implications for nursing practice, *J Clin Nurs* 13(8):934, 2004.

McSherry W, Ross L: Dilemmas of spiritual assessment: considerations for nursing practice, *J Adv Nurs* 38(5):479, 2002.

Moorhead S, Johnson M, Maas M: *Nursing outcomes classification (NOC),* ed 3, St. Louis, 2004, Mosby.

Musgrave CF, Allen CE, Allen GJ: Spirituality and health for women of color, *Am J Public Health* 92(4):557, 2002.

Narayanasamy A: Spiritual coping mechanisms in chronic illness: a qualitative study, *J Clin Nurs* 13(1):116, 2004.

Narayanasamy A and others: Responses to the spiritual needs of older people, *J Adv Nurs* 48(1):6, 2004.

Newlin K, Knafl K, Melkus GD: African-American spirituality: a concept analysis, *ANS Adv Nurs Sci* 25(2):57, 2002.

North American Nursing Diagnosis Association International: *NANDA nursing diagnoses: definitions and classifications 2003-2004,* Philadelphia, 2003, The Association.

O'Brien ME: *Prayer in nursing: the spirituality of compassionate caregiving,* Sudbury, 2003, Jones & Bartlett Publishers.

Otis-Green S and others: An integrated psychosocial-spiritual model for caner pain management, *Cancer Pract* 10(S1):S58, 2002.

Perry DJ: Self-transcendence: Lonergan's key to integration of nursing theory, research, and practice, *Nurs Philos* 5(1):67, 2004.

Phillips JS and others: African American women's experiences with breast cancer screening, *J Nurs Scholarsh* 33(2):135, 2001.

Roberts D: Alternative therapies for arthritis treatment: part II, *Holist Nurs Pract* 18(3):167, 2004.

Smith J, McSherry W: Spirituality and child development: a concept analysis, *J Adv Nurs* 45(3):307, 2004.

Tanyi R: Towards clarification of the meaning of spirituality, *J Adv Nurs* 39(5):500, 2002.

Taylor EJ: *Spiritual care: nursing theory, research, and practice,* Upper Saddle River, NJ, 2002, Prentice Hall.

Taylor EJ: Spiritual needs of patients with cancer and family caregivers, *Cancer Nurs* 26(4):260, 2003.

Theis SL and others: Spirituality in caregiving and care receiving, *Holist Nurs Pract* 17(1):48, 2003.

Wallace DC and others: Client perceptions of parish nursing, *Public Health Nurs* 19(2):128, 2002.

Wong FKY and others: Health problems encountered by dying patients receiving palliative home care until death, *Cancer Nurs* 27(3):244, 2004.

Wright LM: *Spirituality, suffering, and illness: ideas for healing,* Philadelphia, 2005, FA Davis Co.

Young C, Koopsen C: *Spirituality, health, and healing,* Thorofare, NJ, 2005, SLACK Inc.

# CHAPTER 19

# Growth and Development

## MEDIA RESOURCES

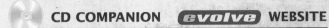
CD COMPANION *evolve* WEBSITE

http://evolve.elsevier.com/Potter/basic

- **NCLEX® Review**
- **Audio Glossary**
- **English/Spanish Audio Glossary**

## OBJECTIVES

- Compare the frameworks for growth and development as described by major developmental theorists.
- Describe the growth and development changes that occur in individuals from conception through old age.
- Identify factors that facilitate or interfere with normal growth and development of individuals at each stage of life.
- Specify the physical and psychosocial health concerns of infants, children, adolescents, and adults.

- Use knowledge of growth and development to enhance use of the nursing process for individuals across the life span.
- Identify specific nursing interventions for the health promotion of patients across the life span.
- Use critical judgment to determine appropriate teaching topics for individual patients across the life span.

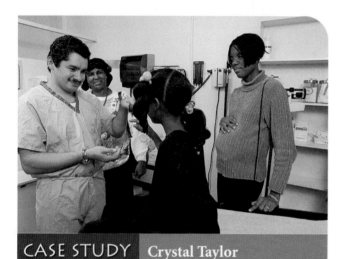

## CASE STUDY   Crystal Taylor

Crystal Taylor, a 25-year-old black young adult, is the single parent of 2½-year-old Zachary and 6-year-old Monica and is in the sixth month of a current pregnancy. She lives with her 44-year-old mother and 15-year-old brother. Crystal's 68-year-old maternal grandmother and aunt live next door and often help care for Zachary and Monica. Crystal's family has used the city clinic for years, and she now brings her children to the neighborhood clinic for their health care. Today she has brought Monica to the clinic for her checkup before beginning school.

Louis Ruiz is a 28-year-old student assigned to the clinic, where he is to select a family to follow throughout the semester. Louis, who is married and has a 4-year-old son who attends day care, was a medical technician in the army for 4 years. The clinic is Louis's first clinical experience as a nursing student, and he is eager to become involved in health promotion activities but also anxious about his new role as a professional nurse.

As a nurse you will care for individuals of all ages. Human growth and development are orderly, predictable processes beginning with conception and continuing until death. Knowledge of these patterns helps you in assisting your patients to reach their full potential (Behrman and others, 2004).

## KEY TERMS

adolescence, p. 537
Alzheimer's disease, p. 545
associative play, p. 534
attachment, p. 531
climacteric, p. 541
critical period of development, p. 529
delirium, p. 545
dementia, p. 545
depression, p. 546
development, p. 529
egocentric, p. 534
geriatrics, p. 544
gerontology, p. 544

growth, p. 529
maturation, p. 529
menarche, p. 538
menopause, p. 541
neonate, p. 532
parallel play, p. 534
polypharmacy, p. 548
preadolescence, p. 537
puberty, p. 538
reality orientation, p. 548
regression, p. 534
reminiscence, p. 546
teratogens, p. 532
trimester, p. 532

## Scientific Knowledge Base

### Growth and Development Theory

The terms *growth* and *development* used together include all of the many changes that take place throughout an individual's lifetime (Hockenberry and others, 2003). **Growth** is the measurable aspect of a person's increase in physical dimensions. Measurable growth indicators include changes in height, weight, teeth and skeletal structures, and sexual characteristics. **Development** occurs gradually and refers to changes in skill and capacity to function. These changes are qualitative in nature and difficult to measure in exact units. There are, however, certain predictable characteristics that are measurable, such as development proceeds from simple to complex. An example of this is learning to walk before learning to run.

**Maturation** is the biological plan for growth and development. Physical growth and motor development are a function

| TABLE 19-1 | Comparison of Major Development Theories | | | |
|---|---|---|---|---|
| Developmental Stage (Approximate Age) | Freud (Psychosexual Development) | Erikson (Psychosocial Development) | Piaget (Logical and Cognitive Development and Moral Development) | Kohlberg (Development of Moral Reasoning) |
| Infancy (birth to 18 months) | Oral stage | Trust versus mistrust (Stage 1) Ability to trust others | Sensorimotor period Progress from reflex activity to simple repetitive actions | |
| Early childhood/ toddler (18 months to 3 years) | Anal stage | Independence versus shame and doubt (Stage 2) Self-control and independence | Preoperational period— thinking using symbols; egocentric | Preconventional level Punishment-obedience orientation |
| Preschool (3-5 years) | Phallic stage | Initiative versus guilt (Stage 3) Highly imaginative | Use of symbols; egocentric | Preconventional level Premoral Instrumental orientation |
| Childhood (6-12 years) | Latent stage | Industry versus inferiority (Stage 4) Engaged in tasks and activities | Concrete operations period Logical thinking | Conventional level Good-boy, nice-girl orientation |
| Adolescence (12-19 years) | Genital stage | Identity versus role confusion (Stage 5) Sexual maturity, "Who am I?" | Formal operations period Abstract thinking | Postconventional level Social contract orientation |

of maturation. Examples of age-related behaviors that follow a specific sequence are sitting, walking, and reading, which are a result of maturation.

A **critical period of development** refers to a specific phase or period when the presence of a function or reasoning has its greatest effect on a specific aspect of development. For example, if a child does not walk by 20 months, there is delayed gross motor ability, which slows exploration and manipulation of the environment. The success or failure experienced within a phase affects the child's ability to complete the next phases.

**THEORIES OF HUMAN DEVELOPMENT.** Human development theories are models intended to account for how and why people become what they are (Thomas, 1997). Useful theories explain behavior, as well as predict behavior that is testable and observable (Table 19-1). Some theories view development as a continuous process, moving from the simple to the more complex. Others consider it as discontinuous, with alternating periods of relative equilibrium and disequilibrium.

**Sigmund Freud.** Sigmund Freud (1856-1939) provided the first formal structured theory of personality development. Freud's psychoanalytic model of personality development is grounded in the belief that two internal biological forces drive the psychological change in a child: sexual (libido) and aggressive energies (Freud, 1949). Each of the five stages is associated with a pleasurable zone, serving as the focus of gratification. In the first stage, oral stage, sucking and oral satisfaction are not only vital to life, but are also very pleasurable. During the anal stage, the focus of pleasure changes to the anal zone. In Stage 3, phallic stage, the genital organs become the focus of pleasure. In the latency stage, Freud believed that the sexual urges from the earlier phallic stage are

repressed and channeled into productive activities that are socially acceptable. The genital stage occurs during adolescence and is a turbulent time for the child and the family. The child's sexual urges reawaken, and social activities begin to occur outside the family circle.

**Erik Erikson's Eight Stages of Development.** Erik Erickson (1902-1994) expanded Freud's psychoanalytic stages into a psychosocial model that covered the whole life span (Erikson, 1963, 1997). In this theory, Erickson divided life into eight stages, known as Erickson's eight stages of development. According to this theory, individuals need to accomplish a particular task before successfully completing the stage. Each task is framed with opposing conflicts, such as trust versus mistrust. Each stage builds upon the successful attainment of the previous developmental conflict. In addition to the five stages in Table 19-1, three additional stages occur from young adulthood to the older adulthood years. Stage 6, intimacy versus isolation, occurs as young adults develop a sense of identity and deepen their capacity to love others and care for them. Generatively versus self-absorption and stagnation (Stage 7) occurs during the middle adult years. The last stage, ego integrity versus despair, occurs through the aging process. As the adult ages, he or she begins to struggle with losses, such as the loss of loved ones, changes in family, or losses in functional status. These changes challenge the person to adjust while continuing to live a full and rich life.

**Piaget's Theory of Cognitive Development.** Jean Piaget (1896-1980) developed the theory of cognitive development, which describes children's intellectual organization and how they think, reason, and perceive the world (Piaget, 1952). The theory includes four periods: sensorimotor, preoperational, concrete operations, and formal operations (see Table 19-1). As the child grows from infancy into adolescence, the

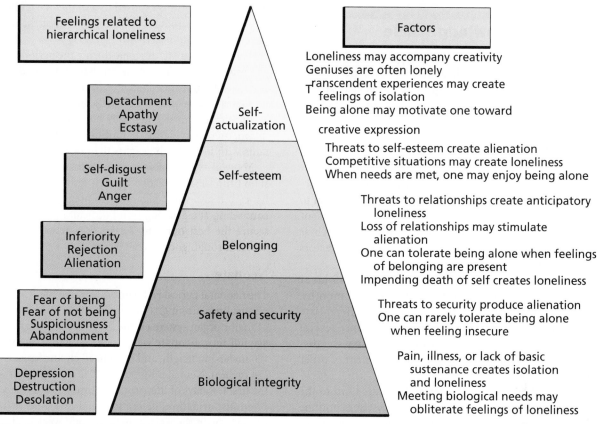

FIGURE **19-1** Loneliness in relation to Maslow's hierarchy of needs. (Modified from Ebersole P, Hess P: *Toward healthy aging: human needs and nursing responses,* ed 6, St. Louis, 1998, Mosby.)

intellectual development progresses, starting with reflex and repetitive motion responses, to the use of symbols and objects from the child's point of view, to logical thinking, and finally to abstract thinking.

**Kohlberg's Moral Developmental Theory.** Lawrence Kohlberg (1927-1987) expanded on Piaget's work. According to Kohlberg (1964, 1969), moral development is one component of psychosocial development. It involves the reasons an individual makes a decision about right and wrong behaviors within a culture. Moral development depends on the child's ability to accept social responsibility and to integrate personal principles of justice and fairness. In addition, the child's knowledge of right and wrong and behavioral expression of this knowledge must be founded on respect and regard for the integrity and rights of others. Cognitive development underlies the progression of a person's morality from level to level.

**Abraham Maslow.** Abraham Maslow (1908-1970) developed a theory of human needs from his study of individuals without physical or mental illness (Figure 19-1). He described an ordering (hierarchy) of needs that motivate human behavior. This ordering is often depicted as a pyramid composed of five levels (Maslow, 1970). When the most basic needs for hunger, thirst, and so on have been met, the person strives to satisfy those needs for safety and security on the next highest level. Disturbances at lower levels interfere with the highest

level, self-actualization or the realization of one's potential. This theory has made a valuable contribution to understanding human development through its positive viewpoint and recognition of needs that motivate all humans. It has also been criticized for not differentiating needs according to ages.

**Carol Gilligan.** Carol Gilligan (1982) compared male and female personality development and highlighted the differences. She believes that there are parallel ways that men and women develop, with one not being superior to the other. Gilligan's perspective is basically that there are developmental differences in relationships and issues of dependency between women and men (Berk, 2003; Gilligan, 1982). Separation and individualization are critically tied to male development. Separation refers to the child's recognition of biological distinctness and is based on his emergence from a dependent relationship with his mother.

Gilligan (1982) identified **attachment** within relationships as the most important factor in successful female development. Females learn to value relationships and become interdependent at an earlier age. Women also struggle with the issues of care and responsibility. As women progress toward adulthood, the moral dilemma changes from how to exercise their rights without interfering in the rights of others to "how to lead a moral life," which includes obligations to themselves, their families, and people in general.

## Nursing Knowledge Base

A strong body of knowledge about growth and development gives you good insight regarding how individuals perceive an event or behave in response to a given situation at a particular age or stage of life. The following is an overview of the stages of life and related health concerns.

### Conception and Fetal Development

From the moment of conception, human development proceeds rapidly. The ovum and sperm each carry half the genetic material that guides biochemical processes essential to the developing organism. Abnormalities in the genes or chromosomes alter health. Other health problems, such as fetal alcohol syndrome, result from environmental factors (e.g., the mother's diet or tobacco use).

Intrauterine life generally lasts 9 calendar or 10 lunar months. The first **trimester** is the first 3 calendar months. After implantation the fetal cells continue to differentiate and develop into essential organ systems. Because several organ systems are developing at the same time, the disruption of one system can affect the development of other systems.

The second trimester is the period from the third to the sixth prenatal months of life. Some organ systems continue basic development during this time, and the functional capabilities of others are refined. By the end of the second trimester most organ systems are complete and able to function. The fetus weighs about 0.7 kg (1½ lb) and is approximately 30 cm (12 inches) long.

During the last 3 months of intrauterine life the fetus grows to approximately 50 cm (20 inches) in length. Weight increases to approximately 3.2 to 3.4 kg (7 to 7½ lb). The skin thickens, lanugo (soft, downy hair) begins to disappear, and the fetal body becomes rounder and fuller. A tremendous spurt in brain growth begins during this trimester and lasts well into the first few years of life. The central nervous system has established its total number of neurons and connections between neurons, and myelination of nerve fibers progresses rapidly. Damage to the central nervous system during the third trimester can potentially alter higher-level cognitive functions. Exposure to toxic agents and the absence of essential nutrients are the most common causes of damage during this trimester.

**HEALTH PROMOTION.** Because the placenta is extremely porous, teratogens pass easily from mother to fetus. **Teratogens** are chemical or physiological agents capable of having adverse effects on the fetus. Some examples of teratogens are viruses, drugs (prescribed, over-the-counter, and street drugs), alcohol, and environmental pollutants, such as lead. The fetal effect of these harmful agents depends on the developmental stage in which exposure takes place. Some teratogens produce defects only if the fetus is exposed to the agent at a critical time when the vulnerable organ is developing. For example, the rubella or measles virus is primarily dangerous if a fetus is exposed to it in the first trimester. This virus can cause spontaneous abortion, stillbirth, or defects of the eyes, ears, and heart.

Many drugs are teratogenic during the period of rapid organ growth in the first trimester. Barbiturates, alcohol, anticonvulsants, and anticoagulants have caused fetal abnormalities. Health care providers weigh the benefits of prescribed medications against potentially harmful fetal effects. In addition, there is evidence that mothers who smoke deliver infants with lower birth weights than nonsmoking mothers.

You will explore lifestyle changes that can help women abstain from tobacco, alcohol, and drugs not only during pregnancy but also while planning for pregnancy. Preconception counseling is a growing trend in health care. The goal is to secure the best outcome for mother, fetus, and significant others through good prenatal care.

### Neonate

The neonatal period is the first 28 days of life. The newborn's physical functioning is primarily reflexive, and stabilization of major organ systems is the body's primary task. The average full-term **neonate** weighs 3.4 kg (about 7½ lb), is 50 cm (20 inches) in length, and has a head circumference of 35 cm (14 inches). Neonates lose up to 10% of their birth weight in the first few days of life, primarily through fluid losses by respirations, urination, defecation, and low fluid intake. They usually regain the weight by the second week of life.

Physically, the neonate may have lanugo on the skin of the back; cyanosis of the hands and feet (acrocyanosis), especially during activity; and a soft, protuberant abdomen. Behaviorally, the newborn has periods of sucking, crying, sleeping, and activity. The newborn's movements are generally sporadic, but they are symmetrical and involve all extremities. Newborns respond to sensory stimuli, particularly the caregiver's face, voice, and touch.

Early cognitive development begins with innate behaviors, reflexes, and sensory functions. For example, neonates instinctively turn to the nipple. Newborns are able to focus on objects 20 to 25 cm (8 to 10 inches) from their faces and respond to auditory stimuli. Therefore you need to teach parents the importance of talking to their babies and providing appropriate visual stimulation.

**HEALTH PROMOTION.** Parental concerns during the neonatal period most frequently center on the baby's crying, feeding, eliminating, and sleeping behaviors (Box 19-1). New parents are not always aware of the newborn's immature immune system and need information about how to protect the baby from infection (e.g., not taking the infant to church or the grocery store until at least 4 weeks old).

The American Academy of Pediatrics (AAP) recommends placing healthy infants on their backs while they sleep to decrease the risk of sudden infant death syndrome (SIDS). Side sleeping is not advised because it is not as safe as back sleeping. The academy also recommends not placing infants on thick bedding, sheepskins, waterbeds, or cushions. Research has associated these measures with a decreased incidence of

BOX 19-1 **Health Promotion Guidelines for Parents of Newborns**

- Selection of a crib with slats less than 2⅜ inches (approximately 6 cm) apart (Hockenberry and others, 2003)
- Mattress fitting snugly against the slats
- No pillows or bumper pads in baby's crib
- Positioning infants on their backs in the crib, "face up to wake up" (American Academy of Pediatrics, n.d.)
- Expected physiological newborn behaviors
- Variability of behavioral cycles (sleep-awake states)
- Principles and techniques for feeding method chosen
- Appropriate stimulation techniques and support for parents' attempts to provide sensory stimulation to the newborn
- Feeding patterns and behaviors
- Schedule of well-baby visits and immunization schedule
- Care measures, including hygiene, dressing, comfort
- Not to expose newborn to drafts or cool air during bathing process
- Protective measures, including asepsis, safety, cardiopulmonary resuscitation (CPR), thermoregulation
- Cleansing of umbilical cord stump with alcohol until it falls off
- Signs and symptoms of the newborn requiring evaluation by a health care professional
- Recommended health care guidance

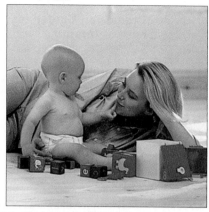

FIGURE **19-2** Playing with blocks helps to develop infant's motor skills. (From Wong DL and others: *Whaley and Wong's nursing care of infants and children,* ed 6, St. Louis, 1999, Mosby.)

sudden infant death syndrome (SIDS) (AAP, n.d.). Nurses assist parents in attaining the knowledge and skills required to foster the newborn's physical, psychosocial, and cognitive well-being and development. You help new parents by teaching the phrase "face up to wake up" as a reminder to always place children on their backs.

## Infant

Growth and development are more rapid during the first 12 months of life than they will ever be again. The infant depends completely on caretakers to provide for basic needs of food and sucking, warmth and comfort, love and security, and sensory stimulation.

Typically infants double their birth weight by 5 months and triple it by 12 months. Their length increases about 1 inch per month during the first 6 months and then ½ inch per month to the end of their first year. Play provides opportunities for the infant to develop many motor skills. Rattles, plastic stacking rings, and wooden blocks are just a few examples of toys that promote fine motor development of the hands and fingers (Figure 19-2).

**HEALTH PROMOTION.** In addition to those health promotion activities regarding feeding, crying, eliminating, and sleeping for the newborn, new health promotion activities for the 1- to 12-month-old infant are often related to dentition, immunizations, and safety.

The first tooth to erupt is usually one of the lower central incisors at the average age of 7 months. Most babies have six teeth by their first birthday (Hockenberry and others, 2003).

The use of a frozen teething ring and medication to numb the gums is helpful to comfort the irritable infant during teething episodes. Tooth decay is preventable by providing adequate fluoride through formula or otherwise, cleaning inside the baby's mouth at least once a day with a wet washcloth, and not allowing the baby to take the bottle to bed (Hockenberry and others, 2003).

The quality and quantity of nutrition influence the infant's growth and development. Breast-feeding is recommended for infants. It is associated with a decreased frequency of gastroenteritis, otitis media, and food allergies (Behrman and others, 2004; Hockenberry and others, 2003; U.S. Department of Health and Human Services [USDHHS], 2000). However, when breast-feeding is not possible or desired by the parent, an acceptable alternative is iron-fortified commercially prepared formula. All types of cow's milk (skim, 2%, or whole) or imitation milk (soy products) are not recommended in the first year because of the infant's decreased ability to digest fat.

The use of immunizations has resulted in a dramatic decline of infectious diseases over the past 50 years. However, recently complacency and fears regarding side effects of vaccines have resulted in inadequate immunization of children less than 2 years (Behrman and others, 2004). Nurses play a major role in assisting community organizations in promoting immunizations and eliminating preventable childhood disease.

Infants' quickly developing motor skills increase their mobility and their ability to place all types of objects in their mouths. Infants need constant supervision when not sleeping. You need to help parents raise their level of awareness regarding potential hazards in their homes. Common accidents during infancy include automobile accidents, aspiration, burns, drowning, falls, poisoning, and suffocation (Box 19-2).

**ACUTE CARE.** When an infant becomes ill, it is important that you maintain the infant's routine daily care. Whenever this is impossible, limit the number of caregivers

BOX 19-2 **Health Promotion Guidelines for Parents of Infants**

- Keeping crib away from radiators, the blast of air ducts, and cords from drapes or blinds
- Expected growth and developmental norms
- Play activities to stimulate gross and fine motor development
- Techniques to encourage development of language
- Readiness for weaning from breast or bottle to cup
- Addition of solid foods and other fluids by introducing only one new food at a time to assess for food allergies
- Need for immunizations and immunization schedule
- Safety measures related to use of approved car seats, falls, drowning, and use of mouth to explore everything in environment
- Development of attachment, stranger awareness, and separation anxiety
- Use of voice, eyes, and facial gestures as disciplinary measures
- Signs of illness, measures for assessment (temperature taking), and appropriate action
- Criteria to use when choosing day care

who have contact with the infant, and follow the parents' directions for care. If hospitalization is necessary, infants sometimes have difficulty establishing physical boundaries because of repeated bodily intrusions and painful sensations. Limiting these negative experiences and providing pleasurable sensations support early psychosocial development.

## Toddler

The toddler period ranges from 12 to 36 months of age. The rapid development of motor skills allows the child to participate in feeding, dressing, and toileting. Toddlers walk in an upright position with a broad-stance gait, bowed legs, protuberant abdomen, and arms flung out to the sides for balance. Soon the child begins to navigate stairs, run, jump, stand on one foot for several seconds, and kick a ball.

Because moral development is closely associated with cognitive ability, the moral development of toddlers is just beginning. It is also **egocentric.** Toddlers do not understand concepts of right and wrong. However, they do grasp that some behaviors bring pleasant results and others bring unpleasant results.

Toddlers are generally able to speak in short sentences. Common questions they ask are, "Who's that?" and "What's that?" By 3 years of age, toddlers have a beginning mastery of speech, are possessive of their toys, and are often heard to say, "That's mine!" They begin to learn that sharing is a desirable behavior when they offer parents toys to hold and the parents express pleasure. Play is frequently solitary in nature. However, toddlers often participate in **parallel play,** playing beside another child with a similar toy or object but not actively interacting through their play. Gradually play begins to include the exchanging or sharing of objects when playing beside another toddler engaged in a similar activity. An example of this **associative play** is sharing a shovel when playing in a sand pile.

**HEALTH PROMOTION.** Slower growth rates are accompanied by a decrease in caloric needs and a smaller food intake.

Confirming the child's pattern of growth with standard growth charts is reassuring to parents concerned about their toddler's decreased appetite (physiological anorexia). Encourage parents to offer a variety of nutritious foods, in reasonable servings, for mealtime and snacks. Special dietary considerations are necessary for the toddler who is ill, is going to have surgery, or is on a vegetarian diet. Finger foods allow the toddler to be independent and "eat on the run." Toilet training is a major task of toddlerhood. The success of toilet training is based on three primary factors: physical ability to control anal and urethral sphincters (after the child learns to walk), the child's ability to recognize urge and communicate it to the parent, and the desire to please the parent by holding on and letting go at appropriate times. The average age for achieving control is 2 years for daytime and 3 years for nighttime control. Girls usually toilet train earlier than boys (Hockenberry and others, 2003).

The natural curiosity and the mobility of the toddler, without good reasoning abilities, make him or her an accident waiting to happen. Toddlers seem to want to put everything into their mouths (e.g., bugs, bleach, or electrical cords) or place their hands, feet, or entire bodies into dangerous sites (e.g., electrical outlets, clothes dryers, tubs with very hot water, or pools). They need constant supervision unless they are in a totally child-proofed area such as their bed. Toddlers have little awareness of physical safety, and accidents continue to be the leading cause of death and injury. The most common accidents are burns, drowning, falls, motor vehicle accidents, and poisoning (Behrman and others, 2004). You will often help parents anticipate the safety needs of their toddlers and make appropriate suggestions (Box 19-3).

**ACUTE CARE.** Whenever toddlers are ill, it is important to provide care consistent with the child's developmental needs. Use the responses of children and their parents to determine children's specific care. Being separated from one's family in an unfamiliar environment when not feeling well is a great stress for a young child to experience. Parents are more likely to remain with their young child when the nurse and members of the health care team create a comfortable environment for them. If a significant caretaker does not remain with the toddler, it is especially important that one nurse assume responsibility for providing the toddler with consistent and appropriate care. Limiting the number of strange caretakers will help establish trust and reduces separation anxiety for the toddler. During times of stress or illness children often return to behaviors of an earlier time that provide them comfort and security. This **regression** of behavior is often disturbing to parents, and they need reassurance that this behavior is normal and that the child will return to more mature behavior patterns when the stressful situation is resolved.

Toddlers cannot clearly identify where they feel pain and often find anything that causes pressure intrusive or extremely painful. You reduce physical discomfort by keeping periods of restraint or immobility to a minimum. A soft voice, physical contact, and a security item will also comfort the child.

| BOX 19-3 | **Health Promotion Guidelines for Parents of Toddlers** |
|---|---|

- Expected growth and developmental norms
- Play activities to stimulate gross and fine motor development (e.g., push/pull, nesting toys)
- Physiological anorexia; good nutritional habits and feeding of self
- Techniques to encourage development of language
- Readiness and appropriate methods for toilet training
- Need for autonomy and setting limits on behavior
- Need to set limits and provide firm, gentle discipline to resolve negativism and temper tantrums
- Continued separation anxiety and development of ritualism
- Safety measures, including child-proofing the home environment (e.g., storage of cleaning products and medication, use of car seats, selection of appropriate safe toys, pool and water precautions, outdoor play, placing plants out of reach and getting rid of poisonous ones)
- Keeping electrical cords out of reach and covering unused electrical outlets
- Blocking stairways and balconies and not leaving infant unsupervised near water
- Reducing the risk for injuries: not leaving iron on ironing board, turning handles of saucepans and frying pans to the inside of the stove when cooking
- Continued need for immunization and developmental assessments

| BOX 19-4 | **Health Promotion Guidelines for Parents of Preschool Children** |
|---|---|

- Expected growth parameters and developmental tasks
- Encouraging parents to support their child's sense of initiative and recognizing they will be unable to complete all activities begun
- Nutritional requirements for optimal growth
- Methods to stimulate continued progress in the development of motor skills, language, cognitive skills, and social skills: reading to the child, using play groups, encouraging the child to do small chores and activities for the family
- Signs of common childhood communicable diseases and measures to reduce their risk and spread
- Beginning instruction for children for personal safety (e.g., do not talk to strangers; tell an adult about inappropriate touching, strangers in the area)
- Criteria to use when evaluating preschool education programs:
  - Teaching methods used to help preschoolers learn about their health, including nutrition, exercise, and rest
  - Safety measures and education related to motor vehicles, tricycles, and fire
- Increased sexual curiosity and need for use of correct anatomical terminology
- Child abuse, including how to protect children, identify signs of abuse, and know community agencies available for assistance
- Great sense of imagination and development of fears, particularly in regard to bodily harm
- Development of conscience

## Preschool Child

Early childhood is a period between the ages of 3 and 5 years when children refine the mastery of their bodies and eagerly await the beginning of formal education. Many parents find this age-group more enjoyable than toddlerhood because children are more cooperative, share thoughts with greater accuracy, and interact and communicate more effectively. Physical development continues to slow, whereas cognitive and psychosocial development accelerates.

Three-year-olds are able to recognize persons, objects, and events by their outward appearance. For example, they prefer having two nickels over a dime because it appears to be more. The continued egocentricity of early thinking makes it difficult to suggest acceptable alternatives to the preschooler. When they are hungry they expect others also to be hungry, and they think they must eat now!

In addition, preschoolers are increasingly able to solve problems intuitively on the basis of one aspect of a situation. For example, they can classify objects either according to size or to color, but not both. They also ask questions such as, "Why do they call it the thirty-first day of the month instead of the thirty-last?" They also have a great sense of imagination. Adults often misinterpret preschoolers' "tall tales" as lying; however, they are actually presenting their own reality. Their imagination also contributes to the development of fears, the greatest of which in this age-group is the fear of bodily harm. For example, this manifests as fear of various

animals, the dark, or of procedures such as having their blood pressure measured.

If two events are related in time or space, children link them causally. The hospitalized child, for example, reasons, "I cried last night and that's why the nurse gave me the shot." As children near age 5, they begin to use rules to understand cause and effect. They then begin to reason from the general to the particular.

**HEALTH PROMOTION.** Ingestion of large amounts of carbohydrates and fats from junk foods results in overweight and undernourishment. Encourage parents to role model good eating habits and to offer their children a varied diet that prevents deficiencies and excesses. Children enjoy helping prepare healthy snacks such as fruit slices, carrot sticks, celery stuffed with peanut butter, and popcorn.

Preschoolers require role modeling and instruction to develop good hygiene measures such as brushing their teeth after meals and sugary snacks, covering their mouths and noses when coughing or sneezing, keeping their fingers out of their noses and eyes, and washing their hands before eating and after using the toilet.

Accidents are the major cause of mortality for this age-group, and motor vehicle accidents (usually as a pedestrian) are the major cause of death. Parents need education to assist in meeting the health promotion needs of their child (Box 19-4). This is a good time for you to teach children to learn what to do in case of fire, safety regulations for crossing the street, the necessity of riding in the back seat of the car, and how to get help when someone is hurt.

**ACUTE CARE.** When preschoolers become ill, their beginning abilities to reason and understand make illness less stressful. Although preschoolers have developed object permanence and recognize their parents still exist when out of sight, most tolerate only short absences without becoming distressed. Encourage parents to tell the child when they are leaving and when they will return in terms the child can understand (e.g., I am leaving and will be back after lunch). Be present when parents leave to provide distraction and support for the child. The following are some strategies for reducing children's fears: allowing the child to sit up for assessments and procedures when possible, demonstrating procedures on another person or doll, allowing the child to see and handle equipment, and allowing the child to assist with a procedure as appropriate. Encouraging parents to be present during procedures and leaving the room door open at night if the child requests it reduce fear as well. Simple and factual information is especially important to this age-group because of their great sense of imagination (Hockenberry and others, 2003).

## School-Age Child

The foundation for adult roles in work, recreation, and social interaction is laid during the "middle years" of childhood (ages 6 to 12). Great developmental strides are made in physical, cognitive, and psychosocial skills. Children become "better" at things. For example, they run faster and farther as proficiency and endurance develop.

Educational experience in school expands the child's world and transitions the child from a life of relatively free play to a life of structured play, learning, and work. The school and home influence growth and development. For optimal development to occur, the child has to learn to cope with the rules and expectations of school and peers.

School-age children become more graceful as they gain increasing control over their bodies (Figure 19-3). Strength doubles, and large muscle coordination improves. Participation in the basic gross motor skills of running, jumping, balancing, throwing, and catching refines neuromuscular function and skills. Holding a pencil and printing letters and words are evidence of fine motor coordination improvement in 6-year-olds. By age 12 the child makes detailed drawings and writes sentences in script, or cursive. Assessment of neurological development is often based on fine motor coordination. Teachers often ask school nurses to conduct fine motor assessment of children with questionable ability.

The middle childhood years are often referred to as the "age of the loose tooth," because children often lose all of their primary teeth during this period. The secondary teeth are much larger in proportion and are often referred to as "tombstone teeth." Regular dental visits will confirm that children are brushing their teeth with regularity and good technique. As children begin to move away from their family and into the

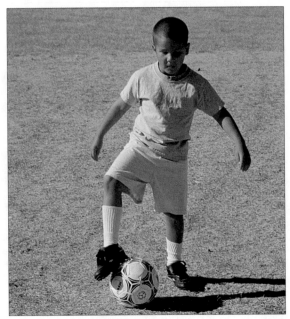

FIGURE **19-3** Coordination improves in school-age children as they gain control over their bodies.

world of school, there are many opportunities for them to gain a sense of competence as they learn reading, writing, and other academic skills. They also have the ability to follow the rules of a new authority person and to compete and cooperate with peers in play and work. The recognition that a child receives at home for achievements also improves the child's developing self-esteem and provides reason to put forth further good efforts. Children's success in work and play leads to an increasing sense of independence and a need to participate in any decisions that involve them. As children move through these middle years of childhood, they confront a number of stressors in the school, in their home, and from peers.

The school-age child prefers same-sex peers to opposite-sex peers. In general, girls and boys view the opposite sex negatively. Peer influence becomes diverse during this stage.

**HEALTH PROMOTION.** Accidents and injuries are major health problems affecting school-age children and are the causative factor in 51% of deaths in this age-group. Motor vehicle accidents, followed by drowning, fires, burns, and firearms are the most frequent fatal accidents. Other major causes of accidents involve recreational activity, most frequently involving bicycles, swings, skateboards, and contact sports. Encourage parents of school-agers to have their children assume some responsibility for their own safety by establishing rules and acting as good role models (Box 19-5).

Blood pressure elevation in childhood is the single best predictor of adult hypertension. This recognition has reinforced the significance of making blood pressure measurement a part of every annual assessment of the child (Behrman and others, 2004; Hockenberry and others, 2003; National

| BOX 19-5 | **Health Promotion Guidelines for School-Agers and Their Parents** |

- Expected growth parameters and developmental tasks, including the middle childhood growth spurt and puberty
- Measures to enhance adjustment to school and reduce school-related stressors
- Promotion of child's sense of industry through opportunities for achievement
- Influence and importance of peers as they learn to follow rules and be competitive
- Development and expression of sexuality, including sex play (e.g., masturbation)
- Parental modeling of safety practices
- Instruction for children for personal safety (e.g., do not talk to strangers, tell an adult about inappropriate touching, strangers in the area)
- Monitoring the time the child spends on the computer, especially alone on the computer
- Limiting recreational screen time (computer, video games, television) to 1 to 2 hours a day (American Academy of Pediatrics, 2001)
- Educate parent to read violence and sexual language ratings on video and computer games and media (American Academy of Pediatrics, 2001)
- Begin instruction regarding Internet safety (e.g., inappropriate e-mail messages, pop-up messages, the need to tell an adult when there is "something funny" on the screen or in the e-mail)
- Recreational safety, including helmets for sports, bicycling, and skateboarding
- Substance abuse (tobacco, alcohol, drugs), including dangers, signs of use, and available community agency support
- Measures to facilitate development of cognitive skills (reading out loud, appropriate use of television, family discussions regarding school performance and homework) and decision-making skills, including weighing the consequences of actions taken
- Responsibility for health-promoting activities, including nutrition, exercise, and safety

High Blood Pressure Education Program [NHBPEP], 2003). Measure on at least three separate occasions with the appropriate-size cuff and in a relaxed situation before concluding that the child's blood pressure is elevated and needs further medical attention. Daily exercise and maintaining normal body weight are important as both interventions and prevention.

**ACUTE CARE.** During illness, school-agers usually tolerate the absence of their parents better than the younger child because of their reasoning abilities. Although they understand their parents often need to be elsewhere, they want and expect daily visits and intervening phone calls. The items school-agers often bring from home, such as their own pillows and favorite books, give them a sense of security and independence. Honesty, factual information, and interest in their concerns are helpful in establishing a trusting relationship with this age-group.

School-agers are usually able to pinpoint their pain, describe it with moderate assistance, and sometimes attempt to explain its cause. They often use play to cope with their pain or withdraw in an attempt to deal with their discomfort. They are usually aware that they receive medication for pain but sometimes do not ask for it until the pain is intense. They are quick to learn to use a scale to assess their discomfort. Most school-agers are eager learners who enjoy learning to find their various pulses, read a thermometer, or operate the blood pressure machine during hospitalization. Many school-agers are able to assist in checking their urine for sugar or protein or to learn to do their own finger sticks for blood samples. School-agers who become ill are often threatened by a loss of their recently developed independence by needing to use a bedpan, having help with bathing, bed rest, or having someone else select their menus.

## Preadolescent

At present, children experience more emotional and social pressures than youngsters 30 years ago. As a result, children 10 to 12 years of age are now having experiences that were once unique to 13- and 14-year-old youths. This transitional period between childhood and adolescence is **preadolescence.** Others refer to this period as late childhood, early adolescence, pubescence, and transescence. Physically it refers to the beginning of the second skeletal growth spurt, when the physical changes such as the development of pubic hair and female breasts begin. Children also become more social, and their behavioral patterns become much less predictable.

## Adolescent

**Adolescence** is the transition from childhood to adulthood, usually between 13 and 18 years of age but sometimes extending until graduation from college. The term *adolescence* refers to the psychological maturation of the individual, whereas *puberty* refers to the point when reproduction is possible. A steady progression of physical, social, cognitive, psychological, and moral changes all characterize this period. The adaptations required by these changes push adolescents to develop individualized coping mechanisms and styles of behaviors, which they will continue to use or adapt throughout life. Most teenagers successfully meet the challenges of this period.

**PHYSICAL DEVELOPMENT.** Although timing varies greatly, physical changes occur rapidly during adolescence. Sexual maturation occurs with the development of primary and secondary sexual characteristics. Primary characteristics are physical and hormonal changes necessary for reproduction. Secondary characteristics externally differentiate males from females.

Height and weight increases accelerate during the prepubertal growth spurt. The growth spurt for girls generally begins between 8 and 14 years of age, with height increases of 2 to 8 inches (5 to 20 cm) and weight increases of 15 to 55 lb. The male growth spurt usually takes place between 10 and 16 years of age, with height increases of approximately 4 to 12 inches (10 to 30 cm) and weight increases of 15 to 65 pounds.

Girls attain 90% to 95% of their adult height by **menarche** (the onset of menstruation) and reach their full height by 16 to 17 years of age. Boys continue to grow taller until 18 to 20 years of age. Adolescents are sensitive about physical changes that make them different from peers. Thus they are generally interested in the normal pattern of growth, as well as in their personal growth curves.

**PUBERTY.** A wide variation exists between the sexes and within the same sex as to when the physical changes of **puberty** begin. Use the ranges of normal growth to assess the progress of growth for an adolescent patient. As with increases in height and weight, the pattern of sexual changes is more significant than their time of onset. Large deviations from normal time frames require attention. Visible and invisible changes take place during puberty as a result of hormonal change.

Language development is fairly complete by adolescence, although vocabulary continues to expand. The primary focus becomes developing diverse communication skills to use effectively in many situations, which will be refined later in life. Adolescents need to communicate thoughts, feelings, and facts to peers, parents, teachers, and other persons of authority.

Developing moral judgment depends on cognitive and communication skills and peer interaction. Moral development, begun in early childhood, matures. Adolescents learn to understand that rules are cooperative agreements that can be changed to fit the situation, rather than absolutes. Adolescents learn to apply rules by using their own judgment rather than simply to avoid punishment as in the earlier years. They judge themselves by internalized ideals, which often leads to conflict between personal and group values.

The search for personal identity is the major task of adolescent psychosocial development. Teenagers establish close peer relationships or remain socially isolated. Erickson (1963) sees identity (or role) confusion as the prime danger of this stage. Teenagers have to become emotionally independent from their parents and yet retain family ties. They also need to develop their own ethical systems based on personal values.

The physical changes of puberty enhance achievement of sexual identity. These changes encourage the development of masculine and feminine behaviors. If these physical changes involve deviations, the person has more difficulty developing a comfortable sexual identity. Adolescents depend on these physical clues because they want assurance of maleness or femaleness and because they do not wish to be different from peers. Cultural attitudes, expectations of sex role behavior, and available role models also influence sexual identity. The masculine and feminine behaviors teenagers see and the ex-

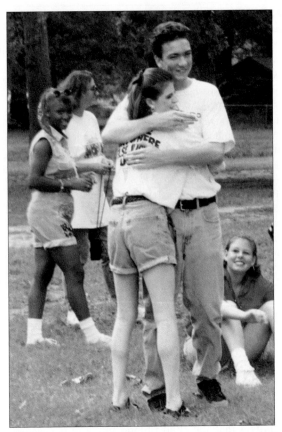

FIGURE **19-4** Heterosexual relationships are an important part of adolescence. (From Hockenberry and others: *Whaley and Wong's nursing care of infants and children,* ed 7, St. Louis, 2003, Mosby.)

pectations they perceive for behaving as a man or woman affect how they express sexuality. Adolescents master age-appropriate sexuality when they feel comfortable with sexual behaviors, choices, and relationships (Figure 19-4).

**HEALTH PROMOTION.** A component of personal identity is perception of health. Healthy adolescents evaluate their own health according to feelings of well-being, ability to function normally, and absence of symptoms. Health problems causing severe or long-term alteration of these factors permanently alter self-identity. Along with parents, you will assist adolescents in taking responsibility for their own health status and practices (Box 19-6).

The major causes of mortality in the adolescent age period are injuries, homicide, and suicide (Hockenberry and others, 2003). Motor and other vehicular accidents, pregnancy, sexually transmitted diseases (STDs), and substance abuse are major causes of morbidity. Mental disorders, chronic illness, and eating disorders are other causes.

Females are more likely to have eating disorders and emotional distress, and males are more often involved in vehicular accidents (Behrman and others, 2004). Homicide is the most frequent cause of death among older black adolescents, whereas vehicular accidents are the leading cause of death among white males (Edelman and Mandel, 2002).

| BOX 19-6 | Health Promotion Guidelines for Adolescents and Their Parents |
|---|---|

- Clear, reasonable limits for acceptable behavior and consequences for breaking the rules
- Automobile safety, including driver's education course; use of seat belts; risks to self and others associated with drinking, drugs, and driving; use of helmet by bicyclists and motorcyclists
- Developing a mutual plan so that the adolescent never gets into a car when the driver has been drinking or the adolescent never drives if he has been drinking; plan to include whom to call to pick up the child
- Awareness of warning signs of depression and suicide, alternatives to suicide, and methods to deal with a suicidal peer
- Potential of social isolation and the excessive use of computer for recreational activities (e.g., searching the Internet, solitary computer games)
- Discuss threats to safety from the Internet (e.g., identify theft, sexual predators)

- Dealing with peer pressure, school-related stressors, anger, and violent feelings through decision-making skills, conflict resolution, and positive coping strategies
- Prevention of unintentional injuries (e.g., classes on use of firearms, danger of swimming alone or under the influence of alcohol or drugs)
- Sexual experimentation and measures to prevent STDs and pregnancy, including abstinence, transmission of infection, symptoms of disease, prophylactic measures, and community organizations that provide assistance
- Importance of routine HIV testing for adolescents who have placed themselves at risk
- Allowing increasing independence within limits of safety and well-being
- Providing privacy and unconditional love
- Listening to and respecting the adolescent's viewpoint

Health services for adolescents need to be readily available, affordable, and approachable if parents and communities expect teens to use them. Adolescents tend to use school-based programs, where instituted. Health care workers need skills in interviewing adolescents and identifying those more at risk. Successful health promotion activities actively involve teenagers at all times. The involvement of teens in organizations that promote responsible behaviors such as Drug Abuse Resistance Education (DARE) and Students Against Destructive Decisions (SADD, formerly Students Against Drunk Driving) is a key element. Through your efforts in the school and community, you will make a contribution in meeting the *Healthy People 2010* objectives (USDHHS, 2000).

Substance abuse is a major concern to those who work with teenagers. All adolescents are at risk for experimental or recreational substance use. You assess those at risk, educate them to prevent accidents related to substance abuse, and counsel those in rehabilitation.

Suicide is the third leading cause of death in persons between 15 and 24 years of age and the second leading cause of death for white males in this age-group (Edelman and Mandel, 2002). Depression and social isolation commonly precede a suicide attempt, but suicide most likely results from a combination of several factors. Be alert to the following warning signs, which often occur for at least 1 month before a suicide attempt (Behrman and others, 2000; Hockenberry and others, 2003):

1. Decrease in school performance
2. Withdrawal from family and friends
3. Loss of initiative
4. Drug or alcohol abuse
5. Personality changes such as boredom, anger, apathy, anxiety, panic, and neglect of appearance
6. Appetite and sleep disturbances
7. Verbalization of suicidal thought

Make immediate referrals to mental health professionals when your assessment suggests an adolescent is considering suicide. Guidance helps focus on the positive aspects of life and strengthen coping abilities.

Sexual experimentation is common among adolescents. Peer pressure, physiological and emotional changes, and societal expectations contribute to heterosexual and homosexual relations. More than 50% of adolescent students have had sexual intercourse during their lifetime, and two thirds of these sexually active teenagers are inconsistent in their use of safe sex. The risk-taking behaviors of adolescent sexual activity and drug use make adolescents vulnerable to the threat of human immunodeficiency virus (HIV) and acquired immunodeficiency syndrome (AIDS). AIDS is the sixth leading cause of death among individuals between 15 and 24 years of age (USDHHS, 2000).

The United States has one of the highest rates of teenage pregnancy in the world. Pregnancy rates are higher among older adolescents than they are among younger adolescents (Hockenberry, and others, 2003). Adolescent pregnancy occurs across socioeconomic classes, in public and private schools, among all ethnic and religious backgrounds, and all parts of the country.

**ACUTE CARE.** Hospitalization imposes rules and separates adolescents from their usual support system, restricts their independence, and threatens their personal identity. Adolescents who are forced into dependency or have their need for privacy ignored respond with frustration, anger, or self-assertion. Although most hospitals allow peers to visit, some adolescents will isolate themselves until they are able to compete on an equal basis with peers. The telephone is often the lifeline between adolescents and their friends and helps them maintain their place in their social group. Many adolescents welcome peer visitors, and hospitals often allow the patient to go to a lounge or cafeteria with them.

Adolescents who are more independent from their parents usually do well with intermittent visiting but expect

| TABLE 19-3 | Common Physical Changes of Aging |
|---|---|

| System | Normal Findings |
|---|---|
| **Integumentary** | |
| Skin color | Brown age spots and spotty pigmentation in areas exposed to sun; pallor even in absence of anemia |
| Moisture | Dry, scaly |
| Temperature | Extremities cooler; perspiration decreased |
| Texture | Decreased elasticity; wrinkles; folding, sagging |
| Fat distribution | Decreased on extremities; increased on abdomen |
| Hair | Thinning and graying on scalp; axillary and pubic hair and hair on extremities sometimes decreased; facial hair in men decreased; chin and upper lip hair is present in women |
| Nails | Decreased growth rate |
| **Head and neck** | |
| Head | Nasal and facial bones sharp and angular; loss of eyebrow hair in women; men's eyebrows become bushier |
| Eyes | Decreased visual acuity; decreased accommodation; reduced adaptation to darkness; sensitivity to glare; diminished light reflex |
| Ears | Decreased pitch discrimination; diminished hearing acuity |
| Nose and sinuses | Increased nasal hair; decreased sense of smell |
| Mouth and pharynx | Use of bridges or dentures; decreased sense of taste; atrophy of papillae of lateral edges of tongue; occasionally change in voice pitch |
| Neck | Thyroid gland nodular; slight tracheal deviation resulting from muscle atrophy |
| **Thorax and lungs** | Increased anterior-posterior diameter; increased chest rigidity; increased respiratory rate with decreased lung expansion |
| **Heart and vascular system** | Blood pressure (BP) remains within normal limits <120/80 (NHBPEP, 2003); BP between values 120-139/80-89 are considered prehypertension; elevations in BP are not a normal aspect of aging and older adults need minor elevations monitored (NHBPEP, 2003); peripheral pulses easily palpated; pedal pulses weaker and lower extremities colder, especially at night; orthostatic hypertension common |
| **Breasts** | Diminished breast tissue; pendulous |
| **Gastrointestinal system** | Decreased salivary secretions, which make swallowing more difficult; decreased peristalsis; decreased production of digestive enzymes, hydrochloric acid, pepsin, and pancreatic enzymes, leading to indigestion and constipation |
| **Reproductive system** | |
| Female | Decreased estrogen; decreased uterine size; decreased secretions; atrophy of epithelial lining of the vagina; vaginal dryness |
| Male | Decreased testosterone; decreased sperm count; erections less firm and slower to develop; decreased testicular size |
| **Urinary system** | Decreased renal filtration and renal efficiency; subsequent loss of protein from kidney; nocturia |
| Female | Urgency and stress incontinence from decrease in perineal muscle tone |
| Male | Frequent urination resulting from prostatic enlargement |
| **Musculoskeletal system** | Decreased muscle mass and strength; bone demineralization (more pronounced in women); shortening of trunk from intervertebral space narrowing; decreased joint mobility; decreased range of joint motion; kyphosis (usually in women); slowed reaction time |
| **Neurological system** | Decreased rate of voluntary or automatic reflexes; decreased ability to respond to multiple stimuli; insomnia; shorter sleeping periods |

Modified from Ebersole P and others: *Toward healthy aging: human needs and nursing response,* ed 6, St. Louis, 2004, Mosby.

tire at 50, and others work into their 80s and 90s. It is not unusual for those who write about older adults to divide them into the "young old," who are vital, vigorous, and active, and the "old old," who are frail and infirm. The fastest growing subset is the nearly 3 million people over the age of 85, whose growth rate is nearly three times that of the overall older adult population (Ebersole and others, 2004).

**Geriatrics** is the branch of health care dealing with the physiology and psychology of aging and with the diagnosis and treatment of diseases affecting older adults. **Gerontology** is the study of all aspects of the aging process and its consequences.

Nursing care of older adults poses special challenges because of diversity in patients' physical, cognitive, and psychosocial health. Older adults vary in level of function and productivity. Before making a health assessment, be aware of the normal expected findings of physical and psychosocial assessment for an older adult and consider the normal changes of aging.

**PHYSICAL DEVELOPMENT.** The older adult must adjust to the physical changes of aging. These changes are not associated with a disease state but are the normal changes anticipated with aging. The physiological changes that occur with advancing age vary with the patient. Table 19-3 describes the common types of physiological changes to expect with older adults. Some are visible to the eye, and others are not. They occur in all persons but take place at different rates and depend on accompanying circumstances in an individual's life. As the nurse assessing the older adult patient, you need to consider the potential for sensory changes that will influence data gathering.

**COGNITIVE DEVELOPMENT.** Older adults often remain alert and highly perceptive until the time of their death. Nevertheless, the misconception that older adults always have cognitive impairments and suffer from memory loss and confusion persists. Because cognitive impairment occurs in this age-group, be aware of the nature and type of these impairments.

Intelligence testing in late adulthood seems to indicate that fluid intelligence, the ability to solve new problems, declines during late adulthood, but crystallized intelligence, based on learning and experience, increases or at least is maintained. Practical thinking, specialized knowledge and skills, and wisdom continue to increase, although the mechanics of intelligence often decline. Certain aspects of short-term memory (e.g., numbers) decrease with age, but visual memory, which allows a person to remember how to read, remains strong. Long-term memory for newly learned information decreases significantly with age, but recall for distant experiences and procedural experiences (e.g., driving) do not seem to be affected in the later years of life. Both intelligence and memory vary greatly among individuals. Most older people who want and need to learn new skills and information do so when it is presented more slowly over a long period. Continuing mental activity is essential to keeping older adults alert, and older people do benefit from memory training (Ebersole and others, 2004; Edelman and Mandel, 2002).

Three common conditions affect cognition in older adults; delirium, dementia, and depression (Box 19-8). It is important that you learn how to distinguish between these three conditions in order to select appropriate nursing interventions for your patients (Foreman and others, 1996).

**Delirium** is an acute confusional state. It is a potentially reversible cognitive impairment that is often due to physiological causes. Some of these causes include electrolyte imbalance, hypoglycemia, infection, and hemorrhage. In addition, very slight body temperature alterations cause delirium in older adults. This condition often accompanies infections, such as pneumonia. The characteristics of delirium usually include fluctuations in cognition that develop over a short time. This change in cognition also includes a reduced ability to focus, sustain, or shift attention (Cacchione and others, 2003). In addition, there are acute changes in mood, arousal, and self-awareness. Other signs are hallucinations, transient incoherent speech, disturbed sleep pattern, and disorientation. Presence of delirium requires prompt assessment, identification of etiology, and etiology-specific treatment, such as antibiotics in the presence of pneumonia.

**Dementia** is a broad category of disorders that refers to a generalized impairment of intellectual functioning, which in-

---

| BOX 19-8 | USING EVIDENCE IN PRACTICE |

**Research Summary**

Understanding the cognitive and neurological function in older adults is important when caring for this population. Altered thought processes occur with cognitive decline or disturbances in cognitive function. Because of the interaction between physical illness and cognitive changes, it is important to accurately assess for the causes of cognitive change, specifically acute confusion. Acute confusion is a common geriatric syndrome in older adults who reside in long-term care facilities. Sensory impairments, specifically vision and hearing impairment, are even more common in this population.

This study investigated the relationship between sensory impairments and the development of acute confusion in older adults who resided in rural long-term care facilities. One hundred fourteen residents participated in the study and underwent sensory screening. Of this population, 52% were visually impaired, 44.1 % were hearing impaired, and 24.6 % had both visual and hearing impairments. The investigators noted a significant relationship between visual impairment and dual sensory impairment and the development of acute confusion in this population.

**Application to Nursing Practice**

Older adults living in long-term care facilities are at risk for acute confusion. Nurses in this setting need to be aware of the residents' sensory status and correctly assess for sensory functioning. Residents should have routine visual acuity examinations and obtain the best-corrected visual acuity glasses. Staff should ensure that the residents wear the correct glasses and that proper lighting be used. For some residents magnification devices for reading are helpful. There must be routine assessment of ear canals and use of cerumen softening agents or referrals for cerumen removal as needed. Identifying the presence of and providing treatment for visual and hearing impairments are simple interventions to reduce the risk of acute confusion.

Data from Cacchione PZ and others: Risk for acute confusion in sensory-impaired, rural long-term care elders, *Clin Nurs Res* 12(4): 340, 2003.

---

terferes with social and occupational functioning. Cognitive function impairments lead to a decline in the ability to perform basic and instrumental activities of daily living (Ebersole and others, 2004). Dementia differs from delirium in that it is a gradual, progressive, irreversible dysfunction. Early recognition is thus important, requiring you to make thorough observations of patient behavior, neurological function (see Chapter 13), and laboratory diagnostic studies. Family and friends are valuable resources in detecting behavioral changes.

**Alzheimer's disease** is the most common form of dementia. Alzheimer's disease is a progressive loss of memory (amnesia), loss of ability to recognize objects (agnosia), loss of the ability to perform familiar tasks (apraxia), and loss of language skills (aphasia). As the disease progresses some patients also experience changes in personality and behavior, such as anxiety, suspiciousness, or agitation, as well as delusions or hallucinations (Alzheimer's Association, 2004). The disease progresses in three stages: an early stage involving memory loss; a middle stage involving loss of language skills and motor function; and the final stage involving incontinence, inability to ambulate, and a complete loss of language skills.

**Depression** among older adults is increasing. This diagnosis was once overlooked; it was assumed to be a normal response to aging, physical losses, or other life events. About 25% of older adults living in the community have depressive symptoms (Raj, 2004). Depression reduces overall happiness and well-being, contributes to physical and social limitations, complicates the treatment of other medical conditions, and increases the risk for suicide (National Institutes of Mental Health [NIMH], 2003). Like delirium, depression is reversible, and with individualized collaborative care that includes appropriate medication, treatment of underlying conditions, control for polypharmacy, physical rehabilitation when needed, and individualized psychotherapeutic techniques the patient's depression improves (NIMH, 2003; Raj, 2004).

**PSYCHOSOCIAL DEVELOPMENT.** The older adult has to adapt to many psychosocial changes that occur with aging. Among the more common transitions that occur with aging include retirement, volunteerism, and loss of spousal roles (Ebersole and others, 2004). Many older adults also have experienced occupational success and spend their later years forming independent businesses (e.g., consulting, travel agencies, or sales). Despite the changes that occur, the older adult has the potential for developing new and fulfilling life patterns.

Most older adults desire to work as long as they are physically able (Ebersole and others, 2004). The time a person chooses to retire is often based on type of work, status achieved, and length of time employed. When a patient describes retirement, it is important to know whether the individual is fully retired, partially retired, or retired from one position to assume another.

Retirement represents a developmental stage that occupies 30 years of one's life. It also represents a highly productive and fulfilling period of life. Help patients and their families prepare for retirement by gathering information as to why the patient is considering retirement. Retirement also affects more individuals than the retired person; it affects spouses, adult children, and grandchildren. In addition, the retired person may be spending more time alone for the first time in his or her life.

Thirty-five percent of the population age 65 and older engages in some type of volunteer work. This includes offering assistance for religious and charitable organizations and government and community service programs.

**Death.** The majority of older adults experience death of spouses, friends, and in some cases children. These losses require individuals to go through a process of grieving (see Chapter 23). Losing a partner that one has lived with for many years in a satisfying relationship is like losing oneself (Ebersole and others, 2004). For many older adults the grief associated with loss of a spouse lasts for many years. Experiencing the grieving process requires support from family, nurses, and other health professionals. You lend support by showing warmth and caring to help patients feel they are not alone. Helping the patient understand the normal process of grief is important (see Chapter 23).

A common misconception is that the death of an older adult is always a blessing and the culmination of a full and rich life. Many dying older adults still have life goals and are not emotionally prepared to die. **Reminiscence,** or life review, is a technique that facilitates the individual's preparation for the end of life. It is an adaptive function of older adults that allows them to recall the past for the purpose of assigning new meaning to past experiences. Reminiscence is the natural way older adults revive their past in an attempt to establish order and meaning and to reconcile conflicts and disappointments as they prepare for death. You support reminiscence by sharing some of your own conflicts or uncertainties so as to encourage patients to participate in the process (Ebersole and others, 2004). It takes time to help patients truly explore how they feel. The sharing of personal memories requires you and the patient to trust one another. Be patient, and recognize that it will take several weeks or months for a patient to review past hopes and future expectations.

**Aloneness and Loneliness.** With advancing age, more people live alone. This is particularly common for older white women. The growing percentage of unmarried individuals, the likelihood of widowhood for women, and the support of families in allowing older adults to maintain their independence all contribute to more individuals living by themselves. However, living alone is not equivalent to the feeling of loneliness. A person can be surrounded by others yet still feel lonely. Ebersole and others (2004) define loneliness as an affective state of longing and emptiness, whereas being alone is to be solitary, apart from others, and undisturbed. Many patients choose to be alone or isolated simply because of the desire for privacy or an opportunity for self-reflection and creativity. Loneliness, on the other hand, is sometimes a passive and painful emotion, influenced by psychological, economic, sociological, and physiological factors (see Figure 19-1).

It is important to understand the differences between aloneness and loneliness and to be able to recognize which condition is affecting a patient. Too often the two concepts are confused. When you see a patient spending time alone, it is important to share observations with the patient and to determine why the patient chooses privacy. Some patients desire to be left alone to have time to think about existing concerns or about an illness. It is necessary to help these patients find more time for privacy and to find ways to minimize disturbances (especially for the hospitalized patient).

**Housing and Environment.** Changes in social roles, family responsibilities, and health status influence the older patient's choice of living arrangements. An older adult sometimes need to change living arrangements because of the death of a spouse or a change in health status. A change in an older patient's living arrangements requires an extended period of adjustment during which assistance and support will be needed from health care professionals and the patient's family.

Housing and the environment as a whole are important because they have a major effect on the health of the older adult. Nurses are often asked to help patients and their families determine appropriate living arrangements. It is important for you to assess patients' activity level, financial status, access to public transportation and community activities, environmental hazards, and support systems. For example, certain physical problems make it difficult to live on the second floor or have laundry facilities in the basement. Because falls commonly occur in older adulthood, caregivers need to use preventive measures to decrease their incidence. Making changes in the home environment to reduce the patient's fear of falling is helpful. Physical assessment of older adults reveals risk factors that predispose to falls, such as neuropathy of the feet, severe joint problems, abnormal gait, changes in posture, poor vision, loss of muscle control, and affected memory. Chapter 36 summarizes changes that provide a safer environment for older adults.

**HEALTH PROMOTION.** The possibility of an individual being reasonably healthy and fit in later life often depends on the person's lifestyle. Older adults need to continue the same recommended health practices introduced in the young adult section. Some older adults will need encouragement to maintain a pattern of physical exercise and activity. It is not too late for an older person to begin an exercise program; however, older adults need to have a complete physical examination, which usually includes a stress cardiogram or stress test. Assessment of activity tolerance will help you and the patient plan a program that meets physical needs while allowing for physical impairments (Box 19-9).

Most older adults are in good health; however, chronic medical conditions increase dramatically with age. The effect of a particular chronic health problem on mobility and independence depends greatly on the individual. Most older adults are capable of taking charge of their lives and assume responsibility for preventing disability. Coronary artery disease (CAD) remains the leading cause of death in those 65 years of age or older.

Hypertension contributes to both strokes and heart attacks. Hypertension is no longer considered part of the aging process, and it is important to keep the blood pressure at or below 120/80 mm Hg (NHBPEP, 2003). African-Americans are at greater risk than whites, and men are at greater risk than women. The relationship between hypertension and CAD (including myocardial infarction, congestive heart failure, peripheral vascular disease, and stroke) is well documented (NHBPEP, 2003). Lifestyle modifications including weight reduction; adequate physical activity; salt restriction (1 to 2 g per day); limiting alcohol intake; reducing dietary saturated fat and cholesterol; adequate intake of potassium, calcium, and magnesium; and smoking cessation will lower the blood pressure and reduce the incidence of CAD (NHBPEP, 2003).

Malignant neoplasms are the second most common cause of death among older adults. They commonly affect the lung, prostate, colon, rectum, pancreas, bladder, skin, breast, and uterus (ACS, 2005). Early detection and treatment are

| BOX 19-9 | CARE OF THE OLDER ADULT |

- Inform patient about preretirement planning, to ease the transition from a full-time work schedule.
- Provide information from the American Association of Retired Persons, www.aarp.org, regarding supplemental health insurance, group discounts for older adults, and medical and legal information.
- Discuss housing alternatives to help the older adult make a decision regarding the sale of the home, relocation to another area of the country, or retirement communities.
- Instruct patient about health maintenance programs, such as exercise activities, that are designed to increase exercise tolerance, flexibility, and socialization.
- Teach patient that the need for annual influenza and routine pneumonia vaccines increases, especially when chronic illness is present.
- Teach patient about safe and appropriate administration of prescribed drugs: purpose; effect; possible other prescription, over-the-counter, or dietary interactions; and reportable side effects.
- Instruct patient regarding environmental safety issues (e.g., home lighting, floor coverings, stairs, shoes, electrical cords) to reduce the risk of falling.
- Discuss changes in sleep patterns with age and methods to promote adequate rest and energy.
- Instruct patient about nutritional aspects related to disease (e.g., a low-fat diet with hypertension, the need for a balanced diet with reduced total calories because of aging changes and lower energy expenditures).
- Teach an individual exercise program based on an assessment of the patient's overall health status and lifestyle.

important. Older adults need to continue cancer risk reduction practices and screenings recommended for the middle-age adult.

Sensory impairments are common in the older adult (see Chapter 36). These changes are frequently the result of the normal aging process. You aid the older adult in identifying resources to help correct visual and auditory problems. The sense of touch usually remains strong. Older adults who often become victims of social isolation are often deprived of touching and holding, which convey affection and friendliness. The touch of nurses and all caregivers who work with older adults serves to provide sensory stimulation, reduce anxiety, relieve physiological and emotional pain, orient the person to reality, and provide comfort, particularly during the dying process.

Dental problems are common in older adults. They lead to changes in taste and a decrease in nutritional intake. Because of missing teeth or poorly fitting dentures, older adults often restrict their diet to soft foods. Help prevent dental and gum disease through health education. In addition to teaching the older adult to maintain routine dental care, teach specific measures to reduce the risk of gum disease.

As a group, adults over 65 years of age are the greatest users of prescription drugs. Many drugs interact with one another, potentiating or negating the effect of another drug. Some drugs cause confusion; affect balance; cause dizziness, nausea, or vomiting; or promote constipation or urinary frequency. **Polypharmacy,** the prescription, use, or administration of more medications than are indicated clinically, is a common problem of older adults. The combined use of multiple drugs causes serious problematic effects.

**Health Care Services.** A variety of health care services are available to the population. Chapter 2 outlines a variety of services such as day care centers and respite care used frequently by older adults and their families. Home care services and homemaker services prevent or delay institutionalization for older adults who need assistance with self-care and activities of daily living.

Situations of declining health, decreased physical and human resources, and increased dependence necessitate the older adult's institutionalization in a long-term care facility. Such a facility provides extended residential, intermediate, or skilled nursing care, medical care, and personal and psychosocial services. The decision for institutional care is not easy to make, and the family requires a great deal of support. In addition, the family will need your help in locating the proper facility to meet the needs of the patient. When possible, a facility close to the patient's and family's home is best to provide accessibility for visits.

**ACUTE CARE.** Hospitalization of older adults is often disturbing to them because they are not accustomed to the environment and routines. Even those who are able to live independently with some assistance from their families become temporarily disoriented by the strange surroundings of a hospital. Monitor the patient for confusion, and encourage frequent visitation by family members. In addition, use reality orientation techniques to help reorient the older adult who has been disoriented by a change in environment, surgery, illness, or emotional stress.

**Reality orientation** is a communication modality used for making the patient aware of time, place, and person. The major purposes of reality orientation include:

- Restoring patients' sense of reality
- Improving their level of awareness
- Promoting socialization
- Elevating patients to a maximal level of independent functioning
- Minimizing confusion, disorientation, and physical regression

Environmental changes within a hospital, such as the bright lights and lack of windows in intensive care and the noise from nearby roommates, often lead to disorientation and confusion. The patient's environment and the nursing personnel are constantly changing in the hospital, and the immediate environment is unstable, making coping and adaptation difficult. Anticipate disorientation and confusion as a consequence when older adults are hospitalized, and incorporate reality orientation interventions into their care.

When an older adult is hospitalized or has an acute or chronic illness, the related physical dependence makes it difficult for the person to maintain a positive body image. You are able to have an influence on the older adult patient's appearance. Help the patient maintain a pleasant appearance, and present a socially acceptable image.

# Critical Thinking

## Synthesis

When caring for an individual patient or family, a variety of factors will influence your care. You and your patients bring unique backgrounds and personal experiences to each care setting. Although you do not always discuss these individual perspectives openly, they do influence your care. Both you and your patients will have preexisting ideas as to how to best meet their developmental needs. You will use your knowledge, experience, attitudes, and standards to best meet the individual needs of each patient and his or her family.

**KNOWLEDGE.** Before assessing your patient, review the developmental theories that relate to the patient. In addition, as you work with your patients in attaining an optimal level of health, it is essential that you know the expected physical developmental milestones, psychosocial developmental crises, cognitive development, and health concerns for each age-group.

Another important area of knowledge to consider when caring for a patient's developmental needs is that of cultural diversity (see Chapter 17). Together with the patient, explore the cultural variations in family roles and relationships as they influence an individual's development, to have a clear understanding of patient needs.

**EXPERIENCE.** If you are a parent or have been involved in the teaching of children, you are aware that the thinking abilities of individuals of different ages differ, and it is necessary to change your approach to gain their cooperation. In addition, your family, social, and educational experiences with individuals of various ages will make it easier for you to determine age-specific appropriate or inappropriate behaviors and health concerns.

**ATTITUDES.** Humility is an important attitude for you to apply when collecting data about a patient's developmental history. It is easy to form opinions about patients' developmental needs on the basis of developmental theory and related psychosocial principles. However, as is the case in any nursing situation, do not assume you know what the patient's needs are without gathering a clear picture of a patient's physical and psychosocial health concerns. Often information about the patient's health practices will reflect the patient's cultural background, which is sometimes very different from yours. Creativity is a valuable critical thinking attitude when you conduct an assessment of an infant or child. Often you will incorporate play or other activities into the assessment to better visualize the child's physical developmental capacities.

**STANDARDS.** Critical thinking standards help to ensure that you are making the right decisions. When developing a plan of care that incorporates growth and development principles and approaches, strive to apply the intellectual standards of relevance and completeness. It is important that you employ a developmental approach that fits with the patient's level of maturation. For example, having a preschooler attempt a motor skill, such drawing a detailed picture, that is not within his or her ability is irrelevant and inappropriate for promoting developmental enrichment. When selecting a plan of care, you need to be sure the plan uses psychosocial, cognitive, and physical approaches that complement and strengthen the patient's developmental abilities.

Also use professional standards when providing care to patients of various age-groups. For example, when supporting parents' health promotion practices, it is important to refer to standards for immunizations. These standards help to determine not only the required immunizations for certain age-groups but also the parents' success in ensuring a child is immunized. Similarly, a variety of standards have been established for health screening of adult age-groups, and you will refer to these standards when providing patient education.

## Nursing Process

### Assessment

Nursing assessment of individuals across the life span requires you to be familiar with the physiological, cognitive, and psychosocial changes that occur during each stage of development and the health concerns for each age-group. Table 19-4 is an example of a focused assessment for a school-age child, like Crystal's daughter, Monica. A number of assessment tools facilitate concise but comprehensive data collection for individuals of various ages. During the health history, physical assessment, and developmental assessment, observe the interactions between the individual and any family member present. Data gathered will provide information regarding the patient's lifestyle, level of functioning, family relationships, health concerns, and health promotion activities.

Throughout life, illness and hospitalization are stressful experiences. Many factors affect the ability of individuals to cope, such as their level of development, their coping skills, their previous experiences with illness and hospitalization, and the seriousness of the diagnosis. The degree to which the illness interferes with activities of daily living and lifestyle and the availability of a support system also have an impact on how individuals cope. Your assessment needs to demonstrate an awareness of specific patient concerns at various stages of life.

**PATIENT EXPECTATIONS.** During your assessment it is important to determine what patients and/or their families expect from the caregiver. At the beginning of a home visit ask, "What do you think is most important for us to accomplish today?" or when preparing to leave, ask, "Have I met your expectations for this visit?" In the outpatient setting ask what expectation(s) the patient and/or family have for the visit. In the hospital setting it is wise to determine if family members want to participate in the care of the patient and how members of the health team can help. As the patient's primary nurse, you will begin each day with a brief assessment to determine any change in condition and the patient's perceptions of the care received.

## FOCUSED PATIENT ASSESSMENT

TABLE 19-4

| Factors to Assess | Questions and Approaches | Physical Assessment Strategies |
|---|---|---|
| Home safety | Ask patient about the location of household cleaners, medications. | Observe patient's home environment. Observe child's play area. |
| | Ask about history of home-based accidents. | |
| | Ask parent and child about home evacuation plans and a meeting place. | Along with parent play out a situation when the home needs to be evacuated (e.g., fire), and observe the evacuation and congregation of the family at the meeting place. |
| | Ask about the child's use of the Internet. Are there parental controls that block unsafe sites? Does the child use the computer in a common room or in the bedroom? | If able, observe the child's use of a home computer if a home visit is made. |
| Health promotion activities | Ask mother about childhood immunizations. | Obtain actual immunization history. |
| | Review child's usual food intake. | Obtain serial weight and height measurements, and compare with standards. |
| | Review child's usual play activities. | Ask child to color, draw, skip, and jump. |
| Sibling interaction | Ask parent about child's interactions with siblings. | Observe child playing and interacting with sibling. |
| | Ask parent about any change in child's behavior, independence when sibling was born. | |

## SYNTHESIS IN PRACTICE

Louis has selected Crystal Taylor and her family to follow throughout this semester of his nursing program. As he prepares to begin an assessment, he focuses on 6-year-old Monica, who Crystal has brought to the clinic for a checkup before beginning school. Louis will recall the physical, psychosocial, and cognitive developmental characteristics that are typical of the older preschool child and prepare to use this information as a basis for his observations. He will engage Monica in play activities with dolls to ensure that observations of her physical abilities are relevant and complete. He is also interested in any concerns Crystal has regarding Monica's health. In preparation for doing anticipatory guidance with Monica and her mother, he reviews types of accidents common among her age-group and appropriate health promotion activities. He is also interested in observing the quality of the interaction between Monica and her mother and assessing how Crystal copes with being a single parent.

As the parent of a 4-year-old, Louis knows the importance of immunizations in keeping children free of many contagious diseases with serious consequences, and he is aware that children are not admitted to school without the completion of certain immunizations. His own child has made him very conscious of the great fear young children have for bodily harm and the fact that

Monica may have difficulty cooperating with an injection. He recalls the approach he has used to help his own son cooperate with and recover from the discomfort of an injection. Louis refers to the standards for immunizations that the American Academy of Pediatrics, the American Academy of Family Physicians, and the Centers for Disease Control and Prevention (CDC) update twice yearly to determine Monica's immunization needs. Louis knows that the key to having a positive effect on the practice of health promotion activities by Crystal Taylor's family members is the development of trust through positive interactions.

Louis's nursing instructors have informed him that he is responsible for encouraging health promotion activities among his patients. Louis recognizes that *Healthy People 2010: National Objectives for Improving Health* is a guide for choosing health promotion activities for Crystal's family (see Chapter 1). Louis knows he cannot be judgmental of Ms. Taylor as a single parent. He knows he needs to assess the resources she has to support health promotion in her family. Understanding that Crystal probably has some definite ideas about parenting and health promotion will ensure that Louis is complete in assessing patient needs and in offering appropriate suggestions to support Crystal and her family.

## Nursing Diagnosis

Your nursing assessment of the patient, and when appropriate the family, reveals clusters of data from the nursing history, physical examination, and developmental assessment. These data include defining characteristics, which you analyze through critical thinking to select the nursing diagnoses that apply. Accuracy is important because the defining characteristics help to differentiate the nursing diagnosis that applies to the clinical situation. For example, *parental role conflict* and *impaired parenting* are two distinctly different nursing diagnoses. Carefully review all information before selecting the nursing diagnosis that applies to the patient's and family's needs. Defining characteristics for the nursing diagnosis of *ineffective sexuality patterns* include factors such as difficulties or limitations in sexual functioning, expressions of concern about sexuality, and inappropriate verbal and nonverbal sexual behavior. The following are some examples of nursing diagnoses for patients with developmental problems throughout the life span:

- Impaired adjustment
- Caregiver role strain
- Risk for caregiver role strain
- Decisional conflict
- Parental role conflict
- Compromised family coping
- Delayed growth and development
- Health-seeking behaviors
- Risk for injury
- Impaired parenting
- Risk for poisoning

- Ineffective sexuality patterns
- Impaired social interaction
- Social isolation

The second part of the nursing diagnostic statement states suspected causes or related factors for the patient's response to the health problem. Revealed in the assessment data, the related factors allow you to target specific interventions toward the patient's diagnosis. For example, the nursing diagnosis of *ineffective sexuality patterns* might be related to the stress of an impaired relationship with a significant other, fear of pregnancy, or lack of a significant other. The related factors are different, and each requires different nursing strategies.

## Planning

**GOALS AND OUTCOMES.** The plan addresses each identified nursing diagnosis by determining goals, patient outcomes, and interventions for the alleviation or resolution of the diagnosis. The goal for each nursing diagnosis identifies a specific and measurable patient outcome that is realistic and reflects the patient's highest level of wellness and independence in function. An example of a goal is "Patient acquires healthy psychosocial behavior within 3 months." An example of an outcome is "Patient participates in health promotion activities within 6 weeks." See the care plan for detailed examples of goals and outcomes.

Collaboration with patients and their families is essential when determining goals and outcomes. Patients' degree of participation in planning depends on their developmental

## CARE PLAN  Health-Seeking Behaviors

### ASSESSMENT

Louis's physical assessment reveals that Monica's weight of 45 lb places her between the 50th and 75th percentiles, and her height of 46 inches places her in the 75th percentile for age 6 years on the growth grid. In comparison with her 2½-year-old brother, she appears thinner with longer legs. She has a gap-toothed grin from the loss of a front tooth. Monica is able to do all of the items for a 6-year-old on the Denver II (Denver Developmental Screening Test). This includes the gross motor skill of balancing on each foot for 6 seconds; the language ability to define seven words such as house and banana; the fine motor skill of copying a square; and the reported personal/social skills of brushing teeth and dressing without assistance, preparing her own cereal, and playing a board game. It was also noted that she does not squint or hold the storybook at an unusual distance from her eyes. She enjoys showing and telling Louis about the pictures she is coloring and often giggles. **Her mother reports that Monica is very protective of and bossy with her brother, and she always wants to sit on Crystal's lap when she is holding Zachary.** Crystal denies that Monica has ever been involved in any accident that required a visit to the physician or health care provider, but **she did say she had found Monica playing with her father's cigarette lighter one day.** Crystal reports that Monica rides a tricycle with ease but has no experience with a bicycle.

When Louis inquires, Crystal tells him that she is feeling tired but well during this pregnancy and that her obstetrician/gynecologist told her during her prenatal clinic appointments that she is doing well. **Crystal wants to be sure that Zachary and Monica have all their health care up-to-date before the baby comes, because she knows the baby will keep her busy and she wants them to be healthy.** Louis asks Crystal how she plans to prepare Monica and Zachary for the new sibling. She tells him that other than informing them of the event, she has not done anything in particular. Monica did ask her mother why she was getting so fat, and Crystal told her that she has a baby brother or sister growing in a special place inside her tummy. She is expecting that Monica will soon want to know how the baby will get out, but so far she has not asked. **Crystal asks Louis what suggestions he has for preparing her children for the arrival of the new baby.**

*Defining characteristics are shown in bold type.

---

**NURSING DIAGNOSIS** Health-seeking behaviors related to a lack of knowledge regarding age-related health promotion activities.

---

### PLANNING
#### GOAL

• Crystal will become more knowledgeable about health concerns related to her children's ages within the next 3 months.

#### EXPECTED OUTCOMES*
#### Knowledge: Health Promotion

• Crystal will begin to discuss the safety needs of her children with all other family members who participate in their care before her next clinic visit.
• Crystal will talk to other family caregivers and Monica about protecting Monica from the danger of playing with fire before the next clinic visit.
• Crystal will begin to prepare Monica and Zachary for the birth of a sibling before the next clinic visit.

#### Health Promotion Behavior

• Crystal will keep her children's appointments for well-baby or well-child checkups and have the children receive appropriate immunizations.

*Outcomes classification label from Moorhead S, Johnson M, Maas M: *Nursing outcomes classification (NOC)*, ed 3, St. Louis, 2004,

---

### INTERVENTIONS†
#### Health Education

• Provide Crystal with handouts that describe safety measures according to age of child.
• Discuss with Crystal measures to decrease Monica's risk for playing with fire.


• Provide Crystal with a list of books about preparing children for a new sibling.

### RATIONALE

Handouts provide initial information and allow for a quick review of information whenever needed (Bass, 2005).
Adults need to remember to keep potentially hazardous items out of reach of children; a lighter, like a match, is an adult tool (Hockenberry and others, 2003).
The list will assist Crystal in finding these books in a bookstore or at the local library.

†Intervention classification labels from Dochterman JM, Bulechek GM, editors: *Nursing interventions classification (NIC)*, ed 4, St. Louis, 2004, Mosby.

## CARE PLAN Health-Seeking Behaviors—cont'd

| INTERVENTIONS† | RATIONALE |
|---|---|
| **Decision-Making Support** | |
| • Encourage Crystal to write appointment dates for well-child checkups on a pocket calendar she carries in her purse and to keep a copy of her children's immunization records with the calendar. | Immunization education that includes immunization schedules, appointment reminder methods, and the importance for routine immunizations is essential. Vaccinations are the major preventive measure to control many communicable diseases (Goldrick, 2005). |

†Intervention classification labels from Dochterman JM, Bulechek GM, editors: *Nursing interventions classification (NIC)*, ed 4, St. Louis, 2004, Mosby.

**EVALUATION**

- Ask Crystal to report on success of holding a discussion about child safety with the family.
- Ask Monica to talk about the arrival of a new baby in the family.

- Observe Monica during the next clinic visit to see if she continues to play with the lighter.
- Monitor adherence to return visits and immunizations.

---

### BOX 19-10 PATIENT TEACHING

Louis knows that he is developing a therapeutic nurse-patient relationship with Crystal. Crystal told Louis that she wants to provide good health care for her children, but she does not understand the suggested immunization schedule for her children.

**Outcome**

At the end of the teaching session Crystal will be able to state the routine immunization schedule for her children.

**Teaching Strategies**

- Provide Crystal with a laminated schedule for routine immunizations for her children.
- Using Crystal's personal calendar, highlight the dates when the immunizations are due.

- Provide Crystal with the phone contact for the appropriate clinic for immunizations.
- Show Crystal how to safely keep a permanent record of the immunizations.
- Tell Crystal to provide only copies to the children's school and provide resources to obtain copies.

**Evaluation Strategies**

- Ask Crystal when the next immunizations are due.
- Review Crystal's personal calendar for a scheduled appointment for immunizations.
- Ask Crystal where she keeps the children's' immunization records.

---

status, as well as physiological and psychological condition. For example, because young children are often unable to articulate feelings and needs, their parents need to become involved in establishing goals. The participation of patients and their families in this process will increase their motivation for achievement of identified goals and outcomes.

**SETTING PRIORITIES.** During the planning phase of the nursing process, you formulate a plan of care that is directed toward the identified nursing diagnoses for the patient. You then address the nursing diagnoses in order of priority, giving the most pressing problems immediate attention. Base your priorities of nursing diagnoses on such factors as the nature of the problem (e.g., whether it is life threatening, interferes with activities of daily living, or affects level of comfort) and the degree of importance attributed to the problem by the patient or family. Maslow's theory of human needs is helpful as a guide when arranging nursing diagnoses in order of priority. A high priority nursing diagno-

sis is not always a physiological problem. For example, in the case study Louis has concerns over Monica's fear of injections, so he views fear as a priority for care in the initial clinic visit, especially when immunizations are necessary.

**CONTINUITY OF CARE.** Collaboration and consultation with other members of the health care team provide valuable resources for care for patients throughout the life span. Such collaboration will help identify community resources to help parents of a child with developmental disabilities or help a family find adult day care activities for an older adult. In addition, these resources will assist in providing continuity in discharge planning.

You begin discharge planning at the time of admission to the hospital because the length of stay is usually very brief. Effective planning involves the health care team, the patient, and the patient's support system. Make sure you individualize nursing interventions for the patient and modify them accordingly for home- or hospital-based nursing care. Make

## EVALUATION

Louis sees Crystal 1 month later when she returns to the clinic for a scheduled prenatal visit. She has left the children at home with their grandmother. While she waits to see her primary caregiver, Louis takes the opportunity to evaluate the progress she has made in meeting expected outcomes. Louis asks Crystal if she has been able to find any of the list of books he had given her about preparing young children for the birth of a sibling. Crystal reports that the librarian helped her locate two books, one appropriate for her toddler and the other one for Monica. She adds that the children loved the books and want her to read them every night at bedtime. Louis asks her if she thinks the content of the books was the kind of information she wanted to share with her children, and she replies that they explained childbirth so simply it really made it easy for her to talk about the new baby with both children.

During the previous clinic visit, Louis had also given Crystal pamphlets that described important safety measures for infants and young children. He asks her if she has discussed any of this information with any family members. Crystal tells him that her mother and grandmother have looked at the pamphlets and have told her it is a big responsibility to watch those two grandchildren and that they are very hard to keep up with. She also reports that they have all talked to Monica about not playing with candles, matches, or lighters. She tells Louis about the evening news on TV talking about a child who hid in her bedroom playing with a lighter and caught herself and the mattress on fire and almost died. The story seemed to scare Monica, and they talked about what young children should do if anything caught fire around them. She says Monica has often brought up the situation and asked what happened to the little girl on TV.

Crystal asks Louis if he will be there for her next prenatal appointment, and he tells her that he plans to be. He asks if there is anything in particular that she would like to talk about next time, and Crystal replies, "Just tell me how I can manage a new baby and my other two at the same time!" Before leaving, Crystal again tells Louis she likes having him be with her at each clinic visit and that he has given her helpful information. Louis is satisfied that they are developing a therapeutic relationship and that he has assisted her in developing her knowledge base for managing health promotion activities for her children.

**Documentation Note**

After the primary caregiver has documented Crystal's prenatal visit, Louis adds the following documentation in Crystal's clinic chart:

"While waiting for primary caregiver, patient reports that she has begun to prepare her two children for the birth of a new sibling through reading books and talking about the event. States she has shared safety measures for children, particularly in regard to fire, with family caregivers. Has requested additional information pertaining to child rearing; will assess further during next visit."

needed referrals to community agencies coincide with the patient's arrival home.

## Implementation

You will provide developmental interventions in collaboration with the patient and the family or significant others. It is important that you keep patients and their families as active in this process as possible. Interventions are appropriate for both the patient's developmental level and the patient's unique needs and thus support and promote normal developmental processes. Collaboration with a variety of health team members facilitates the provision of optimal care for patients.

Many of the interventions related to your patients' developmental stage include a component of patient education (see Chapter 10). Patient education is an effective tool to teach your patients about health promotion practices, desired behavioral changes, and the need for age-appropriate screening practices. However, patients from different cultures or countries have different languages and beliefs that affect their ability to understand or talk to a health care provider (Edmunds, 2005). Effective patient education must consider your patient's health literacy, and it is planned according to the patient's needs (Box 19-10).

Earlier in this chapter, nursing strategies for health promotion and acute care were discussed for each age-group. Restorative care measures for older adults were also outlined. You will refer to each of the developmental age-groups for specific interventions regarding age-related health concerns. It is important to remember that a patient's developmental needs should be incorporated into any plan of care, regardless of the nature of the patient's health problem. Whether the patient has serious physiological alterations or merely is seeking health promotion information, developmental care considerations ensure a more individualized and thorough nursing approach.

## Evaluation

**PATIENT CARE.** During evaluation, measure the patient's progress and the degree to which the planned interventions were effective in meeting the expected outcomes and goals of care (see case study). Evaluate the patient's behavioral response to the interventions, and thus determine the success or failure of the nursing action. This includes observing family members interact, having the patient describe health promotion habits, or visiting the home to see if your patient followed suggestions for improving child safety. Both you and the patient and/or family evaluate if the expected outcomes were met in the manner anticipated. When outcomes are not met, a review will determine if they were realistic and appropriate, or if there is a need to modify an approach. Ongoing evaluation is necessary to ensure that progress toward defined goals is achieved (Table 19-5).

| OUTCOME EVALUATION | | TABLE 19-5 |
|---|---|---|
| **Nursing Action** | **Patient Response/Finding** | **Achievement of Outcome** |
| Crystal received handouts describing safety measures. | Crystal locked up medicines and cleaning agents. She was able to get grandmother to move medicines and cleaning agents to a locked cabinet. | Crystal is beginning to modify home and home of grandmother for safety risks. |
| Crystal received an appointment book for next visit and an up-to-date immunization schedule. | Crystal kept next appointment. Crystal provided child's school with an up-to-date record of immunizations. | Crystal needs to continue to keep appointments for well-baby or well-child checkups and receive appropriate immunizations. |
| Crystal received list of books and tapes to prepare children for arrival of new sibling. | Children were able to talk about the "almost new baby." "Baby is coming for Halloween." | Preparation for new sibling is progressing, but remains ongoing. |

**PATIENT EXPECTATIONS.** Nurse-patient relationships are often long term when you start a developmental plan of care. Always remember to determine if the patient's expectations of care are continuing to be met. Over time the patient's expectations sometimes change. To add to the complexity of evaluation, expectations are sometimes varied when family members are involved. Basic to understanding the patient's and family members' expectations is trust. When you and the patient have established trust, it becomes easier to evaluate on a frequent basis how your relationship with the patient is proceeding and whether the patient senses his or her health care needs are being adequately and professionally addressed.

## KEY CONCEPTS

- Growth and development are orderly, predictable, interdependent processes that continue throughout the life span.
- Growth is most rapid during the prenatal and infancy stages and continues to slow until the second skeletal growth spurt announces that puberty is approaching.
- People progress through similar stages of growth and development but at an individual pace and with individual behaviors.
- Theories of growth and development, such as those of Freud, Erickson, and Piaget, provide nurses with a framework for understanding individual behaviors.
- Physiological, cognitive, and psychosocial development continue across the life span, and you must be familiar with normal expectations to determine potential problems and promote normal development.
- Accidental injuries occur at any developmental stage, but they are the major cause of death in individuals between 1 and 25 years of age, and their prevention is a focus of many health promotion activities.

- Patients need specific immunizations throughout life, not just in childhood. These immunizations help to protect individuals against illness and infections.
- All adult age-groups need to practice healthy habits regarding nutrition, exercise, medical screening practice, lifestyle, and so on.
- Young adults have few health problems but need to develop positive health habits to avoid many health problems in middle and late adulthood.
- The health concerns of the middle adult commonly involve hormonal changes, stress-related illnesses, situational stressors, screening for health problems, and adoption of positive health habits.
- The health concerns of older adults are related to chronic illnesses, lifestyle changes, functional ability changes, accidents, and infectious diseases, such as the flu.

## CRITICAL THINKING IN PRACTICE

*As indicated in the case study, Monica, 6 years old, is having a checkup in preparation for beginning school. The nurse needs to perform a number of procedures, which Monica may perceive as threatening because of their intrusive or invasive nature (e.g., measure her blood pressure, check her throat, and look in her ears).*

1. What nursing approaches can Louis use to gain the child's cooperation?

2. During the checkup Monica was able to help with the examination by answering questions and reading the eye chart. She also had the opportunity to play with the equipment and has had her blood pressure and other vital signs taken. During the review of immunizations Louis has noted that up to now Monica is up-to-date, but she will need two shots at this visit. How should Louis approach this?

3. Crystal is also concerned that her 15-year-old brother may soon become sexually active and wants to be sure that he knows the risks involved and how to protect himself from STDs (including AIDS) and from becoming a father before he is ready for the responsibility. How should Louis advise her?

4. As you noted in the case study, Crystal is pregnant with her third child; she is a single parent as well. After you do the well-child examination on the children you are able to turn your attention to Crystal. What information would you like to obtain from Crystal?

## NCLEX® REVIEW

1. While assessing for a toddler's growth and developmental status, it is important to remember that:
   1. Each toddler has the same set of communication skills
   2. Each toddler progresses at the same rate of development
   3. The toddler may have sufficient motor skills to assist in self-care activities
   4. The toddler does not have sufficient motor skills to assist in self-care activities

2. When teaching safety tips to the parents of a preschooler, you need to tell the parents that the major cause of mortality is:
   1. Violence
   2. Poisonings
   3. Infectious illness
   4. Motor vehicle accidents

3. During an assessment a patient indicates that the school performance of her 16-year-old daughter has declined and the girl is withdrawn, appears bored, and no longer takes pride in caring for possessions. You feel that these assessment findings indicate:
   1. A dislike of school
   2. An increased risk for suicide
   3. Normal adolescent changes
   4. A breakup with her boyfriend

4. You are working in an adolescent health clinic. A 16-year-old girl enters the clinic and is concerned that she might have a sexually transmitted disease because she had unprotected sex 6 weeks ago. You perform a pregnancy test, which is negative. At the patient's request you obtain appropriate specimens and requests for STD testing, including HIV and hepatitis. What is your next priority of care?
   1. Notify the young girl's parents
   2. Initiate education regarding safe sex
   3. Obtain a prescription for birth control pills
   4. Ask the girl's sexual partner to make a clinic appointment

5. When assessing young adults, you will find that this population usually has a high level of wellness. However, it is important to direct health care education toward activities related to:
   1. Health promotion
   2. Primary prevention
   3. Tertiary prevention.
   4. Secondary prevention

6. When you suspect that your patient is a victim of domestic violence, you need to know that patients' risk for violence increases when:
   1. They seek medical treatment
   2. They experience their first violent attack
   3. They seek law enforcement intervention
   4. They initiate a plan to remove themselves from the abusive environment

7. Women need to increase their daily calcium intake to 1000 to 1500 mg to prevent:
   1. Arthritis
   2. Osteoporosis
   3. Hypertension
   4. Coronary artery disease

## REFERENCES

Administration on Aging: *Statistics on the aging population*, Washington, DC, 2005, US Department of Health and Human Services, http://www.aoa.gov/prof/Statistics/statistics.asp, accessed May 27, 2005.

Alzheimer's Association: *Alzheimer's disease fact sheet*, Chicago, 2004, The Association, www.alz.org, accessed May 27, 2005.

American Academy of Pediatrics: A childcare provider's guide to safe sleep, http://www.healthychildcare.org/pdf/SIDSchildcaresafesleep.pdf.

American Academy of Pediatrics, Task Force on Infant Sleep Position and Sudden Infant Death Syndrome: Changing concepts of sudden infant death syndrome: implications for infant sleeping environment and sleep position, *Pediatrics* 105(3):650, 2000.

American Cancer Society: *ACS cancer detection guidelines*, New York, 2005, The Society, http://www.cancer.org, accessed May 27, 2005.

Bass L: Health literacy: implications for teaching the adult patient, *J Infus Nurs* 28 (1):15, 2005.

Behrman RE and others: *Nelson textbook of pediatrics*, ed 17, Philadelphia, 2004, WB Saunders.

Berk L: *Child development*, ed 6, Boston, 2003, Allyn & Bacon.

Cacchione PZ and others: Risk for acute confusion in sensory-impaired, rural, long-term-care elders, *Clin Nurs Res* 12(4):340, 2003.

Dochterman JM, Bulechek GM, editors.: *Nursing interventions classification (NIC)*, ed 4, St. Louis, 2004, Mosby.

Ebersole P, Hess P: *Toward healthy aging: human needs and nursing responses*, ed 6, St. Louis, 1998, Mosby.

Ebersole P, Hess P, Luggen AS: *Toward healthy aging: human needs and nursing response*, ed 6, St. Louis, 2004, Mosby.

Edelman C, Mandel C: *Health promotion throughout the lifespan*, ed 5, St. Louis, 2002, Mosby.

Edmunds M: Health literacy: a barrier to patient education, *Nurse Pract* 30(3):54, 2005.

Erikson E: *Childhood and society,* New York, 1963, WW Norton.

Erikson E: *The lifecycle completed,* New York, 1997, WW Norton.

Foreman M and others: Assessing cognitive function, *Geriatr Nurs* 17(5):239, 1996.

Freud S: *An outline of psychoanalysis,* New York, 1949, Norton.

Gilligan C: *In a different voice: psychological theory and women's development,* Cambridge, Mass, 1982, Harvard University Press.

Goldrick B: Pertussis on the rise: clinicians should be aware of its signs and symptoms until vaccination recommendations are changed, *Am J Nurs* 105(1):69, 2005.

Hockenberry M and others: *Whaley and Wong's nursing care of infants and children,* ed 7, St. Louis, 2003, Mosby.

Kohlberg L: Development of moral character and moral ideology. In Hoffman ML, Hoffman LNW, editors: *Review of child development research,* vol 1, New York, 1964, Russell Sage Foundation.

Kohlberg L: Stages and sequence: the cognitive-developmental approach to socialization. In Goslin DA, editor: *Handbook of socialization theory and research,* Chicago, 1969, Rand McNally.

Lewis SM and others: *Medical/surgical nursing: assessment and management of clinical problems,* ed 6, St. Louis, 2004, Mosby.

Maslow AH: *Motivation and personality,* Upper Saddle River, NJ, 1970, Prentice Hall.

Moorhead S, Johnson M, Maas M: *Nursing outcomes classification (NOC),* ed 3, St. Louis, 2004, Mosby.

National High Blood Pressure Education Program; National Heart, Lung, and Blood Institute; National Institutes of Health: The seventh report of the Joint National Commission on Detection, Evaluation, and Treatment of High Blood Pressure, *JAMA* 289(19):2560, 2003.

National Institute of Mental Health: *Older adults: depression and suicide facts,* Bethesda, Md, 2003, National Institutes of Health, http://www.nimh.nih.gov/publicat/elderlydepsuicide.cfm, accessed May 27, 2005.

Phillips JM and others: African American women's experiences with breast cancer screening, *J Nurs Scholarsh* 33(2):135, 2001.

Piaget K: *The origin of intelligence in children,* New York, 1952, International Universities Press.

Raj A: Symposium on geriatric psychiatry: depression in the elderly, *Postgrad Med* 115(6):26, 2004, http://www.postgradmed.com/issues/ 2004/06_04/raj.html.

Stuart G, Laria M: *Principles and practice of psychiatric nursing,* ed 7, St. Louis, 2001, Mosby.

Thomas RM: Moral development theories: secular and religious: a comparative study, Westport, Conn, 1997, Greenwood Press.

U.S. Department of Health and Human Services, Public Health Service: *Healthy people 2010 objectives,* Washington, DC, 2000, Office of Disease Prevention and Health Promotion.

Wong DL and others: *Whaley and Wong's nursing care of infants and children,* ed 6, St. Louis, 1999, Mosby.

# CHAPTER 20

# Self-Concept and Sexuality

## MEDIA RESOURCES

**CD COMPANION**  **evolve** **WEBSITE**

http://evolve.elsevier.com/Potter/basic

- **NCLEX® Review**
- **Audio Glossary**
- **English/Spanish Audio Glossary**

## OBJECTIVES

- Discuss factors that influence the following components of self-concept: identity, body image, and role performance.
- Identify stressors that affect self-concept, self-esteem, and sexuality.
- Describe the components of self-concept as each relates to Erikson's developmental stages.
- Discuss ways in which your self-concept and nursing actions affect your patient's self-concept and self-esteem.
- Discuss your role in maintaining or enhancing a patient's sexual health.
- Apply the nursing process to promote a patient's self-concept and sexual health.

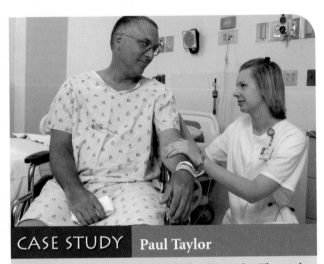

### CASE STUDY  Paul Taylor

Paul Taylor, a 48-year-old man, suffered a stroke. The stroke was unexpected and sudden. He did not know that he had hypertension, because he had not been getting yearly checkups. Mr. Taylor woke up in the hospital bed to find that he could not move his hand. He was not able to care for himself or to turn himself for days. With his nurses' constant encouragement, he is finally able to transfer from his bed into a chair. Mr. Taylor wonders what lies ahead for him. His body image has dramatically changed from that of a man of strength to that of a helpless individual. Mr. Taylor worries about his family and what will happen. He and his wife, Meredith, are terrified. Although Mrs. Taylor works, they have not saved enough money to meet monthly expenses or to educate their children without both incomes. Mr. Taylor's role as primary breadwinner for the family will be drastically changed if his condition does not improve.

Mr. Taylor's self-esteem lessens as his recovery and rehabilitation move slowly. His self-concept has changed from that of a strong laborer, one who did his own plumbing and car repairs, to a man who must rely on others. Although he is now at home in the rehabilitation process, Mr. Taylor is not able to perform tasks for the family and waits until his wife and son get home to help him with things that require strength. Moreover, because of the sexual side effects of the antihypertensive medication he is taking, his sexual health has been dramatically altered, and the lack of intimacy with his wife is affecting their relationship. Mr. Taylor's adaptation capabilities are stretched to the maximum. Mr. Taylor's identity is not clear to him anymore. He has no clear role within the family, his body image has been drastically

altered, his sexual health has suffered, and his self-esteem has never been lower.

Maria Kendal is a 27-year-old first-year nursing student assigned to care for Mr. Taylor. Ms. Kendal is divorced, has two school-age children, and works part-time as a certified nursing assistant (CNA) at a local long-term care facility while in school. She recognizes that changes in health status often result in stressors that affect a person's self-concept and sexuality. Such stressors influence a person's ability to interact with others and to function effectively. Ms. Kendal's knowledge of self-concept and sexuality will aid in identifying stressors that affect Mr. Taylor and promote effective planning to support the patient's growth and adaptation to change.

### KEY TERMS

body image, p. 559
identity, p. 559
role performance, p. 560
self-concept, p. 558
self-esteem, p. 560
sexual dysfunction, p. 563

sexual orientation, p. 560
sexuality, p. 560
sexually transmitted disease, p. 563

## Scientific Knowledge Base

**Self-concept** is your view of who you are. It is a combination of unconscious and conscious thoughts, attitudes, and perceptions. Self-concept, or how you think about yourself, directly affects your self-esteem, or how you feel about yourself. What you think and how you feel about yourself affect the way in which you care for yourself physically and emotionally. It also influences the way in which you are able to care for others. As a nurse you need to have knowledge of factors that affect self-concept and self-esteem. Being sensitive to ethnic and cultural differences in self-concept and self-esteem is important to individualize your approach to patient care (see Chapter 17).

## Development of Self-Concept

The development of self-concept is a complex process that involves many factors. Erikson's psychosocial theory of development (1963) is helpful in understanding key tasks that individuals face at various stages of development. Each stage builds on the tasks of the previous stage. Completing each developmental stage successfully leads to a solid sense of self. The development of self-concept and self-esteem begins at a young age and continues throughout life.

As a nurse you will use Erikson's theory to identify the stage of psychosocial development a patient is in based on his or her biological age. You will also assess where the patient actually is and determine how the patient is handling the tasks of that stage. Awareness of these developmental tasks (Box 20-1) will allow you to select appropriate nursing actions.

## Components and Interrelated Terms of Self-Concept

A positive self-concept gives a sense of meaning and wholeness to a person. The components of self-concept frequently considered by nurses are identity, body image, and role performance. Sexuality also has an impact on self-concept. Identity, body image, role performance, and self-esteem affect sexual health. Although overlap exists between concepts, this chapter will present each one separately.

**Identity** involves the sense of individuality and completeness of a person over time and in various circumstances. Identity implies being distinct and separate from others. Being "oneself," or living a life that is genuine and authentic, is the basis of true identity.

The achievement of identity is necessary for intimate relationships because you express your identity in relationships with others. Sexuality is a part of your identity. Gender identity is a person's private view of maleness or femaleness, and gender role is the feminine or masculine behavior exhibited.

Racial or cultural identity develops from identifying and socializing within an established group and through incorporating the responses of individuals who do not belong to that group into one's self-concept. The opinion or approval of others does not constitute the basis for self-esteem in the same way for all racial and cultural groups. When racial identity is central to self-concept and is positive, self-esteem tends to be high (Twenge and Crocker, 2002).

**Body image** involves attitudes related to the body, including physical appearance, femininity and masculinity, youthfulness, health, and strength. These views are not always the same as the person's actual physical structure or appearance. When a change in health status occurs, as in the case of Mr. Taylor, exaggerated disturbances in body image sometimes occur. The way others view a person's body and the feedback offered is also influential. For example, a controlling, violent husband tells his wife that she is ugly and that no one else would want her. Over the years of marriage, this criticism is incorporated into her self-concept.

Normal developmental changes such as puberty and aging have a more obvious effect on body image than on other aspects of self-concept. Hormonal changes during puberty and menopause in later adulthood influence body image. The development of secondary sex characteristics and changes in body fat distribution have a tremendous impact on the self-

---

| **BOX 20-1** | **Erikson's Developmental Tasks and Impact on Self-Concept and Sexuality** |

**Trust Versus Mistrust (Birth to 1 Year)**

Develops trust following consistency in caregiving and nurturing interactions
Distinguishes self from environment

**Autonomy Versus Shame and Doubt (1 to 3 Years)**

Begins to communicate likes and dislikes
Increasingly independent in thoughts and actions
Appreciates body appearance and function (including dressing, feeding, talking, and walking)

**Initiative Versus Guilt (3 to 6 Years)**

Takes initiative
Identifies with a gender
Enhances self-awareness
Increases language skills including identification of feelings

**Industry Versus Inferiority (6 to 12 Years)**

Incorporates feedback from peers and teachers
Increases self-esteem with new skill mastery (e.g. reading, math, sports, music)
Sexual identity strengthens
Aware of strengths and limitations

**Identity Versus Role Confusion (12 to 20 Years)**

Accepts body changes/maturation
Examines attitudes, values, and beliefs; establishes goals for the future
Feels positive about expanded sense of self
Interacts with those whom he or she finds sexually attractive or intellectually stimulating

**Intimacy Versus Isolation (Mid-20s to Mid-40s)**

Has intimate relationships with family and significant others
Has stable, positive feelings about self
Experiences successful role transitions and increased responsibilities

**Generativity Versus Self-Absorption (Mid-40s to Mid-60s)**

Is able to accept changes in appearance and physical endurance
Reassesses life goals
Shows contentment with aging

**Ego Integrity Versus Despair (Late 60s to Death)**

Feels positive about one's life and its meaning
Interested in providing a legacy for the next generation

concept of an adolescent. Changes associated with aging (i.e., wrinkles; graying hair; decrease in visual acuity, hearing, and mobility) affect body image in an older adult.

Cultural and societal attitudes and values also influence body image. Culture and society influence the accepted norms of body image and affect one's attitudes. Values such as ideal body weight and shape, as well as attitudes toward body markings, piercing, and tattoos are culturally based. American society typically emphasizes youth, beauty, and wholeness. This is apparent in television programs, movies, and advertisements. Western cultures have been socialized to dread the normal aging process. In contrast, Eastern cultures view aging very positively and respect the older adult.

Body image depends only partly on the reality of the body. When physical changes occur, individuals may or may not incorporate these changes into their body image. For example, people who have experienced significant weight loss do not perceive themselves as thin and may still tell you there is still a "fat person" inside. Body image issues are often associated with negative self-concept and self-esteem. The majority of men and women experience some degree of body dissatisfaction, which can affect body image and overall self-concept. As a nurse you are in an ideal position to influence a patient's body image.

**Role performance** is the way in which a person views his or her ability to carry out significant roles. Common roles include mother or father, wife or husband, daughter or son, sister or brother, employee or employer, and nurse or patient. For example, stating, "I am a good mother" or "I am a caring and competent nurse" reflects a positive self-concept and self-esteem. Each role involves meeting certain expectations. Fulfillment of these expectations leads to an enhanced sense of self. Difficulty or failure in meeting role expectations leads to decreased self-esteem or altered self-concept.

**Self-esteem** is an individual's overall sense of self-worth or the emotional evaluation of self-concept. It represents the overall judgment of personal worth or value. Self-esteem is positive when one feels capable, worthwhile, and competent (Rosenberg, 1965). Once established, basic feelings about the self tend to be constant, even though there is sometimes a little fluctuation. A situational crisis, like a hospitalization, often temporarily affects one's self-esteem.

Self-evaluation is an ongoing mental process. A positive sense of self-worth, or self-esteem, is an important factor in determining how an individual functions in the world. A person's ability to contribute in a meaningful way to society often affects self-concept and self-esteem. Some individuals who are chronically ill feel a sense of worthlessness. Your acceptance of a patient as an individual with worth and dignity will help maintain and improve the patient's self-esteem.

**Sexuality** is a broad term that refers to all aspects of being sexual. It is a part of who a person is and is important for overall health. It is possible for people to be sexually healthy in numerous ways. Sex is considered a basic physiological need, and sexual intimacy throughout the life span is equally important for sexual health. Healthy sexuality enables a per-

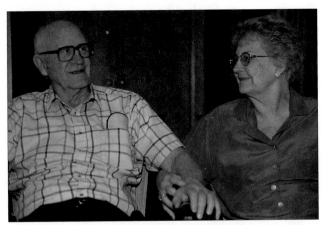

FIGURE **20-1** Sexuality is important across the life span.

son to develop and maintain one's fullest potential. Sexuality includes a person's thoughts and feelings about their bodies, a sense of femaleness or maleness, romantic and erotic attachments toward others, and attitudes toward sexual functioning. Our sexual health is based on our ability to form healthy relationships with others (Figure 20-1).

As a person grows and develops, so does his or her sexuality. Each stage of development brings changes in sexual functioning, sexual focus, and sexual relationships (see Chapter 19). Knowledge of sexual development and changes throughout the life span is essential for a nurse. The adult has achieved physical maturation but is continuing to explore and define emotional maturation in relationships. Even into adulthood, we continue to struggle with questions of who we are, how we want to present ourselves, and what type of partners we find most attractive. A clear sense of your sexual orientation and the ability to form open relationships also influences sexual health. You will provide care to individuals whose **sexual orientation** is heterosexual (attracted to different-sex partners), homosexual (same-sex partners), or bisexual (both male and female partners). Also, you will care for patients who are involved in intimate relationships with several partners and for patients whose sexual relationships occur outside of marriage.

## Stressors Affecting Self-Concept and Sexuality

A self-concept stressor is any real or perceived change that threatens identity, body image, or role performance (Figure 20-2). The individual's perception of the stressor is the most important factor in determining his or her response. For example, a man who has had a heart attack believes that he will no longer be able to be the aggressive businessman he has prided himself as being. This perception of what the heart attack will mean to his lifestyle will possibly lead to depression. However, another man views his heart attack as a message to slow down and enjoy his life.

Any change in health is a stressor that potentially affects self-concept. A physical change in the body leads to an altered body image, affecting identity and self-esteem. Chronic

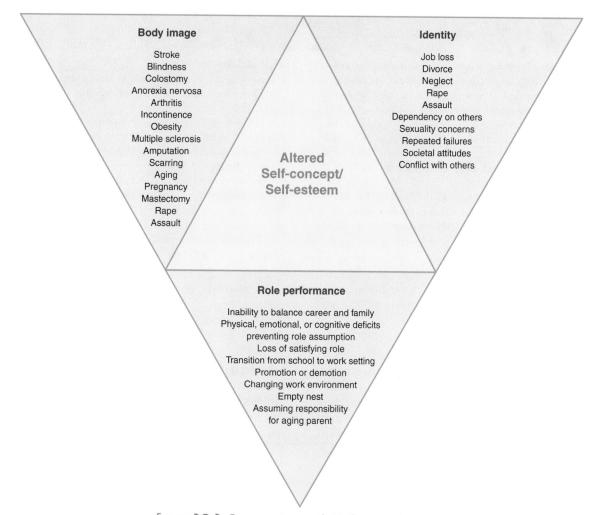

Body image

Stroke
Blindness
Colostomy
Anorexia nervosa
Arthritis
Incontinence
Obesity
Multiple sclerosis
Amputation
Scarring
Aging
Pregnancy
Mastectomy
Rape
Assault

Altered
Self-concept/
Self-esteem

Identity

Job loss
Divorce
Neglect
Rape
Assault
Dependency on others
Sexuality concerns
Repeated failures
Societal attitudes
Conflict with others

Role performance

Inability to balance career and family
Physical, emotional, or cognitive deficits
preventing role assumption
Loss of satisfying role
Transition from school to work setting
Promotion or demotion
Changing work environment
Empty nest
Assuming responsibility
for aging parent

FIGURE 20-2 Common stressors that influence self-concept.

illnesses often alter role performance, which often alter a person's identity and self-esteem. Living with a chronic illness requires a person to cope with a lost sense of self while a new self emerges. After the adjustment to loss, the person has to develop a new self-concept. For example, the loss of a partner sometimes leads to a loss of identity and a lower self-esteem (Van Baarsen, 2002).

A crisis occurs when a person cannot cope with stressors with usual methods of problem solving and adaptation. Any crisis potentially threatens self-concept and self-esteem. Some crises, like the one with Paul Taylor in the case study, directly affect all components of self-concept. If people are unable to adapt to such stressors, their health may be at risk and illness may result.

**IDENTITY STRESSORS.** Stressors throughout life affect an individual's identity, but identity is particularly vulnerable during adolescence, which is a time of great change. Adolescents are trying to adjust to the physical, emotional, and mental changes of increasing maturity, which results in insecurity and anxiety. For example, an adolescent who wants to be identified as part of the popu-

lar crowd at school develops a poor self-concept if not included in that group. Family and cultural factors sometimes influence negative health practices, such as cigarette smoking (Box 20-2). Promoting a change in self-concept demands an evidence-based practice approach, supported by the entire health care team. This means the team uses the best knowledge available about self-concept to drive patient care decisions.

An adult generally has a stable identity and thus a more firmly developed self-concept. Once a person has established his or her identity, the adult is better able to handle stressors such as marriage, divorce, menopause, aging, and retirement. Retirement for some means the loss of an important means of achievement. Some people at retirement begin to reevaluate their identities and accomplishments. More and more older people are working past the traditional retirement age or change careers following retirement. Some do so because of a financial need, whereas others have a desire to remain involved and productive (Ebersole and others, 2005). Sometimes loss of a significant other also leads a person to reexamine aspects of his or her identity.

| BOX 20-2 | CULTURAL FOCUS |
|---|---|

Cigarette smoking by young women is a growing health concern. The decision to smoke is reflective of self-concept issues and is often culturally influenced. Over a period of 10 years, researchers studied 1,213 African-American girls and 1,166 white girls. They discovered that whites were at higher risk of becoming daily smokers than African-Americans. Early predictors of daily smoking included parental education, single family home, drinking alcohol at ages 11 to 12, higher drive for thinness at ages 11 to 12, poor behavioral conduct at ages 11 to 12, and a perceived increase in stress from ages 10 to 11 to ages 12 to 13. Nurses need to be aware of risk factors and early predictors of daily smoking in young women for implementation of preventative health care in a variety of nursing settings.

**Implications for Practice**

- Body weight concerns, as well as family, social environment, and behavioral factors are important issues the nurse needs to address during preadolescence.
- Implement effective, healthy, and realistic weight management methods for young adolescent girls. Techniques include promoting fun, family-oriented physical activity and the elimination of dieting.
- A priority nursing action is the assessment of child and adolescent coping strategies. Appropriate techniques including effective communication, conflict resolution, and stress management.
- Identification of risk factors for early drug and alcohol use, including genetic predisposition and family environment, need to be a priority for nurses and other health care providers.

Data from Voorhees CC and others: Early predictors of daily smoking in young women: the National Heart, Lung, and Blood Institute growth and health study, *Prev Med* 34:616, 2002.

**BODY IMAGE STRESSORS.** Changes in the appearance or function of a body part will require an adjustment in body image. An individual's perception of the change and the relative importance placed on body image in the individual's self-concept will affect the significance of the loss or change. For example, if a woman considers her breasts key to her femininity, a mastectomy will negatively affect her body image. Changes in the appearance of the body, such as an amputation, facial disfigurement, or burns, are obvious stressors affecting body image. Surgical procedures, potentially undetected by others, have a significant impact on the individual. Elective changes such as breast augmentation or reduction also affect body image. Chronic illnesses such as heart and lung disease involve a change in function, in which the body no longer performs at an optimal level. Physical changes associated with aging or treatment for medical conditions negatively affect body image as well. In addition, the effects of pregnancy, significant weight gain or loss, medication management of an illness, or radiation therapy all change body image. Negative body image sometimes leads to adverse health outcomes.

Many people associate success with a specific body part or function. For example, some athletes consider their bodies and physical activities to be the focus of personal success. If they are never again able to participate in athletics because of an accident or injury, this can affect their adaptation and rehabilitation. Body image changes require reevaluation of long-accepted self-perceptions, as well as alterations in lifestyle.

**ROLE PERFORMANCE STRESSORS.** Throughout life a person undergoes many role changes. Normal changes associated with maturation result in changes in role performance. For example, when a woman has a child, she becomes a mother. The new role of mother will involve many changes in

behavior if the woman is going to be successful. Another shift is necessary when a middle-age woman with teenage children assumes responsibility for the care of her older parents. Acute and chronic illnesses alter a person's ability to carry out various roles, which will affect self-esteem and identity.

All people must adapt to two major changes that occur with aging: changes in the work role and in the role of spouse or partner (Ebersole and others, 2005). Role performance changes associated with retirement differ for men and women. Many women have adjusted to several different roles throughout their lifetime and are more likely than men to have developed friendships that are not work-related. Adjusting to changes in role performance has an impact on the marital relationship. Changes in role performance following the loss of a spouse or partner, too, affect self-concept. A widow who has never paid bills or one who needs to learn to cook will need assistance in changing roles.

**SELF-ESTEEM STRESSORS.** Individuals with high self-esteem are generally better able to cope with demands and stressors than those with low self-esteem. Low self-worth contributes to feeling unfulfilled and misunderstood and results in depression and anxiety. Illness, surgery, or accidents that change life patterns also influence feelings of self-worth. The more that chronic illnesses, such as diabetes, arthritis, and heart disease, interfere with the ability to engage in activities contributing to feelings of worth or success, the more they affect self-esteem.

Self-esteem stressors vary with developmental stages. If a child believes that he is unable to meet his parents' expectations or if his parents harshly criticize or inconsistently discipline him, this will reduce his level of self-worth. The self-esteem of an adolescent is also vulnerable because the adolescent directs so much energy to worrying about appearance, searching for identity, and being overly concerned

| BOX 20-3 | CARE OF THE OLDER ADULT |

Self-concept is negatively affected in older adulthood because of life changes such as spousal loss or decline in health. However, in some individuals, aging promotes improved coping strategies that protect against the declining feelings of self-esteem, despite all the physical and emotional changes associated with aging. Nursing interventions aimed at enhancing self-concept and self-esteem in older adults are essential.

- Clarify what the life changes mean and the impact on self-concept for the older adult.
- Be alert to preoccupation with physical complaints. Assess complaints thoroughly and if no physical explanation exists, encourage older adult to verbalize needs (fear, insecurity, loneliness) in a nonphysical way.
- Identify positive and negative coping mechanisms. Support effective strategies.
- Encourage the use of storytelling and review of old photographs.
- Communicate that the older adult is worthwhile by actively listening to and accepting the person's feelings, being respectful, and praising healthy behaviors.
- Allow additional time to complete tasks. Reinforce the older adult's efforts at independence.

Data from Ebersole P and others: *Gerontological nursing and healthy Aging,* ed 2, St. Louis, 2005, Mosby; Robins RW and others: Global self-esteem across the life span, *Psychol Aging* 17(3):423, 2002.

about what others think. Stressors affecting the self-esteem of an adult include failures at work and failures in relationships. Potential self-esteem stressors in older adults are discussed in Box 20-3.

**SEXUALITY STRESSORS.** As a nurse you will work with patients who are making decisions or dealing with issues related to sexuality on a regular basis. For example, people of all ages face reproductive health issues including contraception, infertility, sexual dysfunction, and sexual satisfaction. Understanding some of the decisions and issues patients face increases your effectiveness in helping patients to reach their maximum level of health in the area of sexuality.

Alterations in sexual health occur from a variety of situations such as illness, infertility, trauma, and abuse. **Sexual dysfunction** interferes with sexual health and is a problem with desire, arousal, or orgasm. Erectile dysfunction is a common problem among older men. It is generally related to chronic diseases such as diabetes, kidney disease, alcohol dependence, depression, neurological disorders, vascular insufficiency, and diseases of the prostate (Ebersole and others, 2005). In addition, side effects of medications also contribute to sexual dysfunction. Although we take medications to stay healthy, the side effects sometimes negatively affect sexuality. The causes of sexual dysfunction are physiological or psychological. Sometimes the cause of a dysfunction cannot be identified or is a result of a combination of several factors.

Because sexual dysfunction sometimes results from the use of medications like antidepressants and antihypertensives, it is important to include sexual side effects in patient teaching. Your patient is more likely to adhere to a treatment plan if you discuss side effects of medications that alter sexual function with both partners and the patient is able to make an informed decision. Our current state of health greatly influences sexual response (from desire to arousal to orgasm). The availability of sexual performance–enhancing medication like Viagra (sildenafil) and Cialis (tadalafil) has changed the lives of many couples. These medications treat erectile dysfunction but are contraindicated in men with coronary artery disease or those taking common cardiac drugs.

Changing physical appearance and concerns about physical attractiveness affect sexual functioning. The loss of sexual activity and the absence of a self-concept that includes being a sexual person is not an inevitable aspect of aging. Some older people face health concerns and societal attitudes that make it difficult for them to continue sexual activity. Although declining physical abilities sometimes make sex as they knew it painful or impossible, with intervention, older adults are able to experiment with and learn alternative ways of sexual expression.

Hormonally stimulated changes brought on by developmental maturation are also stressors that affect sexuality across the life span. Menarche, the onset of menstrual cycle in girls, is occurring at an earlier age in the United States with the average age of 12.2 years for African-Americans and 12.7 to 12.8 years for whites (Graber and Brooks-Gunn, 2002). Some adolescent girls are unaware that it is normal to grow pubic, underarm, and body hair and deposit more fat on their hips and breasts, all of which will also affect body image. As boys approach puberty, physical changes include nocturnal emissions and ejaculation, increasing sexual desire, and increased hygiene needs. Older women experiencing menopause, or the cessation of menstrual periods, experience changes in vaginal lubrication and sexual interest. Additional patient teaching needs include the use of latex condoms to prevent **sexually transmitted disease** and unintended pregnancy and instruction on breast and testicular self-examinations.

Sexual abuse, assault, and rape are also stressors that affect self-concept. Be alert to clues that suggest abuse (Box 20-4). In addition, observe the interaction between the patient and partner for additional clues. Controlling behaviors such as speaking for the person or refusing to leave them alone with a caregiver are suggestive of emotional and perhaps physical or sexual abuse. If you suspect abuse, interview the patient privately. A patient will probably not admit to problems of abuse with the abuser present. Some of the following questions are useful: "Are you in a relationship in which someone is hurting you?" or "Have you ever been forced to have sex when you didn't want to?" When you recognize or report abuse, mobilize treatment immediately for the victim and the family. The most important factor to consider is the safety of the suspected victim. Often, all family members require therapy to promote healthy interactions and relationships.

| **BOX 20-4** | **Signs and Symptoms That Indicate Current Sexual Abuse or a History of Sexual Abuse** |
| --- | --- |

Unexplained bruises, lacerations, or abrasions especially around breasts, genital, or anal areas
Unexplained vaginal or anal soreness or bleeding
Unexplained venereal disease or genital infection
Frequent visits to health care providers
Headaches
Gastrointestinal problems
Abdominal pain
Dysmenorrhea
Premenstrual syndrome
Sleep pattern disturbances
Nightmares

Repetitive dreams
Depression
Social withdrawal
Anxiety
Eating disorders
Substance abuse
Decreased self-esteem
Difficulty developing trust
Difficulties with intimate relationships
Impaired school or work performance
Reports of being sexually assaulted or raped
NOTE: No physical symptoms may be present

Modified from Meiner SE, Lueckenotte A: *Gerontologic nursing,* ed 3, St. Louis, 2006, Mosby; Stuart GW, Laraia MT: *Principles and practice of psychiatric nursing,* ed 8, St. Louis, 2005, Mosby.

## The Nurse's Influence on the Patient's Self-Concept and Sexuality

As a nurse you have the ability to positively influence a patient's self-concept. Your acceptance of a patient with an altered self-concept helps promote positive change. Your words and actions convey sincere interest and acceptance and have a profound impact on the patient. When a patient's physical appearance has changed, both the patient and the family will watch your verbal and nonverbal responses and reactions to the changed appearance. A positive and matter-of-fact approach to care provides a model for the patient and family to follow.

How you respond to patients who have experienced changes in body appearance sets the stage for how they come to see themselves. The patient with a change in body functioning or appearance is often extremely sensitive to your verbal and nonverbal responses (Figure 20-3). General nursing interventions, such as building a trusting nurse-patient relationship and appropriately including the patient in decision making, supports most patients' self-concept. Sometimes, individualized approaches including supporting the use of alternative healing techniques or methods of spiritual expression will help a patient adapt to changes in self-concept.

As a nurse, you can affect your patient's body image. For example, you will influence the body image of a woman who has had a mastectomy in a positive way by showing acceptance of the mastectomy scar. On the other hand, a shocked or disgusted facial expression will contribute to the woman's developing a negative body image. It is very important to monitor your responses toward the patient. Matter-of-fact statements such as "This wound is healing nicely" or "This looks healthy" enhance the body image of the patient.

Inadvertently frowning or grimacing when performing procedures has a profound effect on the patient. Your nonverbal behavior conveys the level of caring that exists for a patient and affects your patient's self-esteem. For example, when an incontinent patient perceives that you find the situation un-

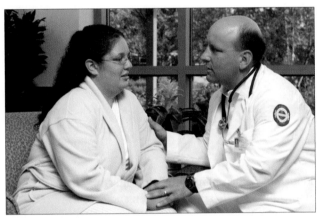

FIGURE **20-3** Nurses use touch and eye contact to enhance a patient's self-esteem.

pleasant, this threatens the patient's self-concept. Anticipate your own reactions, acknowledge them, and focus on the patient instead of the unpleasant task or situation. If you put yourself in the patient's position, this will lessen the patient's embarrassment, frustration, and anger.

When you consider the sexuality of patients, think about your own knowledge regarding sexual development, sexual orientation, sexual response, sexually transmitted diseases, contraception, and alterations in sexual health. Your own sexuality and sexual experience provide a valuable resource for understanding a patient's experiences. Attempts at self-exploration teach us about our bodies and the potential for providing pleasure. Your attitude about masturbation may have stemmed from personal experience or from values or beliefs communicated by other people. Games like "doctor" and "nurse" may have provided other early sex play and exploration. In addition, your own sexual experiences add to understanding about what a first sexual encounter may have been like or what it is like to introduce the topic of sexually transmitted diseases or intercourse. In addition to personal experiences related to sexuality, use what you have learned through working with other patients as you assess and work with current patients. Communication is another important knowledge base to consider when caring for patients with sexuality problems (see Chapter 9).

It is important that you understand the reason for changes in the patient's sexual health. The response to changes in sexuality and intimacy following an illness depends on the person's self-concept, support of sexual partner, and attitudes regarding sexuality. Many health professionals fail to address sexual needs of their patients. Understanding the impact of a diagnosis, treatment, and medications on your patient's perception of sexuality or sexual performance results in a treatment plan that promotes sexual health. For example, when caring for an older man who has had a heart attack, you say, "Following a heart attack, many older men have questions about sexuality, such as when they are able to resume sexual intercourse. Do you have questions like this that I can answer?" A professional specializing in altered sexual health is sometimes necessary to help the patient and partner resume a satisfying sexual relationship. Before making a referral, though, use therapeutic communication techniques to open the discussion about sexual concerns and provide information about sexual health.

## Critical Thinking in Patient Care

### Synthesis

Your nursing expertise will allow you to anticipate and respond to stressors that affect your patient's self-concept. Consider changes in your patient's identity, body image, role performance, and self-esteem as important aspects of care. While using the nursing process, you will apply knowledge, experience, attitudes, and standards in providing appropriate care to promote your patient's self-concept and sexual health.

**KNOWLEDGE.** In addition to considering the various aspects of a patient's self-concept, use knowledge of how various medications and chronic pain influence your patient's ability to perform self-care and function at an optimal level. Many medications have actions and side effects that influence a patient's self-concept and sexuality. When you care for patients who have alterations in self-concept, be particularly alert to the patient who is experiencing chronic pain. Chronic pain predisposes a person to decreased ability to function, irritability, and decreased sleep. These changes negatively affect self-concept. Another area of knowledge to consider is the patient's cultural background. Culture influences the importance people place on such things as appearance, role performance, and acceptance by others (see Chapter 17).

**EXPERIENCE.** Throughout life all individuals, including nurses, have experience with self-concept issues. Personal memories of changes in appearance or times when you were unable to carry out usual roles because of a temporary illness will help you become empathetic with patients who are experiencing

---

**BOX 20-5** USING EVIDENCE IN PRACTICE

**Research Summary**
As low-income women struggle to become self-sufficient, they encounter many barriers. The women in this study did not identify inadequate child care and transportation as obstacles; however, the women did view them as socially acceptable reasons for not working. The researchers explored low-income women's perceptions of barriers to self-sufficiency.

Women attending an occupational skills training center designed to assist low-income, unemployed or underemployed women in their transition to the workforce identified eight obstacles to self-sufficiency. Perceived barriers of self-sufficiency that emerged in this qualitative study were lack of self-esteem, especially about returning to school; "bad" relationships with men; lack of support from family and friends; limited life options; lack of training; lack of quality programs; criminal histories; and fear of success.

**Application to Nursing Practice**
The results from this study reveal that to ensure family health, nurses need to match their approach to needs of women. Nurses must individualize the plan of care for low-income women returning to work and focus nursing interventions on improving patients' self-concepts. The promotion of empowerment, self-esteem building, and the development of self-efficacy are more important nursing interventions to promote behavioral change in low-income women than removing child care and transportation barriers. Therefore aim nursing resources at addressing fundamental self-concept deficits. In addition, follow-up services, including home care and community health, are necessary to promote family health.

Data from Brown SG, Barbosa G: Nothing is going to stop me now: low-income women as they become self-sufficient, *Public Health Nurs* 18(5):364, 2001.

---

stressors to their self-concept or sexuality. Past experiences with patients who have undergone changes in self-concept or experienced self-concept stressors also provide useful insight into how to work effectively with a current patient.

**ATTITUDES.** Attitudes to adopt when caring for patients with threats to self-concept and sexuality are acceptance, respect, and compassion. Some patients will have values, attitudes, or behaviors that differ from your own (Box 20-5). Developing a therapeutic nurse-patient relationship based on mutual respect, professional compassion, and unconditional acceptance promotes positive patient outcomes.

**STANDARDS.** There are several codes of professional conduct for nurses, but each reflects a commitment to the principle of respect for patient autonomy. Autonomy means that individuals have the freedom to choose their own life plan. Supporting your patients' autonomy to make choices and live in an authentic way consistent with personal values and beliefs supports the development and maintenance of a strong and positive self-concept.

| BOX 20-6 | **Behaviors Suggestive of Altered Self-Concept and Sexuality** |
| --- | --- |

| | |
| --- | --- |
| Avoidance of eye contact | Excessively dependent |
| Slumped posture | Hesitant to express views or |
| Unkempt appearance | opinions |
| Overly apologetic | Lack of interest in what is |
| Hesitant speech | happening |
| Overly critical or angry | Passive attitude |
| Frequent or inappropriate | Difficulty in making |
| crying | decisions |
| Negative self-evaluation | |

## Nursing Process

### Assessment

In assessing self-concept and self-esteem, you focus on each component of self-concept (identity, body image, and role performance), behaviors suggestive of altered self-concept (Box 20-6), and actual and potential self-concept stressors (see Figure 20-3). Determining the patient's current and past coping patterns is also important. In addition to direct questioning, you will effectively gather much of the data regarding self-concept through observation of the patient's nonverbal behavior and by paying attention to what a patient says. Take note of the manner in which patients talk about the people in their lives, because this provides clues to both stressful and supportive relationships. It also suggests key roles the patient assumes.

Using knowledge of developmental stages (see Box 20-1) to determine what areas are likely to be important to the patient, inquire about these aspects of the person's life. For example, you ask a 65-year-old male patient about his life and what has been important to him. This is the stage of development in life in which individuals are examining their lives and considering the impact they have had in the world. The individual's conversation will likely provide data relating to role performance, identity, self-esteem, stressors, and coping patterns. At appropriate times, specific questions are useful (Table 20-1).

You also need to assess all relevant factors to determine a patient's sexual well-being. Assessment of sexuality involves physical, psychological, social, and cultural variables. In approaching patients about their sexuality and sexual functioning, it is sometimes unnerving to inquire about another person's sexual functioning. You may worry that the patient will not appreciate being asked about sexuality and sexual practices. However, patients want to know how medications, treatments, and surgical procedures influence their sexual relationship. With experience you will come to recognize that many patients welcome the opportunity to talk about their sexuality. When patients are experiencing difficulty in sexual functioning, they will appreciate it when you bring up the subject. Once you approach the topic, the patient is able to talk about concerns and explore possible ways to resolve

the problem. When you address sexuality in a sensitive, relaxed, matter-of-fact manner, patients will feel safe enough to bring up areas of concern. The intimacy of the nurse-patient relationship, whether it is involved in providing physical care or discussing the impact of a recent diagnosis, provides a unique opportunity for discussing a person's sexual concerns. The acronym PLISSIT is a helpful format for discussing sexuality with patients (Box 20-7).

Every complete nursing history needs to include a few questions related to sexual functioning. Start with a general statement such as "Sex is an important part of life and can be affected by our health status" or "To better understand your health, it is useful to know if you have concerns about your sexual functioning." Explore sexual decision making, including the patient's use of contraception and safe sex practices. Adolescents best respond to a question such as "Many teenagers have questions about sexually transmitted diseases or whether their bodies are developing at the right rate. What questions about sex can I answer?"

In gathering a sexual history, consider physical, functional, relationship, lifestyle, and self-esteem factors that influence sexual functioning. A variety of physical factors can positively or negatively influence sexual desire and function. For example, sexual intercourse sometimes results in pain or discomfort from arthritis, angina, endometriosis, or lack of vaginal lubrication. Even anticipation that sex may hurt, such as during the postpartum period or postoperatively, will lessen sexual desire. Learn to what extent these physical factors affect a patient's sexual performance. Also, perceptions of body image are related to adherence to medical and treatment regimens. Therefore you need to assess a patient's sexual concerns and ask questions about body image changes and effects on sex life. For example, begin a discussion with, "It's common for women to be self-conscious and concerned they are not sexually attractive after losing a breast. Have you and your partner talked about how this change will affect your sexual intimacy?"

Some medications affect sexual desire or cause physical changes that affect performance. Drinking alcohol or using drugs clouds judgment and results in sexual intercourse or other activities that lead to sexually transmitted diseases or pregnancy. Gather a complete history of any medications or illicit drugs the patient is taking or has taken in the past. You will also need to obtain the same information for the patient's partner.

Reviewing sexuality changes associated with aging is also important. Women experience a reduction in vaginal secretions, and the vagina becomes shorter and does not expand as well to accommodate the penis (Meiner and Lueckenotte, 2006). Orgasmic contractions are fewer and are sometimes accompanied by painful uterine contractions. In men, the penis does not become firm as quickly and is not as firm as it is at a younger age. Ejaculation takes longer to achieve and is shorter in duration, and the erection often diminishes more quickly. When assessing sexual changes, you need to ask about the patient's past sexual experiences, perceptions, and difficulties.

## FOCUSED PATIENT ASSESSMENT

TABLE 20-1

| Assessment Questions* | Responses Reflecting Difficulties With Self-Concept and Sexuality |
|---|---|
| **Identity** | |
| "How would you describe yourself?" | Derogatory answers (e.g., "I don't know; there's not too much worth mentioning") raise concern. |
| **Body Image** | |
| "What aspects of your appearance do you like?" "Are there any aspects of your appearance that you would like to change? If yes, describe the changes you would make." | Most people are able to identify something about their appearance that they like (e.g., "People have always told me I have nice eyes"). If a person does not identify any appreciated characteristic, this is suggestive of a negative body image and poor self-esteem. Most people have one or two areas that they would like to change (e.g., "My nose is too big" or "My hips are too large"), but a long list of problem areas leads you to consider difficulties with self-concept. |
| **Self-Esteem** | |
| "Tell me about the things you do that make you feel good about yourself." "How do you feel about yourself?" | Statements about not having any strengths or being able to do anything well raise concern. |
| **Role Performance** | |
| "Tell me about your primary roles (for example, partner, parent, friend, sister, professional role, volunteer). How effective are you at carrying out each of these roles?" | Listen for the number of primary roles identified. A large number of primary roles will put the patient at risk for role conflicts and role overload. As with questions above, if the patient indicates that he or she does not feel that these roles are adequately covered, the patient may be experiencing alterations in self-concept. Although most people carry out many roles and often feel as though some of them are not adequately addressed, listen for the person's perception about his or her overall role competency. |
| **Sexuality** | |
| "How has your illness, medication, or impending surgery affected your sex life?" "Are your needs for intimacy being met?" "Do you have any concerns about your sexual functioning?" | Assess this area in an overall assessment of self-concept and sexual health, because some patients are hesitant to bring up issues of sexuality. Listen for concerns about sexual functioning (e.g., erectile dysfunction in men, changes in vaginal lubrication in women) or overall change in sex drive. |

*In addition to the verbal content of the patient's answer, note the patient's nonverbal behaviors. Watch for hesitant speech, poor eye contact, and slumped posture.

The nursing assessment includes consideration of previous coping behaviors; the nature, number, and intensity of stressors; and the patient's internal and external resources. Knowing how a patient has dealt with self-concept stressors in the past provides insight into the patient's style of coping. Not all patients address issues in the same way, but often a person uses a familiar coping pattern for newly encountered stressors. As you identify previous coping patterns, it is useful to determine whether these patterns have contributed to healthy functioning or created more problems. For example, the use of drugs or alcohol during times of stress often creates additional stressors.

Exploring resources and strengths, such as availability of significant others or prior use of community resources, is important when formulating a realistic and effective plan. You also need to determine how the patient views the situation. For example, some women grow accustomed to changes in

---

**BOX 20-7  PLISSIT Assessment of Sexuality**

**P**ermission to discuss sexuality issues
**L**imited **I**nformation related to sexual health problems being experienced
**S**pecific **S**uggestions—only when the nurse is clear about the problem
**I**ntensive **T**herapy—referral to professional with advanced training if necessary

Modified from Annon J: The PLISSIT model: a proposed conceptual scheme for the behavioral treatment of sexual problems, *J Sex Educ Ther* 2(2):1, 1976.

## SYNTHESIS IN PRACTICE

As Maria prepares to care for Mr. Taylor, she thinks about what she knows about self-concept and sexuality. She realizes that Mr. Taylor's stroke and resulting neurological deficits along with the sexual side effects of his antihypertensive medications are significant stressors in regard to his self-concept and sexuality. Mr. Taylor's independence is threatened because he is in the hospital and is dependent upon the nurses for most of his care. He may never be able to go back to work again, and he does not consider himself a strong man any more. Therefore his family role as provider is threatened. Maria recognizes the significance of these changes and their potential influence on his self-concept and sexuality.

Maria's father experienced a stroke 2 years ago. Although his neurological symptoms finally improved enough to allow him to go back to work, Maria remembers the struggle her father went through as he coped with the physical and emotional changes the stroke created. Maria's experience as a single mother also provides insight into what it is like to assume a new role within a family. Maria uses these two different experiences to guide her assessment of Mr. Taylor's concerns.

Maria needs to learn as much as she can about Mr. Taylor's thoughts and feelings about his self-concept and sexuality. In order to do this, she realizes that she must first establish a trusting relationship with Mr. Taylor and his wife, Meredith. Because Maria feels uncomfortable in discussing sexuality with her patients, she reviews the PLISSIT assessment of sexuality the night before she cares for Mr. Taylor and writes out some questions that she wants to ask him. Maria also plans to talk with both Mr. and Mrs. Taylor about their relationship before and after the stroke.

their health status as they get older. For these women, experiencing heart disease is one more aspect of growing older. For others, a cardiac event is less expected and more problematic, especially for middle-age women who still have family and career responsibilities. As a nurse, be aware of women's changing roles in society such as increased caregiving responsibilities. You are in a unique position to reinforce the need for women to make lifestyle changes after a myocardial infarction and to identify and remove barriers to attending cardiac rehabilitation classes (McSweeney and Coon, 2004).

Valuable assessment data often evolve out of conversations with family and significant others. Sometimes significant others have insights into the person's way of dealing with stressors and have knowledge about what is important to the person's self-concept. The way in which the loved one talks about the patient, including his or her nonverbal behaviors, will provide information about what kind of support is available for the patient. Ask patients if they feel comfortable when they are relating to their partner and whether there is openness in the interaction.

**PATIENT EXPECTATIONS.** The patient's expectations are also important to assess. Asking the patient how he or she believes medical and nursing interventions will make a dif-

ference will provide useful information regarding the patient's expectations. This provides an opportunity to discuss the patient's goals. For example, when working with a patient who is experiencing anxiety related to an upcoming diagnostic study, ask the patient about his expectations of the relaxation exercise that you have been practicing together. The patient's response provides valuable information about his beliefs and attitudes regarding the effectiveness of the interventions, as well as the potential need to modify the nursing approach. When nursing care involves consideration of the patient's sexuality, you need to be sensitive and understanding and always maintain the patient's confidentiality.

## Nursing Diagnosis

You need to carefully consider assessment data to identify a patient's actual or potential problem areas. You rely on knowledge and experience, apply appropriate critical thinking attitudes and professional standards, and look for clusters of defining characteristics that indicate a nursing diagnosis. Possible nursing diagnoses (North American Nursing Diagnosis Association [NANDA International], 2005) related to self-concept and sexual functioning include:

- Disturbed body image
- Disturbed personal identity
- Ineffective role performance
- Readiness for enhanced self-concept
- Chronic low self-esteem
- Situational low self-esteem
- Sexual dysfunction
- Ineffective sexuality patterns

Forming nursing diagnoses about self-concept is complex. Often, isolated data are defining characteristics for more than one nursing diagnosis. If the person who has recently been laid off from work expresses a predominantly negative self-appraisal, including inability to handle situations or events and difficulty making decisions, these characteristics suggest a nursing diagnosis of *situational low self-esteem related to inability to fulfill previous roles.* Assessing information regarding recent events in the patient's life and how the patient has viewed himself in the past would be important. Likewise, identifying a nursing diagnosis regarding sexuality often requires you to clarify that defining characteristics exist and that the patient perceives difficulty with regard to sexuality. Clues to help you identify defining characteristics of a possible nursing diagnosis include surgery of reproductive organs or changes in appearance, chronic fatigue or pain, past or current physical abuse, chronic illness, and developmental milestones such as puberty or menopause. Determining the contributing factors is important. Interventions depend on selecting the correct related factors. When you include all relevant contributing factors, you plan effectively. For example, the nursing diagnosis *ineffective sexuality patterns related to difficulty with accep-*

*tance of recent loss and fear of pain* is appropriate for a woman who has recently undergone a mastectomy. Further expanding the "related to" section to include more about how the mastectomy is affecting sexuality is helpful. For example, altered sexuality is possibly related to postoperative pain or fear of pain, fear of diminished attractiveness, and/or difficulty in moving.

## Planning

**GOALS AND OUTCOMES.** You develop an individualized plan of care for each nursing diagnosis and help the patient set realistic expectations for care. You individualize goals and set realistic and measurable outcomes. In establishing goals, consult with the patient about whether the goals are perceived as realistic (see care plan). Consult with significant others to develop a more comprehensive and workable plan. Once you have formulated a goal, consider how the data that illustrated the problem would change if the problem were diminished. These changes should be reflected in the outcome criteria. As an example, you diagnose a patient with *situational low self-esteem related to a recent job layoff.* The patient has verbalized not being able to do anything right lately and has expressed shame about losing her job. These are the defining characteristics. You formulate the goal that the patient's self-esteem will improve within 1 week. Expected outcomes include that the patient will discuss a minimum of three areas of her life where she is functioning well and voice the recognition that losing her job is not reflective of her worth as a person.

With the nursing diagnosis *ineffective sexuality patterns related to recent mastectomy and fear of pain*, you explore with the patient what she sees as a satisfactory recovery after her mastectomy. This gives the patient the opportunity to share that she wants to return to her presurgical sexual relationship with her partner. She specifies that she wants to feel comfortable having her remaining breast caressed and to engage in intercourse within 2 weeks, without experiencing pain.

**SETTING PRIORITIES.** The care plan presents the goals, expected outcomes, and interventions for a patient with an alteration in self-concept. Your interventions focus on helping the patient adapt to the stressors that led to the self-concept disturbance and on supporting and reinforcing the development of coping methods. The patient often needs time to adapt to physical changes. Self-concept priorities include maximizing the patient's ability to address physical and psychological needs. Priorities for sexual health typically include resuming sexual activities. You look for strengths in both the individual and the family and provide resources and education to turn limitations into strengths. Patient teaching communicates the normalcy of certain situations (e.g., nature of a chronic disease, change in relationships, effect of a loss). It is important that you determine if this is your patient's need and plan accordingly. For example, when caring for a patient whose sexual health is altered, include private time for your patient and partner to quietly sit in the room and have dinner and watch a movie without any interruptions.

**CONTINUITY OF CARE.** The perceptions of significant others are important to incorporate into the plan of care. Sometimes individuals who have experienced deficits in self-concept before the current episode of treatment have established a system of support including mental health clinicians, clergy, and other community resources. Before involving the family, you need to consider the patient's desires for significant others to be involved and cultural norms regarding who most frequently makes decisions in the family. Sexual conflict in marriage or intimacy issues stemming from past sexual assault or incest often requires intensive treatment with mental health professionals. Resolving self-concept issues is a long-term goal and includes referrals to a clinical psychologist, advanced practice psychiatric nurse, social worker, or counselor.

## Implementation

As with all the steps of the nursing process, a therapeutic nurse-patient relationship is central to the implementation phase. Once you have developed goals and outcomes, you need to consider nursing interventions that will help move the patient toward the goals. To develop effective nursing interventions, consider the nursing diagnosis and broad interventions that address the diagnosis. Tailor these broad, standard interventions to the individual patient. You develop additional nursing interventions based on the "related to" component of the nursing diagnosis. Developing interventions that affect the "related to" factors will often decrease the problem reflected in the nursing diagnosis. In the case of Mr. Taylor (see care plan), the "related to" component of the nursing diagnosis focuses on the areas to explore when talking with the patient.

Nursing interventions are designed to promote a patient's healthy self-concept and sexuality. Strategies help patients regain or restore the elements that contribute to a strong and secure sense of self. The approaches that you choose will vary according to the level of care required. Good nursing care includes promoting sexual health in acute and restorative settings. You promote sexual health by helping patients understand their problems and by exploring methods to deal with them effectively.

**HEALTH PROMOTION.** You work with patients to help them develop healthy lifestyle behaviors that contribute to a positive self-concept. Measures that support adaptation to stress, such as proper nutrition, regular exercise within the patient's capabilities, adequate sleep and rest, and stress-reducing practices will contribute to a healthy self-concept. As a nurse you are in a unique position to identify lifestyle practices that put a patient's self-concept at risk or are suggestive of altered self-concepts. For example, a college student visits an outpatient clinic with complaints of being unable to sleep and anxiety attacks. In gathering the patient history, you learn of lifestyle practices such as too little rest, a large num-

## CARE PLAN Self-Esteem

### ASSESSMENT

After Mr. Taylor's physical condition has been stabilized, Maria Kendal sits down with Mr. and Mrs. Taylor to engage in a discussion of how the stroke has affected Mr. Taylor's self-concept and sexual health. When Maria asks about how the stroke has affected his identity and sexual health, Mr. Taylor **looks away, shakes his head,** and states, **"I feel like less of a man.** My wife says she's just thankful I'm alive, but that's not enough for me." When Maria asks Mrs. Taylor about her husband's mood, Mrs. Taylor reports that Mr. Taylor demonstrates **intermittent eye contact, frequent crying when alone, blank staring** at his flaccid hand, and **superficial conversations** with family members. Maria assesses that Mr. Taylor **refuses to bathe or comb hair.** He **eats less** than 50% of meals and **demonstrates avoidance** of the prescribed rehabilitation activities.
*Defining characteristics are shown in bold type.

### NURSING DIAGNOSIS Situational low self-esteem related to negative view of self as less than whole following stroke and uncertainty of future personal, family, and professional roles.

### PLANNING
#### GOAL

- Mr. Taylor will experience fewer reduce alterations in self-concept including low self-esteem, disturbed body image, altered role performance, and impaired sexuality with staff members and significant others before discharge.

#### EXPECTED OUTCOMES*
##### Self-Esteem
- Mr. Taylor will verbalize feelings of self-acceptance and self-worth within 4 days.
- Mr. Taylor will demonstrate maintenance of basic grooming and hygiene needs within 2 days.

##### Role Performance
- Mr. Taylor will describe role changes associated with his stroke and will verbalize commitment to participating in rehabilitation and community resources to fulfill role performance by day of discharge.

##### Body Image
- Mr. Taylor will demonstrate adjustment to changes in body function and appearance within 1 week.

##### Sexual Identity
- Mr. Taylor will challenge negative images of sexual self within 1 week.

*Outcomes classification label from Moorhead S, Johnson M, Maas M: *Nursing outcomes classification (NOC),* ed 3, St. Louis, 2004, Mosby.

### INTERVENTIONS†
#### Self-Esteem Enhancement
- Facilitate an environment and activities that will increase self-esteem (e.g., writing in a journal, reflection, or praying), and use silence and active listening to promote communication.
- Monitor patient's statements of self-worth.

- Encourage increased responsibility for self, and assist patient with accepting dependence on others (e.g., son and wife), as appropriate.

#### Role Enhancement
- Encourage patient to identify a realistic description of change in role and to accept new challenges brought on by the stroke.

- Assist patient with identifying specific role changes required due to illness or disability.

### RATIONALE

Patients need a therapeutic nurse-patient relationship to promote positive patient outcome, including the patient's assuming responsibility for his own care.

Evaluation of a patient's overall self-concept and self-esteem and his expressions of thoughts and feelings, including depression, grief, resentment, fear of rejection, and envy of "healthy" people, indicate how the patient feels about himself.

Promoting self-care will enhance self-concept, including improving role performance.

Having an accurate perception of physical functioning and accepting new challenges will allow the patient to initiate health-promoting behaviors.

Assessment of role performance is necessary to modify behavior and promote optimal functioning. Injuries often disrupt role performance.

†Intervention classification labels from Dochterman JM, Bulechek GM, editors: *Nursing interventions classification (NIC),* ed 4, St. Louis, 2004, Mosby.

## CARE PLAN Self-Esteem—cont'd

### INTERVENTIONS†

#### *Body Image Enhancement*

- Assist patient with discussing changes in physical appearance caused by the stroke.

- Identify support groups and other professionals, including home care and support systems, available to the patient.

#### *Sexual Counseling*

- Inform patient early in the relationship that sexuality is an important part of life and that illness, medications, and stress often alter sexual functioning.
- Include the spouse/sexual partner in the counseling as much as possible, as appropriate.

### RATIONALE

The impact on body image influences other aspects of self-concept and self-esteem, including perception of identity and role performance. This sometimes affects sexuality.

Outpatient support will assist the patient with feeling normal again and integrating a new body image and role performance into his self-concept.

Patients benefit from sexual health teaching. Many patients are uncomfortable initiating a discussion about sexual concerns and often need the nurse to begin.

Family involvement is an essential element of comprehensive care. Sexuality is a basic need and concern for both men and women, yet is one of the most difficult discussions for patients

†Intervention classification labels from Dochterman JM, Bulechek GM, editors: *Nursing interventions classification (NIC)*, ed 4, St. Louis, 2004, Mosby.

### EVALUATION

- Ask Mr. Taylor how effective he feels in his ability to identify and express feelings verbally and nonverbally.
- Monitor changes in Mr. Taylor's statements about himself.

- Observe Mr. Taylor's participation in self-care related to stroke.
- Assist Mr. Taylor in the identification of resources outside the hospital; secure a commitment to use resources.

---

ber of life changes occurring simultaneously, and excessive use of alcohol. These data are suggestive of actual or potential self-concept disturbances. You then talk with the patient to determine how she views the various lifestyle elements, to facilitate the patient's insight into behaviors, and to make appropriate referrals or provide needed health teaching.

Exploring a person's sexuality and providing useful sex education require good communication skills. Make sure the environment and timing provide privacy, uninterrupted time, and patient comfort. For example, discuss contraception methods with a woman in an office rather than in the examination room when she is only partially clothed. Plan the discussion so there are no interruptions, and sit down while showing your interest and readiness to support her needs.

Teaching topics on sexuality vary based on the age of the patient. Education offers explanation of normal developmental changes. For example, you talk to a school-age child about the appearance of breast buds or pubic hair. When discussing sexual health with patients of childbearing age, always consider your patient's cultural and religious beliefs regarding contraception. The discussion may include their desire for children, usual sexual practices, and acceptable methods of contraception. Review all methods of contraception to provide necessary information for an informed patient choice. Reinforce that the best method is the one the patient will use consistently. Teaching needs for an adult in-

clude details of physiological changes resulting from illness or from treatment effects. Box 20-8 summarizes special considerations for promoting sexual health in the older adult.

Individuals who have more than one sex partner or whose partner had other sexual experiences need to learn more about safe sex practices. Provide information on sexually transmitted disease transmission and symptoms, use of condoms, and high-risk sexual activities. Safe sex also means considering the patient's emotional risks within a relationship. Role play is a useful teaching tool to help the patient learn to say "no" or to negotiate with a partner to use a condom.

**ACUTE CARE.** In the acute care setting you are likely to encounter patients who are experiencing potential threats to their self-concept because of the nature of the treatment and diagnostic procedures. Threats to a patient's self-concept result in anxiety and/or fear. Numerous stressors, including unknown diagnoses, the need to make changes in lifestyle, and change in functioning, are present, and you need to address them. In the acute care setting there is often more than one stressor, thus increasing the overall stress level for the patient and the family.

You will also care for patients who are faced with the need to adapt to an altered body image as a result of surgery or other physical change. Often a visit by someone who has experienced similar changes and adapted to them is helpful. The timing of such a visit is important. Because addressing these needs are often difficult to do while in an acute care

BOX 20-8   PATIENT TEACHING

**Promoting Sexual Function for the Older Adult**

**Outcome**
- Patient attains satisfactory level of sexual activity as evidenced by resumption of sexual activity at a level acceptable to the patient and partner.

**Teaching Strategies**
- Provide teaching on normal sexual changes that occur with aging.
- Encourage partners to discuss what types of intimate behavior provide the most sexual stimulation and satisfaction.
- Discuss side effects of medications that commonly alter sexual function and response.
- Encourage selection of a time of day when the patient feels most rested.
- Explain that safe sex involves avoidance of multiple or anonymous partners, prostitutes, and other people with multiple sex partners; avoidance of sexual contact with a person who has a genital discharge or lesions or a medical diagnosis of human immunodeficiency virus (HIV) or hepatitis B; avoidance of genital contact with oral sores; and use of latex condoms and spermicides.
- Instruct females to use a water-based lubricant during intercourse to promote comfort.
- Encourage alternative positions for intercourse (e.g., side-lying, lying on a bed with legs over the side) that will decrease discomfort during intercourse.
- Inform partners that a longer period of foreplay helps the male to achieve penile firmness.
- Instruct couples to conserve strength by not working hard at the beginning of intercourse, so as to avoid tiring before climax.
- Discuss the use of foreplay and time for touching and talking.

**Evaluation Strategies**
- Ask patient and partner to verbalize plan for improved sexual health.
- Have patient verbalize when to consult primary care provider for additional options.

Modified from Meiner S, Lueckenotte A: *Gerontologic nursing* ed 3, St. Louis, 2006, Mosby.

setting, appropriate follow-up and referrals, including home care, are essential. You need to be sensitive to the patient's level of acceptance of the change. Forcing confrontation with the change before the patient is ready will delay the patient's acceptance. Signs that a person is receptive to such a visit include the patient's asking questions related to how to manage a particular aspect of what has happened or looking at the changed area. As the patient expresses readiness to integrate the body change into his or her self-concept, you either let the patient know about groups that are available or ask the patient if he or she wants you to make the initial contact. In addition, you facilitate adjustment to a change in physical appearance through your own response to the wound or change. As you respond with acceptance, you model acceptance for both the patient and the family.

Both physical and psychological aspects of illness have the potential to affect sexuality. Never assume that sexual functioning is not a concern merely because of an individual's age or severity of prognosis. After identifying concerns, address them in the context of the patient's value system. When a patient experiences physical limitations to sexual performance, provide the following suggestions: planning sexual activity when the patient is rested, experimenting with positions that are more comfortable, encouraging partners to give one another more time, and encouraging the use of foreplay to achieve arousal.

**RESTORATIVE AND CONTINUING CARE.** If you work in a home care or restorative care environment, you will have the opportunity to work with a patient to attain a more positive self-concept. Interventions designed to help a patient reach the goal of adapting to changes in self-concept or attaining a positive self-concept are based on the premise that the patient first develops insight and self-awareness concerning problems and stressors and then acts to solve the problems and cope with the stressors. You can incorporate this approach, outlined by Stuart and Laraia (2005), into patient teaching for alterations in self-concept, including situational low-self esteem, which is sometimes present in the home care setting (Box 20-9).

You increase the patient's self-awareness by establishing a trusting relationship that allows the patient to openly explore thoughts and feelings. A priority nursing intervention continues to be the expert use of communication skills to clarify the expectations of the patient and family. Open exploration will make the situation less threatening for the patient and encourages behaviors that expand self-awareness. You encourage the patient's self-exploration by accepting the patient's thoughts and feelings, by helping the patient to clarify interactions with others, and by being empathetic. You encourage self-expression and stress the patient's self-responsibility.

Promoting the patient's self-evaluation involves helping the patient define problems clearly and identify positive and negative coping mechanisms. You work closely with the patient to help analyze adaptive and maladaptive responses, consider alternatives, and discuss outcomes. Collaborating with the patient in establishing realistic goals involves helping the patient identify alternative solutions and develop realistic goals based on them. This facilitates real change and encourages further goal-setting behaviors. You design opportunities that result in success, reinforce the patient's skills and strengths, and assist the patient in getting needed assistance.

Helping the patient become committed to decisions and actions to achieve goals involves teaching the patient to move away from ineffective coping mechanisms and develop successful coping strategies. Supporting attempts that are health promoting is essential because with each success, the patient is more motivated to make another attempt at promoting health. Supporting adaptive, flexible coping is critical to inter-

## BOX 20-9 PATIENT TEACHING

### Alterations in Self-Concept

A home care nurse sees Mr. Taylor following discharge to his home. After meeting with Mr. and Mrs. Taylor, the home health nurse develops the following teaching plan:

### Outcome

- Mr. Taylor will reduce his risks for situational low self-esteem in the home care setting.

### Teaching Strategies

- Reinforce Mr. Taylor's expression of thoughts and feelings; clarify meaning of verbal and nonverbal communication.
- Encourage opportunities for Mr. Taylor to care for himself.
- Elicit Mr. Taylor's perceptions of strengths and weaknesses.
- Convey verbally and behaviorally that Mr. Taylor is responsible for his behavior.
- Identify relevant stressors, and ask for appraisal of them.
- Explore with Mr. Taylor his adaptive and maladaptive coping responses to problems.
- Collaboratively identify alternative solutions; encourage alternatives not previously tried.
- Continue to reinforce strengths and successes.

### Evaluation

- Confirm perception of and actual use of improved communication skills.
- Observe gradual increase in participation in decisions that affect care.
- Confirm with Mr. and Mrs. Taylor that the increase in activities and tasks has been a positive experience.
- Observe Mr. Taylor's establishment of a simple routine.
- Observe Mr. Taylor as he changes maladaptive coping responses and maintains adaptive ones.
- Confirm with Mr. and Mrs. Taylor how they will apply new coping resources during this time of change.

Modified from Stuart GW, Laraia MT: *Principles and practice of psychiatric nursing*, ed 8, St. Louis, 2005, Mosby.

vening in self-concept alterations. Patients who are experiencing threats to or alterations in self-concept often benefit from collaboration with mental health and community resources to promote increased awareness. Knowledge of available community resources allows you to make appropriate referrals.

You will frequently be in a position to establish relationships with couples that encourage honest and open discussions about sexual health. You address sexuality issues by taking a sexual health history and implementing a basic model such as PLISSIT to provide options for patients (see Box 20-7). Assessment and management of sexuality concerns is important as you promote sexual intimacy and provide closeness and closure between partners at the end of life (Stausmire, 2004). Give priority to patients in middle and older adulthood when you address sexuality concerns due to

illness, medications, or physical changes. Provide information on how the specific illness will limit sexual activity and ideas for adapting or facilitating sexual activity. Interventions range from giving permission for a partner to lie in bed and hold a patient to coordinating nursing care and medications in a way that provides opportunity for privacy and intimacy. In the home environment it is important to help patients create an environment comfortable for sexual activity. This sometimes involves making recommendations for ways to rearrange the patient's bedroom to accommodate any limitations. Patients and partners need to know how to accommodate barriers such as Foley catheters or drainage tubes that make sexual positioning difficult.

In the long-term care setting, facilities need to make proper arrangements for privacy during an older patient's sexual experience (Meiner and Lueckenotte, 2006). The ideal situation is to set up a pleasant room that is used for a variety of activities that the older adult is able to reserve for private visits with a spouse or partner. This is not always possible. Another option is to use the patient's room and make other arrangements for the patient's roommate. Although privacy of patients is important, do not leave patients alone in a situation in which they will injure themselves (Meiner and Lueckenotte, 2006).

Establishing a therapeutic relationship is critical to successfully intervening with patients who have alterations in self-concept, whether care is focused on health promotion, dealing with an acute process, or addressing restorative care. To support the development of a positive self-concept in a patient, convey genuine caring for the patient (see Chapter 16). Then, and only then, will you establish a partnership with the patient to address underlying problems.

## Evaluation

**PATIENT CARE.** Expected outcomes for a patient with a self-concept disturbance include nonverbal behaviors indicating a positive self-concept, statements of self-acceptance, and acceptance of change in appearance or function (Table 20-2). For example, a patient who has had difficulty making eye contact will demonstrate a more positive self-concept by making more frequent eye contact and smiling during conversation. Adequate self-care and acceptance of the use of prosthetic devices indicate progress. A positive attitude toward rehabilitation and increased movement toward independence facilitate a return to preexisting roles at work or at home. Patterns of interacting will often reflect changes in self-concept. For example, a patient who has been hesitant to express his or her views will more readily offer opinions and ideas as self-esteem increases.

Sometimes initial goals are unrealistic or require modification as the patient's condition changes. You and the patient will need to revise the plan. Patient adaptation to major changes sometimes take a year or longer, but the fact that this period is long does not suggest problems with adaptation. Look for signs that the patient has reduced some stressors and that some behaviors have become more adaptive.

## EVALUATION

Because Mr. Taylor was in the hospital for 2 weeks, Maria was able to care for Mr. Taylor and watch him recover from his stroke. On the last day Maria cares for Mr. Taylor, he reports that he has been accepted to a rehabilitation center that specializes in helping people who have had strokes. Mr. Taylor is able to do most of his bath independently, and although his gait is a little unsteady, he is able to walk short distances with a walker. During his bath he jokes, "I think my new haircut has made me look a lot younger!" This improvement in function and acceptance of self has helped Mr. Taylor become more satisfied with himself and his progress in therapy. He is hopeful that he will be able to return to work after he leaves the rehabilitation center. Both Mr. and Mrs. Taylor have worked with a therapist who specializes in helping couples who have sexual problems. Mr. Taylor states that the therapy sessions have helped him grow closer to his wife and have strengthened their relationship. Several of his bowling friends visited him last night. Mr. Taylor states, "I can't wait to get better. I have a lot of things to do, and I have a lot to live for."

**Documentation Note**

"Ability to perform ADLs improving. Only needs help to wash his back during the bath. Improvements in function have led to reports of enhanced self-esteem and acceptance of body image. Actively participates in sexual therapy with spouse and maintains relationships with friends. States is highly motivated to get better. Plans to continue to work on improving neurological deficits at the stroke rehabilitation center."

## OUTCOME EVALUATION

**TABLE 20-2**

| Nursing Action | Patient Response/Finding | Achievement of Outcome |
|---|---|---|
| Have Mr. Taylor verbalize his feelings about himself. | Mr. Taylor is frustrated with the slow recovery from his stroke. However, he improves a little each day. With each improvement, he states he feels better about his health and his abilities. | Self-esteem is improving, and he is beginning to accept himself despite his neurological deficits. |
| Ask Mr. Taylor to wash his face, brush his teeth, and comb his hair during his bath. | Mr. Taylor is able to wash his face and brush his teeth during his bath. He continues to struggle with combing his hair. He states, "I really need to get a better haircut to make it easier to comb my hair." | Ability to demonstrate basic grooming and hygiene needs met. |
| Ask Mr. Taylor to describe how his role has changed in his family and in his social life since his stroke; ask about his plans for rehabilitation after discharge from the hospital. | Mr. Taylor describes a conversation he had with his wife last night. He stated, "Although I can't work right now, Meredith is going to pick up some extra hours at her job to help make ends meet. Even though this is going to be a tough time, I know we will make it through this experience. I may not be able to bring home any money right now, but I can do other things around the house to help out. Meredith and I are committed to each other. We are so lucky to have each other." | Relationship with wife is strengthened. Is beginning to accept change in family role. |
| | Mr. Taylor describes how his friends have worked out a plan to take him to the bowling alley with them so he can "get out with my friends." | Social roles with friends are maintained. |
| | Mr. Taylor states, "I am determined to get better, so I will keep going to my rehabilitation classes until I have completely recovered." | Shows strong desire to continue with rehabilitation and to get better. |

This will require a follow-up discussion with the patient to determine if the level of satisfaction with sexual performance or sexual function has improved. Sometimes the patient has achieved the goal and outcome criteria, but sexual functioning is still not ideal. Consider what other steps will be appropriate. Changes in self-concept and sexuality take time. Although change is slow, care of the patient with a self-concept disturbance is rewarding.

**PATIENT EXPECTATIONS.** In evaluating care provided to patients with alterations in self-concept and sexual health, determine if the patient's expectations are met. After determining the achievement of targeted outcomes, ask if the patient thinks that nursing care was effective and supportive. Remain aware of any personal limitations in being able to counsel the patient. In some cases, referrals to other health care providers will still be necessary.

## KEY CONCEPTS

- Self-concept is an integrated set of conscious and unconscious attitudes and perceptions about the self.
- Components of self-concept are identity, body image, and role performance. Self-esteem and sexuality are closely related terms.
- Each developmental stage involves factors that are important to the development of a healthy, positive self-concept.
- Identity is particularly vulnerable during adolescence.
- Body image is the mental picture of one's body and is not necessarily consistent with a person's actual body structure or appearance.
- Body image stressors include changes in physical appearance, structure, or functioning caused by normal developmental changes or illness.
- Self-esteem is the emotional appraisal of self-concept and reflects the overall sense of being capable, worthwhile, and competent.
- Self-esteem stressors include developmental and relationship changes, illness (particularly chronic illness involving changes in what were normal activities), surgery, accidents, and the responses of other individuals to changes resulting from these events.
- The nurse's self-concept and nursing actions often have an effect on a patient's self-concept.
- Planning and implementing nursing interventions for self-concept disturbance involve expanding the patient's self-awareness, encouraging self-exploration, aiding in self-evaluation, helping formulate goals in regard to adaptation, and assisting the patient in achieving those goals.
- Sexuality is related to all dimensions of health. Therefore address sexual concerns or problems as part of nursing care.
- Sexual health involves physical and psychosocial aspects and contributes to an individual's sense of self-worth and positive interpersonal relationships.
- Development and life changes, ethical decisional issues, fertility, personal and emotional conflicts, illness, and hospitalization all affect a patient's sexuality.

## CRITICAL THINKING IN PRACTICE

*Mr. Cheng, a 23-year-old Asian-American patient, was in a motor vehicle accident and sustained multiple fractures to his face and a fractured femur (which was fixated through surgery on the evening of admission 4 days ago). He has been in the United States for 3 years and works as a janitor for a local university. He lives with his girlfriend and their 7-month-old daughter. You have been with him for most of the morning and find he is in moderate pain, which has been treated with morphine. The morphine has decreased his pain rating from a 7 to a 3 on a 10-point scale but has left him somewhat drowsy.*

*During the morning he has shared with you some of his concerns about when he will be able to return to work. He says to you, "I just want to get back to my normal self."*

- - - - - - - - - - - - - - - - - - - - - - - -

1. Describe how you would respond to Mr. Cheng's comment regarding "getting back to normal."
2. As you are teaching Mr. Cheng, you suspect he does not understand information about his rehabilitation. Describe the modifications you need to make in patient teaching.

## NCLEX® REVIEW

1. When developing an individualized treatment plan for a 15-year-old girl, you consider that a primary developmental task of adolescence is to:
   1. Form a sense of identity
   2. Create close intimate relationships with members of the opposite sex
   3. Achieve positive self-esteem through experimentation
   4. Separate from parents and live independently
2. No additional teaching is needed if your patient identifies normal changes in female sexual responses associated with aging as:
   1. Loss of sex drive
   2. Less clitoral response
   3. Less vaginal lubrication
   4. Loss of orgasm
3. Your teaching plan for a 70-year-old man includes discussing which normal change in male sexual response associated with aging?
   1. Loss of firm erection
   2. Loss of sex drive

   3. Increase in semen production
   4. Loss of ability to ejaculate
4. A depressed patient verbalizes feelings of low self-esteem and self-worth such as "I'm such a failure . . . I can't do anything right." The best nursing response is to:
   1. Tell the patient that is not true and that every person has a purpose in life
   2. Remain with the patient and sit in silence until the patient verbalizes his feelings
   3. Reassure the patient you know how he is feeling and that things will get better
   4. Review recent behaviors or accomplishments that demonstrate skill ability
5. The following involves the internal sense of individuality, wholeness, and consistency of a person over time and in various circumstances:
   1. Body image
   2. Self-concept
   3. Role performance
   4. Identity

6. Sexual health refers to:
   1. Having no sexually transmitted diseases
   2. Open and positive attitudes toward sexual functioning
   3. Consistent use of contraception
   4. Sexual activity with a member of the opposite sex

7. When you ask the patient, "How do you feel about yourself?" you are assessing the patient's:
   1. Sexual health
   2. Self-esteem
   3. Role performance
   4. Body image

## REFERENCES

Annon J: The PLISSIT model: a proposed conceptual scheme for the behavioral treatment of sexual problems, *J Sex Educ Ther* 2(2):1, 1976.

Brown SG, Barbosa G: Nothing is going to stop me now: low-income women as they become self-sufficient, *Public Health Nurs* 18(5):364, 2001.

Dochterman JM, Bulechek GM: *Nursing interventions classification (NIC),* ed 4, St. Louis, 2004, Mosby.

Ebersole P and others: *Gerontological nursing and healthy aging,* ed 2, St. Louis, 2005, Mosby.

Erikson E: *Childhood and society,* ed 2, New York, 1963, WW Norton.

Graber JA, Brooks-Gunn J: Adolescent girls' sexual development. In Winwood GM, DiClemente RJ, editors: *Handbook of women's sexual and reproductive health,* New York, 2002, Kluwer Academic/Plenum.

McSweeney JC, Coon S: Women's inhibitors and facilitators associated with making behavioral changes after myocardial infarction, *Medsurg Nurs* 13(1):49, 2004.

Meiner S, Lueckenotte A: *Gerontologic nursing,* ed 3, St. Louis, 2006, Mosby.

Moorhead S, Johnson M, Maas M: *Nursing outcomes classification (NOC),* ed 3, St. Louis, 2004, Mosby.

North American Nursing Diagnosis Association: *NANDA nursing diagnoses: definitions and classifications,* 2005-2006, Philadelphia, 2005, The Association.

Robins RW and others: Global self-esteem across the life span, *Psychol Aging* 17(3):423, 2002.

Rosenberg M: *Society and the adolescent self-image,* Princeton, NJ, 1965, Princeton University Press.

Sorrentino SA: *Mosby's textbook for nursing assistants,* ed 6, St. Louis, 2004, Mosby.

Stausmire J: Sexuality at the end of life, *Am J Hosp Palliat Care* 21(1):33, 2004.

Stuart GW, Laraia MT: *Principles and practice of psychiatric nursing,* ed 8, St. Louis, 2005, Mosby.

Twenge JM, Crocker J: Race and self-esteem: meta-analyses comparing whites, blacks, Hispanics, Asians, and American Indians, *Psychol Bull* 128(3):371, 2002.

Van Baarsen B: Theories on coping with loss: the impact of social support and self-esteem on adjustment to emotional and social loneliness following a partner's death in later life, *J Gerontol* 57(1):S33, 2002.

Voorhees CC and others: Early predictors of daily smoking in young women: the national Heart, Lung, and Blood Institute growth and health study, *Prev Med* 34:616, 2002.

# CHAPTER 21

# Family Context in Nursing

## MEDIA RESOURCES

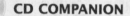

**CD COMPANION** *evolve* **WEBSITE**

http://evolve.elsevier.com/Potter/basic

- **NCLEX® Review**
- **Audio Glossary**
- **English/Spanish Audio Glossary**

## OBJECTIVES

- Examine current trends in the American family.
- Discuss how the term *family* is defined to reflect family diversity.
- Discuss common family forms and their health implications.
- Assess the way family structure and patterns of functioning affect the health of family members and the family as a whole.

- Interpret external and internal factors that promote family health.
- Compare family as context to family as patient and explain the way that these perspectives influence nursing practice.
- Use the nursing process to provide for the health care needs of the family.

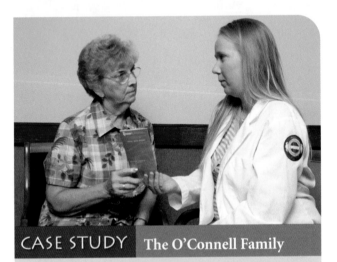

### CASE STUDY The O'Connell Family

Patrick and Michelle O'Connell have been married 9 years and live in Auburn, Maine. Patrick is 38 years old, and he has worked in the Department of Public Safety for the past 8 years. Recently he has learned that he is in danger of being laid off in the next round of cuts. Patrick has been diagnosed with borderline hypertension and admits his stress level is an 8 on a scale of 0 to 10. He enjoys watching TV, playing war games on the computer, and playing with the family's pet dogs and cats. The family has health insurance through Patrick's job. Michelle is 32 years old, is employed part-time as a receptionist at a building supply company, and attends nursing school. They are a childfree couple by choice. Michelle received a diagnosis of cervical cancer 3 months after their wedding and had a hysterectomy. Michelle is very worried about their financial problems and her grandmother's health problems, and she fears needing to work full-time. She describes herself as spiritual and attends church occasionally.

Michelle plays the role of keeping the couple connected to their blended and extended families. Because each of their parents divorced and have since either remarried or are cohabitating, they have four sets of parents and 28 step-, half, and whole brothers and sisters between them. Michelle manages the household duties and finances, works, and goes to school. She is the oldest daughter in her family and is the only one of the siblings to maintain routine contact with her 80-year-old grandmother, Lois. Michelle has learned from the visiting nurse that Lois's condition has worsened. She is becoming more forgetful and less tolerant of physical activity related to severe heart disease. Michelle worries about what she will do about this because

she lives 2 hours away. Lois needs support, and it is probable that this needed support will increase over time. Michelle worries that the only alternative is for Lois to move in with the O'Connells. If so, Michelle would have to rid the house of pets, which Lois is allergic to, and her home would require major renovations to accommodate her 80-year-old grandmother.

Bethany, age 28, is the nursing student assigned to Lois in her community health rotation. She sees Lois living alone in a clean mobile home in a nice park. She understands that Lois has been widowed 17 years and that she receives Social Security and has Medicare. However, she cannot afford supplemental insurance to pay for her medications. Bethany is concerned about Lois's financial situation, especially in light of the fact the visiting nurse has said Lois will soon need different living arrangements.

### KEY TERMS

family, p. 579
family as context, p. 583
family as patient, p. 583
family diversity, p. 579
family durability, p. 579
family forms, p. 579
family functioning, p. 582
family hardiness, p. 583
family health, p. 583
family resiliency, p. 579
family structure, p. 581

The family continues as a central institution in American society. The concept, structure, and functioning of the family unit continue to change over time. Although the family is in transition and looks very different from the families of the 1950s, the family unit is here to stay. Families face many challenges, including the impact of health and illness, childbearing and childrearing, changes in family structure and dynamics, and caring for an older parent. However, family characteristics or attributes, such as durability, resiliency, and diversity, assist in adapting to these challenges.

**Family durability** is the term for the intrafamilial system of support and structure that sometimes extends beyond the walls of the household. For example, Patrick and Michelle are part of a large extended family. Through divorce, remarriages, or cohabitation new members are added to their family. In addition, the extended family also includes contact with former spouses or partners. Michelle keeps the couple connected to this family. The players may change, the parents may remarry, the children may or may not leave home as adults, but the "family" transcends long periods and inevitable lifestyle changes.

**Family resiliency** is the ability to cope with expected and unexpected stressors. One stressor on the O'Connell family is Patrick's potential job loss. Not only does Patrick's job provide income and insurance benefits, it defines part of Patrick's role in the family. Both Patrick's and Michelle's resiliency will be shown in the way they adjust to this stressor. For example, if Michelle needs to resume full-time work with benefits, will Patrick be able and willing to take over household tasks and care for Lois? The family's ability to adapt to role changes, developmental milestones, and crises shows resilience (see Chapter 22). The goal of the family is not only to survive "the challenge" but also to thrive and grow as a result of the newly gained knowledge.

**Family diversity** is the attention to uniqueness. Some families will be experiencing marriage for the first time and having children in later life, whereas others are grandparents at the same age. Every person within a familial unit has specific needs, strengths, and important developmental considerations.

As nurses we are responsible for first understanding the makeup (configuration), structure, function, and coping capacity of the family and then building on the family's relative strengths and resources (Feeley and Gottlieb, 2000). The goal of family-centered nursing care is to promote, support, and provide for the well-being and health of the family and individual family members (Astedt-Kurki and others, 2002).

## Scientific Knowledge Base

### Concept of Family

For some the term *family* evokes a visual image of adults and children living together in a satisfying, harmonious manner. For others this term has the exact opposite image. Families represent more than a set of individuals, and a family is more than a sum of its individual members (Astedt-Kurki and others, 2001). Families are, however, as diverse as the individuals that compose them, and patients have deeply ingrained values about their families that deserve respect. Thus each individual defines the family. In other words, think of the **family** as a set of relationships that the patient identifies as family or as a network of individuals who influence each other's lives whether there are actual biological or legal ties (Figure 21-1).

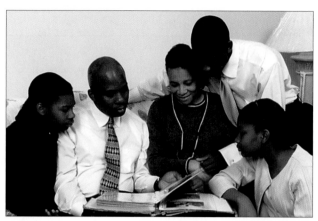

FIGURE **21-1** Family celebrations and traditions strengthen the family.

### Definition: What Is Family?

Defining *family* may at first seem simple. However, different definitions have resulted in heated debates among social scientists and legislators. The definition of family has a significant impact on who is included on health insurance policies, who has access to children's school records, who files joint tax returns, and who has eligibility for sick-leave benefits or public assistance programs. A family is a set of interacting individuals related by blood, marriage, or adoption, who are interdependent in carrying out the relative roles and responsibilities of the family unit (Astedt-Kurki and others, 2004). Your personal beliefs do not have to coincide with those of the patient. To provide individualized family care, you understand that families take many forms and have diverse cultural and ethnic orientations. In addition, no two families are alike. Each has its own strengths, weaknesses, resources, and challenges (Bell and others, 2001).

### Family Forms

**Family forms** are patterns of people who are considered to be family members. Although all families have some things in common, each family form has unique problems and strengths. As a nurse keep an open mind about what makes up a family so that you do not overlook potential resources and concerns. Box 21-1 describes several family forms.

**CURRENT TRENDS AND NEW FAMILY FORMS.** Families are smaller today. People are marrying later, women are delaying childbirth, and couples are choosing to have fewer children or none at all. The number of people living alone is expanding and accounts for approximately 26% of households. Divorce rates have tripled since the 1950s, and although the rate appears to have stabilized, it is estimated that 55% of all marriages will end in divorce (U.S. Bureau of the Census, 2001).

The number of single-parent families doubled from the 1970s to the 1990s but now appears to be stabilizing at about 26% of all families with children. Although mothers head 83% of single-parent families, father-only families are on the

<br>

**BOX 21-1** | **Family Forms**

**Nuclear Family**

This family consists of husband and wife (and perhaps one or more children).

**Extended Family**

This family includes relatives (aunts, uncles, grandparents, and cousins) in addition to the nuclear family.

**Single-Parent Family**

This family is formed when one parent leaves the nuclear family because of death, divorce, or desertion or when a single person decides to have or adopt a child.

**Blended Family**

This family is formed when parents bring unrelated children from prior or foster parenting relationships into a new, joint living situation.

**Alternate Patterns of Relationships**

These relationships include multiadult households, "skip-generation" families (grandparents caring for grandchildren), and communal groups with children, "nonfamilies" (adults living alone), cohabiting partners, and homosexual couples.

---

rise. Forty-one percent of children are living with mothers who have never married; many of these children are a result of an adolescent pregnancy (U.S. Bureau of the Census, 2001).

Adolescent pregnancy is an ever-increasing concern. The majority of these adolescents continue to live with their families. A teenage pregnancy tends to have long-term consequences for the mother and often severely stresses family relationships and resources. In addition, there is an increased risk for continued poverty for these families (SmithBattle, 2000). Teenage fathers also have stressors placed on them when their partner becomes pregnant. These young men have poorer support systems and fewer resources to teach them how to parent (James-Childs, 2000). As a result, both of these adolescents are often struggling with the normal tasks of development and identity but now are also forced to accept a responsibility that they are not ready for physically, emotionally, socially, and/or financially.

Although unable to marry by law in many states, homosexual couples define their relationship in family terms. Approximately half of all gay male couples live together, compared with three fourths of lesbian couples. Individuals in same-sex relationships have become more open about their sexual preference and more vocal about their legal rights.

The fastest-growing age-group is 65 years and older. For the first time in history the average American has more living parents than children, and children are more likely to have living grandparents and even great-grandparents. This "graying" of America has affected the family life cycle; it is perhaps most significant for the middle generation. These individuals are finding that they need to balance their own needs with those of their offspring and the needs of their aging parents. This balance often occurs at the expense of their own well-being and resources. In addition, many of these caregivers report that support received from professional health professionals is often lacking (Isaksen, Thuen, and Hanestad, 2003). The majority of these caregivers are women, who frequently provide an average of 18 hours of care per week (Farran, 2002). Caring for a frail or chronically ill relative is a primary concern for a growing number of families.

**FACTORS INFLUENCING FAMILY FORMS.** Families face many challenges, including changing structures and roles related to the changing economic status of society. There are family challenges related to divorce and the aging of its older members. There are three additional trends that social scientists identify as threats or concerns facing the family: (1) changing economic status (e.g., declining family income, need for dual incomes), decreased health insurance, or lack of access to health care; (2) homelessness; and (3) domestic violence (Voydanoff and Donnelly, 1999).

**Economic Factors.** Making ends meet is a daily concern for many people because of the declining economic status of families. Economics have particularly affected families at the lower end of the income scale, and single-parent families are especially vulnerable. Even though two-income families have become the norm, real family income has not increased since 1973. As a result, many families have inadequate or no health insurance and they have difficulty accessing health care.

**Homelessness.** Another factor influencing family forms is homelessness. The fastest growing segment of the homeless population is families with children. This includes complete nuclear families and single-parent families. In 2000, families with children accounted for 36% of the homeless population (National Coalition for the Homeless, 2001). Poverty, lack of affordable housing, chronic mental illness, and substance abuse are primary causes. Homelessness severely affects the functioning, health, and well-being of the family and its members. Children of homeless families are often in fair or poor health and have higher rates of asthma, ear infections, stomach problems, and mental illness. As a result, usually the only access to health care for these children is through the emergency department (Kushel and others, 2002).

In addition, these children face barriers, such as meeting residency requirements for public schools and inability to obtain previous enrollment records, when enrolling and attending school. As a result, these children are more likely to drop out of school and become unemployable (Shinn and others, 1998). Homeless families and their children are at serious risk for developing long-term health, psychological, and socioeconomic problems, thus posing a major challenge for our entire society (Kushel and others, 2002; Shinn and others, 1998).

**Domestic Violence.** Domestic violence may include not only the intimate partner relationships of spousal, live-in partners, and dating relationships, but also familial, elder, and child abuse may be present in a violent home. Abuse

| BOX 21-2 | USING EVIDENCE IN PRACTICE |
|---|---|

### Research Summary

In recent years domestic violence has become a significant problem in many families. In domestic violence, the abuser controls his or her victim. It affects both genders and all age-groups; children, spouses, and older adults are the direct recipients of the abuse. This same population also experiences the rippling effect of violence on other members of the family. Exposure to violence in a family affects a person's ability to concentrate and function. The symptoms of domestic violence are not always visible wounds. Other symptoms include but are not limited to altered sleep patterns, eating disorders, nightmares, flashbacks, depression, anxiety, and a fatalistic view of the future and intimate relationships. Children who observe domestic violence often place themselves at risk by protecting the victim, and they physically place themselves between the abuser and the victim. Victims of abuse cope in different ways; some victims become abusers, others become withdrawn and passive, still others cannot identify their own goals or needs. In addition, victims of abuse often unknowingly transfer some of the coping strategies to future relationships. For example, a child who witnessed abuse in the home may not become an abusive adult but may always assume the role of "peacekeeper" and go to lengths to avoid conflict. The woman who suffers abuse may not be able to develop any type of trusting relationships. Older adults who are victims of abuse often have no mechanism to report the abuse because they are often dependent on the abuser for basic needs, transportation to and from physician's or health care provider's visits, and financial support. It is important to note that when the abuse victim is finally able to leave the abusive situation, the risk for further and even fatal abuse increases significantly.

### Application to Nursing Practice

Data from these studies identify effective screening procedures during initial assessment and treatment, especially in emergency department and urgent care facilities. It is during this time that the abuse victim has the most privacy and the abuser is not present. Child abuse must always be reported; in addition, many states have mandatory reporting laws for domestic violence. When abuse is disclosed, it is important to protect the victim, which in many cases necessitates a call to law enforcement and initially removing the victim from the home until the abuser can be located, arrested, and removed from the home. The victim also needs compassion and reinforcement that he or she is not the cause of the abuse; no one should feel that the abuse was his or her fault. Social service specialists in health care organizations are skillful in placing victims in safe houses and identifying appropriate community, emotional, and financial resources. When the wounds of abuse are present, skillful documentation of the wounds with a camera or videotape is essential. It is important to protect the victim's privacy and dignity during photo documentation. The use of gender-congruent care providers is often preferred to access, document, and initiate treatment for the abuse. When a victim is discharged from health care, it is important to educate the victim as to how best to protect himself or herself and what options are available and to provide phone numbers for referral agencies.

Data from Alpert EJ and others: "Challenges and strategies" and "evidence-based care," *Violence Against Women* 8(6):639, 2002; Dienemann J and others: Developing a domestic violence program in an intercity academic health center emergency department: the first 3 years, *J Emerg Nurs* 25(2):110, 1999; Lewis-O'Connor A: 'Dying to Tell?': Do mandatory reporting laws benefit victims of domestic violence? *Am J Nurs* 104(10):75, 2004.

---

generally falls into one or more of the following categories: physical battering, sexual assault, and emotional or psychological abuse; and it generally escalates over a period of time (National Coalition Against Domestic Violence [NCADV], 2005). The statistics regarding family violence are disturbing and difficult to calculate because researchers do not use a common definition of abuse. Some only count victims of physical abuse, whereas others include data for both physical and sexual abuse. Still other investigators also include emotional abuse (Lewis-O'Connor, 2004). In 1991 27 million children were reported abused or neglected, up from 1.1 million in the preceding 11 years. The need for foster care increased by almost 50% (Stanhope and Lancaster, 2004). The inflicting of emotional and physical pain on family members occurs in more than half of all households in the United States; approximately 50 million people are victimized each year. Emotional, physical, and sexual abuse occurs toward spouses, children, older adults, and across all social classes. The cause of family violence is complex and multidimensional. Stress, poverty, social isolation, psychopathology, and learned family behavior are all factors associated with violence (Box 21-2).

In addition, other factors such as alcohol and drug abuse, pregnancy, sexual orientation, and mental illness increase the incidence of abuse within a family (Robrecht, 1998). Although abuse sometimes ends when a person leaves a specific family environment, there are often negative long-term physical and emotional consequences. One of these consequences includes moving from one abusive situation to another (Richardson and others, 2002). For example, a child sees marriage as a way to leave an abusive home and in turn marries a person who will continue the abuse within the marriage (Wathen and MacMillan, 2003).

**STRUCTURE AND FUNCTION.** Each family has a unique structure and way of functioning. **Family structure** is based on organization (i.e., the ongoing membership of the family and the pattern of relationships). Relationships are often numerous and complex. For example, a woman's relationships include wife-husband, mother-son, and mother-daughter and employee-boss, boss-employee, and work colleague-colleague, each with different demands, roles, and expectations.

Although the definitions of structure vary, you can assess family structure by asking the following questions: "Who is included in the family?" "Who performs which tasks?" and "Who makes which decisions?" Structure either enhances or detracts from the family's ability to respond to the expected and unexpected stressors of daily life. Structures that are too rigid or flexible can threaten family functioning. Rigid structures specifically dictate who accomplishes different tasks and also limits the number of persons outside the immediate family allowed to assume these tasks. For example, in a rigid family the mother is the only acceptable person to provide emotional support for the children and/or to perform all of the household chores. The husband is the only acceptable person to provide financial support, maintain the vehicles, do the yard work, and/or do all of the home repairs. A change in the health status of the person responsible for a task places a burden on a rigid family because no other person is available, willing, or considered acceptable to assume

that task (Call and others, 1999). An extremely flexible structure also presents problems for the family. There is sometimes an absence of stability that would otherwise lead to automatic action during a crisis or rapid change.

Vaughan-Cole and others (1998) describe functioning as "what the family does." **Family functioning** involves the processes used by the family to achieve its goals. These processes include communication among family members, goal setting, conflict resolution, nurturing, and use of internal and external resources. The reproductive, sexual, economic, and educational goals once considered central family goals no longer apply to all families. Although many families pursue these goals at various times during their development, the provision of psychological support remains an important goal throughout the life span.

**DEVELOPMENTAL STAGES.** Families, like individuals, change and grow over time. Although families are far from identical to one another, they have a basic pattern and similarity in experiences resulting in predictable stages. Each of these developmental stages has its own challenges, needs,

| TABLE 21-1 | Stages of the Family Life Cycle | |
|---|---|---|
| **Family Life Cycle Stage** | **Emotional Process of Transition: Key Principles** | **Changes in Family Status Required to Proceed Developmentally** |
| Unattached young adults | Accepting parent-offspring separation | Differentiation of self in relation to family of origin<br>Development of intimate peer relationships<br>Establishment of self in work |
| Joining of families through marriage: newly married couple | Commitment to new family system | Formation of marital system<br>Realignment of relationships with extended families and friends to include spouse |
| Family with young children | Accepting new generation of members into system | Adjusting marital system to make space for children<br>Taking on parenting roles<br>Realignment of relationships with extended family to include parenting and grandparenting roles |
| Family with adolescents | Increasing flexibility of family boundaries to include children's independence | Shifting of parent-child relationships to permit adolescents to move into and out of system<br>Refocus on midlife marital and career issues<br>Beginning shift toward concerns for older generation |
| Launching children and moving on | Accepting multitude of exits from and entries into family system | Renegotiation of marital system as couple or unit of only two<br>Development of adult-to-adult relationships between grown children and their parents<br>Realignment of relationships to include in-laws and grandchildren<br>Dealing with disabilities and death of parents (grandparents) |
| Family in later life | Accepting shifting of generational roles | Maintaining own or couple functioning and interests in the face of physiological decline; exploration of new familial and social role options<br>Support for more central role for middle generation<br>Making room in system for wisdom and experience of older adults; supporting older generation without overfunctioning for them<br>Retirement; change in role<br>Dealing with loss of spouse, siblings, and other peers, and preparation for own death; life review and integration |

Data from Vaughan-Cole B and others: *Family nursing practice,* St. Louis, 1998, Mosby.

and resources and includes tasks that need to be completed before the family is able to successfully move on to the next stage (Table 21-1).

**FAMILY AND HEALTH. Family health** influences family functioning. The family is the primary social context in which health promotion and disease prevention take place. The family's beliefs, values, and practices strongly influence health-promoting behaviors of its members (Hartrick, 2000). When the family satisfactorily meets its goals through adequate functioning, its members tend to feel positive about themselves and their family. Conversely, when they do not meet goals, families view themselves as ineffective. Constant stress resulting from inadequate functioning adversely affects an individual family member's health (Voydanoff and Donnelly, 1999). Constant stress disrupts cardiovascular function, blood pressure, and circulating neuroendocrine substances, and these disruptions cause poor health (see Chapter 22).

Good health is not always highly valued; in fact, harmful practices are acceptable in some families. A long-term illness in one of the family member's affects the well-being and health of the entire family (Tarkka and others, 2003). Although illness strains relationships, research indicates that family members have the potential to be a primary force for coping.

Although a family is often a source of stress, a family's hardiness and resiliency are factors that moderate a family's stress. **Family hardiness** is defined as the internal strengths and durability of the family unit. Some characteristics of family hardiness are a sense of control over the outcome of life, a view of change as beneficial and growth-producing, and an active rather than passive orientation in adapting to stressful events (McCubbin, McCubbin, and Thompson, 1996). Resiliency helps to evaluate healthy responses when individuals and families are experiencing stressful events. Resources and techniques a family or individuals within the family use to maintain a balance or level of health assist in understanding a family's level of resiliency (Svavarsdottir, McCubbin, and Kane, 2000).

and maintain maximum health throughout and beyond the illness experience (Tapp, 2004).

A family nursing focus includes both **family as context** and **family as patient** (Figure 21-2). Both approaches recognize that a nursing intervention for one member influences all members and affects family functioning. Families are continually changing. As a result, the need for family support changes over time, and it is important for you to understand that the family is more complex than simply a combination of individual members (Newby, 1996; Tapp, 2004).

**FAMILY AS CONTEXT.** When you view the family as context, your primary focus is on the health and development of an individual member existing within a specific environment (i.e., the patient). Although you focus the nursing process on the individual's health status, you will also assess the extent to which the family provides the individual's basic needs. These needs vary, depending on the individual's developmental level and situation. Because families provide more than just material essentials, you need to consider their ability to help the patient meet psychological needs.

**FAMILY AS PATIENT.** When you view the family as patient, the family processes and relationships (e.g., parenting or family caregiving) are your primary focus of care. Your nursing assessment focuses on family patterns versus individual characteristics. The nursing process concentrates on the extent to which these patterns and processes are consistent with reaching and maintaining family and individual health.

**FAMILY AS SYSTEM.** It is important to understand that although you will make theoretical and practical distinctions between the family as context and the family as patient, they are not necessarily mutually exclusive. You will use both simultaneously, such as with the perspective of the family as system. When you view the family as a system, you will see that the impact one member has creates a "trickle-down" effect. This affects all members of the family, including the extended family members (Duhamel and Talbot, 2004).

## Nursing Knowledge Base

To begin work with families, you need a scientific knowledge base in family theory and an adequate knowledge base in family nursing. The two concepts interact to affect the care that you deliver to the family. All practice settings and all health care environments emphasize family nursing.

### Family Nursing: Family as Context, as Patient, and as System

In caring for a family, your goal is to help the family and its individual members reach and maintain maximum health in any given situation. Family nursing is based on the assumption that all people regardless of age are a member of some type of family form (see Box 21-1). The goal of family nursing is to help the family and its individual members reach

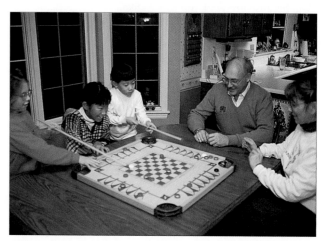

FIGURE **21-2** Observing family interactions assists in understanding family functioning.

## Critical Thinking

Critical thinking is crucial in the care of patients and their families. As a nurse you must synthesize all aspects of critical thinking to give appropriate family care. The care of a family is an ongoing mutually acceptable relationship. As you begin to provide family-centered care, you will continually assess, analyze, and reflect on the changing needs and health care goals of your patients and their families.

### Synthesis

A scientific and family nursing knowledge base enables you to identify the needs of both patients and their families. Synthesis of this knowledge enables you to assess the family as context, as patient, or as a system and to gain information about the family life-cycle perspective, family structure and functioning, and family health. Combine knowledge about the family and its functioning with nursing knowledge of holistic practice.

**KNOWLEDGE.** The health and functioning of each member in the family to some degree depends on the health of the family system as a whole. Family care draws on knowledge from growth and development, psychology, family theories, sociology, and the family life-cycle. When a family is in a transitional phase of the life-cycle perspective (e.g., birth of a first child) or there is an additional stressor to the family unit (e.g., chronic illness), it creates considerable anxiety within the family system. Knowledge of stress and coping will assist in family care.

**EXPERIENCE.** Your past experiences in a related situation often helps you to problem solve. We all draw on life experience even if we are not able to draw on nursing knowledge. Experiences with your own family members will assist you in designing family-centered care. For example, you remember how illness brought family members closer together because they all shared duties, roles, and responsibilities, or perhaps such an event pulled families apart. Consider carefully your use of experience-related information, because no two families are alike.

**ATTITUDES.** You will identify the patient's needs and begin to solve problems by keeping an open mind and applying creativity, perseverance, and risk taking. Respect for your patient's family structure and function, beliefs, values, and expectations enables you to develop a comprehensive, multidisciplinary plan *in partnership with* the patient and family.

**STANDARDS.** As a nurse you will apply nursing standards (e.g., critical care, obstetrical, or gerontological) in a variety of health care settings, such as home care, acute care, or long-term care. In addition, it is important to apply ethical principles when supporting family decisions, such as assisting family members with accepting the advanced directives of their loved ones. Because you will provide a portion of family-centered care in community-based, clinic, or restorative care settings, as well as in the acute care setting,

any information about the family must be kept confidential. In family-centered care there may be many health care providers, so be sure to document the pertinent information accurately and consistently.

## Nursing Process

The nursing process is the same whether the focus is family as patient or family as context or family as system. It is also the same as that used with individuals and incorporates the needs of the family and those of the patient.

 ### Assessment

It is essential for you to assess the patient and family (Table 21-2). The family as a whole differs from individual members. The measure of family health is more than a summation of the health of all members. Areas included in family assessment are the form, structure, and function of the family; its developmental stage, and its progress toward or accomplishment of developmental tasks. Begin assessment by considering the views of the patient toward the family. To determine the family form and membership, ask the patient to tell you about the family: "Who do you consider your family?" or "Who do you share your concerns with?" If the patient is unable to express a concept of family, ask with whom the patient lives, spends time, and shares confidences. Then ask the patient to confirm that people mentioned are his or her family: "Do you consider this person to be family or like family to you?"

It is also important to assess family structure and function. Family structure provides information about composition of the family, for example, is it a nuclear or extended family. To assess family structure it is helpful to determine who is the head of the household, who is the wage earner, and who maintains the household. To assess the family functioning, ask questions that determine the power structure and patterning of roles and tasks. For example, "How are financial decisions made?" "Who makes decisions for the family?" "How are the tasks divided in your family (e.g., who does the laundry, who mows the lawn)?" and "Who decides on where to go on vacation?"

A family's cultural background (see Chapter 17) is an important variable when assessing the family because race and ethnicity affect structure, function, health beliefs, values, and the way they perceive events (Box 21-3). The United States is increasingly more diverse. A large number of immigrants enter the country daily, adding to both the number and the variety of the many ethnic groups that make up the population. American health care institutions tend to operate from a white, middle-class perspective, and immigrant populations often have particular difficulty understanding and "fitting into" the system.

Forming conclusions about families' needs based on cultural backgrounds requires critical thinking and careful con-

## FOCUSED PATIENT ASSESSMENT

**TABLE 21-2**

| Factors to Assess | Questions and Approaches | Physical Assessment Strategies |
|---|---|---|
| Family resources | Ask if there are significant relatives and friends not occupying immediate residence.<br>What are the family's strengths and coping skills?<br>How does the family obtain health services? | When possible, observe family member interaction.<br>Review past medical experiences of the family.<br>Observe communication patterns with individual family members. |
| Family patterns | Ask who works outside the home, type of work, and hours worked.<br>Determine how they do household chores (e.g., housekeeping, shopping, repairs).<br>Ask how they divide child-rearing responsibilities.<br>Determine **decision-making strategies** (e.g., day-to-day decisions, financial decisions, health care decisions). | Observation of family members as they make decisions (e.g., regarding health care, discharge planning) will help obtain this information. Obtaining family pattern information requires long-term interaction with the family unit. |
| Family function | Ask about family's short- and long-term goals regarding a variety of subjects (e.g., child rearing, retirement, health care).<br>Ask individual members about their own short and long-term goals.<br>Ask if they changed their realization of goals as a result of current health problems. | Observe communication and interaction patterns within the family. |

## SYNTHESIS IN PRACTICE

Bethany assesses Lois's health care demands and basic physiological needs. She analyzes the role strain on Michelle and how this affects her relationship with Patrick. She also is aware of the impact of stress on Patrick's hypertension. She operates under the ethical principle of beneficence and tries to do the most good for the most people in this case. She understands that Lois wants to stay in her home and Michelle wants Lois to do what will make her happiest. Patrick wants Michelle to do whatever will not aggravate Michelle's stress level or force her to quit school, because soon they will have to depend on more income from her.

If the Bethany views the family as the context, she will focus on the each member of the family. Lois's changes in health affect the family greatly, and care is directed toward improving Lois's level of health as much as possible and maximizing her independence. Bethany helps Michelle to reduce stress by teaching her relaxation and meditation techniques, helping her to plan "down time," and giving her some time management techniques. Bethany assesses Patrick's knowledge of ways to manage his blood pressure (e.g., strategies for reducing the number of high-sodium foods in the diet, realistic opportunities to reduce the number and extent of perceived stressors in work and family environments, and knowledge and skill in stress management such as re-laxation or biofeedback techniques). She teaches him the same meditation technique she gave to Michelle, and she encourages the couple to do relaxation exercises and meditation together.

If she views the family as a patient, Bethany will assess the family's goals for Lois's care and independence. She will assess the resources available to the family as they assume the role of caregiver. She must also determine what the family perceives as their caregiving strengths and needs, as well as the demands of caregiving. In working with the family Bethany will observe the impact that caregiving will have on Lois, Michelle and Patrick, and the extended family. She will also assess the family's capabilities to support Lois and each other as Lois's health care needs increase and her independence declines.

If Bethany views the family as a system, she will use elements of family as context and family as patient. Bethany will need to work with the entire family to help Lois transition from her own home. One solution to this problem may be to help the family select an assisted living community located half-way between the O'Connell home and the homes of the other members of the extended family. Bethany helps the family make this difficult decision based on several factors, including expendable time and financial resources.

sideration. It is imperative to remember that categorical generalizations are often misleading (e.g., Asian-Americans consume low-fat diets). Overgeneralizations in terms of racial and ethnic group characteristics do not lead to greater understanding of the culturally diverse family. Culturally different families vary in meaningful and significant ways; however, neglecting to examine similarities will lead to inaccurate assumptions and stereotyping (see Chapter 17).

To determine the influence of culture on a family, you might want to ask the patient about his or her cultural background. Then ask questions concerning cultural practices. For example, "What type of foods do you eat?" "Who cares

**BOX 21-3** CULTURAL FOCUS

Bethany knows that families have their unique perspectives and characteristics. Families have differences in values, beliefs, and philosophies. The differences range from traditional nuclear families, to single-parent families, to extended families. The cultural heritage of the family or member of the family affects religious, child-rearing, and nutritional practices; recreational activities; and health promotion behaviors. As she studies and reviews the literature Bethany learns that nurses need to have cultural competence and sensitivity when caring for culturally diverse patients. Incorporating cultural preferences into the plan of care increases the patient's adherence to therapy, assists in transition from hospital to home, and provides a unique aspect to the patient's care.

**Implications for Practice**

- Perception of certain events varies across cultural groups and has particular impact on families. For example, the care of the grandmother has a great significance to the extended family.
- Caregiving values and practices vary across cultures. Bethany knows that in some cultures it is a sign of disrespect to your elders to place them in nursing homes, even those older adults with severe dementia. Bethany knows that Lois's family wants to assist her in living as independently as possible.
- Intergenerational support and patterns of living arrangements are related to cultural background. For example, older Chinese, African-American, Japanese, and Hispanic persons are more likely to live in extended family households than whites.
- Health beliefs differ among various cultures, which affect the decision of a family and its members about when and where to seek help. For example, Asians rarely consider symptoms as psychological and are not likely to go to mental health clinics.

Data from Cox C, Monk A: Strain among caregivers: comparing the experiences of African-American and Hispanic caregivers of Alzheimer's relatives, *Int J Aging Hum Dev* 43(2):93, 1996; Kamo Y, Zhou M: Living arrangements of elderly Chinese and Japanese in the United States, *J Marriage Fam* 56(3):544, 1994; Feeley N, Gottlieb LN: Nursing approaches for working with family strengths and resources, *J Fam Nurs* 6(1):9, 2000.

for sick family members?" "Have you or anyone in your family been hospitalized?" "Did family members remain at the hospital?" "Do you use some of your culture's health practices, such as acupuncture or meditation?" "What role do grandparents play in raising your children?"

A comprehensive, culturally sensitive family assessment is critical to forming an understanding of family life, current changes in family life, and overall goals and expectations. These data provide the foundation for future family-centered nursing care (Anderson, 2000).

Assessment of family functions include the ability to provide emotional support for members, the ability to cope with their current health problem or situation, the appropriateness of their goal setting, and progress toward achievement of tasks of the developmental stage. Because families' goals vary,

make sure measures of family health are flexible. During assessment, assess whether the family is able to provide and distribute sufficient economic resources and if the family's social network is extensive enough to provide support.

The family's home environment and community are also assessed. When assessing the patient's home, determine the size of the home, provision for privacy, and safety factors, such as safe bathrooms, stairwells, and smoke detectors (see Chapter 26). When assessing the community, determine the presence of health care resources, proximity of emergency services, and municipal services (see Chapter 3). If there is a strong extended family, what is the proximity of that extended family to the patient? Do they live together, in the same neighborhood, or the same city? If the family lives together, how large is the space?

**PATIENT EXPECTATIONS.** Families, like individual patients, have certain expectations for care. Some families expect to be consulted as a whole unit when discussing care of their loved one. Others wish to have a designated decision maker. The family sometimes expects the health care system to meet all of their needs, not only those related to health issues. When assessing the family's expectations, be clear whether the family is the patient and receiver of care or whether the family member is the patient and receiver of care. Determining these expectations early in the assessment will help to avoid problems resulting from misunderstandings in the future.

## Nursing Diagnosis

Nursing assessment results in clustering relevant data that support nursing diagnoses and identifying areas in which functioning is inadequate or deficient and intervention is needed. The nursing diagnoses selected often include the family's health needs, current and potential health problems, level of wellness, or a combination of these areas. Some examples of nursing diagnoses for family-focused care include:

- Risk for caregiver role strain
- Compromised family coping
- Disabled family coping
- Readiness for enhanced family coping
- Interrupted family processes
- Impaired parenting
- Ineffective role performance
- Readiness for enhanced spiritual well-being
- Risk for other-directed violence

The nursing diagnosis often focuses on the family's ability to cope with its current situation, whether it is an acute illness, an anticipated developmental transition, or negative behaviors that threaten short-term or long-term health. Appropriate use of internal and external resources allows the family to cope with day-to-day challenges and with unexpected occurrences that threaten health and equilibrium. The nursing diagnosis also focuses on changes in family processes or roles of members. During times of acute illness the family becomes extremely distressed and focuses solely on the ill member, neglecting the needs of the other family members. For example, you will always consider the diagnosis of *risk for caregiver role strain* a possibility when long-term care of a family member is necessary.

In addition, the diagnostic statement indicates possible related factors. For example, *unrealistic expectations* is a possible related factor, because in the case study Michelle initially wanted to assume responsibility for Lois. However, as the scenario evolved, Michelle became more stressed when trying to handle all the demands of care. In this case the nursing diagnosis *risk for caregiver role strain related to unrealistic expectations* is appropriate. Another potential nursing diagnosis, *interrupted family processes related to caregiving demands,* is due to a change in the relationship between Michelle and Patrick. Because of the caregiving demands, Michelle and Patrick are not able relax and spend time together as a couple.

## Planning

**GOALS AND OUTCOMES.** After you develop nursing diagnoses, the next step is to plan care with the family. Goal setting is mutual, and the goals need to be concrete, realistic, compatible with the family's developmental stage, and acceptable to the family.

A family-focused approach enhances nursing practice. Goals for a care plan that incorporates a family approach include those that view the family as patient or the family as context or a combination of the two. The patient situation and availability of family members dictate the type of goals that are feasible. A broad goal is "The family functions at its optimal level," with the expected outcome being "Communication between family members is appropriate, direct, and clear." Family members are able to confront and resolve conflict in a healthy way. *The broader the goals, however, the less measurable and practical they become.* For specific examples, see the care plan.

**SETTING PRIORITIES.** Setting priorities focuses on the patient, the patient/family unit, or the family alone. It is imperative that the family and the patient clearly understand and agree on the plan of care and priorities. The priorities for the patient and family are sometimes different. For example, the priority for your patient is to obtain physiological or emotional stability, self-care, or progress to a rehabilitation facility. However, the family priorities include obtaining temporary housing so they are near their ill family member, spiritual support, assistance with decision making, or understanding the complexities of the health care delivery system. In some instances the priorities of the family and patient are different but require simultaneous interventions.

**CONTINUITY OF CARE.** Collaboration with family members is essential, whether the family is the patient or the context of care. You base a positive collaborative relationship on mutual respect and trust (Figure 21-3 ). The nurse's ability to care facilitates the building of trust. The family needs to feel "in control" as much as possible. By offering alternative

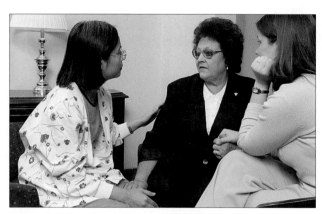

FIGURE **21-3** Nurse and family members.

actions and asking family members for their own ideas and suggestions, you will help to reduce the family's feelings of powerlessness. For example, offering options for how to prepare a low-fat diet or how to rearrange the furnishings of a room to accommodate a family member's disability gives the family an opportunity to express their preferences, make choices, and ultimately feel as though they have contributed. Collaborating with other disciplines, such as physical therapy and social service, increases the likelihood of a comprehensive approach to the family's health care needs, and it ensures better continuity of care. Using other disciplines is particularly important when discharge planning from a health care facility to home or an extended care facility is necessary (Neabel, Fothergill-Bourbonnais, and Dunning, 2000).

## Implementation

Whether you are caring for a patient with the family as context, as patient, or as system, you direct your nursing interventions to increase family members' abilities in certain areas, to remove barriers to health care, and to do things that the family cannot do for itself. You need to guide the family in problem solving, provide practical services, and convey a sense of acceptance and caring by listening carefully to family members' concerns and suggestions.

For example, as a health educator, you provide accurate health information about diagnosis and prognosis that helps the family caregiver to understand and anticipate needs and concerns of a care recipient. Caregivers are not born with the knowledge of how to be caregivers, and older adults are not born with the knowledge of how to accept dependency (Box 21-4). A moderately flexible structure is generally most beneficial to the family. Nursing interventions will therefore involve changing the family patterns away from extremely rigid or flexible structures if either extreme causes problems related to the health of an individual or the family as a whole. Work within the family structure when providing care, and do not attempt to change the structure.

**HEALTH PROMOTION.** It is important to include health promotional activities as part of your family-centered

## CARE PLAN  Compromised Family Coping

**ASSESSMENT**

Patrick and Michelle are **caregivers to Michelle's grandmother,** Lois, who has heart disease, and who is still living in her own home. Lois suffers fatigue and forgetfulness and poses numerous caregiving demands. She frequently **complains about how Michelle offers assistance** with household chores. Michelle and Patrick have frequent arguments over how to best help Lois, because they live 2 hours away. Patrick has been experiencing **an increase in his blood pressure,** he **complains about the time Michelle spends with her grandmother, and the amount of time she spends worrying about her grandmother,** and he admits to **doing less around the home to help Michelle.** Michelle is **not eating regularly** and has **difficulty sleeping, is fearful of "not doing things well for her grandmother,"** and **feels anxious.** They both share concerns as to what will happen to Lois.

*Defining characteristics are shown in bold type.

**NURSING DIAGNOSIS** Caregiver role strain related to increasing needs and unrealistic expectations.

**PLANNING**

**GOAL**

- Michelle and Patrick will gain improved understanding of stress and adaptive management techniques within 1 month.



- Patrick will accept Michelle's household role limitations.



- Patrick and Michelle will seek out and use additional resources if needed within 1 month.

**EXPECTED OUTCOMES***
**Caregiver Well-Being**

Michelle and Patrick will be able to identify and share four caregiving activities within 1 week.

Michelle and Patrick will demonstrate correct meditation techniques within 1 month.

Michelle and Patrick will meditate together 4 nights a week within 6 weeks.

Patrick will assume responsibility for laundry and groceries within 2 weeks.

Patrick will not demonstrate impatient behavior (if tasks are not done at home) while wife performs some caregiving activities within 1 week.

Michelle and Patrick will obtain a biweekly house-cleaning service within 3 weeks.

*Outcomes classification label from Moorhead S, Johnson M, Maas M: *Nursing outcomes classification (NOC),* ed 3, St. Louis, 2004, Mosby.

**INTERVENTIONS†**

*Caregiver Support*
- Discuss with Patrick and Michelle the effects of stress on themselves and the family.
- Teach them techniques, relaxation exercises, and meditation to reduce their response to stress.



- Provide a list of support services, such as hospice volunteers and respite care, for Patrick and Michelle.



- Contact community support groups, such as hospice or American Heart Association, to obtain a list of reputable housecleaning services.
- Consult with Patrick and Michelle to establish a list of community resources, assisted living facilities, and family support to assist with caregiver tasks.

**RATIONALE**

Identification of specific stressors and the effects of the stress on an individual or group need to occur before techniques to reduce the stress will be effective (Vaughan-Cole and others, 1998). Caring and support through listening and accepting the needs and expectations of the members of the family enhance coping (Maijala and others, 2004).

Intergenerational assistance is complex and at times requires some support. Identification of community-based support groups is one means to provide assistance to the caregiver in adjusting to the increased responsibilities (Voydanoff and Donnelly, 1999).

Community service groups frequently maintain lists of reputable household service providers. Such a listing assists the family in identifying the service in a timely manner.

A potential list of resources provides the family with an organized system of providing supportive, safe care for an older adult who is living in the community (Abbott, Shaw, and Bryar, 2004).

†Intervention classification labels from Dochterman JM, Bulechek GM, editors: *Nursing interventions classification (NIC),* ed 4, St. Louis, 2004, Mosby.

**EVALUATION**
- Observe Michelle and Patrick during their meditation exercises.
- Ask Patrick and Michelle to describe caregiving activities they performed.
- Observe Patrick interacting with Michelle during home visit for signs of frustration and violent temper that will frustrate Michelle's functioning and her caregiving activities for Lois.

- Ask how the biweekly house-cleaning service is working out.
- Ask Patrick and Michelle to describe visits to community resources or assisted living facilities.

## CARE OF THE OLDER ADULT

- Consider caregiver role strain; caregivers are usually either spouses, who are sometimes older adults with declining physical stamina, or middle-age children, who often have other responsibilities.
- Later-life families have a different social network than younger families because friends and same-generation family members have died or become ill themselves.
- Identify social support for the family within the community and church affiliation.
- Greater physical health impairment increases the risk of the older adult's depression.
- The demands of caregiving increase the caregiver's risk for social isolation.
- As in the other stages of life, members of later-life families need to be working on developmental tasks. For example, it may be important for the patient to reminisce about the past. Reinforce to the caregiver that repetition of the reminiscence is normal (see Chapter 19).

nursing care. When implementing family nursing, you will need health promotion interventions to improve or maintain the physical, social, emotional, and spiritual well-being of the family unit and its members (Ford-Gilboe, 2002). Encourage patients and families to reach their optimum level of wellness. "Strong" families that adapt to transitions, crises, and change tend to have clear communication, problem-solving skills, a commitment to each other and to the family unit, and a sense of cohesiveness and spirituality. Prevention programs aimed at enhancing or developing these attributes are available for families and children in many communities. You need to be aware of family-oriented offerings so that you are able to refer patients as needed. Often health promotion behaviors that you need to encourage are tied to the developmental stage of the family. For example, the childbearing family needs effective prenatal care, and the child-rearing family needs encouragement to follow immunization schedules.

One approach for meeting goals and promoting health is the use of family strengths. Families do not look at their own system as one that has inherent, positive components. The nurse helps the family become aware of its own unique strengths, thereby increasing its potential and capabilities. Family strengths include clear communication, adaptability, healthy child-rearing practices, support and nurturing among family members, and the use of crisis for growth. The nurse helps the family focus on these strengths instead of its problems and weaknesses. For example, the nurse points out that a couple's 10-year marriage has endured many crises and transitions. Therefore they are likely to have the capabilities to adapt to this latest challenge.

**ACUTE CARE.** The family is becoming more of the focus within the context of health care delivery in a managed care environment. Acute care settings discharge patients very quickly. Thus you need to take more of a role in under-

standing and supporting family and patient needs. Family members often have to maintain their jobs while also providing assistance during the patient's recovery. It is a challenge to prepare family members to assist with health care or to locate appropriate community resources. When family members assume the role of caregiver, they sometimes lose support from significant others. In the acute care setting, you must teach family members how to safely and efficiently assume care responsibilities (Box 21-5). Patient education must be efficient and demonstrate to the family how to provide the care, when to contact the physician or health care provider or home care nurse, and under what conditions to contact emergency services.

**RESTORATIVE AND CONTINUING CARE.** Family nursing emphasizes maintenance of a patient's functional abilities. This means working closely with the family in making sure the home environment is adaptive to the patient's strengths and limitations. Referral to home care nursing is essential. The home care nurse will assist in educating family members about providing ongoing care and making changes in the home so that the patient becomes self-sufficient.

One way you best provide family care is through support of family caregivers. Family caregiving involves the routine provision of services and personal care activities for a family member by spouses, siblings, or parents. Caregiving activities include personal care (bathing, feeding, grooming), monitoring for complications or side effects of medications, performing instrumental activities of daily living (shopping or housekeeping), and providing ongoing emotional support and decision making that is necessary. Whenever an individual becomes dependent on another family member for care and assistance, there is significant stress affecting both the caregiver and the care recipient. In addition, the caregiver needs to continue to meet the demands of his or her normal lifestyle (e.g., raising children, working full time, or dealing with personal problems or illness). Caregiving is more than simply a series of tasks and often occurs within the context of a family. Whether it is a wife caring for a husband or a daughter caring for a mother, caregiving is an interactional process. The interpersonal dynamics between family members influence the ultimate quality of caregiving. Thus you will play a key role in helping family members develop better communication and problem-solving skills to build the relationships needed for caregiving to be successful.

## Evaluation

**PATIENT CARE.** When the patient's family functions as context, evaluation focuses on attainment of patient needs. Thus evaluation is patient centered, although nursing measures have involved assisting the patient in adapting to the family environment. You will compare the response of the patient with predetermined outcomes (Table 21-3).

When the family is the patient, the measure of family health is more than an evaluation of the health of all family members. For example, the family's attainment of family de-

---

**BOX 21-5** PATIENT TEACHING

Michelle tells Bethany that Lois's medications were changed. Now some medications given for Lois's cardiovascular and renal conditions are given 3 times a day, and some of these medications may need to be "held" if Lois's pulse and blood pressure change. Michelle is fearful of giving her grandmother the wrong medication or giving the medication incorrectly.

**Outcomes**

At the end of the teaching sessions, Michelle and Patrick will be able to do the following:

- Correctly place all Lois's medications in the weekly medication dispenser
- Correctly obtain an apical pulse
- State that if Lois's pulse rate is 60 beats per minute or less or 100 beats per minute or greater, she should not be given the Digoxin 0.25 mg and notify the home care nurse
- Correctly obtain a brachial blood pressure
- State that if Lois's blood pressure is less than 100/60 mm Hg, she should not be given the Captopril 25 mg and notify the home care nurse

**Teaching Strategies**

- Provide Michelle and Patrick with a laminated card that lists all medications: include action, side effects, precautions, and premedication assessments (e.g., need for pulse measurement).
- Post a laminated card on the refrigerator that organizes medications to be given in the morning, afternoon, evening, and before bed.

- Demonstrate to both Michelle and Patrick how to fill the weekly medication dispenser.
- Show Michelle and Patrick how to record pulse, blood pressure, and medication administration.
- Demonstrate how to take an apical pulse.
- Have both Michelle and Patrick practice apical pulse measurement on each other.
- Demonstrate how to take a brachial blood pressure.
- Have both Michelle and Patrick practice brachial blood pressure measurement on each other.

**Evaluation Strategies**

- Ask Patrick and Michelle to state actions of Lois's medications.
- Ask Michelle and Patrick to identify which medications have preadministration assessments and when the medication should not be given.
- Observe weekly medication dispenser.
- Review pulse, blood pressure, and medication administration record.
- Observe and validate Michelle and Patrick obtaining an apical pulse.
- Observe and validate Michelle and Patrick obtaining a brachial blood pressure.

---

## OUTCOME EVALUATION

**TABLE 21-3**

| Nursing Action | Patient Response/Finding | Achievement of Outcome |
|---|---|---|
| Ask Patrick and Michelle to describe how they will divide caregiving activities. | Patrick and Michelle describe the new activities they assumed responsibility for and those activities that remained shared. | Patrick was able to perform an increased share of caregiving activities. |
| Ask Michelle and Patrick if they have noticed changes in their behavior and interactions. | Michelle stated that Patrick "doesn't lose his temper or become impatient as often." | Patrick has decreased impatience. |
| | Patrick feels less stressed. | Patrick rates stress as 6 on a scale of 1 to 10. |
| | Patrick has noticed improvement in Michelle's eating and sleeping. | Michelle rates stress as 5. |
| Ask them to evaluate use of a professional house-cleaning service. | Both Patrick and Michelle report satisfaction and relief that someone else is doing housework. | Both partners appear satisfied with assistance from non–family members with regard to housework. |
| | Both note that freedom from housework gives them more time for each other. | |

---

velopmental tasks is a useful criterion. You evaluate the family's change in functioning and its satisfaction with the new level of functioning.

When you care for the family as a system, evaluation focuses on the effects interventions have on the entire family, including extended family. For example, if you are caring for

an older adult who has begun chemotherapy for a new cancer diagnosis, you evaluate how the frequent trips to the oncology clinic and the cancer diagnosis affect the patient, the spouse, the children, and the grandchildren.

Evaluation is an ongoing process. You modify goals and interventions as needed. Evaluation comes not only from

## EVALUATION

Recently Lois's health status declined, and she needed more supervision with medication administration and her activities. As a result, she needed to move in with Michelle and Patrick. Bethany visits Lois periodically throughout the semester and checks to see how the family's short-term goals are coming along for caregiving and maintaining their own family life. She checks to see how Lois's goals are being fulfilled regarding her care in her granddaughter's home, activity tolerance, and forgetfulness. Bethany assesses Michelle's stress level with school, home, and meeting her grandmother's health care needs. To assess Michelle and Patrick, she requests that the family arrange a meeting once a month. This ongoing evaluation requires a multidisciplinary effort from the home care nurse who knows the family best, the family members themselves, their physician, the chaplain, the social worker, and the nutritionist. The nurse is the true coordinator and evaluator of care provided, and Bethany knows this.

Bethany learns through the course of the semester that Patrick has been able to begin implementing some of the more positive coping strategies he has learned. He is also able to help Michelle around the house with some of the daily chores and finances. He assumes responsibility for cleaning Lois's mobile home and preparing it for sale. When he realized how important his help was, he felt more needed and wanted to help. Michelle has more free time to concentrate on her studies every other night so she is able to "hurry through school to get a better job to help their financial future plans," as she and Patrick have wanted. One evening a week another family member comes to Michelle and Patrick's home to stay with Lois so the couple can have an evening out.

Bethany discussed the long-term goals of including the community in Lois's care. A registered nurse visits for 1 hour per week, a hospice volunteer takes Lois to the Senior Enrichment Program on Mondays, and a clergyman visits once per week. Lois sees the nurse practitioner one month and the physician the next. They use the CNA overnight service 3 nights during the week, and the family divides the cost among all the family members who live too far away to help with Lois's care. Michelle has found family members willing to take turns caring for Lois one weekend a month.

### Documentation Note

"Patrick and Michelle are participating in family meetings; both report that sitting down together helps them deal with the stress of their jobs, school, and the care of Lois. Michelle feels that she and Patrick are partners in the work of the family. The overnight care of Lois by the CNA has helped relieve some of the stress. Both Patrick and Michelle know that Lois will eventually need nursing home care and have begun looking at placements together along with other family members."

---

your observations, but also from the patient's and family's perspectives. This comprehensive evaluation helps to determine that the health care team is meeting the expectations of family members, as well as family members' meeting the expectations of the health care team.

Use critical thinking skills and clinical decision making to evaluate your patient's responses to interventions. Often the patient and/or family does not know the best way to deliver care. For example, the family thinks a pain medication does not work at all; however, an adjustment in scheduling is all that is required. Each patient and family is unique. Family nursing requires the use of therapeutic communication skills, scientific and family nursing knowledge, critical think-ing skills, knowledge of oneself, and extensive learning about the patients and their families.

**PATIENT EXPECTATIONS.** It is important to obtain the family's perspective of nursing care: how you planned and delivered the care with them, whether you delivered it satisfactorily, whether it met the family's goals, and if not, what they think was needed instead. With a truly trusting relationship between you and your patient, you will obtain this information to create an even more positive atmosphere. This evaluation is continuous throughout the care planning to modify or adjust care delivery techniques (e.g., how soon the home care nurse was able to make a visit, adequacy of comfort measures, or timeliness of care) or even to adjust care delivery personnel.

## KEY CONCEPTS

- The family has a significant impact on the lives of its members.
- Because the concept of family is highly individualized, base care on the patient's attitude toward family.
- Families are as diverse as the individuals that compose them, and patients have deeply ingrained values about their families that deserve respect.
- Family structure is based on organization (i.e., the ongoing membership of the family and the pattern of relationships).
- Family functioning involves the processes used by the family to achieve its goals.

- The goal of family nursing is to help the family and its individual members reach and maintain maximum health throughout and beyond the illness experience.
- The nurse views the family as an important context for the individual family member or views the family unit as the patient, or as a system. The approach for any family depends in part on the situation.
- Families face many challenges, including changing structures and roles, especially as the economic status of society changes.
- The family is the primary social context in which health promotion and disease prevention take place.

- The cause of family violence is complex and multidimensional. Stress, poverty, social isolation, psychopathology, and learned family behavior are all factors associated with violence.
- As you begin to provide family-centered care, you will continually assess, analyze, and reflect on the changing needs and health care goals of patients and their families.
- Goals for a care plan that incorporate a family approach include those that view the family as patient, as context, as system, or as a combination of the three.

- Whether you are caring for a patient with the family as context, family as patient, , or as system, you direct your nursing interventions to increase family members' abilities in certain areas, to remove barriers to health care, and to do things that the family cannot do for itself.
- The interpersonal dynamics between family members influence the ultimate quality of caregiving.

## CRITICAL THINKING IN PRACTICE

*You are caring for an intergenerational family that consists of an 80-year-old grandmother, who is in the last stages of heart and kidney failure, and a married couple in their 40s, Jane and Harry. Both Jane and Harry are teachers and take additional summer jobs. Jane and Harry have three children: Rachael (16 years old), Harry Jr. (13 years old), and Kathy (11 years old).*

1. What are the stressors placed on this family?
2. When the grandmother's health status changes, what additional stressors do you anticipate?

3. What resources will you provide to the family to help the grandchildren cope with the grandmother's changing health status?
4. Think of the family in which you grew up. Describe the values and attitudes you learned in this environment and the influence they have on how you view this family.
5. What family experiences do you bring to this situation?

## NCLEX® REVIEW

1. Family functioning involves:
   1. The process used by the family to achieve its goals
   2. The patterns of people who are considered to be family members
   3. The ongoing membership of the family and the pattern of relationships
   4. The intrafamilial system of support and structure extending beyond the walls of the household
2. Family structure is:
   1. The process used by the family to achieve its goals
   2. The patterns of people who are considered to be family members
   3. The ongoing membership of the family and the pattern of relationships
   4. The intrafamilial system of support and structure extending beyond the walls of the household
3. Family assessment includes:
   1. Assessing individual family members separately
   2. Assessing only those members living in the household
   3. Assessing only the patient's perception of family interaction
   4. Assessing individual family members and their interactions with one another and the patient
4. When planning care for the family as a patient, you need to:
   1. Consider the developmental stage of the family
   2. Include only the ill family member and the significant other

3. Understand that the family will always help to achieve the health goals of an ill member of the family
4. Understand that cultural background is an important variable to consider when developing nursing interventions
5. You are caring for an intergenerational family. The family consists of a single parent with 2 school-age children (5 and 8 years old) and a grandfather who is 65 with end-stage kidney disease. The family enters the clinic for a follow-up visit to evaluate the grandfather's renal failure. During the course of the history, you notice that the mother has a black eye, which she attributes to a fall. However, the oldest child states that the mother's boyfriend did it. What is your priority?
   1. Continue with the evaluation of the grandfather's kidney disease
   2. Assume that the 8-year-old does not have all the facts
   3. Tell the mother to terminate the relationship with the boyfriend
   4. Refer the mother to a battered victims resource center
6. When working with a family with a rigid family structure, you design interventions to:
   1. Attempt to change the family structure
   2. Include only the most flexible family member
   3. Create interventions that require minimal change
   4. Provide solutions for problems only when they arise

## REFERENCES

Abbott S, Shaw S, Bryar R: Family-centered public health practice: is health visiting ready? *Community Pract* 77(9):338, 2004.

Alpert EJ and others: "Challenges and strategies" and "evidence-based care," *Violence Against Women* 8(6):639, 2002.

Anderson KH: The family health system approach to family systems nursing. *J Fam Nurs* 6(2):103, 2000.

Astedt-Kurki P and others: Methodological issues in interviewing families in family nursing research, *J Adv Nurs* 35(2):288, 2001.

Astedt-Kurki P and others: Development and testing of a family nursing scale, *West J Nurs Res* 24(5):567, 2002.

Astedt-Kurki P and others: Determinants of perceived health in families of patients with heart disease, *J Adv Nurs* 48(2):115, 2004.

Bell JM and others: Learning to nurse the family, *J Fam Nurs* 7(2):117, 2001, (editorial).

Call KT and others: Caregiver burden from a social exchange perspective: caring for older people after hospital discharge, *J Marriage Fam* 61:688, 1999.

Cox C, Monk A: Strain among caregivers: comparing the experiences of African-American and Hispanic caregivers of Alzheimer's relatives, *Int J Aging Hum Dev* 43(2):93, 1996.

Dienemann J and others: Developing a domestic violence program in an intercity academic health center emergency department: the first 3 years, *J Emerg Nurs* 25(2):110, 1999.

Dochterman JM, Bulechek GM, editors: *Nursing interventions classification (NIC)*, ed 4, St. Louis, 2004, Mosby.

Duhamel F, Talbot LR: A constructivist evaluation of family systems nursing interventions with families experiencing cardiovascular and cerebrovascular illness, *J Fam Nurs* 10(1):12, 2004.

Farran CJ. Family caregivers: a critical resource in today's changing healthcare climate, *Chart* 99(4):4, 2002.

Feeley N, Gottlieb LN: Nursing approaches for working with family strengths and resources, *J Fam Nurs* 6(1):9, 2000.

Ford-Gilboe M: Developing knowledge about family health promotion by testing the developmental model of health and nursing, *J Fam Nurs* 8:140, 2002.

Hartrick G: Developing health-promoting practice with families: one pedagogical experience, *J Adv Nurs* 3:27, 2000.

Isaksen AS, Thuen F, Hanestad B: Patients with cancer and their close relatives: experiences with treatment, care, and support, *Cancer Nurs* 26(1):68, 2003.

James-Childs EY: *Adolescent and young adult male parenting: the forgotten half*, doctoral dissertation, Denver, 2000, University of Colorado Health Sciences Center.

Kamo Y, Zhou M: Living arrangements of elderly Chinese and Japanese in the United States, *J Marriage Fam* 56(3):544, 1994.

Kushel M and others: Emergency department use among the homeless and marginally housed: results from a community-based study, *Am J Public Health* 92:778, 2002.

Lewis-O'Connor A: 'Dying to Tell?': Do mandatory reporting laws benefit victims of domestic violence? *Am J Nurs* 104(10):75, 2004.

Maijala H and others: Caregiver's experiences of interaction with families expecting a fetally impaired child, *J Clin Nurs* 13(3):376, 2004.

McCubbin MA, McCubbin HI, Thompson AI: Family Hardiness Index (FHI). In HI McCubbin HI, Thompson AI, McCubbin MS, editors: *Family assessment: resiliency, coping, and adaptation, inventories for research and practice*, Madison, 1996, University of Wisconsin Press.

Moorhead S, Johnson M, Maas M: *Nursing outcomes classification (NOC)*, ed 3, St. Louis, 2004, Mosby.

National Coalition Against Domestic Violence: *Position paper: The problem: what is battering?* http://www.ncadv.org/learn/TheProblem.

National Coalition for the Homeless: *Homeless families with children: NCH fact sheet # 7*, Washington, DC, 2001, The Association, http://www.nationalhomeless.org/families.html.

Neabel B, Fothergill-Bourbonnais F, Dunning J: Family assessment tools: a review of the literature from 1978-1997, *Heart Lung* 29:196, 2000.

Newby NM: Chronic illness and the family life-cycle, *J Adv Nurs* 23(4):786, 1996.

Richardson J and others: Identifying domestic violence: cross sectional study in primary care, *Br Med J* 324:274, 2002.

Robrecht LC: Interpersonal violence and the pregnant homeless woman, *J Obstet Gynecol Neonatal Nurs* 27:684, 1998.

Shinn M and others: Predictors of homelessness among families in New York City: from shelter request to housing stability, *Am J Public Health* 88:1651, 1998.

SmithBattle L. The vulnerabilities of teenage mothers: challenging prevailing assumptions, *Adv Nurs Sci* 23(1):29, 2000.

Stanhope M, Lancaster J: *Community and public health nursing*, ed 6, St. Louis, 2004, Mosby.

Svavarsdottir EK, McCubbin MA, Kane JH: Well-being of parents of young children with asthma, *Res Nurs Health* 23:346, 2000.

Tapp DM: Dilemmas of family support during cardiac recovery: nagging as a gesture of support, *West J Nurs Res* 26(5):561, 2004.

Tarkka MT and others: In-hospital social support for families of heart patients, *J Clin Nurs* 12(5):736, 2003.

U.S. Bureau of the Census: *Population profile of the United States: 2000 (Internet release)*, Washington, DC, October 2001, The Bureau, http//:www.census.gov.

Vaughan-Cole B and others: *Family nursing practice*, St. Louis, 1998, Mosby.

Voydanoff P, Donnelly BW: Multiple roles and psychological distress: the intersection of the paid worker, spouse, and parent roles with the role of the adult child, *J Marriage Fam* 61:725, 1999.

Wathen CN, MacMillan HL: Interventions for violence against women: scientific review, *JAMA* 289:589, 2003.

# CHAPTER 22

# Stress and Coping

## MEDIA RESOURCES

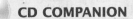 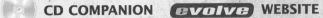 **CD COMPANION** *evolve* **WEBSITE**

http://evolve.elsevier.com/Potter/basic

- **NCLEX® Review**
- **Audio Glossary**
- **English/Spanish Audio Glossary**

## OBJECTIVES

- Describe the three stages of the general adaptation syndrome.
- Discuss the integration of stress theory with nursing theories.
- Formulate nursing diagnoses based on assessment data.
- Describe stress management techniques beneficial for coping with stress.
- Discuss the process of crisis intervention.
- Develop a care plan for patients experiencing stress.
- Discuss how stress in the workplace affects nurses.

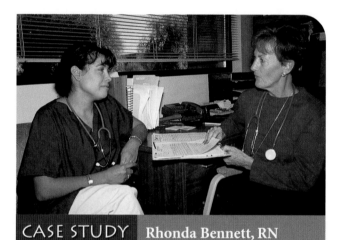

## CASE STUDY  Rhonda Bennett, RN

Rhonda Bennett, a 35-year-old married mother of three children, has worked as a registered nurse for City Hospital since her graduation from a community college 15 years ago. She began her career on a general medical unit and through the years has earned a reputation as a skilled and compassionate nurse. She presently works as the nurse manager in the medical intensive care unit and has always felt very happy with her job.

Rhonda values her family life immensely. She serves as a Girl Scout leader and a soccer coach. Until last year she also enjoyed playing tennis with her husband, who was self-employed as a contractor. Within the past year, however, he has had several hospitalizations related to chest pain, panic attacks, and, finally, a spontaneous pneumothorax. As a result, he has been much less involved in his work and has a decreased income. He has bouts of depression that result in Rhonda's shouldering responsibility for the family alone. Hoping to help her husband overcome his depression by spending more time with him, Rhonda has reduced her community involvement, but chose to take the manager's job for a year for an increase in salary to help pay the family's accumulated debt. Because of Rhonda's employment, the Bennetts have been able to maintain their home and standard of living.

In the nursing shortage environment Rhonda confronts scheduling problems and must employ temporary nurses from an outside staffing agency to adequately staff the unit. Rhonda has seen evidence of decreased quality of patient care. Based on comments that the administration has made, Rhonda knows that patient satisfaction surveys reveal lower patient satisfaction. Furthermore, she feels overwhelmed by the burden of being breadwinner, mother, wife, and nurse to her family. She will not ask for help, but she wishes that someone could take care of *her*. She has tried to "put on a face" of confidence, but every day gets harder for her. She feels defeated and hopeless, has no energy, and has difficulty organizing her thoughts. Her boss has noticed that Rhonda often complains of severe headaches and has become especially concerned since Rhonda tearfully confided that she does not sleep and therefore has begun having couple of glasses of wine at night to help herself "unwind." Because of these behaviors, her boss referred her to the hospital's employee health office. One of this department's duties is to help employees cope with the stress.

Becky Howard, a nurse in the employee health office, does preliminary screening and crisis intervention with staff members experiencing stress and potential substance abuse problems. She has a bachelor's degree in nursing and extensive experience working both in acute care hospitals and on a crisis intervention telephone hot line. A 52-year-old divorced mother of four children, the health office hired Becky as a contract employee, paid by the behavioral health company included in the employee health benefit package.

## KEY TERMS

alarm reaction, p. 596
coping, p. 597
crisis, p. 597
crisis intervention, p. 601
developmental crises, p. 598
distress, p. 597
endorphins, p. 596
eustress, p. 597
exhaustion stage, p. 596
fight-or-flight response, p. 596
flashback, p. 599
general adaptation syndrome (GAS), p. 596
primary appraisal, p. 596
resistance stage, p. 596
secondary appraisal, p. 597
situational crises, p. 598
stress, p. 596
stressor, p. 596

Stress interests all of us. **Stressors** are disruptive forces operating within or on any system (Neuman and Fawcett, 2002). We need to know about **stress,** not only so we recognize stress in patients and families and intervene effectively, but also because stressful events that occur in the course of clinical practice affect us as health care professionals. You need to recognize in your own life the signs and symptoms of stress. It also helps to be knowledgeable about stress management techniques to aid personal coping in yourself, as well as with your patients and their families.

Stress stimulates thinking processes and helps you stay alert to your environment. How you react to stress depends on how you view and evaluate the impact of the stressor, its effect on your situation and support at the time of the stress, and your usual coping mechanisms. Stress provides stimulation and motivation, as well as causing discomfort and retreat. However, when stress overwhelms a person's existing coping mechanisms, a crisis results (Aguilera, 1998).

## Scientific Knowledge Base

Over 60 years ago Walter Cannon proposed the **fight-or flight-response** to stress, an arousal of the sympathetic nervous system (Aldwin, 2000). This reaction prepares a person for action by increasing heart rate; diverting blood from the intestines to the brain and striated muscles; and increasing blood pressure, heart rate, respiratory rate, and blood glucose levels. In the 1930s, 40s, and 50s Hans Selye enlarged on Cannon's fight-or-flight hypothesis to describe the **general adaptation syndrome (GAS),** a three-stage reaction to stress (Selye, 1991). The GAS reflects how the body responds to stressors through the alarm reaction, the resistance stage, and the exhaustion stage. The GAS is triggered either directly by a physical event or indirectly by a psychological event (Lazarus, 1999).

### General Adaptation Syndrome

The GAS is an immediate physiological response of the body to stress. It involves several body systems, especially the autonomic nervous system and the endocrine system (Table 22-1). When an injury or some physical demand occurs, the pituitary gland initiates the GAS. In addition, the hypothalamus, another part of the brain, secretes **endorphins.** Endorphins are hormones that act on the mind like morphine and opiates, and they produce a sense of well-being and reduce pain (Lazarus, 1999). In this way the GAS defends us against stress both by activating the neuroendocrine system and by providing endorphins that decrease our awareness of the pain.

During the **alarm reaction** rising hormone levels result in an increased blood volume, blood glucose levels, epinephrine and norepinephrine amounts, heart rate, blood flow to muscles, oxygen intake, and mental alertness (Selye, 1991). In addition, the pupils of the eyes dilate to produce a greater visual field. This change in body systems prepares an individual for fight or flight and lasts from 1 minute to many hours. If the stressor poses an extreme threat to life or remains for a long time, the person progresses to the second stage, resistance.

During the **resistance stage** the body stabilizes and responds in an opposite manner to the alarm reaction. Hormone levels, heart rate, blood pressure, and cardiac output return to normal, and the body repairs any damage that occurred. However, if the stressor remains and adaptation does not happen, the person enters the third stage, exhaustion.

The **exhaustion stage** occurs when the body is no longer able to resist the effects of the stressor and the struggle to maintain adaptation drains all available energy. The physiological response intensifies, but the person has so little energy left that adaptation to the stressor diminishes. The body can no longer defend itself against the impact of the event, physiological regulation diminishes, and, if the stress continues, illness and death result.

Physiological responses to stress also include immunological responses. The immune system differentiates between self and nonself. This means that under normal conditions your immune system does not treat your own cells as threats but treats bacteria, viruses, parasites, or toxins as threats. Problems occur when the immune system makes a too vigorous response and an autoimmune illness develops. The mechanisms through which stress affects the immune system are unclear (Aldwin, 2000).

Selye (1991) noted that a prolonged state of stress causes disease. Stress makes people ill as a result of (1) increased levels of powerful hormones that change our bodily processes; (2) coping choices that are unhealthy, such as not getting enough rest or a proper diet or use of tobacco, alcohol, or caffeine; and (3) neglect of warning signs of illness or prescribed medicines or treatments (Monat and Lazarus, 1991).

On the other hand, physical exercise, relaxation strategies, and letting go of excess anger reduce a person's level of arousal and stress. Exercise improves circulation and triggers the release of endorphins. The relaxation response, elicited by meditation or progressive muscle relaxation, lowers blood pressure, pulse rate, and respiratory rate. Forgiveness, or letting go of excess anger, has been shown to reduce stress-provoking hormone levels. Anger, a feeling that serves people well as a protective mechanism, for example, overcomes people if they continually seek revenge rather than forgive. If living with anger becomes a daily experience, the burden of carrying the anger results in continuous stress and arousal (Enright and North, 1998).

**REACTION TO PSYCHOLOGICAL STRESS.** The GAS activates indirectly for psychological threats, which differ for each person and influence a variety of responses to stress (Box 22-1). Lazarus (1999) maintains that a person experiences stress only if the person evaluates the event or circumstance as personally significant. Evaluating an event for its personal meaning, or **primary appraisal,** happens very quickly and automatically in the person's mind. If primary appraisal results in the person's identifying the event or cir-

| TABLE 22-1 | Indicators of Stress |
|---|---|

| System | Assessment Findings | Psychological | |
|---|---|---|---|
| **Physical** | | Cognitive | Forgetfulness/preoccupation |
| Cardiovascular | Tightness of chest | | Denial |
| | Increased heart rate | | Poor concentration |
| | Elevated blood pressure | | Inattention to detail |
| Respiratory | Breathing difficulty | | Orientation to past instead of present |
| | Tachypnea | | Decreased creativity |
| Neuroendocrine | Headaches, migraines | | Slower thinking, reactions |
| | Fatigue, exhaustion | | Learning difficulties |
| | Insomnia, sleep disturbances | | Apathy |
| | Feeling uncoordinated | | Confusion |
| | Restlessness, hyperactivity | | Decreased attention span |
| | Tremors (lips, hands) | | Calculation difficulties |
| | Profuse sweating (palms) | | Memory problems |
| | Dry mouth | Emotional | Disruption of logical thinking |
| | Cold hands and feet | | Blaming others |
| Gastrointestinal/ | Urinary frequency | | Lack of motivation to get up in the morning |
| genitourinary | Nausea, diarrhea, vomiting | | Crying tendencies |
| | Weight gain or loss of more than 10 lb | | Lack of interest |
| | Change in appetite | | Irritability |
| | Gastrointestinal bleeding | | Isolation |
| Diagnostic | Blood in stools/vomitus | | Diminished initiative |
| | Elevated blood glucose level | Behavior/lifestyle | Worrying |
| | Elevated cortisol levels | | Decreased involvement with others |
| Musculoskeletal | Backaches, muscle aches | | Withdrawal |
| | Bruxism (clenched jaw) | | Change in interactions with others |
| | Slumped posture | | Increased or decreased food intake |
| Reproductive | Amenorrhea | | Increased smoking or alcohol intake |
| | Failure to ovulate | | Overvigilance to environment |
| | Impotency in men | | Excessive humor or silence |
| | Loss of libido | | No exercise |
| Immunological | Frequent or prolonged colds/flu | | |

cumstance as a harm, loss, threat, or challenge, the person has stress. Following the recognition of stress, **secondary appraisal** focuses on possible coping strategies.

A person manages psychological stress by **coping** (Lazarus, 1999). Effectiveness of coping strategies depends on the individual's needs. For this reason no single coping strategy works for everyone or for every stressor. The same person copes differently from one time to another. In stressful situations people use a combination of problem-focused coping and emotion-focused coping. In other words, when under stress, we obtain information and take action to change the situation, as well as regulate our emotions tied to the stress. In some cases we avoid thinking about the situation or change the way we think about it, without changing the actual situation itself (Lazarus, 1999).

## Types of Stress

Selye identified two types of stress, **distress,** or damaging stress, and **eustress,** stress that protects health. However, the idea of healthy stress has become controversial because researchers cannot readily determine whether a person has

benefited from stress or has coped with the stress by denying it (Aldwin, 2000). Stress includes work stress, family stress, chronic stress, acute stress, daily hassles, trauma, and crisis. "Work and family stress interact, family being the background for work stress, and work the background for family stress" (Lazarus, 1999). One person looks at a stimulus and sees it as a challenge, leading to mastery and growth. Another sees the same stimulus as a threat, leading to stagnation and loss. Lazarus suggests a spillover of stresses between work and home. The individual with family responsibilities and a full-time job outside the home sometimes experiences chronic stress. Chronic stress occurs in stable conditions, from stressful roles, or from living with a long-term illness. Conversely, time-limited major or minor events that are threatening for a relatively brief period of time provoke acute stress. Recurrent daily hassles, such as commuting to work, maintaining a house, dealing with difficult people, and managing money, further complicate chronic or acute stress.

A **crisis** occurs when a person's emotional equilibrium is upset and "customary problem-solving techniques cannot be used to meet the daily problems of living" (Aguilera,

---

| BOX 22-1 | Factors Influencing the Response to Stressors |
|---|---|

**Intensity**

Minimal, severe, or somewhere in between. The greater the perceived magnitude of the stressor, the greater the stress response.

**Scope**

The pervasiveness with which a stressor affects a person's total being. The greater the scope of a stressor, the greater the stress response.

**Duration**

The length of time the person perceives the stressor. The greater the duration of the stressor, the greater the stress response.

**Number and Nature of Other Stressors Present**

Multiple stressors experienced simultaneously or a succession of single stressors with no opportunity for the person to rest and regroup results in a greater stress response.

**Predictability**

Being able to anticipate the occurrence of an event, even if you are unable to control it, generally results in a reduced experience of stress.

**Level of Personal Control**

Believing that you have control over an unpleasant experience, even if you never exercise that control, lessens the level of associated stress and anxiety.

**Feelings of Competence**

Greater self-confidence in your ability to manage a stressful event results in less tension and anxiety.

**Cognitive Appraisal**

The greater the personal meaning of an event, the greater the stress associated with it. Thus the same event sometimes causes differing levels of stress in different people.

**Availability of Social Supports**

The emotional concern and support of other people reduce the negative effects of stressful events.

---

1998). Caplan distinguished two types of crises, those associated with changing developmental levels that require role changes, or **developmental crises,** and **situational crises** that occur when a life event upsets the person's equilibrium (as cited in Benter, 2005). Crisis theory assumes that a person either advances or regresses as a result of a crisis, depending upon how one manages the crisis (Lazarus, 1999).

## Nursing Knowledge Base

### Nursing Theory and the Role of Stress

Concepts of stress and reaction to stress constitute Betty Neuman's systems model. Because the Neuman model uses a systems approach, you will use it to understand your patients' individual responses to stressors and also families' and communities' responses. A systems approach explains that a stressor at one place in a system affects other parts of the system; a system is a person, a family, or a community. Events are multidimensional and not caused or affected by only one thing. Every person has developed a set of responses to stress that constitute the "normal line of defense" (Neuman and Fawcett, 2002). This line of defense helps to maintain health and wellness. "Physiological, psychological, sociocultural, developmental, or spiritual influences" buffer stress. When this does not happen, the normal line of defense breaks, and disease results. In this belief, Neuman's systems model coincides with Selye's general adaptation syndrome.

Neuman's systems model stresses the importance of accuracy in assessment and interventions that promote optimal

wellness using primary, secondary, and tertiary prevention strategies (Neuman and Fawcett, 2002). Primary prevention promotes patient wellness by stress prevention and reduction of risk factors. Secondary prevention occurs after symptoms appear. Tertiary prevention begins when the patient system becomes more stable and recovers. Neuman's model of nursing views the patient, family, or community as constantly changing in response to the environment and stressors.

Pender's health promotion model proposes that health promotion centers on increasing the level of well-being of an individual or group. Primary, secondary, and tertiary prevention focus on avoiding negative events (Pender, Murdaugh, and Parsons, 2002). Pender considers stress reduction strategies important to reduce threats to well-being, to help people fulfill their potential, and to shape and maintain health behaviors. To change behavior, your patient initiates the change and behaves differently in interactions. People want to live in ways that enable them to be as healthy as possible and to be capable of assessing their own abilities and assets. Based on these assumptions of the capability and desire of people to be healthy, Pender suggests strategies for prevention and health promotion related to stress management (see Chapter 1).

### Situational, Maturational, and Sociocultural Factors

Potential stressors and coping mechanisms vary across the life span. For example, adolescence, adulthood, and old age bring different stressors. Appraisal of stressors, amount and type of social support, and coping strategies are balancing

- Coping ability of older adults derives from their previous lifestyle, adaptation to retirement, adjustments to minor ailments, openness to both feelings and ideas, and maintenance of social activities and contacts (Aguilera, 1998).
- Older adults with multiple losses, including job status, mobility, health, vision, spouse, mental acuity, and home, experience more need for institutional support (Aguilera, 1998).
- Depression in later adulthood is a common problem (Aguilera, 1998).
- Avoid the tendency to stereotype the person's appearance and symptoms of stress as part of the normal aging process (Aguilera, 1998).
- Differentiate signs of stress and crisis from dementia and from acute confusion, a condition that is often life threatening.
- Examine the person's current medical history as part of the assessment.

factors when assessing stress, and all depend on previous life experiences (Aguilera, 1998). Furthermore, environmental and social stressors place people who are vulnerable at higher risk for prolonged stress.

**SITUATIONAL FACTORS.** Situational stress arises from job changes, either your own or that of a family member, and relocation. Stressful job situations include promotions, transfers, downsizing, restructuring, changes in supervisors, staffing shortages, and additional responsibilities. Adjusting to chronic illness results in situational stress. Common diseases, such as obesity, hypertension, diabetes, depression, asthma, and coronary artery disease, provoke stress. Furthermore, being a family caregiver for someone with a chronic illness such as Alzheimer's disease causes stress (Aguilera, 1998).

**MATURATIONAL FACTORS.** Stressors vary with life stage (see Chapter 19). Preadolescents experience stress related to self-esteem issues, changing family structure due to divorce or death of a parent, or hospitalizations. As adolescents search for their identity with peer groups and separate from their families, they undergo stress. In addition, they face questions about using mind-altering substances, sexuality, jobs, school, and career choices that cause stress. Stress for adults centers around major changes in life circumstances (Aguilera, 1998). These include the many milestones of beginning a family and a career, losing parents, seeing children leave home, and accepting physical aging. In the older adult, stressors include multiple losses: concerns about income, nutrition, and transportation; the effects of aging and chronic illness; and confronting societal stereotypes about old age (Box 22-2).

**SOCIOCULTURAL FACTORS.** Environmental and social stressors lead to developmental problems. Potential stressors that affect any age-group, but that are especially stressful for young people, include prolonged poverty, physical handicap, and chronic illness. The vulnerability of children escalates when they lose relationships with parents and caregivers through divorce, imprisonment, or death or when parents have mental illness or substance abuse disorders. Furthermore, living under conditions of continuing violence, disintegrated neighborhoods, or homelessness damages people of any age, but especially young people (Pender and others, 2002).

Cultural variations produce stress, particularly if the person's values differ from the dominant culture in aspects of gender roles, family relationships, and religious beliefs. Other aspects of cultural variations are beliefs about causes of illness, rituals related to death and dying, values associated with community involvement versus privacy, and child-rearing practices. Uncertainty about immigration status and citizenship increases stress (Benter, 2005).

## Posttraumatic Stress Disorder

Posttraumatic stress disorder (PTSD) affects people who have experienced accidents, violent events such as rape or domestic abuse, war, and natural disasters (Aguilera, 1998). PTSD symptoms appear to be a normal response to a traumatic event; however, if the symptoms persist beyond 3 months, health care providers make the diagnosis of PTSD. Nevertheless, symptoms may first appear months or years after the traumatic event. People with PTSD sometimes experience a **flashback,** or "a recollection so strong that the individual thinks he is actually experiencing the trauma again or seeing it unfold before his eyes" (Aguilera, 1998).

## Critical Thinking

### Synthesis

When examining your role with a patient experiencing stress, consider your patient's perception of the stress and examine your own frame of reference as a nurse. You will be entering into the nurse-patient relationship with your own past experiences and your views about your responsibilities related to helping the patient cope with his or her stress.

In addition, the patient will also have expectations of you. Interacting with a patient in stress requires you to have confidence in yourself and integrity in dealing with a patient who is temporarily vulnerable. Assess the patient's situation accurately and objectively, and be especially aware of your ethical responsibility in caring for someone who has less independence due to stress.

**KNOWLEDGE.** Physiological changes occur in the patient experiencing the alarm reaction, resistance stage, and exhaustion stage of the general adaptation syndrome. Apply knowledge of those physiological changes. Your knowledge of communication principles helps you to assess the patient's behaviors. Determine the ability of the patient to cope with the stress. If the patient does not succeed with his or her usual coping skills, you need to use crisis intervention counseling.

**EXPERIENCE.** Your experience teaches you to understand the patient's unique perspective. View every person as an individual, recognizing that no two people are exactly alike. Experience with patients also helps you to recognize responses to stress. In addition, your own personal experiences with stress and coping increases your ability to empathize with a patient temporarily immobilized by stress. Understanding the patient's position enables you to intervene more effectively.

**ATTITUDES.** Be confident in the belief that you and the patient are able to manage stress effectively. Patients who feel overwhelmed and who perceive events as being beyond their capacity to cope will rely on you as an expert. Patients respect your advice and counsel and gain confidence from your belief in their ability to move past the stressful event or illness. Patients overwhelmed by life events often lack the ability, at least initially, to act on their own behalf. They require either direct intervention or guidance. You need to have an attitude of integrity through which you respect the patient's perception of or perspective about the stressor. Make the effort to have patients explain their unique viewpoint and situation.

**STANDARDS.** Make accurate assessment of a patient's stress, coping mechanisms, and support system before intervening. Clearly and precisely understand a patient's perception of the stress and focus on factors significant to the patient's well-being. In addition, select interventions that respect the individuality of the patient.

## Nursing Process

### Assessment

Assessment of a patient's stress level and coping resources requires that you first establish a trusting nurse-patient relationship. You will be asking the patient and family to share personal and sensitive information (see Chapter 6). You learn from the patient both by asking questions and by making observations of nonverbal behavior, interactions with the family, and the patient's environment. Synthesize the information you obtain, and adopt a critical thinking attitude while observing and analyzing patient behaviors. Often the patient has difficulty describing the most bothersome aspects of the situation until someone else has time to listen and encourage the patient to explore it.

**SUBJECTIVE FINDINGS.** When you assess a patient's stress level and coping resources, sit with the patient in comfortable chairs in a private setting facing one another. Assume a listening posture, establish eye contact, and allow time for the patient to talk to you. Gather information about the health status of the patient from the patient's perspective, and begin the process of developing a trusting relationship with the patient. Use the interview to determine the patient's view of the stress, coping resources, any possible maladaptive coping, and adherence to prescribed medical recommendations, such as medication or diet (Monat and Lazarus, 1991) (Table 22-2). If the patient uses denial as a coping mechanism, be alert to whether the person overlooks necessary information. Listen for any recurrent themes in

**SYNTHESIS IN PRACTICE**

Becky talks briefly on the phone with Rhonda to set up her appointment. She learns that Rhonda worries about losing her job because of the declining quality of patient care. Rhonda provides sole support for her family at this time. She also learns about Mr. Bennett's recent illness and the effect it has on Rhonda's overall well-being. Becky has also talked with Rhonda's director and knows that Rhonda has been having headaches and difficulty concentrating when making decisions. Becky sets aside some time to plan for her meeting with Rhonda.

Becky takes time to reflect on other employees she has recently seen in the employee health office. Many of the registered nurses have had physical complaints of stress including headaches, sleep problems, changes in eating habits, and flare-ups of existing medical problems. Becky knows she wants to be thorough in assessing the responses and symptoms Rhonda has been experiencing. Previous experience with other employees also has taught Becky the importance of learning about the employee's family and the type of support they offer and the person's appraisal of the situation.

After talking with Rhonda on the phone, Becky detects a great deal of anxiety but also some anger. Becky knows it is important to build trust with Rhonda as quickly as possible. As a single parent, Becky identifies with Rhonda's crisis of being the sole financial support for the family. Yet Becky decides not to tell her life history to Rhonda because she recognizes that no two persons have exactly the same experience or use the same coping strategies to get through difficult times. Becky wants to conduct an accurate assessment of Rhonda's problems, and she reminds herself that Rhonda's perspective of life will be unique. Becky plans to allow Rhonda time to fully describe her feelings and to listen carefully to the message she conveys. Becky wants to be able to work closely with Rhonda and establish priorities that are realistic for her to achieve.

the patient's conversation. As in all interactions with the patient, respect the confidentiality and sensitivity of the information shared.

**OBJECTIVE FINDINGS.** Obtain objective findings related to stress and coping through your observation of the appearance and nonverbal behavior of the patient. Observe grooming and hygiene, gait, characteristics of the patient's handshake, actions of the patient while sitting, quality of speech, eye contact, and the attitude of the patient toward you during the interview (see Chapter 13). Before the interview begins or at the end of the interview, depending upon the anxiety level of the patient, take basic vital signs to assess for physiological signs of stress such as elevated blood pressure, heart rate, or respiratory rate.

**PATIENT EXPECTATIONS.** Recognize the importance of the meaning of the precipitating event to the patient and the ways in which stress affects the patient's life. Allow time for the patient to express priorities for coping with stress. For example, a woman has just found out that a breast mass was identified on a routine mammogram. It is important for you to know what the patient wants and needs most from you. Ask the patient what she wants to know about a surgi-

## FOCUSED PATIENT ASSESSMENT

TABLE 22-2

| Factors to Assess | Questions and Approaches | Physical Assessment Strategies |
|---|---|---|
| Perception of stressor | Ask the patient to identify the stressor. Ask the patient what the stressor means to him or her.<br>Ask the patient about problems sleeping, eating, working, and concentrating.<br>Ask whether the patient has had accidents in the home, in the car, or on the job. | Observe for indicators of anxiety, anger, or tension. For example, you may observe nonverbal behaviors, such as irritability, crying, and inappropriate laughing. |
| Available coping resources | Ask the patient about current friendships and contacts with family members.<br>Ask what the patient has done in the past to cope with similar problems or stress.<br>Ask how the patient spends leisure time. | Observe whether the person is alone or with others.<br>Observe grooming and hygiene.<br>Observe the person's communication skills.<br>Observe if the person is able to ask for help.<br>Observe developmental level and sociocultural circumstances. |
| Maladaptive coping used | Ask about use of tobacco, alcohol, drugs, medications, and caffeine, as well as herbal remedies and over-the-counter medications | Observe for effects of smoking, alcohol, drugs, and caffeine, for example, difficulty sleeping, nervousness, or difficulty concentrating. |
| Adherence to healthy practices | Ask if the patient sees a physician or health care provider regularly for checkups.<br>Ask about nutritional habits, exercise, use of seat belts, helmets (if applicable), and safe sex. | |

cal or diagnostic procedure. Although some persons in this situation identify their need for information about biopsy or mastectomy as their personal priority, other women need guidance and support in discussing how to share the news with family members. Remember also that in some cases, when nothing will change or improve the situation, allowing the patient to use denial as a coping mechanism is helpful. Gaining an understanding of patient expectations does not mean that you will exclude certain types of care that are important simply because a patient does not identify them as needs. However, by inquiring about patient expectations and priorities, you will be better able to ensure that *all* the patient's needs will be addressed in some way. You can add this to the care planning process.

### 🌸 Nursing Diagnosis

Nursing diagnoses for people experiencing stress generally focus on coping. Examples of stress-related nursing diagnoses include:

- Anxiety
- Caregiver role strain
- Compromised family coping
- Ineffective coping
- Ineffective community coping
- Fear
- Chronic pain
- Post-trauma syndrome
- Relocation stress syndrome
- Situational low self-esteem
- Disturbed sleep pattern
- Impaired social interaction

Specifically, major defining characteristics of *ineffective coping* include verbalization of an inability to cope and an inability to ask for help. Identify defining characteristics by asking the patient what concerns him or her most at the time of the interview, and, importantly, allow the patient sufficient time to answer. Observe for psychological indicators of stress (see Table 22-1) and nonverbal signs of anxiety, fear, anger, and irritability. Identify these behaviors as part of your subjective and objective data collection.

Crisis differs from stress in the degree of severity, although stress and crisis share many characteristics (Shontz, 1975). A patient with stress so severe that the patient is not able to cope in any ways that have worked before experiences a crisis. A crisis devastates a person and requires use of all resources available. Unlike stress, which ends when the stressor disappears, the effects of a crisis sometimes last for years (Shontz, 1975).

### 🌸 Planning

**GOALS AND OUTCOMES.** Desirable goals for persons experiencing stress are (1) coping, (2) family coping, (3) caregiver emotional health, and (4) psychosocial adjustment: life change (Moorhead, Johnson, and Maas, 2004). Expected outcomes are behavioral markers that show progress toward goal achievement. For example, if a patient is to cope with stress, outcomes may include increasing interaction and improved sleep. After setting goals and outcomes, you select interventions for managing stress and improved coping (e.g., coping enhancement and **crisis intervention**) (Dochterman and Bulechek, 2004).

Nursing interventions are designed within the framework of primary, secondary, and tertiary prevention. At the primary level of prevention, nursing interventions might include preparing patients for life's turning points, such as the birth of a baby or the death of a parent. Nursing interventions at the secondary level include actions directed at symptoms, such as protecting the patient from self-harm. Tertiary-level interventions assist your patient in readapting and often include relaxation training and time management training. According to Pender's health promotion model (2002), you and the patient assess the level and source of the existing stress and determine the appropriate points for intervention to reduce the stress.

Your assessment of the patient's stress and coping depends on the patient's perception of the problem and coping resources. Similarly, selecting appropriate interventions requires a partnership with the patient and support system, usually the family. In the case of a family or community stressor and impaired family or community coping, your view of the situation and resources would be broader.

**SETTING PRIORITIES.** Prioritizing needs has special meaning for a person experiencing stress or crisis (see care plan). First, ask "What has happened that caused you to come for help today?" or "What happened in your life that is *different?*" This requires some focusing by the patient. Next, learn about the patient's perception of the event, available situational supports, and what the patient usually does about a problem the patient is not able to solve (Aguilera, 1998). As in all areas of nursing, make the safety of the patient and others in the patient's environment the highest priority. Determine if the patient plans to kill himself or someone else by asking directly about suicidal or homicidal thoughts. For example, ask, "Are you thinking of killing yourself or someone else?" If the answer is yes, ask for more information such as whether or not the person has attempted suicide previously, has a plan for committing suicide, and has the means to carry out the specific plan. For example, if the person plans to shoot himself, does he or she have a gun? These questions are sometimes difficult to ask, but a patient who is highly stressed has thought about suicide at some point and is usually relieved when someone else brings up the subject.

After you eliminate suicide or homicide from consideration, examine other potential threats to the safety of vulnerable people for whom the patient is a caregiver. Provide for their temporary care or supervision if necessary. Determine the degree of disruption in the person's life with work, school, home, and family. After completing the immediate assessment and ensuring the safety of the patient and his or her dependents, begin the problem-solving process (Aguilera, 1998).

**CONTINUITY OF CARE.** An effective plan requires you to collaborate with occupational therapists, dietitians, or pastoral care professionals. There will be times when nursing practice alone does not meet all of the patient's needs. Patients experiencing stress from medical conditions or psychiatric disorders will present needs that will make it necessary for you to consult with advanced practice mental health nurses, psychiatrists, psychologists, or psychiatric social workers. Such a multidisciplinary approach to care addresses the holistic needs of the patient. Recognize the need for collaboration and consultation, inform the patient about potential resources, and make arrangements for consultations, group sessions, or therapy as needed.

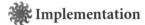 **Implementation**

**HEALTH PROMOTION.** Intervention for stress has a three-pronged approach: (1) decrease stress-producing situations, (2) increase resistance to stress, and (3) learn skills that reduce physiological response to stress (Pender and others, 2002). As a nurse you educate patients and families about the importance of health promotion (Box 22-3).

**Regular Exercise.** A regular exercise program improves muscle tone and posture, controls weight, reduces tension, improves circulation, triggers release of endorphins, and promotes relaxation. In addition, exercise reduces the risk of cardiovascular disease and improves cardiopulmonary functioning. Patients who have a history of a chronic illness, who are at risk for developing an illness, or who are older than 35 years of age begin a physical exercise program only after discussing the plan with a physician or health care provider. In general, for a fitness program to have positive physical effects, a person needs to exercise at least 3 or 4 times a week for 50 to 60 minutes.

**Support Systems.** A support system of family and friends who will listen, offer advice, share recreation time, and provide emotional support benefits a patient experiencing stress (Figure 22-1). People with strong networks of friends, neighbors, and family tend to be healthier than those without support systems. Many organizations, such as the American Heart Association, the American Cancer Society, local hospitals and churches, and mental health organizations offer support group services to individuals. Acceptable support systems vary by cultural group. For example, one cultural group relies heavily upon church members for support. Another cultural group values individual privacy and prefers to avoid a self-help group with "strangers."

**Progressive Muscle Relaxation.** In the presence of anxiety-provoking thoughts and events, muscles tense. Physiological tension diminishes through a systematic approach to releasing tension in major muscle groups. Typically the patient achieves a relaxed state through deep chest breathing, and then the facilitator directs the patient to alternately tighten and relax muscles in specific groupings (see Chapter 30).

**Cognitive Therapy.** Cognitive therapy teaches patients how certain thinking patterns cause symptoms of stress or depression. Cognitive therapy focuses on changing ways of thinking so that the patient feels empowered and in control of his or her own life.

**Assertiveness Training.** Assertiveness training teaches individuals to communicate effectively regarding their needs and desires. The ability to resolve conflict with others through assertiveness training reduces stress. When a group leader teaches assertiveness, the effects of interacting with other people increase the benefits of the experience.

**Stress Management in the Workplace.** The interventions described above address activities and responses that you will make in your personal life or teach your patients to use. Dealing with stress in the workplace requires a different approach, however. Rapid changes in health care technology, diversity in the workforce, organizational restructuring, and

## CARE PLAN Stress and Individual Coping

### ASSESSMENT

When Becky Howard first meets Rhonda, she is immediately struck by Rhonda's appearance. She observes Rhonda showing signs of being nervous, **frequently licking her lips, picking at her fingernails, and being easily startled.** Rhonda's **vital signs show changes in response to stress:** pulse 120, respirations 24, blood pressure 168/84. Rhonda appears thin and pale and reports that she has **lost 15 lb in the last 3 months.** Her appetite has been poor, and she has stopped cooking meals, instead picking up fast food for her family at night. She also reports **difficulty in falling and remaining asleep at night.** In discussing her situation, including both fear of losing her job and being unable to support her family, Rhonda **uses poor eye contact** and then **bursts into tears and expresses feelings of being overwhelmed.** Rhonda admits to having started **drinking at night to help herself "unwind."** During the discussion, Rhonda also talks about **feelings of shame and embarrassment.** She has always been the one to care for other people, and she is ashamed that she cannot "get a grip" on her own life. She cannot easily accept herself in a "patient" role and **thinks of herself as a failure for not coping better.** Rhonda has high expectations of herself as a wife, mother, and nurse.

*Defining characteristics are shown in bold type.

---

**NURSING DIAGNOSIS** Ineffective coping related to increased pressure at work and multiple family stresses and responsibilities.

---

### PLANNING

**GOAL**

- Patient will demonstrate coping strategies in adjusting to increased job pressure and achieving family security within 1 month.

**EXPECTED OUTCOMES***
**Coping**

- Patient will return to normal sleep pattern, requiring less than 1 hour to fall asleep and staying asleep all night within 2 weeks.
- Patient will have three meals a day, joining family during evening meals within 1 week.
- Patient will gain 5 lb within 1 month.
- Patient will report a decrease in stress in 2 weeks.

*Outcomes classification label from Moorhead S, Johnson M, Maas M: *Nursing outcomes classification (NOC)*, ed 3, St. Louis, 2004, Mosby.

---

### INTERVENTIONS†

**Coping**

- Set appointment at employee assistance program clinic with patient 2 times a week. Provide an atmosphere of acceptance.

- During counseling, define the problem from the information given by patient. Explore possible alternative solutions, and give specific directions as needed. At the next session evaluate results with patient. If none of the solutions has been effective, work together to find others.
- Explore with patient previous methods of dealing with life problems.
- Explore patient's previous achievements.

- Encourage patient to identify own strengths and abilities.

- Provide information on cost-free counseling and support groups.
- Instruct the patient in strategies to increase her resistance to stress (see Box 22-3)

### RATIONALE

In order for treatment goals to be accomplished in a short time, patient will see therapist as being likable, reliable, and understanding (Aguilera, 1998).

Patient's primary appraisal of the stressor and her secondary appraisal of her coping strategies define the stressful situation (Benter, 2005).

A problem-solving approach will empower the patient and improve her self-confidence (Benter, 2005).

Emphasizing the positive helps a person feel more optimistic, which leads to positive actions and results.

To manage stress and cope with change, people need to know their strengths and abilities and what is important to them.

Talking with others relieves tension for a person, and helping others, as in a support group, reduces self-absorption and stress.

Increasing resistance to stress is one of the primary modes for intervention for stress management (Pender and others 2002).

†Intervention classification labels from Dochterman JM, Bulechek GM, editors: *Nursing interventions classification (NIC)*, ed 4, St. Louis, 2004, Mosby.

---

### EVALUATION

- Ask patient to report over the course of a week ability to fall asleep and hours slept per night.
- Weigh patient regularly.
- Obtain a 2-day diary of food intake.
- Observe patient's attitude toward therapy, expressions of despair, and increasing depression.

- Continue to monitor patient's suicide potential.
- Ask patient about her perceptions of the counseling sessions and support group.

PATIENT TEACHING

Becky recognizes that Rhonda wants to learn how to increase her resistance to stress (Pender and others, 2002). Becky develops the following teaching plan for Rhonda:

**Outcome**
- At the end of the teaching session, Rhonda will list five ways to increase her resistance to stress.

**Teaching Strategies**
- Meet with Rhonda in a quiet and private setting at a time when Rhonda has about 1 hour to talk without interruptions.
- Schedule a follow-up hour about a week after the first session.
- Based upon Rhonda's identified needs in the areas of physical exercise, assertiveness skills, coping resources, self-esteem, and insight about personal and professional responsibilities, encourage Rhonda to select one aspect of stress resistance upon which to focus.
- For a goal of increasing physical exercise, ask Rhonda to discuss and explore her reasonable alternatives for exercise. Ask her to maintain a daily record of her physical exercise.
- For increasing assertiveness skills, explain assertive behavior and suggest Rhonda keep a log of her assertive, aggressive, or passive responses for the next week.

- For coping resources, explore with Rhonda her support system, possibilities for continuing education, financial status, and her personal appearance, depending upon her identified needs (Pender and others, 2002). Ask her to explore these resources and prepare a summary of her findings.
- For self-esteem describe cognitive skills such as positive self-talk and becoming successful in a particular skill (Pender and others, 2002). Ask her to keep a daily log of her experiences with positive self-talk and her thoughts about a skill at which she excels.
- For developing insight about maintaining appropriate boundaries between work and personal space, explore with Rhonda ways she will increase awareness of her feelings of anger, pain, hurt, sadness, and joy. Discuss with her how she will recognize the limits of her responsibilities. Ask her to keep a personal journal of her feelings for the next week.

**Evaluation Strategies**
- During the follow-up meeting ask Rhonda to report her progress in the chosen area of teaching.
- Ask Rhonda to verbally review her log or record of the week's activities.
- Ask Rhonda to evaluate her progress toward her goal of increased resistance to stress.

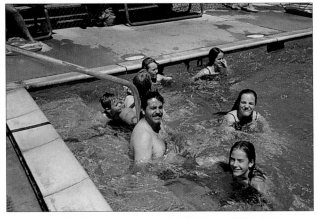

FIGURE **22-1** Sharing recreation with family and friends promotes relaxation. (Courtesy Michael S. Clement, MD, Mesa, Ariz.)

CULTURAL FOCUS

Nurses universally experience job stress. Researchers have studied the job stress, coping, and health perceptions of Hong Kong nurses who work in outpatient clinics, maternal and child health centers, health education centers, and tuberculosis and chest clinics. They concluded that the nurses in these outpatient settings in Hong Kong experience less stress than nurses in acute care and specialized clinical settings. Their main sources of stress are workload, conflict with physicians, and conflict with other nurses. Over half of the nurses use the coping methods of "be as organized as possible" and "attend to important matters." About 45% of the nurses use coping strategies "maintain social communication" and "try to be more tolerant." Finally, the researchers found that the higher the job stress the nurses feel, the worse they believe their health status to be. Based upon this study of Hong Kong nurses, nurse researchers need to study job stress in other countries and cultures to describe job stress as a universal experience.

Data from Lee JKL: Job stress, coping and health perceptions of Hong Kong primary care nurses, *Int J Nurs Pract* 9:86, 2003.

changing work systems place stress on nurses. Additional causes of job stress include particular job assignments, difficult schedules, shift work, fear of failure, and inadequate support services (Box 22-4). Burnout occurs as a result of chronic stress. Burnout is "a syndrome of emotional exhaustion, depersonalization of others, and perceptions of reduced personal accomplishment, resulting from intense involvement with people in a care-giving environment" (Aguilera, 1998).

If you recognize feelings of burnout, make changes in your behavior to cope with workplace stress. Identify the limits and scope of your responsibilities at work (Aguilera, 1998). Recognize the areas over which you have control and the ability to change and those for which you do not have responsibility. Make a clear separation between work and

home life as well. Strengthening friendships outside of the workplace, socially isolating oneself for personal "recharging" of emotional energy, and spending off-duty hours in interesting activities all help reduce burnout (Box 22-5).

**ACUTE CARE**

**Crisis Intervention.** When stress overwhelms a person's usual coping mechanisms and demands mobilization of all available resources, the stress becomes a crisis (Shontz, 1975).

| BOX 22-5 | USING EVIDENCE IN PRACTICE |

**Research Summary**

The stress of working with chronically ill children and their families leads to compassion fatigue. If not treated, compassion fatigue leads to job burnout, which has symptoms of emotional exhaustion and difficulty relating to patients. Ultimately, burnout leads to nurses' leaving the profession. For this reason, nurses need to recognize causes of compassion fatigue, signs of its appearance when they have it, and ways to deal with compassion fatigue before it progresses to burnout. Two researchers interviewed 20 pediatric nurses to learn the triggers to compassion fatigue for them and their coping strategies. From these nurses' experiences, other nurses can identify their own potential triggers to compassion fatigue and coping strategies that work for them.

Triggers for compassion fatigue reported by pediatric nurses are:

- Seeing the pain, sadness, and death that happened to their young patients
- Unreasonable expectations of families who became angry with the nurses
- Unreasonable policies in the job setting
- A perceived lack of support
- Excessive demands of work, including overtime and double shifts
- A sense of overinvolvement with patients and crossing professional boundaries

**Application to Nursing Practice**

The results from this study help nurses recognize their own triggers to compassion fatigue. A variety of personal coping strategies are used. Some of the most effective coping methods include taking care of oneself through exercise, meditation, and journaling; balancing work and personal life with supportive personal relationships; and recognizing the need to seek counseling.

In addition, work-related coping strategies are equally important. These strategies can help nurses recognize the limits of their own responsibility and know what they had the ability to control and what they were not able to control. It is important to maintain supportive relationships within the workplace and to develop a planned approach for dealing with compassion fatigue. Developing a professional philosophy about caring for patients who are chronically ill and dying helps the nurse cope with compassion fatigue.

As a nurse, you learn what you are able to do and what you are not able to do to help a patient. You learn to care for patients while you are working and to care for yourself and your family when you are away from work. You develop an awareness of your feelings of sadness, anger, hurt, fear, and joy. You recognize when you are overidentifying with patients or their family members. Plan coping strategies that help you address your stress. You need a supportive network and time to reflect on your own philosophy of work and personal life.

Data from: Maytum JC and others: Compassion fatigue and burnout in nurses who work with children with chronic conditions and their families, *J Pediatr Health Care* 18:171, 2004.

A crisis creates a turning point in a person's life because it changes the direction of a person's life in some way. According to Aguilera (1998), the precipitating event usually occurs from 1 to 2 weeks before the individual seeks help, but sometimes it has occurred within the past 24 hours. Generally a crisis resolves in some way within approximately 6 weeks. Crisis intervention aims to return the person to a precrisis level of functioning and to promote growth.

Because an individual's or family's usual coping strategies do not help manage the stress of the precipitating event, they need to learn to use new coping mechanisms. This experience, which forces the use of unfamiliar strategies, results either in a heightened awareness of previously unrecognized strengths and resources or in deterioration in functioning. Thus a crisis becomes a situation of both danger and opportunity. Some persons or families will emerge from a crisis state functioning more effectively, whereas others find themselves weakened, and still others completely dysfunctional.

Crisis intervention, a brief psychotherapy with prescribed steps, provides more direction than traditional psychotherapy or counseling. Any member of the interdisciplinary health care team who has been trained in its techniques is able to initiate crisis intervention (Aguilera, 1998). Crisis intervention primarily uses problem solving and focuses only on the problem presented by the crisis.

When using crisis intervention, help the patient make the mental connection between the stressful event and the patient's reaction to it. You need to do this because the person is sometimes unable to see the whole situation clearly. Help the person become aware of present feelings, such as anger, grief, or guilt, to their feelings of tension. In addition, help the patient explore coping mechanisms, perhaps identifying ways of coping the patient had not thought of. Finally, help increase the scope of the person's social contacts if the person is internally focused and isolated (Aguilera, 1998).

**RESTORATIVE AND CONTINUING CARE.** A person under stress recovers when the stress disappears or coping strategies succeed. However, a person who has experienced a crisis has changed, and the effects sometimes last for years or for the rest of the person's life. In the final stage of adapting to a crisis, the patient acknowledges the long-term implications of the crisis. If a person has successfully coped with a crisis and its consequences, he or she becomes a more mature and healthy person. When a person has recovered from a stressful situation, you will introduce stress management skills to reduce the number and intensity of stressful situations in the future.

## Evaluation

**PATIENT CARE.** By evaluating the goals and expected outcomes of care, you know if your nursing interventions were effective and if the patient copes with the identified stress. Assess the patient's perception of the effectiveness of the plan. Review the behaviorally stated, measurable goals, and evaluate

## OUTCOME EVALUATION

**TABLE 22-3**

| Nursing Action | Patient Response/Finding | Achievement of Outcome |
|---|---|---|
| Ask Rhonda about suicidal thoughts. | Rhonda states that she wants to continue to live and to find solutions for her problems. | Demonstrates coping through ability to discuss feelings openly; she needs further counseling. |
| Discuss with Rhonda her ability to ask for assistance when she needs it. | Rhonda has set an appointment with a self-help group offered by an employee assistance program. | Willing to call on others for help; needs to feel comfortable seeking help from friends. |
| Observe Rhonda's personal hygiene, attitude toward therapy, and expressions of loss and powerlessness. | Rhonda will begin to verbally express feelings of loss and powerlessness. | Confidence related to past experience with health behavior. |
| Ask Rhonda to identify areas in her life that she is able to change to reduce stress. | Rhonda will ask friend to consider being the soccer coach. | Verbalizes sense of control over personal life. |
| Ask Rhonda to identify own strengths and abilities. | Rhonda will establish a career plan. | Modifies lifestyle as needed. |
| Ask Rhonda to report over the course of a week ability to fall asleep and hours slept per night. | Rhonda reports improved appetite; she still takes an hour to fall asleep but only awakens once. | Quality of sleep improving. |

## EVALUATION

Three weeks after their initial discussion, Rhonda makes her routine appointment at the employee health office to see Becky. Becky is relieved to see that Rhonda is less anxious and looking better. Her blood pressure is 140/82 and pulse is 88. Her weight reflects a gain of 3 lb since her last visit. The nervous behaviors previously assessed are no longer present. Rhonda is sleeping through the night. Feeling less drained, Rhonda has begun to make progress on developing professional and personal boundaries. She has withdrawn temporarily from her soccer coaching duties to reduce the demands on her time. As a result, her situation has become known among other mothers, and many have offered to help drive her husband to his therapy sessions or to provide casseroles for the family to eat. Rhonda has now accepted this help by reminding herself that it will only be temporary. Furthermore, Rhonda and her husband are going together to a family support group meeting held every week at his rehabilitation facility. She is finding the encouragement of that group to be of benefit to her and an important addition to her in-dividual counseling sessions with her employee assistance program counselor. Although the Bennett family has not yet found full resolution for their stress, they are making progress toward achievable, short-term goals.

**Documentation Note**

"Patient reports feelings of increased hopefulness and return to normal sleep and eating patterns. She is taking Zoloft, 100 mg daily, as prescribed by her personal physician, Dr. Smith, and is returning to see him for follow-up in 1 week. She is attending weekly counseling with Dr. Moody and also a rehabilitation support group with husband. Her blood pressure today is 140/82, pulse 88, and she had a weight gain of 3 lb in the last 3 weeks. She has requested instruction in relaxation techniques. The therapist demonstrated guided imagery in a 15-minute session, and patient reported feeling relaxed. She will practice this at home. We will continue to follow the present plan, and she will return for follow-up in 2 weeks."

whether or not the patient has met the criteria for success as stated in the outcomes. If the nursing interventions have not been effective in helping the patient achieve targeted goals, you must reevaluate the strategies implemented and revise the plan of care in light of the patient's current health status.

To evaluate the patient experiencing stress, observe patient behaviors and talk with the patient and family, if appropriate. Remember that coping with stress takes time. If you are in a setting where contact with a patient ends before achieving goals or resolution, refer your patient to appropriate resources so as not to delay or interrupt progress.

**PATIENT EXPECTATIONS.** Maintain ongoing communication with patients regarding the plan of care. Patients under severe stress often experience feelings of powerlessness, vulnerability, and loss of control. Actively involve patients and families in problem identification (assessment), prioritizing, and goal setting and evaluation (Table 22-3). Involving patients in these processes gives them an opportunity to direct their energy in a positive way and moves them toward taking greater responsibility for health maintenance and promotion.

Engaging the patient as a partner in health care sets the stage for open communication. This gives the patient a sense of control and begins to promote independence, which are both crucial to the patient's successful resolution of the situation. In such an environment the patient feels more freedom to give important feedback to you about interventions that are successful. This helps you better understand why some interventions fail to meet the established goals.

## KEY CONCEPTS

- The general adaptation syndrome, an immediate physiological response to stress, involves several body systems, especially the autonomic nervous system and the endocrine system. Physiological responses to stress also include immunological changes.
- Stress makes people ill as a result of (1) increased levels of powerful hormones that change our bodily processes; (2) coping choices that are unhealthy, such as not getting enough rest or a proper diet or use of tobacco, alcohol, or caffeine; and (3) neglect of warning signs of illness or prescribed medicines or treatments.
- A person experiences psychological stress only if the person evaluates the event or circumstance as personally significant, called primary appraisal.
- Stress includes work stress, family stress, chronic stress, acute stress, daily hassles, trauma, and crisis. Rapid changes in health care technology, diversity in the work-

force, organizational restructuring, staffing shortages, and changing work systems places stress on nurses.
- Potential stressors and coping mechanisms vary across the life span, from childhood through adolescence, adulthood, and old age, and from one culture to another.
- Coping, a process that constantly changes to manage demands on a person's resources, means making an effort to manage psychological stress.
- Posttraumatic stress disorder affects people who have experienced accidents, violent events, war, and natural disasters.
- A patient with such severe stress that the person is unable to cope in any ways that have worked before is experiencing a crisis. A crisis marks a turning point in life, either developmental or situational.
- Generally a crisis resolves in some way within approximately 6 weeks. Crisis intervention aims to return the person to a precrisis level of functioning and to promote growth.

## CRITICAL THINKING IN PRACTICE

*Mrs. Smith, a 75-year-old woman, is at the hospital with a fractured hip. Before her injury she lived with her husband, who suffers from advancing Alzheimer's disease. While she is hospitalized, he is staying with a niece who lives 100 miles away, but this is not a permanent situation because her niece is also in frail health. The patient has no children to help her when she returns home. She is concerned not only about who will care for her after she is discharged but also about her husband.*

- - - - - - - - - - - - - - - - - - - - - -

1. List three potential nursing diagnoses for this woman.
2. Which of the following is an appropriate goal for crisis intervention for Mrs. Smith and her husband?
   a. Mrs. Smith will relocate her husband to a nursing home near her home.

   b. Mrs. Smith will have in-home assistance with her husband until she can resume caring for her husband.
   c. Mrs. Smith will enter a nursing home with her husband.
3. List three cultural factors to assess when meeting with Mrs. Smith.
4. The type of crisis that Mrs. Smith is experiencing is called:
   a. Developmental crisis
   b. Situational crisis

## NCLEX® REVIEW

1. While assessing a person for effects of the general adaptation syndrome, be aware that:
   1. Heart rate increases in the resistance stage
   2. Blood volume increases in the exhaustion stage
   3. Vital signs return to normal in the exhaustion stage
   4. Blood glucose level increases during the alarm reaction stage
2. While teaching a person with hypertension about how stress causes illness, you explain that:
   1. Hypertension causes stress by suppressing immunity
   2. Some antihypertensive medications cause stress and illness
   3. A person who takes antihypertensive medication has an immunity to stress
   4. Stress causes a person to forget to take medication and thereby cause illness

3. Another nurse is talking with you about the stress she feels on the job. You recognize that:
   1. Nurses who feel stress usually pass the stress along to their patients
   2. A nurse who feels stress is ineffective as a nurse and should not be working
   3. Nurses who talk about feeling stress are unprofessional and should calm down
   4. Nurses frequently experience stress with the rapid changes in health care technology and organizational restructuring
4. When assessing a child for the effects of stress, you observe that:
   1. Children are resilient and cope with stress better than adults
   2. Children provoke more stress in others than they experience themselves

3. Stressors and coping methods are different for children than older people
4. Ways of coping that will be effective for a child are similar to those of the child's parents

5. You are evaluating the coping success of a patient experiencing stress from being newly diagnosed with multiple sclerosis and psychomotor impairment. You realize that the patient is coping successfully when the patient says:
   1. "I am going to learn to drive a car so I can be more independent."
   2. "My sister says she feels better when she goes shopping, so I will go shopping."
   3. "I have always felt better when I go for a long walk. I will do that when I get home."
   4. "I am going to attend a support group to learn more about multiple sclerosis and what I will be able to do."

6. When doing an assessment of a young woman who was in an automobile accident 6 months before, you learn that the woman has vivid images of the crash whenever she hears a loud, sudden noise. You recognize this as:

1. Social phobia
2. Acute anxiety
3. Posttraumatic stress disorder
4. Borderline personality disorder

7. A family tells the community mental health nurse that their adult mentally retarded son is experiencing hallucinations. This has begun very recently and had not happened before. They are frightened for him and do not know what to do. In addition, they are living below the poverty level on their pensions and have only enough money to last from one month to the next. The nurse helps them set the following goal:
   1. After a psychiatric evaluation, investigate a group home for the son
   2. With help from the nurse, obtain suitable housing and additional financial resources
   3. Develop a plan to take in a renter so that they can have a better income
   4. Obtain a psychiatric evaluation and stabilization on antipsychotic medication to be covered by Medicaid

## REFERENCES

Aguilera D: *Crisis intervention: theory and methodology,* St. Louis, 1998, Mosby.

Aldwin C: *Stress, coping, and development,* New York, 2000, Guilford.

Benter SE: Crisis intervention. In Stuart GW, Laraia MT: *Principles and practice of psychiatric nursing,* ed 8, St. Louis, 2005, Mosby.

Dochterman JM, Bulechek G, editors: *Nursing Interventions Classification (NIC),* ed 4, St. Louis, 2004, Mosby.

Enright, RD, North, J, editors: *Exploring forgiveness,* Madison, 1998, University of Wisconsin Press.

Lazarus R: *Stress and emotion: a new synthesis,* New York, 1999, Springer.

Lee JKL: Job stress, coping and health perceptions of Hong Kong primary care nurses, *Int J Nurs Pract* 9:86, 2003.

Maytum JC and others: Compassion fatigue and burnout in nurses who work with children with chronic conditions and their families, *J Pediatr Health Care* 18:171, 2004.

Monat A, Lazarus R: *Stress and coping: an anthology,* New York, 1991, Columbia University Press.

Moorhead S, Johnson M, Maas M, editors: *Nursing outcomes classification (NOC),* ed 3, St. Louis, 2004, Mosby.

Neuman B, Fawcett J: *The Neuman systems model,* ed 4, Upper Saddle River, NJ, 2002, Prentice Hall.

Pender NJ, Murdaugh CL, Parsons MA: *Health promotion in nursing practice,* ed 4, Upper Saddle River, NJ, 2002, Prentice Hall.

Selye H: History and present status of the stress concept. In Monat A, Lazarus R, editors: *Stress and coping: an anthology,* New York, 1991, Columbia University Press.

# CHAPTER 23

# Loss and Grief

## MEDIA RESOURCES

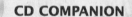 CD COMPANION 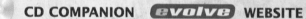 evolve WEBSITE

http://evolve.elsevier.com/Potter/basic

- **NCLEX® Review**
- **Audio Glossary**
- **English/Spanish Audio Glossary**

## OBJECTIVES

- Describe and compare the phases of grieving from Kübler-Ross, Bowlby, and Worden.
- List and discuss the five basic categories of loss.
- Describe the types of grief.
- Describe characteristics of a person experiencing grief.
- Discuss variables that influence a person's response to grief.
- Identify your role in assisting patients with problems related to loss, death, and grief.

- Develop a care plan for a patient or family experiencing loss and grief.
- Explain reasons for the need for improved end-of-life care for patients.
- Discuss principles of palliative care.
- Describe how to involve family members in palliative care.
- Discuss the procedure for care of the body after death.
- Discuss the nurse's own loss experience when caring for dying patients.

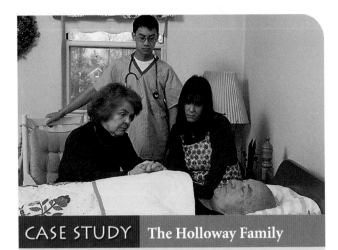

## CASE STUDY  The Holloway Family

Mr. Holloway is a 73-year-old man with a history of colon cancer diagnosed 18 months ago and treated with surgery and chemotherapy. As a result of surgery he experienced incontinence and chronic diarrhea. Chemotherapy caused oral ulcers and loss of appetite. He was recently admitted to the hospital for evaluation and treatment of severe anemia and dehydration. When studies showed widespread metastases of the cancer to his liver and lungs, his oncologist decided to stop all chemotherapy. Medical treatment now includes pain management, blood replacement, and rehydration. The discharge plan is for Mr. Holloway to receive hospice care at home.

Living in the household with Mr. Holloway are his wife of 53 years and their only child, a single daughter who is 38 years old. Mr. Holloway's daughter has taken a leave of absence from her teaching job and moved back home to help care for him during his final illness. His wife, however, is unwilling to accept that he is near death. She continues to insist, "If he would only eat right, take vitamins, and go to a gym, he would regain his strength and recover." Mr. Holloway's wife and daughter argue often about how best to help him. He becomes visibly upset when they argue and often is very withdrawn and tearful. The Holloways have few ties to the community and very limited social support. The health care team is concerned about how they will cope now that Mr. Holloway is ready for discharge.

Peter Wong is a 22-year-old nursing student completing a rotation in community health. He considers himself fortunate

to have never lost a family member and has never cared for a terminally ill patient. When he learns that he will be providing home care for Mr. Holloway and his family, he becomes anxious. He feels unprepared to intervene effectively with the sadness and conflict in the Holloway household. Peter arranges a time to talk with his instructor about his concerns. The instructor assures him that he is competent and that this will be a good opportunity to learn.

## KEY TERMS

acceptance, p. 612
actual loss, p. 611
anger, p. 612
anticipatory grief, p. 613
anxiolytics, p. 624
bargaining, p. 612
bereavement, p. 612
denial, p. 612
depression, p. 612
disorganization and despair, p. 613
grief, p. 612
grieving process, p. 614
hope, p. 615
hospice, p. 625

maturational loss, p. 611
mourning, p. 612
necessary losses, p. 611
numbing, p. 612
palliative care, p. 623
perceived loss, p. 611
postmortem care, p. 626
reorganization, p. 613
situational loss, p. 611
yearning and searching, p. 612

Loss and grief are experiences that affect not only patients and their families but the nurses who care for them as well. The ultimate loss, death, is one that most patients and families have great difficulty accepting and managing. America is a death-denying society (End-of-Life Nursing Education Consortium [ELNEC], 2000). This means that Americans often deny the need to express grief and to feel the pain associated with a loss, both of which promote heal-

| TABLE 23-1 | Types of Loss |
| --- | --- |
| **Definition** | **Implications of Loss** |
| Loss of external objects (e.g., loss, misplacement, theft, destruction by nature) | Extent of grieving depends on object's value, sentiment attached to it, and its usefulness. |
| Loss of a known environment (e.g., moving from a neighborhood, hospitalization, a new job, moving out of intensive care unit) | Loss occurs through maturational or situational events and through injury or illness. Loneliness or newness of unfamiliar setting threatens self-esteem and makes grieving difficult. |
| Loss of a significant other (e.g., being promoted, moving, loss of a family member, friend, trusted nurse, or animal companion) | Significant other typically meets another person's need for psychological safety, love and belonging, and self-esteem. |
| Loss of an aspect of self (e.g., body part, psychological or physiological function) | Illness, injury, or developmental changes result in a loss that causes grief and permanent changes in body image, self-concept, and level of independence. |
| Loss of life (e.g., death of family member, friend, or acquaintance; own death) | Loss of life creates grief for those left behind. Person facing death often fears pain, loss of control, and dependency on others. |

ing. Grief affects individuals physically, psychologically, socially, and spiritually as a result of real, concrete losses. As a nurse you will have the opportunity to help patients and families face devastating losses and accept the reality of impending death. Providing care for patients in crisis and at the end of life requires knowledge and caring to help bring comfort to patients and families even when hope for cure is gone.

## Scientific Knowledge Base

### Loss

Throughout our lives, from birth to death, we form attachments and suffer losses. We become independent from our parents, start and leave school, begin careers, and form relationships. Growing up is natural and positive, yet as we live our lives, losses do occur. **Necessary losses** are a part of each person's life. We expect our losses to be recovered and replaced by something different or better, but there are other losses that change our safety and security. Losses such as death of a loved one, divorce, or loss of a friend are significant and have long-term effects on our health.

Loss comes in many forms based on our values and priorities, which are influenced by our family, friends, society, and culture. A person experiences loss in the absence of an object, person, body part or function, emotion, or idea that was formerly present (Table 23-1). Losses are actual or perceived. An **actual loss** is any loss of a person or object that the individual can no longer feel, hear, know, or experience. Examples include the loss of a body part, child, relationship, or role at work. Lost objects that a person might value include any possession that is worn out, misplaced, stolen, or ruined by disaster. For example, a child grieves over the loss of a favorite toy or pet. A **perceived loss** is any loss that is uniquely defined by the grieving patient. It is sometimes less obvious to others. An example is the loss of confidence or prestige. It is easy to overlook or misunderstand perceived

losses, yet the process of grief follows the same order and progression as actual losses. Individual interpretation makes a difference in how the perceived loss is uniquely valued and the response that a person will have during grieving.

Losses are also maturational, situational, or both. A **maturational loss** is any change in the developmental process that is normally expected during a lifetime. One example is a mother's feeling of loss as a child goes to school for the first time. Events associated with maturational loss are part of normal life transitions, but the feelings of loss persist as grieving helps a person cope with the change. **Situational loss** includes any sudden, unpredictable, external event. Often this type of loss includes multiple losses rather than a single loss, such as an automobile accident that leaves a driver paralyzed, unable to return to work, and grieving over the loss of the passenger in the accident.

The type of loss and the perception of the loss influence the degree of grief a person experiences. Each individual responds to loss differently. This is important for you to remember as a nurse. It is incorrect to assume that the loss of an object does not generate the same level of grief as loss of a loved one. The value an individual places on the lost object (e.g., a family pet) determines the emotional response to the separation. As a nurse you will assess the special meaning that a loss has for a patient and its effect on the patient's health and well-being.

Hospitalization and chronic illness or disability usually have multiple associated losses. When persons enter a hospital, they lose their privacy, control over body functions and daily routines, their modesty, and any ideas that they are indestructible. A chronic or debilitating illness adds concern about one's finances. Furthermore, long-term illness often requires a job change, threatens independence, and forces changes in lifestyle. Even a brief illness or hospitalization requires temporary shifts in family role functioning. Chronic or debilitating illnesses pose a major threat to the stability of relationships.

Death is the ultimate loss. Although death is part of the continuum of life and a universal part of being human, it is also a mystical event that creates anxiety and fear. Death ends relationships with family and friends and separates people from the physical presence of persons who influence their lives. Even in the presence of a strong spiritual grounding, facing death is difficult for the dying person, as well as for the person's family, friends, and caregivers. A person's terminal illness reminds close friends and associates of their own mortality. A person with an advanced, progressive, ultimately fatal illness such as chronic renal failure, lung disease, or metastatic cancer, faces many levels of suffering. It is difficult to be sick, and many people dislike seeking help from others, yet nearly all want companionship in the face of death (Finucane, 2002).

Talking and thinking about death is not something we normally do. Feelings of guilt, anger, and fear arise when we must finally face death. It causes some family members and caregivers to withdraw at a time when the dying person needs their love and support. Personal fundamental beliefs and values, culture, spirituality, and the quality of the emotional support available, all influence the way a person and his or her family approach dying.

As a nurse you will provide grief support to the patient and members of the family affected by a loss. Each individual will require your attentive response and compassionate understanding.

## Grief

**Grief** is the emotional response to a loss. Individuals express grief in a variety of ways that are unique to an individual and based on personal experiences, cultural expectations, and spiritual beliefs (Farber and others, 1999) (see Chapters 17 and 18). Coping with grief after a loss involves **mourning,** the outward, social expression of a loss (ELNEC, 2000). It involves working through the grief until an individual accepts and adapts to his or her expectations to go on in life without that which was lost. **Bereavement** includes grief and mourning—the inner feelings and outward reactions of a survivor (ELNEC, 2000). Survivors go through a bereavement period that is not linear. It does not proceed in sequential stages that you are able to predict precisely. Rather, an individual will move back and forth through a series of stages and/or tasks many times, possibly extending over a period of several years, before the process is over. However, no one really "gets over" a loss, but instead heals and learns to live with a loss (ELNEC, 2000). Many theorists have studied the grief process (Table 23-2). Theories of grief apply to all forms of loss including death, a chronic illness, or sudden loss of body function. Although each theorist uses different terms, the grief process that all of them outline is basically the same (Varcarolis, 2002). Each describes commonly experienced psychological and behavioral characteristics that follow a pattern or stage of response.

**KÜBLER-ROSS'S STAGES OF DYING.** Kübler-Ross's theory (1969) is behavior-oriented and includes five stages (see Table 23-2). During **denial** an individual acts as though nothing has happened and refuses to believe or understand that a loss has occurred. In the **anger** stage, the individual resists the loss and sometimes strikes out at everyone and everything. During **bargaining,** the individual postpones awareness of the reality of the loss and tries to deal with it in a subtle or overt way as though the loss can be prevented. A person realizes the full impact and significance of the loss during the **depression** stage, when the individual feels overwhelmingly lonely and withdraws from interpersonal interaction. However, it is common for the individual to think or talk about memories of the deceased. The memories are usually positive but expressed with sadness. Finally, during the stage of **acceptance,** the individual accepts the loss and begins to look to the future.

**BOWLBY'S PHASES OF MOURNING.** Bowlby's attachment theory (1980) is the foundation for his theory on mourning. Attachment is an instinctive behavior that leads to the development of affection between children and their primary caregiver. These bonds are present and active throughout life. Later the bonds are generalized to other persons with whom individuals form close relationships. Attachment behavior ensures our survival because it keeps us in close contact with persons who offer us protection and support.

Bowlby describes four phases of mourning (see Table 23-2). As in the other grief theories, a person moves back and forth between any two of the phases while responding to the loss. The phase of **numbing** lasts from a few hours to a week or more and is sometimes interrupted by periods of extremely intense emotion. It is the briefest phase of mourning. The grieving person reports feeling "stunned" or "unreal." The second phase of **yearning and searching**

| TABLE 23-2 | **The Grief Process** | |
|---|---|---|
| **Kübler-Ross's Five Stages of Dying** | **Bowlby's Four Phases of Mourning** | **Worden's Four Tasks of Mourning** |
| Denial | Numbing | Accepting the reality of loss |
| Anger | Yearning and searching | Working through the pain of grief |
| Bargaining | Disorganization and despair | Adjusting to the environment without the deceased |
| Depression | Reorganization | Emotionally relocating the deceased and moving on with life |
| Acceptance | | |

arouses emotional outbursts of tearful sobbing and acute distress in most persons. Parkes (1972) has explained that it is necessary for the bereaved person to experience the pain of grief in order to get grief work done. Common physical symptoms include tightness in the chest and throat, shortness of breath, a feeling of weakness and lethargy, and insomnia and loss of appetite. This phase lasts for months or years. During the phase of **disorganization and despair** an individual endlessly examines how and why the loss occurred. It is common for the person to express anger at anyone who is possibly responsible. Gradually this phase gives way to an acceptance that the loss is permanent. During the final phase of **reorganization,** which sometimes requires a year or more, the person begins to accept unaccustomed roles, acquire new skills, and build new relationships. Encourage persons experiencing this phase to untie themselves from the old relationship while not devaluing it or feeling that in doing so they are lessening its importance.

**WORDEN'S FOUR TASKS OF MOURNING.** Worden's four tasks of mourning (1982) suggest that individuals who mourn are able to be actively involved in helping themselves and outside intervention can assist them. Although time varies in individuals, the tasks typically require a minimum of a full year to work through.

- Task I: *To accept the reality of the loss.* Even when a person expects death, there is always some period of disbelief and surprise that the event has really happened. This task involves the processes required to accept that the person or object is gone and will not return.
- Task II: *To work through the pain of grief.* Even though people respond to loss differently, it is impossible to experience a loss and work through grief without emotional pain. Individuals who deny or shut off the pain prolong their grief.
- Task III: *To adjust to the environment in which the deceased is missing.* A person does not realize the full impact of a loss for at least 3 months. At this point visitors and friends stop calling and the person is left to ponder the full impact of loneliness. People completing this task take on roles formerly filled by the deceased, including some tasks that they never fully appreciated.
- Task IV: *To emotionally relocate the deceased and move on with life.* The goal of this task is not to forget the deceased or give up the relationship with the deceased but to have the deceased take a new, less important place in a person's emotional life. This is often the most difficult task to complete. People fear that if they make other attachments they will forget their loved one or become disloyal. A person completes this stage after realizing that it is possible to love other people without loving the deceased person less.

**TYPES OF GRIEF.** Knowledge of the types of grief will assist you in the selection of appropriate nursing therapies.

**Normal Grief.** Normal or uncomplicated grief consists of the normal feelings, behaviors, and reactions to a loss. These include resentment, sorrow, anger, crying, loneliness, and temporary withdrawal from activities. Helping your patients to mature and develop as persons will make the normal grief response positive.

**Anticipatory Grief.** The process of "letting go" that occurs before an actual loss or death has occurred is called **anticipatory grief.** For example, once a person or family receives a terminal diagnosis, they begin the process of saying good-bye and completing life affairs. The process becomes more stressful when the patient is unable to make decisions due to worsening health. Unless guided by a patient's explicit decisions regarding end-of-life care (EOLC), the family assumes responsibility for deciding whether to continue life-sustaining measures. The family weighs factors such as the patient's values and choices, the medical facts and probabilities, the burden of treatment, the expected future quality of life for the patient, and the limitations of their own emotional resources (Tilden and others, 2001). When the process of dying lasts for a long time, members of the patient's family sometimes have few symptoms of grief once the death occurs. This seeming absence of grief symptoms is explainable. By the time the actual moment of death arrives, the family has already experienced much of the shock, denial, and tearfulness.

There are risks in anticipatory grieving. Some family members withdraw emotionally from the patient too soon, leaving the patient with no emotional support as death approaches. There are also complications if a person who was thought to be near death survives. Family members then have difficulty reconnecting and are sometimes resentful that the person has lived past life expectancy.

**COMPLICATED GRIEF.** When a person has difficulty progressing through the normal stages of grieving, bereavement becomes complicated. In these cases, bereavement appears to "go wrong" and loss never resolves. This threatens a person's relationships with others. Complicated grief includes four types:

- *Chronic grief:* Active acute mourning characterized by normal grief reactions that do not decrease and continue over long periods of time (ELNEC, 2000). Persons verbalize an inability to "get past" the grief.
- *Delayed grief:* Characterized by normal grief reactions that are suppressed or postponed and the survivor consciously or unconsciously avoids the pain of the loss (ELNEC, 2000). Active grieving is held back, only to resurface later, usually in response to a trivial loss or upset. For example, a wife only grieves a few weeks after the death of her spouse, only to become hysterical and sad a year later when she loses her car keys. The extreme sadness is a delayed response to the death of her husband.
- *Exaggerated grief:* Persons become overwhelmed by grief, and they cannot function. This is reflected in the form of severe phobias or self-destructive behaviors such as alcoholism, substance abuse, or suicide.
- *Masked grief:* Survivors are not aware that behaviors that interfere with normal functioning are a result of their loss

(ELNEC, 2000). For example, a person who has lost a pet develops changes in sleeping or eating patterns.

**DISENFRANCHISED GRIEF.** Individuals experience grief when they experience a loss and they cannot openly acknowledge it, or when it is not socially accepted or publicly shared (ELNEC, 2000). Examples include the loss of a partner from acquired immunodeficiency syndrome (AIDS), the friend who becomes a drug addict, or a mother whose child dies in utero.

## Nursing Knowledge Base

As a nurse you will help patients deal with loss in every situation. Nursing interventions are validated through research and evidence-based practice to support patients experiencing grief and loss.

### Factors Influencing Loss and Grief

Many factors influence the way an individual feels a loss and responds to it during bereavement.

**HUMAN DEVELOPMENT.** Persons of differing ages and stages of development will display different and unique symptoms of grief. For example, toddlers are unable to understand loss or death, but they feel anxiety over loss of objects and separation from parents. School-age children experience grief over the loss of a body part or function. Middle-age adults usually begin to reexamine life and are sensitive to their own physical changes. Older adults often experience anticipatory grief because of aging and the possible loss of self-care abilities. Aging is frequently associated with losses such as physical changes; loss of employment, social respect, and relationships; loss of self-care ability; and threat to a sense of contributions made in life. A person's level of growth and development helps to explain the individual's ability to understand loss and what it means in life (see Chapter 19). It also influences how an individual chooses to react.

**PSYCHOSOCIAL PERSPECTIVES OF LOSS AND GRIEF.** Everyone experiences loss and death. An individual's expression of grief evolves as the person matures. Personal experiences shape the coping mechanisms that the individual uses to deal with stressors associated with loss and grief. Psychologists explain that individuals repeat coping mechanisms that were effective in the past as a first response to loss. When former coping strategies are unsuccessful, individuals try new coping mechanisms (see Chapter 22). When faced with a loss, a patient learns what is needed for his or her own coping through repetition that is based on the successes and failures of different coping mechanisms. Sometimes the number or depths of losses become overwhelming, and familiar coping strategies are not successful.

**SOCIOECONOMIC STATUS.** Socioeconomic status influences a person's ability to obtain options and use support mechanisms when coping with loss. Generally, an individual feels greater burden from a loss when there is a lack of financial, educational, or occupational resources. For example, a patient with limited financial resources is not able to replace a home lost in a fire or is not able to purchase necessary medications to manage a newly diagnosed disease. These patients require referral to community agencies that are able to provide needed resources.

**PERSONAL RELATIONSHIPS.** When loss involves a loved one, the quality and meaning of the relationship are critical in understanding a person's grief experience. It has been said that to lose your parents is to lose your past, to lose your spouse is to lose your present, and to lose your child is to lose your future. When a relationship between two people has been very close and well connected, it is often very difficult for the one left behind to cope. The support that patients receive from family and friends is based in part on their relationships with members of their social network and the manner and circumstances of their loss. When patients do not receive supportive understanding from others, they become unable to handle grief and look to the future.

**Nature of the Loss.** The ability to resolve grief depends on the meaning of the loss and the situation surrounding it. The ability to accept help from others influences whether the bereaved will be able to cope effectively. The visibility of the loss influences the support a person receives. For example, the total loss of one's home from a tornado will bring support from the community, whereas a private loss of an important possession brings less support. The suddenness of a loss often causes slower resolution from grief. For example, a sudden and unexpected death is generally more difficult for a family to accept that one following a long-term chronic disease.

**CULTURE AND ETHNICITY.** Interpretation of a loss and the expression of grief arise from cultural background and family practices (Box 23-1). Persons' basic belief systems are the part of their culture that they can and often do hold on to when they lose control over aspects of their life due to illness (Thomas, 2001). Culture affects how a support system or family respond to loss. For example, in Western societies the **grieving process** is usually personal and private, with individuals showing restrained emotion. However, the ceremonies surrounding a person's death offer time for grief resolution and reminiscing. Among Chinese, death is taboo and discussion of the topic is associated with bad luck (Yick and Gupta, 2002). Muslims view illness as penance for their sins and death as part of life destined by God (Rassoul, 2000). Despite cultural trends, members of the same ethnocultural background often respond to loss and death differently. As a nurse you need to gain an understanding and appreciation of each patient's cultural values as they apply to the experience of loss, death, and grieving. Culturally sensitive practices are needed to guide the development of effective nursing interventions.

Research has shown that ethnicity is strongly related to attitudes toward life-sustaining treatments during terminal illness (Blackhall and others, 1999). The challenge you face is to explore realistically and practically the desires of patients and their support systems to clearly identify concepts and approaches for effective guidance through the loss experience.

| BOX 23-1 | CULTURAL FOCUS |
|----------|----------------|

**Loss, Death, and Grieving**

At the end of life, rituals, mourning practices, and specific expressions of grief are necessary for a survivor of any culture to have a sense of acceptance and inner peace. Not everyone agrees as to whether appropriate care at the end of life achieves a "good death" or an "acceptable death" for patients. Do patients gain a sense of comfort and peace during death? Most hospital policies and procedures support an "acceptable death" for the patient who is dying. This means providing basic standard levels of care, which sometimes take into account a patient's cultural beliefs and practices. A "good death" is one that allows social adjustments and personal preparations for the transition of death. A "good death" allows time for the patient and family to make private and public preparations and for the patient to complete unfinished tasks. A nurse needs to understand patients' culture-specific practices surrounding end-of-life care.

- European Americans perceive that a "good death" has the attributes of affirming one as a whole person and gives a sense of completion.
- Orthodox Jews will not leave a dying patient alone and will have groups of community members (minyan) praying at the bedside with the patient.

- The family supports a Hindu elder's refusal of nourishment and pain medications to improve his or her change for a better life in the next cycle.
- Among devout Muslims and Jews, religious leaders play a key role in resolving conflicts between medical practices and religious beliefs. These collectivistic groups sometimes object to an ill member being informed of a terminal prognosis.
- Catholics usually arrange for a priest to anoint the patient and give Holy Communion.

**Implications for Practice**

- Providing end-of-life care requires a sensitivity to the timing, form, and type of support provided to grieving patients and families.
- Cultural care requires knowing who makes decisions in a family.
- Care provided at the end of life within the patient and family's cultural context draws on the resources of their whole lives.

Data from Crowley LM and others: Strategies for culturally effective end-of-life-care, *Ann Intern Med* 136(9):673, 2002; Kagawa-Singer M: The cultural context of death rituals and mourning practices, *Oncol Nurs Forum* 25(10):1752, 1998; Schwartz E: Jewish Americans. In Giger JN, Davidhizar RE: *Transcultural nursing: assessment and intervention*, ed 4, St. Louis, 2003, Mosby; Steinhauser K and others: Factors considered important at the end of life by patients, family, physicians, and other care providers, *JAMA* 284:2476, 2000.

**SPIRITUAL BELIEFS.** Individuals' spirituality significantly influences their ability to cope with loss. A person's faith in a higher power or influence, the community of fellowship with friends, the sources of hope and meaning in life, and the use of religious rituals and practices are just some of the spiritual resources the individual uses during loss. Murray and others (2004) found that whether or not patients and their family caregivers held religious beliefs, they expressed needs for love, meaning, and purpose. Loss causes conflicts about spiritual values and the meaning of life. Patients with a strong faith in a higher power are often very resilient and able to face death with relatively minimal discomfort.

## Coping With Grief and Loss

As a nurse, it is important that you learn to understand how people normally cope with grief and loss. Your nursing interventions will involve reinforcement of patients' successful coping strategies or introduction of new coping approaches (see Chapter 22).

**HOPE. Hope** is the anticipation of a continued good, an improvement or lessening of something unpleasant. It is a concept that energizes and provides comfort as a person faces life threats and personal challenges (Bierman and others, 1998; Nowotny, 1991). Hope enhances one's coping skills. A person often reveals hope through an expression of expecta-

tions for life, the present, and the future. A terminally ill patient often focuses hope on milestones (e.g., a child's high school graduation or the completion of a work project), significant events (e.g., an upcoming anniversary), or for the relief of pain or other disabling symptoms (Weissman and others, 1999). Spiritual distress is often tied to one's definition of hope or lack of hope. Some view hope as encouragement to work toward recovery. Others view hope more negatively by not being able to see any future favorable outcomes.

Hope has purpose and direction and gives reason for being (Post-White and others, 1996). The existence and maintenance of hope depend on a person having strong relationships and a sense of emotional connectedness to others. As a nurse you will provide that personal connectedness essential to hope. Hope is often the basis in which patients find meaning in their illness. Hopefulness offers an ability to see life as enduring or having sustained meaning or purpose (Chochinov, 2002).

## Critical Thinking

### Synthesis

When you care for a patient who experiences a loss, successful critical thinking requires a synthesis of knowledge and experiences with loss and grief. In addition, you will apply

I have the right to be treated as a living human being until I die.

I have the right to maintain a sense of hopefulness, however changing its focus may be.

I have the right to be cared for by those who can maintain a sense of hopefulness, however changing this might be.

I have the right to express my feelings and emotions about my approaching death in my own way.

I have the right to participate in decisions concerning my care.

I have the right to expect continuing medical and nursing attention even though "cure" goals must be changed to "comfort" goals.

I have the right not to die alone.

I have the right to be free from pain.

I have the right to have my questions answered honestly.

I have the right not to be deceived.

I have the right to have help from and for my family in accepting my death.

I have the right to die in peace and dignity.

I have the right to retain my individuality and not be judged for my decisions that may be contrary to beliefs of others.

I have the right to discuss and enlarge my religious and/or spiritual experiences, whatever these may mean to others.

I have the right to expect that the sanctity of the human body will be respected after death.

I have the right to be cared for by caring, sensitive, knowledgeable people who will attempt to understand my needs and will be able to gain some satisfaction in helping me face my death.

From Barbus AJ: The dying person's bill of rights, *Am J Nurs* 75:99, 1975.

for patients experiencing loss or those who have died, the lessons are invaluable. Reflect upon those experiences, and consider how to apply what you have learned to caring for your next patient.

**ATTITUDES.** Risk taking, self-confidence, and humility are examples of critical thinking attitudes that will help you to make accurate judgments and decisions about your patients (see Chapter 6). Many nurses become anxious when caring for patients who grieve. Being with a patient or family who is mourning requires a personal risk. You will learn to accept patients' discomfort in the interest of being supportive.

Self-confidence goes hand in hand with risk taking. Confidence helps you to understand that in the absence of something to do or say, what a patient needs most is the personal connection with someone who cares. By silently sharing a moment of sadness with a patient or family, you communicate caring and send the message that you respect and accept the patient's feelings and emotions. You cannot know everything there is to know about a patient's loss. Humility helps you to put aside personal assumptions about how the patient interprets loss and to remain open to hearing and understanding the patient's beliefs, thoughts, and concerns.

**STANDARDS.** The use of appropriate intellectual standards such as significance and relevance guide you during assessment to gather information pertinent to the patient's situation. Professional standards, including those of bioethics (see Chapter 5), the dying person's bill of rights (Box 23-2), and clinical standards such as the American Pain Society's guidelines for managing cancer pain, provide evidence-based guidelines for appropriate and compassionate nursing care.

# Nursing Process

## Assessment

Begin with an open mind and accepting attitude as you assess a patient or family who has experienced a loss. Grief assessment is ongoing throughout the course of an illness for the patient and family and for the bereavement period after the death for the survivors (ELNEC, 2000). Do not assume to know how or if the patient and family experience grief. Also do not assume a particular behavior indicates grief. Allow patients to share what is happening in their own way. You will be very effective by having patients tell their stories. A focused assessment will allow you to determine what phase of grief the patient or family member is experiencing (Table 23-3). Help patients and families find a time and place to express their grief and describe their experience (Figure 23-1). It is recommended that you interview patients and families separately unless a patient requests having family members present.

Begin your interviewing by using honest and open communication. Listen carefully, and observe the patient's responses and behaviors. Assume a neutral perspective and remain alert for nonverbal cues such as facial expressions, voice tones, and avoidance of topics. Your use of critical

critical thinking attitudes and intellectual and professional standards to provide appropriate and responsive nursing care. Each patient enters the health care setting at a different developmental, spiritual, and cultural place and with different expectations. You will learn to consider all of these factors when providing a comprehensive plan of care.

**KNOWLEDGE.** Knowledge of the grief process will help you understand the responses and needs of your patient and family. You also need to have a clear understanding of the nature of the loss, how the patient and family perceive the loss, and how the loss affects their lives. Applying knowledge of therapeutic communication principles (see Chapter 9) allows you to explore the loss thoroughly with a patient and family to understand all influential factors. When loss is tied to an illness, knowledge of pathophysiology will help you offer patients and families a realistic explanation of what to expect about the course of the illness. Understanding the cultural meanings loss and death pose for a specific family allows you to individualize your approach. Finally, principles of caring (see Chapter 16) and an understanding of family dynamics (see Chapter 21) enable you to provide compassionate care.

**EXPERIENCE.** Most of us have experienced some type of loss. Personal experience with loss prepares you to understand what loss means and to anticipate the emotional experience a patient is feeling. When you have previously cared

## FOCUSED PATIENT ASSESSMENT

**TABLE 23-3**

| Factors to Assess | Questions and Approaches | Physical Assessment Strategies |
|---|---|---|
| Phase of grief | Mr. Holloway, tell me how you are feeling now. Validate patient's feelings: You seem (angry/sad); tell me more about that . . . This can be a bewildering time . . . | Observe patient's behaviors: Presence of crying Frequent sighing Poor eye contact Unwillingness to talk about feelings |
| Family member's response to loss | It is so difficult to deal with an illness of this type. What has your husband meant to you in your life? What are your feelings right now? Are you feeling guilty because . . . ? Could you really have prevented this? | Observe nonverbal behaviors as members of family interact together: Tone of conversation Detaches or walks away from members of family Seeks physical closeness from member of family |

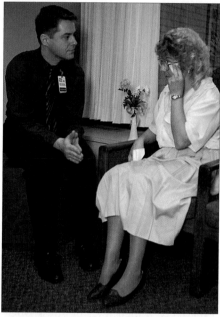

FIGURE **23-1** Nurses assist family members in finding resources to help with the grieving process.

BOX 23-3 **Symptoms of Normal Grief**

**Feelings**

Sadness
Anger
Guilt or self-reproach
Anxiety
Loneliness
Fatigue
Helplessness
Shock/numbness (lack of feeling)
Yearning
Relief

**Cognitions (Thought Patterns)**

Disbelief
Confusion
Preoccupation about the deceased
Sense of the presence of the deceased
Hallucinations
Hopelessness ("I'll never be OK again")

**Physical Sensations**

Hollowness in the stomach
Tightness in the chest
Tightness in the throat
Oversensitivity to noise
Sense of depersonalization ("Nothing seems real")
Feeling short of breath
Muscle weakness
Lack of energy
Dry mouth

**Behaviors**

Sleep disturbances
Appetite disturbances
Dreams of the deceased
Sighing
Crying
Carrying objects that belonged to the deceased

thinking will allow you to review data, interpret patterns of meaning, and eventually make appropriate nursing diagnoses. Other health care workers will contribute to your database, including physicians or health care providers, social workers, and members from pastoral care.

**TYPE AND STAGES OF GRIEF.** Focus on assessing how a patient is reacting to loss rather than how you think the patient should react. Remember, no two people grieve the same way, and most people have some signs and symptoms of grief (Box 23-3). The sequence of stages of grief sometimes occurs in order, out of sequence, or reoccurs. A single behavior represents any number of types of grief. As you identify the type and/or stage of grief, your assessment will have more direction. Application of a theorist's phase of grief will

help you to accurately assess a situation. For example, if a patient is complaining of loneliness and difficulty falling asleep, does this possibly indicate Bowlby's yearning and searching? Probe further by asking questions such as, "When did the loss occur?" or "Tell me how you are feeling." Have patients describe their losses and how loss has affected them.

**FACTORS THAT AFFECT GRIEF.** You will gain a better understanding of the patient's grief by assessing factors that influence grieving in detail (Table 23-4). As you learn more about the patient's situation, use assessment skills from appropriate specialty areas including spiritual and family as-

| TABLE 23-4 | Assessment of Factors Influencing Grieving |
|---|---|
| **Factors** | **Areas/Suggested Questions to Explore** |
| Hope | Goals, worth, adaptations to future changes<br>*Examples:*<br>Tell me what you think about your treatment plan.<br>What do you expect will happen to you?<br>What do you expect to help you through this? |
| Nature of relationships | Functions of family, community, society<br>*Examples:*<br>What role has your parent/friend played in your family?<br>What is your relationship with your parent/spouse? Will it change? |
| Social support system | Availability of health care workers, timing, family needs<br>*Examples:*<br>What do family/friends do that is most helpful?<br>Are family/friends actually available or do they just say, "Call me if you need me"?<br>Are they helpful, or do they avoid the issues offered for discussion by the patient? |
| Nature of loss | Actual versus perceived; death issues; impact on roles<br>*Examples:*<br>How is the loss affecting what is going on in your life?<br>What factors help/interfere with grieving?<br>What past experiences/outcomes have you had with loss? |
| Cultural and spiritual beliefs | Values, practices, customs, attitudes, clergy, spiritualist<br>*Examples:*<br>What are your beliefs about death?<br>How should the body (or part) be treated when removed?<br>What traditions are required to show value of all life?<br>Who has the right to say "yes" or "no"? Legally? Ethically? |
| Loss of personal life goals | Actual or perceived individual losses affecting future decisions and options<br>*Examples:*<br>How has this changed as a result of your diagnosis? Surgery?<br>How will your role change your personal goals?<br>What planning have you and your family made for your own life? |

sessment (see Chapters 18 and 21) to gain a thorough understanding of the patient's loss.

**COPING RESOURCES.** Determine what behaviors and outside resources typically help patients cope with difficulties. Ask open-ended questions or statements to enable the patient to provide details: "Tell me how you find ways to adjust when times get difficult" or "Tell me who you go to when you are experiencing difficult times." Use of direct questions will help you determine if activities such as relaxation exercises, massage, meditation, reading, or exercise help patients deal with stressors. These coping resources will become invaluable in your plan of care.

Assess the entire family's response to loss, recognizing that family members are often dealing with different aspects of grief than the patient. A change in role can become very stressful for a family member. For example, if the mother of a young family dies, the husband must take on more parenting and household management responsibilities. The children's relationship with the father changes, as he becomes the primary source for discipline and guidance. Referral of the family to a counselor or social worker will be helpful.

**END-OF-LIFE DECISIONS.** When a patient has a terminal illness, family members face end-of-life decisions. Families experience a high level of stress when deciding whether to withdraw life-sustaining treatments (Tilden and others, 2001). Although some patients have living wills, it is important for family members to know a patient's wishes in regard to life-sustaining measures. The Study to Understand Prognoses and Preferences for Outcomes and Risks of Treatments (SUPPORT Principal Investigators, 1995) found that more patients received prolonged aggressive treatments rather than palliative therapies, even when patients and families had indicated preference for palliative care rather than life extension measures. Unfortunately, physicians or health care providers and nurses often have difficulty helping patients die with dignity. Many organizations have identified needed improvements in the areas of advance planning, respecting patient and family preferences for location of death and amount of life-sustaining treatment, pain management, and life-sustaining resources (Tolle and others, 2000).

As a nurse, assess the patient's and family's wishes for end-of-life care (EOLC), including the preferred place for

## SYNTHESIS IN PRACTICE

As Peter Wong prepares to meet the Holloway family for the first time, he mentally reviews all of the information that will be essential in making an accurate assessment. He has read about colon cancer and has tried to anticipate key symptoms to look for in a patient who has metastases to the lungs and liver. He will try to be sensitive to any embarrassment Mr. Holloway feels about his incontinence. He has read that family members experience grief in their own way, with roles and responsibilities shifting. Mr. Holloway is facing his own death and has become very dependent. Regardless of Mrs. Holloway's seeming denial, she is forced to assume new responsibilities as her husband's health declines. Mr. Holloway's daughter has already given up her home and job to care for her father. The conflict between these two women as the needs of the family change is a possible source of more stress for Mr. Holloway.

Peter has no past experience with death, but he has cared for seriously ill patients. Humility and the willingness to take risks will be key attitudes to use in caring for this family. If they ask him what he knows about death, he will honestly tell them that he thinks it is very difficult to live through so many stresses. He will ask them to discuss their perceptions and feelings with him, and he will try to understand their feelings and accept them. If family members express emotions, Peter will try to show confidence that he knows he does not need to "fix" things. He just needs to be there to share their sadness. If they ask questions he cannot answer, he will have the humility to admit that he does not know and will try to obtain the information for them or put them in contact with a more experienced nurse.

Peter will be especially careful to attend to Mr. Holloway's complaints of pain and discomfort and teach family members how to position him and medicate him when no nurses are in the home. He will respect Mr. Holloway's privacy, modesty, and need for dignity, especially in the face of problems such as incontinence. At school and at hospice, he will take care to protect Mr. Holloway's confidentiality. He will help the family discuss important subjects such as preparation for death and will be sensitive to Mr. Holloway's need and desire to discuss his wishes regarding his death.

death, the use of and the level of life-sustaining measures, and expectations about pain control and symptom management. Family members face complex decisions with unresolved burdens and guilt, limited knowledge, and an inability to know how a person's final days of life will be experienced (Forbes and others, 2000).

You will play an important role in determining a patient's or family's needs and preferences. Teno and others (2004) have found that families whose loved ones died in hospitals or nursing homes reportedly received insufficient emotional support at the time of death. If you feel uncomfortable in assessing a patient's wishes, find a health care provider who has experience discussing EOLC issues. Also remember, patients' cultural beliefs will significantly influence their choices for EOLC.

**NURSE'S EXPERIENCE WITH GRIEF.** When caring for patients experiencing grief, it is important for you to assess your own emotional well-being. Self-reflection, which is a part of critical thinking, is a valuable tool in asking whether your personal sadness is related to caring for the patient or to unresolved personal experiences from the past. It is normal to have personal feelings and emotions about certain illnesses and death. However, do not put your personal family situation or values before the patient. Part of being a professional is knowing when to get away from a situation and take care of oneself.

**PATIENT EXPECTATIONS.** Always assess your patient's and family's expectations for nursing care. The patient's perceptions and expectations will influence how you prioritize nursing diagnoses. For example, if patients perceive that their level of pain and discomfort are severe, they will be less attentive to any attempts you make to discuss what their other needs are. Symptom management is a priority before beginning any meaningful discussion or counseling about grief. Be sure to assess the patient's and family's expectations within the context of the loss by asking questions such as "How can we help you cope with your loss?" and "What do you feel is necessary from us for you to be able to resolve the grief you feel?" "What is the most important thing we can do for your spouse/friend?" Teno and others (2004) note that family members expect patients to receive relief from pain and dyspnea and that physician and health care provider communication be adequate in helping them to make decisions.

Give family members the chance to explain how they perceive your role as a nurse and what their goals are for the health care team. This part of the assessment helps you to clarify any misunderstanding that might exist. Taking time to assess what patients and families expect and desire from nursing care helps to ensure an individualized and comprehensive plan of care.

### Nursing Diagnosis

After reviewing and interpreting the data you collect, identify the nursing diagnoses and collaborative problems that apply to your patient's and family's situation. Cluster defining characteristics to identify the nursing diagnoses most applicable. The clustering of patient or family behaviors, actual or potential losses, the patient's attempts at coping, and data involving the nature and meaning of the loss will lead to individualized nursing diagnoses such as the following:

- Anxiety
- Caregiver role strain
- Compromised family coping
- Ineffective community coping
- Ineffective denial
- Fear
- Anticipatory grieving
- Dysfunctional grieving
- Hopelessness

- Powerlessness
- Social isolation
- Spiritual distress
- Readiness for enhanced spiritual well-being

The presence of one or two defining characteristics is usually insufficient to make an accurate diagnosis. Carefully review the data you have, and consider if competing diagnoses exist. For example, if a patient who is dying manifests crying or tearfulness, displays anger, and reports nightmares, this points to several possible nursing diagnoses because these characteristics are common to more than one diagnosis. Possibilities include *pain, ineffective coping,* and *spiritual distress*. Examine all available data, and inquire about the presence of other behaviors and symptoms until you feel comfortable in selecting an accurate diagnosis.

Identify the appropriate related factor for each diagnosis. For example, *dysfunctional grieving related to loss of the ability to walk from paralysis* will require different interventions than *dysfunctional grieving related to the loss of a job*. Clarification of the related factor will ensure that you select appropriate interventions for the patient's care.

When a patient is seriously ill, as in the case of a terminal illness, several nursing diagnoses will likely apply (Figure 23-2). In addition to diagnoses pertinent to grieving, you will likely diagnose problems reflecting the patient's physical and psychological condition. Some of these diagnoses are common to grieving, such as *pain* or *imbalanced nutrition*. In such a situation, your interventions will focus on pain relief before you can help to support or resolve the patient's grief.

## ✳ Planning

Grieving is the natural response to loss and has a therapeutic value. Plan your nursing care to meet the physical, emotional, developmental, and spiritual needs of your patient and family (see care plan). Support the patient's self-esteem and right to autonomy by including the patient in decisions about the plan of care. When caring for a dying patient, develop a plan that helps a patient to die with dignity and offers family members the assurance that you are caring for their loved one properly.

**GOALS AND OUTCOMES.** Establish realistic goals and expected outcomes based on the patient's nursing diagnoses. Consider the patient's available resources, such as supportive family members, methods for coping, spiritual faith, and physical energy, and integrate them into the goals of care. For example, if a terminally ill patient has the diagnosis of *powerlessness related to planned cancer therapy*, a goal of "Patient will be able to discuss expected course of disease" will be realistic if the patient is able to remain attentive and participate in educational discussions without becoming fatigued. An expected outcome of "Patient will participate in series of short planned teaching discussions about disease"

accounts for the patient's need to have short teaching sessions so as to avoid exhaustion.

Goals of care for a patient dealing with loss are long or short term, depending on the nature of the loss and the patient's phase of grieving. Because a patient sometimes moves back and forth between phases of grief, you will need to revise goals and outcomes to ensure they are still relevant. Having a patient partner in deciding which goals are relevant is important. General nursing care goals for patients with a loss include accommodating grief, accepting the reality of a loss, and renewing regular relationships.

**SETTING PRIORITIES.** When a patient has multiple nursing diagnoses, it is not possible to address all of the problems at the same time. Always consider the patient's most urgent physical or psychological needs that will require immediate attention. Then consider the patient's expectations and preferences in regard to the priorities of care. If the patient is progressing as desired, you refocus priorities to address unmet needs. For example, Mr. Holloway has begun to tolerate eating, but he continues to have bowel incontinence, which threatens his self-image and comfort level. Nursing interventions focus on revising his diet so that he will manage the incontinence better. Remember, the patient's expectations and preferences influence how you set priorities. If a terminally ill patient places more emphasis on comfort or spiritual support versus other priorities such as mobility or learning about planned treatments, attend to the patient's priorities first. Meeting the patient's priorities first allows you to meet other needs more effectively with less effort.

**CONTINUITY OF CARE.** Interdisciplinary teams help to identify and meet the needs of those who experience losses. For example, pastoral care professionals, social workers, and psychologists are able to assist a patient and family in their grief. A coordinated group approach ensures that little is left to chance and that the patient's plan of care will be managed well. Often, terminally ill patients will return home and require continued intense nursing care. In that situation, home care and hospice nurses will collaborate closely with family members to ensure the patient's ongoing needs are met.

## ✳ Implementation

**HEALTH PROMOTION.** A person experiencing grief requires support to cope with the stressors in his or her life and to move towards healthy grief resolution. In the case of a terminally ill patient or even a person who experiences significant disability or other loss of function, there is the additional goal of enabling the individual to return to optimal physical and emotional functioning. This does not mean the patient and family will not experience sadness or other disturbing emotions but that they will cope with the stressors in their lives. You will assist patients in learning to deal with their loss, to make effective decisions about their health care,

## CONCEPT MAP

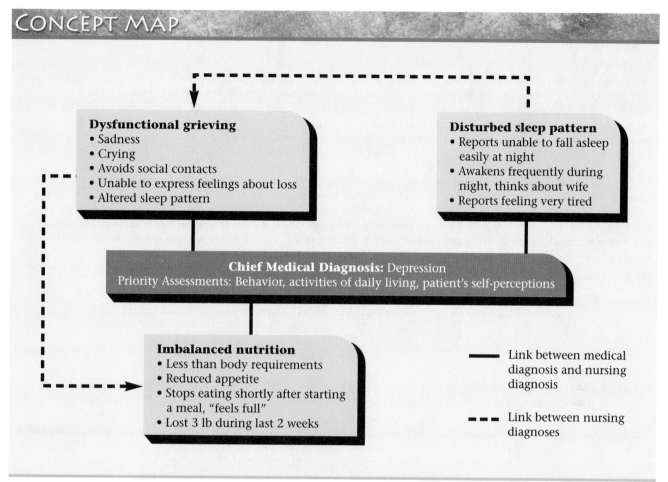

FIGURE 23-2 Concept map for a patient with depression following death of spouse.

and to adjust to any disappointment, frustration, and anxiety created by their loss.

**Therapeutic Communication.** Nursing care of the grieving patient and family begins with establishing the significance of their loss. This is difficult if the patient is unwilling or unable to express feelings or is experiencing shock or denial. Use therapeutic communication strategies that enable the patient to discuss the loss and to work with you in finding ways to resolve it. Use open-ended questions that allow patients to freely share their thoughts and tell their stories. Too often the use of closed-ended questions results in the patient's discussing only what you presume is the problem. Use active listening, be comfortable in silence, and use prompts (e.g., "go on," "tell me more") that urge a patient to continue talking about his or her concerns. Acknowledge the patient's grief, and show caring behaviors such as establishing presence and use of touch (see Chapter 16). You will gain the patient's trust by showing a desire to become involved with the patient at a level that encourages open communication.

If a patient chooses not to share feelings or concerns, convey a willingness to be available when needed. If you are reassuring and respectful of the patient's need for dignity, re-

spect, and privacy, a therapeutic relationship will likely develop. Sometimes patients need to begin resolving their grief before they discuss their loss.

Always recognize that some patients will not discuss feelings about their loss. Be observant for expressions of anger, denial, depression, or guilt. Remember, it is important to know your own feelings before encouraging patients to express their anger. Some individuals retaliate against the family or health care staff. They also become demanding and accusing. Remain supportive by letting patients and family members know that feelings such as anger are normal. For example, say, "You are obviously upset. I just want you to know I am available to talk if you want." Always be sure to avoid barriers to communication (see Chapter 9) such as denying the patient's grief, providing false reassurance, or avoiding discussion of sensitive issues.

Do not avoid any topic that a dying patient wishes to discuss. When you sense that patients want to talk, it is important to find time to let them discuss their concerns. This is very challenging in a busy acute care setting. Respond to questions openly and honestly. Provide information that helps them and their families to understand their condition, the future course

## CARE PLAN Loss and Grief

### ASSESSMENT

During Peter's home visit, he finds Mr. Holloway, who is in reasonably good physical condition 1 week after discharge. He has become very unsteady while walking and says he "feels weak." One night he fell while getting out of bed and badly bruised his face. Mr. Holloway is easy to talk with and very receptive to Peter's questions. Mr. Holloway becomes tearful when talking about his situation, yet he is more relaxed when talking with Peter about memories of his younger years. He confides that his wife **disappears for hours every day** and **does not seem to realize how ill he really is.** Mr. Holloway states, "I know this is very **hard for her to accept,** but I also know I need her help." When asked about his daughter, Mr. Holloway reports that she appears tired and has not been sleeping well. "I think she feels as though she doesn't know what to do."

During Peter's visit, Mrs. Holloway comes into the room. She begins to **describe plans for their summer vacation, still 9 months away.** She avoids Peter's question about what she and her daughter have done to deal with Mr. Holloway's symptoms. Instead she suggests that her husband will benefit from "getting some exercise and eating a more balanced diet." Peter asks to talk with Mrs. Holloway alone for a few minutes. During this time, Mrs. Holloway begins to cry and voices her **fear of being unable to support her husband** appropriately. Mrs. Holloway states, **"I still can't believe this is happening to us."** She collects her thoughts and asks Peter what the family should do; both she and her daughter want to be more helpful.

*Defining characteristics are shown in bold type.

---

### NURSING DIAGNOSIS  Compromised family coping related to stress of impending death of father/husband.

---

### PLANNING
#### GOAL

- Patient's family understands patient's terminal condition and its implications within 1 month.
- Family is able to provide palliative care measures within 2 weeks.

- Patient acquires a sense of completion in affirming relationship with family within 1 month.

#### EXPECTED OUTCOMES*
##### Caregiver Performance: Direct Care
- Wife is able to describe disease process and symptoms husband will have during terminal stage of illness within 2 weeks.
- Wife and daughter describe supportive care measures that Mr. Holloway will require within the next 2 weeks.
- Wife and daughter assist with husband's hygiene and safety care within 2 weeks.

##### Caregiver-Patient Relationship
- Mr. Holloway shares feelings about his life and relationship with wife and daughter within 1 month.

*Outcomes classification label from Moorhead S, Johnson M, Maas M: *Nursing outcomes classification (NOC),* ed 3, St. Louis, 2004, Mosby.

---

### INTERVENTIONS†
#### Reminiscence Therapy†
- Ask Mr. Holloway to participate in process of life review, by sharing his stories with his family during mealtimes.

- Discuss with Mrs. Holloway and daughter the value of reminiscence as part of looking back and evaluating life and its meaning.

#### Caregiver Support†
- Involve Mrs. Holloway and daughter in discussion between home care nurse and Mr. Holloway, focusing instruction on symptom management.
- Offer time for Mrs. Holloway and daughter to ask questions and discuss course of cancer, the expected course of the disease, and desires for life-sustaining treatment.
- Explain to family that setting easily achievable goals helps give hope. Enlist their help to establish goals for the next week.

### RATIONALE

Encouraging patient to talk and tell his story of anecdotes and events in relationships allows patient to sense life was meaningful and worth living (Meiner and Lueckenotte, 2006).
Engaging in this process will help move the family along the process of anticipatory grieving (Worden, 1982).

Even with a poor prognosis, quality of life can be improved through discussion and planning for possible problems (Poncar, 1994).

Clarifying expectations better prepares individuals to face changes that will develop as cancer progresses (Tolle and others, 2000).
Restructuring goals to be more short-term and achievable is a means of supporting and sustaining hope in terminally ill patients (Nowotny, 1991).

†Intervention classification labels from Dochterman JM, Bulechek, GM, editors: *Nursing interventions classification (NIC)* ed 4, St. Louis, 2004, Mosby.

---

### EVALUATION
- Have Mr. Holloway describe feelings felt after sharing stories and life review with family.
- Observe Mrs. Holloway's and daughter's behavior and level of involvement in care.
- Use caregiving scenarios to test wife's and daughter's knowledge of symptom management approaches.

- Two weeks after family instruction, ask family to discuss if any problems exist in providing care to Mr. Holloway.
- Ask family about their progress in locating a support group and about their plans to attend.

of their disease, the benefits and burdens of treatment, and clarification of values and goals (Forbes and others, 2000).

**Promoting Hope.** Hope is an energizing resource for patients experiencing loss. For each dimension of hope, there are nursing strategies that promote a patient's hope:

- **Affective dimension.** Show empathic understanding of the patient's strengths. Reinforce expressions of courage, positive thinking, and realistic goal setting.
- **Cognitive dimension.** Offer information about the illness or health problem, and correct any misinformation. Provide information on self-care strategies. Clarify or modify patient's perceptions.
- **Behavioral dimension.** Assist the patient in returning to healthy behaviors: using personal resources and making use of external supports, establishing a structure for each day and sticking to it, adopting good self-care practices (eating well, talking with friends, getting rest).
- **Affiliative dimension.** Encourage patients to develop supportive relationships.
- **Temporal dimension.** Focus on short-term goals, especially for the terminal patient whose life expectancy diminishes.
- **Contextual dimension.** Encourage development of achievable goals. Reminisce about achievements or positive moments in time so patient will get meaning from suffering.

**Facilitating Mourning.** There are strategies you will use to help patients move through uncomplicated grief (Worden, 1982). These guidelines are helpful for persons who are mourning a death, facing death, and grieving over an actual situational loss.

- **Help the patient accept that the loss is real.** Discuss how the loss or illness occurred or was discovered, when, under what circumstances, who told them about it, and other similar topics to help make the event more real and place it in perspective.
- **Support efforts to live without the deceased person or in the face of disability.** Using a problem-solving approach is often helpful. Have patients or family make a list of their problems, help them prioritize them, and then lead them step by step through a discussion of how they will handle each one. Encourage them to make use of family members, community resources, or others who are able to help.
- **Encourage establishment of new relationships.** Many people will fear that in doing so they will be disloyal. Reassure them that new relationships do not mean that they are replacing the person who has died. Encourage participation in relationships that are nonthreatening (e.g., religious gatherings or volunteer activities).
- **Allow time to grieve.** It is common to have "anniversary reactions" around the time of the loss in subsequent years. Some people worry that they are going crazy when sadness or other signs of grief recur after a period of relative calm. Encourage reminiscence.
- **Interpret "normal" behavior.** The normal behavioral responses to grief do not mean an individual has an emo-

tional problem or is becoming ill in some way. Reinforce that these behaviors are normal and will resolve over time.

- **Provide continuing support.** Patients and their families will need to talk and will look to you for support for many months or years following a loss. If you have occasion to see the patient or family after an extended time, it is appropriate to inquire about how they are coping. This gives them the opportunity to talk if needed.
- **Be alert for signs of ineffective coping.** Be aware of coping mechanisms that are harmful, such as alcohol or substance abuse, which includes excessive use of over-the-counter painkillers and sleep aids.

### ACUTE CARE

**Palliative Care.** For patients with serious life-limiting illness, it is important for health care providers to find ways to help patients approach their end of life. Such is the goal of **palliative care,** the prevention, relief, reduction, or soothing of symptoms of disease or disorders without effecting a cure (Field and Cassel, 1997). Palliative care is for any age, any diagnosis, at any time, and not just during the last months of life. It helps patients to make more informed choices, achieve better alleviation of symptoms, and have more opportunity to work on issues of life closure. When health care providers deliver palliative care, they do the following (World Health Organization [WHO], 2006):

- Affirm life and regard dying as a normal process
- Neither hasten nor postpone death
- Provide relief from pain and other distressing symptoms
- Integrate psychological and spiritual aspects of patient care
- Offer a support system to help patients live as actively as possible until death
- Offer a support system to help families cope during the patient's illness and their own bereavement
- Enhance the quality of life
- Use a team approach to meet the needs of patients and families.

Palliative care is a philosophy of total care. The approach to care usually involves an interdisciplinary team of physicians or health care providers, nurses, social workers, pastoral care professionals, and pharmacists. Sometimes holistic therapists, who offer alternative medicine approaches such as massage or music/art therapy, are a part of the team. A palliative care approach ensures that a patient experiences a "good death," free of avoidable pain and suffering, in accord with the patient's and family's wishes, and reasonably consistent with clinical, cultural, and ethical standards (Tolle and others, 2000).

*Symptom Control.* Comfort for a dying patient requires management of symptoms of disease and therapies. Symptom distress is the experience of discomfort or anguish related to disease progression. Worry or fear are common in many patients, and these heighten their perception of symptoms such as discomfort. The common symptom of fatigue in the terminally ill is one that interferes with a person's abil-

**BOX 23-4** USING EVIDENCE IN PRACTICE

**Research Summary**

Nurses benefit terminally ill patients the most by helping them live with fatigue instead of trying to treat the symptom. One group of researchers interviewed four patients with cancer who were in a palliative care program. The purpose of the study was to gain an understanding of the meanings of fatigue that cancer patients experienced. The study participants, including three women and one man of Swedish descent, participated in hour-long interviews held in their homes.

The cancer patients described a complex relationship between cancer, fatigue, and death. Patients found themselves struggling in vain against fatigue and hoping but not expecting to overcome fatigue. The body is putting a stop to things, signaling that death is coming closer, and yet the individual still longs for a healthy life. To come to terms with fatigue involves listening to one's body and to admit that one is dying.

**Application to Nursing Practice**

How should health care professionals talk to patients with incurable cancer about fatigue? Be humble in your conversations with patients. Do not force a patient into realizing the implications, which he or she may not yet be ready to accept, that death is approaching. However, talking about fatigue gives patients a chance to talk about death without using the difficult and painful words of death. Talking about fatigue borrows the patient's language that makes it possible to discuss death.

Data from Lindquist O and others: Meanings of the phenomenon of fatigue as narrated by four patients with cancer in palliative care, *Cancer Nurs* 27(3):237, 2004.

ity to function in a normal capacity (Box 23-4). Assess the character of the patient's symptoms carefully, and individualize therapies. Chapter 30 provides a detailed discussion of pain management strategies

The terminally ill frequently experience dyspnea, or air hunger. Air hunger causes great panic in the patient and significant stress in the caregiver (Tarzian, 2000). As the patient panics, unable to get a breath, the air hunger simply worsens. Tarzian (2000) interviewed nurses who cared for the terminally ill and found that surrendering and sharing control help reduce panic and anxiety in these patients. Self-beliefs offer hope and peace. When there are options in respiratory therapy, give the patient a choice. Management of air hunger also involves the judicious administration of morphine and **anxiolytics** for relief of respiratory distress. Table 23-5 summarizes nursing care measures for additional symptoms of terminal disease.

*Maintaining Dignity and Self-Esteem.* You help patients maintain dignity and self-esteem by providing spiritual comfort (see Chapter 18). You also promote a patient's self-esteem and dignity by attending to the patient's appearance. Cleanliness, absence of body odors, attractive clothing, and personal grooming all add to a sense of worth. When caring for a patient's bodily functions, always show an attitude of respect, even when the patient becomes dependent. Keep the patient's immediate surroundings pleasant. Open curtains, and let the light change from the bright of day to the dark of night. Remove any unpleasant odors from liquid stool or vomitus as soon as possible.

Disabilities experienced by the patient threaten dignity, especially when caregivers take control of the patient's life. Allow the patient to make nursing care decisions (e.g., how to administer personal hygiene, diet preferences, and timing of nursing care activities). Keep the patient well informed about planned therapies and anticipated effects. Provide the patient privacy during nursing care procedures and when the patient and family need time together.

*Preventing Abandonment and Isolation.* A terminally ill patient often fears dying alone. Thus it is important to answer the call light quickly and to explain when staff will give care and perform assessments throughout the day and night. Establish presence, and use appropriate touch when providing care. Be available often to answer questions. Avoid placing the patient in a private room unless family members visit and plan to stay around the clock. Patients feel a sense of involvement when sharing a room and interacting with staff. Patients share conversation and companionship with roommates and visitors.

If family members have difficulty accepting the patient's impending death, they sometimes avoid visitation. When family members do visit, it is important to talk with them. It is useful to give family members helpful hints about what to discuss with patients. For example, role model attentive listening, and offer reassurance to improve their communication skills. Encourage family to discuss activities other family members are involved in, to reminisce about enjoyable times, and to inquire about the patient's concerns. Also help them find simple and appropriate tasks to perform when they visit in the hospital such as feeding the patient, washing the patient's face, or filling out the patient's menu. Older adults often become particularly lonely at night and feel more secure if a family member stays at the bedside during the night. Allow visitors to remain with dying patients at any time if the patient wants them. Also know how to contact family members at any time if the patient requests a visit or if the patient's condition worsens.

*Providing a Comfortable and Peaceful Environment.* Keep a patient comfortable through frequent repositioning, keeping bed linens dry, and controlling environmental noise. Pictures, cherished objects, cards or letters from family, and plants and flowers create an environment that is more familiar and comforting. Offer the patient frequent back massage, and allow the patient to listen to preferred types of music. Aromatherapy combined with massage has been shown to improve patients' ability to sleep (Soden and others, 2004). A comfortable environment helps patients to relax, which promotes their ability to sleep and minimizes severity of symptoms.

**Support for the Grieving Family.** Some families are the primary caregivers when the patient chooses to be at home

| TABLE 23-5 | Promoting Comfort in the Terminally Ill Patient | |
|---|---|---|

| Symptoms | Characteristics or Causes | Nursing Implications |
|---|---|---|
| Discomfort | Any source of physical irritation (e.g., dehydration) that worsens pain.<br>As patient approaches death, mouth remains open, tongue becomes dry and edematous, and lips become dry and cracked.<br>Blinking reflexes diminish near death, causing drying of cornea. | Provide thorough skin care including daily baths, lubrication of skin, and dry, clean bed linens to reduce irritants.<br>Provide oral care at least every 2 to 4 hours.<br>Use soft toothbrushes or foam swabs for frequent mouth care. Apply a light film of petroleum jelly to lips and tongue (see Chapter 27).<br>Eye care removes crusts from eyelid margins.<br>Artificial tears reduce corneal drying. |
| Fatigue | Metabolic demands of a cancerous tumor cause weakness and fatigue.<br>Exhaustion phase of the general adaptation syndrome causes energy depletion. | Help patient to identify valued or desired tasks; then help patient to conserve energy for only those tasks.<br>Promote frequent rest periods in a quiet environment.<br>Time and pace nursing care activities. |
| Nausea | Occurs as a side effect of medications and as a result of severe pain. | Give antiemetics: provide oral care at least every 2 to 4 hours; offer clear liquids and ice chips; avoid liquids that cause stomach acidity such as coffee, milk, and citric juices. |
| Constipation | Narcotic medications and immobility slow peristalsis.<br>Lack of bulk in diet or reduced fluid intake occurs with appetite changes.<br>Constipation adds to discomfort. | Give preventive care, which is most effective: increase fluid intake; include bran, whole grain products, and fresh vegetables in diet; encourage exercise.<br>Give prophylactic stool softeners. |
| Diarrhea | Diarrhea results from disease process (e.g., colon cancer) and complications of treatment or medications. | Assess for fecal impaction.<br>Confer with physician or health care provider to change medication if possible.<br>Provide low-residue diet. |
| Urinary incontinence | Incontinence results from progressive disease (e.g., involvement of spinal cord, reduced level of consciousness). | Protect skin from irritation or breakdown.<br>Use indwelling urinary catheter or condom catheters. |
| Inadequate nutrition | Nausea and vomiting decrease appetite.<br>Depression from grieving causes anorexia. | Serve smaller portions and bland foods, which may be more palatable.<br>Allow home-cooked meals, which some patients prefer. This also gives the family a chance to participate. |
| Dyspnea or shortness of breath | Disease progression involves lung tissue (e.g., pneumonia, pulmonary edema).<br>Anemia reduces oxygen-carrying capacity.<br>Anxiety increases oxygen demands.<br>Fever increases oxygen demands. | Treat or control underlying cause.<br>Maximize oxygenation (e.g., position patient upright, provide supplemental oxygen, maintain a patent airway, reduce anxiety or fever).<br>Give medications (e.g., bronchodilators, inhaled steroids, narcotics) to suppress cough and ease breathing.<br>Provide antipyretics as ordered. |

during the last days of life. The family requires your support and benefits when you teach them ways to care for their loved one (Box 23-5). Caregiving is emotionally stressful and physically exhausting for family members. In the home setting, provide the opportunity for the family to be temporarily relieved of their duties so they will obtain needed rest and support. Respite care is a resource available through hospice programs. Families also need to know about home care, hospice, and community service options. In some cases, families will need assistance and support in making the very difficult decision about nursing home placement.

Keep the family informed so that they will anticipate the type of symptoms the patient will likely experience and the implications for care. Encourage family members to express their grief openly with the patient and to give the patient the chance to discuss any remaining concerns or requests. The family also needs personal time to share their concerns with you. In the hospital setting, plan a visitation schedule for family members to prevent the patient and family from excessive fatigue. Allow young children to visit dying parents. At the time of death, help the family to stay in communication with the patient through frequent visits, caring silence, touch, and telling the patient of their love. After death, help the family make decisions such as notification of a mortician, transportation of family members, and collection of the patient's belongings.

**Hospice Care.** Hospice care is an alternative for the terminally ill. It is one phase of palliative care. Generally patients accepted into a hospice program have less than 6 months to live. Hospice is not a facility but a concept for family-centered care designed to assist the patient in being comfortable and

**Preparing the Dying Patient's Family**

Peter establishes a teaching plan for Mrs. Holloway and her daughter to learn palliative care measures.

**Outcome**

At the end of the teaching session the Holloways will demonstrate ways to provide comfort measures safely.

**Teaching Strategies**

- Describe and demonstrate feeding techniques and selection of foods to facilitate ease of chewing and swallowing.
- Demonstrate bathing, mouth care, and other hygiene measures, and allow family to perform return demonstration.
- Show video on simple transfer techniques to prevent injury to themselves and the patient; help family to practice.
- Describe ways the family is able to promote the patient's comfort, such as frequent rest periods, giving massage, and repositioning.
- Teach family to recognize signs and symptoms to expect as the patient approaches death and information on whom to call in an emergency.
- Invite questions from family, and provide information as needed.

**Evaluation Strategies**

- Observe family provide direct care activities to Mr. Holloway.
- Have family describe approaches used in caring directly for Mr. Holloway.

maintaining a satisfactory lifestyle until death. Components of hospice care programs include:

- Patient and family as the unit of care
- Coordinated home care with access to inpatient and nursing home beds when needed
- Symptom management
- Physician-directed services
- Provision of an interdisciplinary care team
- Medical and nursing services available at all times
- Bereavement follow-up after a patient's death
- Use of trained volunteers for visitation and respite support

A nurse's role in hospice is to meet the primary wishes of dying patients and to be open to their individual desires by supporting a patient's choice in maintaining comfort and dignity. A hospice program emphasizes palliative care with the patient and family as active participants. Patient care goals are mutually set, and all participants fully understand the options and desires of the patient. Some patients in hospice may become hospitalized, but in this case the health care team coordinates care between the home and inpatient setting. There must be a primary caregiver in the home for a patient to have hospice services. There is always the effort to keep patients at home for as long as possible. The family pro-

vides basic supportive care. However, if the family is unable to meet the patient's needs, a home care aide or nurse becomes available to assist. The interdisciplinary team has a goal of 24-hour accessibility as needed.

**Care After Death.** At the time of a patient's death, a nurse is responsible for **postmortem care.** You care for a patient's body with dignity and sensitivity and in a manner consistent with the patient's religious or cultural beliefs. After death the body undergoes many physical changes. Therefore you provide postmortem care as soon as possible to prevent tissue damage or disfigurement of body parts.

Federal and state legislation require hospitals to formulate policies and procedures based on current laws to validate death, identify potential organ or tissue donors, and to provide postmortem care. For transplantation of organs, remember that the need for ventilatory and circulatory support is necessary for harvesting vital organs. The family needs to understand that the patient is "brain dead" and that the equipment (i.e., ventilator) is not keeping the patient alive but keeping the physical body in a state so that the organs will not be damaged before harvesting.

Provide a private area for the family discussing organ donation. The staff member designated to make a request, such as a transplant coordinator or social worker, will offer the family clarification of what defines brain death because support systems remain in place even after the patient is pronounced "dead" for vital organ retrieval (i.e., heart, lungs, kidneys, and liver). Reinforce your explanations throughout the organ retrieval process. The family must know who can legally give consent, the options for organ or tissue donation, whether there are costs, and how donation will affect burial or cremation. Nonvital tissues such as corneas, skin, long bones, and middle ear bones can be harvested when the patient is pronounced dead without maintaining vital functions. The family must agree on organ and tissue donation if the patient made no specific documented requests before death. Review your state's organ retrieval laws regarding the formal consent process.

As the nurse you are responsible for coordination of all aspects of care surrounding a patient's death. Box 23-6 summarizes nursing and medical responsibilities for care of the body after death. If a patient dies while in a semiprivate room, temporarily transfer the roommate out of the room if possible to prevent that individual from having to listen to the activities surrounding postmortem care. Prepare the body for postmortem care by making it look as natural and comfortable as possible.

The family becomes the primary patient when the actual death has occurred. At this time it becomes important to appropriately use the resources available. For example, pastoral care staff is a valuable resource to help the family deal with grief and to begin to make burial arrangements. However, it is important to know if the family desires to have spiritual counselors present. Some families prefer to grieve alone. Social workers and counselors also offer valuable support.

Documentation of all of the events surrounding death is important to avoid misunderstandings and to clarify final

## BOX 23-6 Care of the Body After Death

**Physician or Health Care Provider Responsibilities**

1. Certify the death—time pronounced, therapy used, actions taken.
2. Request an autopsy, especially for unusual circumstances.
3. Specially trained staff member provides an option for donation of organs or tissue—personal, religious, and cultural needs should be included during this process.

**Nurse Responsibilities**

1. Provide dignity and sensitivity to the patient and the family.
2. Check orders for any specimens or special orders needed by the physician.
3. Make arrangements for staff, minister, or others to stay with the family while preparing the body for viewing; ask for special requests for viewing (e.g., shaving, a special gown, Bible in hand, rosary at the bedside).
4. Determine if the family wishes patient to remain unshaven if it was his custom to wear a beard. Determine if patient's religion or culture has a preference to facial hair.
5. Remove all equipment, tubes, supplies, and dirty linens according to protocol (unless organ donation or autopsy is to take place; in that case leave in place).
6. Cleanse the body thoroughly, apply clean sheets, and remove all trash from the room.
7. Brush and comb patient's hair. Apply any personal hairpiece.
8. Position according to protocol—the eyes should be closed by gently holding them down a few minutes; dentures should be in the mouth to maintain facial alignment.
9. Cover with a clean sheet up to the chin with arms outside covers if possible.
10. Lower the lighting, and spray a deodorizer if possible to remove unpleasant odors.
11. Give the family the option to view or not to view, and go with them.
12. Clarify that either option is acceptable.
13. Encourage the family to say goodbye through both touch and talk.
14. Do not rush this process. Once the family is more comfortable, *ask* if they would like to be left alone. Remind them they can call you if needed.
15. Clarify personal belongings that are to stay with the body or who has taken personal items; documentation will require both a descriptor of the objects and the name of who received them, with the time and date.
16. Discard nothing if items are found after the family is gone—call the family and tell them what was found, and ask who might pick it up—describing the articles will be helpful in the decision-making process for the patient's family.
17. Apply name tags according to protocol—such as at the wrist, right big toe, or outside a shroud.
18. Complete documentation in the nursing notes.
19. Remain sensitive to other hospitalized patients or visitors when transporting the body, such as covering the body with a clean sheet and watching to avoid visitors when moving the body to another part of the hospital or to the exit for the funeral home.
20. Follow all protocol and policies to meet all legal requirements in caring for the body.

---

event's in a patient's life. Your notes need to reflect time of death (pronounced by a physician or health care provider), the name of the person who pronounced the death, any preparation and type of organ or tissue donation, preparation of the body, stipulation of what equipment was left in place, what valuables or possessions were either given to the family or left with the patient, and the time of discharge and destination of the body. There are legal guidelines that each facility follows for care of the body. Complete and accurate documentation offers a summary of activities that become the focus for risk management or legal investigations.

**The Grieving Nurse.** When you have cared for a patient for a period of time, it is possible to have deep personal feelings of loss and sadness for the family when the patient dies. In these instances some choose to cope with their own grief by attending the viewing at the mortuary or the funeral. It is natural for you to go through the grieving process. If you work in an area where you experience multiple losses and fail to process them, you will experience bereavement overload. You will possibly feel frustration, anger, guilt, sadness, or other feelings of being overwhelmed. It is important to develop your own support systems that allow time away from the care setting and opportunities for you to share your feel-

ings. Stress management techniques will help to restore your energy and continued enjoyment in your work.

 **Evaluation**

**PATIENT CARE.** You will care for patients and families at every phase of the grief process. This requires you to remain aware of signs and symptoms of grief. These same signs and symptoms are criteria to evaluate whether a patient is able to deal with a loss and progress through the grief process. Critical thinking ensures that the evaluation process is thorough and relevant to the patient's situation.

Refer to the goals and expected outcomes in your plan of care and then use evaluative measures to identify actual behavioral outcomes (Table 23-6). Compare the actual behaviors with expected outcomes to determine the patient's health status and the need to revise the plan of care. For example, your goal is to have the patient be able to share his feelings about death through reminiscing, so you evaluate the verbal and nonverbal communication for cues that reflect normal grieving and healthy coping. Your patient's responses will determine if the problem is resolved, if the patient needs new therapies, or if you need to revise existing therapies. It is important for the patient

## OUTCOME EVALUATION

TABLE 23-6

| Nursing Action | Patient Response/Finding | Achievement of Outcome |
|---|---|---|
| During home visit ask Mrs. Holloway to describe her involvement in care of her husband. | Wife continues to have difficulty helping Mr. Holloway with incontinence but reports that she is regularly assisting daughter during bathing. | Outcome partially met. Provide further encouragement to wife, discuss her continued concerns about providing incontinence care. |
| Observe Mr. Holloway's daughter provide a bath for her father. | Daughter is able to keep her father involved in conversation during the bath. She bathes him effectively; skin is clean and intact. There are no safety risks observed in her approach. | Outcome met. Reinforce daughter's success in bathing her father. Remain available to answer questions or clarify how to perform any bathing techniques. |

## EVALUATION

Two weeks after discussing his proposed interventions with the Holloway family, Peter observes Mrs. Holloway helping Mr. Holloway with his bath. She explains that her daughter is "out taking a break, reading a book in the park." Mrs. Holloway has obtained a walker from the hospital supply store, and Mr. Holloway states that he feels much more secure when he uses it and is less fearful of walking. Mr. Holloway explains that he and his daughter have enjoyed looking through old photo albums together, and in the last day or two Mrs. Holloway has "wanted to join in the fun, too." They are enjoying their time as a family. Mrs. Holloway tells Peter that although Mr. Holloway's incontinence appears to be less, she remains uncomfortable with cleaning up after an accident. She also tells Peter that she and her daughter have inquired about a support group sponsored by the cancer society.

**Documentation Note**

"Uses walker to ambulate in the home. States he feels more secure. Wife more involved in bathing and interaction with patient. Wife and daughter working together in care activities. Bath in progress at time of visit. Skin has no redness, tenderness, or evidence of tissue breakdown. Reportedly continues to have incontinent episodes daily. States has recurrent right side pain every 3 to 4 hours, rapidly relieved with current pain medication. Is sleeping at night, waking only once for pain meds. Vital signs: T 98.0, pulse 68, resp. 18, BP 110/60. Family contacted cancer society regarding support group. Plan is to continue supportive care and current medication management."

and family to share experiences and be active participants in evaluation.

**PATIENT EXPECTATIONS.** Maintain open communication with patients to allow them to evaluate their nursing care. Patients who have developed a good relationship with a nurse will feel comfortable in discussing their perceptions of "how things are going." When caring for a terminally ill patient, take the time to frequently ask the family about their level of satisfaction. When a patient offers feedback or suggestions, consider this a sign of a satisfactory relationship. Such suggestions indicate that the patient and family perceive that they can approach you with their concerns. Once the patient identifies new approaches or problems, revise the plan of care to meet these emerging needs. Similarly, be encouraged when the patient's feedback reflects that he or she is making progress toward achieving the goals of care.

## KEY CONCEPTS

- Assist grieving patients by helping them feel the loss, express the loss, and move through the tasks of the grief process.
- The type of loss and the perception of the loss influence the degree of grief a person experiences.
- The bereavement period is not linear; rather, individuals will move back and forth through stages of grief, possibly extending over a period of several years.
- Several theorists have identified stages of grief and a series of tasks for survivors to successfully complete in order to adapt to a loss.
- Knowledge of the types of grief allows for implementation of appropriate bereavement interventions.

- Many factors influence the individual's reaction to loss, including developmental stage, beliefs, roles, culture, relationships, and socioeconomic status.
- Assessment of the grieving patient considers behavioral characteristics that suggest the patient's stage of grieving.
- When assessing patients in grief, does not assume how a patient experiences grief; rather allow patients to tell their stories.
- Therapeutic communication is an important nursing intervention to assist the grieving patient and family in coping with loss.

- Nursing care of the grieving and dying patient promotes the patient's sense of identity, dignity, and self-esteem, and improves the quality of remaining life.
- Palliative care is for any age, any diagnosis, at any time, and not just during the last months of life.
- Palliative care allows patients to make more informed choices, achieve better symptom relief, and have more opportunity to work on issues on life closure.

- Assess whether family members are willing to be involved in a dying patient's care before using them as resources.
- Care after death involves caring for the body with dignity and sensitivity.
- The evaluation of nursing care for the grieving and dying patient is ongoing and is based on identifiable behavioral changes through the grieving process.
- Stress management skills help you deal with feelings of loss when your patients die.

## CRITICAL THINKING IN PRACTICE

*Two months have passed, and Mr. Holloway's condition has worsened. He is having increased pain, requiring a morphine drip. He remains in the home, but his wife has decided to have a nurse assistant from home care come to help with daily hygiene activities. Mr. Holloway is still responsive and able to talk with his family, but he becomes fatigued very easily. He has also developed shortness of breath. Mr. Holloway's daughter tells Peter, "I still keep thinking over and over, why this had to happen. Mom and Dad were really enjoying retirement. If only Dad had taken care of himself better."*

- - - - - - - - - - - - - - - - - - - - - -

1. Explain how you can promote hope in the family, along the following dimensions:
   Affective
   Temporal

2. Describe the stage of grief, according to Bowlby's phases of mourning, that best describes the daughter's response. Provide a rationale.
3. Which of the following is the best response for the nurse to give Mr. Holloway's daughter?
   a. Why do you think he did not take care of himself?
   b. It's hard to find meaning in an illness like this; it must be very difficult for you.
   c. So, how is your mother feeling? This has been stressful for her.
   d. Tell me, are you angry with your Dad?
4. Identify a goal of care and expected outcome for helping to manage Mr. Holloway's fatigue.

## NCLEX® REVIEW

1. A middle-age man comes to the community clinic for his annual flu shot. In your discussion you learn that he still works at a local law firm; however, he has recently lost two important cases, and his boss has been applying pressure on him "to turn it around." The patient is experiencing:
   1. An actual loss
   2. A perceived loss
   3. A situational loss
   4. A maturational loss
2. Your patient has been diagnosed with terminal brain cancer. When you visit him during rounds, he asks you whether the cancer could have been caused by something he ate or perhaps following exposure to some chemical toxin. Your patient is likely experiencing:
   1. Bowlby's phase of numbing
   2. Kübler-Ross's stage of acceptance
   3. Worden's task of emotionally relocating
   4. Bowlby's phase of disorganization and despair
3. As a community health nurse your job is to provide grief counseling for the citizens of your town, where a major flood has occurred. The loss associated with flooding is best described as:
   1. An actual loss
   2. A perceived loss
   3. A situational loss
   4. A maturational loss

4. Since the death of his wife, your patient has assumed full responsibility for the care of his children. He has noticed over the last few weeks that friends are calling less often. He is most likely in which phase of mourning:
   1. Anticipatory grieving
   2. Worden's task III of mourning
   3. Kübler Ross's phase of bargaining
   4. Bowlby's disorganization and despair
5. A factor that uniquely influences an older adult's grief response is:
   1. Cultural background
   2. Socioeconomic resources
   3. Sense of contributions in life
   4. Support available from family members
6. A 16-year-old has been admitted to the intensive care unit (ICU) after suffering a closed head injury in a head-on car collision. The physician and nurse are preparing to approach the family to consider donation of heart and lungs. When working with families in this situation, it is important to explain that:
   1. The ventilator is being used to prevent brain death
   2. The ventilator maintains organ perfusion until time for harvesting
   3. Tissues such as corneas can be harvested only if the patient remains ventilated
   4. Organ donation can occur only if the patient has made a prior request to donate organs

# REFERENCES

Barbus AJ: The dying person's bill of rights, *Am J Nurs* 75:99, 1975.

Bierman E and others: Assessing access as a first step towards improving the quality of care for very old adults, *J Ambul Care Manage* 21(3):17, 1998.

Blackhall LJ and others: Ethnicity and attitudes towards life sustaining technology, *Soc Sci Med* 48:1779, 1999.

Bowlby J: *Attachment and loss,* vol 3, Loss, sadness, and depression, New York, 1980, Basic Books.

Chochinov HM: Dignity-conserving care: a new model for palliative care—helping the patient feel valued, *JAMA* 287(17):2253, 2002.

Crowley LM and others: Strategies for culturally effective end-of-life-care, *Ann Intern Med* 136(9):673, 2002.

Dochterman JM, Bulechek GM, editors: *Nursing interventions Classification (NIC),* ed 4, St. Louis, 2004, Mosby.

End-of-Life Nursing Education Consortium, American Association of Colleges of Nursing and City of Hope National Medical Center, 2000.

Farber SJ and others: Issues in end-of-life care: family practice faculty perceptions, *J Fam Pract* 48(7):525, 1999.

Field MJ, Cassel CK: *Approaching death: improving care at the end of life,* Washington, DC, 1997, (Institute of Medicine Committee on Care at the End of Life), National Academy Press.

Finucane TE: Care of patients nearing death: another view, *J Am Geriatr Soc* 50(3):551, 2002.

Forbes S and others: End-of-life decision making for nursing home residents with dementia, *J Nurs Scholarsh* 32(3):251, 2000.

Kagawa-Singer M: The cultural context of death rituals and mourning practices, *Oncol Nurs Forum* 25(10):1752, 1998.

Kübler Ross E: *On death and dying,* New York, 1969, Macmillan.

Lindquist O and others: Meanings of the phenomenon of fatigue as narrated by four patients with cancer in palliative care, *Cancer Nurs* 27(3):237, 2004.

Meiner SE, Lueckenotte AG: *Gerontologic nursing,* ed 3, St. Louis, 2006, Mosby.

Moorhead S, Johnson M, Maas M: *Nursing outcomes classification (NOC),* ed 3, St. Louis, 2004, Mosby.

Murray SA and others: Exploring the spiritual needs of people dying of lung cancer or heart failure: a prospective qualitative interview study of patients and their carers, *Palliative Med* 18(1):39, 2004.

Nowotny M: Every tomorrow a vision of hope, *J Psychosoc Oncol* 9(3):117, 1991.

Parkes CM: *Bereavement: studies of grief in adult life,* London, 1972, Tavistock.

Poncar PJ: Inspiring hope in the oncology patient, *J Psychosoc Nurs Mental Health Serv* 32(1):33, 1994.

Post-White J and others: Hope, spirituality, sense of coherence, and quality of life in patients with cancer, *Oncol Nurs Forum* 23(10):1571, 1996.

Rassoul GH: The crescent and Islam: healing, nursing and the spiritual dimension, *J Adv Nurs* 32(6):1476, 2000.

Schwartz E: Jewish Americans. In Giger JN, Davidhizar RE: *Transcultural nursing: assessment and intervention,* ed 4, St. Louis, 2003, Mosby.

Soden K and others: A randomized controlled trial of aromatherapy massage in hospice setting, *Palliat Med* 18(2)87, 2004.

Steinhauser K and others: Factors considered important at the end of life by patients, family, physicians, and other care providers, *JAMA* 284:2476, 2000.

SUPPORT Principal Investigators: A controlled trial to improve care for seriously ill hospitalized patients, *JAMA* 274:1591, 1995.

Tarzian AJ: Caring for dying patients who have air hunger, *Image J Nurs Sch* 32:137, 2000.

Teno and others: Family perspectives on end-of-life care at the last place of care, *JAMA* 291(1):88, 2004.

Thomas ND: The importance of culture throughout all of life and beyond, *Holist Nurs Pract* 15(2):40, 2001.

Tilden VP and others: Family decision-making to withdraw life sustaining treatments from hospitalized patients, *Nurs Res* 50:105, 2001.

Tolle SW and others: Family reports of barriers to optimal care of the dying, *Nurs Res* 49:310, 2000.

Varcarolis EM: *Foundations of psychiatric mental health nursing,* Philadelphia, 2002, Saunders.

Weissman DE and others: Pain assessment and management in the long-term care setting, *Theor Med Bioeth* 20(1):31, 1999.

World Health Organization: *Palliative care,* 2006, http://www.who.int/hiv/topics/palliative/care/en.

Worden JW: *Grief counseling and grief therapy,* New York, 1982, Springer.

Yick AG, Gupta R: Chinese cultural dimensions of death, dying and bereavement: focus group findings, *J Cult Divers* 9(2):32, 2002.

# CHAPTER 24

# Managing Patient Care

## MEDIA RESOURCES

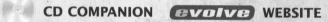

**CD COMPANION** | **evolve** WEBSITE

http://evolve.elsevier.com/Potter/basic

- **NCLEX® Review**
- **Audio Glossary**
- **English/Spanish Audio Glossary**

## OBJECTIVES

- Discuss the importance of education in professional nursing practice.
- Describe the purpose of professional standards of nursing practice.
- Differentiate among the types of nursing care delivery models.
- Describe the elements of decentralized decision making.
- Discuss the ways in which a nurse manager supports staff involvement in a decentralized decision-making model.

- Discuss ways to apply clinical care coordination skills in nursing practice.
- Discuss principles to follow in the appropriate delegation of patient care activities.
- Differentiate among structure, process, and quality outcomes.
- Describe an example of a quality improvement project on a nursing unit.

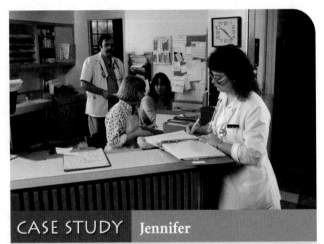

## CASE STUDY  Jennifer

Jennifer is a nursing student assigned to care for two patients. Her first patient is Mrs. Sinclair, who will have surgery at 1 PM to repair her fractured right hip. It is the first time she has had surgery. It is now 11:30 AM. The operating room (OR) has notified Jennifer that they will pick up Mrs. Sinclair in 30 minutes. Jennifer enters Mrs. Sinclair's room to complete the preoperative checklist and to make final preparations for surgery. She finds Mrs. Sinclair moving about restlessly in bed and reluctant to talk. At the same time, the call light system at the bedside comes on and the unit clerk notifies Jennifer that her second patient, Mr. Timmons, has finished his lunch and is ready for his pain medication and to have Jennifer change his dressing so he is able to ambulate down the hall. Mr. Timmons had abdominal surgery 2 days ago for removal of a colon tumor. What should Jennifer do in this situation?

In setting her priorities, Jennifer remembers the categories of priority needs she learned in school and prioritizes her care according to these. Jennifer asks the unit clerk to send John, another nursing student, to Mr. Timmons's room to check on him and tell him that Jennifer is preparing a patient for surgery and will be with Mr. Timmons as soon as she finishes. Jennifer stays with Mrs. Sinclair and begins an assessment of her to determine the cause of the restlessness. She also asks Mrs. Sinclair if she has any questions or concerns about surgery. Mrs. Sinclair voices her concerns about pain after surgery. Jennifer reinforces the earlier teaching she did on patient-controlled analgesia

pumps. This seems to relax Mrs. Sinclair. Jennifer completes her preoperative preparation and checklist. She tells Mrs. Sinclair that the OR staff will be here in 15 minutes to get her. Jennifer then goes to assess Mr. Timmons's pain. She then prepares and administers the prescribed pain medication for Mr. Timmons. Jennifer then gathers the supplies for his dressing change. After completing the dressing change, Jennifer assists Mr. Timmons with his walk.

## KEY TERMS

accountability, p. 639
authority, p. 639
benchmarking, p. 644
code of ethics, p. 634
decentralized management, p. 639
delegation, p. 643
functional nursing, p. 638
licensed practical nurse (LPN), p. 634
licensed vocational nurse (LVN), p. 634
outcome, p. 644

primary nursing, p. 638
quality improvement, p. 644
quality indicator, p. 645
registered nurse (RN), p. 633
responsibility, p. 639
root cause analysis, p. 644
team nursing, p. 638
total patient care, p. 638

As a nursing student, it is important for you to acquire the necessary knowledge and competencies that ultimately allow you to practice as an entry-level staff nurse (Box 24-1). Regardless of the type of setting you eventually choose to work in as a staff nurse, you will be responsible for practicing professional standards of care, using organizational resources, and participating in organizational routines. While doing this you will provide direct patient care, use your time

> **BOX 24-1  Entry-Level Staff Nurse Competencies**
>
> Identify organizational resources (people, equipment, services), and determine when you will need them.
>
> Work within various nursing care delivery models.
>
> Use position descriptions to establish the scope and limitations of your own and other nursing team members' practices.
>
> Manage time purposefully and productively.
>
> Prioritize patient needs and plan related care.
>
> View patient holistically.
>
> Exhibit flexibility in providing care within available time constraints.
>
> Show initiative and creativity as leadership qualities.
>
> Use nursing process to make clinical decisions.
>
> Show accountability for own nursing actions.
>
> Communicate effectively with patients and other health team members.
>
> Resolve conflicts within the health team.
>
> Delegate care activities appropriately.
>
> Exhibit a sense of professionalism.
>
> Serve as a role model.
>
> Participate in lifelong learning.
>
> Modified from Wywialowski E: *Managing patient care*, ed 3, St. Louis, 2004, Mosby.

productively, collaborate with all members of the health care team, and use certain leadership characteristics to manage others on the nursing team (Wywialowski, 2004). The delivery of nursing care within the health care system is a challenge because of the changes that are influencing health professionals, patients, and health care organizations (see Chapter 2). However, change offers opportunities. As you develop the knowledge and skills to become a staff nurse, you will learn what it takes to effectively manage the patients you care for and to take the initiative in becoming a leader among your professional colleagues.

## Professionalism

Nursing is a profession. A person who acts professionally is conscientious in actions, knowledgeable in the subject, and responsible to self and others. Professions possess the following characteristics:

- An extended education of members and a basic liberal education foundation
- A theoretical body of knowledge leading to defined skills, abilities, and norms
- Provision of a specific service
- Autonomy in decision making and practice
- A code of ethics for practice

Nursing shares each of these characteristics, offering an opportunity for the growth and enrichment of all its members.

### Registered Nurse Education

As a profession, nursing requires that its members possess a significant amount of education. There are various educational routes for becoming a **registered nurse (RN)**. Currently in the United States an individual becomes an RN by completion of an associate degree, diploma, or baccalaureate degree program. In Canada there are currently only diploma and baccalaureate degrees. The Canadian Nurses Association (2004) has identified the baccalaureate degree as the entry to practice standard for RNs. Nursing education provides the solid foundation for practice, and it responds to changes in health care created by scientific and technological advances.

After completion of the professional education program, RN candidates in the United States must pass the National Council Licensure Examination for Registered Nurses (NCLEX-RN), which the individual state boards of nursing administer. Regardless of candidates' educational preparation, the examination for RN licensure is the same in every state, ensuring a standardized minimum knowledge base for the patient population nurses serve. In all Canadian provinces except Quebec, new graduates must pass the Canadian Registered Nurse Examination (CRNE) to become an RN. Whether nurses are able to practice in a state or province other than their own depends on the agreement between the states or provinces involved.

The opportunities in the nursing profession are limitless, but often they require a professional nurse to pursue additional education. A nurse has the opportunity to choose to work toward certification in a specific area of clinical nursing practice. Minimum practice requirements are set based on the certification the nurse is seeking, such as in critical care, oncology, or gerontology. National nursing organizations, such as the American Nurses Association (ANA), have many types of certifications for nurses to work toward. After passing the initial examination, the nurse maintains certification by ongoing continuing education and clinical practice.

### Advanced Education

There are roles for registered nurses in nursing that require advanced educational degrees. A master's degree in nursing (e.g., master of arts in nursing [MA], master in nursing [MN], master of science in nursing [MSN]) is for RNs seeking roles as nurse educator, clinical nurse specialist, nurse administrator, or nurse practitioner. The degree provides the advanced clinician with strong skills in nursing science and theory with emphasis in the basic sciences and research-based clinical practice. There are also roles within nursing that require doctoral degrees. Expanding clinical and research roles, new areas of nursing, such as nursing informatics, and the influential presence of nursing in public policy and health care planning are just a few reasons for increasing the number of nurses with doctoral degrees. The health care industry needs doctorally prepared nurses to educate beginning nurses and those seeking advanced academic and clinical preparation. Nurses with doctorates advance the profession by conducting and disseminating research and developing and testing theory.

## Licensed Practical Nurse Education

A licensed practical or vocational nurse is educated in basic nursing techniques and direct patient care. The **licensed practical nurse (LPN)** or **licensed vocational nurse (LVN)** practices under the supervision of a registered nurse in a hospital or community health practice setting. An LPN, or in Canada a registered nurse's assistant (RNA), generally receives 1 year of education and clinical preparation in a community college or other agency. There are some RN programs that allow an LPN to enter the program at an advanced level. A board licenses the LPN or LVN after the LPN or LVN completes the educational program and passes the licensure examination.

## Theory

The practice of professional nursing and nursing knowledge have been developed through nursing theories, global views that help to describe, predict, or prescribe activities for the practice of nursing. Theoretical models provide frameworks for how nurses practice. Typically a nursing school's curriculum integrates a theoretical model. Examples of theories used in education and practice include Orem's self-care deficit theory, Benner's primacy of caring, and Roy's adaptation theory. There are also nursing organizations that adopt a nursing theory to serve as the foundation for the organization's standards of nursing care. The ongoing development of nursing theory or nursing science involves generating knowledge to advance and support nursing practice and health care (Chinn and Kramer, 1999).

## Service

Nursing is a service profession and a vital and indispensable component of the health care delivery system. Nurses in practice today maintain a consumer and service-based focus. Patients are more aware and knowledgeable about their health care problems, their options, and their rights. As a nurse you will work with the patient and family, individualizing care while incorporating their preferences and expectations. Show respect for patients by providing care on time, displaying a caring attitude, considering patients' cultural and social differences, and collaborating with necessary health care providers to ensure a smooth continuation of care from one setting to the next.

## Autonomy

Autonomy is essential to professional nursing. Autonomy means that a person is reasonably independent and self-governing in decision making and practice. You reach autonomy through experience, advanced education, and the support of an organization that values the independent role of the nurse. With increased autonomy comes greater responsibility and accountability for the performance of nursing care activities.

## Code of Ethics

Nursing has a **code of ethics** that defines the principles by which nurses function (see Chapter 5). In addition, nurses incorporate their own values and ethics into practice. The ANA's *Code of Ethics for Nurses With Interpretive Statements* provides a guide for carrying out nursing responsibilities to ensure quality nursing care and to provide for the ethical obligations of the profession (ANA, 2001).

## Standards of Nursing Practice

Nursing is a helping, independent profession that provides services that contribute to the health of people. Three essential components of professional nursing are care, cure, and coordination. The care aspect is more than "to take care of"; it is also "caring about." Caring is relational and requires you as a nurse to understand the patient's needs at a level that permits individualization of nursing therapies (see Chapter 16). When you promote health and healing, you are practicing the cure aspect of professional nursing. To cure is to assist patients in understanding their health problems and to help them to cope. The cure aspect involves the administration of treatments and the use of clinical nursing judgment in determining, on the basis of patient outcomes, whether the plan of care is effective. Coordination of care involves organizing and timing medical and other professional and technical services to meet the holistic needs of a patient. Often a patient requires many services simultaneously in order to be well cared for. A professional nurse also supervises, teaches, and directs all of those involved in nursing care.

As an independent profession, nursing has increasingly set its own standards for practice. Standards of nursing practice are guidelines for how nurses perform professionally and how they exercise the care, cure, and coordination aspects of nursing. Clinical, academic, and administrative nurse experts have developed standards of nursing practice. As an example, the ANA has published *Nursing: Scope and Standards of Practice* (2004). Within this document are Standards of Professional Performance (Table 24-1) and Standards of Practice (Table 24-2).

### Standards of Care

In the practice setting it is important to have objective guidelines for providing and evaluating nursing care. Standards of nursing care are developed and established on the basis of strong scientific research and the work of clinical nurse experts. The purpose of a standard of care is to describe the common level of professional nursing care in order to judge the quality of nursing practice (Dean Baar, 2001). An organization sometimes adopts a general set of standards for nursing care, such as organizational protocols, policies, or procedures. For example, an organization has a written nasogastric tube protocol based on research findings. This protocol spells out the expected nursing care for patients with nasogastric tubes in that organization. Individual nursing

| TABLE 24-1 | ANA Standards of Professional Performance | |
|---|---|---|
| **Standard** | **Definition** | **Measurement Criteria** |
| I: Quality of practice | The nurse systematically enhances the quality and effectiveness of nursing practice. | Participates in quality activities<br>Practice changes are a result of quality-of-care activities<br>Uses quality improvement activities to initiate changes in nursing practice and the health care delivery system<br>Uses creativity and innovation to improve nursing care delivery |
| II: Education | The nurse attains knowledge and competency that reflects current nursing practice. | Participates in ongoing educational activities related to clinical knowledge and professional issues<br>Demonstrates commitment to lifelong learning<br>Seeks experiences to maintain clinical skills<br>Seeks knowledge and skills appropriate to the practice setting |
| III: Practice evaluation | The nurse evaluates one's own nursing practice in relation to professional practice standards and guideline, relevant statutes, rules and regulations. | Engages in self-evaluation on a regular basis<br>Seeks constructive feedback regarding one's own practice<br>Takes action to achieve goals identified during the evaluation process<br>Participates in systematic peer review as appropriate<br>Practice reflects knowledge of current professional practice standards, laws, and regulations<br>Provides age-appropriate care in culturally and ethnically sensitive manner |
| IV: Collegiality | The nurse interacts with and contributes to the professional development of peers and other health care providers as colleagues. | Shares knowledge and skills with peers and colleagues<br>Provides peers with feedback regarding their practice<br>Interacts with peers and colleagues to enhance one's own professional nursing practice<br>Maintains compassionate and caring relationships with peers and colleagues<br>Contributes to an environment that is conducive to clinical education of nursing students as appropriate<br>Contributes to a supportive and healthy work environment |
| V: Collaboration | The nurse collaborates with patient, family, and others in the conduct of nursing practice. | Communicates with the patient, significant others, and health care providers regarding patient care and nursing's role in the provision of care<br>Collaborates with the patient, family, and other health care providers in the formulation of overall goals and the plan of care and in the decisions related to care and delivery of services<br>Partners with others to effect change and generate positive outcomes<br>Documents referrals, including provisions for continuity of care, as needed |
| VI: Ethics | The nurse integrates ethical provisions in all areas of practice. | Practice is guided by the *Code of Ethics for Nurses with Interpretive Statements*<br>Maintains patient confidentiality<br>Serves as a patient advocate<br>Maintains therapeutic and professional patient-nurse relationship<br>Delivers care in a manner that preserves patient autonomy, dignity, and rights<br>Seeks available resources in formulating ethical decisions<br>Reports illegal, incompetent, or impaired practice |
| VII: Research | The nurse integrates research findings in practice. | Utilizes best available evidence including research findings to guide practice decisions<br>Participates in research activities as appropriate to the nurse's education and position, such as the following:<br>  Identifying clinical problems suitable for nursing research<br>  Participating in data collection<br>  Participating in a unit, organization, or community research committee<br>  Sharing research activities with others<br>  Conducting research<br>Critiquing research for application to practice<br>Uses research findings in the development of policies, procedures, and practice guidelines for patient care<br>Incorporates research as a basis for learning |

*Continued*

| TABLE 24-1 | ANA Standards of Professional Performance—cont'd |
|---|---|

| Standard | Definition | Measurement Criteria |
|---|---|---|
| VIII: Resource utilization | The nurse considers factors related to safety, effectiveness, cost, and impact on practice in the planning and delivery of nursing services. | Evaluates factors related to safety, effectiveness, availability, and cost when practice options would result in the same expected patient outcome<br>Assists the patient and family in identifying and securing appropriate and available services to address health-related needs<br>Assigns or delegates tasks as defined by the state nurse practice acts and according to the knowledge and skills of the designated caregiver<br>Assigns or delegates tasks based on the needs and condition of the patient, the potential for harm, the stability of the patient's condition, the complexity of the task, and the predictability of the outcome<br>Assists the patient and family in becoming informed consumers about the cost, risks, and benefits of treatment and care |
| IX: Leadership | The nurse provides leadership in the professional practice setting and the profession. | Engages in teamwork<br>Works to create and maintain healthy work environments<br>Teaches others to succeed through mentoring<br>Exhibits creativity and flexibility during change<br>Directs coordination of care across settings and caregivers<br>Serves in key roles in the work setting<br>Promotes advancement of the profession |

Reprinted with permission from American Nurses Association: *Nursing: scope and standards of practice*, Washington, DC, 2004, The Association.

| TABLE 24-2 | ANA Standards of Practice |
|---|---|

| Standard | Measurement Criteria |
|---|---|
| **Assessment**<br>The nurse collects comprehensive data pertinent to the patient's health or the situation. | Data collection involves the patient, significant others, and health care providers, when appropriate.<br>The patient's immediate condition or needs determine the priority of data collection.<br>Collects pertinent data using appropriate assessment techniques.<br>Documents relevant data in a retrievable form.<br>The data collection process is systematic and ongoing. |
| **Nursing Diagnosis**<br>The nurse analyzes the assessment data to determine the diagnoses or issues. | Derives diagnoses from the assessment data.<br>Validates the diagnoses with the patient, significant others, and health care providers, when possible.<br>Documents diagnoses in a manner that facilitates the determination of expected outcomes and plan of care. |
| **Outcomes Identification**<br>The nurse identifies expected outcomes for a plan individualized to the patient or the situation. | Derives outcomes from the diagnoses.<br>Formulates outcomes mutually with the patient and health care providers, when possible.<br>Outcomes are culturally appropriate and realistic in relation to the patient's present and potential capabilities.<br>Outcomes are attainable in relation to resources available to the patient.<br>Outcomes include a time estimate for attainment.<br>Outcomes provide direction for continuity of care.<br>Documents outcomes as measurable goals. |

| TABLE 24-2 | ANA Standards of Practice—cont'd |
|---|---|

| Standard | Measurement Criteria |
|---|---|
| **Planning** | |
| The nurse develops a plan that prescribes strategies and alternatives to attain expected outcomes. | The plan is individualized to the patient and patient's condition or needs. |
| | Develops the plan with the patient, significant others, and health care providers, when appropriate. |
| | The plan reflects current nursing practice. |
| | The plan provides for continuity of care. |
| | Considers economic impact of the plan. |
| | Establishes priorities for care. |
| | Documents the plan. |
| **Implementation** | |
| The nurse implements the identified plan of care. | Interventions are consistent with the established plan of care. |
| | Implements interventions in a safe and appropriate manner. |
| | Documents interventions. |
| | Collaborates with nurse colleagues to implement the plan. |
| | Utilizes community resources and systems to implement the plan. |
| **Evaluation** | |
| The nurse evaluates progress toward attainment of outcomes. | Evaluation is systematic, ongoing, and criterion-based. |
| | Involves the patient, significant others, and health care providers in the evaluation process, when appropriate. |
| | Uses ongoing assessment data to revise diagnoses, outcomes, and the plan of care as needed. |
| | Documents revisions in diagnoses, outcomes, and the plan of care. |
| | Evaluates the effectiveness of interventions in relation to outcomes. |
| | Documents the patient's responses to interventions. |

Reprinted with permission from American Nurses Association: *Nursing: scope and standards of practice*, Washington, DC, 2004, The Association.

units or work groups also establish standards of care to address the unique needs of patients for whom they care. For example, an oncology nursing unit develops standards of care for pain management and palliative care. Standards of care are important if a legal dispute arises over whether a nurse practiced appropriately in a particular case (see Chapter 4). More importantly standards of care establish the guidelines for nursing excellence within an organization.

## Building a Nursing Team

Nurses want to work within an institutional culture that promotes autonomy and quality (Wywialowski, 2004). Your education and the commitment you make in practicing within established standards and guidelines will ensure a rewarding professional career. It is also important to work as a member of a cohesive and strong nursing team that values mentoring, integrity, and respect for their teamwork. An empowering work environment brings out the best in a professional. It concentrates on effective patient care systems (e.g., patient assessment, referral mechanisms, and collaboration between nurses and physicians or health care providers), supports risk taking and innovation, focuses on results and rewards, and offers professional opportunities for growth and advancement.

One way of creating an empowering work environment is through the Magnet Recognition Program. The American Nurses Credentialing Center Magnet Recognition Program recognizes excellence in nursing service and quality. The Magnet Recognition Program recognizes nursing services that build programs of excellence for the delivery of nursing care, promote quality in environments that support professional nursing practice, and promote achievement of positive patient outcomes (American Nurses Credentialing Center, 2005). A Magnet hospital has a culture that is dynamic and positive for nurses. Typically a Magnet hospital has clinical promotion systems, research programs, and evidence-based practice. The nurses have professional autonomy over their practice and control over the practice environment (Bolton and Goodenough, 2003). A Magnet hospital empowers the nursing team to make changes and be innovative. This culture and empowerment combine to produce a strong collaborative relationship among team members and improve patient quality outcomes.

It takes an excellent nurse manager and an excellent nursing staff to achieve an enriching work culture. Together a manager and the nursing staff share a philosophy of care for their work unit. A philosophy of care incorporates the professional nursing staff's values and concerns for the way that they view and care for patients. For example, a philosophy addresses the nursing unit's purpose, how staff will work with patients and families, and the standards of care for the work unit. A philosophy is a vision for how to practice nursing. Integral to the philosophy of care is the selection of a nursing care delivery model and management structure that support professional nursing practice.

## Nursing Care Delivery Models

A nursing care delivery model allows you as a nurse to achieve desirable outcomes for your patients. Historically, economic issues, political issues, the focus on quality and patient satisfaction, and the social environment are factors that contribute to the development of models of nursing care delivery (Tiedeman and Lookinland, 2004). There are a variety of nursing care delivery models. All of the nursing care delivery models are used in acute care settings. Case management and primary nursing are the common nursing care delivery models used in the home care setting.

**FUNCTIONAL NURSING. Functional Nursing** is a model of care that evolved in the 1940s and is task focused, not patient-focused. In this model you divide tasks, with one nurse assuming responsibility for specific tasks. For example, one nurse does the hygiene and dressing changes, whereas another nurse assumes responsibility for medication administration. Typically a lead nurse responsible for a specific shift assigns available nursing staff members according to their qualifications, their particular abilities, and tasks to be completed. Nurses become highly competent with tasks that are repeatedly assigned to them. The major disadvantages of functional nursing are problems with continuity of care, fragmentation of care, absence of a holistic view of patients, and the possibility that care will become mechanical (Tiedeman and Lookinland, 2004). In other words, a task-focused approach does not ensure that patient care needs are met shift to shift. Communication is not always clear, because a single nurse is not responsible for the overall care of the patient. This model place more emphasis on nurses' following rules, regulations, and policies and does not promote nurses' decision making, autonomy, or professional development.

**TEAM NURSING.** Team nursing was developed during the 1950s. In **team nursing** an RN leads a team composed of other RNs, LPNs or LVNs, and nurse assistants or technicians. The team members provide direct patient care to groups of patients, under the direction of the RN team leader. In this model, the RN gives the nurse assistants patient assignments rather than assigning particular nursing tasks. The team leader provides strong leadership and is a clear communicator (Tiedeman and Lookinland, 2004). When team leading was popular, there were generally fewer RNs than LPNs and other staff.

The team leader develops patient care plans and coordinates care delivered by the nursing team. The team leader also provides care requiring complex nursing skills, problem solves with physicians and members of other disciplines, and assists the team in evaluating the effectiveness of their care (Wywialowski, 2004). Limitations to the model include the task orientation of the model that leads to fragmentation of patient care and the lack of time the team leader spends with patients (Ritter-Teitel, 2002). Depending on the mix of staff members, this sometimes means that patients see an RN infrequently. Risks exist if an RN is unable to make necessary patient assessments and be involved in important clinical decision making. Nurses are not always assigned to the same patients each day, which potentially causes lack of continuity of care. Another disadvantage some perceives is that the model is expensive because of the increased number of personnel needed (Tiedeman and Lookinland, 2004). An advantage of team nursing is the collaborative style that encourages each member of the team to help the other members.

**TOTAL PATIENT CARE. Total patient care** delivery was the original care delivery model developed during Florence Nightingale's time. The model disappeared in the 1930s but gained popularity again in the 1980s (Tiedeman and Lookinland, 2004). An RN is responsible for all aspects of care for one or more patients during an assigned shift. The RN delegates aspects of care to an LPN or unlicensed staff, but retains accountability for care of all assigned patients. The nurse works directly with the patient, family, physician or health care provider, and health care team members. The model has a shift-based focus. The same nurse does not necessarily care for the same patient over successive days or visits. Continuity and coordination of care from shift to shift or day to day is a problem if staff members do not clearly communicate patient needs to one another. Patient satisfaction with this model tends to be high but the model is not cost-effective because of the high number of RNs needed to deliver care (Tiedeman and Lookinland, 2004).

**PRIMARY NURSING.** The **primary nursing** model of care delivery was developed in the 1960s with the aim of placing RNs at the bedside and improving the professional relationships among staff members (Tiedeman and Lookinland, 2004). The model became more popular in the 1970s and early 1980s as hospitals began to employ more RNs. Primary nursing supports a philosophy regarding nurse and patient relationships. Primary nursing is a model of care delivery whereby an RN assumes responsibility for a caseload of patients over time (e.g., a length of stay in a hospital or a series of home care visits). Typically the RN selects the patients for his or her caseload and cares for the same patients during their hospitalization or stay in the health care setting. The RN assesses patient needs, develops a care plan, and ensures that the designated caregiver delivers the appropriate nursing interventions to the patient.

Primary nursing maintains continuity of care across shifts, days, or visits. The model increases nursing autonomy and improves collaboration between nurses and physicians or health care providers (Ritter-Teitel, 2002). It is applied in any health care setting. When a primary nurse is off-duty, associate nurses, including LPNs or other RNs, follow through with the developed plan of care. If there are differences in opinion as to patient needs, associates and primary nurses collaborate to redefine the plan as needed.

Although primary nursing requires the presence of more professional staff members, this does not mean that the model is more costly. Care consistently managed by a single professional minimizes delays in therapies, improves collaboration with other professionals, and improves the patient-nurse relationship.

**CASE MANAGEMENT.** Case management is a delivery of care approach that emerged in the 1980s as health care institutions needed to provide complex cost-effective care. Case management coordinates and links health care services to patients and their families (see Chapter 2). Case management requires an RN to maintain responsibility for patient care from admission to after discharge (Wywialowski, 2004). What is unique about case management is that clinicians, either as individuals or as part of a collaborative group, oversee the management of patients with specific case types (e.g., patients with specific diagnoses presenting complex nursing and medical problems). They are usually held accountable for some standard of cost management and quality. A case manager coordinates a patient's acute care in the hospital, for example, and then follows the patient after discharge home. For example, the case manager calls a meeting of the patient, family, social services, dietician, and physical therapist to plan the discharge of a patient following a stroke. Case managers do not always provide direct care. Instead, they collaborate with and supervise the care delivered by other staff members and actively coordinate patient discharge planning. Many organizations use critical pathways, which are multidisciplinary treatment plans, in a case management delivery system (see Chapter 2). Advantages of case management include cost-effectiveness, focus on patients' complex health needs, efficiency in planning discharge, and multidisciplinary collaboration (Wywialowski, 2004).

## Decentralized Decision Making

**Decentralized management,** in which decision making is moved down to the level of staff, is very common within health care organizations. It is clear that progressive organizations achieve more when they involve employees at all levels actively. As a result, the role of a nurse manager has become critical in the management of effective nursing units or groups. Box 24-2 highlights the diverse responsibilities assumed by nursing managers. To make decentralized decision making work, managers know how to move decision making down to the lowest level possible. On a nursing unit, it is important for all staff members (RNs, LPNs, and LVNs), nurse assistants, and unit secretaries to feel involved particularly with issues affecting their ability to care for patients. Key elements of the decision-making process are responsibility, authority, and accountability (Marriner Tomey, 2004).

**Responsibility** refers to the duties and activities that an individual is employed to perform. A position description outlines a professional nurse's responsibilities in patient care and in participating as a member of the nursing unit. Responsibility reflects ownership; the individual who oversees the employee gives responsibility, and the employee ac-

---

**BOX 24-2** **Responsibilities of the Nurse Manager**

Assist staff in establishing yearly goals for the unit and the systems needed to accomplish goals.

Monitor professional nursing standards of practice on the unit.

Develop an ongoing staff development plan, including one for new employees.

Recruit new employees (interview and hire).

Conduct routine staff evaluations.

Establish self as a role model for positive customer service (customers include patients, families, and other health care team members).

Serve as an advocate for the nursing staff to the administration of the institution.

Submit staffing schedules for the unit.

Conduct regular patient rounds and help to solve patient or family complaints.

Establish and implement a quality improvement (QI) plan for the unit.

Review and recommend new equipment needs for the unit.

Conduct regular staff meetings.

Conduct rounds with physician or health care provider.

Establish and support necessary staff and interdisciplinary committees.

---

cepts it. For example, a primary nurse is responsible for completing a nursing assessment of all assigned patients and for developing a plan of care that addresses each of the patient's nursing diagnoses. As the staff delivers the plan of care, the primary nurse is responsible for evaluating whether the plan is successful and what to do when it is not successful. This responsibility becomes a work ethic for the nurse in delivering excellent patient care.

**Authority** refers to the official power to act in areas where an individual has been given and accepts responsibility (Marriner Tomey, 2004). For example, a primary nurse, managing a caseload of patients, discovers that members of the nursing team did not follow through on a discharge teaching plan for an assigned patient. The primary nurse has the authority to consult other nurses to learn why they did not follow recommendations on the plan of care and to choose appropriate teaching strategies for the patient that all members of the team will follow. The primary nurse has the final authority in selecting the best course of action for the patient's care.

**Accountability** refers to individuals being answerable for their actions. It involves follow-up and a reflective analysis of your decisions to evaluate their effectiveness. A primary nurse delegates responsibility but is accountable for his or her patients' outcomes (Marriner Tomey, 2004). In the example above, the primary nurse is accountable for ensuring that the patient learns the information necessary to improve self-care. By using authority in bringing the nursing team together, the primary nurse determines if collaboration was successful, if continuity in teaching occurred, and if the patient and family understood and related the information.

A successful decentralized nursing unit exercises the three elements of decision making on an ongoing basis. An effective manager sets the same expectations for the staff in how to make decisions. Staff members must feel comfortable in expressing differences of opinion and in challenging ways in which the team functions. Staff does this while recognizing their own responsibility, authority, and accountability. Ultimately, decentralized decision making is the way to realize a nursing unit's vision of what professional nursing care should be.

**STAFF INVOLVEMENT.** When decentralized decision making exists on a nursing unit, all staff members actively participate in unit activities (Figure 24-1). Because the work environment promotes participation, all staff members benefit from the knowledge and skills of the entire work group. If the staff learns to value knowledge and the contributions of colleagues, better patient care becomes an outcome. The nursing manager supports staff involvement through a variety of ways:

1. *Establishment of nursing practice or problem-solving committees.* Staff committees establish and maintain professional nursing practice on a unit. Practice committees become involved in activities such as the review and revision of standards of care, development of policy and procedure, and resolution of repeated patient satisfaction issues. These activities ensure the delivery of quality care on the unit. A senior staff member usually chairs a committee. Managers do not always sit on the committee, but they receive regular reports of committee progress. The nature of work on the nursing unit determines committee membership. At times, members of other disciplines, for example, pharmacy, respiratory therapy, or clinical nutrition, participate on practice committees.
2. *Nurse and physician or health care provider collaborative practice.* The unit's delivery of care model influences how to strengthen nurse and physician or health care provider collaboration. If the unit practices team nursing, it is important for team leaders to regularly participate in physician or health care provider rounds. If the unit practices primary nursing, the physician or health care provider communicates either with each primary nurse or the associate nurse who is assuming care for the patient on that day. The manager avoids taking care of problems for the staff. Instead, staff members learn to keep physicians or health care providers informed on important information about their patients. Open communication is critical for the success of the unit.
3. *Interdisciplinary collaboration.* The emphasis on efficiency in health care delivery brings all members of the health care team together. The staff recognizes the importance of prompt referrals and timely communication. Interdisciplinary collaboration involves bringing representatives of the various disciplines together in practice projects, in-services, conferences, and staff meetings.

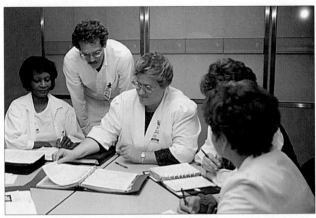

FIGURE **24-1** Nursing staff collaborating on practice issues.

4. *Staff communication.* In the present health care environment, it is difficult for a manager to get a clear, accurate, and timely message to all members of a nursing staff. Staff members quickly become uneasy and distrusting if they fail to hear about planned changes on their unit. However, a manager does not assume total responsibility for all communication. Instead, the manager establishes a variety of approaches to ensure the quick and accurate communication of information to all staff members. For example, many managers distribute biweekly or monthly newsletters of ongoing unit or health care agency activities. They also post minutes of staff and practice committee meetings in an accessible location for all staff members to read. When the manager needs to discuss important issues regarding the operations of the unit or the organization with the staff, the manager conducts staff meetings. When the unit has practice or quality improvement committees, the manager assigns each member responsibility to communicate directly to a select number of staff members. In that way all staff members are contacted and given the opportunity to comment.
5. *Staff education.* A professional nursing staff always grows in knowledge. It is impossible to remain knowledgeable of current medical and nursing practice trends without ongoing education. The nurse manager is responsible for giving staff members the necessary opportunities to remain competent in their practice. This involves planning in-services, sending staff members to professional conferences, and having members present case studies or practice issues during staff meetings.

## Leadership Skills for Nursing Students

As you begin to assume clinical assignments, it is important for you not only to learn how to care for patients but also to become a responsible and productive team member. Start by always being responsible and accountable for the care you provide your patients. Learn to become a leader by making good clinical decisions and by learning from your mistakes. Seek guidance, collaborate closely with professional nurses, and strive to improve your performance during each patient interaction. Use the following skills to become a competent professional.

**CLINICAL CARE COORDINATION.** Learn to acquire the skills necessary to deliver patient care competently and in a timely and effective manner. In the beginning you may care for only one patient, but eventually you will care for groups of patients. Clinical care coordination includes clinical decision making, priority setting, organizational skills, use of resources, time management, and evaluation.

**Clinical Decisions.** When you begin a patient assignment, always conduct a focused but complete assessment of the patient's condition and ask what outcomes the patient expects in his or her care. This will allow you to know the patient so that you can get a grasp of the patient's situation, helping you to recognize the patient's responses and patterns during care. Your assessment will also direct you in making accurate clinical decisions as to your patient's needs (see Chapter 6). Failing to make accurate clinical judgments about a patient has undesirable outcomes. The patient's condition will worsen or remain the same when you lose the potential for improvement. An important lesson in clinical care is being thorough. Always attend to the patient, look for any cues (obvious or subtle) that point to a pattern of findings, and direct your assessment to explore the pattern further. Accurate clinical decision making keeps you focused on the proper course of action. Never hesitate to ask for assistance when a patient's assessment reveals a changing clinical condition.

**Priority Setting.** As you begin to make clinical judgments (including nursing diagnoses), a picture of the patient's total needs begins to form. While planning care, decide what patient needs or problems to address first (see Chapter 7). To make this decision, use Maslow's hierarchy of patient needs. According to Maslow, meet the patient's physiological needs such as oxygen, food, water, sleep, and elimination first. After meeting the physiological needs, you meet the patient's higher-level needs of safety, security, belonging, esteem, and self-actualization (Marriner Tomey, 2004). Wywialowski (2004) describes categories of priority nursing needs of individual patients that you will use to set priorities:

- *First-order priority needs:* An immediate threat to a patient's survival or safety, such as a physiological episode of obstructed airway, loss of consciousness, or a psychological episode of an anxiety attack
- *Second-order priority needs:* Actual problems for which the patient or family has requested immediate help, such as comfort measures, nausea, or a full bladder
- *Third-order priority needs:* Relatively urgent actual or potential problems that the patient or family does not recognize, such as monitoring for postoperative complications or anticipating teaching needs of a patient who is unaware of side effects of a drug
- *Fourth-order priority needs:* Actual or potential problems with which the patient or family needs help in the future, such as teaching for self-care in the home

Many patients have all four types of priorities, requiring you to make careful judgments in choosing your course of action. Obviously, first-order priority needs demand your immediate attention. When a patient has diverse priority needs, sometimes it helps to focus on the patient's basic needs. For example, you have a patient in traction who reports being uncomfortable from being in the same position. The dietary assistant arrives in the room to deliver a meal tray. Instead of immediately assisting the patient with the meal, you reposition the patient and offer basic hygiene measures. The patient will likely become more interested in eating after you make him or her feel comfortable. The patient will also then be more receptive to any instruction you provide.

Over time you will also be required to meet the priority needs of a group of patients. This requires you to know the priority needs of each patient within the group: assess each patient's needs as soon as possible while addressing first- and second-priority needs in a timely manner (Wywialowski, 2004). To identify which patients require assessment first, you rely on information from the change-of-shift report, the agency's classification system that identifies patient acuity, and information from the medical record. Over time you will learn to spontaneously rank patients' needs by priority or urgency. Remember to think about the resources you have available, be flexible in recognizing that priority needs change, and consider how you will use your time wisely. The case study provides an example of how to prioritize your patient care.

Priorities must also be set on the basis of patient expectations. Sometimes you have an excellent plan of care established, but if your patient is resistant to certain therapies or disagrees with your approach, you will gain very little success. Working closely with the patient and family is important. Share the priorities you define with the patient to establish a level of agreement and cooperation.

**Organizational Skills.** Implementing a plan of care requires you to be effective and efficient. Effective use of time entails doing the right things, whereas efficient use of time entails doing things right (Wywialowski, 2004). As you address your patient's priorities, certain organizational skills will ensure that you become more efficient. Efficient care conserves effort and minimizes interruptions. One way to be efficient is by combining various nursing activities, in other words, doing more than one thing at a time. This of course takes practice. For example, during medication administration or while obtaining a specimen, combine therapeutic communication skills, teaching interventions, and assessment and evaluation. Always try to establish and strengthen relationships with patients, and use any patient contact as an opportunity to convey important information. Always attend to the patient's behaviors and responses to therapies to assess if any new problems are developing and to evaluate responses to interventions.

A nursing procedure is easier to perform if you are well organized. Prepare in advance by having all necessary equipment and supplies available and making sure to prepare the patient. Be sure the patient is comfortable, positioned correctly for the procedure, and well informed to increase the likelihood the procedure will go smoothly. Sometimes you will require the assistance of colleagues to perform or complete a procedure (e.g., helping to turn a patient for an enema or handing supplies during a dressing change). It is always wise to have the work area organized and preliminary steps completed before asking colleagues for assistance.

When you try to deliver care based on established priorities, events sometimes occur that interfere with your plans. For example, just as you begin to provide a patient's bath, the x-ray technician enters to do a portable chest film. Once the technician completes the x-ray film, the phlebotomist arrives to draw a sample of blood. Your priorities seem to conflict with the priorities of other health care personnel. It is important to always keep the patient's needs as the center of attention. The patient experienced symptoms earlier that required a chest film and laboratory work. In such a case it is important to be sure to complete the diagnostic tests. In another example, a patient is waiting to visit family and the chest film was a routine order from 2 days ago. The patient's condition has since stabilized, and the x-ray technician is willing to return later to shoot the film. Attending to the patient's hygiene and comfort so that the family is able to visit is more of a priority at this time.

**Use of Resources.** Another important aspect of clinical care coordination is appropriate use of resources. Resources in this case include members of the health care team. In any setting the administration of patient care occurs more smoothly when staff members work together. As a student always look for opportunities to help other staff members. For example, answer a call light, help a staff member make a bed, or offer to sit and talk with another nurse's patient. Also, never hesitate to ask staff members to assist you, especially when there is the opportunity to make a procedure or activity more comfortable and safer for the patient. For example, assistance in turning, positioning, and ambulating patients is frequently necessary when patients experience impaired mobility. Having a staff member assist with handling equipment and supplies during more complicated procedures, such as catheter insertion or a dressing change, helps make procedures more efficient. This is an excellent way for you to learn how to delegate aspects of care activities and to work with assistive personnel.

There are also times when you will recognize personal limitations and use professional resources for assistance. For example, you assess a patient and find relevant clinical signs and symptoms but are unfamiliar with the patient's underlying physical condition. Consulting an RN leads you to confirm findings and ensures that you take the proper course of action for the patient. Throughout your professional career there are always new experiences. A leader knows his or her limitations and seeks professional colleagues for guidance and support.

**Time Management.** A nurse's attitude and how a nurse values time affect time management (Wywialowski, 2004).

Changes in health care and increasing complexity of patients creates stress for nurses as they work to meet patient needs (Marriner Tomey, 2004). One way to manage this stress is through the use of time management skills. These skills involve learning how, where, and when to use your time. Because you have a limited amount of time with patients, it is essential to remain goal oriented and focused on your patients' priorities. For example, priorities of care help you determine what procedures you will perform first, patient assessments that you will do on an ongoing basis, and the anticipated response of your patient to care activities.

One useful time management skill involves keeping a to-do list. When you first begin working with a patient or patients, make a list that sequences the nursing activities you will perform. The change-of-shift report may help you sequence activities based on what you learn about your patient's condition and the care provided before your arrival to the unit. Consider activities that have specific time limits in terms of addressing patient needs, such as administering a pain medication before a scheduled procedure or instructing patients before their discharge home. Also, analyze the items on your list that agency policies or routines will schedule. Note which activities need to be done on time and which activities you are able to do at your discretion (Wywialowski, 2004). For instance, you need to administer medications within a specific schedule, but you can also perform other activities while you are in the patient's room. Finally, estimate the amount of time needed to complete the various activities. Activities requiring the assistance of other staff members usually take longer because you will plan around their schedule.

Good time management also involves completing one task before starting another. Complete the activities you begin with one patient before moving on to the next if possible. Your care will then become less fragmented, and you will better focus on what you are doing for each patient. As a result, it is less likely that you will make errors in your care.

**Evaluation.** One of the most important aspects of clinical care coordination is evaluation (see Chapter 7). It is a mistake to think that evaluation occurs at the end of an activity. Evaluation is an ongoing process. Once you assess a patient's needs and begin therapies directed at a specific problem area, immediately evaluate if therapies are effective and the patient's response. The process of evaluation compares actual patient outcomes with expected outcomes. When expected outcomes are not being met, evaluation reveals the need to continue current therapies for a longer period, revise approaches to care, or introduce new therapies. Throughout the day as you care for a patient anticipate when you need to return to the bedside to evaluate your care. For example, you decide to return 30 minutes after you administered a medication, 15 minutes after an intravenous (IV) line has begun infusing, or 60 minutes after discussing discharge instructions with the patient and family.

Keeping a focus on evaluation of the patient's progress lessens the chance of becoming distracted by the tasks of care. It is common to assume that staying focused on planned activities ensures that you perform care appropriately. However, task orientation does not ensure good patient outcomes. The competent nurse learns that at the heart of good organizational skills is the constant inquiry into the patient's condition and progress toward an improved level of health.

**TEAM COMMUNICATION.** As a part of a nursing team, each nurse is responsible for open, professional communication. Regardless of the setting, nurses learn that an enriching, professional environment is one in which staff members respect one another's ideas, share information, and keep one another informed. On a busy nursing unit this means keeping the nurse in charge of the unit and colleagues informed about patients with emerging problems. This also includes informing physicians or health care providers who have been called for consultation. In a clinic setting it means sharing unusual diagnostic findings or conveying important information regarding a patient's source of family support. One way of fostering good team communication is by setting expectations of one another. Always treat colleagues with respect. Listen to the ideas of other staff members without interruption. Be honest and direct in what you say. Clarify what others are saying, and build on the merits of co-workers ideas (Marriner Tomey, 2004). An efficient team counts on all members when needs arise. Sharing expectations of what, when, and how to communicate is a step toward establishing a strong work team.

**DELEGATION.** The art of effective delegation is a skill you as a student need to observe and practice to improve your management skills. Delegation is the process of assigning part of one person's responsibility to another qualified person in a specific situation (National Council of State Boards of Nursing, 1995). One purpose of delegation is to improve efficiency. Asking a staff member to obtain an ordered specimen while you attend to a patient's pain medication request effectively prevents a delay in the patient's gaining pain relief. Delegation also provides job enrichment. A nurse shows trust in colleagues by delegating tasks to them and showing staff members that they are important players in the delivery of care. Never delegate a task that you dislike doing or would not do yourself because this creates negative feelings and poor working relationships. Remember that even though the delegation of a task transfers the responsibility and authority to another person, the delegator retains accountability for the delegated tasks.

Professional nurses are finding themselves in situations where they need more support to do the daily, repetitive tasks of care, such as basic hygiene, specimen collection, and feeding patients. The RN needs time to coordinate care delivery for groups of patients, to conduct individual assessments, and to make professional judgments about a patient's health and therapeutic needs. The RN also needs time to deliver complex therapies and to provide patient counseling and education. An LPN in acute care benefits from acquiring support to deliver care to a group of patients whose needs are complex. In long-term care settings the LPN directs care and relies on assistive personnel to provide basic care measures. A nurse is simply not able to do all the work necessary to care for groups of patients.

To be able to perform your professional responsibilities as a nurse, learn how to work effectively with other staff members. Each health care member has a set of job responsibilities that contribute to the overall care of patients. As a nurse your job will be to help the care team work efficiently. Because you will oversee the care of groups of patients, it will become necessary at times for you to delegate work to others.

The American Nurses Association (1997) defines **delegation** as transferring responsibility for the performance of an activity or task while retaining accountability for the outcome. For example, you delegate catheter care to a competent and trained patient care technician after you have assessed the condition of the patient's catheter and perineal tissues. However, you are ultimately accountable for having the patient receive catheter care. When delegating responsibilities to a competent individual, you as the RN still remain accountable for the overall nursing care of the patient (Marriner Tomey, 2004). Thus exercise good judgment at all times in deciding what tasks to delegate and in what situations. The National Council of State Boards of Nursing offers guidelines for delegation of tasks in accordance with an RN's legal scope of practice (Box 24-3).

It is important to recognize that in regard to delegation to assistive personnel, you delegate tasks, not patients. Further, do not automatically delegate a task because it is a task but because it is appropriate for someone else to perform the

---

**BOX 24-3** **The Five Rights of Delegation**

**Right Task**

The task is delegable for a specific patient, such as tasks that are repetitive, require little supervision, and are relatively noninvasive.

**Right Circumstances**

Consider the appropriate patient setting, available resources, and other relevant factors.

**Right Person**

The right person is delegating the right tasks to the right person to be performed on the right person.

**Right Direction/Communication**

Give a clear, concise description of the task, including its objective, limits, and expectations.

**Right Supervision**

Provide appropriate monitoring, evaluation, intervention as needed, and feedback.

Modified and reprinted with permission from National Council of State Boards of Nursing, Inc: *Delegation: concepts and decision-making process,* Chicago, 1995, The Council.

task. For example, as the nurse you are always responsible for the assessment of a patient's ongoing status, but if a patient is stable, you delegate vital sign monitoring to assistive personnel. Leah Curtin (1994), a well-known nurse administrator, wrote that assistive personnel should not be at the bedside but at the nurse's side. It is important for you to have assistive personnel work as your assistants or partners and take on tasks that you determine are safe and appropriate for them to provide. Know how to give clear instructions, effectively prioritize patient needs and therapies, and be able to give staff members timely and meaningful feedback.

Here are a few tips on appropriate delegation (Keeling and others, 2000):

- *Assess the knowledge and skills of the delegate:* Determine what assistive personnel know and what they are able to do by asking open-ended questions that will elicit conversation and details on what the person knows. For example, "How do you usually put the cuff on when you measure a blood pressure?" or "Tell me how you prepare the tubing before you give an enema."
- *Match tasks to the delegate's skills:* Know what skills the training program includes for assistive personnel at your facility. Determine if personnel have learned critical thinking skills, such as knowing when a patient is in danger or knowing what changes to report.
- *Communicate clearly:* Always provide unambiguous and clear directions by describing a task, the desired outcome, and the time period within which the person is to complete the task. Never give instructions through another staff member. Make the person feel as though he or she is part of the team. For example, "I'd like you to help me by getting Mr. Floyd up to ambulate before lunch. Be sure to check his blood pressure before he stands, and write your finding on the graphic sheet. OK?"
- *Listen attentively:* Listen to the response of assistive personnel after you provide directions. Do they feel comfortable in asking questions or requesting clarification? If you encourage a response, listen to what the person has to say. Be especially attentive if the staff member has been given a deadline to meet by another nurse. Help sort out priorities.
- *Provide feedback:* Always give assistive personnel feedback regarding performance, regardless of outcome. Let them know when a job was well done. If an outcome is undesirable, find a private place to discuss what occurred, any miscommunication, and how to achieve a better outcome in the future.

## Quality Improvement

Managing patient care involves your active participation not only in clinical care management activities but also in quality improvement (QI). The Joint Commission on Accreditation of Healthcare Organizations (JCAHO) (2002) defines **quality improvement** as an approach to the continuous study and improvement of the processes of providing health care services to meet the needs of patients and others. Quality improvement of an institution focuses on improvement of performance related to processes. Among the processes that most directly influence patients are those that make up nursing practice. Nurses achieve quality and patient safety by "doing the right thing the right way the first time" (Caramanica and others, 2003). Typically in health care, however, many individuals are involved in a single process of care. For example, medication delivery involves the nurse who prepares and administers the drug, the physician or health care provider who prescribes the medication, the pharmacy that prepares the dosage, the secretary who communicates orders and changes, and the transporter who delivers medications. With so many individuals involved, it is important for you as a professional to become involved in finding ways to make processes more efficient and effective for better quality patient care. When you or others identify problems in processes, it is helpful to do a root cause analysis. A **root cause analysis** is a process of data collection and analysis that helps you find the real cause of the problem and work on dealing with it rather than just dealing with the effects of the problem. Root cause analyses are beneficial in repeated, unwanted situations that use up resources (Bellinger, 2004).

Another component of quality improvement is performance measurement. Performance measurement means what an institution does and how well it does it (JCAHO, 2004). In performance measurement, an organization analyzes and evaluates current performance to use results to develop focused improvement actions. Organizations use benchmarking as a part of performance improvement. **Benchmarking** consists of identifying best practices and comparing them to the organization's current practices for the purpose of improving performance. This process helps to support the institution's claims of quality care delivery. Groups who make decisions on where to go for quality health care use this information during their decision-making process.

A key component of quality improvement is analysis of outcomes (Moorhead, Johnson, and Maas, 2004; Titler, 2001). Outcomes are the conditions the patient achieves as a result of care delivery. An **outcome** tells whether interventions are effective, whether patients progress, how well the facility meets standards, and whether changes are necessary. When nursing staff members think in terms of outcomes, their actions become much more purposeful and more focused on improving the condition of their patient's health. Patient outcomes are either generic or condition specific. Facilities assess effects of treatment on overall health status with generic outcomes such as mortality or health-related quality of life. Condition-specific outcomes focus on specific aspects of health related to medical condition such as dyspnea severity for a person with chronic obstructive pulmonary disease (Titler, 2001). A new development in quality improvement is standardized performance measures such as report cards (Moorhead and others, 2004). A balanced scorecard is an example of a report card used to manage change within an organization. The focus of the balanced scorecard is on achievement of the organization's mission, strategic planning and management, and quality improvement of programs and services. A balanced scorecard that measures nursing performance focuses on collaboration, strategic thinking, and continuous improvement (Zelman and others, 2003). Open communication is a critical component to creating a culture of quality (Caramanica and others, 2003).

A well-organized QI program focuses on processes or systems that significantly contribute to outcomes. Facilities need a systematic approach organizationally to ensure that everyone supports a continuous QI philosophy. This begins with the organizational culture, where all staff members understand their responsibility toward maintaining and improving quality. On a unit level the nursing manager is responsible for supporting a unit-based QI program. As a member of the nursing team you will participate in recognizing trends in nursing practice, identifying when recurrent problems develop, and initiating opportunities to improve the quality of care. For example, after reviewing patients who have undergone hip surgery, a nursing staff member asks, "Are our patients regaining functional mobility without severe pain?" "Are we administering the proper analgesic being administered?" "Are we delaying rehabilitation?" The QI process begins at the staff level, where problems are defined. This requires staff members to know the standards or guidelines that define quality. In order to judge whether patients with hip surgery have functional mobility impaired by poor pain management, there needs to be an agreement as to how patients normally function after surgery and how to manage pain. Figure 24-2 outlines an organization's framework for quality by showing the relationship of the mission, vision, and values of a nursing organization to its professional standards and standard of care guidelines. The mission, vision, and values of a health care organization serve as the framework for defining professional standards and nursing care guidelines. You find these guidelines in the workplace in the form of policies, protocols, and procedures. Ultimately a nursing organization with a strong foundation of practice is able to provide quality care and achieve excellent patient outcomes.

Unit practice committees review activities or services considered most important in providing quality care to patients. To identify the greatest opportunity for improving quality, the committees consider those activities that are high volume (greater than 50% of a unit's activity), high risk (potential for trauma or death), and problem areas (potential problem for patient, staff, or institution). For example, on the orthopedic unit, hip surgery is high volume, older adults over age 80 years have more postoperative complications, and a recurrent problem has been family dissatisfaction with patients' pain control. Staff members will review all available information and then select a **quality indicator** as the focus of their QI project. The three types of indicators are structure, process, and outcome. Structure indicators evaluate the structure or systems for delivering care: an example is whether staff delivers patient-controlled analgesic pumps in a timely manner. Process indicators evaluate the

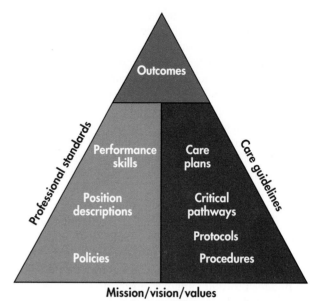

FIGURE **24-2** Framework for quality. (Data from Peters DA: Outcomes: the mainstay of a framework for quality care, *J Nurs Care Qual* 10[1]:61, 1995.)

manner in which staff delivers care: an example is the process of pain assessment. Outcome indicators, as described earlier, evaluate the end result of care: an example is a patient's report of pain severity and use of analgesics.

After selecting a quality indicator, staff members determine ways to quantitatively measure the indicator. The occurrence of an indicator or the percentage of times staff members observe the indicator (e.g., the number of patients who have their pain assessed on return from the operating room) is a common measure. A threshold is a standard set by staff members for determining if a problem exists. In the example of pain assessment, anything below 100% indicates a problem. Lower thresholds are tolerated depending on the indicator; for example, staff members may set an 80% threshold for patients they refer to a community resource after discharge. In many cases, expect variations in quality indicators. Staff members decide what level of variation is tolerable.

Once staff members have chosen indicators, they will collect data and analyze their findings. Depending on the indicator, this process sometimes includes patient observations or interviews, medical record review, or staff interviews. It is important in data collection to collect data on the right criteria and to then have adequate data from which to make decisions. Many organizations have made QI so important that they conduct formal research studies. In this case the process of data collection and analysis is very formal. When conducting simple evaluation studies, staff members will collect and analyze data, determine if problems exist, and then analyze their possible causes.

Monitoring of quality indicators evaluates whether a specifically defined process reaches desired outcomes. If results exceed or meet a threshold, there is no identifiable problem and the process is performing well. When indicators do not meet thresholds for satisfactory care, staff members try to find the cause of problems. For example, if there is a proven delay in patient-controlled analgesic pumps arriving on the nursing unit, thus preventing proper orientation of patients to the use of the pump before surgery, the unit practice committee must recommend solutions. When a process is not working well, staff members use one of the models for QI (e.g., Focus-PDCA). This allows staff members to structure problem analysis and resolution in order to improve the process of care and outcomes and improve patient safety (Robinson, 2004). It is often appropriate to organize an expert team who knows the process well. For example, the committee working on patient-controlled analgesia includes staff nurses, colleagues from pharmacy, and staff members from the equipment supply area. Focus-PDCA is an acronym for the following: **f**ind the process to improve, **o**rganize a team that knows the process, **c**larify current knowledge of the process, **u**nderstand causes of process variation, and **s**elect a process improvement. Once the committee selects the improvement, they will then **P**lan, **D**o, **C**heck, **A**ct (Marriner Tomey, 2004).

It often takes several meetings before a group agrees on the proper actions to take. After reviewing all options the committee eventually selects the best approach for improving the process and achieving desired outcomes. It is important to establish actions likely to be successful. For example, the orthopedic unit decides that because they have a large number of patients receiving patient-controlled analgesia, the nearby satellite pharmacy will begin to prepare the pumps instead of the central pharmacy. Nursing staff members will be able to order the pumps directly through the satellite center, reducing delivery time significantly.

After implementing an action plan, staff members reevaluate its success. The change may be positive or negative. For example, the new pump delivery process reduces waiting time by 50%. However, if the problem remains, a new plan of action is necessary. The QI process is similar to the nursing process (see Chapter 7) in that when you do not meet desired outcomes, the staff reinstitutes the QI process.

Communicate the results of QI activities to staff members in all appropriate organizational departments. If no one communicates the findings and results, practice changes will likely not occur. Revision of policies and procedures, modification of standards of care, and implementation of system changes are examples of ways that an organization responds. Over time, incorporation of a QI program benefits the patient, the professional staff, and the organization.

## KEY CONCEPTS

- A profession possesses the characteristics of extended education, theory, service, autonomy, and a code of ethics.
- The essential components of professional nursing are care, cure, and coordination.
- Standards of care offer objective guidelines for nurses to provide care and to evaluate care.
- A manager sets a philosophy for a work unit, ensures appropriate staffing, and mobilizes staff and institutional resources to achieve objectives. A manager also motivates staff members to carry out their work, sets standards of performance, and makes the right decisions to achieve objectives.
- Empowering staff members brings out the best in a manager and allows him or her to concentrate on effective patient care systems, to support risk taking and innovation, and to focus on results and rewards.
- Nursing care delivery models vary by the responsibility of the RN in coordinating care delivery and the roles other staff members play in assisting with care.
- Critical to the success of decentralized decision making is making staff members aware that they have the responsibility, authority, and accountability for the care they give and the decisions they make.
- A nurse manager fosters decentralized decision making by establishing nursing practice committees, supporting nurse–physician or health care provider and interdisciplinary collaboration, setting and implementing QI plans, and maintaining timely staff communication.
- Clinical care coordination involves accurate clinical decision making, establishing priorities, efficient organizational skills, appropriate use of resources and time management skills, and an ongoing evaluation of care activities.
- Each member of a nursing work team is responsible for open, professional communication.
- When done correctly, delegation improves job efficiency and job enrichment.
- Exercise good judgment at all times in deciding what tasks to delegate and in what situations.
- QI initiatives are designed to maintain or improve the outcomes of nursing practice.
- Communicate the results of QI activities to staff members in all appropriate organizational departments.

## CRITICAL THINKING IN PRACTICE

*Don, the evening RN, is preparing to assess Mr. Sequera and Mrs. Lennox. Mr. Sequera, who experienced a myocardial infarction 3 days ago, is ready to ambulate down the hall for his evening walk. Mrs. Lennox is a patient newly admitted with gastrointestinal bleeding. Don finds that Mr. Sequera is resting comfortably and visiting with his daughter. He is eager to go for his walk. Mrs. Lennox is very restless and experiencing discomfort from her nasogastric tube. The physician has ordered stool specimens to be collected.*

- - - - - - - - - - - - - - - - - - - - - - - -

1. Which of these tasks for the two patients should Don delegate to the nurse technician, Linda? Explain your answer.
2. Which activities by Don indicate that he practiced appropriate delegation when delegating the task of taking Mrs. Tomison to the bathroom to Linda? (Mark all that apply.)
   a. Don mentally reviewed Mrs. Tomison's condition and determined that she could ambulate to the bathroom with the assistance of one person.
   b. Don instructed Linda to take Mrs. Tomison to the bathroom as soon as possible.
   c. Don told Linda he would answer her question about Mrs. Tomison later because he had to administer a stat medication.
   d. Don asked Linda if she thought that she could get Mrs. Tomison out of bed on her own and walk her to the bathroom.
   e. Don told Linda in the break room that she did not save Mrs. Tomison's urine for the 24-hour urine that was in progress.
   f. Don told Linda he would come in and see if she needed assistance with Mrs. Tomison right after he administered a medication.
3. Don completes the following activities for Mrs. Lennox. For each activity, identify whether it is a first-order, second-order, third-order, or fourth-order priority need.
   a. Don makes a referral to the home health department for home care when Mrs. Lennox is discharged.
   b. Don administers the pain medication that Mrs. Lennox requested because her pain rating was 8 (scale of 0 to 10, with 10 being the worst pain).

c. Don notifies the physician of Mrs. Lennox's decreased hemoglobin and hematocrit levels.
   d. Don explains the potential side effects of the newly prescribed medication to Mrs. Lennox.
4. Don is a member of his nursing unit's practice committee. The committee is investigating the problem of completing the documentation of the nursing history taken on admission. Which type of quality indicator—structure, process, or outcome—will the committee focus the quality improvement project on? Explain your answer.
5. Don is mentoring a new graduate nurse, Sandy, in orientation. Sandy tells Don that she has a hard time telling others to do a job and asks Don how he developed his delegation skills. Don talks to Sandy and gives her helpful tips on how to improve her delegation skills. What are the five rights of delegation that Don should review with Sandy?
6. Don tells Sandy that he really enjoys working on this unit because he likes having a caseload of patients. He says that being responsible for their care during the entire hospitalization allows him to get to know patients well. On his days off, other caregivers follow the care plans he develops. What type of nursing care delivery system is found on Don's floor?
   a. Functional nursing
   b. Case management
   c. Primary nursing
   d. Team nursing

## NCLEX® REVIEW

1. While administering medications, June realizes she has given the wrong dose of a medication to a patient. June acts by completing an occurrence report and notifying the patient's physician or health care provider. This is an example of June exercising:
   1. Authority
   2. Responsibility
   3. Accountability
   4. Decision making
2. During morning rounds, Rhea assesses Mr. Nile's condition. The patient had major heart surgery 2 days ago. His vital signs are stable. Rhea finds that Mr. Nile's incision is clean and healing well. Mr. Niles complains of pain in his lower leg where the vein graft was removed. Rhea finds that the IV infusion is running on time but only 100 ml remains before the infusion runs out. An order exists for the IV infusion to continue. The patient is likely to be discharged in 2 days if he continues to progress. A second-order priority is:
   1. To replace the IV bag with a new one
   2. To administer an analgesic for Mr. Niles' leg pain.
   3. To provide instruction on complications of wound healing
   4. To determine if the pharmacy has delivered IV solutions ordered for the day

3. Sharon checks her patient, Mr. Rawls, a 62-year-old man admitted to the hospital with pneumonia. Mr. Rawls has been coughing profusely and has required nasotracheal suctioning. He also has an IV infusion of antibiotics. Mr. Rawls is febrile with a temperature of 101° F (38.3° C). Mr. Rawls asks Sharon if he can have a bed bath because he has been perspiring profusely. The task for Sharon to delegate to the nurse assistant working with her today is:
   1. Vital signs
   2. Changing IV dressing
   3. Nasotracheal suctioning
   4. Administering a bed bath
4. Jennifer, an RN, is working with Ken, a nurse assistant. Jennifer has completed morning rounds on her assigned patients and is giving Ken directions for what he needs to do for the next hour. An appropriate way to communicate directions when delegating nursing care is:
   1. "Ken, why don't you go to room 20A and see what Mr. Wilson needs."
   2. "Ken, I would like you to take all the vital signs for rooms 12 and 13 and let me know if there are any problems."
   3. "Ken, would you start Mrs. McNamara's bath while I check on the IV line in room 14? I will help you with

turning her so I can assess her skin and decide on the turning schedule we will need to follow."

4. "Ken, I want you to help Mr. Nelson off the bedpan, and while you are at it get a specimen if he passed any stool. I don't think I can go in his room one more time, so I would appreciate your help."

5. The nurse is teaching the patient about the action, side effects, and correct way to take the Coumadin that he will be taking after discharge. This type of nursing care is an example of what type of priority nursing need of a patient?
   1. First-order priority need
   2. Second-order priority need
   3. Third-order priority need
   4. Fourth-order priority need

6. You are an RN providing care to a group of patients with an LPN and nurse assistant. You are the leader and assign individual patients to the LPN and nurse assistant. You are responsible for developing the patient care plan and interacting with other members of the health care team. What type of nursing care delivery model are you participating in?
   1. Case management
   2. Functional nursing
   3. Primary nursing
   4. Team nursing

7. Sam, the RN, is working with Tina, a nurse assistant, to provide care for four patients. After Tina completed her cares and walking of Mr. Sands, Sam told her that Mr. Sands had expressed his appreciation to Sam for the hair washing, shave, and bathing assistance that Tina had provided. Sam thanked Tina for doing these cares for Mr. Sands. Sam's interaction with Tina is an example of which of the five rights of delegation?
   1. Right supervision
   2. Right task
   3. Right direction
   4. Right circumstances

8. The nursing unit committee is working on a project with the pharmacy to ensure that newly prescribed medications have the initial dose administered to the patient within 1 hour of being prescribed. This is an example of which type of quality improvement indicator?
   1. Structure
   2. Process
   3. Outcome
   4. Patient

## REFERENCES

American Nurses Association: *Definitions related to ANA 1992 position statement on unlicensed assistive personnel*, 1997, http://www.nursingworld.org/readroom/position/uap/uapuse.htm.

American Nurses Association: *Code of ethics for nurses with interpretive statements*, Washington, DC, 2001, The Association.

American Nurses Association: *Nursing: scope and standards of practice*, Washington, DC, 2004, The Association.

American Nurses Credentialing Center: *ANCC Magnet program: recognizing excellence in nursing series*, 2005, http://www.nursingworld.org/ancc/magnet/index.htm.

Bellinger G: *Root cause analysis*, 2004, http://www.systems-thinking.org/rca/rootca.htm.

Bolton LB, Goodenough A: A magnet nursing service approach to nursing's role in quality improvement, *Nurs Admin Q* 27(4):344, 2003.

Canadian Nurses Association: *Education preparation for entry into practice*, Ottawa, 2004, The Association, http://www.cna-nurses.ca/frames/policies/policiesmainframe.htm.

Caramanica L and others: Four elements of a successful quality program: alignment, collaboration, evidence based practice, and excellence, *Nurs Admin Q* 27(4):336, 2003.

Chinn PL, Kramer MK: *Theory and nursing: integrated knowledge development*, ed 2, St. Louis, 1999, Mosby.

Curtin L: The heart of patient care, *Nurs Manage* 25(5):7, 1994.

Dean-Baar SL: Standards and guidelines: have they made any difference? In Dochterman JM, Grace HK, editors: *Current issues in nursing*, ed 6, St. Louis, 2001, Mosby.

Joint Commission on Accreditation of Healthcare Organizations: *Comprehensive accreditation manual for hospitals: the official handbook*, Chicago, 2002, The Commission.

Joint Commission on Accreditation of Healthcare Organizations: *Performance measurement in healthcare*, 2004, http://www.jcaho.org/pms/index.htm.

Keeling B and others: Appropriate delegation, *Am J Nurs* 100(12):24, 2000.

Marriner Tomey A: *Guide to nursing management and leadership*, ed 7, St. Louis, 2004, Mosby.

Moorhead S, Johnson M, Maas M: *Nursing outcomes classification (NOC)*, ed 3, St. Louis, 2004, Mosby.

National Council of State Boards of Nursing, Inc: *Delegation: concepts and decision-making process*, Chicago, 1995, The Council.

Peters DA: Outcomes: the mainstay of a framework for quality care, *J Nurs Care Qual* 10(1):61, 1995.

Ritter-Teitel J: The impact of restructuring on professional nursing practice, *J Nurs Adm* 32(1):31, 2002.

Robinson P: Master the steps to performance: plan, do, study, act to enhance your facility's patient care initiatives, *Nurs Manage* 35(5):45, 2004.

Tiedeman ME, Lookinland S: Traditional models of care delivery: what have we learned, *J Nurs Adm* 34(6):291, 2004.

Titler M: Outcomes management for quality improvement. In Dochterman JM, Grace HK, editors: *Current issues in nursing*, ed 6, St. Louis, 2001, Mosby.

Wywialowski E: *Managing patient care*, ed 3, St. Louis, 2004, Mosby.

Zelman WN and others: Use of balanced scorecard in health care, *J Health Care Finance* 29(4):1, 2003.

# Exercise and Activity

## MEDIA RESOURCES

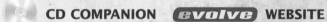 **CD COMPANION** 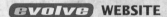 **WEBSITE**

http://evolve.elsevier.com/Potter/basic

- **NCLEX® Review**
- **Audio Glossary**
- **English/Spanish Audio Glossary**
- **Video Clips**

## OBJECTIVES

- Describe the role of the skeleton, skeletal muscles, and nervous system in the regulation of movement.
- Discuss physiological and pathological influences on body alignment and joint mobility.
- Assess patients for impaired body alignment, exercise, and activity.
- Formulate nursing diagnoses for patients experiencing problems with exercise and activity.

- Write a nursing care plan for a patient with impaired body alignment and activity.
- Describe the interventions for maintaining proper alignment, assisting a patient in moving up in bed, repositioning a patient needing assistance, and transferring a patient from a bed to a chair.
- Evaluate the nursing care plan for maintaining body alignment and activity.

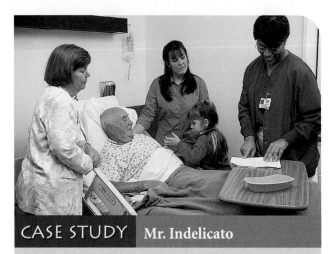

## CASE STUDY   Mr. Indelicato

Mr. Indelicato is a 72-year-old man who is going to be hospitalized for surgery on his right knee. His general level of health is good. He does not have any underlying chronic illnesses, such as cardiovascular illness, diabetes mellitus, or other musculoskeletal illnesses. He relates the problem with his knees to previous sports injuries. He repeatedly "twisted the knee" while playing racquetball. He knows that he hurt his knee at least six times over the last 30 years while playing the sport. He first sought medical advice and treatment about 6 years ago. His last injury to his knee was approximately "5 or 6 years ago, and it hasn't worked the same since." He has tried various treatments, including physical therapy, rest, and pain medication. His only preoperative medication is ibuprofen 600 mg every 6 to 8 hours. He has not taken his ibuprofen for the past few days because of the impending surgery. He chooses to have surgery so he can get back to being active. He and his wife are very active and enjoy golf, tennis, and bike riding. In addition, they have an active social life of attending the theater, dinner with friends, and visiting their children and grandchildren. Mr. Indelicato's wife is in good health as well. He feels they are very fortunate in that neither one has any illnesses or takes any prescribed medication.

Marilyn Sweeney is a 40-year-old nursing student completing her second clinical semester. She has just finished rotating through a general surgical unit and is spending the remaining 6 weeks in the orthopedic/rehabilitation division of the agency. Her assignment is to follow this patient through his surgery and rehabilitation.

## KEY TERMS

abduction, p. 660
active range-of-motion exercises, p. 678
activity tolerance, p. 656
adduction, p. 660
balance, p. 653
bed boards, p. 660
body mechanics, p. 653
center of gravity, p. 651
crutch gait, p. 680
dorsiflexion, p. 670
extension, p. 652
foot boots, p. 660
footdrop, p. 659
friction, p. 651
gait, p. 656
hand rolls, p. 660
hand-wrist splints, p. 660
Hoyer lift, p. 671
hyperextension, p. 670

joints, p. 652
logroll, p. 668
muscle tone, p. 651
orthostatic hypotension, p. 678
passive range-of-motion exercises, p. 678
plantar flexion, p. 670
posture, p. 651
prone, p. 670
proprioception, p. 652
range of motion (ROM), p. 656
sandbags, p. 660
side rails, p. 660
supine, p. 655
trapeze bar, p. 660
trochanter rolls, p. 660

The actions of walking, turning, lifting, or carrying are all common in the provision of nursing care. Such activities require muscle exertion. To reduce the risk of injury, know and practice proper body mechanics and remain knowledgeable of current research, standards, and guidelines concerning safe transfer and positioning techniques (Box 25-1). This includes knowledge of the actions of various muscle groups, understanding of the factors involved in the coordination of body movement, and familiarity with the integrated functioning of the skeletal, muscular, and nervous systems.

BOX 25-1 ## USING EVIDENCE IN PRACTICE

### Research Summary

Musculoskeletal disorders are the most prevalent and debilitating occupational health hazards among nurses (Trinkoff and others, 2002). You will need preventive interventions to avert the hazards and economic burdens associated with patient handling tasks (Nelson and others, 2003). The American Nurses Association (ANA) put forth a position statement calling for the use of assistive equipment and devices to promote a safe health care environment for nurses and their patients (ANA, 2003). The use of assistive equipment and continued use of proper body mechanics significantly reduce the risk of musculoskeletal injuries (ANA, 2003). In addition, the Occupational Safety and Health Administration (OSHA) recommends that you minimize or eliminate manually lifting patients in all cases when possible (2003). Many facilities are moving toward limited lift policies (LLP) that minimize patient handling by nurses and instead use lift devices to reduce on-the-job injuries (Moreno, 2003). For example, a comprehensive program initiated by the Veterans Health Administration was designed to reduce job-related musculoskeletal injuries in nurses. The program included an algorithm for each major patient transfer and repositioning task and the purchase of lift devices. One year after the inception of the program, preliminary data projected a cost savings of approximately $5 million over the next 9 years due to reduction in job-related musculoskeletal injuries (Nelson and others, 2003).

### Application to Nursing Practice

Health care facilities are required to provide employees with safety information and training concerning the transfer, positioning, and lifting of patients. OSHA has identified recommendations on back safety and guidelines on the prevention of musculoskeletal injuries (OSHA, 2003). By becoming knowledgeable about the current research, standards, and guidelines regarding safe positioning and transfer of patients, you will safely transfer patients without causing injury to the patient or yourself.

Data from American Nurses Association: *Position statement on elimination of manual patient handling to prevent work-related musculoskeletal disorders,* 2003, http://www.nursingworld.org/readroom/position/workplac/pathand.htm; Moreno J: Limit liability with lift programs, *Provider* 29(1):41, 2003; Nelson A and others: Safe patient handling and movement: preventing back injury among nurses requires careful selection of the safest equipment and techniques, *Am J Nurs* 103(3), 2003; Trinkoff AM and others: Musculoskeletal problems of the neck, shoulder, and back and functional consequences in nurses, *Am J Ind Med* 41(3):170, 2002.

## Scientific Knowledge Base

The coordinated efforts of the musculoskeletal and nervous systems to maintain balance, posture, and body alignment during lifting, bending, moving, and performing activities of daily living provide the foundation for body mechanics.

Proper implementation of these activities decreases the risk of musculoskeletal system injury and allows physical mobility without muscle strain and excessive use of muscle energy.

### Body Alignment

Body alignment refers to the relationship of one body part to another body part along a horizontal or vertical line. Correct alignment reduces strain on musculoskeletal structures, maintains adequate **muscle tone,** and contributes to balance.

### Body Balance

You achieve body balance when you balance a relatively low **center of gravity** over a wide, stable base of support. A vertical line falls from the center of gravity through the base of support. The base of support is the foundation. When the vertical line from the center of gravity does not fall through the base of support, the body loses balance.

Posture also enhances body balance. The term **posture** means maintaining optimal body position. It means a position that most favors function, requires the least muscular work to maintain, and places the least strain on muscles, ligaments, and bones (Thibodeau and Patton, 2003).

You maintain proper body alignment and posture by using two simple techniques. First, widen your base of support by separating your feet to a comfortable distance. Second, bring the center of gravity closer to your base of support to increase balance. You achieve this by bending the knees and flexing the hips until squatting and maintaining proper back alignment by keeping the trunk erect.

### Coordinated Body Movement

Weight is the force exerted on a body by gravity. When you lift an object , you must overcome the object's weight and be aware of its center of gravity. In symmetrical objects, the center of gravity is located at the exact center of the object. The force of weight is always directed downward. An object that is unbalanced has its center of gravity away from the midline and falls without support. Like unbalanced objects, patients who fail to maintain a balance with their center of gravity are unsteady, placing them at risk for falling. Be able to identify such patients and intervene in such a way to maintain safety.

### Friction

**Friction** is the effect of rubbing or the resistance that a moving body meets from the surface on which it moves. As you turn, transfer, or move a patient up in bed, you need to overcome friction. You reduce friction by following some basic principles. The greater the surface area of the object you are moving, the greater the friction.

A passive or immobilized patient produces greater friction to movement. Thus, when possible, use some of the patient's strength and mobility when lifting, transferring, or moving the patient up in bed. You do this by explaining the procedure and telling the patient when to move. For instance, you decrease friction if the patient is able to bend his or her knees while being moved up in bed. You also reduce friction by lifting rather than pushing a patient. Lifting has an upward component and decreases the pressure between the patient and the bed or the chair. The use of a drawsheet reduces friction because you are able to move the patient more easily along the bed's surface.

## Regulation of Movement

Coordinated body movement involves the integrated functioning of the skeletal, muscular, and nervous systems. Because these three systems cooperate so closely in mechanical support of the body, they are often considered as a single functional unit.

**SKELETAL SYSTEM.** Bones perform five functions in the body: support, protection, movement, mineral storage, and hematopoiesis (blood cell formation). Two of these functions, support and movement, are most important during activity and exercise. In support, bones serve as the framework and contribute to the shape, alignment, and positioning of the body parts. In movement, bones with their **joints** constitute levers for muscle attachment. When muscles contract and shorten, they pull on bones, producing joint movement (Thibodeau and Patton, 2003).

**Joints.** An articulation, or joint, is the connection between bones. Each joint is classified according to its structure and degree of mobility. On the basis of connective structures, joints are classified as fibrous, cartilaginous, and synovial (Huether and McCance, 2004). Fibrous joints fit closely together and are fixed, permitting little if any movement. The cartilaginous joint has little movement but is elastic and uses cartilage to unite separate body surfaces.

The synovial or true joint is a freely moveable joint and the body's most mobile, numerous, and anatomically complex joint. There are seven structural characteristics of synovial joints: joint capsule, synovial membrane, articular cartilage, joint cavity, menisci, ligaments, and bursae (Thibodeau and Patton, 2003).

**Ligaments.** Ligaments are white, shiny, flexible bands of fibrous tissue that bind joints and connect bones and cartilages. Ligaments are elastic and aid joint flexibility and support. In some areas of the body, ligaments also have a protective function. For example, ligaments between vertebral bodies prevent damage to the spinal cord during back movement.

**Tendons.** Tendons are white, glistening, fibrous bands of tissue that connect muscle to bone. Tendons are strong, flexible, and inelastic and occur in various lengths and thicknesses.

**Cartilage.** Cartilage is nonvascular, supporting connective tissue with the flexibility of a firm, plastic material. The gristlelike nature of cartilage permits it to sustain weight and serve as a shock-absorber pad between articulating bones. It is located chiefly in the joints and in the thorax, trachea, larynx, nose, and ear (Thibodeau and Patton, 2003).

**SKELETAL MUSCLE.** In addition to facilitating movement, muscles determine body form and contour. Muscles span at least one joint and attach to both articulating bones. When contraction occurs, one bone is fixed while the other moves. The origin is the point of attachment that remains still; the insertion is the point that moves when the muscle contracts (Thibodeau and Patton, 2003).

**Muscles Concerned With Movement.** The muscles of movement are near the skeletal region, where a lever system causes movement (Thibodeau and Patton, 2003). The lever system makes the work of moving a weight or load easier. It occurs when specific bones, such as the humerus, ulna, and radius, and the associated joints, such as the elbow, act as a lever. Thus the force applied to one end of the bone to lift a weight at another point tends to rotate the bone in the opposite direction of the applied force. Muscles that attach to bones of leverage provide the necessary strength to move the object.

**Muscles Concerned With Posture.** Gravity pulls on parts of the body all the time; the only way the body stays in position is for muscles to exert pull on bones in the opposite direction. Muscles accomplish this counterforce by maintaining a low level of sustained contraction. Poor posture places more work on muscles to counteract the force of gravity. This leads to fatigue and will eventually interfere with bodily functions and cause deformities.

**Muscle Groups.** The nervous system coordinates the antagonistic, synergistic, and antigravity muscle groups that maintain posture and initiate movement. Antagonistic muscles bring about movement at the joint. During movement the active mover muscle contracts while its antagonist relaxes. For example, during **extension** of the arm, the active mover, the triceps brachii, contracts, and the antagonist, the biceps brachii, relaxes.

Synergistic muscles contract to accomplish the same movement. When you flex your arm, you increase the strength of the contraction of the biceps brachii by contraction of the synergistic muscle, the brachialis.

Antigravity muscles are involved with joint stabilization. These muscles continuously oppose the effect of gravity on the body and permit a person to maintain an upright or sitting posture. In an adult the antigravity muscles are the extensors of the leg, the gluteus maximus, the quadriceps femoris, the soleus muscles, and the muscles of the back.

Skeletal muscles support posture and carry out voluntary movement. The muscles are attached to the skeleton by tendons, which provide strength and permit motion.

**NERVOUS SYSTEM.** The nervous system regulates movement and posture. The major voluntary motor area, located in the cerebral cortex, is the motor strip (precentral gyrus). A majority of motor fibers descend from the motor strip and cross at the level of the medulla. The motor fibers from the right motor strip initiate voluntary movement for the left side of the body, and motor fibers from the left motor strip initiate voluntary movement for the right side of the body. Transmission of the impulse from the nervous system to the musculoskeletal system is an electrochemical event that requires a neurotransmitter, a chemical that transfers the electric impulse from the nerve to the muscle.

**Proprioception.** The nervous system also regulates posture. Posture requires coordination of proprioception and balance. **Proprioception** is the awareness of the position of the body and its parts and is dependent on impulses from the inner ear and from receptors in joints and ligaments (Huether and McCance, 2004). Proprioceptors located on nerve endings in muscles, tendons, and joints monitor proprioception. While a person carries out activities of daily living, proprioceptors monitor muscle activity and body position. When a person walks, the proprioceptors on the bottom of the feet monitor pressure changes. Thus when the bottom of the moving foot comes in contact with the walking surface, the individual automatically moves the stationary foot forward.

**Balance.** The cerebellum and the inner ear control **balance** through the nervous system. The major function of the cerebellum is to coordinate all voluntary movement. Within the inner ear are the fluid-filled semicircular canals. When you rotate your head suddenly in one direction, the fluid remains stationary for a moment, whereas the canal turns with the head. This allows a person to change position suddenly without losing balance.

## Principles of Body Mechanics

Using principles of **body mechanics** during routine activities also prevents injury. Teach colleagues and patients' families to lift, transfer, or position patients properly. For example, teaching a patient's family how to transfer the patient from bed to chair increases and reinforces the family's knowledge and provides opportunity to consistently demonstrate proper body mechanics (Box 25-2).

## Pathological Influences on Body Alignment, Exercise, and Activity

Many pathological conditions affect body alignment, exercise, and activity. A few of these conditions include congenital defects; disorders of bones, joints, and muscles; central nervous system damage; and musculoskeletal trauma.

**CONGENITAL DEFECTS.** Congenital abnormalities affect the efficiency of the musculoskeletal system in regard to alignment, balance, and appearance. Osteogenesis imperfecta is an inherited disorder that affects bone. Some characteristics of this are fractures and bone deformity (Hockenberry and others, 2003). Bones are porous, short, bowed, and deformed; as a result, children experience curvature of the spine and shortness of stature. Scoliosis is a structural curvature of the spine associated with vertebral rotation. Muscles, ligaments, and other soft tissues become shortened. This affects balance and mobility in proportion to the severity of abnormal spinal curvatures (Huether and McCance, 2004).

**DISORDERS OF BONES, JOINTS, AND MUSCLES.** Osteoporosis is a well-known and well-publicized disorder of aging in which the density or mass of bone is reduced. The bone remains biochemically normal but has difficulty maintaining integrity and support. There are many factors that cause this, varying from hormonal imbalances to insufficient intake of nutrients (Huether and McCance, 2004).

Inflammatory and noninflammatory joint diseases and articular disruption all alter joint mobility. Some characteristics of inflammatory joint disease (e.g., arthritis) are in-

---

**BOX 25-2** | **Principles of Body Mechanics**

A wide base of support increases stability.
A lower center of gravity increases stability.
You maintain the equilibrium of an object as long as the line of gravity passes through its base of support.
Facing the direction of movement prevents abnormal twisting of the spine.
Dividing balanced activity between arms and legs reduces the risk of back injury.
Leverage, rolling, turning, or pivoting requires less work than lifting.
When you reduce friction between the object and the surface, it requires less force to move it.
Reducing the force of work reduces the risk of injury.
Maintaining good body mechanics reduces fatigue of the muscle groups.
Alternating periods of rest and activity helps to reduce fatigue.

---

flammation or destruction of the synovial membrane and articular cartilage and systemic signs of inflammation. Noninflammatory diseases have none of these characteristics, and the synovial fluid is normal (Huether and McCance, 2004).

**CENTRAL NERVOUS SYSTEM DAMAGE.** Damage to any component of the central nervous system that regulates voluntary movement results in impaired body alignment and mobility. For example, your patient has experienced head trauma that has damaged the motor strip in the cerebrum. The amount of voluntary motor impairment is directly related to the amount of destruction of the motor strip. A patient with a right-sided cerebral hemorrhage and damage to the right motor strip sometimes has left-sided hemiplegia.

**MUSCULOSKELETAL TRAUMA.** Trauma to the musculoskeletal system sometimes results in bruises, contusions, sprains, and fractures. A fracture is a disruption of bone tissue continuity. Fractures most commonly result from direct external trauma. They also occur because of some deformity of the bone, as with pathological fractures of osteoporosis.

## Nursing Knowledge Base

Knowledge from areas of nursing practice enables you to meet the activity and exercise needs of the patient. Growth and development changes, behavioral aspects, and cultural and ethnic origin are a few areas of knowledge that you will incorporate into the plan of care.

### Growth and Development

Throughout the life span the body's appearance and functioning undergo change. Knowledge of growth and development (see Chapter 19) enables you to anticipate types of activities patients will be able to perform. The newborn infant's spine is flexed and lacks the anteroposterior curves of the adult. As growth and stability increase, the thoracic spine straightens, and the lumbar spinal curve appears, which allows sitting and standing. As the baby grows, musculoskeletal development permits support of weight for standing and walking. The toddler's posture is awkward because of the slight swayback and protruding abdomen (Hockenberry and others, 2003). From the third year through the beginning of adolescence, the musculoskeletal system continues to grow and develop. Greater coordination enables the child to perform tasks that require fine motor skills. With aging changes in musculoskeletal function limit patient activity.

## Behavioral Aspects

It is important to take into consideration the patient's knowledge of exercise and activity, barriers to a program of exercise and physical activity, and current exercise behavior or habits. Patients are more open to developing an exercise program if they are at the stage of readiness to change their behavior (Prochaska and others, 1994). Patients' decisions to change behavior and include a daily exercise routine in their lives often occur gradually with repeated information individualized to their needs and lifestyle (Box 25-3).

## Cultural and Ethnic Origin

Exercise and physical fitness is beneficial to all people. When developing a physical fitness program for culturally diverse populations, consider what motivates individuals to exercise and what activities will be appropriate and enjoyable (Box 25-4).

## Critical Thinking

### Synthesis

It is important for you to synthesize knowledge, experience, attitudes, and standards when providing care for a patient with activity intolerance or improper body mechanics. Doing so will help prevent complications, promote rehabilitation, and promote a timely return of patients to their homes.

**KNOWLEDGE.** When you begin the process of problem solving for patient care, you need to consider a variety of concepts and weave them together to provide the best outcome for your patient. Knowledge of the musculoskeletal system, exercise physiology, and health alterations that create problems for the patient in the area of exercise and activity provide the foundation for decision making and planning care.

**EXPERIENCE.** Your past experiences with exercise or caring for patients with problems related to activity and exercise help you anticipate patients' needs such as pain control, positioning, transferring, and support of activities of daily living. Visits to a physical or occupational therapy unit in a hospital or community setting will increase your experiential base.

**ATTITUDES.** You need to possess creativity because problems with activity and exercise are often prolonged. The more creative your approach for improving activity tolerance and

---

| BOX 25-3 | **General Guidelines for Initiating and Maintaining an Exercise Program** |

The patient will most likely initiate and maintain an exercise program if the individual:

Perceives a net benefit

Chooses an enjoyable activity

Feels competent doing the activity

Feels safe doing the activity

Has easy access the activity on a regular basis

Is able to fit the activity into the daily schedule

Feels that the activity does not generate financial or social costs that he or she is unwilling to bear

Experiences a minimum of negative consequences such as injury, loss of time, negative peer pressure, and problems with self-identity

Is able to successfully address issues of competing time demands

Recognizes the need to balance the use of labor-saving devices and sedentary activities with activities that involve a higher level of physical exertion.

Data from National Institutes of Health Consensus Development Panel on Physical Activity and Cardiovascular Health: Physical activity and cardiovascular health, *JAMA* 276(3):241, 1996; Schlicht J and others: Build self-efficacy to promote exercise adherence, *ACSM's Health Fitness Journal* 3(6):27, 1999.

---

| BOX 25-4 | CULTURAL FOCUS |

As Marilyn studies about activity and exercise, she learns that physical inactivity is one of the risk factors associated with type 2 diabetes. In the United States, type 2 diabetes is more common in African-American and Native American populations. Physical activity plays an important role in the prevention and treatment of type 2 diabetes, yet these two ethnic groups have a disproportionate number of poor, unemployed, and disadvantaged individuals who lack access to the health care systems and recreational facilities.

**Implications for Practice**

• Support promotion of physical activity through formal programs in schools, churches, and government agencies within African-American and Native American communities.

• Incorporate motivational factors into the exercise program such as providing a healthy snack or meal for the participants and furnishing each with a log to monitor weight loss and blood glucose levels.

• Develop an exercise/prevention program that removes barriers such as transportation and cost to facilitate commitment to the program.

Data from O'Brien-Gillespie H: Exercise. In Edelman CL, Mandle CL editors: *Health promotion throughout the lifespan*, ed 5, St. Louis, 2006, Mosby; Lee ET and others: Incidence of diabetes in American Indians of three geographic areas, *Diabetes Care* 25:49, 2002; Rimmer JH and others: Feasibility of a health promotion intervention for a group of predominantly African American women with type 2 diabetes, *Diabetes Educ* 28(4):571, 2002.

mobility skills, the greater chance for success. This is especially important with children. Creating a game that incorporates the goal of improving activity tolerance will elicit better cooperation and participation from the child. Also, providing colorful stickers to symbolize success is a creative approach to enhance cooperation (Hockenberry and others, 2003).

**STANDARDS.** The use of professional standards and guidelines, such as those from the American Nurses Association (ANA) (2003) and Occupational Safety and Health Administration (OSHA) (2003) concerning the use of assistive equipment and devices to transfer and position patients, provide valuable guidelines for patient and your safety. In addition, these standards help you promote the patient's independence while adhering safely to the prescribed rehabilitation plan, for example, the National Institutes of Health guidelines on physical activity and cardiovascular health (1996).

## Nursing Process

### Assessment

The assessment includes the patient's present activity tolerance and information about pre-illness functioning. You are able to assess body alignment and posture with the patient standing, sitting, or lying down. Table 25-1 presents factors to assess related to activity intolerance, questions and approaches, and physical assessment strategies.

Through assessment you are able to determine normal physiological changes in growth and development; deviations related to poor posture, trauma, muscle damage, or nerve dysfunction; and any learning needs of patients. In addition, assessment provides opportunities for patients to observe their posture and obtain important information about other factors that contribute to poor alignment, such as fatigue, malnutrition, and psychological problems.

**BODY ALIGNMENT.** The first step in assessing body alignment is to put the patient at ease, so he or she does not assume unnatural or rigid positions. Remove pillows and positioning supports from the bed (if not contraindicated) and place the patient in the **supine** position.

**Standing.** Assessment of the patient includes the following:

- The head is erect and midline.
- Body parts are symmetrical.
- The spine is straight with normal curvatures (cervical concave, thoracic convex, and lumbar concave).
- The abdomen is comfortably tucked.
- The knees are in a straight line between the hips and ankles and slightly flexed.
- The feet are flat on the floor and pointed directly forward and slightly apart to maintain a wide base of support.
- The arms hang comfortably at the sides (Figure 25-1).

The patient's center of gravity is in the midline, and the line of gravity is from the middle of the forehead to a midpoint between the feet. Laterally the line of gravity runs vertically from the middle of the skull to the posterior third of the foot (Wilson and Giddens, 2005).

**Sitting.** Assess your patient for the following: the head is erect, and the neck and vertebral column are in straight alignment; the body weight is distributed on the buttocks and thighs; the thighs are parallel and in a horizontal plane (be careful to avoid pressure on the popliteal nerve and blood supply); the feet are supported on the floor; and the forearms are supported on the armrest, in the lap, or on a table in front of the chair.

Assessment of alignment in the sitting position is particularly important for the patient with neuromuscular disorders, muscle weakness, muscle paralysis, or nerve damage. A patient with these alterations has diminished sensation in affected areas and is unable to perceive pressure or decreased

## FOCUSED PATIENT ASSESSMENT

**TABLE 25-1**

| Factors to Assess | Questions and Approaches | Physical Assessment Strategies |
|---|---|---|
| Range of motion (ROM) | Ask if patient has limited movement in joints.<br>Ask if patient has a history of connective tissue disorders, fractures, and/or damage to ligaments or tendons. | Observe patient's gait and ability to carry out activities of daily living (ADLs).<br>Inspect joints for deformity.<br>Measure ROM of affected joints. |
| Pain | Ask if patient experiences pain or discomfort upon movement.<br>Ask if patient needs pain medication before ambulating (with assistance), particularly after surgical procedure.<br>Ask patient to rate pain on a scale of 0 to 10 with 10 representing the worst pain. | Inspect joints for redness or swelling indicating potential inflammatory process.<br>Observe for objective signs of pain such as grimacing, moaning, increasing respiratory rate, pulse, and blood pressure. (NOTE: These objective signs are not always present, and it is best to ask patient if pain is present.) |
| Activity tolerance | Ask if patient feels fatigued.<br>Ask if patient is experiencing difficulty with ADLs because of muscle weakness.<br>Ask if patient feels short of breath, palpitations, light-headed, or dizzy. | Observe for signs of fatigue.<br>Observe patient's performance of ADLs.<br>Observe patient for paleness, obtain vital signs, and compare to baseline measures. |

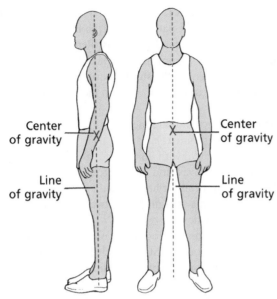

FIGURE **25-1** Correct body alignment with standing.

circulation. Proper sitting alignment reduces the risk of musculoskeletal system damage in such a patient.

**Recumbent.** Position your patient in the lateral position with all but one pillow and all positioning supports removed from the bed. Make sure the vertebrae are in straight alignment without observable curves. This assessment provides baseline data concerning the patient's body alignment.

Conditions that create a risk of damage to the musculoskeletal system when lying down include impaired mobility (e.g., spinal curvature), use of immobilization devices (e.g., traction), decreased sensation (e.g., hemiparesis from a stroke), impaired circulation (e.g., diabetes), and lack of voluntary muscle control (e.g., spinal cord injuries).

When a patient is unable to change position voluntarily, assess the position of body parts while the patient is lying down. Make sure the vertebrae are in straight alignment without any observable curves. Normally the extremities are in alignment and do not cross over one another. The head and neck are aligned without excessive flexion or extension.

**MOBILITY.** The adequacy of your patient's mobility determines the patient's coordination and balance while walking, the ability to carry out activities of daily living, and the ability to participate in an exercise program. The assessment of mobility has three components: range of joint motion, gait, and exercise.

**Range of Motion.** Observing **range of motion (ROM)** is one of the first assessment techniques used to determine the degree of limitation or injury to a joint. Assess ROM to collect data to answer questions about joint stiffness, swelling, pain, limited movement, and unequal movement. Chapter 34 covers a thorough ROM assessment. Limited range of motion indicates inflammation such as arthritis, fluid in the joint, altered nerve supply, or contractures. Increased mobility (beyond normal) of a joint indicates connective tissue disorders, ligament tears, and possible joint fractures.

**Gait. Gait** is the manner or style of walking, including rhythm, cadence, and speed. Assessing gait allows for conclusions about balance, posture, and the ability to walk without assistance (see Chapter 13). Note conformity, a regular smooth rhythm, symmetry in the length of leg swing, smooth swaying related to the gait phase, and a smooth, symmetrical arm swing (Wilson and Giddens, 2005).

**Exercise.** Exercise is physical activity for conditioning the body, improving health, maintaining fitness, or providing therapy for correcting a deformity or restoring the body to a maximal state of health. When a person exercises, physiological changes occur in body systems (Box 25-5).

During exercise, you improve muscle tone, size, and strength and cardiopulmonary conditioning. As a result, you are able to exercise longer with each strengthening of the muscles. Exercise also enhances joint mobility because the exercise itself requires movement of body parts.

**Activity Tolerance. Activity tolerance** is the kind and amount of exercise or work a person is able to perform without undue exertion or injury (Box 25-6). Observe patients after ambulation, self-bathing, or sitting in a chair for several hours, and assess their verbal report of fatigue and weakness. Assess heart rate and blood pressure response to activity.

**PATIENT EXPECTATIONS.** In assessing the patient's expectations concerning body alignment and joint mobility, determine your patient's perception of what is normal or acceptable in regard to mobility. For example, if exercising is painful or tiresome to patients, they may lack adherence and commitment to desired interventions. Some patients are content with their present range of motion or mobility and do not perceive a need for improvement. Unless there is a real threat to health maintenance, forcing patients to accept perspectives not in accordance with their own beliefs is a breach of standards of care.

## BOX 25-5 Effects of Exercise

**Cardiovascular System**

Increased cardiac output

Improved myocardial contraction, thereby strengthening cardiac muscle

Decreased resting heart rate

Improved venous return

**Pulmonary System**

Increased respiratory rate and depth followed by a quicker return to resting state

Improved alveolar ventilation

Decreased work of breathing

Improved diaphragmatic excursion

**Metabolic System**

Increased basal metabolic rate

Increased use of glucose and fatty acids

Increased triglyceride breakdown

Increased gastric motility

Increased production of body heat

**Musculoskeletal System**

Improved muscle tone

Increased joint mobility

Improved muscle tolerance to physical exercise

Possible increase in muscle mass

Reduced bone loss

**Activity Tolerance**

Improved tolerance

Decreased fatigue

**Psychosocial Factors**

Improved tolerance to stress

Reports of "feeling better"

Reports of decrease in illness (e.g., colds, influenza)

Data from Huether SE, McCance KL: *Understanding pathophysiology,* ed 3, St. Louis, 2004, Mosby; Hoeman SP: *Rehabilitation nursing: process, application, and outcomes,* ed 3, St. Louis, 2002, Mosby.

## BOX 25-6 Factors Influencing Activity Tolerance

**Physiological Factors**

Skeletal abnormalities

Muscular impairments

Endocrine or metabolic illnesses (e.g., diabetes mellitus, thyroid disease)

Hypoxemia

Decreased cardiac function

Decreased endurance

Impaired physical stability

Pain

Sleep pattern disturbance

Prior exercise patterns

Infectious processes and fever

**Emotional Factors**

Anxiety

Depression

Chemical addictions

Motivation

**Developmental Factors**

Age

Sex

Pregnancy

Physical growth and development of muscle and skeletal support

Modified from Phipps WJ and others: *Medical surgical nursing,* ed 7, St. Louis, 2003, Mosby.

Alterations in body alignment and joint mobility result from developmental changes, postural and bone formation abnormalities, impaired muscle development, damage to the central nervous system, or direct trauma to the musculoskeletal system. In some cases alterations in joint mobility or alignment are one of the defining characteristics of a separate nursing diagnosis and not the actual nursing diagnosis. Nursing diagnoses often focus on the individual's ability to move. Make sure the diagnostic label directs nursing interventions. For example, the diagnostic label *impaired physical mobility* related to pain and muscle weakness will direct you to initiate pain relief and exercise measures.

## Planning

During planning for your patient, use data gathered during assessment and critical thinking to develop an individualized plan of care. You will identify patient needs and, in collaboration with the patient and family, integrate these needs with the goals and outcomes of care, care priorities, and restorative and continuing care needs. This will enable you to develop a plan of care to optimize the patient's exercise and activity levels.

**GOALS AND OUTCOMES.** Once you define the nursing diagnoses, work with the patient to set goals and expected outcomes, which then direct nursing interventions. For example, the goal of achieving optimum ROM in the right knee will have the outcome of achieving 90-degree flexion in the right knee by discharge. Nursing therapies will include ROM and muscle strengthening. The plan considers risks for injury to the patient and preexisting health concerns. It is especially important to have knowledge of your patient's previous functional status and home environment.

**SETTING PRIORITIES.** You will individualize care planning for your patient, taking into consideration your

## Nursing Diagnosis

The pateint's assessment provides related clusters of data or defining characteristics that lead to the identification of the following nursing diagnoses:

- Activity intolerance
- Risk for activity intolerance
- Disturbed body image
- Fatigue
- Risk for injury
- Impaired physical mobility
- Acute pain
- Chronic pain
- Impaired skin integrity
- Risk for impaired skin integrity

## CARE PLAN Impaired Physical Mobility

### ASSESSMENT

Joseph Indelicato is a 72-year-old man hospitalized for surgery on his right knee. Over the past 5 years, he has continued to experience pain and decreased mobility. He is now 2 days *postoperative* following right total knee replacement. His incision is healing, and there is no edema or erythema. He rates his **pain as 6 to 7 on a 10-point scale** and is using a **patient-controlled analgesia pump.** He uses a **continuous passive motion (CPM) machine.** His degree of **knee flexion is now 70 degrees.** He is able to **ambulate 10 feet with a walker** but states, **"I can't go any further."** The nurse observes Mr. Indelicato **using the walker incorrectly.** In addition, he further describes his muscle strength in his right leg as **feeling weak and tired after walking a short distance.** He states, **"I can't put all my weight on my right leg, it is just too painful."**

*Defining characteristics are shown in bold type.

---

### NURSING DIAGNOSIS Impaired physical mobility related to pain, muscle weakness, and limited joint motion.

---

### PLANNING

**GOAL**
- Patient will gain optimal functioning of the right knee with independent, purposeful movement.

**EXPECTED OUTCOMES***
- Patient will gain a minimum of 90 degrees flexion in right knee by discharge.
- Patient will ambulate 50 to 75 feet with aid of a walker by discharge.
- Patient's pain will be 2 to 3 on a 10-point scale by discharge.
- Patient will verbally report pain controlled by oral analgesics.

*Outcomes classification labels from Moorhead S, Johnson M, Maas M: *Nursing outcomes classification (NOC)*, ed 3, St. Louis, 2004, Mosby.

---

### INTERVENTIONS†

**Ambulation**
- Provide analgesics 30 minutes before ambulation.

**Endurance**
- Consult physical therapist to obtain prescription for muscle-strengthening exercises.
- Teach patient and family ROM and muscle-strengthening exercises

**Safety**
- Teach patient and family proper use of walker.

### RATIONALE

Peak actions of analgesic will occur as patient begins activity, promoting greater tolerance to discomfort (Gahart and Nazareno, 2002).

Exercise improves circulation to the area and strengthens extremity for ambulation (Vincent and others, 2002).

Prevents injury and loss of function until patient achieves full weight bearing.

†Intervention classification labels from Dochterman JM, Bulechek GM, editors: *Nursing interventions classification (NIC)*, ed 4, St. Louis, 2004, Mosby.

---

### EVALUATION

- Measure degree of flexion in right knee with goniometer.
- Ask Mr. Indelicato to rate the quality of pain control before attempting ambulation.
- Ask Mr. Indelicato to demonstrate muscle-strengthening exercises.

- Observe Mr. Indelicato's use of the walker during ambulation.
- Ask Mr. Indelicato to state safety guidelines while using the walker.

---

patient's most immediate needs. You determine the immediacy of any problem by the effect the problem has on the patient's mental and physical health. For example, if a patient is in acute pain, relieving pain is a priority before you are able to initiate exercise. Because of the many skills associated with the care of patients with activity intolerance, improper body mechanics, and/or impaired mobility, such as turning, transferring, and positioning, it is easy to overlook the complications associated with these nursing and medical diagnoses. Therefore you need to be vigilant in monitoring your patients and supervising assistive personnel in carrying out activities to prevent complications and potential injury.

**CONTINUITY OF CARE.** Planning also involves an understanding of the patient's need to maintain motor function and independence. Collaborate with other members of the health care team, such as physical or occupational therapists. Long-term rehabilitation is sometimes necessary, and you begin discharge planning when a patient enters the health care system. In addition, always individualize a plan of care directed at meeting the actual or potential needs of the patient (see care plan).

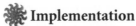 Implementation

**HEALTH PROMOTION.** In recent years the rate of injuries in occupational settings has increased dramatically (Trinkoff and others, 2002). The most common back injury is strain on the lumbar muscle group, which includes the muscles around the lumbar vertebrae. Injury to these areas affects the ability to bend forward, backward, and side to side. This also decreases the ability to rotate the hips and lower back. You and your patients need to learn and master proper body mechanics to prevent injury to your patient and yourself.

**Lifting Techniques.** Before lifting, assess the weight you will lift and what assistance, if any, you will need. If you need help, assess if a second person is adequate or if you will need mechanical assistance. Once you determine the amount of needed assistance you need, follow these steps:

1. Keep the weight you are lifting as close to the body as possible; this action places the object in the same plane as the lifter and close to the center of gravity for balance.
2. Bend at the knees; this helps to maintain the center of gravity and uses the stronger leg muscles to do the lifting (Figure 25-2). Avoid twisting. Twisting overloads the spine and leads to serious injury.
3. Tighten abdominal muscles and tuck the pelvis; this provides balance and helps protect the back.
4. Maintain the trunk erect and knees bent so that multiple groups work together in a coordinated manner.

However, note that injuries are not only related to lifting. You spend time in many activities bending and twisting that also cause injury. Examples of such activities include bathing, feeding, dressing, and undressing patients (Nelson, Fragala, and Menzel, 2003).

### ACUTE CARE

**Positioning Techniques.** Patients with impaired nervous or musculoskeletal system functioning, patients with increased weakness, or those restricted to bed rest benefit from therapeutic positioning (Hoeman, 2002). During patient positioning determine areas of bony prominences where pressure, friction, and shear cause the most wear and tear. Through the use of proper positioning and pressure-relief methods, you are able to protect these areas (see Chapter 35).

In general, you reposition patients as needed and at least every 2 hours if they are in bed and every 20 to 30 minutes if they are sitting in a chair. Those patients with contractures or who are at greater risk for skin breakdown over bony prominences need repositioning more frequently. The following also influence the frequency of position changes: level of comfort, amount of spontaneous movement, presence of edema, loss of sensation, and overall physical and mental status (Hoeman, 2002).

Several devices are available for you to use in maintaining good body alignment for your patients (Table 25-2). The following paragraphs describe various positions. Skill 25-1 describes the methods of positioning patients.

*Fowler's Position.* Elevate the head of the patient's bed 45 to 60 degrees, and slightly elevate the patient's knees, avoiding pressure on the popliteal vessels. The head rests against the mattress or a small pillow for support. Use pil-

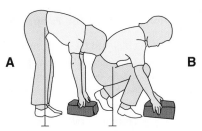

FIGURE **25-2** Incorrect (**A**) and correct (**B**) body position for lifting.

lows to maintain natural alignment of the hands, wrists, and forearms. In semi-Fowler's position the head of the bed is at a 30-degree angle; you will use this position for patients who will not tolerate a supine position, such as those with cardiac and respiratory problems. The following are common trouble areas for the patient in the Fowler's position:

- Increased cervical flexion because the pillow at the head is too thick and head thrusts forward
- Extension of the knees, allowing the patient to slide to the foot of the bed
- Pressure on the posterior aspect of the knees, decreasing circulation to the feet
- External rotation of the hips
- Arms hanging unsupported at the patient's sides
- Unsupported feet or pressure on the heels
- Unprotected pressure points at the sacrum and heels
- Increased shearing force on the back and heels when you raise the head of the bed greater than 60 degrees

*Supine Position.* In the supine position the patient rests on the back. A small, flat pillow supports the head, neck, and upper shoulders (Hoeman, 2002). You use pillows, trochanter rolls (see Table 25-2), and hand rolls or arm splints to increase comfort and reduce injury to the skin or musculoskeletal system. The risk of aspiration is greater with this position; thus avoid the supine position when the patient is confused, agitated, experiencing a decreased level of consciousness, or at risk for aspiration.

Make sure the mattress is firm enough to support the cervical, thoracic, and lumbar vertebrae. Avoid pressure on the back of the legs. Use a foot support to prevent **footdrop,** maintain proper alignment, and provide freedom of movement for the feet. The following are some common trouble areas for patients in the supine position:

- Pillow at the head that is too thick, increasing cervical flexion
- Head flat on the mattress
- Shoulders unsupported and internally rotated
- Elbows extended
- Thumb not in opposition to the fingers
- Hips externally rotated
- Unsupported feet
- Unprotected pressure points at the vertebrae, coccyx, elbows, heels, and the occipital region of the head

*Text continued on p. 670*

| TABLE 25-2 | Devices Used for Proper Positioning |
| --- | --- |
| **Devices** | **Uses and Descriptions** |
| Pillows | Make sure pillows are appropriate size for the body part you will position. They provide support, elevate body parts, and splint incisional areas. |
| Foot boots | **Foot boots** maintain feet in dorsiflexion. Remove boots at least 2 to 3 times per day to assess skin integrity and joint mobility. |
| Trochanter rolls | **Trochanter rolls** prevent external rotation of legs when patients are in the supine position. To form a trochanter roll, fold a cotton bath blanket or a sheet lengthwise to a width extending from the greater trochanter of the femur to the lower border of the popliteal space (Figure 25-3). Place the roll under the buttocks, and then roll it away from the patient until the thigh is in a neutral position or an inward position with the patella facing upward. |
| Sandbags | **Sandbags** provide support and shape to body contours; they immobilize extremities and maintain specific body alignment. You use them in place of or in addition to the trochanter roll. |
| Hand rolls | **Hand rolls** maintain the thumb slightly adducted and in opposition to the fingers; they maintain fingers in a slightly flexed position (Figure 25-4). You make hand rolls by folding a washcloth in half, rolling it lengthwise, and securing the roll with tape. Place the roll against the palmar surface of the hand. Evaluate the position of the hand to make certain the hand is in a functional position. |
| Hand-wrist splints | **Hand-wrist splints** are individually molded for the patient to maintain proper alignment of the thumb in slight **adduction** and the wrist in slight dorsiflexion. Use these splints only for the patient for whom they were made. |
| Trapeze bar | The **trapeze bar** descends from a securely fastened overhead bar attached to the bed frame (Figure 25-5). The trapeze allows the patient to use upper extremities to raise the trunk off the bed, to assist in transfer from bed to wheelchair, or to perform upper arm–strengthening exercises. |
| Side rails | **Side rails** are bars positioned along the sides of the length of the bed. They are designed to increase patient's ability to move and turn in bed, for example, rolling from side to side or sitting up in bed. |
| Bed boards | **Bed boards** are plywood boards placed under the entire surface of the mattress. They are useful for increasing back support and alignment, especially with a soft mattress. |
| Wedge pillow | A wedge or abductor pillow is a triangular-shaped pillow made of heavy foam. You use it to maintain the legs in **abduction** following total hip replacement surgery. |

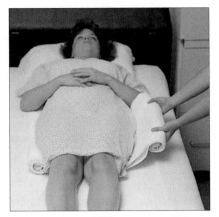

FIGURE **25-3** Trochanter roll.

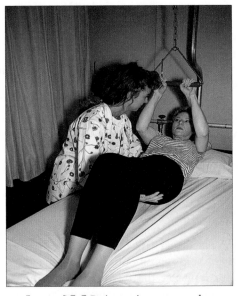

FIGURE **25-5** Patient using a trapeze bar.

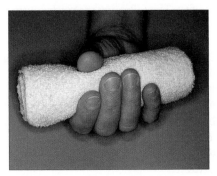

FIGURE **25-4** Hand roll.

## SKILL 25-1 Moving and Positioning Patients in Bed

### Delegation Considerations

The skill of moving and positioning patients in bed to can be delegated to assistive personnel. Before delegation, instruct the assistive personnel about:

- Any limitations affecting movement and positioning of patient in bed
- Scheduled times to reposition patient throughout the shift
- Maintaining proper body mechanics
- When to request assistance, such as when the patient is unable to assist the nurse or has a lot of equipment or is confused, etc.

### Equipment

- Pillows
- Footboard (optional)
- High-top sneakers
- Trochanter roll
- Sandbag
- Hand rolls
- Side rails

| STEP | RATIONALE |
|---|---|

### ASSESSMENT

1. Assess patient's body alignment and comfort level while patient is lying down.

Provides baseline data for later comparisons. Determines ways to improve position and alignment.

2. Assess for risk factors that will contribute to complications of immobility:

Increased risk factors require you to reposition the patient more frequently (Buss, Halfens, and Abu-Sand, 2002).

   a. *Paralysis:* hemiparesis resulting from cerebrovascular accident (CVA); decreased sensation

Paralysis impairs movement; muscle tone changes; affects sensation. Because of difficulty in moving and poor awareness of involved body part, patient is unable to protect and position body part for self.

   b. Impaired mobility: traction or arthritis or other contributing disease processes

Traction or arthritic changes of affected extremity result in decreased ROM.

   c. Impaired circulation

Decreased circulation predisposes patient to pressure ulcers.

   d. *Age:* very young, older adult

Premature and young infants require frequent turning because their skin is fragile. Normal physiological changes associated with aging predispose older adults to greater risks for developing complications of immobility.

   e. Level of consciousness and mental status

Comatose or semicomatose patients are unable to verbalize areas of skin pressure, increasing the risk for skin breakdown.

3. Assess patient's physical ability to help with moving and positioning:

Use patient's mobility and strength. Determines need for additional help. Ensures the patient's and the nurse's safety.

   a. Age

Some older adult patients move more slowly with less strength. Determines need for special aids or devices.

   b. Level of consciousness and mental status

Patients with altered levels of consciousness do not always understand instructions and are often unable to help.

   c. Disease process

Cardiopulmonary disease requires patient to have head of bed elevated.

   d. Strength, coordination

Determines amount of assistance provided by patient during position change.

   e. ROM

Limited ROM contraindicates certain positions.

4. Assess health care provider's orders. Clarify whether patient's condition contraindicates any positions (e.g., spinal cord injury; respiratory difficulties; certain neurological conditions; presence of incisions, drain, or tubing).

Placing patient in an inappropriate position causes injury.

5. Assess for tubes, incisions, and equipment (e.g., traction).

Will alter positioning procedure and affect patient's ability to independently change positions.

6. Assess ability and motivation of patient, family members, and primary caregiver to participate in moving and positioning patient in bed in anticipation of discharge to home.

Determines ability of patient and caregivers to assist with positioning.

## SKILL 25-1 Moving and Positioning Patients in Bed—cont'd

| STEP | RATIONALE |
|---|---|

### PLANNING

1. Collect appropriate equipment.
2. Perform hand hygiene. — Reduces transfer of microorganisms.
3. Correctly identify patient, and explain procedure. — Decreases anxiety and increases patient cooperation.
4. Position patient flat in bed if tolerated. — Repositioning from a flat position decreases friction and possible shear on patient's skin.
5. Keep patient aligned.

---

• *Critical Decision Point:* Before flattening bed, account for all tubing, drains, and equipment to prevent dislodgement or tipping if caught in mattress or bed frame as bed is lowered.

---

### IMPLEMENTATION

1. Position patient in bed.
   **A. Assist Patient in Moving Up in Bed (Two Nurses)** — This is not a one-person task. Assisting a patient in moving up in bed without help from other co-workers or with the aid of an assistive device (i.e., friction-reducing pad) is no longer recommended or considered safe for the patient or nurse (ANA, 2003; Nelson and others, 2003).

   (1) Remove pillow from under head and shoulders, and place pillow at head of bed. — Prevents striking patient's head against head of bed.

   (2) Face head of bed. — Facing direction of movement prevents twisting of your body while moving patient.

   (3) Each nurse has one arm under patient's shoulders and one arm under patient's thighs.

   (4) Alternative position: position one nurse at patient's upper body. Nurse's arm nearest head of bed is under patient's head and opposite shoulder; other arm is under patient's closest arm and shoulder. Position other nurse at patient's lower torso. The nurse's arms are under patient's lower back and torso. — Prevents trauma to patient's musculoskeletal system by supporting shoulder and hip joints and evenly distributing weight.

   (5) Place feet apart, with foot nearest head of bed behind other foot (forward-backward stance). — Wide base of support increases balance. Stance enables you to shift body weight as you move patient up in bed, thereby reducing force needed to move load.

   (6) When possible, ask patient to flex knees with feet flat on bed. — Decreases friction and enables patient to use leg muscles during movement.

   (7) Instruct patient to flex neck, tilting chin toward chest. — Prevents hyperextension of neck when moving patient up in bed.

   (8) Instruct patient to assist moving by pushing with feet on bed surface. — Reduces friction. Increases patient mobility. Decreases workload.

   (9) Flex knees and hips, bringing forearms closer to level of bed. — Increases balance and strength by bringing your center of gravity closer to patient. Uses thighs instead of back muscles.

   (10) Instruct patient to push with heels and elevate trunk while breathing out, thus moving toward head of bed on count of three. — Prepares patient for move. Reinforces assistance in moving up in bed. Increases patient cooperation. Breathing out avoids Valsalva maneuver.

| STEP | RATIONALE |
|---|---|
| (11) On count of three, rock and shift weight from front to back leg. At the same time patient pushes with heels and elevates trunk. | Rocking enables you to improve balance and overcome inertia. Shifting weight counteracts patient's weight and reduces force needed to move load. Patient's assistance reduces friction and workload. |

**B. Move Immobile Patient Up in Bed With Drawsheet (Two Nurses)**

| STEP | RATIONALE |
|---|---|
| (1) Place drawsheet under patient by turning side to side. Extend sheet from shoulders to thighs. Return to supine position. | Supports patient's body weight and reduces friction during movement. |
| (2) Position one nurse at each side of the patient's hips. | Distributes weight equally between nurses. |
| (3) Grasp drawsheet firmly near the patient. | |
| (4) Place feet apart with forward-backward stance. Flex knees and hips. Shift weight from front to back leg, and move patient and drawsheet to desired position in bed. | Facing direction of movement ensures proper balance. Shifting weight reduces force needed to move load. Flexing knees lowers center of gravity and thighs instead of back muscles. |
| (5) Realign patient in correct body alignment. | Prevents injury to musculoskeletal system. |

**C. Position Patient in Supported Fowler's Position**
(See illustration)

| STEP | RATIONALE |
|---|---|
| (1) Elevate head of bed 45 to 60 degrees. | Increases comfort, improves ventilation, and increases patient's opportunity to socialize or relax. |
| (2) Rest head against mattress or on small pillow. | Prevents flexion contractures of cervical vertebrae. |
| (3) Use pillows to support arms and hands if patient does not have voluntary control or use of hands and arms. | Prevents shoulder dislocation from effect of downward pull of unsupported arms, promotes circulation by preventing venous pooling, and prevents flexion contractures of arms and wrists. |
| (4) Position pillow at lower back. | Supports lumbar vertebrae and decreases flexion of vertebrae. |
| (5) Place small pillow or roll under thigh. | Prevents hyperextension of knee and occlusion of popliteal artery from pressure from body weight. |
| (6) Place small pillow or roll under ankles. | Prevents prolonged pressure of mattress on heels. |

---

• *Critical Decision Point:* To keep feet in proper alignment and prevent footdrop, place footboard at bottom of patient's feet.

---

**D. Position Hemiplegic Patient in Supported Fowler's Position**

| STEP | RATIONALE |
|---|---|
| (1) Elevate head of bed 45 to 60 degrees. | Increases comfort, improves ventilation, and increases patient's opportunity to relax. |
| (2) Position patient in sitting position as straight as possible. | Counteracts tendency to slump toward affected side. Improves ventilation, cardiac output, and decreases intracranial pressure. Improves patient's ability to swallow and helps to prevent aspiration of food, liquids, and gastric secretions (Glenn-Molali, 2002). |

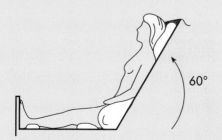

60°

STEP **1C** Fowler's position with footboard in place.

# SKILL 25-1 Moving and Positioning Patients in Bed—cont'd

| STEP | RATIONALE |
|---|---|
| (3) Position head on small pillow with chin slightly forward. If patient is totally unable to control head movement, avoid hyperextension of the neck. | Prevents hyperextension of neck. Too many pillows under head causes or worsens neck flexion contracture. |

• *Critical Decision Point:* If the patient has a paralyzed extremity, provide support for involved arm and hand on over-bed table in front of patient. Place arm away from patient's side, and support elbow with pillow.

• *Critical Decision Point:* Position flaccid hand in normal resting position with wrist slightly extended, arches of hand maintained, and fingers partially flexed; use section of rubber ball cut in half; clasp patient's hands together.

• *Critical Decision Point:* Position spastic hand with wrist in neutral position or slightly extended; extend fingers with palm down or leave fingers in relaxed position with palm up. At times it is difficult to position spastic hands without the use of specially made splints for the patient.

| STEP | RATIONALE |
|---|---|
| (4) Flex knees and hips by using pillow or folded blanket under knees. | Ensures proper alignment. Flexion prevents prolonged hyperextension, which impairs joint mobility. |
| (5) Support feet in dorsiflexion with firm pillow or footboard. | Prevents footdrop. Stimulation of ball of foot by hard surface has tendency to increase muscle tone in patient with extensor spasticity of lower extremity. |
| **E. Position Patient in Supine Position** | |
| (1) Be sure patient is comfortable on back with head of bed flat. | Some patients' physical conditions will not tolerate supine position. |
| (2) Place small rolled towel under lumbar area of back. | Provides support for lumbar spine. |
| (3) Place pillow under upper shoulders, neck, or head. | Maintains correct alignment and prevents flexion contractures of cervical vertebrae. |
| (4) Place trochanter rolls or sandbags parallel to lateral surface of patient's thighs. | Reduces external rotation of hip. |
| (5) Place small pillow or roll under ankle to elevate heels (see illustration for step 1C). | Reduces pressure on heels, helping to prevent pressure ulcers. |
| (6) Place footboard or firm pillows against bottom of patient's feet. *Optional:* Apply high-top sneakers. | Maintains dorsiflexion and prevents footdrop. |
| (7) Place pillows under pronated forearms, keeping upper arms parallel to patient's body (see illustrations). | Reduces internal rotation of shoulder and prevents extension of elbows. Maintains correct body alignment. |
| (8) Place hand rolls in patient's hands. Consider physical therapy referral for use of hand splints. | Reduces extension of fingers and abduction of thumb. Maintains thumb slightly adducted and in opposition to fingers. |
| **F. Position Hemiplegic Patient in Supine Position** | |
| (1) Place head of bed flat. | Necessary for positioning in supine position. |
| (2) Place folded towel or small pillow under shoulder or affected side. | Decreases possibility of pain, joint contracture, and subluxation. Maintains mobility in muscles around shoulder to permit normal movement patterns. |

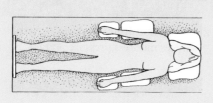

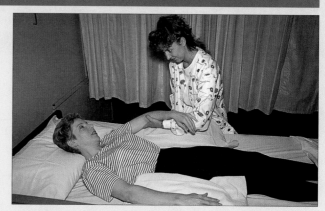

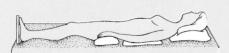

STEP 1E(8) Supine position with pillows in place.

| STEP | RATIONALE |
|---|---|
| (3) Keep affected arm away from body with elbow extended and palm up. (Alternative is to place arm out to side, with elbow bent and hand toward head of bed.) | Maintains mobility in arm, joints, and shoulder to permit normal movement patterns. (Alternative position counteracts limitation of ability of arm to rotate outward at shoulder [external rotation]. Need external rotation to raise arm overhead without pain.) |

• *Critical Decision Point:* Position affected hand in one of the recommended positions for flaccid or spastic hand.

| STEP | RATIONALE |
|---|---|
| (4) Place folded towel under hip of involved side. | Diminishes effect of spasticity in entire leg by controlling hip position. |
| (5) Flex affected knee 30 degrees by supporting it on pillow or folded blanket. | Slight flexion breaks up abnormal extension pattern of leg. Extensor spasticity is most severe when patient is supine. |
| (6) Support feet with soft pillows at right angle to leg. | Maintains foot in dorsiflexion and prevents footdrop. Pillows prevent stimulation to ball of foot by hard surface, which has tendency to increase muscle tone in patient with extensor spasticity of lower extremity. |
| **G. Position Patient in Prone Position** | |
| (1) With patient supine, roll patient over arm positioned close to body, with elbow straight and hand under hip. Position on abdomen in center of bed. | Positions patient correctly to maintain alignment. |
| (2) Turn patient's head to one side, and support head with small pillow (see illustration). | Reduces flexion or hyperextension of cervical vertebrae. |
| (3) Place small pillow under patient's abdomen below level of diaphragm (see illustration). | Reduces pressure on breasts of some female patients and decreases hyperextension of lumbar vertebrae and strain on lower back. |
| (4) Support arms in flexed position level at shoulders. | Maintains proper body alignment. Support reduces risk of joint dislocation. |

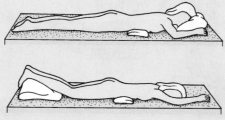

STEP 1G(2-3) Prone position with pillows in place.

## SKILL 25-1 | Moving and Positioning Patients in Bed—cont'd

| STEP | RATIONALE |
|---|---|
| (5) Support lower legs with pillow to elevate toes (see illustration). | Prevents footdrop. Reduces external rotation of hips. Reduces mattress pressure on toes. |

**H. Position Hemiplegic Patient in Prone Position**

• *Critical Decision Point:* Increase frequency of positioning if pressure areas begin to appear, joint mobility becomes impaired or worsened, or patient demonstrates signs of discomfort. Consult with physical and occupational therapists as needed.

| | |
|---|---|
| (1) With patient lying supine, move patient toward unaffected side. | Creates room for proper patient alignment in center of bed when patient is rolled onto abdomen. |
| (2) Roll patient onto affected side. | |
| (3) Place pillow on patient's abdomen. | Prevents sagging of abdomen when patient is rolled over; decreases hyperextension of lumbar vertebrae and strain on lower back. |
| (4) Roll patient onto abdomen by positioning involved arm close to patient's body, with elbow straight and hand under hip. Roll patient carefully over arm. | Prevents injury to affected side. |
| (5) Turn head toward involved side. | Promotes development of neck and trunk extension, which is necessary for standing and walking. |
| (6) Position involved arm out to side, with elbow bent, hand toward head of bed, and fingers extended (if possible). | Counteracts limitation of arm's ability to rotate outward at shoulder (external rotation). Need external rotation to raise arm over head without pain. |
| (7) Flex knees slightly by placing pillow under legs from knees to ankles. | Flexion prevents prolonged hyperextension, which impairs joint mobility. |
| (8) Keep feet at right angle to legs by using pillow high enough to keep toes off mattress. | Maintains feet in dorsiflexion. |

**I. Position Patient in Lateral (Side-Lying) Position**

| | |
|---|---|
| (1) Lower head of bed completely or as low as patient tolerates. | Provides position of comfort for patient and removes pressure from bony prominences on back and buttocks. |
| (2) Position patient to one side of bed. | Provides room for patient to turn to side. |
| (3) Prepare to turn patient onto side. Flex patient's knee that will not be next to mattress. Place one hand on patient's hip and one hand on patient's shoulder. | Positioning will set up leverage for easy turning. |

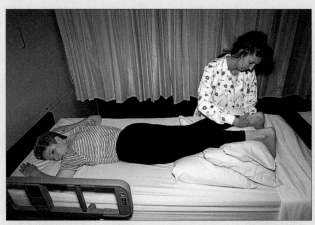

STEP **1G(5)** Prone position with pillows supporting lower legs.

| STEP | RATIONALE |
|------|-----------|

• *Critical Decision Point:* Patients at risk for pressure ulcer development require the 30-degree lateral position (see Chapter 35).

| | |
|---|---|
| (4) Roll patient onto side toward you. | Rolling patient towards you decreases trauma to tissues. In addition, positioning patient so leverage is on hip makes turning easy. |
| (5) Place pillow under patient's head and neck. | Maintains alignment. Reduces lateral neck flexion. Decreases strain on sternocleidomastoid muscle. |
| (6) Bring shoulder blade of dependent arm forward. | Prevents patient's weight from resting directly on shoulder joint. |
| (7) Position both arms in slightly flexed position. A pillow level with shoulder, other arm, or mattress supports upper arm. | Decreases internal rotation and adduction of shoulder. Supporting both arms in slightly flexed position protects joints. Improves ventilation because chest is able to expand more easily. |
| (8) Place tuck-back pillow behind patient's back. (Make by folding pillow lengthwise. Smooth area is slightly tucked under patient's back.) | Provides support to maintain patient on side. |
| (9) Place pillow under semiflexed upper leg level at hip from groin to foot (see illustrations). | Maintains leg in correct alignment. Prevents pressure on bony prominence. |
| (10) Place sandbag parallel to plantar surface of dependent foot. | Maintains dorsiflexion of foot. Prevents footdrop. |

**J. Position Patient in Sims' (Semiprone) Position**

| | |
|---|---|
| (1) Lower head of bed completely. | |
| (2) Be sure patient is comfortable in supine position. | Provides for proper body alignment while patient is lying down. |
| (3) Position patient to one side of bed, then roll over one arm positioned close to body. Roll patient to lateral position, lying partially on abdomen. Position dependent arm out from body. | Facilitates turning onto side. Avoids injury to arm; semiprone position places less pressure on abdomen. |
| (4) Place small pillow under patient's head. | Patient is rolled only partially on abdomen. |
| (5) Place pillow under flexed upper arm, supporting arm level with shoulder. | Maintains proper alignment and prevents lateral neck flexion. Prevents internal rotation of shoulder. Maintains alignment. |
| (6) Place pillow under flexed upper legs, supporting leg level with hip. | Prevents internal rotation of hip and adduction of leg. Flexion prevents hyperextension of leg. Reduces mattress pressure on knees and ankles. |

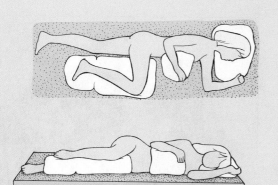
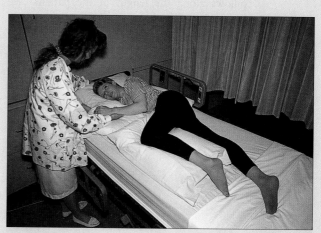

STEP 11(9) Lateral position with pillows in place.

## SKILL 25-1  Moving and Positioning Patients in Bed—cont'd

| STEP | RATIONALE |
|---|---|

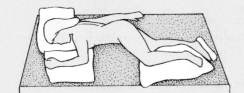

STEP **1J(7)** Sandbag supporting foot in dorsiflexion.

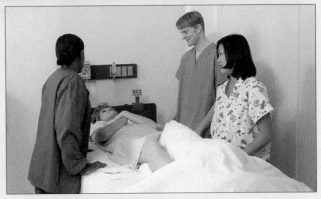

STEP **1K(3)** Position nurses on each side of patient.

| | |
|---|---|
| (7) Place sandbags parallel to plantar surface of foot (see illustration). | Maintains foot in dorsiflexion. Prevents footdrop. |

**K. Logrolling the Patient (Three Nurses)**

---

• *Critical Decision Point:* Supervise and aid assistive personnel when there is a health care provider's order to **logroll** a patient. Patients who have suffered from a spinal cord injury or are recovering from neck, back, or spinal surgery often need to keep the spinal column in straight alignment to prevent further injury.

---

| | |
|---|---|
| (1) Place pillow between patient's knees. | Prevents tension on the spinal column and adduction of the hip. |
| (2) Cross patient's arms on chest. | Prevents injury to arms. |
| (3) Position two nurses on side of bed to which the patient will be turned. Position third nurse on the other side of bed (see illustration). | Distributes weight equally between nurses. |
| (4) Fanfold or roll the drawsheet. | Provides strong handles in order to grip the drawsheet without slipping. |
| (5) Move the patient as one unit in a smooth, continuous motion on the count of three (see illustration). | This maintains proper alignment by moving all body parts at the same time, preventing tension or twisting of the spinal column. |
| (6) Nurse on the opposite side of the bed places pillows along the length of the patient (see illustration). | Pillows keep patient aligned. |

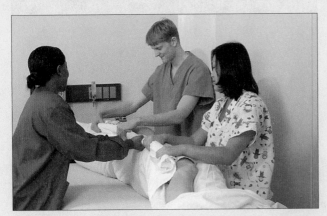

STEP **1K(5)** Move patient as a unit, maintaining proper alignment.

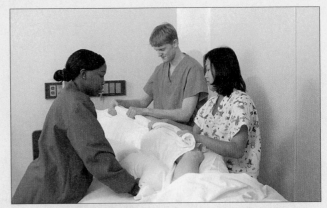

STEP **1K(6)** Place pillows along patient's back for support.

| STEP | RATIONALE |
|------|-----------|

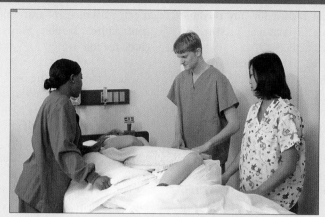

STEP **1K(7)** Gently lean patient as a unit against pillows.

| | |
|---|---|
| (7) Gently lean the patient as a unit back toward the pillows for support (see illustration). | Ensures continued straight alignment of spinal column, preventing injury. |
| **2.** Perform hand hygiene. | Reduces transmission of microorganisms. |

## EVALUATION

| | |
|---|---|
| **1.** Evaluate patient's body alignment, position, and level of comfort. | Determines effectiveness of positioning. Add or remove additional supports (e.g., pillows, bath blankets) to promote comfort and correct body alignment. |
| **2.** Measure ROM (see Chapter 34). | Determines if joint contracture is developing. |
| **3.** Observe for areas of erythema or breakdown involving skin. | Indicates complications of immobility or improper positioning of body part. Determines if need for increasing frequency of repositioning patient. |

## RECORDING AND REPORTING

■ Record procedure and observations (e.g., condition of skin, joint movement, patient's ability to assist with positioning).

■ Report observations at change of shift and document in nurses' notes.

■ Report turning schedule and frequency of repositioning patient at change of shift.

■ Patient avoids moving.
  • Medicate for pain as ordered by a health care provider to ensure patient's comfort before moving.
  • Allow pain medication to take effect before proceeding.

## UNEXPECTED OUTCOMES AND RELATED INTERVENTIONS

■ Joint contractures develop or worsen.
  • Ensure patient is positioned properly.
  • Consider referral to physical or occupational therapy.

■ Skin shows areas of erythema and breakdown.
  • Increase frequency of repositioning.
  • Place turning schedule above patient's bed.
  • Initiate skin care protocol (check agency's policy).

***Prone Position.*** When prone, the patient is in the face-down position. Before placing a patient in the **prone** position, assess the patient's medical record for any possible complications such as increasing intracranial pressure or cardiopulmonary disease (Hoeman, 2002).

Assist the patient in lying on the abdomen. Have the patient turn the head to the side. This facilitates respiration and drainage of oral secretions. Place a pillow under the head for comfort and relief from pressure. As an alternative, place a wedge under the patient's chest, or arms flexed over the head, if it is more comfortable. Place a pillow under the lower leg; this promotes relaxation. If a pillow is unavailable, make sure the patient's ankles are in **dorsiflexion** over the end of the mattress. Body alignment is poor when the ankles are continuously in **plantar flexion** and the lumbar spine remains in **hyperextension**. Sometimes lung expansion is compromised in this position, especially in the obese. Monitor your patient for signs of respiratory distress. You assess for and correct any of the following potential trouble points:

- Neck hyperextension
- Hyperextension of the lumbar spine
- Plantar flexion of the ankles
- Unprotected pressure points at the chin, elbows, hips, knees, and toes

***Lateral Position.*** In the lateral (or side-lying) position, the patient is supported on the right or left side with the opposite arm, thigh, and knee flexed and resting on the bed. You place a pillow under the patient's head to keep the head, neck, and spine in alignment. The upper arm is flexed and supported with a pillow. The upper leg is flexed at the hip and knee and positioned on a small pillow (Hoeman, 2002). Patients who are obese or older are often not able to tolerate this position for any length of time. The following trouble points are common in the side-lying position:

- Lateral flexion of the neck
- Spinal curves out of normal alignment
- Shoulder and hip joints internally rotated, adducted, or unsupported
- Lack of support for the feet
- Lack of protection for pressure points at the ear, shoulder, anterior iliac spine, trochanter, and ankles
- Excessive lateral flexion of the spine if the patient has large hips and a pillow is not placed superior to the hips at the waist

***Sims' Position.*** In the Sims' position the patient is semiprone on the right or left side with the opposite arm, thigh, and knee flexed and resting on the bed. The Sims' position differs from the side-lying position in the distribution of the patient's weight. In this position you place the patient's weight on the anterior ilium, humerus, and clavicle.

Improper positioning causes unnecessary harm to patients, such as pressure ulcers and joint contractures, especially if they have certain preexisting conditions (e.g., peripheral vascular disease, diabetes). Positions that compromise peripheral blood flow damage nerves as well. Every time you reposition the patient, make certain to check total body alignment, placement of extremities, skin breakdown, and joint contractures. Trouble points common in Sims' position include the following:

- Lateral flexion of the neck
- Internal rotation, adduction, or lack of support to the shoulders and hips
- Lack of support for the feet
- Lack of protection for pressure points at the ilium, humerus, clavicle, knees, and ankles

**Transfer Techniques.** You often provide care for immobilized patients who need a position change, who need to be moved up in bed, or who need to be transferred from a bed to a chair or a bed to a stretcher. Proper use of body mechanics enables you to move, lift, or transfer patients safely and also protects you from injury to your musculoskeletal system (Skill 25-2).

You will follow these general guidelines in any transfer procedure:

- Mentally review the transfer steps before beginning to ensure both the patient's and your safety.
- Assess the patient's mobility and strength to determine the assistance he or she is able to offer during transfer.
- Determine the amount and type of assistance you require.
- Explain the procedure, and describe what you expect of the patient.
- Raise the side rail on the side of the bed opposite of where you are standing to prevent the patient from falling out of bed on that side.
- Position the level of the bed to a comfortable and safe height.
- Arrange equipment (e.g., intravenous [IV] lines, feeding tube, Foley catheter) so it will not interfere with the transfer.
- Evaluate patient for correct body alignment and pressure areas after the transfer.

Transferring is a skill that helps the dependent patient regain optimal independence as quickly as possible. Physical activity maintains and improves joint motion, increases strength, promotes circulation, relieves pressure on skin, and improves urinary and respiratory functions. It also benefits the patient psychologically by increasing social activity and mental stimulation and providing a change in environment. Thus mobilization plays a crucial role in the patient's rehabilitation.

One of the major concerns during transfer is the safety of you and your patient. You prevent self-injury by using correct posture, minimal muscle strength, and effective body mechanics and lifting techniques. Always be aware of the patient's motor deficits, ability to aid in transfer, and body weight. As a rule of thumb, GET HELP to transfer a patient.

You will need to consider many special problems in transfer. A patient who has been immobile for several days or longer is often weak or dizzy or sometimes develops

*Text continued on p. 678*

# SKILL 25-2 | Using Safe and Effective Transfer Techniques

## Delegation Considerations

The skill of transfer techniques can be delegated to assistive personnel. Patients whom you are transferring for the first time after prolonged bed rest, extensive surgery, critical illness, or spinal cord trauma require supervision by professional nurses. Before delegation, instruct assistive personnel about:

• Seeking assistance when moving or lifting a patient, for example, when the patient is overweight or confused
• Patient limitations that affect safe transfer techniques

## Equipment

• Transfer belt, sling, or lapboard (as needed), nonskid shoes, bath blankets, pillows
• Wheelchair: position chair at 45-degree angle to bed, lock brakes, remove footrests, lock bed brakes
• Stretcher: position at right angle (90 degrees) to bed, lock brakes on stretcher, lock brakes on bed
• Mechanical/hydraulic lift: use frame, canvas strips or chains, and hammock or canvas strips

| STEP | RATIONALE |
|------|-----------|

## ASSESSMENT

**1.** Assess the patient for the following:

Provides information relative to the patient's abilities, physical status, ability to comprehend, and the number of individuals needed to provide safe transferring.

a. Muscle strength (legs and upper arms)

Immobile patients have decreased muscle strength, tone, and mass. Affects ability to bear weight or raise body.

b. Joint ROM and contracture formation

Immobility or inflammatory processes (e.g., arthritis) lead to contracture formation and impaired joint mobility.

c. Paralysis or paresis (spastic or flaccid)

Patient with central nervous system damage sometimes has bilateral paralysis (requiring transfer by swivel bar, sliding bar, or **Hoyer lift**) or unilateral paralysis, which requires belt transfer to "best" side. Weakness (paresis) requires stabilization of knee while transferring. Flaccid arm needs support with sling during transfer.

d. Risk for orthostatic (postural) hypotension (e.g., previously on bed rest, first time arising from supine position following surgical procedure, history of dizziness when arising)

Determines risk of fainting or falling during transfer. Immobile patients have decreased ability for autonomic nervous system to equalize blood supply, resulting in drop of 15 mm Hg or more in blood pressure when rising from sitting position (Phipps and others, 2003).

e. Activity tolerance

Determines ability of patient to assist with transfer.

f. Level of comfort

Pain reduces patient's motivation and ability to be mobile. Pain relief before transfer enhances patient participation.

g. Vital signs

Vital sign changes such as increased pulse and respiration and change in blood pressure indicate activity intolerance (see Chapter 12).

**2.** Assess patient's sensory status:
a. Adequacy of central and peripheral vision
b. Adequacy of hearing
c. Loss of peripheral sensation

Determines influence of sensory loss on ability to make transfer. Visual field loss decreases patient's ability to see in direction of transfer. Peripheral sensation loss decreases proprioception. Patients with visual and hearing losses need transfer techniques adapted to deficits. Patients with CVA sometimes lose area of visual field, which profoundly affects vision and perception.

---

• *Critical Decision Point:* Patients with hemiplegia also often "neglect" one side of the body (inattention to or unawareness of one side of body or environment), which distorts perception of the visual field. If patient experiences neglect of one side, instruct patient to scan all visual fields when transferring.

---

**3.** Assess patient's cognitive status:

Determines patient's ability to follow directions and learn transfer techniques.

---

• *Critical Decision Point:* Patients with head trauma or CVA have perceptual cognitive deficits that create safety risks. If patient has difficulty in comprehension, simplify instructions and maintain consistency.

---

| STEP | RATIONALE |
|---|---|
| 4. Assess patient's level of motivation:<br>  a. Patient's eagerness versus unwillingness to be mobile<br>  b. Whether patient avoids activity and offers excuses | Altered psychological states reduce patient's desire to engage in activity. |
| 5. Assess previous mode of transfer (if applicable). | Determines mode of transfer and assistance required to provide continuity. Use of transfer belts is necessary with all patients being transferred. |
| 6. Assess patient's specific risk of falling when transferred: Neuromuscular deficits, motor weakness, calcium loss from long bones, cognitive and visual dysfunction, and altered balance. | Certain conditions increase patient's risk of falling or potential for injury. |
| 7. Assess special transfer equipment needed for home setting. Assess home environment for hazards. | Prior teaching of family and support persons, assessment of home for safety risks and functionality, and provision of applicable aids greatly enhance transfer ability at home. |

## PLANNING

| | |
|---|---|
| 1. Gather appropriate equipment. | |
| 2. Perform hand hygiene. | Reduces transmission of microorganisms. |
| 3. Explain procedure to patient. | Increases patient participation. |

## IMPLEMENTATION

| | |
|---|---|
| 1. Transfer patient.<br>  **A. Assist Patient to Sitting Position (Bed at Waist Level)**<br>    (1) Place patient in supine position. | Enables you to assess your patient's body alignment continually and to administer additional care, such as suctioning or hygiene needs. |
|     (2) Face head of bed at a 45-degree angle, and remove pillows. | Proper positioning reduces twisting of your body when moving the patient. Pillows cause interference when the patient is sitting up in bed. |
|     (3) Place feet apart with foot closest to bed behind other foot. | Improves balance and allows transfer of body weight as you move patient to sitting position. |
|     (4) Place hand farther from patient under shoulders, supporting patient's head and cervical vertebrae. | Maintains alignment of head and cervical vertebrae and allows for even lifting of patient's upper trunk. |
|     (5) Place other hand on bed surface. | Provides support and balance. |
|     (6) Raise patient to sitting position by shifting weight from front to back leg. | Improves balance, overcomes inertia, and transfers weight in direction in which you move patient. |
|     (7) Push against bed using arm that is placed on bed surface. | Divides activity between arms and legs and protects back from strain. By bracing one hand against mattress and pushing against it as you lift the patient, you transfer weight away from your back muscles through your arm onto the mattress. |
|   **B. Assist Patient to Sitting Position on Side of Bed With Bed in Low Position**<br>    (1) Turn patient to side, facing you on side of bed on which patient will be sitting (see illustration). | Decreases amount of work needed by you and your patient. |
|     (2) With patient in supine position, raise head of bed 30 degrees. | Prepares patient to move to side of bed and protects from falling. |

| STEP | RATIONALE |
|------|-----------|

(3) Stand opposite patient's hips. Turn diagonally so you face your patient and far corner of foot of bed.

Places your center of gravity nearer patient. Reduces twisting of your body because you are facing the direction of movement.

(4) Place feet apart with foot closer to head of bed in front of other foot.

Increases balance and allows you to transfer weight as you bring patient to sitting position on side of bed.

(5) Place arm nearer head of bed under patient's shoulders, supporting head and neck.

Maintains alignment of head and neck as you bring your patient to a sitting position.

(6) Place other arm over patient's thighs (see illustration).

Supports hip and prevents patient from falling backward during procedure.

(7) Move patient's lower legs and feet over side of bed. Pivot toward rear leg, allowing patient's upper legs to swing downward.

Decreases friction and resistance. Weight of patient's legs when off bed allows gravity to lower legs, and weight of legs assists in pulling upper body in sitting position.

(8) At same time, shift weight to rear leg and elevate patient (see illustration).

Allows you to transfer weight in direction of motion.

(9) Remain in front until patient regains balance, and continue to provide physical support to weak or cognitively impaired patient.

Reduces patient risk for falling. Immobilized patients experience light-headedness or dizziness when assuming a sitting position.

**C. Transferring Patient From Bed to Chair With Bed in Low Position**

(1) Assist patient to sitting position on side of bed. Have chair in position at 45-degree angle to bed on the patient's strong side.

Positions chair within easy access for transfer. Placing the chair on the patient's stronger side will allow the patient to assist when transferring.

(2) Apply transfer belt or other transfer aids.

Transfer belt maintains stability of patient during transfer and reduces risk of falling (Nelson and others, 2003). Put patient's arm in sling if flaccid paralysis is present.

(3) Ensure that patient has stable nonskid shoes. Place weight-bearing or strong leg forward, with weak foot back.

Nonskid soles decrease risk of slipping during transfer. Always have patient wear shoes during transfer; bare feet increase risk of falls. Patient will stand on stronger, or weight-bearing, leg.

(4) Spread your feet apart.

Ensures balance with wide base of support.

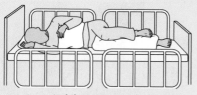

STEP **1B(1)** Side-lying position.

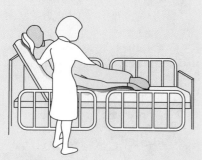

STEP **1B(6)** Nurse places arm over patient's thighs.

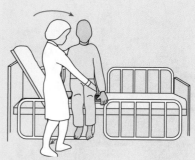

STEP **1B(8)** Nurse shifts weight to rear leg and elevates patient.

## SKILL 25-2 | Using Safe and Effective Transfer Techniques—cont'd

| STEP | RATIONALE |
|---|---|
| (5) Flex your hips and knees, aligning knees with patient's knees (see illustration). | Flexion of knees and hips lowers the center of gravity to object to be raised; aligning knees with patient's allows for stabilization of knees when patient stands. |
| (6) Grasp transfer belt from underneath. | Grasping transfer belt at patient's side provides movement of patient at center of gravity. Never lift patients by or under arms (Nelson and others, 2003). |

---

• *Critical Decision Point:* Use a transfer belt or walking belt with handles in place of the under-axilla technique. The under-axilla technique is physically stressful for nurses and uncomfortable for patients (Owens and others, 1999).

---

| STEP | RATIONALE |
|---|---|
| (7) Rock patient up to standing position on count of three while straightening hips and legs and keeping knees slightly flexed (see illustration). Unless contraindicated, instruct patient to use hands to push up, if applicable. | Rocking motion gives patient's body momentum and requires less muscular effort to lift patient. |
| (8) Maintain stability of patient's weak or paralyzed leg with knee. | Often patient maintains ability to stand on paralyzed or weak limb with support of knee to stabilize. |
| (9) Pivot on foot farther from chair. | Maintains support of patient while allowing adequate space for patient to move. |
| (10) Instruct patient to use armrests on chair for support, and ease into chair (see illustration). | Increases patient stability. |
| (11) Flex hips and knees while lowering patient into chair (see illustration). | Prevents injury from poor body mechanics. |
| (12) Assess patient for proper alignment for sitting position. Provide support for paralyzed extremities. Lapboard or sling will support flaccid arm. Stabilize leg with bath blanket or pillow. | Prevents injury to patient from poor body alignment. |
| (13) Praise patient's progress, effort, or performance. | Continued support and encouragement provide incentive for patient perseverance. |

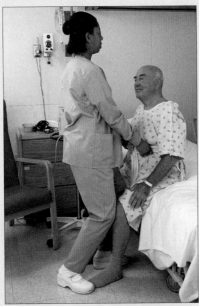

STEP **1C(5)** Nurse flexes hips and knees, aligning knees with patient's knees.

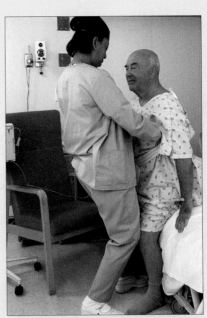

STEP **1C(7)** Nurse rocks patient to standing position.

| STEP | RATIONALE |
|---|---|

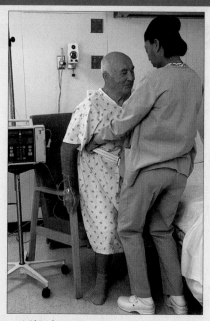

STEP **1C(10)** Patient uses armrests for support.

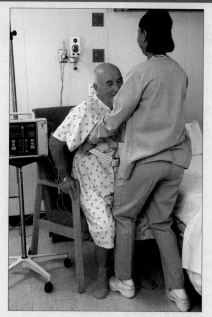

STEP **1C(11)** Nurse eases patient into chair.

**D. Perform Three-Person Carry From Bed to Stretcher (Bed at Stretcher Level)**

Use transfer boards (if available) to transfer a patient from bed to stretcher. These boards reduce friction and significantly reduce the force required to move the patient (Nelson and others, 2003).

(1) Three nurses stand side by side facing side of patient's bed.

Prevents twisting of nurses' bodies. Maintains patient's alignment.

(2) Each person assumes responsibility for one of three areas: head and shoulders, hips and thighs, and ankles.

Distributes patient's body weight evenly.

(3) Each person assumes wide base of support with foot closer to stretcher in front and knees slightly flexed.

Increases balance and lowers center of gravity of person lifting.

(4) Lifters place arms under patient's head and shoulders, hips and thighs, and ankles, with fingers securely around other side of patient's body (see illustration).

Distributes patient's weight over forearms of lifters.

---

• *Critical Decision Point:* Verify that patients with spinal cord injuries are stabilized before transfer. Make sure the inexperienced care provider does not attempt to move the spinal cord–injured patient.

---

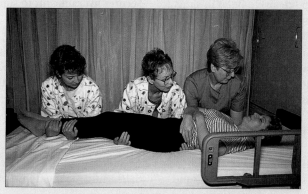

STEP **1D(4)** Proper positioning of lifters during three-person transfer.

## SKILL 25-2 ¦ Using Safe and Effective Transfer Techniques—cont'd

| STEP | RATIONALE |
|---|---|
| (5) Lifters roll patient toward their chests. On count of three, lift patient and hold against nurses' chests. | Moves workload over lifters' base of support. Enables lifters to work together and safely lift patient. |
| (6) On second count of three, nurses step back and pivot toward stretcher, moving forward if needed. | Transfers weight toward stretcher. |
| (7) Gently lower patient onto center of stretcher by flexing knees and hips until elbows are level with edge of stretcher. | Maintains nurses' alignment during transfer. |
| (8) Assess patient's body alignment, place safety straps across body, and raise side rails. | Reduces risk of injury from poor alignment or falling. |

**E. Use Hoyer (Mechanical/Hydraulic) Lift to Transfer Patient From Bed to Chair**

| STEP | RATIONALE |
|---|---|
| (1) Bring lift to bedside. | Ensures safe elevation of patient off bed. (Before using lift, be thoroughly familiar with its operation.) |
| (2) Position chair near bed, and allow adequate space to maneuver lift. | Prepares environment for safe use of lift and subsequent transfer. |
| (3) Raise bed to high position with mattress flat. Lower side rail. | Maintains center of gravity. |
| (4) Keep bed side rail up on the side opposite of you. | Maintains patient safety. |
| (5) Roll patient away from you. | Positions patient for use of lift sling. |
| (6) Place hammock or canvas strips under patient to form sling. With two canvas pieces, lower edge fits under patient's knees (wide piece), and upper edge fits under patient's shoulders (narrow piece). | Two types of seat are supplied with mechanical/hydraulic lift: hammock style is better for patients who are flaccid, weak, and need support; use canvas strips for patients with normal muscle tone. Hooks face away from patient's skin. Place sling under patient's center of gravity and greatest portion of body weight. |
| (7) Raise bed rail. | Maintains patient safety. |
| (8) Go to opposite side of bed, and lower side rail. | |
| (9) Roll patient to opposite side, and pull hammock (strips) through. | Completes positioning of patient on mechanical/hydraulic sling. |
| (10) Roll patient supine onto canvas seat. | Sling extends from shoulders to knees (hammock) to support patient's body weight equally. |
| (11) Remove patient's glasses, if appropriate. | Swivel bar is close to patient's head and could break eyeglasses. |
| (12) Place lift's horseshoe bar under side of bed (on side with chair). | Positions lift efficiently and promotes smooth transfer. |
| (13) Lower horizontal bar to sling level by releasing hydraulic valve. Lock valve. | Positions hydraulic lift close to patient. Locking valve prevents injury to patient. |
| (14) Attach hooks on strap (chain) to holes in sling. Short chains or straps hook to top holes of sling; longer chains hook to bottom of sling. | Secures hydraulic lift to sling. |
| (15) Elevate head of bed. | Positions patient in sitting position. |
| (16) Fold patient's arms over chest. | Prevents injury to paralyzed arms. |
| (17) Pump hydraulic handle using long, slow, even strokes until you raise patient off bed (see illustration). | Ensures safe support of patient during elevation. |
| (18) Use steering handle to pull lift from bed and maneuver to chair. | Moves patient from bed to chair. |
| (19) Roll base around chair. | Positions lift in front of the chair. |
| (20) Release check valve slowly (turn to left), and lower patient into chair (see illustration). | Safely guides patient into back of chair as seat descends. |

| STEP | RATIONALE |
|---|---|

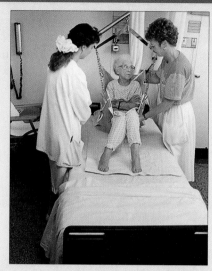

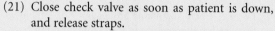

STEP **1E(17)** Patient is raised off bed after being properly placed in the sling.

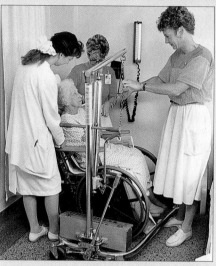

STEP **1E (20)** Use of hydraulic lift to lower patient into chair.

| | |
|---|---|
| (21) Close check valve as soon as patient is down, and release straps. | If valve is left open, boom continues to lower and injure patient. |
| (22) Remove straps and mechanical/hydraulic lift. | Prevents damage to skin and underlying tissues from canvas or hooks. |
| (23) Check patient's sitting alignment, and correct if necessary. | Prevents injury from poor posture. |
| **2.** Perform hand hygiene. | Reduces transmission of microorganisms. |

## EVALUATION

| | |
|---|---|
| **1.** Evaluate vital signs. Ask if patient feels fatigued. | Evaluates patient's response to postural changes and activity. |
| **2.** Observe for correct body alignment and presence of pressure points on skin. | Minimizes risk of immobility complications. |
| **3.** Ask if patient experienced pain during transfer. | Determines need for additional pain control or alternation of technique of transferring. |

## RECORDING AND REPORTING

- Record procedure, including pertinent observations: weakness, ability to follow directions, weight-bearing ability, balance, ability to pivot, number of personnel needed to assist, and amount of assistance (muscle strength) required.
- Report any unusual occurrence to nurse in charge. Report transfer ability and assistance needed to next shift or other caregivers. Report progress or transfer difficulties to rehabilitation staff (physical therapist or occupational therapist).

## UNEXPECTED OUTCOMES AND RELATED INTERVENTIONS

- Patient unable to comprehend and follow directions for transfer.
  - Reassess continuity and simplicity of instructions.
- Patient sustains injury on transfer.
  - Evaluate incident that caused injury (e.g., assessment inadequate, change in patient status, improper use of equipment).
  - Complete occurrence report according to institution policy.
- Patient's level of weakness does not permit active transfer.
  - Obtain increased assistance from nursing personnel.
  - Increase bed activity and exercise to heighten tolerance.

## SKILL 25-2 | Using Safe and Effective Transfer Techniques—cont'd

| STEP | RATIONALE |
|---|---|
| ■ Patient continues to bear weight on non–weight-bearing limb.<br>• Reinforce information about weight-bearing status.<br>■ Patient transfers well on some occasions, poorly on others.<br>• Assess patient for factors that affect ability to transfer (e.g., pain, fatigue, confusion) before transfer.<br>• Allow for a rest period before transferring, medicate for pain if indicated or reorient patient.<br>• Periodic confusion also alters performance. | ■ Patient is unable to stand for time required in transfer.<br>• Provide for adequate assistance during transfer.<br>• Assess for orthostatic changes in blood pressure when transferring patient.<br>■ Localized areas of erythema develop that do not disappear quickly (see Chapter 35).<br>• Establish individualized skin care regimen.<br>• Position patient in 30-degree lateral position. |

**orthostatic hypotension** (a drop in blood pressure of 15 mm Hg or more when rising from a sitting position) when transferred (Phipps and others, 2003). A patient with neurological deficits sometimes has paresis (muscle weakness) or paralysis unilaterally or bilaterally, which complicates safe transfer. A flaccid arm sustains injury during transfer if unsupported. As a general rule, use a transfer belt and obtain assistance for mobilization of such patients.

### Joint Mobility and Ambulation

*Range-of-Motion Exercises.* The easiest intervention to maintain or improve joint mobility for patients and one that you are able to coordinate with other activities is the use of range-of-motion exercises. In **active range-of-motion exercises,** the patient is able to move his or her joints. In contrast, the nurse moves the patient's joints in **passive range-of-motion exercises.** The use of these exercises enables you to systematically assess and improve the patient's joint mobility (see Chapter 34).

Joints that are not moved periodically develop contractures, a permanent shortening of a muscle followed by the eventual shortening of associated ligaments and tendons. Over time the joint becomes fixed in one position, and the patient loses normal use of the joint. For the patient who does not have voluntary motor control, passive range-of-motion exercises are the exercises of choice.

The older adult often experiences a decline in physical activity and changes in joints that predispose to problems with mobility and limit joint flexibility. You will recommend approaches that help older adults to use proper body mechanics and prevent injury (Box 25-7).

Mechanical devices are available for specific joints, which place these joints through continuous passive motion (CPM). You will usually use these CPM machines postoperatively to place joints through a selective repetitive range of motion. You set the machine to certain degrees of joint mobility with increasing joint mobility or flexion as the goal. The most common patients who use the CPM machine are those who have undergone some form of total joint replacement surgery.

| BOX 25-7 | CARE OF THE OLDER ADULT |
|---|---|

• Encourage the older adult patient to avoid prolonged sitting and to get up and stretch. Frequent stretching decreases joint contractures.
• Be sure patient maintains proper body alignment when sitting. Proper alignment minimizes joint and muscle stress.
• Teach patients how to use stronger joints or larger muscle groups to manipulate spray cans, container lids, etc. Efficient distribution of workload decreases joint stress and pain.
• Provide resources for planned exercise programs. Proper exercise activities slow further bone loss and prevent fractures in the older adult with osteoporosis (Burbank and others, 2002; Phipps and others, 2003).
• It is never too late to begin an exercise program (Burbank and others, 2002; O'Brien-Gillespie, 2006). Consult a health care provider before beginning an exercise program, particularly in the presence of heart or lung disease and other chronic illnesses.

Unless contraindicated, the nursing care plan includes exercising each joint through as nearly a full range of motion as possible. Initiate passive range-of-motion exercises as soon as the patient loses the ability to move the extremity or joint (see Chapter 34).

*Walking.* Walking also increases joint mobility. In the normal walking posture the head is erect; the cervical, thoracic, and lumbar vertebrae are aligned; the hips and knees have appropriate flexion; and the arms swing freely in alternation with the legs. Illness or trauma reduces activity tolerance, necessitating a need for assistance with walking or the use of mechanical devices such as crutches, canes, or walkers.

*Assisting a Patient in Walking.* Assisting the patient in walking requires preparation. Assess the patient's activity tolerance, strength, coordination, and balance to determine the type of assistance needed. Also assess the patient's orientation, and determine if there are any signs of distress. This precludes attempts at ambulation.

Evaluate the environment for safety before ambulation. Remove obstacles, be sure the floor is clean and dry, and establish rest points in case the patient's activity tolerance decreases or if the patient becomes dizzy. Also, make sure the patient wears supportive, nonslip shoes.

When preparing a patient for ambulation, dangling is an important technique. You assist the patient to a sitting position with the legs dangling off the side of the bed and have the patient rest for 1 to 2 minutes before standing. The longer the period of immobility, the greater the physiological changes. This is especially true with changes in circulation. When the patient has been flat for extended periods, blood pressure drops when the patient stands. Dangling helps to prevent this. After standing, have the patient remain stationary for a minute or two before moving. If the patient becomes dizzy, the bed is still nearby and you are able to quickly ease him or her back to bed.

You can use several methods for assisting a patient with ambulation. Provide support at the waist by using a gait belt so the patient's center of gravity remains midline. Make sure patients do not lean to one side because their center of gravity is no longer midline, which distorts their balance and increases their risk of falling.

Return the patient who appears unsteady or complains of dizziness to the closest bed or a chair. If the patient has a syncopal episode or begins to fall, you assume a wide base of support with one foot in front of the other, thus supporting the patient's body weight. Gently lower the patient to the floor, protecting the patient's head. Although lowering a patient to the floor is not difficult, practice this technique with a friend or classmate before attempting it in a clinical setting (Figure 25-6).

Patients with hemiplegia (one-sided paralysis) or hemiparesis (one-sided weakness) need assistance in ambulating. Stand by the patient's affected side, and support the patient by holding onto the gait belt around the patient's waist and placing the other arm around the inferior aspect of the patient's upper arm so that your hand is supporting the patient's axilla. The patient's unaffected arm is left free to enable the patient to assist. Providing support by holding the patient's arm is incorrect because, if the patient experiences syncope or fall, it is not easy to support the weight and lower the patient to the floor. In addition, if the patient falls with you holding the arm, you risk dislocating the shoulder joint.

The two-nurse method helps to distribute the patient's weight evenly. The two nurses stand on either side of the patient. Each nurse holds onto the gait belt, and the other arm is around the inferior aspect of the patient's arm so that the hands of both nurses are supporting the patient's axillae.

**RESTORATIVE AND CONTINUING CARE.** Restorative and continuing care involving activity and exercise involves implementing strategies to assist the patient in activities of daily living (ADLs) after the patient's need for acute care is no longer warranted. In collaboration with other health care professionals such as physical therapists, you promote activity

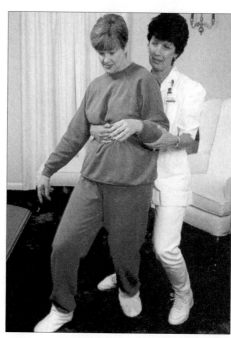

FIGURE **25-6** Ease the patient down to the floor by bending the nurse's knees, keeping the nurse's back straight. (From Birchenall M, Streight ME: *Mosby's textbook for the home care aide*, St. Louis, 1997, Mosby.)

and exercise by teaching the use of canes, walkers, or crutches, depending on the assistive device most appropriate for the patient's condition. Restorative and continuing care includes activities and exercises that restore and improve optimal functioning in the patient with chronic musculoskeletal illnesses, such as arthritis, trauma, and other chronic illnesses, such as coronary artery disease (CAD).

### Assistive Devices for Walking

*Walkers.* Walkers are extremely light, moveable devices, about waist high and made of metal tubing (Figure 25-7). They have four widely placed, sturdy legs. The patient holds the handgrips on the upper bars, takes a step, moves the walker forward, and takes another step.

*Canes.* Canes are lightweight, easily moveable devices about waist high, made of wood or metal. Two common types of canes are the single straight-legged cane and the quad cane. The single straight-legged cane is more common and is used to support and balance a patient with decreased leg strength. Make sure the patient keeps the cane on the stronger side of the body. For maximum support when walking, the patient places the cane forward 15 to 25 cm (6 to 10 inches), keeping body weight on both legs. The patient moves the weaker leg to the cane, which divides body weight between the cane and the stronger leg. The patient then advances the stronger leg past the cane so the weaker leg and the body weight is supported by the cane and weaker leg. During walking, the patient continually repeats these three steps. Teach the patient that two points of support, such as both feet or one foot and the cane, are present at all times.

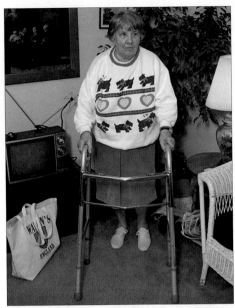

FIGURE **25-7** Patient using a walker.

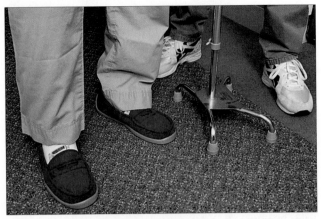

FIGURE **25-8** Base of quad cane.

The quad cane provides the most support and is used when there is partial or complete leg paralysis or some hemiplegia (Figure 25-8). You teach the same three steps used with the straight-legged cane to the patient.

*Crutches.* The use of crutches is usually temporary, such as after ligament damage to the knee. However, some patients, such as those with paralysis of the lower extremities, need crutches permanently. A crutch is a wooden or metal staff. The two types of crutches are the double adjustable Lofstrand or forearm crutch (Figure 25-9) and the axillary wooden or metal crutch. The forearm crutch has a handgrip and a metal band that fits around the patient's forearm. The metal band and the handgrip are adjustable to fit the patient's height. The axillary crutch has a padded curved surface at the top, which fits under the axilla. The patient holds a handgrip in the form of a crossbar at the level of the palms to support the body. It is important to measure crutches for the appropriate length and to teach patients to use their crutches safely. This includes teaching the patient to achieve a stable gait, to ascend and descend stairs, and to rise from a sitting position. You or a physical therapist will teach the patient safety measures and guidelines associated with the use of crutches (Box 25-8).

*Measuring for Crutches.* The axillary crutch is the crutch more commonly used. Measurements include the patient's height, the angle of elbow flexion, and the distance between the crutch pad and the axilla. When fitting crutches, the appropriate length of the crutch is from three to four finger widths from the axilla to a point 15 cm (6 inches) lateral to the patient's heel (Hoeman, 2002) (Figure 25-10).

Make sure you position the handgrips so the axillae do not support all patient's body weight. Pressure on the axillae increases risk to underlying nerves, which sometimes results in partial paralysis of the arm. You determine the correct position of the handgrips with the patient upright, supporting

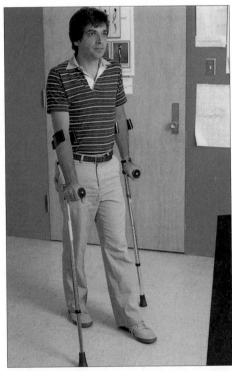

FIGURE **25-9** Double adjustable Lofstrand or forearm crutch.

weight by the handgrips with the elbows slightly flexed (20 to 25 degrees). You verify elbow flexion with a goniometer (Figure 25-11). When you have determined the height and placement of the handgrips, you again verify that the distance between the crutch pad and the patient's axilla is three to four finger widths (Figure 25-12).

*Crutch Gait.* The patient assumes the **crutch gait** by alternatively bearing weight on one or both legs and on the crutches. The health care provider determines the gait by assessing the patient's physical and functional abilities and the disease or injury that resulted in the need for crutches. This section summarizes the basic crutch stance and the four

| BOX 25-8 | PATIENT TEACHING |
| --- | --- |

### Crutch Safety

The physical therapist (PT) told Marilyn that Mr. Indelicato will need crutches for a short period of time because of limited weight bearing on the affected knee. It is important that Mr. Indelicato begin to use the crutches before discharge. Marilyn and the PT work together to develop the following teaching plan:

### Outcomes

- Patient will state the steps needed for safe crutch walking.
- Patient will describe how to identify axillary pressure points.
- Patient will demonstrate safe crutch walking.

### Teaching Strategies

- Tell patient about the dangers of pressure on the axilla and how to identify pressure in the axillary region.
- Instruct patient not to lean on his crutches to support body weight.
- Demonstrate to patient how to inspect the crutch tips routinely. Make sure the rubber tips are securely attached to the crutches. When the tips are worn, they need replacing immediately. Rubber crutch tips increase surface friction and prevent the crutches from slipping.

- Inform patient about the importance of keeping the crutch tips' dry. If the tips become wet, the patient needs to dry them. Water decreases surface friction and increases the risk that the crutches will slip.
- Show patient how to inspect the structure of the crutches routinely. Cracks in a wooden crutch decrease the crutch's ability to support weight. Bends in aluminum crutches alter body alignment, increasing the risk of further damage to the musculoskeletal system.
- Give patients a list of medical suppliers in their community. This allows the patients to obtain repairs, new rubber tips, handgrips, and crutch pads.
- Suggest that patient investigate the possibility of having a set of spare crutches and tips.

### Evaluation Strategies

- Ask patient to describe how he will maintain crutch safety.
- Observe patient inspect his crutch tips and structure.
- Observe patient using the crutches.
- Observe axillae for signs of pressure or skin breakdown.
- Ask patient what he will do if his crutch breaks or he needs additional crutch tips.

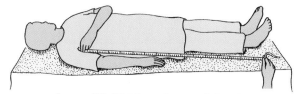

FIGURE **25-10** Measuring crutch length.

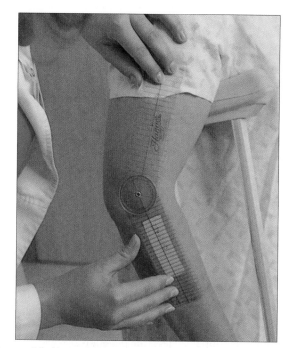

FIGURE **25-11** Using the goniometer to verify correct degree of elbow flexion for crutch use.

standard gaits: four-point alternating gait, three-point alternating gait, two-point gait, and swing-through gait.

The basic crutch stance is the tripod position, formed when the crutches are placed 15 cm (6 inches) in front of and 15 cm to the side of each foot (Figure 25-13). This position improves the patient's balance by providing a wider base of support. The body alignment of the patient in the tripod position includes erect head and neck, straight vertebrae, and extended hips and knees. No weight should be borne by the axillae. The tripod position is used before crutch walking.

Four-point alternating or four-point gait gives stability to the patient but requires weight bearing on both legs. Each leg is moved alternately with each opposing crutch so that three points of support are on the floor at all times (Figure 25-14).

Three-point alternating or three-point gait requires the patient to bear all of the weight on one foot. In a three-point gait, the patient puts weight on both crutches and then on the uninvolved leg, and then repeats the sequence (Figure 25-15). The affected leg does not touch the ground during the early phase of the three-point gait. Gradually the patient progresses to touchdown and full weight bearing on the affected leg.

The two-point gait requires at least partial weight bearing on each foot (Figure 25-16). The patient moves a crutch at the same time as the opposite leg, so the crutch movements are similar to arm motion during normal walking.

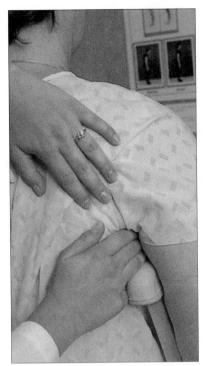

FIGURE **25-12** Verifying correct distance between crutch pad and axilla.

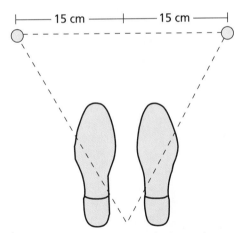

FIGURE **25-13** Tripod position, basic crutch stance.

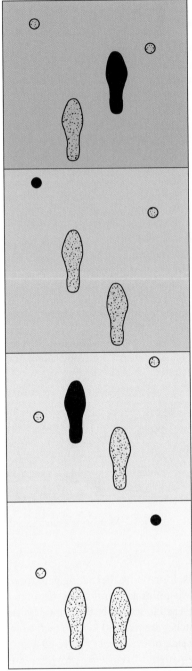

FIGURE **25-14** Four-point alternating gait. Solid feet and crutch tips show foot and crutch tip moved in each of the four phases. (Read from bottom to top).

Paraplegics who wear weight-supporting braces on their legs frequently use the swing-through gait. With weight placed on the supported legs, the patient places the crutches one stride in front and then swings to or through the crutches while they support the patient's weight.

*Crutch Walking on Stairs.* When ascending stairs on crutches, the patient usually uses a modified three-point gait (Figure 25-17). The patient stands at the bottom of the stairs and transfers body weight to the crutches. The patient advances the unaffected leg between the crutches to the stairs. The patient then shifts weight from the crutches to the unaf-

fected leg. Finally, the patient aligns both crutches on the stairs. The patient repeats this sequence until the patient reaches the top of the stairs.

To descend the stairs (Figure 25-18), patients also use a three-phase sequence. The patient transfers body weight to the unaffected leg. The patient places crutches on the stair, and the patient begins to transfer body weight to the crutches, moving the affected leg forward. Finally, the pa-

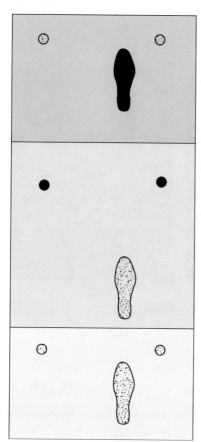

FIGURE **25-15** Three-point gait with weight borne on unaffected leg. Solid foot and crutch tips show weight bearing in each phase. (Read from bottom to top).

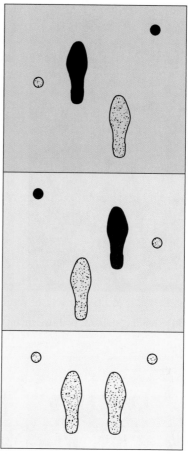

FIGURE **25-16** Two-point gait with weight borne partially on each foot and each crutch advancing with opposing leg. Solid areas indicate leg and crutch tips bearing weight. (Read from bottom to top).

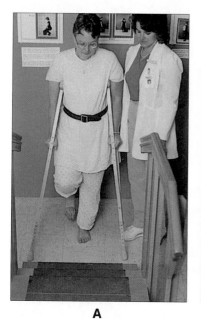
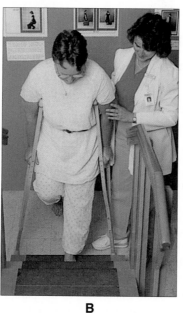
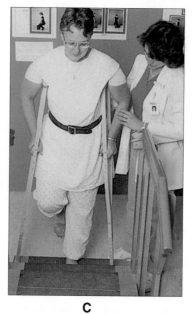

| A | B | C |

FIGURE **25-17** Ascending stairs. **A,** Weight is placed on crutches. **B,** Weight is transferred from crutches to unaffected leg on stairs. **C,** Crutches are aligned with unaffected leg on stairs.

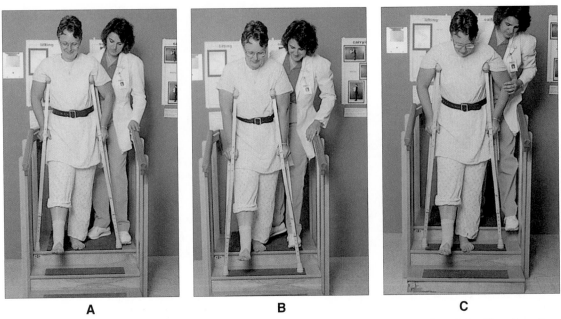

FIGURE **25-18** Descending stairs. **A,** Body weight on unaffected leg. **B,** Body weight transferred to crutches. **C,** Unaffected leg aligned on stairs with crutches.

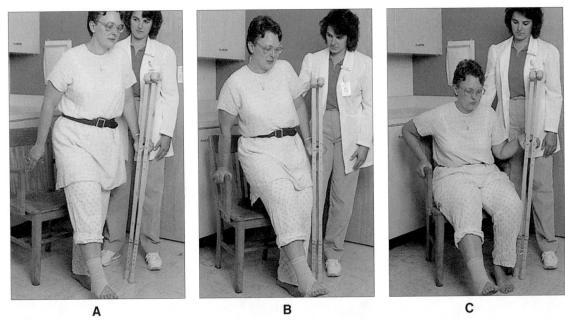

FIGURE **25-19** Sitting on chair. **A,** Both crutches are held by one hand. Patient transfers weight to crutches and unaffected leg. **B,** Patient grasps arm of chair with free hand and begins to lower herself into chair. **C,** Patient completely lowers herself into chair.

tient moves the unaffected leg to the stairs with the crutches. Again, the patient repeats the sequence until reaching the bottom of the stairs.

*Sitting in a Chair With Crutches.* As with crutch walking and crutch walking up and down stairs, the procedure for sitting in a chair involves phases and requires the patient to transfer weight (Figure 25-19). First, the patient gets positioned at the center front of the chair with the posterior aspect of the legs touching the chair. Then the patient holds both crutches in the hand opposite the affected leg. If both legs are affected, as with a paraplegic who wears weight-supporting braces, the patient holds the crutches in the hand on the patient's stronger side. With both crutches in one hand, the patient supports body weight on the unaffected leg and crutches.

## OUTCOME EVALUATION

TABLE 25-3

| Nursing Action | Patient Response/Finding | Achievement of Outcome |
|---|---|---|
| Measure degree of knee flexion. | Able to flex knee to a 70-degree angle. Complains of pain at 75 degrees of flexion. | Outcome partially met. Determine need for analgesic before flexion exercises. |
| Observe Mr. Indelicato's ROM or use of CPM machine. | Able to perform ROM and use CPM machine. | Outcome met. Mr. Indelicato expresses understanding of need for ROM and CPM machine. |
| Observe Mr. Indelicato's ambulation. | Steady gait with aid of walker. | Outcome met. Demonstrates correct use of walker. |
| Ask Mr. Indelicato to rate level of pain on a 10-point scale. | Mr. Indelicato reports a 7 on the pain scale during use of CPM machine. | Outcome not met. Need to provide analgesic before use of CPM machine. |

## EVALUATION

It has been 5 weeks since Marilyn began to care for Mr. Indelicato. For the last 4 weeks she has followed him in the outpatient rehabilitation setting. Mr. Indelicato has progressed steadily to increase both weight bearing and range of joint motion on the affected knee. His pain was more difficult to manage. Mr. Indelicato expected pain to be completely resolved on hospital discharge and did not expect pain to follow his physical therapy. Marilyn and the physical therapist worked with Mr. Indelicato and his orthopedic surgeon to identify pain-control measures following physical therapy. Currently Mr. Indelicato takes 600 mg of ibuprofen 45 minutes before physical therapy and every 8 to 12 hours thereafter. Mr. Indelicato reports that his pain is now almost totally gone. He is now working on increasing strength so he is able to return to golf and bike riding. He says he will probably give up racquetball and tennis.

**Documentation Note**

"Weight bearing and range of motion continue to improve. States takes 600 mg ibuprofen 45 minutes before coming to therapy and every 8 to 12 hours as needed for pain. Rates pain a 1 when exercising. States would like to begin riding bike and playing golf again in next 1 to 2 months."

While still holding the crutches, the patient grasps the arm of the chair with the remaining hand and lowers the body into the chair. To stand, the patient reverses the procedure and when fully erect, assumes the tripod position before beginning to walk.

### 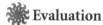 Evaluation

**PATIENT CARE.** You evaluate all nursing interventions by comparing the patient's actual response to the expected outcomes for each goal (Table 25-3). You will evaluate specific outcomes designed to demonstrate improved activity and exercise. If the patient does not achieve the expected outcomes, you will need to revise the care plan. The success in meeting each outcome is based on the use of evaluative measures such as ROM, ability of patient to ambulate, and activity/exercise tolerance.

**PATIENT EXPECTATIONS.** For the patient with alterations in body mechanics or joint mobility, you measure the effectiveness of nursing interventions by the success of meeting the patient's expected outcomes and goals of care. For some patients with altered body mechanics or joint mobility, maintenance of joint mobility will be easily accomplished and will not be a priority goal. For others, return of joint mobility and maintenance of body alignment will be the most important outcome and you will direct all interventions toward its accomplishment.

For you to evaluate the patient's perception of the interventions, first you need to know the patient's expectations concerning joint mobility, posture, or body alignment. What is acceptable or anticipated on your part is sometimes vastly different from what the patient and family members anticipate or accept.

## KEY CONCEPTS

- Muscles primarily associated with movement are located near the skeletal region, where movement results from leverage.
- Muscles primarily associated with posture are located in the lower extremities, trunk, neck, and back.
- The cerebellum and inner ear control balance.
- Body alignment is the positioning of joints, tendons, ligaments, and muscles in various body positions.

- You achieve body balance when there is a wide base of support, the center of gravity falls within the base of support, and vertical line falls from the center of gravity through the base of support.
- Conditions that affect body alignment and mobility include postural abnormalities, altered bone formation or joint mobility, impaired muscle development, central nervous system damage, and musculoskeletal system trauma.

- Assessment of a patient's mobility enables you to determine the patient's coordination, balance, and ability to complete activities of daily living and makes it possible to evaluate or plan an exercise program.
- Assessing gait allows you to draw some conclusions about the patient's balance, posture, and ability to walk without assistance.

- Patients with impaired body alignment require nursing interventions to maintain them in the supported Fowler's, supine, prone, side-lying, and Sims' positions.
- Transfer techniques require the use of correct body mechanics.
- Mechanical devices, such as canes and walkers, require specific nursing interventions to promote walking.

## CRITICAL THINKING IN PRACTICE

*Mr. Timber is 65 years old and had a knee replacement 2 days ago. He has type 2 diabetes mellitus. The nurse tells you that he is "uncooperative" and refuses to use his crutches or get up in the chair. In addition, he continually turns his CPM machine off. He is allowed partial weight bearing on his right leg.*

1. During your assessment of Mr. Timber, what potential barriers is he experiencing that are preventing him from participating in his treatment?
2. Which of the following statements from Mr. Timber do you address first?
   a. "My pain level is 8 out of 10. I just can't take it."
   b. "I don't understand how to use those crutches."
   c. "I've been in this bed for 2 days, and I feel weak."
3. Mr. Timber has agreed to begin crutch training. However, this is his first time out of bed since his surgery. What risk factors does he possess that contribute to orthostatic hypotension, and what interventions do you initiate before attempting to transfer Mr. Timber?
4. You find out that Mr. Timber is anxious about the CPM machine. He states, "I don't think that machine is safe to use." Describe what measures you will take to assess the safety of the CPM machine and how you will help to alleviate Mr. Timber's anxiety.
5. Which is the most appropriate crutch gait for Mr. Timber? Explain your choice.
   a. Two-point
   b. Three-point
   c. Four-point
   d. Swing through

## NCLEX® REVIEW

1. A patient begins to fall during ambulation. To prevent injury to the patient, you:
   1. Call for assistance
   2. Slide her down your body to the floor
   3. Instruct the patient to sit in the nearest chair
   4. Contact the health care provider, and document the fall
2. A principle of good body mechanics includes:
   1. Keeping knees in locked position
   2. Maintaining a wide base of support
   3. Bending at the waist to maintain center of gravity
   4. Holding objects away from the body for better leverage
3. Passive range-of-motion exercises prevent:
   1. Contractures
   2. Osteoporosis
   3. Muscle atrophy
   4. Renal calculi formation
4. A necessary safety precaution when ambulating a patient is to:
   1. Have family members present
   2. Have patient wear well-fitting rubber-soled shoes or slippers
   3. Have at least two people present to assist the patient
   4. Be sure no pain medication was given for at least 3 hours before ambulation

5. The piece of equipment that works best to help ambulate an unsteady patient is:
   1. A walker
   2. Crutches
   3. A wheelchair
   4. A mechanical lift device
6. A device that helps prevent footdrop is the:
   1. Foot roll
   2. Footboard
   3. Trochanter roll
   4. Ankle-foot splint
7. Two nurses are standing on opposite sides of the bed to move a patient up in bed with a drawsheet. In relation to the patient, they stand even with the patient's:
   1. Hips
   2. Chest
   3. Knees
   4. Shoulders
8. A health care provider orders partial weight bearing on the left foot of a patient with a broken ankle and full weight bearing on the right foot. The crutch gait that the patient uses is the:
   1. Two-point
   2. Four-point
   3. Three-point
   4. Swing-through

## REFERENCES

Ackley BJ, Ladwig GB: *Nursing diagnosis handbook: a guide to planning care,* ed 6, St. Louis, 2004, Mosby.

American Nurses Association: *Position statement on elimination of manual patient handling to prevent work-related musculoskeletal disorders,* 2003, http://www.nursingworld.org/readroom/position/workplac/pathand.htm.

Birchenall M, Streight ME: *Mosby's textbook for the home care aide,* St. Louis, 1997, Mosby.

Burbank PM and others: Exercise and older adults: changing behavior with the transtheoretical model, *Orthop Nurs* 21(4):51, 2002.

Buss IC, Halfens RJG, Abu-Sand HH: The most effective time interval for repositioning subjects at risk of pressure sore development: a literature review, *Rehabil Nurs* 27(2):59, 2002.

Dochterman JM, Bulechek GM, editors: *Nursing interventions classification (NIC),* ed 4, St. Louis, 2004, Mosby.

Gahart BL, Nazareno AR: *2002 intravenous medications: a handbook for nurses and allied health professionals,* St. Louis, 2002, Mosby.

Glenn-Molali NH: Nourishment and swallowing. In Hoeman SP, editor, *Rehabilitation nursing: process, application, and outcomes,* ed 3, St. Louis, 2002, Mosby.

Hockenberry DL and others: *Whaley and Wong's nursing care of infants and children,* ed 7, St. Louis, 2003, Mosby.

Hoeman SP: *Rehabilitation nursing: process, application and outcomes,* ed 3, St. Louis, 2002, Mosby.

Huether SE, McCance KL: *Understanding pathophysiology,* ed 3, St. Louis, 2004, Mosby.

Lee ET and others: Incidence of diabetes in American Indians of three geographic areas, *Diabetes Care* 25:49, 2002.

Moorhead S, Johnson M, Maas M: *Nursing outcomes classification (NOC),* ed 3, St. Louis, 2004, Mosby.

Moreno J: Limit liability with lift programs, *Provider* 29(1):41, 2003.

National Institutes of Health Consensus Development Panel on Physical Activity and Cardiovascular Health: Physical activity and cardiovascular health, *JAMA* 276(3):241, 1996.

Nelson A, Fragala G, Menzel H: Myths and facts about back injuries in nursing, *Am J Nurs* 103(2):32, 2003.

Nelson A and others: Safe patient handling and movement: preventing back injury among nurses requires careful selection of the safest equipment and techniques, *Am J Nurs* 103(3):32, 2003.

O'Brien-Gillespie H: Exercise. In Edelman CL, Mandle CL, editors: *Health promotion throughout the lifespan,* ed 6, St. Louis, 2006, Mosby.

Occupational Safety and Health Association: *Ergonomics: guidelines for nursing homes,* 2003, http://www.osha.gov/ergonomics/guidelines/nursinghome/final_nh_guidelines.html.

Owens B and others: What are we teaching about lifting and transferring patients? *Res Nurs Health* 22:3, 1999.

Phipps WJ and others: *Medical surgical nursing,* ed 7, St. Louis, 2003, Mosby.

Prochaska JO and others: *Changing for good,* New York, 1994, William Morrow.

Rimmer JH and others: Feasibility of a health promotion intervention for a group of predominantly African American women with type 2 diabetes, *Diabetes Educ* 28(4):571, 2002.

Schlicht J and others: Build self-efficacy to promote exercise adherence, *ACSM Health Fitness J* 3(6):27, 1999.

Thibodeau GA, Patton KT: *Anatomy and physiology,* ed 5, St. Louis, 2003, Mosby.

Trinkoff AM and others: Musculoskeletal problems of the neck, shoulder, and back and functional consequences in nurses, *Am J Ind Med* 41(3):170, 2002.

Vincent KR and others: Improved cardiorespiratory endurance following 6 months of resistance exercise in elderly men and women, *Arch Intern Med* 162:673, 2002.

Wilson SF, Giddens JF: *Health assessment for nursing practice,* ed 3, St. Louis, 2005, Mosby.

# CHAPTER 26

# Safety

## MEDIA RESOURCES

**CD COMPANION**  *evolve* **WEBSITE**

http://evolve.elsevier.com/Potter/basic

- **NCLEX® Review**
- **Audio Glossary**
- **English/Spanish Audio Glossary**
- **Video Clip**

## OBJECTIVES

- Describe how unmet basic physiological needs of oxygen, nutrition, temperature, and humidity threaten safety.
- Discuss methods to reduce physical hazards and the transmission of pathogens.
- Discuss the specific risks to safety as they pertain to developmental age.
- Identify factors to assess when it becomes necessary to physically restrain a patient.
- Describe four categories of safety risks in a health care agency.

- Describe assessment activities designed to identify a patient's physical, psychological, and cognitive status as it relates to safety.
- State nursing diagnoses associated with risks to safety.
- Develop a nursing care plan for patients whose safety is threatened.
- Describe nursing interventions specific to the patient's age for reducing risk of falls, fires, poisonings, and electrical hazards.
- Describe methods to evaluate interventions designed to maintain or promote safety.

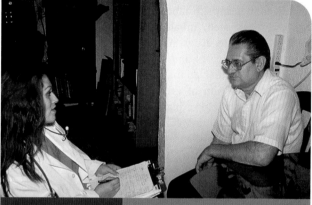

### CASE STUDY   Mr. Gonzales

Mr. Gonzales is a 68-year-old man who has lived alone in a senior apartment building since his wife died 6 months ago. He and his wife were born in Mexico but came to live in the United States shortly after they were married. He is retired from a produce warehouse where he worked for 37 years. He and his wife raised three sons, who are all married and have families of their own. The closest son, Carlos, is 30 minutes away by car. Carlos visits Mr. Gonzales every week to socialize and take him shopping. Mr. Gonzales is generally healthy but has decreased visual acuity, hearing loss from the noisy warehouse job, and some "arthritis." He expects to live at least as long as his father, who lived to be 92 years old. Since his wife's death, Mr. Gonzales has attended Catholic mass every day at his parish church, where his wife had attended daily.

Joani Green, a 25-year-old married mother of two, is currently a senior nursing student at the local college. As part of the clinical requirements for the home care course, she and her partner are conducting health screenings and providing health promotion education for the residents of the apartment building where Mr. Gonzales lives. Part of her screening will include Mr. Gonzales' home environment.

Safety, the freedom from psychological and physical injury, is a basic human need. Health care, provided in a safe manner, and a safe community environment are essential for a patient's well-being. A safe environment reduces the risk of accidents and helps to contain the cost of health care. One of your primary responsibilities as a nurse is to protect patients from harm. Including interventions for a safe environment in your plan of care increase a patient's safety.

### KEY TERMS

AMBULARM, p. 701
carbon monoxide, p. 690
food poisoning, p. 690
grounded, p. 710
heat exhaustion, p. 690

hypothermia, p. 690
immunization, p. 691
pathogen, p. 691
poison, p. 690
poison control center, p. 709
restraint, p. 701

## Scientific Knowledge Base

Vulnerable groups that often require help in achieving a safe environment include infants, children, older adults, the ill, the physically and mentally disabled, the illiterate, and the poor. To be effective, you need to understand factors that contribute to a safe environment in the home or health care agency and thoroughly assess the environment for threats to safety. You also need to understand how alterations in mobility, sensory function, and cognitive function affect a patient's safety (see Chapters 34 and 36). A safe environment includes meeting basic human needs, reducing physical hazards, and reducing transmission of pathogens.

### Basic Human Needs

Basic human needs often at risk from a variety of environmental hazards include the physiological needs of adequate oxygen, nutrition, and favorable temperature and humidity.

**OXYGEN.** A common environmental hazard in the home is an improperly functioning heating system. A furnace that is not properly vented introduces carbon monoxide into the environment. **Carbon monoxide** is a colorless, odorless, poisonous gas produced by the combustion of carbon or organic fuels. This gas binds strongly with hemoglobin, preventing the formation of oxyhemoglobin and thus reducing the supply of oxygen delivered to the tissues (see Chapter 28). Low concentrations cause nausea, dizziness, headache, and fatigue. Higher concentrations are often fatal (National Safety Council, 2002a). Carbon monoxide is responsible for more than half of all fatal inhalation poisonings in the United States (Hockenberry, 2005).

**NUTRITION.** In the home, patients need to properly refrigerate, store, and prepare food. The patient needs a refrigerator with a freezer compartment to keep perishable foods fresh. An adequate, clean water supply is necessary for drinking and to wash fresh produce and dishes. Provisions for garbage collection are necessary to maintain sanitary conditions. Foods need to be adequately cooked to kill any residing organisms. If the patient does not adequately prepare or store foods, this will increase the patient's risk for infections and **food poisoning.** Groups at the highest risk are children, pregnant women, older adults, and people with compromised immune systems (Nix, 2005). Eating food contaminated by bacteria such as *E. coli, Salmonella, Shigella,* or *Listeria* will cause food poisoning. Although most food-borne diseases are bacterial, the hepatitis A virus is spread by fecal contamination of food, water, or milk.

**TEMPERATURE.** A person's comfort zone is usually between 18.3° and 23.8° C (65° and 75° F). Temperature extremes, which often occur during the winter and summer, affect comfort, productivity, and safety. Exposure to severe cold for prolonged periods causes frostbite and accidental **hypothermia** (see Chapter 12). Older adults, the young, patients with cardiovascular conditions, patients who have ingested drugs or excess alcohol, and the homeless are at high risk for hypothermia. Exposure to extreme heat changes the body's electrolyte balance and raises the core body temperature, resulting in heatstroke or **heat exhaustion.** People at risk from high environmental temperatures need to avoid extremely hot, humid environments, or heat exhaustion will result.

**HUMIDITY.** The relative humidity of the air affects a patient's health and safety. Relative humidity is the amount of water vapor in the air compared with the maximum amount of water vapor that the air could contain at the same temperature. Increasing the environmental humidity with the use of a home humidifier has therapeutic benefits for patients with upper respiratory infections. The increase in humidity helps to liquefy pulmonary secretions and improves breathing.

## Physical Hazards

Physical hazards in the environment threaten a person's safety and result in physical or psychological injury or death. Motor vehicle accidents are the leading cause of unintentional death, followed by poisonings, falls, suffocation, and drowning (National Safety Council, 2002b). As a nurse you play an important role by anticipating potential hazards in the health care setting and patient's home and then implementing appropriate nursing interventions.

Common hazards in the home include inadequate lighting, barriers along normal walking paths and stairways, and a lack of safety devices. Inadequate lighting causes eyestrain while the patient carries out daily activities. Poorly illuminated stairs or walkways increase the risk of injury from falls. Injuries frequently result from accidental contact with objects on stairs, floors, bedside tables, closet shelves, refrigerator tops, and bookshelves. Older adults, patients with impaired vision, and patients with impaired mobility are at greater risk of injury due to falls. Observe the patient's home for clutter and the condition of stairways, bathrooms, and limited-access areas to be sure safety devices are in place, such as handrails around toilets and grab bars in showers.

A **poison** is any substance that impairs health or destroys life when ingested, inhaled, or absorbed by the body. Poisoning, due to drugs, medicines, other solid and liquid substances, and gases and vapors, is the leading cause of death in the home (National Safety Council, 2002a). Poisons impair the function of every major organ system. In the home, accidental poisoning is a greater risk for the toddler, preschooler, and young school-age child, who often ingest household cleaning solutions, medications, or personal hygiene products. However, the 25-to-44 age-group has the highest death rate for poisoning. Poisoning is also a risk for health care providers who work around chemicals such as mercury and toxic cleaning agents. Mercury is common in glass thermometers and sphygmomanometers. When there is equipment breakage, health care workers and patients are at risk for exposure to mercury. When a person has ingested a poisonous substance or comes in contact with a chemical that is absorbed through the skin, emergency treatment is a necessity. Specific antidotes or treatments are available only for some types of poisons. A poison control center is the best resource for patients needing information about the treatment of an accidental poisoning.

Home fires are a major cause of death and injury. Smoking materials such as cigarettes, cigars, and pipes are the leading cause of fire deaths in the United States. Roughly one in every four fire deaths in 2001 was caused by smoking materials (National Fire Protection Association, 2004). Many fatal fires are the result of individuals smoking in bed and accidentally falling asleep. Another problem related to fatal fires is a failure to keep fresh batteries in home smoke detectors.

When they strike, natural disasters such as floods, tsunamis, hurricanes, tornadoes, and wildfires are also a major cause of death and injury. These types of disasters kill one million people around the world each decade and leave millions more homeless (FEMA, 2004a). It is important for individuals and communities to focus on preparation and mitigation to avoid losses and to reduce the risk of injury associated with these types of disasters.

A new potential environmental health threat is the possibility of a bioterrorist attack. Threats of this type come in the form of biological, chemical, and radiological. A biological attack involves release of a biological agent, such as anthrax, plague, botulism, smallpox, and typhoid, into the environment. A chemical attack includes spreading a toxic agent such as cyanide, mustard gas, chlorine, or nerve agents (e.g., tabun or sarin). Radiological events threaten the community by dispersal of radioactive materials into the food and water supply, over terrain, or as a "dirty bomb." Although the likelihood is low, disaster can strike quickly and without warning. It forces members of a community to evacuate neighborhoods or be confined to their homes. The Federal Emergency Management Agency's (FEMA's) Family Protection Program and the American Red Cross' Disaster Education Program provide nationwide efforts to help community members prepare for disasters of all types (FEMA, 2004b).

## Pathogen Transmission

Pathogens and parasites pose a threat to patient safety. A **pathogen** is any microorganism capable of producing an illness (see Chapter 11). The most common means of transmission of pathogens is by the hands. For example, if an individual infected with hepatitis A does not wash his or her hands thoroughly after having a bowel movement, the risk of transmitting the disease during food preparation is great. One of the most effective ways to limit the transmission of pathogens is the medical aseptic practice of hand washing.

The human immunodeficiency virus (HIV), the pathogen that causes acquired immunodeficiency syndrome (AIDS), and the hepatitis B virus are transmitted through blood and other body fluids. Drug abusers frequently share syringes and needles, which increases their risk of acquiring these viruses. Some state and many nonprofit organizations fund syringe exchange programs as a means to slow down the spread of infectious diseases obtained through needle sharing (Coalition for Safe Community Needle Disposal, 2005a). Unsafe sexual practices, such as unprotected sexual intercourse or oral sex, also increase the likelihood of contracting AIDS, as well as other sexually transmitted diseases.

Insects and rodents are carriers of pathogens. For example, some mosquitoes are carriers of malaria, and rats and mice carry rat-bite fever. Uncontrolled mosquito and rodent populations increase the risk of these diseases. Persons living at the poverty level sometimes live in homes that landlords do not maintain. Rat and roach infestation are common problems.

Adequate disposal of human waste also controls the transmission of pathogens and parasites. Without a satisfactory sewer and waste system, the population is at risk for illnesses such as typhoid fever and hepatitis.

Immunization often reduces or prevents the transmission of disease from person to person. **Immunization** is the process by which resistance to an infectious disease is produced or increased. The body acquires active immunity by injecting a small amount of weakened or dead organisms and modified toxins from the organism (toxoids) into the body. Passive immunity occurs when antibodies produced by other persons or animals are introduced into a person's bloodstream for protection against a pathogen. Encourage all adults to have their children immunized and to receive regular immunizations for influenza and tetanus.

Health care agencies are concerned with the processing of biohazardous wastes. It is important that you properly dispose of needles, surgical dressings, and syringes to prevent the risk of exposure to the general population and employees. You also need to clean or dispose of bed linens and patient gowns contaminated by body fluids to reduce threats to safety.

## Nursing Knowledge Base

A person's developmental stage, lifestyle habits, mobility status, sensory and cognitive impairments, and safety awareness all influence threats to safety. In the United States accidents are the leading cause of death in people between 1 and 34 years of age and the fifth leading cause overall (Centers for Disease Control and Prevention [CDC], 2001). It is important to be aware of the threats to safety and to teach patients, parents, and other caregivers how to lessen the dangers.

### Developmental Level

**INFANT, TODDLER, AND PRESCHOOLER.** Injuries are the leading cause of death in children over age 1 and cause more death and disability than do all diseases combined (Hockenberry, 2005). The nature of an injury is closely related to normal growth and development. For example, the incidence of lead poisoning is highest in late infancy and toddlerhood because of the ability to explore the environment and the increase in oral activity in which toddlers put environmental objects in their mouths. Accidents involving children are largely preventable, but parents need to be aware of specific dangers at each stage of growth and development. Accident prevention requires health education for parents and the removal of dangers whenever possible.

**SCHOOL-AGE CHILD.** When children enter school, their environment expands to include the school, the means of transportation to and from school, and after-school activities. School-age children are learning how to perform more complicated motor activities and oftentimes are uncoordinated. Instruct parents and teachers about safe practices to follow at school and during play. Teach school-age children involved in team and contact sports rules for playing safely and how to use protective safety equipment, such as helmets. Head injuries are a major cause of death, with bicycle accidents being one of the major causes of such injuries (Hockenberry, 2005). Playground safety is especially important during the summer months. Teach children about safe distances for jumping and climbing, to avoid unsafe and isolated areas, and to keep away from strange dogs.

**ADOLESCENT.** As children enter adolescence, they develop greater independence and a sense of identity. The adolescent begins to separate emotionally from the family, and the peer group begins to have a stronger influence. Wide variations that swing from childlike to mature behavior are characteristic of adolescent behavior (Hockenberry, 2005). To relieve the tensions associated with the physical and psychosocial changes, as well as peer pressure, adolescents often engage in risk-taking behaviors such as smoking and using drugs. This increases the risk of accidents such as drowning and motor vehicle accidents. According to the Insurance Institute for Highway Safety (2002), two out of five deaths among teens in the United States are the result of motor vehicle accidents. To assess for possible substance abuse, have parents look for environmental and psychosocial clues. Environmental clues include the presence of drug-oriented magazines, beer and liquor bottles, drug paraphernalia, blood spots on clothing, and the continual wearing of long-sleeved shirts in hot weather and dark glasses indoors. Psychosocial clues include failing grades, change in dress, increased absenteeism from school, isolation, increased aggressiveness, and changes in interpersonal relationships.

**ADULT.** Threats to an adult's safety are often related to lifestyle habits. The patient who excessively uses alcohol or drugs, for example, is at greater risk for motor vehicle accidents. The adult experiencing a high level of stress is also at a greater risk for accidents and certain stress-related illnesses such as headaches, gastrointestinal disorders, and infections.

**OLDER ADULT.** The physiological changes associated with aging, effects of multiple medications, psychological factors, and acute or chronic disease increase the older adult's risk for falls and other types of accidents. Beginning at about age 70, the death rate from falls increases dramatically and the rate continues to increase with age. In 2001 more than 11,600 people age 65 and older died from fall-related injuries (CDC, 2003b). Most falls occur within the home, specifically in the bedroom, bathroom, and kitchen. Environmental factors such as broken stairs, icy sidewalks, inadequate lighting, throw rugs, and exposed electrical cords cause many of the accidents. Older adults typically fall while transferring from beds, chairs, and toilets; getting into or out of bathtubs; tripping over carpet edges or doorway thresholds; and slipping on wet surfaces or descending stairs.

## Other Risk Factors

**LIFESTYLE.** Lifestyle choices increase safety risks. People who drive or operate machinery while under the influence of chemical substances or work at jobs that are inherently more dangerous are at greater risk of injury. People who are preoccupied by stress or anxiety are more accident-prone because they fail to recognize the source of potential accidents, such as a cluttered stair or a stop sign.

**IMPAIRED MOBILITY.** A patient with impaired mobility has many kinds of safety risks. Immobilization predisposes a patient to physiological and emotional hazards, which in turn further restrict mobility and independence (see Chapter 34). Physically challenged patients are at greater risk for injury when entering motor vehicles and buildings not equipped for the handicapped.

**SENSORY IMPAIRMENTS.** Patients with visual, hearing, tactile, or communication impairments such as aphasia or language barrier are at greater risk for injury. Such patients are not always able to perceive a potential danger or express need for assistance (see Chapter 36).

**COGNITIVE IMPAIRMENTS.** Cognitive impairments associated with delirium, dementia, and depression place patients at greater risk for injury. These conditions contribute to altered concentration and attention span, impaired memory, and orientation changes. Patients with these alterations become easily confused about their surroundings and are more likely to have falls and burns.

**SAFETY AWARENESS.** Some patients are unaware of safety precautions, such as keeping medicine, poisonous plants, or other poisons away from children or reading the expiration date on food products. Your nursing assessment will identify the patient's level of knowledge regarding home safety so that you are able to correct safety problems with an individualized care plan.

## Risks in the Health Care Agency

Environmental safety pertains to the health care agency, as well as to the patient's home and community. However, there are specific risks in health care agencies that you also need to address. Various forms of chemicals used are a source of an environmental risk. Chemicals such as mercury and those found in some medications, anesthetic gases, cleaning solutions, and disinfectants are potentially toxic if ingested or inhaled.

A study by Health Grades Inc reported that nearly 195,000 people in the United States died each year in 2000, 2001, and 2002 as a result of potentially avoidable medical errors (Warner, 2004). Some of the most common preventable errors include bed sores, leaving a foreign object in the body during procedures, infection and other complications following surgery, and failure to diagnose and treat a patient in time. In addition, the Joint Commission on Accreditation of Healthcare Organizations (JCAHO) has identified National Patient Safety Goals (2005) in an effort to reduce the risk of medical mistakes. These evidence-based recommendations require health care agencies to focus their attention on a series of specific actions (Boxes 26-1 and 26-2)

Patients in health care settings are at risk for falls, patient-inherent accidents, procedure-related accidents, and equipment-related accidents. Learn to recognize factors associated with these risks, and take steps to prevent or minimize accidents.

**FALLS.** In 2001 more than 1.6 million older adults were treated in emergency departments for fall-related injuries and nearly 388,000 were hospitalized (CDC, 2003b). The most prevalent causes of falling in nursing homes are stroke, parkinsonism, blindness, arthritis, and drug related hypoten-

## BOX 26-1 JCAHO 2005 National Patient Safety Goals for Hospitals

Improve the accuracy of patient identification:
- Use at least two patient identifiers when administering medications or blood products, taking blood samples and other specimens, or providing any treatment or procedure.
- Conduct a preprocedure time-out verification process before any invasive procedure.

Improve the effectiveness of communication among caregivers:
- Implement a read-back process for taking verbal or telephone orders.
- Standardize a list of abbreviations, acronyms, and symbols used in documentation.
- Improve the timeliness of reporting and receipt of critical test results.

Improve safety of using medications:
- Remove high-risk concentrated electrolyte medications.
- Prevent errors involving the use of look-alike/sound-alike drugs.
- Limit the number of drug concentrations available.

Improve the safety of using infusion pumps:
- Ensure free flow protection on general use and patient-controlled analgesia pumps.

Reduce the risk of health care–associated infections:
- Comply with CDC hand hygiene guidelines.
- Conduct root cause analysis on health care–associated infections resulting in unanticipated death or loss of function.

Accurately and completely reconcile medications across the continuum of care:
- Develop a process for obtaining a complete list of the patient's current medications and comparing those with the medications the organization prescribes.
- Communicate the list of medications to the next provider of service when transferring a patient to another setting, service, practitioner, or level of care.

Reduce the risk of patient harm resulting from falls:
- Assess the patient's risk for falls, including the risks associated with medications, and take actions to address identified risks.

©2005 Joint Commission on Accreditation of Healthcare Organizations. Reprinted with permission.

## BOX 26-2 USING EVIDENCE IN PRACTICE

### Research Summary

Most research on falls has been conducted in samples from the community and in nursing homes, concentrating on the older adult population (Halfon and others, 2001). Less is known about falls among hospital inpatients, and only a few studies conducted used strong methodological design.

Research does show evidence that regardless of clinical setting, fall prevention consists of identifying a patient's risk factors and implementing targeted strategies or interventions aimed at reducing risk. Nurses need to link fall prevention strategies to the patient characteristics that lead to a fall and implement a comprehensive program that targets interventions that are appropriate and effective (Morse, 2002). Assessment of fall risk includes fall history, medication review, acute or chronic medical problems, mobility level, examination of vision, gait and balance, and basic neurological and cardiovascular function (American Geriatrics Society, 2001). Successful interventions, based upon the patient's assessment, include such things as balance and gait training, exercise programs, medication modification, postural hypotension treatment, environmental hazard modification, and behavioral and educational programs (Tinetti, 2003). Although some interventions, such as assistive devices (bed alarms, canes, and walkers) and behavioral and educational programs, do not prevent falls when used in isolation, they do demonstrate benefit as a part of a multifaceted intervention program (American Geriatrics Society, 2001). Nurses need to select fall prevention equipment carefully and base their selection on empirical outcomes rather than on untested consensus (Brush and Capezuti, 2001). It is clear that the combined effect of multiple interventions produces the best outcomes.

### Application to Nursing Practice

Nurses play a key role in fall prevention in any setting. In addition to promoting a safe environment for patients, educating patients about why falls occur and how to prevent them will lead not only to increased awareness and positive attitudes, but most importantly to behavior changes regarding fall prevention.

Data from American Geriatrics Society, British Geriatrics Society, American Academy of Orthopedic Surgeons Panel on Falls Prevention: Guideline for the prevention of falls in older persons, *J Am Geriatr Soc* 49:664, 2001; Brush BL, Capezuti E: Historical analysis of siderail use in American hospitals, *J Nurs Scholarsh* 33(4):381, 2001; Halfon P and others: Risk of falls for hospitalized patients: a predictive model based on routinely available data, *J Clin Epidemiol* 54(12):1258, 2001; Morse JM: Enhancing the safety of hospitalization by reducing patient falls, *Am J Infect Control* 30:376, 2002; and Tinetti ME: Preventing falls in elderly persons, *N Engl J Med* 348:42, 2003.

sion (Ebersole and Hess, 2004). Of those who fall, many suffer moderate to severe injuries such as hip fractures or head trauma that result in reduced mobility and independence and the increase the risk of premature death. Confusion, multiple medical problems, generalized weakness, postural instability, and an unfamiliar environment are major contributors to falling when an older patient is hospitalized (Ebersole and Hess, 2001). A risk assessment tool helps you assess potential risks before accidents and injuries result (Box 26-3).

**BOX 26-3** **Fall Assessment Tool**

Directions: Circle the score for the risk factor that corresponds to the patient. You administer the tool on admission to the facility or agency and again at specified intervals and when warranted by changes in health status. Scores of 15 and higher indicate high risk, and you should implement preventive measures.

| | Date Admit | Initial Score | Date | Reassessed Score |
|---|---|---|---|---|
| **Patient Factors** | | | | |
| History of falls | | 15 | | 15 |
| Confusion | | 5 | | 5 |
| Age (over 65) | | 5 | | 5 |
| Impaired judgment | | 5 | | 5 |
| Sensory deficit | | 5 | | 5 |
| Unable to ambulate independently | | 5 | | 5 |
| Decreased level of cooperation | | 5 | | 5 |
| Increased anxiety/ emotional lability | | 5 | | 5 |
| Incontinence/urgency | | 5 | | 5 |
| Cardiovascular/ respiratory disease affecting perfusion and oxygenation | | 5 | | 5 |
| Medications affecting blood pressure or level of consciousness | | 5 | | 5 |
| Postural hypotension with dizziness | | 5 | | 5 |
| **Environmental Factors** | | | | |
| First week on unit/ facility/services, etc. | | 5 | | 5 |
| Attached equipment (e.g., IV pole, chest tube, appliances, oxygen, tubing) | | 5 | | 5 |

From Funk SG and others, editors: *Key aspects of elder care: managing falls, incontinence, and cognitive impairment*, New York, 1992, Springer.

**PATIENT-INHERENT ACCIDENTS.** Patient-inherent accidents are accidents other than falls in which the patient is the primary factor causing the accident. Examples are self-inflicted cuts, injuries, and burns; ingestion or injection of foreign substances; self-mutilation or setting fires; and pinching fingers in drawers or doors. One of the more common precipitating factors for a patient-inherent accident is a seizure. A seizure leads to sudden, violent, and involuntary muscle contractions that are sometimes paroxysmal and episodic, causing loss of consciousness, falling, tonicity (rigidity of muscles), and clonicity (jerking of muscles). You must place patients with a seizure disorder on seizure precautions, which are designed to protect patients when seizures occur.

**PROCEDURE-RELATED ACCIDENTS.** Procedure-related accidents are caused by health care providers and include medication and fluid administration errors, improper application of external devices, and improper performance of procedures such as dressing changes. Following an organization's policies and procedures and standards of nursing practice helps prevent procedure-related accidents. For example, correct use of body mechanics and transfer techniques reduces the risk of injuries when moving and lifting patients (see Chapter 25).

**EQUIPMENT-RELATED ACCIDENTS.** Accidents that are equipment related result from the malfunction, disrepair, or misuse of equipment or from an electrical hazard. For example, too rapid infusion of intravenous (IV) fluids results from a dysfunctional IV pump. The Joint Commission on Accreditation of Healthcare Organizations (2005) now requires that all general use and patient-controlled analgesia pumps have free flow protection devices (see Box 26-1). To avoid injury, understand how to operate all monitoring or therapy equipment. If you discover faulty equipment, place a tag on it to prevent it from being used on another patient, and promptly report any malfunctions.

## Critical Thinking in Patient Care

### Synthesis

The synthesis of knowledge, experience, and other elements of critical thinking help you to make clinical decisions. To provide for patient safety, you will collect, analyze, and synthesize data to make well-reasoned clinical decisions.

**KNOWLEDGE.** You will need a complete picture of a patient's situation, including physical, cultural, physiological, psychosocial, and environmental information to protect the patient from injury. Consider a wide variety of factors (e.g., the patient's risk for injury, medications being taken, and the environment where most activities of daily living occur) before you develop a plan of care. Because every patient is different, with various strengths and weaknesses, prioritize factors that are threats to safety, and concentrate on the probable threats. After considering a patient's specific strengths and weaknesses, the patient's environment, and the developmental stage, work with the patient and family to determine creative interventions.

**EXPERIENCE.** Use clinical and personal experience to recall incidents that occurred with another patient or family member and the specific circumstances that led to the situation. For example, your grandmother has fallen because her slipper became entangled in a throw rug at the top of the stairs. Use the experience of your grandmother's fall and apply the knowledge gained when you assess a patient's home for safety hazards during a home visit.

**ATTITUDES.** Use of critical thinking attitudes ensures your plan of care for a patient's safety is comprehensive. For

## FOCUSED PATIENT ASSESSMENT

TABLE 26-1

| Factors to Assess | Questions and Approaches | Physical Assessment Strategies |
|---|---|---|
| Environment | Ask patient about recent or past injuries such as falls or burns; when did injury occur, what caused it, where did it happen, was this a recurrence? | Inspect the home environment both inside and outside for potential hazards: focus on the kitchen and bath. |
| Sensory | Ask patient to read label of medication bottle with glasses on. | Observe patient's ability to read printed material accurately. |
| Physical mobility | Ask patient about activity or exercise patterns: type of exercise, location where performed, type of footwear. | Observe patient's posture, gait, and balance during activities of daily living. |

example, show perseverance in identifying all potential safety risks and threats. Be responsible for collecting unbiased, accurate data that is relevant to the patient's safety. It is important to show discipline in conducting a thorough review of a patient's home environment. View all situations as opportunities to protect the patient. Once they occur, injuries cause pain, immobility, loss of income, or even death.

**STANDARDS.** The American Nurses Association's (ANA's) *Nursing: Scope and Standards of Practice* (2004) includes the concept of safety, stating that nurses will implement nursing interventions competently in a safe and appropriate manner. The ANA code of ethics (see Chapter 5) includes safety issues in the statement of the nurse's responsibility to promote, advocate for, and strive to protect the health, safety, and rights of the patient. Regulatory agencies such as JCAHO and the Occupational Safety and Health Administration (OSHA) define standards and guidelines related to safety in health care settings.

## Nursing Process

### Assessment

To conduct a thorough patient assessment, consider possible threats to the patient's safety, including the patient's immediate environment and any individual risk factors. Table 26-1 offers an example of focused assessment questions and assessment strategies. When caring for a patient in the home, a home hazard assessment is necessary (Box 26-4). A thorough hazard assessment covers topics such as adequacy of lighting, presence of safety devices, placement of furniture or other items that will possibly create barriers, condition of flooring, and safety of the kitchen and bathrooms. To assess the home, walk through the rooms with the patient and discuss how the patient normally conducts daily activities and whether the environment poses problems. For example, when assessing adequacy of lighting, inspect areas where the patient moves and works, particularly outside walkways, steps, interior halls, and doorways. Getting a sense of the patient's routines helps you to recognize safety hazards.

---

**BOX 26-4** | **Home Hazard Assessment**

Proper lighting inside and outside
Storage areas within easy reach
Appliances in good working order
Extension cords placed along walls
Presence of smoke detectors and a fire extinguisher
Presence of carbon monoxide detector
Flammable objects away from stove or heaters
Gas pilot lights lit
Hot water thermostat set to 120° F or less
Handrails or grip bars installed
Nonskid surfaces in the bathroom, tub, or shower
Floor coverings secured and floors free of clutter
Furniture and assistive devices promote ease of mobility
Medications stored properly and not outdated
Telephone accessible and includes emergency phone numbers

---

In a health care facility, determine if any hazards exist in the immediate care environment. Does the placement of equipment pose barriers when the patient attempts to ambulate? Does positioning of the patient's bed allow the patient to safely reach items on a bedside table? Are self-care items in a bathroom arranged for accessibility? Be sure to collaborate with the hospital's clinical engineering staff to ensure equipment functions properly.

Your nursing history will include data about the patient's level of wellness to determine if any underlying conditions pose a threat to safety. For example, assess the patient's activity tolerance, gait, muscle strength and coordination, balance, and vision. Consider the patient's developmental level when you analyze your data. Review if the patient is taking any medications or undergoing any procedures that pose risks. For example, using a diuretic increases the frequency of voiding and results in the patient using toilet facilities more often. Falls often occur when patients get out of bed quickly to urinate. When you assess an older adult, recognize the types of physical changes that increase the risk of injury (Box 26-5).

Joani has completed the health screening on Mr. Gonzales. She knows she needs to incorporate knowledge about environmental risks as they relate to her patient's age, level of independence, health status, and expectations. In addition, Mr. Gonzales is the third patient Joani has cared for in the home, and she also has an experiential basis for practice. As Joani integrates knowledge with previous experience, she remembers that the patient values his independence. As a result, Joani is able to develop a plan of care to meet Mr. Gonzales' safety needs while assisting him in maintaining his independence. At his apartment Joani inspects for environmental hazards. She discovers that the lighting is poor and that several throw rugs are near the chairs and the bedside. The health screening has revealed that Mr. Gonzales has decreased visual acuity and has not had a new pair of glasses for 3 years. He fell in his apartment about a month ago without incurring any injuries.

### BOX 26-5 CARE OF THE OLDER ADULT

**Physical Assessment Findings in the Older Adult That Increase the Risk of Accidents**

**Musculoskeletal Changes**
Muscle strength decreases
Joints become less mobile
Brittle bones due to osteoporosis
Posture changes; some kyphosis is common
Range of motion (ROM) is limited

**Nervous System Changes**
Voluntary or autonomic reflexes are slower
Decreased ability to respond to multiple stimuli
Decreased sensitivity of touch

**Sensory Changes**
Peripheral vision and lens accommodation decrease
Decrease in night vision and ability to adjust to changes in light
Lens develops opacity (cataracts)
Stimuli threshold for light touch and pain increases
Hearing is impaired because high-frequency tones are less perceptible

**Genitourinary Changes**
Increased nocturia
Increased occurrence of incontinence

Modified from Ebersole P, Hess P: *Toward healthy aging*, St. Louis, 2004, Mosby

**PATIENT EXPECTATIONS.** When you care for patients with safety needs, ask what they expect from your care. For example, "How can I provide care that will make you feel safe?" or "After we walk through your home, tell me what is important that we do to help you feel safe." In some cases a patient's and family's expectations of what is safe are not al-

ways appropriate. When this happens, intervene and educate both the patient and family regarding safe practices concerning everyday decisions, use of medications and medical equipment, and the environment. When patients are uninformed or inexperienced, this threatens their safety.

### Nursing Diagnosis

Gather data from your nursing assessment, and analyze clusters of defining characteristics to identify relevant nursing diagnoses. Include specific related or contributing factors to individualize your nursing care. Nursing diagnoses for patients with safety risks include:

- Risk for imbalanced body temperature
- Impaired home maintenance
- Risk for injury
- Deficient knowledge
- Risk for poisoning
- Disturbed sensory perception
- Risk for suffocation
- Disturbed thought processes
- Risk for trauma

For example, the nursing diagnosis *risk for injury* could be related to altered mobility, or it could be related to sensory alteration (e.g., visual). Altered mobility leads you to select such nursing interventions as range-of-motion (ROM) exercises or teaching the proper use of safety devices such as side rails, canes, or crutches. Visual impairment as the related factor leads you to select different interventions such as keeping the area well lighted; orienting the patient to the surroundings; or keeping eyeglasses clean, handy, and well protected. When you do not identify the correct related factor, the use of inappropriate interventions increases a patient's risk of injury. For example, not evaluating the home environment for hazards will possibly result in sending a hospitalized patient back home only to return with an additional injury.

### Planning

Patients with actual or potential risks to safety require a nursing care plan with interventions that prevent and minimize threats to safety. Your interventions need to be designed to help a patient feel safe to interact freely within the environment. The total plan of care will address all aspects of patient needs and use resources of the health care team and the community when appropriate.

**GOALS AND OUTCOMES.** Planning and goal setting need to be done in collaboration with the patient, family, and other members of the health care team. Remember to keep goals realistic, within the resources available to the patient. When you involve the patient and family in planning, they will be more alert to safety risks and potential hazards. For example, you develop a goal "Reduce the number of falls" in a patient with Parkinson's disease who falls frequently at home. An expected outcome is "Patient reduces barriers to reaching the bathroom." You then suggest the in-

## CARE PLAN  Risk for Injury

### ASSESSMENT

Mr. Gonzales is a 68-year-old man **with diminished visual acuity** who lives alone in an apartment on the third floor with **throw rugs on the floors and poor lighting.** He states that he **cannot read the labels on his medication bottles** very well and sometimes takes his medication from memory. His son Carlos recently purchased for him a medication organizer that Mr. Gonzales is not yet using. When observed walking, he **does not pick his feet very high up off the floor, and his movements appear stiff.**

*Defining characteristics are shown in bold type.

### NURSING DIAGNOSIS Risk for injury related to altered mobility and decreased visual acuity.

### PLANNING

| GOAL | EXPECTED OUTCOMES* |
|---|---|
| | *Safe Home Environment* |
| • Adapt patient's environment to motor, sensory, and cognitive developmental needs (within 2 months). | • Patient will list hazards within 1 week.<br>• Nurse and patient will reduce modifiable hazards by 100% within 1 month. |

*Outcomes classification label from Moorhead S, Johnson M, Maas M: *Nursing outcomes classification (NOC)*, ed 3, St. Louis, 2004, Mosby.

| INTERVENTIONS† | RATIONALE |
|---|---|
| **Environmental Management: Safety**<br>• Review with patient the potential risks for accidents observed in the home. | An accurate home assessment identifies threats to a patient's safety. |
| a. Remove throw rugs. | Throw rugs often roll up or bunch to create an uneven walking surface. |
| b. Increase lighting to a minimum of 75 watts per light. | Adequate lighting reduces the likelihood of falling over objects or bumping into them. |
| c. Label medication bottles clearly in bold, large print. Use medication organizer for daily medications. | Clearly labeled medication bottles and use of a medication organizer reduces the risk of a medication error. |
| • Stress the importance of making safety modifications in the home, and give specific instructions for prevention of burns, falls, and poisoning. | Advance guidance is important in preventing potential injuries. |
| • Arrange for patient to visit ophthalmologist and have a new prescription written for eyeglasses. | Reduced visual acuity is correctable. Routine eye examinations are recommended annually for all persons after the age of 50 (Ebersole and Hess, 2004). |
| **Exercise Promotion**<br>Encourage patient to take 20-minute walks in the neighborhood at least 3 times per week. | Maintenance of a physically active lifestyle delays age changes associated with cardiovascular, respiratory, and musculoskeletal function (Ebersole and Hess, 2004). |

†Intervention classification labels from Dochterman JM, Bulechek GM, editors: *Nursing interventions classification (NIC)*, ed 4, St. Louis, 2004, Mosby.

### EVALUATION

- Observe environment for elimination of threats to safety.
- Reassess patient's motor, sensory, and cognitive status for appropriate environmental modifications.
- Revisit patient in 2 weeks to determine if patient has made a visit to ophthalmologist and if patient is taking regular walks.

---

tervention that the patient sleep in a bedroom closest to the bathroom. After collaborating with the family, however, you select the alternative of a bedside commode.

**SETTING PRIORITIES.** Prioritize patient nursing diagnoses and interventions that are most important in terms of risk to safety and health promotion. In some situations you need to select more than one nursing diagnosis that best represents a patient's particular needs. For example, the nursing diagnoses *risk for poisoning* and *deficient knowledge* are important for an older patient who takes several medica-

tions and has an impaired memory. Priority nursing interventions include ways to reduce accidental poisoning (e.g., large labels on medication containers, use of dose dispensers, and having a family member prepare medications) and teaching safe methods of taking medications, within a patient's learning capabilities (see care plan).

**CONTINUITY OF CARE.** It is important for you to help patients with safety needs develop a link within their community that helps to maintain a safe environment. Hospitalized patients need to learn how to identify and select resources within their community that will enhance safety once they return home. For example, an older adult may need to go to an adult day care center during weekdays when family members are working and unable to provide regular assistance.

## Implementation

Direct your nursing interventions toward maintaining the patient's safety in all types of settings. Providing a safe environment includes health promotion, developmental interventions, and environmental protection. Each of these areas of implementation is appropriate in acute and restorative care settings.

**HEALTH PROMOTION.** The emphasis in health care today is on health promotion. Edelman and Mandle (2002) describe passive and active strategies aimed at health promotion. Passive strategies are put into practice through government legislation (e.g., sanitation and clean water laws). Active strategies involve the individual and include changes in lifestyle and participation in wellness programs.

Participate in health promotion activities by supporting legislation, by acting as a positive role model, and by recommending safety measures in the home, school, neighborhood, and workplace.

### DEVELOPMENTAL INTERVENTIONS

**Infant, Toddler, and Preschooler.** Growing, curious children depend on adults to protect them from injury. Educate young parents or guardians about reducing risks of injuries to children, and teach ways to promote safety in the home. Some examples are preventing access to poisonous substances; correct use of safety seats; use of safe, age-appropriate toys; and placement of safety covers on electrical outlets (see Chapter 19). Encourage parents to position infants on the back or side ("back to sleep") to prevent sudden infant death syndrome (SIDS). As a pediatric nurse, teach new parents about removing poisonous substances from easy-to-reach storage areas and the importance of supervised play. Educate parents about the importance of immunizations and how they protect a child from life-threatening diseases.

**School-Age Child.** School-age children increasingly explore their environment. They have friends outside their immediate neighborhood, and they become more active in school, church, and the community. Teach children to wear seat belts whenever riding in a car, to wear a helmet when riding a bicycle, skateboard, or scooter, and to keep adults informed of where they are. Also teach children how to cross the street safely and to refrain from talking to or accepting rides or gifts from strangers. Teach them what to do if a stranger approaches.

**Adolescent.** Risks to the adolescent's safety involve many factors outside the home because they spend much of their time away from home and with their peer group. However, adults serve as role models for adolescents and, through providing examples, setting expectations, and providing education, help adolescents minimize safety risks. Because adolescence is a time when sexual physical characteristics develop, adolescents often begin to have physical relationships with others. They need prompt, accurate instructions about ab-

stinence and/or safe sexual practices. When adolescents learn to drive, they need education on complying with rules and regulations regarding the use of a car. Most schools have driver's education programs. Make sure you strictly enforce the regular use of a seat belt. Box 26-6 offers an example of patient teaching for preventing automobile accidents during adolescence.

**Adult.** Risks to young and middle-age adults frequently result from lifestyle factors such as child rearing, high-stress states, inadequate nutrition, use of firearms, and abuse of drugs or alcohol. In this fast-paced society there also appears to be more expression of anger. This anger can quickly precipitate accidents such as "road rage." Help adults understand their safety risks, and guide them in making lifestyle modifications by referring them to resources such as classes to help quit smoking and for stress management and employee assistance programs. Also encourage adults to exercise regularly, to practice relaxation techniques, and to acquire adequate sleep (see Chapter 29).

**Older Adult.** Elimination of threats to the safety of the older adult focuses primarily on accidents. Advancing age and concurrent physiological changes predispose older adults to falls (Box 26-7) (see Chapter 19). Certain disease states common to older adults, such as arthritis or cerebrovascular accidents, increase the chance of injury. The effects of many medications, such as sedatives, diuretics, and laxatives also increase the chance of injury. Table 26-2 lists nursing interventions designed to prevent falls and compensate for the physiological changes of aging.

Provide information about neighborhood resources to help the older adult maintain an independent lifestyle. Older adults frequently relocate to new neighborhoods and must get acquainted with new resources such as modes of transportation, church schedules, and food resources (e.g., Meals on Wheels). Although retired from their jobs, older adults have a wealth of past experiences to aid volunteer organizations. Some retirees even enjoy reentering the work force in a new capacity. Information about assistance resources, such as daily "hello" programs, emergency services, and elder abuse hot lines, is also helpful.

**ENVIRONMENTAL INTERVENTIONS.** To eliminate environmental threats, make sure your nursing interventions include general preventive measures and specific measures to reduce the risk of accidental injuries.

**General Preventive Measures.** Your nursing interventions contribute to a safer environment by helping patients meet their basic physiological needs. To ensure that there are no threats to oxygen availability, encourage patients to have their furnaces inspected each season for proper functioning. Carbon monoxide detectors are available for installation in the home. To achieve a comfortable level of humidity in the home, attach a humidifier to the furnace or, in the case of patients who have upper respiratory tract infections, use a room humidifier while sleeping. Teach patients to follow the manufacturer's directions regarding the cleaning and maintenance of home humidifiers to reduce contamination of the water. Teach basic techniques for food handling and prepa-

---

**BOX 26-6** PATIENT TEACHING

During a follow-up visit to Mr. Gonzales' apartment, Joani meets Carlos, Mr. Gonzales' son, and Carlos' son John. During the visit, Carlos expresses concern to Joani about his 16-year-old son's safety while driving. Carlos wants his son John to learn to drive but knows there are many risks. He asks Joani for advice on how to keep his son safe. Joani develops the following teaching plan for Carlos and his son John.

**Outcome**

At the end of the teaching session, Carlos and John will verbalize understanding of ways to promote safe driving habits.

**Teaching Strategies**

- Establish rapport with Carlos and John, and maintain eye contact.
- Provide a brief description of what will be taught.
- Suggest to Carlos that he enroll John in a driver's education course.
- Explain the importance of using seat belts while driving and as a passenger.
- Stress to Carlos the importance of being a role model by practicing safe driving habits.

- Explain to Carlos the importance of providing John frequent opportunities to practice driving in good and bad weather.
- Explain to John the safety risks associated with driving under the influence of drugs and alcohol.
- Explain the costs associated with traffic violations such as higher insurance premiums and possible loss of driver's license.
- Ask Carlos and John to form a contract regarding not driving and drinking. Instruct John never to enter an automobile when the driver has been using drugs or alcohol.

**Evaluation Strategies**

- Use open-ended questions.
- Ask Carlos to identify when he will provide opportunities for John to practice driving.
- Ask John what he would do if he were drinking at a party and needed to get home.
- Ask John what will happen if he receives a traffic violation.
- Ask Carlos how he will demonstrate safe driving habits to John.
- Ask John what the risks are of driving without a seat belt.

---

**BOX 26-7** CARE OF THE OLDER ADULT

- Because of visual impairments, teach patients to keep living areas well lighted and free of clutter, to keep eyeglasses in good condition, and to avoid night driving.
- Older adults have musculoskeletal changes that make movement difficult and increase the risk of falling. Teach patients to keep assistive devices in proper working order (canes, rails in tub and bathroom, and elevated seats) and to use nonskid strips in bathtubs.
- Advise older adults to avoid smoking in bed, to lower thermostats on water heaters, to avoid overloading electrical outlets, and to install and maintain smoke and carbon monoxide detectors in the house.
- Older adults are more likely to have automobile accidents due to decreased hearing and visual acuity, altered depth perception, slowed reaction time, and poor peripheral vision. Advise older adults to only drive short distances and in the daylight;

avoid driving in inclement weather, such as fog, heavy rain and snow; use side and rear view mirrors carefully; look behind them toward their blind spot before changing lanes; and keep a window rolled down in order to hear sirens and horns.
- Older adults frequently have some impairment of memory. Teach patients about the proper handling and storage of food and safe methods of scheduling and taking medications.
- Older adults have physiological changes that result in slower metabolism of drugs. Teach patients about drug interactions and signs and symptoms of drug toxicity to report to their health care provider.
- Some older adults suffer from an irreversible dementia. Assist family caregivers in understanding the nature of dementia. Teach them ways to match expectations with the patient's capabilities, how to incorporate earlier life skills and interests, and to provide a calm, caring, and structured environment.

---

ration so that patients meet all their nutritional needs safely (e.g., wash hands before and after food preparation, clean cutting surfaces thoroughly with soap and water, cook food thoroughly, refrigerate food after preparation, and label and date when leftovers are saved). To prevent injury from exposure to temperature extremes, educate older adults or patients who enjoy outdoor activities about signs and symptoms of frostbite, hypothermia, heatstroke, and heat exhaustion and how to avoid these conditions.

Adequate lighting and security measures in and around the home, including the use of night-lights, exterior lighting,

and locks on doors and windows, enable patients to reduce the risk of injury from falls or crime. The local police department and community organizations often have safety classes available on how not to become a victim of crime. If patients have a history of falling and live alone, recommend that they obtain an electronic safety alert device to wear. This device, when activated by the wearer, alerts a monitoring site to call emergency services for assistance.

Within the health care setting, eliminate physical hazards by removing clutter, extra equipment, and furniture from traffic areas. Always be sure an ambulatory patient has a

| TABLE 26-2 | Measures to Prevent Falls in Older Adults |
|---|---|

| Measure | Rationale |
|---|---|
| **Home or Health Care Facility** | |
| **Stairs** | |
| Install treads with uniform depth of 9 inches (22.5 cm) and 9-inch risers (vertical face of steps). | If stairs are of uniform size, older adult does not have to continually adjust vision. |
| Install uniform-textured or plain-colored surfaces on each tread, and mark edge of tread with contrasting color. | Uniform textures or color help to decrease vertigo. Marking edge of tread provides obvious visual clue to end of stair. |
| Ensure proper lighting of each tread. Block sun or lightbulb glare with translucent shades or screen, or use lower-wattage bulbs. | Older adults' vision is unable to adjust quickly to changes in lighting. |
| Ensure adequate head room so that users do not have to duck to negotiate stairs. | Sudden changes in head position often result in dizziness. |
| Remove protruding objects from staircase walls. | Decreased peripheral vision prevents patient from seeing object. Moving to avoid protruding objects will disrupt balance. |
| Maintain outdoor walkways and stairs in good condition and free of holes, cracks, and splinters. | Decreased visual acuity prevents patient from seeing any structural defect. |
| **Handrails** | |
| Install smooth but slip-resistant handrail at least 2 inches (5 cm) from wall. | Two-inch distance allows patient to grasp handrail firmly for support. |
| Secure handrail firmly to support user's weight, especially at bottom and top of stairway. | Older adult has greatest risk of falling at top and bottom of stairs because they shift their center of gravity, making balance unstable. |
| Install grab rails in bathroom near toilet and tub. | Enables patient to have support while rising from sitting to standing position. |
| **Floors** | |
| Ensure patients wear properly fitting shoes or slippers with non-skid surface. | Reduces chances of slipping. |
| Secure all carpeting, mats, and tile; place nonskid backing under small rugs. | Sudden slip causes dizziness and inability to regain balance. |
| Place bath mats or nonskid strips on bathtub or shower stall floors. | Wet surfaces increase the risk of falling. |
| Secure electrical cords against baseboards. | Prevents tripping. |
| Maintain proper illumination in areas both inside and outside where the patient moves and walks. | Reduces the risk of falling due to eyestrain. |
| **Health Care Facility** | |
| **Orientation** | |
| Place disoriented patients in room near nurses' station. | Provides for more frequent observation by nursing staff. |
| Maintain close supervision of confused patients. | Confused patient often attempts to wander out of bed or room. |
| Show the patient how to use the call light at the bedside and in bathroom, and place within easy reach. Instruct patient to call for assistance with movement as needed. | Location and use of the call light is essential to patient safety. |
| Place bedside tables and over-bed tables close to the patient. Place articles within easy reach. | Prevents patient from searching or overreaching for items such as eyeglasses, dentures, hearing aid, or telephone. |
| Remove clutter from bedside tables, hallways, bathrooms, and grooming areas. | Eliminates potential hazards and promotes patient independence. |
| Keep the bed in low position. Have the patient rise from the bed or chair slowly. | Prevents dizziness resulting from postural hypotension. |
| Leave one side rail up and one down on the side where the oriented and ambulatory patient gets out of bed. | Patient is able to use the side rail for support when getting in and out of bed and to position self once in bed. |
| **Transport** | |
| Lock beds and wheelchairs when transferring a patient from a bed to a wheelchair or back to bed. | Provides stability and support during transfer. |
| Place side rails in the up position, and secure safety straps around the patient on a stretcher. | Prevents the patient from rolling off the stretcher. |

clear path to the bathroom. Keeping the bathroom light on also helps patients ambulate safely.

To control pathogen transmission, teach patients how and when to wash hands (e.g., following toileting, before food preparation, and before wound care). Patients also need to know how to dispose of infected material such as wound dressings and used needles in the home. For example, heavy plastic containers such as 1-L soda bottles are excellent for needle disposal. The Environmental Protection Agency (EPA) encourages disposal of used needles by way of community drop-off programs, household hazardous waste facilities, sharps mail-back programs, or using home needle destruction devices (Coalition for Safe Community Needle Disposal, 2005a). Encourage patients to contact neighborhood community governments for guidelines on waste disposal methods. Teach patients safe sexual practices, including correct use of condoms and engaging in monogamous relationships to reduce the risk of sexually transmitted diseases. Nurses use standard precautions for all patients to protect themselves from contact with blood and body fluids (see Chapter 11).

**Specific Safety Concerns.** There are specific interventions that you as a nurse implement to ensure patient safety.

*Falls.* Modifying a patient's environment reduces the risk for falls. For example, a heavy patient needs a bed, wheelchair, or commode specifically designed to support the additional weight. A patient with impaired mobility benefits from having the home organized so it becomes unnecessary to walk up or down stairs. In a health care facility, explain to patients how to use the call light or intercom system and make sure you always place the call device close to the patient. For patients needing assistance to ambulate, respond quickly when call lights are on so that the patient does not attempt to get out of bed without help. Removing excess furniture and equipment and providing patients with rubber-soled shoes or slippers for walking or during transfer helps keep the immediate environment safe. Inspect canes, walkers, and crutches to be sure rubber tips are intact and connections are tight and that the assistive devices are at the appropriate height for the patient.

Implementing certain safeguards and teaching the family ways to reduce the risk of falls further minimizes the risk of falls (see Table 26-2). Confused and disoriented patients or patients who repeatedly fall or try to remove medical devices (e.g., oxygen equipment, IV lines, or dressings) often require the temporary use of restraints or side rails to keep them from falling out of bed. Restraints are not a solution to a patient problem, but rather a temporary means to maintain patient safety.

*Restraints.* Restraints are either chemical or physical. Chemical restraints are medications, such as anxiolytics and sedatives, used to control the patient's behavior. A physical **restraint** is any manual method or a physical or mechanical device that the patient is unable to remove. It restricts the patient's physical activity or normal access to the body and is not a usual part of treatment indicated by the patient's condition or symptoms (Centers for Medicare and Medicaid

Services [CMS], 2000). The use of restraints is associated with serious complications due to immobilization, such as pressure ulcers, constipation, and incontinence. In some cases death has resulted because of restricted breathing and circulation. There have been cases where patients have hung themselves in a restraint while trying to get out of bed while restrained. As a result, nursing homes and many health care facilities have banned the use of the jacket (vest) restraint because of this risk. This text discusses proper use of the vest restraint because if you ever use it, you need to know how to apply it correctly. Loss of self-esteem, humiliation, and agitation are also serious concerns. Because of these risks, current legislation emphasizes reducing the use of restraints. Regulatory agencies such as JCAHO and the Centers for Medicaid and Medicare Services (CMS) enforce standards for the safe use of restraint devices. A restraint-free environment, either physical or chemical, is your first goal for all patients. Always try alternatives such as more frequent observation, involvement of family during visitation, frequent reorientation, and the introduction of familiar stimuli (e.g., knitting or crocheting or looking at family photos) within the environment to reduce behaviors that often lead to restraint use.

In keeping with current trends toward health promotion, your assessment techniques and modifications of the environment are effective alternatives to restraints (Box 26-8). For patients who continue to attempt to ambulate without assistance, use electronic bed and chair alarm devices. These devices warn nursing staff that a patient is attempting to leave the bed or chair unassisted. A variety of devices are available and include the use of a knee band, such as the **AMBULARM,** that sounds an alarm when the patient reaches a near-vertical position. Other devices include pressure-sensitive strips placed beneath the patient under the buttocks or a tether alarm that you clip to the patient's gown. These devices help avoid physical restraints and prevent a patient fall.

When restraints are required to protect the patient or others, involve the patient and family in the decision to use restraints. Assist them in adapting to this change by explaining the purpose of the restraint, expected care while the patient is in restraints, and that the restraint is temporary and protective. It is a requirement for nursing homes to obtain informed consent from family members before using restraints. As with other procedures, follow specific guidelines when using physical restraints (Skill 26-1). The overall objectives for restraint use include the following:

1. Reduce the risk of patient injury from falls
2. Prevent interruption of therapy such as traction, IV infusions, nasogastric tube feeding, or Foley catheter
3. Prevent the confused or combative patient from removing life support equipment
4. Reduce the risk of injury to self or others

For legal purposes know agency-specific policies for appropriate use and monitoring of a restrained patient. Some medications, such as sedatives or hypnotics given to calm an

*Text continued on p. 707*

---

**BOX 26-8** | **Alternatives to Restraints**

Involve patients and families in planning care; explain all procedures and treatments to them.

Encourage family and friends to stay, or utilize sitters for patients who need continuous supervision.

Use calm, simple statements and physical cues as needed.

Use a knee band such as the AMBULARM to alert caregivers when the patient reaches a near-vertical position.

Eliminate full side rails. To reduce injury due to falls, use low beds with a floor mat at bedside.

Assign confused or disoriented patients to rooms near the nurses' station. Observe these patients frequently, and institute regular patient checks.

Provide appropriate visual and auditory stimuli (e.g., family pictures, clock, radio).

Eliminate bothersome treatments as soon as possible. For example, discontinue tube feedings and begin oral feedings as quickly as the patient's condition allows.

Camouflage IV lines with clothing, skin sleeves, or Kling dressing. Camouflage a gastrostomy tube (G-tube) with an abdominal binder. Use freedom splints and endotracheal tube (ET) holders to maintain ET tubes.

Provide ongoing pain assessment. Try nonpharmacological interventions first such as positioning and relaxation techniques (e.g., music, massage).

Use diversional activities appropriate for the patient.

Institute exercise and ambulation schedules as the patient's condition allows.

Provide scheduled toileting, especially during peak fall times, such as 6 to 8 AM and 4 to 6 PM.

Consult with physical and occupational therapists to enhance strength, mobility, and exercise.

Use protective devices such as hip pads, helmet, skid-proof slippers, and nonskid strips near bed.

Provide prompt treatment and ongoing evaluation of medical problems (e.g., orthostatic hypotension, constipation, fluid overload, dehydration, infection, drug toxicity, medication side effects).

Modified from GeronurseOnline.org: *Want to know: physical restraints,* 2005, http://www.geronurseonline.org/index.dfm?section_id=30&geriatric_topic_id=10&sub_section_id=74&page_id=156&tab=2.

---

## SKILL 26-1 | Use of Restraints

### Delegation Considerations

You can delegate the skill of applying a restraint to trained assistive personnel. Before delegation, instruct the assistive personnel about:

- The patient's need for restraint
- Appropriate type of restraint to use
- Correct placement of the restraint
- How to check the patient's circulation, skin integrity, and breathing

- When and how to change patient's position, providing ROM, skin care, and opportunities for socialization
- Reporting signs and symptoms of patient's not tolerating the restraint (e.g., increased agitation, constriction of circulation, impaired skin integrity, change in breathing pattern)

### Equipment

- Proper restraint: jacket, belt, extremity, or mitten
- Padding (if needed)

| STEP | RATIONALE |
|------|-----------|

### ASSESSMENT

1. Assess if a patient needs a restraint. Does the patient continually try to interrupt needed therapy? Is the patient repeatedly trying to ambulate independently, creating a serious risk of injury?

   Use restraints only when other less restrictive measures fail to prevent interruption of therapies. This includes traction, endotracheal intubation, IV infusions, or nasogastric tube feedings; preventing a confused or combative patient from self-injury by getting out of bed or falling out of bed; preventing a patient from removing urinary catheters, surgical drains, or life support equipment; and reducing risk of injury to others by patient.

2. Assess patient's behavior, such as confusion, disorientation, agitation, restlessness, combativeness, or inability to follow directions.

   If patient's behavior continues despite attempts to eliminate cause of behavior, use of physical restraint is sometimes necessary.

| STEP | RATIONALE |
|---|---|
| 3. Review agency policies regarding restraints. Check physician's or health care provider's order for purpose and type of restraint, location, and duration of restraint; prn orders for restraint should never be written. Determine if you need a signed consent for use of a restraint. | Physician's or health care provider's order is necessary to apply restraints. The least restrictive type of restraint should be ordered. Because restraints limit patient's ability to move freely, make clinical judgments appropriate to patient's condition and agency policy. A face-to-face physician or health care provider assessment within 1 hour is required when you emergently restrain a patient for violent or aggressive behavior (CMS, 2000). |

## PLANNING

| | |
|---|---|
| 1. Review manufacturer's instructions for restraint application before entering patient's room. | Be familiar with all devices used for patient care and protection. Incorrect application of restraint device will result in patient injury or death. |
| 2. Perform hand hygiene, and collect appropriate equipment. | Reduces transmission of microorganisms and promotes organization. |
| 3. Correctly identify patient by checking armband and having patient state name if possible. | Prevents patient care errors. |
| 4. Introduce self to patient and family, and assess their feelings about restraint use. Explain that restraint is temporary and designed to protect patient from injury. | You need to inform patient and family about the use of restraint. In nursing homes, informed consent is mandatory. |
| 5. Inspect area where you will place restraint. Assess condition of skin underlying area on which you will apply restraint. | Sometimes restraints compress and interfere with functioning of devices or tubes. Assessment provides baseline to monitor patient's skin integrity. |

• *Critical Decision Point:* Make sure restraints do not interfere with equipment such as IV tubes. Do not place them over access devices, such as an arteriovenous (AV) dialysis shunt.

| | |
|---|---|
| 6. Approach patient in a calm, confident manner. Explain what you plan to do. | Reduces patient anxiety and promotes cooperation. |

## IMPLEMENTATION

| | |
|---|---|
| 1. Provide privacy. Position and drape patient as needed. | Prevents lowering of patient's self-esteem. |
| 2. Adjust bed to proper height, and lower side rail on side of patient contact. | Allows use of proper body mechanics and prevention of injury. |
| 3. Be sure patient is comfortable and in correct anatomical position. | Prevents contractures and neurovascular impairment. |
| 4. Pad skin and bony prominences (if necessary) that will be under the restraint. | Reduces friction and pressure from restraint to skin and underlying tissue. |
| 5. Apply appropriate-size restraint: **Always refer to manufacturer's directions.** | |
|   a. **Jacket (vest or Posey) restraint:** Apply jacket or vest over gown, pajamas, or clothes. Jacket restraints have sleeves. Place patient's hands through armholes or sleeves, and secure according to manufacturer's directions. Vest restraints have front and back of garment labeled as such. Some vests secure in the front of the patient, and others secure in the back. Adjust to patient's level of comfort (see illustration). | Restrains patient while lying or reclining in bed and while sitting in chair or wheelchair. Crisscrossing in back will cause risk of death from strangulation. Clothing or gown prevents friction against skin. |

• *Critical Decision Point:* Vest or jacket restraints have caused death due to strangulation. Monitor patients closely while in this device.

---
**SKILL 26-1** | **Use of Restraints—cont'd**
---

| STEP | RATIONALE |
|------|-----------|

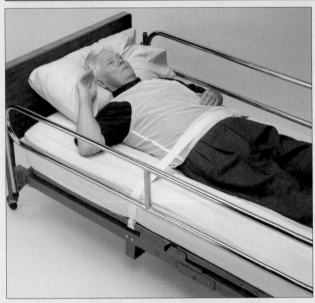

STEP **5a** Vest restraint securely attached to bed frame. (Courtesy JT Posey Co, Arcadia, Calif.)

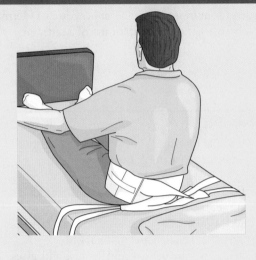

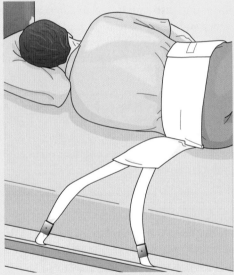

STEP **5b** Roll belt restraint tied to the bed frame and to an area that does not cause the restraint to tighten when the side rail is raised or lowered. (From Sorrentino SA: *Mosby's textbook for nursing assistants,* ed 6, St. Louis, 2004, Mosby.)

b. **Belt restraint:** Have patient in a sitting position. Apply over clothes, gown, or pajamas. Remove wrinkles or creases from front and back of restraint while placing it around patient's waist. Bring ties through slots in belt. Help patient lie down if in bed. Avoid placing belt too tightly across patient's chest or abdomen (see illustrations).

Restrains center of gravity and prevents patient from rolling off stretcher or sitting up while on stretcher or from falling out of bed. Tight application interferes with breathing.

c. **Extremity (ankle or wrist) restraint:** Restraint designed to immobilize one or all extremities. Commercially available limb restraints are made of sheepskin with foam padding (see illustration). Wrap limb restraint around wrist or ankle with soft part toward skin and secured snugly in place by Velcro straps.

Maintains immobilization of extremity to protect patient from injury from fall or accidental removal of therapeutic device (e.g., IV tube, Foley catheter). Tight application interferes with circulation.

| STEP | RATIONALE |
|---|---|

- *Critical Decision Point:* Patient with wrist and ankle restraints is at risk for aspiration if placed in supine position. Place patient in lateral position rather than supine.

---

**d. Mitten restraint:** Thumbless mitten device that restrains patient's hands (see illustration). Place hand in mitten, being sure Velcro strap is around the wrist and not the forearm.

Prevents patients from dislodging invasive equipment, removing dressings, or scratching, yet allows greater movement than a wrist restraint.

6. Attach restraint straps to portion of bed frame that moves when head of bed is raised or lowered (see illustration). **Do not attach to side rails.** You can also attach restraint with patient in chair or wheelchair to chair frame.

You will injure patient if you secure restraint to a side rail and it is lowered.

7. When patient is in a wheelchair, secure jacket restraint by placing ties under armrests and securing at back of chair (see illustration).

Prevents patient from sliding restraint ties up the back of the chair.

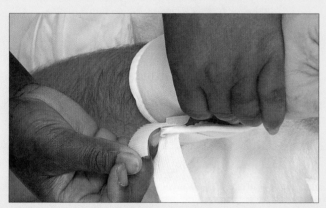

STEP **5c** Placement of wrist restraint.

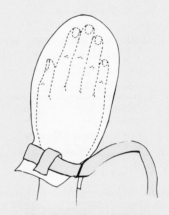

STEP **5d** Mitten restraint.

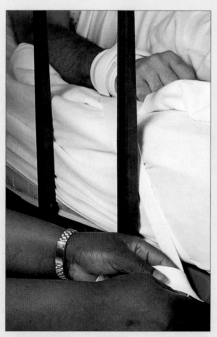

STEP **6** Tie restraint strap to bed frame.

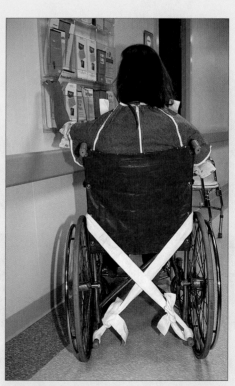

STEP **7** Straps of vest restraint secured at back of chair.

SKILL 26-1 | Use of Restraints—cont'd

| STEP | RATIONALE |
|---|---|
| • *Critical Decision Point:* If ties are not under armrests, patients will be able to slide ties up the back of the chair and free themselves. | |
| 8. Secure restraints with a quick-release tie (see illustrations). **Do not tie in a knot.** | Allows for quick release in an emergency. |
| 9. Insert two fingers under secured restraint (see illustration). | Checking for constriction prevents neurovascular injury. |
| • *Critical Decision Point:* A tight restraint causes constriction and impedes circulation. | |
| 10. Assess proper placement of restraint, skin integrity, pulses, temperature, color, and sensation of the restrained body part according to health status and needs of the patient but **at least every 2 hours** (JCAHO, 2004) or more frequently as determined by agency policy. | Frequent assessments prevent complications, such as suffocation, skin breakdown, and impaired circulation. |
| 11. Remove restraints at least every 2 hours (or more frequently as determined by patient need or agency policy) (JCAHO, 2004). If patient is violent or noncompliant, remove one restraint at a time and/or have staff assistance while removing restraints. | Provides opportunity to change patient's position; to perform full ROM, toileting, and exercise; and to provide food or fluids. |
| • *Critical Decision Point:* Do not leave violent or aggressive patients unattended while restraints are off. | |
| 12. Secure call light or intercom system within reach. | Allows patient, family, or caregiver to obtain assistance quickly. |
| • *Critical Decision Point:* Restraints restrict movement, making patients unable to perform their activities of daily living without assistance. Providing food and/or fluids and assisting with toileting and other activities is essential. | |
| 13. Leave bed or chair with wheels locked. Make sure bed is in the lowest position. | Locked wheels prevent bed or chair from moving if patient attempts to get out. If patient falls when bed is in lowest position, this will reduce chances of injury. |
| 14. Perform hand hygiene. | Reduces transmission of microorganisms. |

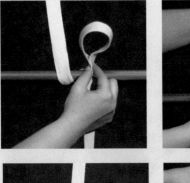
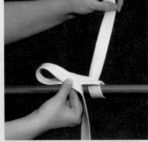
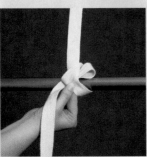
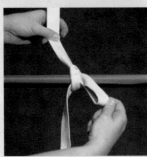

STEP 8 The Posey quick-release tie. (Courtesy JT Posey Co, Arcadia, Calif.)

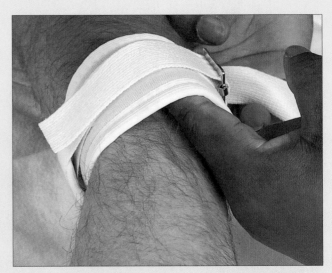

STEP 9 Place two fingers under restraint to check tightness.

## EVALUATION

1. Inspect patient for any injury, including all hazards of immobility, while restraints are in use.

Ensures patient is free of injury and does not exhibit any signs of immobility complications.

2. Observe IV catheters, urinary catheters, and drainage tubes to determine that you positioned them correctly.

Reinsertion is uncomfortable and increases risk of infection or interruption of therapy.

3. Reassess patient's need for continued use of restraint at least every 24 hours with the intent of discontinuing restraint at the earliest possible time (see agency policy) (CMS, 2000; JCAHO, 2004).

Face-to-face reassessment by physician or health care provider is required and new order obtained if continuing restraint.

4. Provide appropriate sensory stimulation, and reorient patient as needed.

Use of restraints further increases disorientation.

## RECORDING AND REPORTING

- Record patient behaviors before you applied restraints.
- Record restraint alternatives you attempted and the patient's response.
- Record patient's and/or family's understanding of and consent to restraint application.
- Record type and location of the restraint and time applied.
- Record times that you performed assessments and releases while patient in restraints.
- Record findings from your assessments related to orientation, oxygenation, skin integrity, circulation, and positioning.
- Record patient's behavior and expected or unexpected outcomes after you applied the restraint.
- Record patient's response when you removed restraints.
- Also see behavioral restraint flow sheet (Figure 26-1).

## UNEXPECTED OUTCOMES AND RELATED INTERVENTIONS

- Skin integrity becomes impaired.
  - Reassess the continued need for the restraint; use a different type of restraint.
  - If restraint is necessary, make sure you apply restraint correctly and provide adequate padding.
  - Assess skin, provide appropriate therapy, or remove restraints more frequently.
  - Change wet or soiled restraints.
- Patient becomes more confused and agitated after you apply restraints.
  - Determine the cause of the behavior and eliminate the cause, if possible.
  - Determine the need for more or less sensory stimulation.
  - Reorient as needed and/or attempt other restraint alternatives.
- Neurovascular status of an extremity is altered, manifested by cyanosis, pallor, edema, or coldness of skin, or patient complains of tingling, pain, numbness, or loss of ROM.
  - Remove the restraint immediately, stay with the patient, and notify the physician or health care provider.
  - Protect extremity from further injury.
- Patient releases the restraint and suffers a fall or other injury.
  - Attend to patient's immediate physical needs.
  - Notify the physician or health care provider.
  - Assess the type of restraint, correct application, and whether alternatives will be useful.

agitated patient, are a chemical restraint when they are not a standard part of that patient's treatment plan. You must have clinical justification for the use of a restraint, and it must be a part of the patient's prescribed medical treatment and plan of care. A physician's or health care provider's order is required and must be based on a face-to-face assessment of the patient. The order must be current and specify the duration and circumstances under which you will use the restraints. Your nursing interventions focus on preventing complications of restraints, such as hazards of immobility, a decreased sense of self-esteem, and increased agitation. Collaborate with other members of the health care team to design fall prevention programs and a restraint-free environment for the patient. The goal is to discontinue the use of restraints as soon as possible.

*Side Rails.* When used properly, side rails increase a patient's mobility and stability in bed when moving from a bed to a chair. Raising only the top two side rails gives the patient room to exit a bed safely and maneuver within the bed. Side rails also help to prevent the unconscious or sedated patient from rolling out of bed. Always check agency policy about the use of side rails; they are a restraint when used to prevent the patient's desired movement or activity, such as getting out of bed. Side rails also have the potential to trap the head and body in gaps and openings between the bed frame and mattress (Brush and Capezuti, 2001). Use side rail netting or protective padding to prevent the mattress from sliding to one side.

The use of side rails alone for a disoriented patient often causes only more confusion and further injury. Frequently a

**Holy Family Hospital and Medical Center**
**70 East Street, Methuen, MA 01844**

# BEHAVIORAL RESTRAINT
# FLOW SHEET

**Behavior Requiring Restraint:** (Check all that apply)

☐ Confusion/disorientation/combative

☐ Self Harm

☐ Harm to others/surroundings

☐ Removing medical devices

☐ Other: _____

**Physician order obtained:** ☐ Yes; ☐ No

**Type of Restraint:** (Check all that apply)

☐ Soft wrist/ankle

☐ Halter type vest

☐ Seat Belt

☐ Mitts

☐ Leather

☐ Other: _____

**Less Restrictive Measures Attempted:** (Check all that apply)

☐ Pain/comfort measures

☐ Schedule position changes

☐ Schedule toileting

☐ Place closer to Nursing Station

☐ Reorient

☐ Encourage family/friends to visit

☐ Other: _____

**Patient/Family Informed:** ☐ Yes; ☐ No

If no, Comment: _____

_____

**Date Restraint Applied:** _____ **Time:** _____

**Date Restraint** ☐ Ended / ☐ Renewed: _____ **Time:** _____

| Date:<br>Time:am/pm | 12 | 2 | 4 | 6 | 8 | 10 | 12 | 2 | 4 | 6 | 8 | 10 |
|---|---|---|---|---|---|---|---|---|---|---|---|---|
| 1. Hydration/Nutrition/Elimination | | | | | | | | | | | | |
| 2. Skin condition | | | | | | | | | | | | |
| 3. Range of motion/turn & position | | | | | | | | | | | | |
| 4. Communication (call light in reach) | | | | | | | | | | | | |
| 5. Circulation/Neurovascular Changes | | | | | | | | | | | | |
| 6. Assess chg. in clinical condition/behavior | | | | | | | | | | | | |
| 7. Assess for early release | | | | | | | | | | | | |
| 8. Restraint reduced/removed* | | | | | | | | | | | | |
| 9. Behavioral/Safety Check done q15" | | | | | | | | | | | | |
| 10. Vital Signs (if applicable)** | | | | | | | | | | | | |
| Initials of assessor: | | | | | | | | | | | | |

Initials/Signature: _____ Initials/Signature: _____ Initials/Signature: _____

Comments: _____

_____

_____

_____

* New order required when restraint removed or reduced.   ** Temperature not required unless indicated.

**KEY:** ✓ = Observation / Intervention;   NN = Nurses' Notes;   O = Patient Off Unit;   R = Restraint Removed

**Note:** It is not necessary to document the Behavioral/Safety Check every 15 minute but nurse must note every 2 hours in the assessment documentation #7 that the observation was performed. *Any changes in behavior require an assessment.*

*Caritas Christi · A Catholic Health Care System · Member*

Written: 7/95; Revised: 29 January 1999

FIGURE **26-1** Behavioral restraint flow sheet. (Courtesy Holy Family Hospital and Medical Center, Methuen, Mass.)

confused patient or one determined to get out of bed because of pain, toileting needs, or anxiety attempts to climb over the side rail or out at the foot of the bed. Either attempt usually results in a fall. To reduce a patient's confusion, focus your interventions first on the cause. Confusion is frequently mistaken for a patient's attempt to explore the environment or to self-toilet. If all efforts to reduce confusion or restlessness fail and the patient is at risk for injury to self or others, a restraint is sometimes necessary. However, remember the goal is to remove the restraint at the earliest possible time.

When you raise side rails, be sure the bed is in the lowest position possible.

*Fires.* A fire is always possible in the home or health care setting. Accidental home fires typically result from smoking in bed, careless extinguishing of cigarette butts in trash cans, grease fires, improper use of candles or space heaters, or electrical fires resulting from faulty wiring or appliances. Institutional fires typically result from a patient smoking in bed or from an electrical or anesthetic-related fire. Regardless of where the fire occurs, it is important to have an evacuation plan in place. Know where fire extinguishers and gas shut-off valves are located, and know how to activate a fire alarm.

To reduce the risk of fires in the home, have patients inspect the condition of cooking equipment and appliances, particularly irons and stoves. For patients with visual deficits, it helps to have dials installed with large numbers or symbols on temperature controls. Make sure smoke detectors are in strategic positions throughout the home (e.g., in a kitchen and near a bedroom) so that the alarms will alert the occupants in a home when a fire breaks out. Make sure all patients, even young children, are familiar with the phrase, "stop, drop, and roll," which describes what to do when a person's clothing or skin is burning.

If a fire occurs in a health care agency, first protect any patients in immediate danger. All personnel help to evacuate patients from the area, especially those patients who are closest to the fire. If a patient requires oxygen but not life support, discontinue the oxygen, which is combustible and will fuel an existing fire. If the patient is on life support, maintain the patient's respiratory status manually with a bag-valve mask (e.g., Ambu-bag) (see Chapter 28) until you move the patient away from the fire. Direct ambulatory patients to walk by themselves to a safe area, or have them assist in moving patients in wheelchairs. Move bedridden patients from the scene by a stretcher, their bed, or a wheelchair, or have one or two rescuers carry them. Use the blanket drag when two or more people are necessary to move a patient. Place the victim on a blanket and drag the victim headfirst along the floor to safety. A variant of the blanket drag is the clothes drag, where the rescuer drags the victim head first by upper body clothing. Another two-rescuer technique is the chair carry, where the victim is seated in a chair and both rescuers carry the chair (Integrated Publishing, 2004). If you must carry a patient, be careful not to overextend your physical limits for lifting because an injury to you will result in further injury to the patient. If fire department personnel are on the scene, they will also help to evacuate patients.

After a fire has been reported and patients are out of danger, you and other personnel need to take measures to contain or put out the fire, such as closing doors and windows, turning off oxygen and electrical equipment, and using a fire extinguisher. Extinguishers are used for three basic types of fires: paper and rubbish (type A), grease and anesthetic gas (type B), and electrical (type C). Use the appropriate extinguisher for each type.

Your best intervention to prevent fires is to comply with the agency's smoking policies and keep combustible materials away from heat sources. Some agencies have fire doors that are held open by magnets and close automatically when a fire alarm sounds. Make sure that you keep equipment away from these doors.

*Poisoning.* You help parents reduce the risk of accidental poisoning by teaching them to keep hazardous substances such as medications, cleaning fluids, and batteries out of the reach of children. With adolescents and adults, insect bites or snakebites are the leading causes of poisoning. Drug and other substance poisonings in these age-groups are commonly related to suicide attempts or drug experimentation. Teach parents that calling a **poison control center** for information before attempting home remedies will save their child's life. There are guidelines for accepted interventions for accidental poisonings that you teach a parent or guardian (Box 26-9). Older adults are also at risk for poisoning because diminished eyesight may cause an accidental ingestion of a toxic substance. In addition, the impaired memory of some older adult patients results in an accidental overdose of prescribed medications. Be sure medications are labeled in large print. Recommend the use of medication organizers that are filled once a week by the patient and/or family. Have patients keep poisonous substances out of the bathroom.

In the health care setting it is important for you to know how to respond when exposure to a poisonous substance occurs. OSHA considers mercury a hazardous chemical. Common exposures in a hospital include broken thermometers or sphygmomanometers. Mercury enters the body through inhalation and absorption through the skin. Exposures that occur in a hospital setting are usually short term, some of which affect the brain or kidney. However, full recovery is likely to occur once the body cleans itself of the contamination. Box 26-10 summarizes steps to take in the event of a mercury spill. Many hospitals are in the process of replacing mercury thermometers and sphygmomanometers with electronic equipment to improve safety.

*Bioterrorism.* Government agencies such as the Department of Homeland Security and the Centers for Disease Control and Prevention have developed plans to protect the health and safety of people at home and abroad in the event of a biological, chemical, or radiological attack (Perry and Potter, 2006). Preparedness is the first focus of these plans and is key to responding to any disaster. Health care facilities need to be prepared to treat mass casualties by having an emergency management plan. This plan details how to respond to a terrorist attack. Health care providers play a very important role in preparing for and responding to all types of disasters. Nurses, as the largest sector of the health care workforce, need to have a basic understanding of types of disasters and key components of a plan to deal with any mass casualty event (CDC, 2003a). When disaster strikes, the first priority is to ensure your own personal safety and that of other team members. Rapid response is crucial; therefore be familiar with agency policies for disaster response and specific roles to follow. In addition, know types of transmission, types of isolation and radiation precautions used, treatment options such as fluid and nutrition therapy, and crisis intervention techniques to manage public alarm and fear of the unknown. Participate in

## BOX 26-9 PROCEDURAL GUIDELINES FOR

### Intervening in Accidental Poisoning

1. Assess for signs or symptoms of accidental ingestion of harmful substances, such as nausea, vomiting, drooling, difficulty breathing, sweating, lethargy.
2. Terminate the exposure by emptying the mouth of pills, plant parts, or other material.
3. If poisoning is due to skin contact or eye contact, irrigate the skin or eye with copious amounts of tap water for 15 to 20 minutes. In the case of an inhalation exposure, safely remove the victim from the potentially dangerous environment.
4. Identify the type and amount of substance ingested to help determine the correct type and amount of antidote needed.
5. **If the victim is conscious and alert, call the local poison control center or the national toll-free poison control center number (1-800-222-1222) before attempting any intervention.** Poison control centers have information needed to treat poisoned patients or to offer referral to treatment centers. The administration of ipecac syrup is no longer recommended for routine home treatment of poisoning (American Academy of Pediatrics, 2003).
6. If the victim has collapsed or stopped breathing, call 911 for emergency transportation to the hospital. Initiate CPR, if indicated, until emergency personnel arrive. Ambulance personnel will be able to provide emergency measures if needed. In addition, parent or guardian is sometimes too upset to drive safely.
7. Position victim with head turned to side to reduce risk of aspiration.
8. Never induce vomiting if the victim has ingested the following poisonous substances: lye, household cleaners, hair care products, grease or petroleum products, and furniture polish, paint thinner, or kerosene.
9. Never induce vomiting in an unconscious or convulsing victim because vomiting increases risk of aspiration.

Modified from Hockenberry MJ: *Wong's Essentials of Pediatric Nursing*, St. Louis, 2005, Mosby and, American Academy of Pediatrics, Committee on Injury, Violence and Poison Prevention: Poison Treatment in the home, *Pediatrics* 112(5): 1182, 2003.

## BOX 26-10 Mercury Spill Cleanup Procedure

In the event of a mercury spill, follow these steps:
1. Evacuate the room except for a housekeeping crew (if available).
2. Cleanup personnel need to wear rubber (latex or vinyl) gloves while handling the mercury.
3. Spray the spill area with a mist of water. This diminishes vaporization of mercury.
4. Ventilate the area. Close interior doors, and open any outside windows.
5. Use a suction device, such as a syringe without a needle, to extract as much of the mercury as possible from the spill site. Put recovered mercury in a leakproof glass or plastic container with a nonmetallic cap or lid. **DO NOT VACUUM THE SPILL.**
6. Mop the floor with a mercury cleaner (see agency policy).
7. Dispose of collected mercury according to local environmental safety regulations.

ground. Teach patients and family how to reduce their risk of electrical injury in the home. For example, discuss prevention of electrical shock by avoiding use of electrical appliances near a water source, the importance of grounding appliances, and avoiding operation of unfamiliar equipment.

### Evaluation

**PATIENT CARE.** Evaluate your nursing interventions for reducing threats to safety by comparing the patient's response to the expected outcomes for each goal of care. When the expected outcomes are not achieved, revise your interventions. It is also possible that new nursing diagnoses have developed. Apply evaluative measures to determine a patient's progress toward outcomes and goals. An example of a goal, outcome, and evaluative measure includes the goal "Patient's environment is adapted to motor, sensory, and cognitive developmental needs." A possible outcome for this goal is "Modifiable hazards in the home are reduced by 100% within 2 weeks." Your evaluative measures would include "Observe environment for elimination of threats to safety" and "Reassess motor, sensory, and cognitive status for appropriate environmental modifications" (Table 26-3).

Evaluate the patient's outcome by comparing what you planned with what resulted, and evaluate how well you implemented the plan. Examine the planned interventions for appropriateness and effectiveness in each situation. By accomplishing goals and outcomes you validate effective care.

**PATIENT EXPECTATIONS.** The patient has come to expect the highest quality care from you and the health care system. Expectations as a result of care include restoration of health, reduction in risks for falling, a safer home environment, and improved recognition of safety risks. Patients are often unaware of the dangers in their homes and workplaces, and many will make the necessary adjustments to keep themselves and loved ones safe and injury free once you identify the dangers.

disaster planning efforts, education and training, and disaster drills to help prepare for a mass casualty event. The best protection in the event of any disaster is a strong and prepared public health system; well-trained medical personnel; coordinated planning between medical, public health, emergency management, and law enforcement personnel; and an informed public. Instruct patients to inquire about emergency plans at schools, day care centers, and places of work (American Medical Association, 2004).

***Electrical Hazards.*** Much of the equipment used in health care settings is electrical and needs to be well maintained. Decrease the risk of electrical injury and fire by using properly **grounded** and functional electrical equipment. The ground prong carries any stray electrical current back to the

## OUTCOME EVALUATION

**TABLE 26-3**

| Nursing Action | Patient Response/Finding | Achievement of Outcome |
|---|---|---|
| Observe environment for elimination of threats to safety. | Throw rugs have been removed or replaced with rubber-backed rugs.<br>Lighting has increased to 75 watts except in bathroom and bedroom.<br>Mr. Gonzales is able to identify potential hazards. | Mr. Gonzales has reduced hazards. Mr. Gonzales verbalizes adaptation to environmental modifications. |
| Reassess motor, sensory, and cognitive status for appropriate environmental modifications. | Mr. Gonzales has obtained new glasses.<br>Mr. Gonzales is able to read medication bottle labels and is using the medication organizer.<br>Mr. Gonzales takes 20-minute walks in the neighborhood at least 3 times per week.<br>Mr. Gonzales reports difficulty getting into bathtub due to stiffness. Bathtub floor is without nonskid strips. | Outcome of reducing hazards 100% has not been fully achieved. Mr. Gonzales will purchase nonskid strips for tub floor and bathtub transfer assist device. |

## EVALUATION

It has been 2 weeks since Joani implemented the plan of care for Mr. Gonzales. She has identified the hazards and made modifications. With regular exercise Mr. Gonzales has found that his walking has improved, and now he feels safer about leaving the apartment. The new medication labels and medication organizer have made it easier for Mr. Gonzales to tell his several medications apart. His new glasses will arrive within a few days. The patient is currently injury free and now feels better about living to a "ripe old age" like his father. He understands that he is able to make changes in his environment that will keep him safe. In the last 2 weeks he has not suffered a fall. Joani Green, the student nurse, has a sense of accomplishment in a job well done.

**Documentation Note**

"Mr. Gonzales' home has improved lighting, and he has removed the throw rugs. During good weather and during daylight hours he takes walks in his neighborhood. He is able to list all medications by name, dose, when taken, and significant side effects. No reports of injury."

## KEY CONCEPTS

- A safe environment in a health care agency is comfortable; maintains the patient's privacy; and reduces the risks of injury, infection, and untoward effects of treatment or medications.
- In the community a safe environment means basic needs are achievable, physical hazards are reduced, transmission of pathogens and parasites is reduced, pollution is controlled, and sanitation is maintained.
- The transmission of pathogens and parasites is reduced through medical and surgical asepsis, food sanitation, insect and rodent control, and disposal of human wastes.
- Every developmental stage involves assessment of specific safety risks.
- The school-age child is at risk for injury at home, at school, and traveling to and from school.
- Adolescents are at risk for injury from the effects of drug and alcohol abuse.
- Threats to an adult's safety are frequently associated with lifestyle habits.
- Risks of injury for older adults are directly related to the physiological changes of the aging process.
- Risks to patient safety within a health care agency include falls and patient-inherent, procedure-related, and equipment-related accidents.
- You individualize nursing interventions for promoting safety for developmental stage, lifestyle, and the environment.
- You continually evaluate the nursing care plan to promote safety in order to identify new or continued risks to the patient.
- Use physical restraints only as a last resort, when patients' behavior places them or others at risk for injury.

## CRITICAL THINKING IN PRACTICE

*You are assigned to care for Mrs. Pruitt, a 73-year-old who recently had a colectomy to remove a mass in her colon. Mrs. Pruitt did very well after her surgery. Although morphine has been effective in relieving her pain, during your initial assessment she appears agitated and restless and is picking at her tubes. You are concerned that Mrs. Pruitt is at risk for removing her nasogastric tube and IV catheter.*

- - - - - - - - - - - - - - - - - -

1. What measures do you take to prevent the use of a restraint with Mrs. Pruitt?
2. What factors about restraints and their safety implications affect your decision to use a restraint on Mrs. Pruitt?

3. If a restraint is necessary to avoid disruption of therapy, what interventions are necessary to ensure Mrs. Pruitt's safety while in restraints?
4. After application of upper extremity restraints, assistive personnel report that Mrs. Pruitt repeatedly tries to remove the restraints. What actions do you take after hearing this report? Select the correct choices. Explain your answers.
   a. Notify the physician or health care provider.
   b. Instruct the assistive personnel to continue hourly checks.
   c. Immediately assess Mrs. Pruitt's behavior.
   d. Instruct the assistive personnel to remove the restraints.

## NCLEX® REVIEW

1. You discover an electrical fire in a patient's room. Your first action is to:
   1. Activate the fire alarm
   2. Evacuate any patients/visitors in immediate danger
   3. Confine the fire by closing all doors and windows
   4. Extinguish the fire by using the nearest fire extinguisher
2. A parent calls the pediatrician's office frantic about the bottle of cleaner that her 2-year-old child drank. Which of the following is the most important instruction you give to this parent?
   1. Contact the local poison control center
   2. Take the child to the nearest emergency department
   3. Give the child milk
   4. Give the child syrup of ipecac
3. During your assessment of a 52-year-old man, he reports increased alcohol consumption secondary to stress at work. One of your expected outcomes for this patient is to:
   1. Provide this patient with resources for stress management classes
   2. Decrease his alcohol intake during stress
   3. Decrease stress in his life
   4. Teach him ways to promote sleep
4. You have just completed a gait assessment on 78-year-old Mrs. Jones. Your assessment reveals shuffling gait, decreased balance, and instability. Based upon this data, which one of the following nursing diagnoses indicates an understanding of the assessment findings?
   1. Activity intolerance
   2. Impaired bed mobility
   3. Disturbed sensory perception
   4. Risk for falls
5. You have just found your 68-year-old female patient wandering in the hallway in a confused pattern. She says she is looking for the bathroom. Which interventions are appropriate to ensure the safety of the patient?
   1. Ask the physician or health care provider to order a vest restraint.
   2. Insert a urinary catheter.
   3. Provide scheduled toileting rounds every 2 to 3 hours.
   4. Assign a nurse to stay with the patient.

5. Keep the bed in low position with the upper side rails up.
6. Keep the pathway from the bed to the bathroom clear.

6. Mrs. Kline, who is 62 years old, is being discharged to home with her husband after surgery for a hip fracture from a fall at home. When providing discharge teaching about home safety to this patient and her husband, you know that:
   1. A safe environment promotes patient independence
   2. Your assessment focuses on environmental factors only
   3. Teaching the patient and her husband about home safety is difficult to do in the hospital setting
   4. Most accidents in the older adult are due to lifestyle factors
7. A fragile 87-year-old nursing home patient has just been admitted to the hospital with increased confusion. The patient has upper limb restraints to prevent her from pulling the nasogastric tube. In delegating care of this patient to the assistive personnel; you would tell the assistive personnel to:
   1. Call the physician or health care provider if the patient becomes more agitated
   2. Check every hour the patient's circulation, skin integrity, and breathing
   3. Move the patient to a room down the hall
   4. Check to see if the patient can have a medication for agitation
8. Terry, the assistive personnel assigned to you, tells you that the portable sphygmomanometer broke while transferring a bed into a patient's room. There is now mercury on the floor of the room. Terry asks you what to do. The best answer to give her is:
   1. Spray the mercury with a fire extinguisher
   2. Pick the mercury up carefully with a towel
   3. Evacuate the room
   4. Tell the patient to remain in bed

9. A pleasantly confused 80-year-old patient was recently admitted to your medical unit. Your assessment reveals that she is at risk for injury due to falls because she continues to get out of bed without help despite frequent reminders. Your initial nursing intervention is to:
   1. Place a bed alarm device on the bed
   2. Place the patient in a vest restraint
   3. Provide one-to-one observation of the patient
   4. Apply wrist restraints

10. The family of your confused, ambulatory patient insists that all four side rails be up when the patient is alone. The best way to handle this situation is to:
    1. Thank them for being conscientious
    2. Restrict their visiting privileges
    3. Report them to the charge nurse
    4. Inform them of the risks associated with side rail use

## REFERENCES

American Academy of Pediatrics, Committee on Injury, Violence and Poison Prevention: Poison treatment in the home, *Pediatrics* 112(5):1182, 2003.

American Geriatrics Society, British Geriatrics Society, American Academy of Orthopedic Surgeons Panel on Falls Prevention: Guideline for the prevention of falls in older persons, *J Am Geriatr Soc* 49:664, 2001.

American Medical Association: *Bioterrorism: frequently asked questions,* 2004, http://www.ama-assn.org/ama/pub/category/6667.html.

American Nurses Association: *Nursing: scope and standards of practice,* Washington, DC, 2004, The Association.

Brush BL, Capezuti E: Historical analysis of siderail use in American hospitals, *J Nurs Scholarsh* 33(4):381, 2001.

Centers for Disease Control and Prevention, National Center for Injury Prevention and Control: *10 leading causes of death by age group—2001,* http://www.cdc.gov/ncipc/osp/charts.htm, accessed January 4, 2005, 2001, CDC.

Centers for Disease Control and Prevention: *Interim guidelines for hospital response to mass casualties from a radiological incident,* Atlanta, 2003a, CDC.

Centers for Disease Control and Prevention, Web-Based Injury Statistics Query and Reporting System (WISQARS), National Center for Injury Prevention and Control, 2003b, http://www.cdc.gov/ncipc/wisqars, accessed November 24, 2003, CDC.

Centers for Medicare and Medicaid Services: *Section 482.13 conditions of participation: patient's rights: interpretive guidelines and survey procedures—hospitals,* U.S. Department of Health and Human Services, 2000, CDC.

Coalition for Safe Community Needle Disposal: *EPA revises needle disposal options,* 2005a, http://www.safeneedledisposal.org/news/041216.html.

Coalition for Safe Community Needle Disposal: *Types of sharps disposal programs,* 2005b, http://www.safeneedledisposal.org/gentypes.html.

Dochterman JM, Bulechek GM: *Nursing interventions classification (NIC),* ed 4, St. Louis, 2004, Mosby.

Ebersole P, Hess P: *Geriatric nursing and healthy aging,* St. Louis, 2001, Mosby.

Ebersole P, Hess P: *Toward healthy aging,* St. Louis, 2004, Mosby.

Edelman CL, Mandle CL: *Health promotion throughout the life span,* ed 5, St. Louis, 2002, Mosby.

Farmer B: *Try this: best practices in nursing care to older adults,* New York, 2000, The Hartford Institute for Geriatric Nursing, New York University.

Federal Emergency Management Agency: *Disaster facts,* 2004a, http://www.fema.gov/library/df_1.shtm, accessed June 8, 2005.

Federal Emergency Management Agency: *Your family disaster plan,* 2004b, http://www.fema.gov/rrr/famplan/shtm, accessed January 4, 2005.

GeronurseOnline.org: *Want to know: physical Restraints,* 2005, http://www.geronurseonline.org/index.dfm?section_id=30&geriatric_topic_id=10&sub_section_id=74&page_id=156&tab=2.

Halfon P and others: Risk of falls for hospitalized patients: a predictive model based on routinely available data, *J Clin Epidemiol* 54(12):1258, 2001.

Hockenberry MJ: *Wong's essentials of pediatric nursing,* ed 7, St. Louis, 2005, Mosby.

Insurance Institute for Highway Safety, *Fatality facts: teenagers,* Arlington, Va, 2002, The Institute, http://www.iihs.org/safetyfacts/fatality/teens.htm, accessed September 15, 2003.

Integrated Publishing Inc: *Rescue drag and carry techniques,* 2004, http://www.tpub.com/corpsman/115.htm.

Joint Commission on Accreditation of Healthcare Organizations: *Comprehensive accreditation manual for hospitals,* 2004, Chicago, Ill.

Joint Commission on Accreditation of Healthcare Organizations: *2005 National Patient Safety Goals,* 2005, http://www.jcaho.org/accredited+organizations/patient+safety/npsg.htm, accessed January 4, 2005.

Moorhead S, Johnson M, Maas M: *Nursing outcomes classification (NOC),* ed 3, St. Louis, 2004, Mosby.

Morse JM: Enhancing the safety of hospitalization by reducing patient falls, *Am J Infect Control* 30:376, 2002.

National Fire Protection Association: *Smoking materials related to fires,* 2004, http://www.nfpa.org/displayContent.asp?categoryID=127, accessed January 4, 2005.

National Safety Council: *Fact sheet: carbon monoxide,* 2002a, Itasca, Ill.

National Safety Council: *Report on injuries in America,* 2002b, http://www.nsc.org/library/report_injury_usa.htm, accessed January 2, 2005.

Nix S: *Basic nutrition and diet therapy,* St. Louis, 2005, Mosby.

Perry A, Potter P: *Clinical nursing skills and techniques,* ed 6, St. Louis, 2006, Mosby.

Sorrentino SA: *Mosby's textbook for nursing assistants,* ed 6, St. Louis, 2004, Mosby.

Tinetti ME: Preventing falls in elderly persons, *N Engl J Med* 348:42, 2003.

Warner J: *Medical errors still plague U.S. hospitals,* 2004, http://my.webmd.com/content/Article/91/101128.htm, accessed June 8, 2005.

# CHAPTER 27

# Hygiene

## MEDIA RESOURCES

**CD COMPANION** *evolve* **WEBSITE**

http://evolve.elsevier.com/Potter/basic

- **NCLEX® Review**
- **Audio Glossary**
- **English/Spanish Audio Glossary**
- **Video Clips**

# OBJECTIVES

- Identify common skin problems and related interventions.
- Describe factors that influence personal hygiene practices.
- Discuss conditions that place a patient at risk for impaired skin integrity.
- Describe the types of bathing techniques used for various physical conditions and for patients of various age-groups.
- Perform a complete bed bath and back rub.
- Discuss factors that influence the condition of the nails and feet.
- Explain the importance of foot care for the diabetic patient.
- Describe the methods used for cleaning and cutting the nails.

- Discuss conditions that place a patient at risk for impaired oral mucous membranes.
- Discuss measures used to provide special oral hygiene.
- Assist with or provide oral hygiene.
- Describe effect of oral hygiene on periodontal disease.
- List common hair and scalp problems and their related interventions.
- Offer hygiene to meet the needs of patients requiring eye, ear, and nose care.
- Describe how hygiene for the older adult differs from that for the younger patient.
- Make an occupied and unoccupied hospital bed.

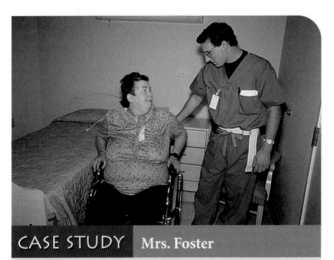

## CASE STUDY    Mrs. Foster

Mrs. Foster is a 55-year-old white woman who has been a resident in a skilled nursing facility for the past 3 years. She has a medical history of multiple sclerosis, a family history of coronary artery disease, and a healing stage I pressure ulcer on her coccyx. Mrs. Foster uses a wheelchair and requires assistance in transferring to the chair. Recently she has developed dental problems and had three root canal procedures. Mrs. Foster is married and has three daughters. Her family lives approximately 2 hours from the facility. Her family rotates visits so every weekend a family member is present. Mrs. Foster also receives telephone calls from her family on Tuesdays and Thursdays. Today she related the "need to feel better about herself."

James Joseph is a freshman nursing student assigned to the skilled nursing facility. James is 20 years old and single. James has had some experience working with patients who have been in a skilled nursing facility. James has a part-time job in a facility near his home. He knows how important it is for patients to feel comfortable and have their basic needs met.

To provide basic hygiene, James needs to learn about what is important to Mrs. Foster's comfort. When hygiene needs are not fulfilled, patients experience low self-esteem and have difficulties dealing with individuals in their environment. Give patients opportunities to maintain self-care needs. At an optimal level of functioning with assistance, this patient is at risk for potential self-care deficits, impaired skin integrity, and altered health maintenance. During hygiene James interacts with the patient to assess the patient's readiness to learn and to teach health promotion practices. James wants to preserve as much of the patient's independence as possible, ensure privacy, and foster physical well-being.

## KEY TERMS

acne, p. 720
buccal cavity, p. 716
complete bed bath, p. 728
dental caries, p. 721
dermis, p. 716
epidermis, p. 716

maceration, p. 733
oral hygiene, p. 721
partial bed bath, p. 728
perineal care, p. 728
subcutaneous, p. 716

## Scientific Knowledge Base

Good physical hygiene is necessary for comfort, safety, and well-being. People are usually capable of meeting their own hygiene needs; however, when ill, some people require assistance. Several factors influence hygiene practice. First deter-

| TABLE 27-1 | Functions of the Skin and Implications for Care |
|---|---|

| Function/Description | Implications for Care |
|---|---|
| **Protection** | |
| The epidermis is the relatively imperme-able skin layer that prevents entrance of microorganisms. Although microorgan-isms reside on skin surface and in hair follicles, relative dryness of surface in-hibits bacterial growth. Sebum removes bacteria from hair follicles. Acidic pH of skin further slows bacterial growth. | Weakening of epidermis occurs by scraping or stripping its surface as by use of dry razors, tape removal, or improper turning or positioning techniques. Excessive dryness causes cracks and breaks in skin and mucosa that allow bacteria to enter. Emollients soften and prevent moisture loss; soaking improves moisture retention; and hydration of mucosa pre-vents dryness. However, constant exposure to moisture causes maceration or softening, which interrupts dermal integrity and promotes ulcers and bacterial growth. Keep bed linen and clothing dry. Misuse of soap, detergents, cosmetics, deodorant, and depilatories causes chemical irritation. Alkaline soaps neutralize protective acid condition of skin. Cleansing removes excess oil, sweat, dead skin cells, and dirt that promote bacterial growth. |
| **Sensation** | |
| The skin contains sensory organs for touch, pain, heat, cold, and pressure. | Minimize friction to avoid loss of stratum corneum, which increases risk of pressure ul-cers. Smoothing linen removes sources of mechanical irritation. Remove rings during bathing to prevent injuring patient's skin. Make sure bath water is not too hot or cold. |
| **Temperature Regulation** | |
| Radiation, evaporation, conduction, and convection control body temperature. | Factors that interfere with heat loss can alter temperature control. Wet bed linen or gowns increase heat loss. Excess blankets or bed coverings interfere with heat loss through radiation and conduc-tion. Coverings conserve heat. |
| **Excretion and Secretion** | |
| Sweat promotes heat loss by evaporation. Sebum lubricates skin and hair. | Perspiration and oil sometimes harbor microorganism growth. Bathing removes excess body secretions, although excessive bathing causes dry skin. |

mine a patient's ability to perform self-care, and then pro-vide hygiene care according to your patient's needs and pre-ferred practices.

The skin and mucosa cells exchange oxygen, nutrients, and fluids with underlying blood vessels. The cells require adequate nutrition, hydration, and circulation to resist in-jury and disease. The skin often reflects a change in a per-son's physical condition by alterations in color, thickness, texture, turgor, temperature, and hydration.

## Skin

The skin is an active organ. The skin protects, secretes, ex-cretes, regulates temperature, and is a sense organ (Table 27-1). The three primary layers of the skin are the **epider-mis, dermis,** and **subcutaneous** tissue. The epidermis shields underlying tissue against water loss and injury and prevents entry of microorganisms. The dermis contains nerve fibers, blood vessels, sebaceous and sweat glands, and hair follicles. Subcutaneous tissue insulates and cushions the skin. Cleanliness of skin is basic for patient comfort.

## Feet and Nails

The feet and nails often require special attention to prevent infection, odor, and injury. Problems result from abuse or poor care. The feet are important to physical and emotional health. Foot pain often changes a walking gait, causing strain on different muscle groups. Discomfort while standing or walking leads to physical and emotional stress.

The nails are epithelial tissues that grow from the root of the nail bed, located in the skin at the nail groove. A nor-mal healthy nail is transparent, smooth, and convex, with a pink nail bed and translucent white tip. Disease causes changes in the shape, thickness, and curvature of the nail (see Chapter 13).

## Oral Cavity and Teeth

The oral cavity is lined with mucous membranes continuous with the skin. The oral or **buccal cavity** consists of the lips surrounding the opening of the mouth, the cheeks running along the side walls of the cavity, the tongue and its muscles, and the hard and soft palate. The oral mucosa is normally light pink and moist.

## Hair

Hair growth, distribution, and pattern indicate general health status (see Chapter 13). Hormonal changes, emo-tional and physical stress, aging, infection, and certain ill-nesses can affect hair characteristics. The hair shaft is an in-ert structure. A lack of hormones and nutrients to the hair follicle cause changes in hair color or condition.

## Care of the Eyes, Ears, and Nose

When you provide hygiene, the patient's eyes, ears, and nose also require careful attention. Chapter 36 describes the structure and function of these organs. You will cleanse these sensitive sensory tissues in a way that prevents injury and discomfort to the patient. For example, when washing your patient's face, be careful not to get soap into the eyes. In addition, the time you spend with your patient during hygiene provides an excellent opportunity to ask if there has been any change in vision, hearing, or sense of smell.

## Nursing Knowledge Base

A number of factors influence personal preferences for hygiene. No two individuals perform hygiene in the same way. As a nurse you will provide individualized care only after knowing about the patient's unique hygiene practices and preferences.

Hygiene care is never routine. Because hygiene care often requires intimate contact with the patient, use communication skills to promote a therapeutic relationship and to learn about the patient's emotional needs. Also use this time to convey caring and respect.

During hygiene care also assess your patient's readiness to learn about health promotion practices. As you bathe your patient, consider the patient's specific physical limitations, beliefs, values, and habits. Individual hygiene preferences do not significantly affect health, and you can usually include them in the plan of care. Preserve as much of the patient's independence as possible, ensure privacy, and foster physical well-being.

### Body Image

A patient's general appearance reflects the importance hygiene holds for that person. Body image is a subjective concept of a person's physical appearance. Body image changes frequently and affects the way in which patients maintain personal hygiene. The patient's body image may change as the result of surgery, illness, or a change in functional status. Because of these factors, make an extra effort to promote the patient's hygienic comfort and appearance.

### Social Practices

Social groups influence hygiene preferences and practices, including the type of hygienic products used and the nature and frequency of personal care. During childhood, family customs, such as the frequency of bathing and the time of day bathing is performed, influence hygiene. As children enter adolescence, dating and peer groups influence hygiene practices. Young girls, for example, become more interested in their personal appearance and begin to wear makeup. Later in life, friends and work groups shape the expectations people have about their personal appearance.

### Personal Preferences

Each patient has individual desires and preferences about when to bathe, shave, and perform hair care. Patients select different hygiene products according to personal preference and needs. These desires will assist you in delivering individualized care for the patient. In addition, assist the patient in developing new hygiene practices or adapting existing ones when indicated by an illness or condition.

| BOX 27-1 | CULTURAL FOCUS |
|---|---|

It is important to provide patients with a culturally competent plan of care. Hygiene is a personal matter; patients from different cultures will vary in the perceptions of who can assist in their care.

**Implications for Practice**
- Maintain privacy, especially for women from cultural groups that value female modesty.
- Avoid uncovering the lower torso and exposing the arms of Middle Eastern and East Asian women.
- Allow family member participation in the care of patients by adapting the schedule of hygiene activities when they are present.
- Provide gender-congruent care for Hindu, Orthodox Jewish, Muslim, and Amish patients.
  - Male patients prefer to be cared for by males; female patients prefer female caregivers.
  - Touching is taboo between unrelated males and females.
  - Have the patient or close kin do personal hygiene involving the lower torso if gender-congruent caregivers are not available.
- Respect cultural and religious practices relevant to hygienic practices.
  - Among Asians (Chinese, Japanese, Koreans, and Hindus), consider the top parts of the body cleaner than the lower parts.
  - Among Hindus and Muslims the left hand is used for cleaning whereas the right hand is reserved for eating and praying.

### Socioeconomic Status

A patient's economic resources influence the type and extent of hygiene practices used. Always be sensitive in considering if a patient's economic status influences his or her ability to regularly maintain hygiene. Determine whether patients are able to afford supplies such as deodorant, shampoo, toothpaste, and so on. In the home, assess if patients can assume the cost of needed modifications to the home environment, including safety devices such as nonskid surfaces in the bath or the addition of a tub chair in order for a patient to perform hygienic self-care. When patients have the added problem of limited socioeconomic resources, it is difficult for them to participate and take responsibility in health promotion activities.

### Cultural Variables

A patient's cultural beliefs and personal values influence hygiene care (Box 27-1). People from diverse cultural backgrounds follow different self-care practices (see Chapter 17). Culturally, maintaining cleanliness may not hold the same importance for some ethnic groups as it does for others. In North America it is common to bathe or shower daily, whereas in some other cultures it is customary to completely bathe only once a week.

### Health Beliefs and Motivation

Knowledge about the importance of hygiene and its implications for a person's well-being influences hygiene practices. However, knowledge alone is not enough. A patient needs to be motivated to maintain self-care. Health motivation is a general state of intent that results in behaviors to maintain or improve health. Studies show that patients' health beliefs or attitudes influence health-related behaviors (Champion, 1984). You must learn to know, for example, if a patient perceives being at risk for dental disease, perceives dental disease to be serious, perceives brushing to be effective in reducing risk, and perceives any negative implications from following recommended hygiene practices. When a patient recognizes there is a risk and reasonable action can be taken with no negative consequence, he or she will be more receptive to your nursing care.

### Physical Condition

People with certain illnesses or trauma or those who have undergone surgery sometimes lack the physical energy and dexterity to perform hygiene. A patient whose arm is in a cast or traction requires assistance with hygiene. Chronic illnesses, such as cardiac disease, cancer, or neurological disorders, often exhaust or incapacitate the patient and require you to perform total hygiene.

## Critical Thinking in Patient Care

### Synthesis

You will synthesize knowledge, draw from experience, use critical thinking attitudes, and be knowledgeable about intellectual and professional standards. Use practical experience and knowledge from scientific and nursing domains to provide individualized nursing care for patients requiring assistance with hygiene. The patient's hygiene needs and practices will differ from your own; therefore you will need to accept and respect these differences.

**KNOWLEDGE.** It is important that you understand the implications of proper hygiene for the patient's total health status. Proper hygiene promotes skin integrity, a sense of well-being, and improved body image. Knowledge about hygiene practices, which include cultural, developmental, and pathophysiological factors, provides a scientific basis for identifying and meeting patients' hygiene needs. For example, the diabetic patient has specialized needs for nail and foot care. The pathophysiology of diabetes and the effect of the illness on the patient's circulation provide you with the scientific knowledge base needed to implement proper foot care practices.

Use knowledge from basic sciences to determine how changes in mobility, aging, exposure to the environment, and pathophysiology affect the skin. To effectively identify the hygiene needs of individual patients, use your knowledge of communication techniques and cultural influences with regard to hygiene. These principles assist you in establishing a trusting relationship and acquiring basic understanding of the principles of self-concept in identifying and meeting your patient's hygiene needs.

Also apply knowledge of physical assessment skills (see Chapter 13) when providing hygiene. A thorough examina-

tion of the skin, oral cavity, peripheral circulation plus motor function or any limitations in range of motion will provide a database to identify hygiene problems and monitor a patient's progress over time.

**EXPERIENCE.** You have your own experiences in meeting specific hygiene needs. In addition, you may have assisted family members with their hygiene. Usually an early clinical experience involves providing hygiene to a patient. As your experience increases, your comfort and expertise in meeting the individualized hygiene needs of your patients increase as well.

**ATTITUDES.** There are multiple critical thinking attitudes that you can apply to hygiene care. For example, you use creativity to collaborate with the patient to determine the best way to meet hygiene needs. Be nonjudgmental and confident when providing care. Because patients' individual physical strength and hygiene practices will differ, it is important that you and the patient mutually establish flexibility in the patient's schedule to identify needs for periods of rest to lessen the chance of exhaustion during hygiene. You need to demonstrate responsibility and accountability when making the plan of care for the patient that will promote the patient's well-being.

**STANDARDS.** The use of critical thinking standards ensures that assessment of hygiene needs is relevant and accurate. You will also apply professional standards of care in your practice. For example, when caring for patients with diabetes, standards from the American Diabetes Association (ADA) will ensure that you give proper foot care.

Also apply standards of professional responsibility to advocate for the patient. During hygiene care, promote your patients' independence as much as possible while still maintaining their safety. Also be mindful of patients' limitations. These concerns for patients establish and maintain self-concept, independence, and mutual respect through advocacy.

## Nursing Process

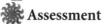 **Assessment**

Nursing assessment is an ongoing process. You do not assess all body regions before providing hygiene; however, you do routinely observe the patient as you give care. You will also assess whether the patient can tolerate hygiene procedures, which are often exhausting.

Most assessment occurs while you care for the patient's hygiene needs. For example, during oral care you are able to observe the condition of the teeth and mucosa. Hygiene care allows you to assess for a variety of health care problems and thus helps to set health care priorities (Table 27-2).

**ASSESSMENT OF THE SKIN.** While assisting a patient with personal hygiene, thoroughly assess all external body surfaces. Using inspection and palpation (see Chapter 13), look for alterations and determine the need for hygiene. Be sure to inspect anterior and posterior surfaces of all body structures. Carefully assess the skin under orthopedic devices (braces, splints) and beneath other applied equipment such as elastic support stockings and tape.

## FOCUSED PATIENT ASSESSMENT

**TABLE 27-2**

| Factors to Assess | Questions and Approaches | Physical Assessment Strategies |
|---|---|---|
| Skin care | Ask patient about hygiene practices, type of bath, frequency, use of soaps, lotions.<br>Ask if patient needs assistance to perform hygiene. | Observe patient during hygiene activities.<br>Inspect condition of skin and bony prominences. |
| Mouth | Ask if patient has difficulty chewing, change in appetite.<br>Ask if patient has dentures (upper, lower, and/or partial).<br>Ask if patient has any mouth sores. | Inspect condition of teeth, gums, and mouth.<br>Observe patient during mouth care or eating to determine presence of oral pain or discomfort that could impair hygiene practices.<br>Observe fit of dentures.<br>Inspect gums for sores or pressure areas. |
| Feet | Determine if patient is at risk for foot problems (e.g., peripheral vascular disease, callus formation).<br>Obtain information about patient's usual practices for foot and nail care. | Watch patient walk; observe for limping, uneven gait.<br>Inspect feet and between toes for pressure or open area.<br>Inspect patient's shoes for unequal wear.<br>Inspect nail beds for open sores, trauma, and proper nail care. |

## SYNTHESIS IN PRACTICE

Before entering Mrs. Foster's room, James reviews and synthesizes knowledge about the impact of chronic illness on body image and independence, reviews principles of communication, and reviews the pathophysiology for pressure ulcers.

When James arrives in Mrs. Foster's room, he finds her in bed facing the wall. Mrs. Foster does not want to talk; in fact, she is having a difficult time trying not to cry. Initially, James begins to straighten up the environment, giving Mrs. Foster some private time.

Previous clinical experience has taught James that patients need to have an opportunity to determine how nurses implement nursing care. By applying the ethical standard of autonomy, James encourages Mrs. Foster to make decisions about how to proceed. James engages Mrs. Foster into some discussion regarding how she would like her morning care. He learns that Mrs. Foster first likes to have face and hands washed and then her teeth brushed

before breakfast. But then she tells him that is not important. She tells him, "I am not going to have breakfast today, I just want to stay in bed because I am just not feeling well." James learns that Mrs. Foster was incontinent of stool during the night, and although the nurses did provide perineal care, Mrs. Foster still feels "dirty" and wants a shower. The night nurses told her she had to wait until her routine shower day, which is 2 days away. Mrs. Foster tells James that she is having more frequent incontinence. At this point in time James feels that assisting Mrs. Foster with a shower is his first priority.

James continues to synthesize knowledge and uses previous clinical experience to appropriately analyze assessment data and make his nursing diagnoses. He maintains accurate information and incorporates good communication skills, which will ensure meeting standards for quality care.

Observe the skin's color, texture, thickness, turgor, temperature, and hydration, giving special attention to the characteristics most influenced by hygiene measures. Is the skin dry from too much bathing? Are there calluses of the feet that will benefit from soaking?

Certain conditions place patients at risk for impaired skin integrity (see Chapter 35). Be particularly alert when assessing patients with reduced sensation, vascular insufficiency, and immobility. These patients are often unaware of skin disorders because they are unable to feel pressure or maneuver to self-inspect the skin. The development of pressure ulcers is a common complication that extends hospital stays.

While inspecting the skin, note the presence and condition of lesions. Certain common skin problems affect how you administer hygiene (Table 27-3). Take special care to assess less obvious surfaces, such as skinfolds, under the female

patient's breasts, or around perineal tissues. When you observe skin problems, explain proper skin care to the patient. Also educate the patient about avoiding irritants, which worsen the skin condition.

**Developmental Changes.** Age influences the normal condition of the skin and the type of hygiene required. The neonate's skin is relatively immature and thin. The epidermis and dermis are loosely bound together. Handle the neonate carefully during bathing to avoid friction, which sometimes results in bruising. A break in the skin will easily cause infection.

The toddler's skin layers are more tightly bound together and thus have a greater resistance to infection and skin irritation. However, because the child is more active and does not have regular hygiene habits, be attentive as a caregiver.

During adolescence, growth and maturation of the skin are increased. Sebaceous glands become more active, result-

| TABLE 27-3 | Common Skin Problems | | |
|---|---|---|---|
| **Problem** | **Characteristics** | **Implications** | **Interventions** |
| Dry skin | Flaky, rough texture on exposed areas such as hands, arms, legs, or face | Skin may become infected if epidermal layer cracks. | Bathe less frequently. Use superfatted soap (e.g., Dove) for cleansing. Rinse body of all soap well because residue left will cause irritation and breakdown. Add moisture to air through use of humidifier. Increase fluid intake when skin is dry. Use moisturizing lotion to aid healing process; lotion forms protective barrier and helps maintain fluid within skin. Use creams to clean skin that is dry or irritated by soaps and detergents. |
| Acne | Inflammatory, papulopustular skin eruption, usually involving bacterial breakdown of sebum; appears on face, neck, shoulders, and back | Infected material within pustule will spread if area is squeezed or picked. Permanent scarring can result. | Wash hair and skin each day with hot water and soap to remove oil. Use cosmetics sparingly because oily cosmetics or creams accumulate in pores and tend to make conditions worse. Implement dietary restrictions if necessary. Eliminate foods from diet that aggravate condition. Use prescribed topical antibiotics for severe acne. |
| Skin rashes | Skin eruption that may result from overexposure to sun or moisture or from allergic reaction; appears flat or raised, localized or systemic, pruritic or nonpruritic | If patient scratches skin, inflammation and infection will occur. Rashes also cause discomfort. | Wash area thoroughly, and apply antiseptic spray or lotion to prevent further itching and aid healing process. Warm soaks sometimes relieve inflammation. |
| Contact dermatitis | Inflammation of skin characterized by abrupt onset with erythema, pruritus, pain, and appearance of scaly oozing lesions; seen on face, neck, hands, forearms, trunk, and genitalia | Dermatitis is often difficult to eliminate because person is usually in continual contact with substance causing skin reaction. Substance may be hard to identify. | Condition usually disappears when patients avoid exposure to causative agents (e.g., cleansers, soaps). |
| Abrasion | Scraping or rubbing away of epidermis; results in localized bleeding and later weeping of serous fluid | Infection occurs easily as result of loss of protective skin layer. | Be careful not to scratch patients with your jewelry or fingernails. Wash abrasions with mild soap and water. Dressing or bandage sometimes increases risk of infection because of retained moisture. |

ing in **acne.** Eccrine and apocrine sweat glands become fully functional during puberty. More frequent bathing and use of antiperspirants become necessary to reduce body odors.

The condition of an adult's skin depends on hygiene practices and exposure to environmental irritants. Normally the skin is elastic, well hydrated, firm, and smooth. With age the skin loses its resiliency and moisture, and sebaceous and sweat glands become less active. This encourages dry, cracked skin. Daily bathing, inadequate fluid and nutrition, and the use of some soap products cause the skin of an older adult patient to become too dry (Box 27-2). The epithelium thins, and elastic collagen fibers shrink, making the skin fragile and subject to bruising and breaking. Use caution when turning and repositioning an older adult patient.

**Cultural Factors.** Each culture is unique in the way members perform personal hygiene. In addition, because

hygiene is a personal matter, patients from different cultures will vary in their perceptions of who can assist in their care. Be mindful of these differences when you assess patients in advance of hygiene care. Ask patients, "How would you prefer we do your bath?" "Are you comfortable with someone assisting you; if not, how can we best help you?" "Would you feel more comfortable having a nurse of the same sex bathe you?"

When caring for patients with dark skin pigmentation, be aware of assessment techniques and skin characteristics unique to highly pigmented skin (see Chapter 35). It is especially important to carefully assess dark skin in patients who are at risk for pressure ulcers. Understanding of normal skin assessment characteristics in patients with darkly pigmented skin assists in early identification of impaired skin integrity (Box 27-3).

| BOX 27-2 | CARE OF THE OLDER ADULT |
| --- | --- |

**Skin Changes With Aging**

- The turnover rate for the stratum corneum declines by 50% as the patient ages, resulting in slower healing, reduced barrier protection, and delayed absorption of medications or chemicals placed on the skin (Meiner and Lueckenotte, 2006).
- Older patients produce less sebum and perspire less and thus generally need to bathe less frequently. However, always consider their personal preferences.
- Older patients' skin is often more fragile; avoid hot water, and use only a mild cleansing agent. Some authorities suggest the use of bath oils; use with caution because this increases the danger of falling in a slippery tub.
- The majority of older patients have some degree of itching and skin sensitivity; hydrocortisone cream, superfatted soaps, and petrolatum offer relief.
- Dryness and redness are a common problem as skin ages. Minimize environmental factors that lead to skin drying such as low humidity (less than 40%) and exposure to cold. (Agency for Health Care Policy and Research [AHCPR], 1992).
- Elder abuse affects between 1 and 2 million persons a year; do not ignore unexplained bruises and skin trauma.

| BOX 27-3 | **Skin Assessment for the Patient With Darkly Pigmented Intact Skin** |
| --- | --- |

Assess localized skin color changes.
　　Any of the following may appear:
- Color darker than surrounding skin, purplish, bluish, eggplant
- Taut
- Shiny
- Indurations
- Assess for edema (nonpitting swelling)
　Use appropriate lighting to illuminate dark skin:
　- Use natural or halogen light.
　- Avoid fluorescent lamps, which give the skin a bluish tone.
　Assess skin temperature:
　- Area of pressure initially feels warmer than surrounding skin.
　- Subsequently area of pressure feels cooler than surrounding skin.
- Use the back of your hand and fingers and, if patient's condition permits, no gloves when doing this assessment.

Data from Bennett MA: Report of the task force on the implications for darkly pigmented intact skin in the prediction and prevention of pressure ulcers, *Adv Wound Care* 8(6):34, 1995.

**Assessment of Self-Care Ability.** When a patient is unable to bathe or perform personal skin care, you need to provide assistance. To determine whether a patient requires a bed bath instead of a tub bath or shower, assess your patient's balance, activity tolerance, and muscle strength and coordination. The degree of assistance needed by a patient during bathing also depends on the patient's vision, the ability to sit without support, hand grasp, and range of motion (ROM) of extremities. If your patient has some impairment in cognitive function, you will need to consult with therapists and specialists from other disciplines. This often requires an order from the physician or health care provider.

**ASSESSMENT OF FEET AND NAILS.** Incorporate foot care into the patient's daily hygiene routine. Often people are unaware of foot or nail problems until pain or discomfort occurs. Problems sometimes result from abuse or poor care of the feet and hands, such as nail biting or trimming nails improperly, exposure to harsh chemicals, and wearing poorly fitting shoes. Assess your patients for nail and foot problems by reviewing developmental factors contributing to alterations, determining the patient's type of footwear, and assessing hygiene care practices. Inspect the condition of the nails, and look for lesions, dryness, inflammation, or cracking (Table 27-4).

Chronic foot problems are common with older adults, who often have dry feet because of a decrease in sebaceous gland secretion, dehydration, or poor condition of footwear. Fissures result in severe itching. One of the more common problems in the older adult population is foot pain (Meiner and Lueckenotte, 2006).

**ASSESSMENT OF THE MOUTH. Oral hygiene** helps to maintain the healthy state of the mouth, teeth, gums, and lips. Brushing cleans the teeth of food particles, plaque, and bacteria. It also massages the gums and relieves discomfort resulting from unpleasant odors and tastes. Complete oral hygiene enhances well-being and stimulates the appetite. Your responsibilities in oral hygiene are maintenance and prevention. Help patients to maintain good oral hygiene by teaching correct techniques or by performing oral hygiene for weakened or disabled patients.

Include a thorough assessment for problems related to oral hygiene in every patient's care (Table 27-5). During the assessment, inform the patient about good oral hygiene habits. If during your assessment you identify any common oral problems (Box 27-4), notify the patient's physician or health care provider. Early identification of poor oral hygiene practices and common oral problems reduces the risk of gum disease and **dental caries** or cavities (Box 27-5).

**ASSESSMENT OF HAIR.** A person's appearance and feeling of well-being often depend on the way the hair looks and feels. Illness or disability sometimes prevents a patient from maintaining daily hair care. An immobilized patient's hair soon becomes tangled. Dressings may leave sticky blood or antiseptic solutions on the hair. Proper hair care is important to the patient's body image. Brushing, combing, and shampooing are basic hygiene measures for all patients.

Before performing hair care, assess the condition of the hair and scalp (Table 27-6). Findings will reveal the frequency and extent of care needed. Conditions such as arthritis, fatigue, and the presence of physical encumbrances (e.g.,

**TABLE 27-4** **Common Foot and Nail Problems**

| Problem | Characteristics | Implications | Interventions |
|---|---|---|---|
| Callus | Thickened portion of epidermis, consisting of mass of horny, keratotic cells; usually flat, painless, and found on undersurface of foot or on palm of hand; caused by local friction or pressure. | Foot calluses may cause discomfort when wearing tight-fitting shoes. | Wear gloves when using tools or objects that create friction on palms. Wear comfortable shoes. Soak callus in warm water and Epsom salts to soften cell layers (soaking of feet is contraindicated with diabetic patients). Use pumice stone to remove callus after it softens. Be careful not to use stone on noncallused skin. Applications of creams or lotions reduce re-formation. Use of orthotic devices (e.g., foam insoles, metatarsal pads, various cushioning devices) redistributes weight and pressure away from callus area. |
| Corns | Keratosis caused by friction and pressure from shoes; mainly on toes, over bony prominence; usually cone shaped, round, and raised; calluses with painful core. | Conical shape compresses underlying dermis, making it thin and tender. Tight-fitting shoes aggravate pain. Tissue will attach to bone if allowed to grow. Patient sometimes suffers alteration in gait because of pain. | Surgical removal may be necessary, depending on location and severity of pain and size of corn. Use oval corn pads carefully, because they increase pressure on toes and reduce circulation. Do not use corn pads for diabetics or patients with impaired circulation. |
| Plantar warts | Fungating lesion that appears on sole of foot; caused by papillomavirus. | Warts are sometimes contagious, painful, and make walking difficult. | Treatment ordered by physician or health care provider may include topical applications of acids, electrodesiccation (burning with electric spark), cryotherapy (freezing with carbon dioxide or liquid nitrogen), or laser therapy (Osterman and Stuck, 1990). |
| Athlete's foot (tinea pedis) | Fungal infection of foot; scaliness and cracking of skin between toes and on soles of feet; small blisters containing fluid appear, apparently induced by constricting footwear (e.g., sneakers). | Athlete's foot can spread to other body parts, especially hands. It is contagious and frequently recurs. | Make sure feet are well ventilated. Drying feet well after bathing and applying powder help prevent infection. Wearing clean socks or stockings reduces incidence. Physician or health care provider may order application of griseofulvin, miconazole nitrate, or tolnaftate. |
| Ingrown nails | Toenail or fingernail growing inward into soft tissue around nail; results from improper nail trimming, poor shoe fit, or heredity. | Ingrown nails cause localized pain in presence of pressure. | Treatment is frequent hot soaks in antiseptic solution and removal of portion of nail that has grown into skin. Instruct patient in proper nail trimming techniques. Recommend professional podiatry if needed. |
| Ram's horn nails | Unusually long, curved nails. | Attempt by nurse to cut nails may damage nail bed and/or cause infection. | Refer patient to podiatrist. |
| Paronychia | Inflammation of tissue surrounding nail after hangnail or other injury; occurs in people who frequently have their hands in water; common in diabetic patients. | Area sometimes becomes infected. | Treatment is hot compresses or soaks and local application of antibiotic ointments. Careful manicuring prevents parenchyma. |
| Foot odors | Result of excess perspiration promoting microorganism growth. Faulty foot hygiene or improper footwear also cause foot odor. | | Frequent washing, use of foot deodorants and powders, and clean footwear will prevent or reduce this problem. |
| Nail fungal infection | Results from excess moisture and use of artificial nails. | Infection requires treatment with a fungicide. | Wear clean, dry footwear (see athlete's foot). |

| TABLE 27-5 | Risk Factors for Hygiene Problems |
|---|---|

| Risks | Hygiene Implications |
|---|---|
| **Oral Problems** | |
| Patients who are unable to use upper extremities due to paralysis, weakness, or restriction (e.g., cast or dressing) | Patient lacks upper extremity strength or dexterity needed to brush teeth. |
| Dehydration, inability to take fluids or food by mouth (NPO) | Causes excess drying and fragility of mucosa; increases accumulation of secretions on tongue and gums. |
| Presence of nasogastric or oxygen tubes; mouth breathers | Causes drying of mucosa. |
| Chemotherapeutic drugs | Drugs kill rapidly multiplying cells, including normal cells lining oral cavity. Ulcers and inflammation develop. |
| Over-the-counter lozenges, cough drops, antacids, and chewable vitamins | Medications contain large amounts of sugar. Repeated use increases sugar or acid content in mouth. |
| Radiation therapy to head and neck | Causes oral mucositis, which affects all the mucosal folds within the oral cavity, resulting in erythema, ulceration, and pain (Scully, 2004). |
| Oral surgery, trauma to mouth, placement of oral airway | Cause trauma to oral cavity with swelling, ulcerations, inflammation, and bleeding. |
| Immunosuppression; alters blood clotting | Predisposes to inflammation and bleeding gums. |
| Diabetes mellitus | Prone to dryness of mouth, gingivitis, periodontal disease, and loss of teeth. |
| Poorly fitting dentures | Food trapped under dentures causes mouth odor. |
| Inadequate brushing and flossing of teeth | Predisposes patients to periodontal disease. |
| Cardiovascular disease | Linked to periodontal disease. |
| **Skin Problems** | |
| Immobilization | Dependent body parts are exposed to pressure from underlying surfaces. The inability to turn or change position increases risk for pressure ulcers. |
| Reduced sensation due to stroke, spinal cord injury, diabetes, local nerve damage | Patient does not receive normal transmission of nerve impulses when excessive heat or cold, pressure, friction, or chemical irritants are applied to skin. |
| Limited protein or caloric intake and reduced hydration (e.g., fever, burns, gastrointestinal alterations, poorly fitting dentures) | Limited caloric and protein intake predispose to impaired tissue synthesis. Skin becomes thinner, less elastic, and smoother with a loss of subcutaneous tissue. Poor wound healing results. Reduced hydration impairs skin turgor. |
| Excessive secretions or excretions on the skin from perspiration, urine, watery fecal material, and wound drainage | Moisture is a medium for bacterial growth and causes local skin irritation, softening of epidermal cells, and skin maceration. |
| Presence of external devices (e.g., casts, restraint, bandage, dressing) | Device exerts pressure or friction against skin's surface. |
| Vascular insufficiency | Arterial blood supply to tissues is inadequate, or venous return is impaired, causing decreased circulation to extremities. Tissue ischemia and breakdown occur. Risk for infection is high. |
| **Foot Problems** | |
| Patient unable to bend over or has reduced visual acuity | Patient is unable to fully visualize entire surface of each foot, making it difficult to adequately assess condition of skin and nails. |
| Decreased sensation | Patient is unable to sense pressure. Patient requires education on importance of regular foot inspection and the potential for referral to podiatrist. |
| **Eye Care Problems** | |
| Reduced dexterity and hand coordination | Physical limitations create inability to safely insert or remove contact lenses. |

---

**BOX 27-4** | **Common Oral Problems**

**Dental Caries (Cavities)**

Caries are most common among young people
Buildup of plaque causes acid destruction of tooth enamel.
  Initially appears as chalky, white discoloration of the tooth

**Periodontal Disease (Pyorrhea)**

Most common after age 35
Involves destruction of gingiva (gums) and other supporting
  structures with bleeding gums, inflammation, and receding
  gum lines

**Other Problems**

Oral mucositis (oral erythema, ulceration, and pain)
Glossitis (inflammation of the tongue)
Gingivitis (inflammation of the gums)
Halitosis (bad breath)
Cheilosis (cracked lips)
Oral malignancy (mouth lumps or ulcers)

---

cast or intravenous [IV] access) often alter a patient's self-care ability. Assess your patient's physical ability to perform hair care. It is also essential to consider a patient's personal hair care practices so you make every effort to maintain the patient's preferred appearance (Box 27-6).

**Cultural Practices.** When caring for patients from different cultures, learn as much as possible about and be sensitive to the patients' customs, beliefs, and practices. Ask the patient about preferred hair care methods or any cultural restrictions. For example, African-Americans usually have dry hair. Use special lanolin conditioners to maintain conditioning.

**ASSESSMENT OF EYES, EARS, AND NOSE.** Give special attention to cleansing the eyes, ears, and nose during the patient's bath. Focus care on preventing infection and maintaining normal organ function. Carefully inspect all external eye structures. Normally the conjunctivae are clear and not inflamed. The eyelid margins are in close approximation with the eyeball, and the lashes are turned outward. The lid margins are normally without inflammation, drainage, or lesions. Flaking skin around the eyebrows sometimes indicates dandruff.

Assessment of the external ear structures includes inspecting the auricle, external ear canal, and tympanic membrane. When performing hygiene, you are most concerned with presence of accumulated cerumen or drainage in the ear canal, local inflammation, or pain. It is easy for cerumen to become impacted, so make sure to irrigate the ear canal routinely, especially in older adults.

Inspect the nares for signs of inflammation, discharge, lesions, edema, and deformity. The nasal mucosa is normally pink, clear, and without discharge. For patients with any form of tubing exiting the nose, observe for tissue sloughing, localized tenderness, inflammation, and even bleeding.

**BOX 27-5** | USING EVIDENCE IN PRACTICE

**Research Summary**

A number of studies have shown institutionalized older adults have a higher prevalence of nosocomial bacteria pathogens causing lower respiratory infections. In this study, researchers suspected that a source for the pathogens was the oral cavity and that dental plaque (DP) served as the reservoir, especially with patients with poor oral hygiene. A sample of 49 older adult patients participated in the study. All patients had poor oral hygiene and high plaque indexes. However, the patients with colonized DP had a significantly lower functional status, less ability to perform activities of daily living, and worse plaque index then the noncolonized patients. Fourteen patients developed pneumonia, and researchers traced the bacteria pathogens of the pneumonia to the bacteria in the patient's initial dental plaque.

**Application to Nursing Practice**

As a nurse you can apply the results of this study by providing more rigorous oral hygiene to patients at risk for respiratory complications, such as older adults and unconscious patients. This study depicted how the presence of dental plaque in institutionalized older adults contributes to bacteria in the oral cavity. The bacteria are easily aspirated, resulting in the development of lower respiratory tract infection or pneumonia. Therefore it is important that nurses complete a thorough assessment of patients, including their ability to perform adequate oral hygiene and the hygiene agents they use. Patients will benefit from a plan of care that increases the frequency of oral hygiene and uses new antimicrobial mouthwashes that attack dental plaque.

Data from El-Solh A and others: Colonization of dental plaques: a reservoir of respiratory pathogens for hospital-acquired pneumonia in institutionalized elders, *Chest* 126(5):1575, 2004.

**Use of Sensory Aids.** For patients who wear eyeglasses, contact lenses, artificial eyes, or hearing aids, assess the patient's knowledge regarding methods used to care for the aids, as well as any problems caused by them. Have patients describe how they typically care for the aids. Compare information gathered with what you know is the proper care technique. Any inconsistencies in findings will indicate a need for patient education.

Assess your patient's physical ability to perform eye, ear, and nose care and care of any sensory aids. Patients who are unable to grasp small objects (e.g., hearing aid battery or contact lens), have limited upper extremity mobility, have reduced vision, or are seriously fatigued will require assistance.

**PATIENTS AT RISK FOR HYGIENE PROBLEMS.** There are patients who present risks that require more attentive and rigorous hygiene care (see Table 27-5). These risks result from side effects of medications, lack of knowledge, an inability to perform hygiene, or a physical condition that potentially injures the skin, integument, or other struc-

| TABLE 27-6 | Hair and Scalp Problems | | |
|---|---|---|---|
| **Problem** | **Characteristics** | **Implications** | **Interventions** |
| Dandruff | Scaling of the scalp accompanied by itching; in severe cases, dandruff on eyebrows. | Dandruff causes embarrassment; if dandruff enters eyes, conjunctivitis may develop. | Shampoo regularly with medicated shampoo; in severe cases seek physician's or health care provider's advice. |
| Ticks | Small gray-brown parasites that burrow into skin and suck blood. | Ticks transmit Rocky Mountain spotted fever, Lyme disease, and tularemia. | Do not pull ticks from skin; sucking apparatus remains and may become infected; place drop of oil or ether on tick, or cover it with petrolatum to ease removal. |
| Pediculosis capitis (head lice) | Tiny grayish white parasitic insects that attach to hair strands; eggs look like oval particles, resemble dandruff; bites or pustules often found behind ears and at hairline. | Head lice are difficult to remove and if not treated will spread to furniture and other people. | Check entire scalp. Use medicated shampoo for eliminating lice or permethrin (Nix) available as a crème rinse. **Caution against use of products containing lindane, because the ingredient is toxic and known to cause adverse reactions** (National Pediculosis Association, 2001). Remove patient's clothing before treatment, and apply new clothing following treatment. Repeat treatment according to product directions. Check the hair for nits and comb with a nit comb for 2 to 3 days until sure all lice and nits have been removed. Manual removal of lice is best option when treatment has failed. Vacuum infested areas of home. Vacuum car upholstery as well. |
| Pediculosis corporis (body lice) | Tend to cling to clothing, making them difficult to see; body lice suck blood and lay eggs on clothing and furniture. | Patient itches constantly; scratches on skin become infected; hemorrhagic spots appear on skin where lice are sucking blood. | Have patient bathe or shower thoroughly; after drying skin, apply lotion for eliminating lice; after 12 to 24 hours have patient take another bath or shower; bag infested clothing or linen until laundered. |
| Pediculosis pubis (crab lice) | Found in pubic hair; crab lice are grayish white with red legs. | Lice spread through bed linen, clothing, furniture, or sexual contact. | Shave hair off affected areas; cleanse as for body lice; if lice were sexually transmitted, patient needs to notify partner. |
| Alopecia | Balding patches in periphery of hair line; hair becomes brittle and broken; caused by improper use of hair curlers and picks, tight braiding, hot styling tools, certain diseases. | Patches of uneven hair growth and loss alter patient's appearance. Alopecia is very distressing for all patients, especially women. Hair care practices do not cause or accelerate male pattern. | Stop hair care practices that damage hair (e.g., teasing hair, hair dyes, excessive heat when blow-drying). |

| BOX 27-6 | Assessment of Hair Care |
|---|---|

**Physical Changes**

Assess condition of hair and scalp (see Chapter 13). Consider age-appropriate changes.
Consider racial or ethnic differences.
Determine reasons for change in distribution or loss of hair.
Check oiliness and texture of hair.
Inspect scalp for lesions, inflammation, infection, or parasites.

**Self-Care Ability**

Assess patient's ability to grasp comb or brush.
Determine patient's ability to physically care for hair.
Does patient become easily fatigued?

**Hair-Care Practices**

Assess patient's preferences in hair styling.
Identify patient's preferences for hair care and shaving products.
Assess adequacy of patient's hygiene practices.
Determine patient's perceptions of own appearance.
Assess patient's socioeconomic background.

ture. For example, an immobilized patient with a fever will become diaphoretic and have difficulty turning independently. The patient will require more frequent bathing, turning, and positioning to reduce the risk for skin breakdown. Also, older adults sometimes need extra assistance because of changes in their sensory status. When the aging process alters vision, touch, and gait in a way that makes common everyday practices difficult, you will be more involved in the patient's care.

Your assessment will include risks for hygiene problems. Timely identification of these risks results in nursing interventions designed to prevent injury to the skin, feet and nails, and oral mucosa.

**PATIENT EXPECTATIONS.** With all nursing care it is important to know the patient's expectations. Hygiene is a very personal aspect of care, and patients will indeed have varying expectations. When providing skin care, determine the patient's preferences for soaps, lotions, showers, or tub bath. How much privacy does the patient wish? Is it important to have hygiene completed before family members visit, or does the patient wish the family to assist with hygiene practices? Incorporate the patient's routine practices into hygiene care whenever possible. You will need extra time to offer the patient a shampoo. However, hygiene is one aspect of care where flexibility is easier to achieve.

## Nursing Diagnosis

Your assessment will reveal the patient's need for and ability to maintain personal hygiene. Review all data gathered (e.g., the patient's risk for physical immobilization, presence of secretions, or altered circulation and sensation). Clustering of defining characteristics allows you to identify the nursing diagnoses related to hygiene. Accurate selection of a diagnosis ensures that you will meet the patient's needs. A nursing diagnosis is accurate only if you select the appropriate related factors, which influence the nursing therapies chosen. For the diagnosis *impaired skin integrity related to decreased mobility,* you will select nursing interventions that will increase the patient's mobility and lower risk of skin breakdown. Frequent turning or repositioning, using a proper support surface, and removing underlying tubing are good measures. In contrast, the diagnosis *impaired skin integrity related to exposure to body excretions* requires you to choose different therapies. Frequent skin cleansing, controlling sources of wound drainage or incontinence, and timely bed linen changes are good measures to control the irritation of excretions. Remember, selecting an incorrect related factor for a diagnosis will result in inappropriate and ineffective nursing care. Use your judgment and critical thinking as you carefully select diagnoses for your patient. Nursing diagnoses for patients with hygiene problems may include:

- Bowel incontinence
- Impaired dentition
- Fatigue
- Ineffective health maintenance
- Functional urinary incontinence
- Risk for infection
- Deficient knowledge
- Impaired physical mobility
- Impaired wheelchair mobility
- Impaired oral mucous membrane
- Risk for powerlessness
- Bathing/hygiene self-care deficit
- Dressing/grooming self-care deficit
- Situational low self-esteem
- Impaired skin integrity
- Impaired tissue integrity
- Ineffective tissue perfusion (peripheral)

## Planning

During planning use critical thinking to ensure that you individualize the plan of care to meet the patient's needs according to the nursing diagnoses identified (see care plan). In planning care it is important that you identify patient goals and outcomes, set priorities for care, and plan for continuity of care.

**GOALS AND OUTCOMES.** After you identify and individualize nursing diagnoses, partner with the patient to set goals and expected outcomes of care. Establish goals with the patient's self-care abilities, risks, and resources in mind. Focus on maintaining or improving the condition of the skin and mucosa. Develop outcomes that are measurable and achievable within patient limitations. Once you establish goals and outcomes, work closely with the patient to select hygiene measures that are appropriate and realistic. Remember, it is important to consider a patient's hygiene preferences.

You will provide hygiene for a variety of patients with different self-care abilities. For example, in the case of the patient who has one-sided paralysis following a cerebral vascular accident (stroke), you might develop the following goal: "Patient's musculoskeletal system remains free of breakdown or contractures." You would then establish a series of realistic individualized expected outcomes that might include:

- Patient's skin is clean, dry, and intact without signs of inflammation.
- Patient's skin remains elastic and well hydrated.
- Patient's range of joint motion remains within normal limits on both affected and unaffected side.
- Patient tolerates bathing without excessive fatigue.

**SETTING PRIORITIES.** The patient's condition influences your priorities for delivering hygiene. For example, a seriously ill patient usually needs a daily bath because body secretions accumulate, and the patient is unable to maintain cleanliness. An older adult patient who is awaiting discharge may sometimes only need a partial bath before leaving the hospital. Set priorities based on the necessary assistance required by patients, the extent of hygiene problems, and the nature of the patient's nursing diagnoses. For example, a pa-

## CARE PLAN Skin Care

### ASSESSMENT

Mrs. Foster is very concerned about her physical appearance. She wants to "look her best." She is in a semiprivate room. She has been alone in her room for the last 3 months, but last week a new patient was admitted and now she has a new roommate. Mrs. Foster is **in a wheelchair** and **does not have the coordination or muscle strength to independently transfer or stand.** Her skin is intact, but when she arises from the wheelchair, there is **prolonged erythema over the ischial pressure areas bilaterally.** Her skin is **dry, her fingernails and toenails are very brittle,** and **she is frequently incontinent of stool and urine.** Once she is in her wheelchair, her main activity is watching TV. Mrs. Foster has her hair cut once a month at the in-house beauty shop. She has two married children and five grandchildren. Members of her family visit every weekend. Her shower is scheduled for Monday, Thursday, and Saturday.

*Defining characteristics are shown in bold type.

---

**NURSING DIAGNOSIS** Risk for impaired skin integrity related to impaired mobility and incontinence.

---

### PLANNING

**GOAL**
- Patient's skin remains intact.

**EXPECTED OUTCOMES***
- Patient's skin is without increased erythema.
- Patient's skin remains dry.
- Patient's skin is odor free.
- Patient reports feeling clean and dry.

*Outcomes classification label from Moorhead S, Johnson M, Maas M: *Nursing outcomes classification (NOC),* ed 3, St. Louis, 2004, Mosby.

---

### INTERVENTIONS†

- Provide perineal care after each incontinence episode.

- Change linen after diaphoresis or incontinence episode.

- Apply lotion to areas that easily become dried and chapped.

- Monitor length of time any area of redness persists. Determine turning and positioning interval. Turning interval – hypoxia time = suggested interval (e.g., 2 hours – 30 minutes = $1\frac{1}{2}$ hours). Instruct patient that while sitting in wheelchair to shift position in chair during commercials.
- Do **not** massage reddened areas.

### RATIONALE

Minimizing skin exposure to moisture decreases irritation and susceptibility to injury (Panel for the Prediction and Prevention of Pressure Ulcers in Adults [PPPUA], 1993).
Moisture from wet linen causes maceration, which increases risk of pressure ulcers.
Lotion reduces drying and chapping of skin. Dry, chapped skin impairs skin integrity and is port of entry for bacteria.
Repositioning reduces pressure and allows for normal hyperemic response (Bennett, 1995).

Massage increases breaks in capillaries in underlying tissues, causing skin breakdown (Maklebust, 1991; U.S. Department of Health and Human Services [USDHHS], 1994).

†Intervention classification labels from Dochterman JM, Bulechek GM, editors: *Nursing interventions classification (NIC),* ed 4, St. Louis, 2004, Mosby.

---

### EVALUATION

- Observe skin for pressure and moisture after each position change, according to turning interval, every $1\frac{1}{2}$ hours.

- Inspect skin for breakdown.
- Ask patient how her skin feels after skin care.

---

tient who has *acute pain* requires a bath but it is necessary to administer pain medications first before giving the bath.

Timing is also important in planning hygiene care. Being interrupted in the middle of the bath for an x-ray procedure can frustrate and embarrass the patient. If a patient is tired after extensive diagnostic tests (e.g., stress test), rest will be an important patient priority. In this situation it is best to delay hygiene and allow the patient to rest.

**CONTINUITY OF CARE.** It is important to plan for care throughout the patient's hospital visit, discharge to a rehabilitation facility, and home in order to achieve a restored

level of wellness. It is sometimes necessary for you to assist the family in developing a plan for providing hygiene care in which the patient gradually takes over some self-care responsibility that he or she is able to manage. Be mindful of the equipment and procedures used in the agency so that the patient and family are knowledgeable about the care, have the skill needed to provide the care, and have access to necessary equipment.

Collaborate with other health care providers such as physical or occupational therapists. For example, physical therapists assist patients with strengthening exercises needed for bathing, and occupational therapists fit patients with useful assist devices that allow patients to pick up toileting items. Use various community resources, such as having home care agencies provide staff to assist with bathing if the patient and/or family are unable to perform hygiene activities.

## 🌸 Implementation

**HEALTH PROMOTION, ACUTE CARE, AND RESTORATIVE AND CONTINUING CARE.** You will use the nursing knowledge and skills needed for performing hygiene care consistently in all health care settings to provide health promotion, acute care, and restorative and continuing care.

**BATHING AND SKIN CARE.** In hospital settings, you will usually bathe patients in the morning when more staff are available, unless the patient's condition contraindicates or the patient strongly prefers a different option. The Panel for Prediction and Prevention of Pressure Ulcers (Agency for Health Care Policy and Research [AHCPR], 1992) made important recommendations for bathing. The panel designed guidelines to prevent and treat pressure ulcers, but these guidelines are also sound principles for good bathing techniques.

- Clean the skin at the time of soiling and at routine intervals. Individualize frequency of cleansing according to patient need and preference. Problems such as incontinence, wound drainage, or excessive diaphoresis require bathing several times a day.
- Avoid hot water, and use a mild cleansing agent that minimizes irritation.
- During cleansing of the skin avoid use of force and friction.
- Minimize environmental factors that lead to skin drying such as low humidity (less than 40%) and exposure to cold.

Additional guidelines to apply in bathing include:

- Protect patients from injury by assessing and controlling the bath water temperature. This is especially important for older adults and others with reduced sensation, such as diabetics with peripheral neuropathy or spinal cord–injured patients.
- Use bathing as a time to interact with and assess a patient. When giving a complete bath, examine a variety of body systems and discuss issues of concern for the patient.
- During bathing assist patients through joint range-of-motion exercises to promote circulation and joint integrity.

For patients who fatigue easily, consider administering a partial instead of a complete bed bath.

When educating patients, instruct them to follow a few general rules for skin health. Have patients routinely inspect their skin for any changes in skin color and texture and re-

---

**BOX 27-7** **Types of Baths**

**Complete bed bath**—Bath administered to totally dependent patient in bed.

**Partial bed bath**—Bed bath that consists of bathing only body parts that would cause discomfort if left unbathed, as well as washing back and a back rub. Give a partial bath to dependent patients in need of partial hygiene or self-sufficient bedridden patients who are unable to reach all body parts.

**Sponge bath at the sink**—Involves bathing from a bath basin or sink with patient sitting in a chair. Patient is able to perform a portion of the bath independently. You will assist patient with hard-to-reach areas.

**Tub bath**—Involves immersion in a tub of water that allows more thorough washing and rinsing than a bed bath.

**Shower**—Patient sits or stands under a continuous stream of water. The shower provides more thorough cleansing than a bed bath but can be fatiguing.

**Bag Bath/Travel Bath**—Developed by Skewes (1994). The Bag Bath contains several soft, nonwoven cotton cloths that are premoistened in a solution of no-rinse surfactant cleanser and emollient.

---

port abnormalities to their primary care provider. Instruct patients to handle the skin gently, avoiding excessive rubbing. Finally, encourage patients to eat nutritious food from all the food groups, as well as those rich in vitamins and minerals.

There are two categories of baths: cleansing and therapeutic. Cleansing baths include the **complete bed bath** and **partial bed bath,** tub bath, shower, sponge bath at a sink, and the Bag Bath/Travel Bath (Box 27-7). The type of cleansing bath you provide depends on the patient's physical capabilities and the degree of hygiene required. You are responsible for deciding what type of bath is most appropriate (see Box 27-7). Stay informed of any new evidence regarding bathing techniques (Box 27-8). Therapeutic baths include sitz baths or medicated baths (e.g., oatmeal, cornstarch, or Aveeno). A sitz bath cleanses and reduces pain and inflammation of perineal and anal areas. Medicated baths relieve skin irritation and create an antibacterial and drying effect.

**Perineal Care.** Perineal care is usually part of the complete bed bath (Skill 27-1). Patients most in need of perineal care are those with perineal secretions (e.g., patients who have indwelling urinary catheters [see Chapter 32] or who are recovering from rectal or genital surgery or childbirth). Excretions that accumulate along the urinary meatus or a suture line sometimes lead to infection. If a patient is able to perform self-care, allow the patient to do so. Many nurses are embarrassed about providing perineal care, particularly to patients of the opposite sex. This should not cause you to overlook the patient's hygiene needs. A professional, dignified attitude will reduce embarrassment and put the patient and you at ease.

If a patient performs self-care, various problems such as vaginal or urethral discharge, skin irritation, and unpleasant

*Text continued on p. 740*

| BOX 27-8 | USING EVIDENCE IN PRACTICE |
|---|---|

**Research Summary**

Recently researchers studied interventions for reducing dry skin in older adults. Sheppard and Brenner (2000) tested the Bag Bath/Travel Bath with traditional bathing techniques for the effects on skin dryness. The Bag Bath/Travel Bath, which contains a no-rinse surfactant, a humectant to trap moisture, and an emollient, significantly reduced overall skin dryness, especially skin flaking and scaling. There are now several commercial body cleansing systems available that contain the same ingredients as the Bag Bath.

Bathing creates high levels of discomfort in some patients who suffer dementia. Bathing tends to increase agitation and aggression in these patients. Dunn and others (2002) measured the frequency of agitated behaviors during bathing in 15 older adult residents with dementia. They compared the conventional tub bath with the Thermal bath (no-rinse bathing with nine washcloths soaked in 300 ml warm water and a nonrinse cleanser). For all behaviors combined, the Thermal bath caused significantly fewer agitated behaviors. In conclusion, bed bath variations such as the Thermal bath reduce agitation in the demented patient.

**Application to Nursing Practice**

Regardless of the type of bath the patient receives, use the following guidelines:

1. Provide privacy. Close the door, or pull room curtains around the bathing area. While bathing the patient, expose only the areas being bathed.
2. Maintain safety. When it is appropriate to use side rails, keep them raised while away from the patient's bedside. (This is particularly important for dependent or unconscious patients.) Remember, **do not use side rails to restrain patients from getting out of bed** unless there is a physician's or health care provider's order (see Chapter 26). Place the call light in the patient's reach if leaving the room.
3. Maintain warmth. Keep the room warm because the patient is partially uncovered and this leads to chilling. Control drafts, and keep windows closed. Keep the patient covered by exposing only the body part being washed during the bath.
4. Promote the patient's independence as much as possible during bathing activities. Offer assistance as needed.
5. Anticipate needs. Bring a new set of clothing and hygiene products to the bedside or bathroom.

Data from Dunn JC and others: Bathing: pleasure or pain? *J Gerontol Nurs* 28(11):6, 2002; Sheppard CM, Brenner PS: The effects of bathing and skin care practices on skin quality and satisfaction with an innovative product, *J Gerontol Nurs* 26(10):36, 2000.

---

| SKILL 27-1 | Bathing and Perineal Care |
|---|---|

**Delegation Considerations**

You can delegate bathing of a patient to assistive personnel. Before delegation, instruct the assistive personnel about:

- Not massaging reddened skin areas and reporting early signs of impaired skin integrity, including redness or pallor
- Proper ways to position male and female patients with musculoskeletal limitations

**Equipment**

- Two washcloths
- Two bath towels
- Bath blanket
- Soap and soap dish
- Toiletry items (deodorant, powder, lotion, cologne)
- Warm water
- Clean hospital gown or patient's own pajamas or gown
- Laundry bag
- Disposable gloves (when risk for contacting body fluids)
- Washbasin

| STEP | RATIONALE |
|---|---|

### ASSESSMENT

| | |
|---|---|
| 1. Assess patient's tolerance for bathing: activity tolerance, comfort level during movement, cognitive ability, musculoskeletal function, and the presence of shortness of breath. | Determines patient's ability to perform bathing and type of bath to administer (e.g., tub bath, partial bed bath). |
| 2. Assess patient's visual status, ability to sit without support, hand grasp, ROM of extremities. | Determines degree of assistance patient will need for bathing. |

• *Critical Decision Point:* Patients whose levels of independence and mobility change frequently will differ in how much assistance they require during bathing.

| | |
|---|---|
| 3. Assess for presence of equipment (e.g., IV line or oxygen tubing, Foley catheter) | Affects how you will plan bathing activities and positioning. |

| STEP | RATIONALE |
|---|---|
| 4. Assess patient's bathing preferences: frequency of and time of day bathing preferred, type of hygiene products used, and other factors related to cultural diversity. | Patient participates in plan of care. Promotes patient's comfort and willingness to cooperate. |

## PLANNING

| | |
|---|---|
| 1. Ask if patient has noticed any problems related to condition of skin and genitalia: excess moisture, inflammation, drainage, or excretions. | Provides you with information to direct physical assessment of skin during bathing. |
| 2. Before or during bath, assess condition of patient's skin. Note the presence of dryness, indicated by flaking, redness, scaling, and cracking. | Provides a baseline for comparison over time in determining if bathing improves condition of skin. |
| 3. Identify risks for skin impairment:<br>  a. Immobilization (e.g., clients with paralysis, traction)<br>  b. Reduced sensation (e.g., paresthesia, decreased circulation)<br>  c. Nutritional and hydration alterations<br>  d. Excessive moisture on skin, particularly on skin surfaces that rub against each other.<br>  e. Vascular insufficiencies<br>  f. External devices applied to or around skin<br>  g. Older adult patients<br>  h. Shear or friction (sliding down in bed)<br>  i. Incontinence (bowel or bladder)<br>  j. Allergies (tape, cleansing agents)<br>  k. Poor score on pressure ulcer risk assessment tool (see Chapter 35) | Risk factors increase the likelihood of injury to the skin because of pressure, impaired tissue synthesis, softening of or friction on tissues, and impaired circulation. |
| 4. Assess patient's knowledge of skin hygiene in terms of its importance, preventive measures to take, and common problems. | Determines patient's learning needs. |
| 5. Check physician's or health care provider's therapeutic bath order for type of solution, length of time for bath, body part to be attended. | Therapeutic baths are ordered for specific physical effect, which usually includes promotion of healing or soothing effects. |
| 6. Review orders for specific precautions concerning patient's movement or positioning. | Prevents accidental injury to patient during bathing activities. Determines level of assistance required by patient. |
| 7. Explain procedure, and ask patient for suggestions on how to prepare supplies. If partial bath, ask how much of bath patient wishes to complete. | Promotes patient's cooperation and participation. |
| 8. Adjust room temperature and ventilation, close room doors and windows, and draw room divider curtain. | Warm room that is free of drafts prevents rapid loss of body heat during bathing. Privacy ensures patient's mental and physical comfort. |
| 9. Prepare equipment and supplies. If it is necessary to leave room, be sure call light is within patient's reach. | Avoids interrupting procedure or leaving patient unattended to retrieve missing equipment. |

## IMPLEMENTATION

| | |
|---|---|
| 1. **Complete or Partial Bed Bath**<br>  a. Offer patient bedpan or urinal. Provide towel and washcloth.<br>  b. Perform hand hygiene. Apply clean disposable gloves | Patient will feel more comfortable after voiding. Prevents interruption of bath.<br>Reduces transmission of microorganisms. |

• *Critical Decision Point:* Apply gloves if there is actual or a risk for drainage or secretions on patient's skin.

| | |
|---|---|
|   c. Place hospital bed at comfortable working height. Lower side rail closest to you, and assist patient in assuming comfortable supine position, maintaining body alignment. Bring patient toward side closest to you. | Helps your access to patient. Maintains patient's comfort throughout procedure. You do not have to reach across bed, thus minimizing strain on back muscles. |

d. Place bath blanket over patient, and then loosen and remove top covers without exposing patient. If possible, have patient hold top of bath blanket. Place soiled linen in laundry bag. Take care to not allow linen to touch your uniform.

Removal of top linens prevents them from becoming soiled or moist during bath. Blanket provides warmth and privacy.

e. Remove patient's gown or pajamas.

Provides full exposure of body parts during bathing. Undressing unaffected side first allows easier manipulation of gown over body part with reduced ROM.

(1) If available, be sure a patient with IV or upper extremity injury has a gown that has either ties or has snaps on the sleeves.

(2) If a snap on gown is not available and a patient has an injured extremity or has an IV access, remove gown from *unaffected side first.*

Manipulation of IV tubing and container may disrupt flow rate.

(3) Remove gown from arm *without* IV first (see illustrations). Then remove gown from arm with IV. Remove IV from pole, and slide IV container and tubing through arm of patient's gown. Rehang IV container, and check flow rate. Regulate if necessary.

(4) If IV pump is in use, turn pump off, clamp tubing, remove tubing from pump, and proceed as in step (3). Insert tubing into pump, unclamp tubing, and turn pump on at correct rate. Observe flow rate and regulate if necessary.

Regulation is necessary to prevent improper infusion of fluids.

f. Pull side rail up. Lower bed temporarily to lowest position, then raise upon return. Fill washbasin two-thirds full with warm water. Place basin and supplies on over-bed table over bed. Check water temperature, and also have patient place fingers in water to test temperature tolerance. Place plastic container of bath lotion in bathwater to warm if desired.

Raising side rail and lowering bed position maintains patient's safety while you leave bedside. Warm water promotes comfort, relaxes muscles, and prevents unnecessary chilling. Testing temperature prevents accidental burns. Bathwater warms lotion for application to patient's skin.

g. Lower side rail, remove pillow, and raise head of bed 30 to 45 degrees if allowed. Place bath towel under patient's head. Place second bath towel over patient's chest.

Aids your access to patient. You do not have to reach across bed, thus minimizing strain on back muscles.

Removal of pillow makes it easier to wash patient's ears and neck. Placement of towels prevents soiling of bed linen and bath blanket.

h. Wash face.

(1) Ask if patient is wearing contact lenses. If so, perform eye care as described on pp. 752 and 754.

Prevents accidental injury to eyes.

(2) Fold washcloth around fingers of your hand to form a mitt (see illustration). Immerse mitt in water, and wring thoroughly.

Mitt retains water and heat better than loosely held washcloth; keeps cold edges from brushing against patient, and prevents splashing.

(3) Wash patient's eyes with plain warm water. Use different section of mitt for each eye. Move mitt from inner to outer canthus (see illustration). Soak any crusts on eyelid for 2 to 3 minutes with damp cloth before attempting removal. Dry around eyes gently and thoroughly.

Soap irritates eyes. Use of separate sections of mitt reduces infection transmission. Bathing eye from inner to outer canthus prevents secretions from entering nasolacrimal duct. Pressure can cause internal injury.

(4) Ask if patient prefers to use soap on face. Otherwise, wash, rinse, and dry forehead, cheeks, nose, neck, and ears without using soap. (Men sometimes wish to shave at this point or after bath.)

Soap tends to dry face, which is exposed to air more than other body parts.

(5) Provide eye care for the unconscious patient.

a. Cleanse the eyelids with a washcloth from the inner to outer canthus using plain warm water.

b. Instill prescribed eye drops or ointment per physician's order (see Chapter 20).

c. In the absence of a blink reflex the eyelids may be kept closed and covered with an eye patch or shield. Do not tape the eyelid.

| STEP | RATIONALE |
|---|---|

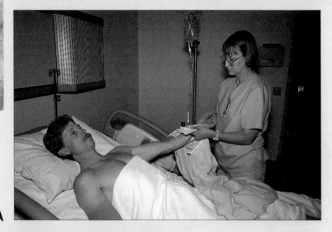

**A**

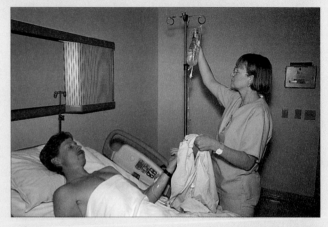

**B**

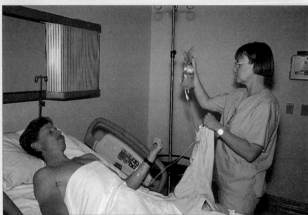

**C**

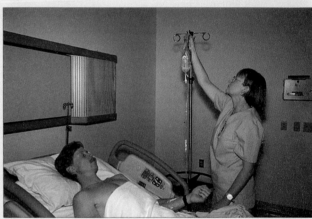

**D**

STEP **1e(3)** **A,** Remove patient's gown. **B,** Remove IV from pole, **C,** Slide IV tubing and bag through arm of patient's gown. **D,** Rehang IV bag.

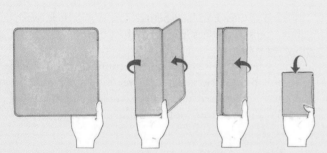

STEP **1h(2)** Steps for folding washcloth to form a mitt.

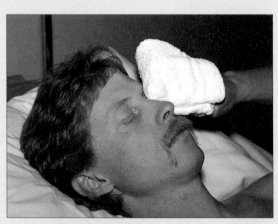

STEP **1h(3)** Wash eye from inner to outer canthus.

i. Wash trunk and upper extremities.

   (1) Remove bath blanket from patient's arm closest to you. Place bath towel lengthwise under arm. Bathe with minimal soap and water using long, firm strokes from distal to proximal (fingers to axilla).

Long, firm strokes promote venous return.

    (2) Raise and support arm above head (if possible) to wash, rinse, and dry axilla thoroughly (see illustration). Apply deodorant or powder to underarms if desired or needed.

Movement of arm exposes axilla and exercises joint's normal ROM. Respect patient's preference in use of hygiene products.

    (3) Move to other side of bed, and repeat steps (1) and (2) with other arm.

    (4) Cover patient's chest with bath towel, and fold bath blanket down to umbilicus. Bathe chest using long, firm strokes. Take special care with skin under female's breasts, lifting breast upward, if necessary, using back of your hand. Rinse and dry well.

Draping prevents unnecessary exposure of body parts. Towel maintains warmth and privacy. Secretions collect easily in areas of tight skinfolds. Skin under breasts is vulnerable to excoriation if not kept clean and dry.

  j. Wash hands and nails.

    (1) Fold bath towel in half, and lay it on bed beside patient. Place basin on towel. Immerse patient's hand in water. Allow hand to soak for 2 to 3 minutes before washing hand and fingernails (see Skill 27-2). Remove basin, and dry hand well. Repeat for other hand.

Soaking softens cuticles and calluses of hand, loosens debris beneath nails, and enhances feeling of cleanliness. Thorough drying removes moisture from between fingers.

  k. Check temperature of bathwater, and change water if necessary.

Warm water maintains patient's comfort.

---

• **Critical Decision Point:** If patient is at risk for falling, be sure two side rails are up before obtaining fresh water. Also lower bed when it is necessary to leave bedside. NOTE: All side rails raised may be considered a restraint.

---

  l. Wash the abdomen.

    (1) Place bath towel lengthwise over chest and abdomen. (Two towels may be needed.) Fold bath blanket down to just above pubic region. Bathe, rinse, and dry abdomen with special attention to umbilicus and skinfolds of abdomen and groin. Keep abdomen covered between washing and rinsing. Dry well.

Keeping skinfolds clean and dry helps prevent odor and skin irritation. Moisture and sediment that collect in skinfolds predispose skin to **maceration.**

    (2) Apply clean gown or pajama top.

Maintains patient's warmth and comfort. Dressing affected side first allows easier manipulation of gown over body part with reduced ROM.

---

• **Critical Decision Point:** If one extremity is injured or immobilized, always dress affected side first for easier manipulation of gown over body.*

---

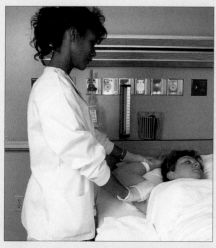

STEP **1i(2)** Positioning the patient's arm to wash the axilla.

*This step may be omitted until completion of bath; gown should not become soiled during remainder of bath.

| STEP | RATIONALE |
|---|---|
| m. Wash the lower extremities. | |
| (1) Cover chest and abdomen with top of bath blanket. Cover legs with bottom of blanket. Expose near leg by folding blanket toward midline. Be sure to drape perineum with blanket. | Prevents unnecessary exposure. |
| (2) Place bath towel under leg, supporting leg at knee and ankle. If appropriate, place patient's foot in the bath basin to soak while washing and rinsing. (Bend patient's leg at knee, and while grasping patient's heel, elevate leg from mattress slightly and place bath basin on towel.) If patient is unable to support leg, cleansing can simply be done by washing feet thoroughly with washcloth. | Towel prevents soiling of bed linen. Support of joint and extremity during lifting prevents strain on musculoskeletal structures. Sudden movement by patient could spill bathwater. Soaking softens calluses and rough skin. |

- *Critical Decision Point:* If patient has diabetes or peripheral vascular disease, do not soak feet.

| | |
|---|---|
| (3) Wash leg using long, firm strokes from ankle to knee, then knee to thigh (see illustration). Do not rub or massage the back of the calf. Dry well. Wash between the toes of foot. Cleanse foot, making sure to bathe between toes. Clean and clip nails as needed (see Skill 27-2). Dry toes and feet completely. Remove and discard towel. | Promotes circulation and venous return. Excess massage of calf could loosen deep vein thrombus. Secretions and moisture may be present between toes, predisposing patient to maceration and breakdown. |
| (4) Raise side rail, move to opposite side of bed, lower side rail, and repeat steps (2) and (3) for other leg and foot. If skin is dry, apply moisturizing lotion (AHCPR, 1992). When finished, cover patient with bath blanket. | Moisturizers are effective in reducing dry skin. |

- *Critical Decision Point:* Do not wash the lower extremities of patients with history of deep vein thromboses or blood-clotting disorders with long, firm strokes. Use short, light strokes.

| | |
|---|---|
| n. Raise side rail for patient's safety, remove contaminated gloves, and change bathwater. | Decreased bathwater temperature causes chilling. Clean water reduces microorganism transmission. |
| o. Provide perineal hygiene | |
| (1) If patient is able to maneuver and handle washcloth, allow to cleanse perineum on own. | Maintains patient's dignity and self-care ability. |

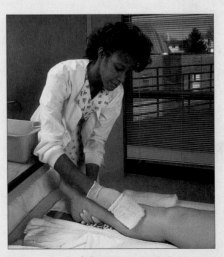

STEP **1m(3)** Wash patient's leg.

(2) Female Patient

(a) Apply new pair of disposable gloves. Lower side rail. Assist patient in assuming dorsal recumbent position. Note restrictions or limitations in patient's positioning. Be sure waterproof pad is positioned under patient's buttocks. Drape patient with bath blanket placed in the shape of a diamond. Lift lower edge of bath blanket to expose perineum (see illustration).

Provides full exposure of female genitalia. If patient is totally dependent, provide assistance to support patient in side-lying position and to raise leg as perineum is bathed. If position causes patient discomfort, reduce degree of abduction in female's hips.

(b) Fold lower corner of bath blanket up between patient's legs onto abdomen. Wash and dry patient's upper thighs.

Keeping patient draped until procedure begins minimizes anxiety. Buildup of perineal secretions soils surrounding skin surfaces.

(c) Wash labia majora. Use nondominant hand to gently retract labia from thigh: with dominant hand, wash carefully in skinfolds. Wipe in direction from perineum to rectum. Repeat on opposite side using separate section of washcloth. Rinse and dry area thoroughly.

Perineal care involves thorough cleansing of the patient's external genitalia and surrounding skin. Skinfolds may contain body secretions that harbor microorganisms. Wiping front to back reduces chance of transmitting fecal organisms to urinary meatus.

(d) Gently separate labia with nondominant hand to expose urethral meatus and vaginal orifice. With dominant hand, wash downward from pubic area toward rectum in one smooth stroke (see illustration). Wash the middle and both sides of the perineum. Use separate section of cloth for each stroke. Cleanse thoroughly around labia minora, clitoris, and vaginal orifice. Avoid placing tension on indwelling catheter if present, and clean area around it thoroughly.

Cleansing method reduces transfer of microorganisms to urinary meatus. (For menstruating women or patients with indwelling catheters, cleanse with cotton balls.)

(e) Provide catheter care as needed (see Chapter 32).

Cleansing along catheter from exit site reduces incidence of nosocomial urinary infection.

(f) Rinse area thoroughly. If patient uses bedpan, pour warm water over perineal area. Dry thoroughly, dry from front to back.

Rinsing removes soap and microorganisms more effectively than wiping. Retained moisture harbors microorganisms.

(g) Fold lower corner of bath blanket back between patient's legs and over perineum. Ask patient to lower legs and assume comfortable position.

(3) Male Patient

(a) Lower side rail. Assist patient to supine position. Note any restriction in mobility.

Provides full exposure of male genitalia. Position patients who are unable to lie supine on their side.

(b) Fold lower half of bath blanket up to expose upper thighs. Wash and dry thighs.

Buildup of perineal secretions soils surrounding skin surfaces.

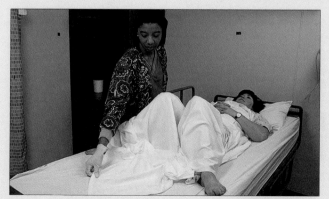

STEP **1o(2)(a)** Drape the patient for perineal care.

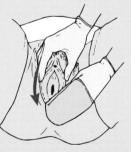

STEP **1o(2)(d)** Cleanse from perineum to rectum (front to back).

## SKILL 27-1 Bathing and Perineal Care—cont'd

| STEP | RATIONALE |
|---|---|
| (c) Cover thighs with bath towels. Raise bath blanket up to expose genitalia. Gently raise penis and place bath towel underneath. Gently grasp shaft of penis. If patient is uncircumcised, retract foreskin. If patient has an erection, defer procedure until later. | Draping minimizes patient anxiety. Towel prevents moisture from collecting in inguinal area. Gentle but firm handling of penis reduces chance of an erection. Secretions capable of harboring microorganisms collect underneath foreskin. |
| (d) Wash tip of penis at urethral meatus first. Using circular motion, cleanse from meatus outward (see illustration). Discard washcloth, and repeat with a clean cloth until penis is clean. Rinse and dry gently. | Direction of cleansing moves from area of least contamination to area of most contamination, preventing microorganisms from entering urethra. |
| (e) Return foreskin to its natural position. This is extremely important in patients with decreased sensation in their lower extremities. | Tightening of foreskin around shaft of penis causes local edema and discomfort. Patients with reduced sensation will not feel tightening of foreskin. |
| (f) Gently cleanse shaft of penis and scrotum by having patient abduct legs. Pay special attention to underlying surface of penis. Lift scrotum carefully, and wash underlying skinfolds. Rinse and dry thoroughly. | Vigorous massage of penis may cause an erection. Underlying surface of penis is an area where secretions accumulate. Abduction of legs provides easier access to scrotal tissues. Secretions easily collect between skinfolds. |
| (g) Avoid placing tension on indwelling catheter if present, and clean area around it thoroughly. Provide catheter care (see Chapter 32). | Cleansing along catheter from exit site reduces incidence of nosocomial urinary infection. |
| p. Dispose of bathwater, and dispose of gloves in receptacle. | Prevents transmission of infection. |
| q. Wash back. | |
| (1) Reapply clean pair of gloves. Lower side rail. Assist patient in assuming prone or side-lying position (as applicable). Place towel lengthwise along patient's side, and keep patient covered with bath blanket. | Exposes back and buttocks for bathing. |
| (2) If fecal material is present, enclose in a fold of underpad or toilet tissue, and remove with disposable wipes. | Skinfolds near buttocks and anus may contain fecal secretions that harbor microorganisms. |
| (3) Keep patient draped by sliding bath blanket over shoulders and thighs during bathing. Wash, rinse, and dry back from neck to buttocks using long, firm strokes. Pay special attention to folds of buttocks and anus. | Cleansing buttocks after back prevents contamination of water. |

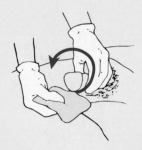

STEP 1o(3)(d) Use circular motion to cleanse tip of penis.

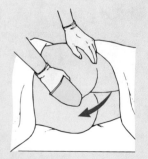

STEP 1q(4) Cleanse buttocks from front to back.

| STEP | RATIONALE |
|---|---|
| (4) Cleanse buttocks and anus, washing front to back (see illustration). Cleanse, rinse, and dry area thoroughly. If needed, place a clean absorbent pad under patient's buttocks. Remove contaminated gloves. | Cleansing motion prevents contaminating perineal area. |
| (5) Give a back rub. | Promotes patient relaxation. Make sure that a back rub is appropriate for your patient. Contraindicated in some cardiac patients. |
| r. Apply additional body lotion or oil to patient's skin as needed. | Moisturizing lotion prevents dry, chapped skin. |
| s. Remove soiled linen, and place in dirty-linen bag. Clean and replace bathing equipment. Wash hands. | Reduces transmission of microorganisms. |
| t. Assist patient in dressing. Comb patient's hair. Women may want to apply makeup. Assist as needed. | Promotes patient's body image. |
| u. Make patient's bed (see Skill 27- 5 and Box 27-12). | Provides clean environment. |
| v. Check the function and position of external devices (e.g., indwelling urethral catheters, nasogastric tubes, IV lines). | Ensures that systems remain functional after bathing activities. |
| w. Place bed in lowest position. | Maintains patient's safety by deceasing height of bed frame from floor. |
| x. Replace call light and personal possessions. Leave room as clean and comfortable as possible. | Prevents transmission of infection. Clean environment promotes patient's comfort. Keeping call light and articles of care within reach promotes patient's safety. |
| y. Perform hand hygiene. | Reduces transmission of microorganisms. |

**2. Commercial Bag Bath or Cleansing Pack**

| STEP | RATIONALE |
|---|---|
| a. The cleansing pack contains 8 to 10 premoistened towels for cleansing (see illustrations). Warm the package contents in a microwave following package directions. | Provides warm soothing heat. |
| b. Use a single towel for each general body part cleansed. Follow the same order of cleansing as the total or partial bed bath. | Reduces transmission of microorganisms. |
| c. Allow the skin to air dry for 30 seconds. It is permissible to lightly cover patient with a bath towel to prevent chilling. | Drying the skin with a towel removes the emollient that is left behind after the water/cleanser solution evaporates. |
| d. NOTE: If there is excessive soiling (e.g., in the perineal region), use an extra Bag Bath or conventional washcloths, soap, water, and towels. | |

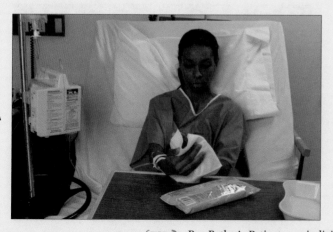
A

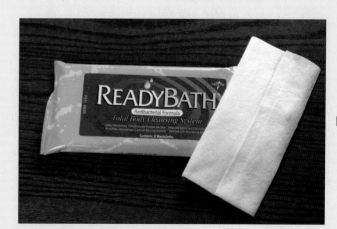
B

STEP **2a** Bag Bath. **A,** Patient uses individual wipes to bathe. **B,** Bag Bath package.

## SKILL 27-1 | Bathing and Perineal Care—cont'd

| STEP | RATIONALE |
|---|---|

**3. Tub Bath or Shower**

a. Consider patient's condition, and review orders for precautions concerning patient's movement or positioning.

Prevents accidental injury to patient during bathing.

b. Schedule use of shower or tub.

Prevents unnecessary waiting that causes fatigue.

c. Check tub or shower for cleanliness. Use cleaning techniques outlined in agency policy. Place rubber mat on tub or shower bottom. Place disposable bath mat or towel on floor in front of tub or shower.

Cleaning prevents transmission of microorganisms. Mats prevent slipping and falling.

d. Collect all hygienic aids, toiletry items, and linens requested by patient. Place within easy reach of tub or shower.

Placing items close at hand prevents possible falls when patient reaches for equipment.

e. Assist patient to bathroom if necessary. Have patient wear robe and slippers to bathroom.

Assistance prevents accidental falls. Wearing robe and slippers prevents chilling.

f. Demonstrate how to use call signal for assistance.

Bathrooms are equipped with signaling devices in case patient feels faint or weak or needs immediate assistance. Patients prefer privacy during bath if safety is not jeopardized.

g. Place "occupied" sign on bathroom door.

Maintains patient's privacy.

h. Fill bath tub halfway with warm water. Check temperature of bath water, then have patient test water, and adjust temperature if water is too warm. Explain which faucet controls hot water. If patient is taking shower, turn shower on and adjust water temperature before patient enters shower stall. Use shower seat or tub chair if needed (see illustration).

Adjusting water temperature prevents accidental burns. Older adults and patients with neurological alterations (e.g., diabetes, spinal cord injury) are at high risk for burn as a result of reduced sensation. Use of assistive devices facilitates bathing and minimizes physical exertion.

i. Instruct patient to use safety bars when getting in and out of tub or shower. Caution patient against use of bath oil in tub water.

Prevents slipping and falling. Oil causes tub surfaces to become slippery.

j. Instruct patient not to remain in tub longer than 10 to 15 minutes. Check on patient every 5 minutes.

Prolonged exposure to warm water causes vasodilation and pooling of blood in some patients, leading to light-headedness or dizziness.

k. Return to bathroom when patient signals, and knock before entering.

Provides privacy.

l. For patient who is unsteady, drain tub of water before patient attempts to get out of it. Place bath towel over patient's shoulders. Assist patient in getting out of tub as needed, and assist with drying.

Prevents accidental falls. Patient may become chilled as water drains.

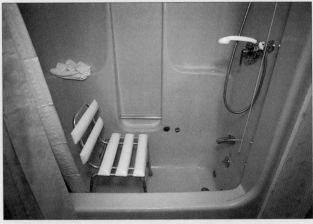

STEP **11h** Shower seat for patient safety.

| STEP | RATIONALE |
|---|---|

• *Critical Decision Point:* Weak or unstable patients need extra assistance in getting out of a tub. Planning for additional personnel is essential before attempting to assist the patient from the tub.

| STEP | RATIONALE |
|---|---|
| m. Assist patient as needed with getting dressed in a clean gown or pajamas, slippers, and robe. (In home setting, patient may put on regular clothing.) | Maintains warmth to prevent chilling. |
| n. Assist patient to room and comfortable position in bed or chair. | Maintains relaxation gained from bathing. |
| o. Clean tub or shower according to agency policy. Remove soiled linen, and place in dirty-linen bag. Discard disposable equipment in proper receptacle. Place "unoccupied" sign on bathroom door. Return supplies to storage area. | Prevents transmission of infection through soiled linen and moisture. |
| p. Perform hand hygiene. | Reduces transfer of microorganisms. |

## EVALUATION

| | |
|---|---|
| 1. Observe skin, paying particular attention to areas previously soiled, reddened, dry, or showing early signs of breakdown. | Techniques used during bathing leave skin clean and clear. Over time dry skin will diminish. If patient shows areas of redness, use a Braden scale to measure risk for pressure ulcers (see Chapter 35). |
| 2. Observe ROM during bath. | Measures joint mobility. |
| 3. Ask patient to rate level of comfort. | Determines patient's tolerance of bathing activities. |
| 4. Ask patient to rate level of fatigue. | Determines patient's tolerance of bathing activities. |

## RECORDING AND REPORTING

■ Record procedure and observations (e.g., breaks in skin, inflammation, ulcerations).

■ Report any breaks in skin or ulcerations to nurse in charge or physician or health care provider. These are serious in patients with altered circulation to the lower extremities. Patient may need special foot care treatments.

## UNEXPECTED OUTCOMES AND RELATED INTERVENTIONS

■ Areas of excessive dryness, rashes, or pressure ulcers appear on skin.
  • Complete pressure ulcer assessment (see Chapter 35).
  • Apply moisturizing lotions or topical skin applications per agency policy.
  • Limit frequency of complete baths.
  • Obtain special bed surface if patient is at risk for skin breakdown.
■ Joint ROM decreases.
  • Increase ROM exercises unless contraindicated.
  • Encourage more self-care by patient.

■ Patient becomes excessively fatigued and unable to cooperate or participate in bathing.
  • Reschedule bathing to a time when patient is more rested.
  • Patients with breathing difficulties require pillow or elevated head of bed during bath.
  • Notify physician or health care provider if this is a change in patient's fatigue level.
■ Patient seems unusually restless or complains of discomfort.
  • Schedule patient rest periods.
  • Consider analgesia if patient complains of pain or discomfort before the bath.
■ The rectum, perineum, or genital area is inflamed, swollen, or has foul-smelling odor.
  • Bathe perineal area frequently enough to keep clean and dry.
  • Obtain an order for a sitz bath.
  • Apply protective barrier ointment or antiinflammatory cream.
  • Report findings to physician or health care provider.

odors sometimes go unnoticed. Stress the importance of perineal care in preventing skin breakdown and infection. Be alert for complaints of burning during urination, localized soreness or excoriation, or perineal pain. Also inspect vaginal and perineal areas and bed linen for signs of discharge.

**Back Rub.** A back rub usually follows the bath (see Chapter 30). It promotes relaxation, relieves muscular tension, stimulates skin circulation, and patients tolerate it well even when critically ill (Labyak and Metzger, 1997). During the back rub, assess skin condition.

An effective back rub takes 3 to 5 minutes. Always ask if the patient wants a back rub because some patients dislike physical contact. Also, consult the patient's record for contraindications, such as spinal cord injury, rib fractures, or other painful conditions.

**NAIL AND FOOT CARE.** Feet and nails require special care to prevent infection, odors, pain, and injury to soft tissues. Often people are unaware of foot or nail problems until discomfort or pain develops. For proper foot and nail care, instruct your patients to protect the feet from injury, keep the feet clean and dry, and wear footwear that fits properly. Help the patient learn the proper way to inspect the feet for lesions, dryness, or signs of infection. The patient, family, or delegated assistive personnel need to report any of these conditions to you. This is especially important in patients with peripheral vascular diseases, diabetes mellitus, older adults, and patients with suppressed immune systems. Finally, to maintain and promote foot and nail health, have patients visit a podiatrist when necessary.

Foot and nail care involves soaking to soften cuticles and layers of horny cells, thorough cleansing, drying, and proper nail trimming. Always check agency policy to determine if you can trim nails independently or if a physician's or health care provider's order is required. You provide foot and nail care in bed for an immobilized patient or have the patient sit in a chair (Skill 27-2). During the procedure is an excellent time to teach the patient proper techniques for cleaning and trimming nails. Stress ways to prevent infection and promote good circulation.

Patients with insensate extremities, such as those with diabetes mellitus, require daily foot care and inspection to prevent the development of foot ulcers and subsequent complications that may lead to amputation (Neil, 2002). The ADA (2005) identifies the following conditions that place patients at risk for amputation: peripheral neuropathy, evidence of increased pressure for callus, foot ulcers, limited joint mobility, bone deformity of feet and toes, nail pathological conditions, and peripheral vascular diseases. Although ongoing good foot care helps prevent amputation, studies have shown that many patients have not learned proper care. Instruct diabetic patients or patients

with peripheral vascular diseases in the following precautions during foot and nail care:

1. Wash the feet daily using lukewarm water; **do not soak.** Thoroughly pat the feet dry, and dry well between the toes.

2. Do not cut corns or calluses or use commercial chemical removers. Consult a physician, health care provider, or podiatrist.

3. If the feet perspire, apply a bland foot powder.

4. If you notice dryness along the feet, apply lanolin, baby oil, or even corn oil, and rub gently into the skin.

5. File the toenails straight across and square; do not use scissors or clippers. Consult a podiatrist as needed, based on orders from physician or health care provider.

6. Do not use over-the-counter preparations to treat athlete's foot or ingrown toenails. Consult a physician, health care provider, or podiatrist.

7. Avoid wearing elastic stockings, knee-high hose, or constricting garters. If these devices are worn, assess skin for pressure points. Do not cross the legs. Both impair circulation to the lower extremities.

8. Inspect the feet daily, including tops and soles of the feet, heels, and the area between the toes. Use a mirror to inspect all surfaces.

9. Wear clean socks or stockings daily. Make sure socks are dry and free of holes or darns that cause pressure.

10. Do not walk barefoot.

11. Wear shoes that fit properly. Make sure soles of shoes are flexible and do not slip. Use lamb's wool between toes that rub or overlap. Wear shoes that are sturdy, closed in, and not restrictive. Patients with increased plantar pressure (e.g., callus, erythema) or foot and toe deformities need to use therapeutic shoes and inserts that cushion and redistribute pressure (ADA, 2005).

12. Exercise regularly to improve circulation to the lower extremities. Walk slowly, elevate, rotate, flex, and extend the feet at the ankle. Dangle the feet over the side of the bed 1 minute, then extend both legs and hold them parallel to the bed while lying supine for 1 minute, and finally rest 1 minute.

13. Avoid applying hot-water bottles or heating pads to the feet; use extra covers instead.

14. Wash minor cuts immediately, and dry thoroughly. Only apply mild antiseptics (e.g., Neosporin ointment) to the skin. Avoid iodine or Mercurochrome. Contact a physician or health care provider to treat cuts or lacerations.

15. If patients smoke, encourage them to stop. Smoking decreases circulation by affecting blood flow in small vessels.

*Text continued on p. 744*

┌──────────────────────────────────────────────────────────────
│ SKILL 27-2 ┆ Performing Nail and Foot Care                [View Video!]

## Delegation Considerations

You can delegate nail and foot care of the nondiabetic patient and patients without circulatory compromise to assistive personnel. Provide assistive personnel with direction, including:

- Proper use of nail clippers (NOTE: Many agencies do not allow assistive personnel or even RNs to use nail clippers; consult policy).
- Cautioning assistive personnel to use warm water
- Instructing assistive personnel to report any changes that may indicate inflammation or injury to tissues

## Equipment

- Washbasin
- Emesis basin
- Washcloth
- Bath or face towel
- Nail clippers
- Orange stick (optional)
- Emery board or nail file
- Unscented body lotion
- Disposable bath mat
- Paper towels

| STEP | RATIONALE |
|---|---|

### ASSESSMENT

| | |
|---|---|
| 1. Inspect all surfaces of fingers, toes, feet, and nails. Pay particular attention to areas of dryness, inflammation, or cracking. Also inspect areas between toes, heels, and soles of feet. | Foot hygiene, especially in patients with diabetes, is important to prevent foot complications. It is important to assess the condition of the skin on feet and toes. Look for skin changes (reddened or discolored) or open areas that require future intervention to prevent complications (ADA, 2005). |

• *Critical Decision Point:* Patients with peripheral vascular diseases, diabetes mellitus, older adults, and patients with a suppressed immune system sometimes require nail care from a specialist to reduce the risk for infection.

| | |
|---|---|
| 2. Assess color and temperature of toes, feet, and fingers. Assess capillary refill of nails. Palpate radial and ulnar pulse of each hand and dorsalis pedis pulse of foot; note character of pulses. | Assess adequacy of blood flow to extremities. Circulatory alterations change integrity of nails and increase patient's chance of localized infection when break in skin integrity occurs (Strauss and others, 1998). |
| 3. Observe patient's walking gait. Have patient walk down hall or walk a straight line (if able). | Painful disorders of feet cause limping or unnatural gait (Armstrong and Lavery, 1998). |
| 4. Ask female patients about whether they use nail polish and polish remover frequently. | Chemicals in these products cause excessive dryness. |
| 5. Assess type of footwear worn by patients: Are socks worn? Are shoes tight or ill fitting? Are garters or knee-high nylons worn? Is footwear clean? | Some types of shoes and footwear predispose patient to foot and nail problems (e.g., infection, areas of friction, ulcerations). |
| 6. Obtain physician's or health care provider's order for cutting nails if agency policy requires it. | Patient's skin may be accidentally cut, creating risk of infection. Certain patients are more at risk for infection, depending on their medical condition. |
| 7. Identify patient's risk for foot or nail problems: | Certain conditions increase likelihood of foot or nail problems. |
| a. Older adult | Poor vision, lack of coordination, or inability to bend over contributes to difficulty among older adults in performing foot and nail care. Normal physiological changes of aging also result in nail and foot problems. |
| b. Diabetes | Vascular changes associated with diabetes reduce blood flow to peripheral tissues. Break in skin integrity places diabetic patient at high risk for skin infection. Lower extremity complications of diabetes involve nerves, muscles, bone, and vasculature, making assessment of and management of foot problems complex (Cooppan and Habershaw, 1995). |
| c. Heart failure, renal disease | Both conditions increase tissue edema, particularly in dependent areas (e.g., feet). Edema reduces blood flow to neighboring tissues. |
| d. Cerebrovascular accident, stroke | Presence of residual foot or leg weakness or paralysis results in altered walking patterns. Altered gait pattern causes increased friction and pressure on feet. |

| STEP | RATIONALE |
|---|---|
| 8. Assess type of home remedies patients use for existing foot problems: | Certain preparations or applications cause more injury to soft tissue than initial foot problem. |
| a. Over-the-counter liquid preparations to remove corns | Liquid preparations sometimes cause burns and ulcerations. |
| b. Cutting of corns or calluses with razor blade or scissors | Cutting of corns or calluses may result in infection caused by break in skin integrity. |
| c. Use of oval corn pads | Oval pads sometimes exert pressure on toes, thereby decreasing circulation to surrounding tissues. |
| d. Application of adhesive tape | Skin of older adult is thin and delicate and prone to tearing when removing adhesive tape. |

• *Critical Decision Point:* Patients with impaired circulation or those with diabetes need to seek health care provider advice for treatment of corns or calluses.

| STEP | RATIONALE |
|---|---|
| 9. Assess patient's ability to care for nails or feet: visual alterations, fatigue, and musculoskeletal weakness. | Extent of patient's ability to perform self-care determines degree of assistance required from you. |
| 10. Assess patient's knowledge of foot and nail care practices. | Level of patient's knowledge determines patient's need for health teaching. |

## PLANNING

| | |
|---|---|
| 1. Explain procedure to patient, including fact that proper soaking requires several minutes. | Patient must be willing to place fingers and feet in basins for 10 to 20 minutes. Patient may become anxious or fatigued. |
| 2. Perform hand hygiene. Arrange equipment on over-bed table. | Easy access to equipment prevents delays. |
| 3. Pull curtain around bed, or close room door (if desired). | Maintaining patient's privacy, reduces anxiety. |

## IMPLEMENTATION

| | |
|---|---|
| 1. Assist ambulatory patient to sit in bedside chair. Help bed-bound patient to supine position with head of bed elevated. Place disposable bath mat on floor under patient's feet or place towel on mattress. | Sitting in chair facilitates immersing feet in basin. Bath mat protects feet from exposure to soil or debris. |
| 2. Fill washbasin with warm water. Test water temperature. | Warm water softens nails and thickened epidermal cells, reduces inflammation of skin, and promotes local circulation. Proper water temperature prevents burns. |
| 3. Place basin on bath mat or towel, and help patient place feet in basin. Place call light within patient's reach. | Patients with muscular weakness or tremors have difficulty positioning feet. Ensures patient's safety. |
| 4. Adjust over-bed table to low position, and place it over patient's lap. (Patient sits in chair or lies in bed.) | Easy access prevents accidental spills. |
| 5. Fill emesis basin with warm water, and place basin on paper towels on over-bed table. | Warm water softens nails and thickened epidermal cells. |
| 6. Instruct patient to place fingers in emesis basin and place arms in comfortable position. | Prolonged positioning causes discomfort unless patient maintains normal anatomical alignment. |
| 7. Allow patient's feet and fingernails to soak for 10 to 20 minutes. Rewarm after 10 minutes. | Softening of corns, calluses, and cuticles ensures easy removal of dead cells and easy manipulation of cuticle. Soaking extremities of diabetic patients contributes to risk of infection. |

• *Critical Decision Point:* Patients with diabetes should never soak hands or feet because of risk of infection. Also, do not put oils or creams between the toes of diabetic patients; the extra moisture leads to infection.

| STEP | RATIONALE |
|---|---|
| 8. Clean gently under fingernails with orange stick while immersing fingers (see illustration). Remove emesis basin, and dry fingers thoroughly. | Orange stick removes debris under nails that harbors microorganisms. Thorough drying impedes fungal growth and prevents maceration of tissues. |
| 9. With nail clippers, clip fingernails straight across and even with tops of fingers (see illustration). Shape nails with emery board or file. If patient has circulatory problems, do not cut nail; file the nail only. | Cutting straight across prevents splitting of nail margins and formation of sharp nail spikes that will irritate lateral nail margins. Filing prevents cutting nail too close to nail bed (Strauss and others, 1998). |

| STEP | RATIONALE |
|------|-----------|

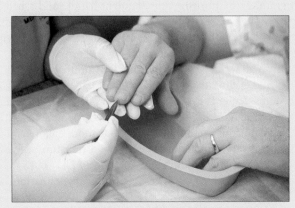

STEP **8** Clean under fingernails with orange stick.

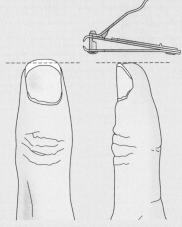

STEP **9** Clip fingernails straight across. Use a nail clipper.

| | |
|---|---|
| 10. Push cuticle back gently with orange stick. | Reduces incidence of inflamed cuticles. |
| 11. Move over-bed table away from patient. | Provides easier access to feet. |
| 12. Put on disposable gloves, and scrub callused areas of feet with washcloth. | Gloves prevent transmission of fungal infection. Friction removes dead skin layers. |
| 13. Clean gently under nails with orange stick. Remove feet from basin, and dry thoroughly. | Removal of debris and excess moisture reduces chances of infection. |
| 14. Clean and trim toenails using procedures in steps 8 and 9. Do not file corners of toenails. | Shaping corners of toenails damages tissues. |
| 15. Apply lotion to feet and hands, and assist patient back to bed and into comfortable position. | After soaking, dry feet and seal in the remaining moisture with a thin coat of plain petroleum jelly or unscented lotion. Do not apply lotion between toes (ADA, 2005). |
| 16. Remove disposable gloves, and place in receptacle. Clean and return equipment and supplies to proper place. Dispose of soiled linen in hamper. Perform hand hygiene. | Reduces transmission of infection. |

## EVALUATION

| | |
|---|---|
| 1. Inspect nails and surrounding skin surfaces after soaking and nail trimming. | Evaluates condition of skin and nails. Allows you to note any remaining rough nail edges. |
| 2. Ask patient to explain or demonstrate nail care. | Evaluates patient's level of learning techniques. |
| 3. Observe patient's walk after toenail care. | Evaluates level of comfort and mobility achieved. |

## RECORDING AND REPORTING

- Record procedure and observations (e.g., breaks in skin, inflammation, ulcerations).
- Report any breaks in skin or ulcerations to nurse in charge or physician or health care provider. These are serious in patients with altered circulation to the lower extremities. Patient may need special foot care treatments.

## UNEXPECTED OUTCOMES AND RELATED INTERVENTIONS

- Nails discolored, rough, and concave or irregular in shape.
  - Increase frequency of nail hygiene because one intervention will not correct long-term problems.

- Cuticles and surrounding tissues are inflamed and tender to touch.
  - Repeated soakings are necessary to help relieve inflammation and remove layers of cells from calluses or corns.
  - Patients with diabetes often require referral to a podiatrist.
- Localized areas of tenderness occur on feet with calluses or corns at point of friction.
  - Patient may need a change in footwear or corrective foot surgery for permanent improvement in corns or calluses.
- Ulcer appears between toes.
  - Provide frequent foot hygiene.
  - Notify physician or health care provider of your assessments.

**ORAL HYGIENE.** Good daily oral hygiene, including brushing, flossing, and rinsing, is necessary for the prevention and control of plaque-associated oral diseases. Proper care prevents inflammation and infection and promotes comfort, nutrition, and verbal communication. Brushing cleanses the teeth of food particles, plaque, and bacteria; massages the gums; and relieves discomfort from unpleasant odors and taste. Flossing removes tartar that collects at the gum line. Rinsing removes dislodged food particles and excess toothpaste. Recent research has shown that twice daily rinsing with an essential oil–containing mouth rinse (e.g., Cool Mint Listerine Antiseptic) is an effective adjunct in reducing plaque and gingivitis (Bauroth and others, 2003).

When patients become ill, many factors influence their need for oral hygiene. Patients in hospitals or long-term care facilities often do not receive the aggressive oral care they need. Base the frequency of care on the condition of the oral cavity and the patient's level of comfort (Skill 27-3). Oral hygiene may be required as often as every 1 to 2 hours.

Once patients return home, instruct them to brush their teeth after each meal and before bedtime and to floss once daily. Acidic fruits in the patient's diet will reduce plaque formation. All patients need to visit a dentist regularly every 6 months for checkups. To prevent tooth decay, patients sometimes have to change eating habits (e.g., reducing intake of carbohydrates, especially sweet snacks between meals). A well-balanced diet ensures the integrity of oral tissues.

**Brushing.** Thorough tooth brushing at least twice a day with a fluoride toothpaste is basic to an effective oral hygiene program. A toothbrush with a straight handle and a brush small enough to reach all areas of the mouth is best. Older adult patients with reduced dexterity and grip require an enlarged handle with an easier grip.

Brush all tooth surfaces thoroughly. Commercially made foam rubber toothbrushes are useful for patients with sensitive gums. Patients can use electric toothbrushes, but check for electrical hazards. Avoid lemon-glycerin sponges because they dry mucous membranes and erode tooth enamel. Moi-Stir is a salivary supplement that improves moisture and texture of the tongue and mucosa (Poland, 1987).

Patients who receive cancer chemotherapy, radiation, or immunosuppression agents develop mucositis and may require certain modifications to oral care. These modifications reduce the discomfort of mucositis. Interventions for patients with mucositis include good oral hygiene, narcotic analgesics, and topical palliative mouth rinses (Scully, 2004).

When teaching patients about mouth care, recommend that they not share toothbrushes with family members or drink directly from a bottle of mouthwash. Cross-contamination occurs easily.

*Text continued on p. 748*

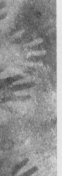

# SKILL 27-3 | Providing Oral Hygiene

## Delegation Considerations

You can delegate oral hygiene to assistive personnel. As the nurse, assess a patient's gag reflex if there is any question that the patient is at risk for aspiration. Instruct assistive personnel in:

- Proper positioning of patient to avoid aspiration
- How to recognize impaired integrity of oral mucosa and the alterations to report

## Equipment

- Tongue depressor
- Soft-bristle toothbrush
- Nonabrasive fluoride toothpaste or dentifrice
- Dental floss
- Water glass with cool water
- 20 ml essential oil–antiseptic mouth rinse
- Emesis basin
- Face towel
- Paper towels
- Disposable gloves

| STEP | RATIONALE |
|---|---|
| **ASSESSMENT** | |
| 1. Perform hand hygiene, and apply disposable gloves. | Reduces transmission of microorganisms. Gloves prevent contact with microorganisms in blood or saliva. |
| 2. Instruct patient to not bite down. Then, using a tongue depressor, inspect integrity of lips, teeth, buccal mucosa, gums, palate, and tongue (see Chapter 13). | Determines status of patient's oral cavity and extent of need for oral hygiene. |
| 3. Identify presence of common oral problems: | Helps determine type of hygiene patient requires and information patient requires for self-care. |
|    a. Dental caries—chalky white discoloration of tooth or presence of brown or black discoloration | |

   b. Gingivitis—inflammation of gums
   c. Periodontitis—receding gum lines, inflammation, gaps between teeth
   d. Halitosis—bad breath
   e. Cheilosis—cracking of lips
   f. Stomatitis—inflammation of the mouth

4. Remove gloves, and perform hand hygiene.

Prevents spread of microorganisms.

5. Assess risk for oral hygiene problems:

Certain conditions increase likelihood of impaired oral cavity integrity and need for preventive care.

   a. Dehydration, inability to take fluids or food by mouth (NPO)

Causes excess drying and fragility of mucous membranes; increases accumulation of secretions on tongue and gums.

   b. Presence of nasogastric or oxygen tubes; mouth breathers

Requires frequent mouth care because drying of mucous membranes.

   c. Chemotherapeutic drugs

Mucositis is the most common oral complication following the administration of chemotherapy, a nonsurgical treatment for cancer. The characteristics are oral erythema, ulceration, and pain (Scully, 2004).

   d. Calcium channel blockers, phenytoin, some amphetamines used to treat hyperactivity in children, and cyclosporine used by organ transplant recipients.

Produces gum overgrowth.

   e. Over-the-counter lozenges, cough drops, antacids, and chewable vitamins.

Medications contain large amounts of sugar. Repeated daily use increases sugar or acid content in mouth.

   f. Radiation therapy to head and neck

Therapy affects the mucosal tissues within the radiation field 100% of the time and results in oral mucositis. Characteristics are oral erythema, ulceration, and pain (Scully, 2004).

   g. Presence of artificial airway

Increases irritation to gums and mucosa. Excess secretions accumulate on teeth and tongue.

   h. Blood-clotting disorders (e.g., leukemia, aplastic anemia)

Predisposes to inflammation and bleeding of gums.

   i. Oral surgery, trauma to mouth

Break in mucosa increases risk of infection. Vigorous brushing disrupts suture lines.

   j. Aging

Results in drying and thinning of mucosa.

   k. Diabetes mellitus

Prone to dryness of mouth, gingivitis, periodontal disease, and loss of teeth.

6. Determine patient's oral hygiene practices and willingness to attend to hygiene needs:
   a. Frequency of tooth brushing and flossing

Identifies errors in patient's technique, deficiencies in preventive oral hygiene, and patient's level of knowledge regarding dental care.

   b. Type of toothpaste or dentifrice used

Toothpaste needs to contain fluoride.

   c. Last dental visit

Provides reference for subsequent visits.

   d. Frequency of dental visits

American Dental Association recommends regular visits to the dentist for professional cleanings and oral examinations at least twice a year (American Dental Association, 2005).

   e. Type of mouth rinse or moistening preparation

Lemon-glycerin preparations are harmful. Glycerin is an astringent that dries and shrinks mucous membranes and gums. Lemon exhausts salivary reflex and erodes tooth enamel (Fitch and others, 1999). Mouthwash provides pleasant aftertaste but dries mucosa after extended use if it has an alcohol base. An essential oil–antiseptic mouthwash such as Cool Mint Listerine is effective in reducing plaque and gingivitis (Bauroth and others, 2003). However, mouthwashes are not a replacement for flossing (American Dental Association, 2005).

| STEP | RATIONALE |
|------|-----------|
| 7. Assess patient's ability to grasp and manipulate toothbrush. Assessment determines level of assistance required from you. | Older adult patients or persons with musculoskeletal or nervous system alterations are sometimes unable to hold toothbrush with firm grip or manipulate brush. |

## PLANNING

| | |
|---|---|
| 1. Place paper towels on over-bed table, and arrange other equipment within easy reach. | Creates organized work space. |

## IMPLEMENTATION

| | |
|---|---|
| 1. Raise bed to comfortable working position. Raise head of bed (if allowed), and lower side rail. Move patient, or help patient move closer. Use side-lying position if needed. | Raising bed and positioning patient prevent you from straining muscles. Semi-Fowler's position helps prevent patient from choking or aspirating. |
| 2. Place paper towel over patient's chest. | Prevents soiling of patient's gown. |
| 3. Apply disposable gloves. | Prevents contact with microorganisms or blood in saliva. |
| 4. Apply enough toothpaste to brush to cover length of bristles (American Dental Association, 2005). Hold brush over emesis basin. Pour small amount of water over toothpaste. | Moisture aids in distribution of toothpaste over tooth surfaces. |
| 5. Patient assists by brushing. Hold toothbrush bristles at 45-degree angle to gum line (see illustration). Be sure tips of bristles rest against and penetrate under gum line. Brush inner and outer surfaces of upper and lower teeth by brushing from gum to crown of each tooth. Clean biting surfaces of teeth by holding top of bristles parallel with teeth and brushing gently back and forth (see illustration). Brush sides of teeth by moving bristles back and forth (see illustration). | Angle allows brush to reach all tooth surfaces and to clean under gum line, where plaque and tartar accumulate. Back-and-forth motion dislodges food particles caught between teeth and along chewing surfaces. |
| 6. Have patient hold brush at 45-degree angle and lightly brush over surface and sides of tongue. Avoid initiating gag reflex. | Microorganisms collect and grow on tongue's surface and contribute to bad breath. Gagging will sometimes cause aspiration of toothpaste. |
| 7. Allow patient to rinse mouth thoroughly by taking several sips of water (may use straw), swishing water across all tooth surfaces, and spitting into emesis basin. Use this time to teach patient importance of brushing teeth twice a day. | Irrigation removes food particles. |

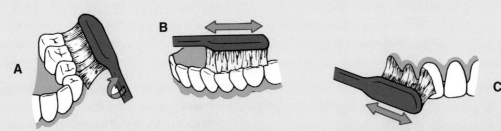

STEP 5 Direction for toothbrush placement. **A,** Forty-five-degree angle brushes gum line. **B,** Parallel position brushes biting surfaces. **C,** Lateral position brushes side of teeth.

| STEP | RATIONALE |
|---|---|
| 8. Have patient rinse teeth with antiseptic mouth rinse for 30 seconds. Then have patient spit rinse into emesis basin. | Using an essential oil–antiseptic mouth rinse a minimum of twice daily is at least as effective as flossing daily in reducing plaque and gingivitis (Bauroth and others, 2003). Mouth rinse also leaves a pleasant taste. |
| 9. Assist in wiping patient's mouth. | Promotes sense of comfort. |
| 10. Allow patient to floss. Floss between all teeth. Hold floss against tooth while moving floss up and down sides of teeth and under gum line. | Reduces tartar on tooth surfaces and prevents gum disease. The American Dental Association (2005) recommends flossing once daily. |
| 11. Allow patient to rinse mouth thoroughly with cool water and spit into emesis basin. Assist in wiping patient's mouth. | Irrigation removes plaque and tartar from oral cavity. |
| 12. Assist patient to comfortable position, remove emesis basin and over-bed table, raise side rail, and lower bed to original position. | Provides for patient comfort and safety. |
| 13. Wipe off over-bed table, discard soiled linen and paper towels in appropriate containers, remove soiled gloves, and return equipment to proper place. | Proper disposal of soiled equipment prevents spread of infection. |
| 14. Perform hand hygiene. | Reduces transmission of microorganisms. |

## EVALUATION

| | |
|---|---|
| 1. Ask patient if any area of oral cavity feels uncomfortable or irritated. | Pain indicates more chronic problem. |
| 2. Apply gloves, and inspect condition of oral cavity. | Determines effectiveness of hygiene and rinsing. |
| 3. Ask patient to describe proper hygiene techniques. | Evaluates patient's learning. |
| 4. Observe patient brushing and flossing. | Evaluates patient's ability to use correct technique. |

## RECORDING AND REPORTING

- Record procedure on flow sheet. Note condition of oral cavity in nurses' notes.
- Report bleeding or presence of lesions to nurse in charge or physician or health care provider.

## UNEXPECTED OUTCOMES AND RELATED INTERVENTIONS

- Mucosa is dry and inflamed. Tongue has thick coating.
  - Increase patient's hydration.
  - Apply protectant to patient's lips.
  - Increase frequency of tongue brushing.
- Gum margins are retracted from teeth, with localized areas of inflammation. Bleeding occurs around gum margins.
  - Report findings because patient may have an underlying bleeding tendency.
  - Switch to a soft-bristle toothbrush.
  - Avoid too vigorous brushing and flossing.
  - Use a swab stick containing an aqueous solution of sorbitol, sodium, carboxymethylcellulose, and electrolytes.
- Teeth show signs of dental caries.
  - Review patient's hygiene routines at home.
  - Refer patient to dentist upon order from physician or health care provider.

**Oral Hygiene for the Unconscious and/or Orally Intubated (Artificial Airway) Patient.** Unconscious or orally intubated patients pose challenges because of their risk for having alterations of the oral cavity. The absence of saliva movement and production in the unconscious or orally intubated (artificial airway) patient has serious implications. If left undisturbed for as little as 3 days, plaque will become a host for hundreds of gram-negative bacteria (Marsh and Martin, 1992). Bacteria cause infection in the oral cavity and directly enter the bloodstream of the vascular mucosa to cause systemic disease. Critically ill patients with endotracheal tubes who are on mechanical ventilation are at high risk for ventilator-associated pneumonia if saliva is aspirated into the tracheobronchial tree. Pathogens found in plaque have the potential for causing pneumonia.

Unconscious patients need special attention because they often do not have a gag reflex. Proper oral hygiene requires keeping the mucosa moist and removing secretions that can lead to infection. While providing hygiene to an unconscious patient, you must protect the patient from choking and aspiration. The safest practice is to have two nurses provide the care. One does the actual cleaning, and the other removes secretions with suction equipment. While cleansing the oral cavity, use a small oral airway or a padded tongue blade to hold the mouth open. Never use your fingers. A human bite is highly contaminated. It is sometimes necessary to perform mouth care at least every 2 hours. Explain the steps of mouth care and the sensations the patient will feel. Also tell the patient when the procedure is completed (Skill 27-4).

Research has resulted in improved standards for oral care of the critically ill (Stiefel and others, 2000). Researchers have found that foam stick applicators, a popular substitute for the toothbrush, stimulate the mucosal tissues but are ineffective in removing debris from the teeth (Grap and others, 2003). A pediatric-size toothbrush is more effective in removing plaque and tartar and fits better around an endotracheal tube. Hydrogen peroxide, once used routinely in intensive care units (ICUs) for mouth care, removes debris and is antiinfective, but if it is not diluted it will easily cause burns of the mucosa (Grap and others, 2003).

**Flossing.** Dental flossing is necessary to remove plaque and tartar between teeth. Flossing involves inserting waxed or unwaxed dental floss between all tooth surfaces, one at a time. The seesaw motion used to pull floss between teeth removes plaque and tartar from tooth enamel. If you apply toothpaste to the teeth before flossing, fluoride comes in direct contact with tooth surfaces, aiding in cavity prevention. Flossing once a day is sufficient. Because it is important to clean all teeth surfaces thoroughly, do not rush to complete flossing. Placing a mirror in front of the patient will help you to demonstrate the proper methods for holding the floss and cleaning between the teeth.

**Denture Care.** Encourage patients to clean their dentures on a regular basis to avoid gingival infection and irritation. When patients become disabled, you or the caregiver assume responsibility for denture care (Box 27-9). Dentures are the patient's personal property and need to be handled with care because they are fragile. Remove dentures at night to give the gums a rest and prevent bacterial buildup. To prevent warping, keep dentures covered in water when they are not being worn, and always store them in an enclosed, labeled cup with the cup placed in the patient's bedside stand. Discourage patients from removing their dentures and placing them on a napkin or tissue because they could be easily thrown away.

*Text continued on p. 752*

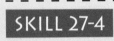 **Performing Mouth Care for an Unconscious or Debilitated Patient**

### Delegation Considerations

The skills of brushing teeth of an unconscious or debilitated patient can be delegated to assistive personnel. As the nurse, assess the patient's gag reflex. Instruct assistive personnel in:
- The proper way to position patients for mouth care.
- Use of oral suction catheter for clearing oral secretions (see Chapter 28, Skill 28-1.)
- How to recognize impaired integrity of oral mucosa.
- To report any abnormal findings to the nurse.
- Signs of aspiration to report.

### Equipment

- Small pediatric soft-bristle toothbrush
- Sponge toothette for edentulous patient
- Fluoridated toothpaste
- Tongue blade
- Small oral airway (optional)
- Face towel
- Paper towels
- Emesis basin
- Water glass with cool water
- Water-soluble lip lubricant
- Small-bulb syringe or suction machine equipment (required for patients with poor or absent gag reflex)
- Disposable gloves

| STEP | RATIONALE |
|---|---|

## ASSESSMENT

1. Perform hand hygiene. Apply disposable gloves.

   Reduces transmission of microorganisms. Gloves prevent contact with microorganisms in blood or saliva.

2. Test for presence of gag reflex by placing tongue blade on back half of tongue.

   Reveals whether patient is at risk for aspiration.

• *Critical Decision Point:* Patients with impaired gag reflex require oral care as well. Determine the type of suction apparatus needed at the bedside to protect the patient's airway against aspiration.

3. Inspect condition of oral cavity (see Chapter 13).

   Determines condition of oral cavity and need for hygiene.

4. Remove gloves. Perform hand hygiene.

   Prevents spread of infection.

5. Assess patient's risk for oral hygiene problems (see Skill 27-3).

   Certain conditions increase likelihood of alterations in integrity of oral cavity structures and require more frequent care.

## PLANNING

1. Unless contraindicated (e.g., head injury, neck trauma), lower side rail and position patient on side (Sims' position) with head turned well toward dependent side and head of bed lowered. Raise side rail.

   Allows secretions to drain from mouth instead of collecting in back of pharynx. Prevents aspiration.

2. Explain procedure to patient, even if patient is unconscious.

   Allows debilitated patient to anticipate procedure without anxiety. Unconscious patients sometimes retain the ability to hear.

## IMPLEMENTATION

1. Apply disposable gloves.

   Reduces transfer of microorganisms.

2. Place paper towels on over-bed table, and arrange equipment. If needed, turn on suction machine, and connect tubing to suction catheter.

   Prevents soiling of table top. Equipment prepared in advance ensures smooth, safe procedure.

3. Pull curtain around bed, or close room door.

   Provides privacy.

4. Raise bed to its highest horizontal level; lower side rail.

   Use of good body mechanics with bed in high position prevents injury to nurse.

5. Position patient close to side of bed; turn patent's head toward mattress.

   Proper positioning of head prevents aspiration.

6. Removes dentures or partial plates if present.

   Allows for thorough cleansing of prosthetics later. Provides clearer access to oral cavity.

7. Place towel under patient's head and emesis basin under chin.

   Prevents soiling of bed linen.

8. If patient is unconscious, uncooperative, or having difficulty keeping mouth open, insert an oral airway. Insert upside down, then turn the airway sideways and then over tongue to keep teeth apart. Insert when patient is relaxed, if possible. Do not use force (see illustration).

   Prevents patient from biting down on your fingers and provides access to oral cavity.

• *Critical Decision Point:* Never place fingers into the mouth of an unconscious or debilitated patient. The normal response is to bite down.

---

# Performing Mouth Care for an Unconscious or Debilitated Patient—cont'd

| STEP | RATIONALE |
|---|---|

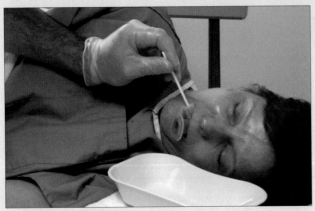

STEP **8** Insertion of oral airway.

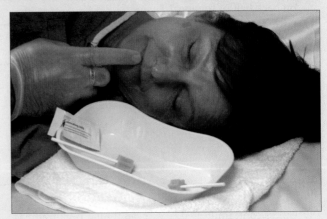

STEP **12** Application of water-soluble moisturizer to lips.

9. Brush teeth with toothpaste using an up-and-down gentle motion. Clean chewing and inner tooth surfaces first. Clean outer tooth surfaces. Brush roof of mouth, gums, and inside cheeks. Gently brush tongue but avoid stimulating gag reflex (if present). Moisten brush with water to rinse. (Bulb syringe may also be used to rinse.) Repeat rinse several times.

   Brushing action removes food particles between teeth and along chewing surfaces. Swabbing helps remove secretions and crusts from mucosa and moistens mucosa. Repeated rinsing removes all debris.

10. For patients without teeth, use a toothette moistened in water or normal saline to clean oral cavity.

   Less traumatic to mucosa of gums.

11. Suction secretions as they accumulate.

   Suction removes secretions and fluid that will collect in posterior pharynx.

12. Apply thin layer of water-soluble jelly to lips (see illustration).

   Lubricates lips to prevent drying and cracking.

13. Inform patient that procedure is completed.

   Provides meaningful stimulation to unconscious or less responsive patient.

14. Raise side rails as appropriate or ordered. Remove gloves, and dispose in proper receptacle.

   Prevents transmission of microorganisms.

15. Lower side rails. Reposition patient comfortably, raise side rail, and return bed to original position.

   Maintains patient's comfort and safety.

16. Clean equipment, and return to its proper place. Place soiled linen in proper receptacle.

   Proper disposal of soiled equipment prevents spread of infection.

17. Perform hand hygiene.

   Reduces transmission of microorganisms.

## EVALUATION

1. Apply gloves, and inspect oral cavity.

   Determines efficacy of cleansing. Once you remove thick secretions, you will see if any underlying inflammation or lesions remain.

2. Ask debilitated patient if mouth feels clean.

   Evaluates level of comfort.

3. Evaluate patient's respirations, and auscultate lung sounds on an ongoing basis.

   Ensures early recognition of aspiration.

| STEP | RATIONALE |
|---|---|

## RECORDING AND REPORTING

■ Record procedure, including pertinent observations (e.g., presence of bleeding gums, dry mucosa, ulcerations, crusts on tongue).

■ Report any unusual findings to nurse in charge or physician or health care provider.

## UNEXPECTED OUTCOMES AND RELATED INTERVENTIONS

■ Secretions or crusts remain on mucosa, tongue, or gums.
  • Patient needs more frequent oral hygiene.
  • Use a pediatric-size toothbrush to provide better hygiene (Fitch and others, 1999).

■ Localized inflammation of gums or mucosa is present.
  • Patient needs more frequent oral hygiene with soft-bristle toothbrush.
  • Apply moisturizing gel to mucosa and massage (Fitch and others, 1999).
  • Chemotherapy and radiation therapy can cause oral stomatitis. Patients should rinse mouth before and after

meals and at bedtime using normal saline or a solution of $\frac{1}{2}$ to 1 teaspoon of salt or baking soda to 1 pint tepid water. Another option is to use chlorhexidine, a broad-spectrum topical antiseptic (Scully, 2004).

  • A daily preventive protocol for leukemia patients consists of (1) elimination of plaque, (2) application of a mouthwash with a nonalcoholic solution of chlorhexidine 0.12%, and (3) topical application of iodopovidone followed by "swish and swallow" with nystatin, 500,000 units (Scully, 2004).

■ Lips are cracked or inflamed.
  • Apply moisturizing gel or water-soluble lubricant to lips.

■ Patient aspirates secretions.
  • If present, suction oral airways as secretions accumulate to maintain patent airway (see Chapter 28).
  • Elevate patient's head of bed to facilitate breathing.
  • Be prepared to have chest x-ray examination ordered by physician or health care provider.

---

### BOX 27-9  PROCEDURAL GUIDELINES FOR

### Cleaning Dentures

**Delegation Considerations:** You can delegate cleaning dentures to assistive personnel.

**Equipment:** soft-bristle toothbrush, denture toothbrush, emesis basin or sink, denture dentifrice or toothpaste, water glass, 4 × 4 inch gauze, washcloth, denture cup, disposable gloves

1. Perform hand hygiene.
2. Clean dentures for patient during routine mouth care. Dentures need to be cleansed as often as natural teeth.
3. Fill emesis basin with tepid water. (If using sink, place washcloth in bottom of sink, and fill sink with approximately 1 inch of water.)
4. Remove dentures: If patient is unable to do this independently, don gloves, grasp upper plate at front with thumb and index finger wrapped in gauze, and pull downward. Gently lift lower denture from jaw, and rotate one side downward to remove from patient's mouth. Place dentures in emesis basin or sink.
5. Apply dentifrice or toothpaste to denture, and brush surfaces of dentures (see illustration). Hold dentures close to water. Hold brush horizontally, and use back-and-forth motion to cleanse biting surfaces. Use short strokes from top of denture to biting surfaces of teeth to clean outer tooth surface. Hold brush vertically, and use short strokes to clean inner tooth sur-

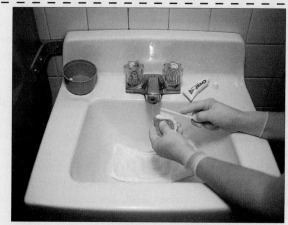

STEP 5 Brush surface of dentures.

faces. Hold brush horizontally, and use back-and-forth motion to clean undersurface of dentures.
6. Rinse dentures thoroughly in tepid water.
7. Return dentures to patient, or store in tepid water in denture cup.

## HAIR CARE

**Brushing and Combing.** Frequent brushing helps to keep hair clean and distributes oil evenly along hair shafts. Combing prevents hair from tangling. Encourage patients to maintain routine hair care. However, patients with limited mobility and poor coordination and those who are confused or seriously weakened by illness require help. Patients in a hospital or extended care facility appreciate the opportunity to have their hair brushed and combed before others see them.

Long hair easily becomes matted when a patient is confined to bed, even for a short period. When lacerations or incisions involve the scalp, blood and topical medications also cause tangling. Frequent brushing and combing keep long hair neatly groomed. Braiding helps to avoid repeated tangles. Ask permission before braiding a patient's hair.

To brush hair, part the hair into two sections and separate each into two more sections. It is easier to brush smaller sections of hair. Brushing from the scalp toward the hair ends minimizes pulling. Moistening the hair with water or an alcohol-free detangle product makes the hair easier to comb. Never cut a patient's hair without written consent.

**Shampooing.** Frequency of shampooing depends on a patient's daily routines. Remind hospitalized patients that staying in bed, excess perspiration, or treatments that leave blood or solutions in the hair may require more frequent shampooing. For patients at home the greatest challenge is to find ways for the patient to shampoo the hair without injury.

If the patient is able to take a shower or bath, he or she will usually be able to shampoo the hair without difficulty. Use a shower chair for the ambulatory patient who becomes tired or faint. Handheld shower nozzles allow patients to wash the hair during a tub bath or shower. If the patient is allowed to sit in a chair, you will usually shampoo the hair in front of a sink. If the patient has to sit at the bedside, shampoo the hair as the patient leans forward over a washbasin.

If a patient is unable to sit but you can move him or her, transfer the patient to a stretcher for transportation to a sink or shower equipped with a handheld nozzle. Place a towel or small pillow under the patient's head and neck, allowing the head to hang slightly over the stretcher's edge. Use caution when shampooing patients with neck injuries because hyperextension of the neck will possibly cause further injury. You will need a physician's or health care provider's order to shampoo the hair of patients with neck injuries.

When patients are unable to move, sit in a chair, be transferred to a stretcher, or tolerate a wet hair-washing procedure, there are various "dry" shampoo products available. It is important to read manufacturer's guidelines carefully. In general, you will massage these products into the patient's hair and scalp. Some products require you to apply a towel to remove excess oil and dirt, whereas other products require you to brush the product through the patient's hair.

A final option is to wash the patient's hair in the bed. Many institutions require a physician's or health care provider's order for the procedure (Box 27-10).

**Shaving.** Shave a patient's facial hair after the bath or shampoo. Women sometimes prefer to shave their legs or axillae while bathing. When assisting a patient, take care to avoid cutting the patient with razor blades. Patients prone to bleeding (e.g., those receiving anticoagulants or high doses of aspirin) need to use an electric razor. Before using an electric razor, check for electrical hazards. Use electric razors on only one patient because of the risk of infection transmission.

When patients use razor blades for shaving, they need to make sure the skin is soft to prevent pulling, scraping, or cuts. Placing a warm washcloth over the male patient's face for a few seconds, followed by application of shaving cream or a lathering of mild soap, softens the skin. If the patient is unable to shave, you will perform the shave. To avoid causing discomfort or razor cuts, gently pull the skin taut and use short, firm razor strokes in the direction the hair grows. Short downward strokes work best to remove hair over the upper lip. A patient will usually explain to you the best way to move the razor across the skin.

***Mustache and Beard Care.*** Patients with mustaches or beards require daily grooming. Keeping these areas clean is important because food particles and mucus easily collect in the hair. If the patient is unable to carry out self-care, do so at the patient's request. Never shave off a mustache or beard without the patient's consent.

***Hair and Scalp Care.*** To best promote and restore hair and scalp health, instruct patients to keep hair clean, combed, and brushed regularly. Patients also need to know how to check for and remove parasites (see Table 27-6). Tell patients to notify their primary health care provider of changes in the texture and distribution of hair.

**CARE OF EYES, EARS, NOSE.** To maintain optimal health, instruct patients in the proper methods of caring for the eyes, ears, and nose. Patients with specific health concerns involving these sensory organs need to see the appropriate specialist regularly for checkups and ongoing care. When active, patients need to know the best ways of protecting these sensitive organs (e.g., eye protective devices). Older adults experience a variety of changes in sensory function (see Chapter 36).

**Basic Eye Care.** Cleansing the eyes simply involves washing with a clean washcloth moistened in water. Soap causes burning and irritation. Never apply direct pressure over the eyeball because it may cause serious injury.

| BOX 27-10 | PROCEDURAL GUIDELINES FOR |
|---|---|

## Shampooing Hair of Bed-Bound Patient

**Delegation:** You can delegate shampooing hair of bed-bound patients to assistive personnel.

**Equipment:** bath towels, washcloths, shampoo and hair conditioner (optional), water pitcher, plastic shampoo trough, washbasin, bath blanket, waterproof pad, disposable gloves if open lesions involve scalp, clean comb and brush, hair dryer (optional)

1. Before washing patient's hair, determine that there are no contraindications to this procedure. Certain medical conditions, such as head and neck injuries, spinal cord injuries, and arthritis, place the patient at risk for injury during shampooing because of positioning and manipulation of patient's head and neck.

2. Perform hand hygiene. Apply disposable gloves if open lesions present.

3. Inspect the hair and scalp before initiating the procedure. This determines the presence of any conditions that require the use of special shampoos or treatments (e.g., for the removal of dried blood, dandruff).

4. Place waterproof pad under patient's shoulders, neck, and head. Position patient supine, with head and shoulders at top edge of bed. Place plastic trough under patient's head and washbasin at end of trough spout (see illustration). Be sure trough spout or tubing extends beyond edge of mattress.

5. Place rolled towel under patient's neck and bath towel over patient's shoulders.

6. Brush and comb patient's hair.

7. Obtain warm water.

8. Ask patient to hold face towel or washcloth over eyes.

9. Slowly pour water from water pitcher over hair until it is completely wet (see illustration). If hair contains matted blood, put on gloves, apply peroxide to dissolve clots, and then rinse hair with saline. Apply small amount of shampoo.

10. Work up lather with both hands. Start at hairline, and work toward back of neck. Lift head slightly with one hand to wash back of head. Shampoo sides of head. Massage scalp by applying pressure with fingertips.

11. Rinse hair with water. Make sure water drains into basin. Repeat rinsing until hair is free of soap.

12. Apply conditioner or cream rinse if requested, and rinse hair thoroughly.

13. Wrap patient's head in bath towel. Dry patient's face with cloth used to protect eyes. Dry off any moisture along neck or shoulders.

14. Dry patient's hair and scalp. Use second towel if first becomes saturated.

15. Comb hair to remove tangles, and dry with dryer if desired.

16. Apply oil preparation or conditioning product to hair, if desired by patient.

17. Assist patient to comfortable position, and complete styling of hair.

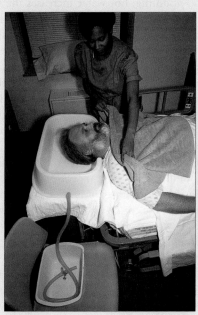

STEP 4 Patient positioned for shampoo.

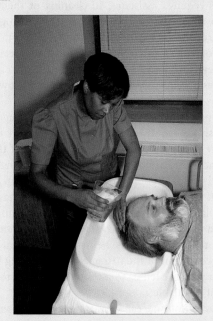

STEP 9 Rinsing of hair.

The unconscious patient requires more frequent eye care. Secretions collect along the lid margins and inner canthus when the blink reflex is absent or when the eye does not totally close. When an eye remains open, it is sometimes necessary to place an eye patch over the involved eye to prevent corneal drying and irritation. Administer lubricating eye drops according to the physician's or health care provider's orders.

*Eyeglasses.* Eyeglasses are made of hardened glass or plastic that is impact resistant to prevent shattering. Nevertheless, because of the cost, be careful when cleaning glasses and protect them from breakage or other damage when the patient is not wearing them. Put eyeglasses in a case and in a drawer of the bedside table when not in use.

Warm water is sufficient for cleaning glass lenses. A soft cloth is best for drying to prevent scratching the lens. Plastic lenses in particular are easy to scratch, and special cleansing solutions and drying tissues are available.

*Contact Lenses.* A contact lens is a thin, transparent, circular disk that fits directly over the cornea of the eye. Contact lenses are designed specifically to correct refractive errors of the eye or abnormalities in the shape of the cornea. They are easy to apply and remove.

Care of contact lenses includes proper cleaning, insertion and removal, and storage. Patients who wear contact lenses usually wear them all day and take care of their own lenses. If patients requires assistance in cleaning of their contact lenses, do so by performing hand hygiene, using contact soap, and rinsing with sterile saline solution. Instruct patient to avoid homemade solutions for cleansing contacts to avoid potential eye infections. Also make sure patients clean contact lens cases frequently with warm water and allow them to air dry.

When patients are admitted to hospitals or agencies in unresponsive or confused states, it is important to determine if the patient is a contact lens wearer and if the lenses are in place. If a seriously ill patient is wearing contact lenses and this fact goes undetected, severe corneal injury will result. If you determine that your patient has contact lenses in place and the patient cannot remove them, seek assistance in removing these lenses from the patient's eyes. Once you remove the lenses, be sure to document removal of lenses, condition of the patient's eyes following removal, and if you gave the lenses to a relative or placed them with the patient's valuables.

**Ear Care.** Routine ear care involves cleansing the ear with the end of a moistened washcloth, rotated gently into the ear canal. When cerumen is visible, gentle, downward retraction at the entrance of the ear canal usually causes the wax to loosen and slip out. Instruct your patient never to use sharp objects such as bobby pins or paper clips to remove cerumen. These objects will cause trauma to the ear canal or rupture of the tympanic membrane. In addition, avoid using cotton-tipped applicators because they cause cerumen wax to become impacted within the ear canal.

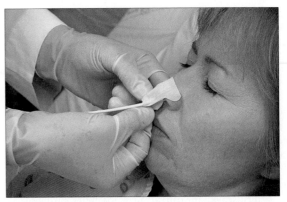

FIGURE **27-1** Apply new fixative device over feeding tube.

When cerumen is impacted, you can usually remove it by irrigation. Irrigate only after you inspect the patient's tympanic membrane to be sure it is intact; a perforated tympanic membrane is a contraindication to irrigation.

Before irrigation, instill 2 to 3 drops of glycerin at bedtime; this assists in softening the wax. Two to three drops of hydrogen peroxide are instilled twice a day to assist in loosening the wax. To irrigate the ear, have patient sit or lie with the affected ear up. Place a curved emesis basin under the affected ear. Using a bulb irrigating syringe, gently wash the ear canal with 250 ml of warm water. Cold water causes dizziness and vomiting; hot water increases the risk to the ear canal. Initiate the flow of solution at the top of the canal, which will assist in loosening the wax from the sides of the canal. After the canal is clear, remove any moisture from the ear and inspect the canal for remaining cerumen.

**Nose Care.** The patient usually removes secretions from the nose by gently blowing into a soft tissue. Caution the patient against harsh blowing that creates pressure capable of injuring the eardrum, nasal mucosa, and even sensitive eye structures. Bleeding from the nares is a key sign of harsh blowing.

If the patient is unable to remove nasal secretions, assist by using a wet washcloth or a cotton-tipped applicator moistened in water or saline. Never insert the applicator beyond the length of the cotton tip. You remove excessive nasal secretions also by gentle suctioning.

When patients have tubes inserted through the nose, change the tape anchoring the tube at least once a day. When tape becomes moist from nasal secretions, the skin and mucosa can easily become macerated. Friction causes tissue sloughing. Know how to anchor tubing correctly with tape or fixative devices to minimize tension or friction on the nares (Figure 27-1). When sloughing occurs, it is often necessary for you to remove the tube and insert one through the other naris.

## Evaluation

The evaluation of hygiene activities includes not only actual patient care but also whether you met the patient's expectations. Combining both of these aspects of evaluation is important in determining the success of hygiene care.

**PATIENT CARE.** During and after hygiene, evaluate the success of interventions. This usually involves careful inspection of those areas cleansed. The process is dynamic because the patient's condition changes (Table 27-7). Always be prepared to revise the care plan based on your evaluation. For example, if a patient's skin is not dried thoroughly after bathing, that area will become reddened and irritated, resulting in breaks in the skin integrity. Systematic evaluation requires you to determine if the patient has met expected outcomes.

**PATIENT EXPECTATIONS.** During assessment you collected data on the patient's expectations of care. After hygiene care you need to determine if you met the patient's expectations. For example, ask the patient if you met hygiene preferences or if family members were able to assist as desired. In addition, ask the patient about the care provided, thus determining if the patient's expectations were met or whether the patient had additional needs. In the case of Mrs. Foster, the patient requires additional teaching (Box 27-11).

## Patient's Room Environment

Attempting to make a patient's room as comfortable as the home is one of your priorities. An acceptable room for a patient is comfortable, safe, and large enough to allow the patient and visitors to move about freely. You will control room temperature, ventilation, noise, and odors to create a more comfortable environment. Keeping the room neat and orderly also contributes to the patient's sense of well-being.

### Maintaining Comfort

The nature of what constitutes a comfortable environment depends on the patient's age, severity of illness, and level of normal daily activity. Depending on the patient's age and physical condition, maintain the room temperature between 20° and 23° C (68° and 74° F). Infants, older adults, and the acutely ill need a warmer room. However, certain critically ill patients benefit from cooler room temperatures to lower the body's metabolic demands.

A good ventilation system keeps stale air and odors form lingering in the room. Protect the acutely ill, infants, and older adults from drafts by ensuring they are adequately dressed and covered with a lightweight blanket.

Good ventilation also reduces lingering odors caused by draining wounds, vomitus, bowel movements, and unemptied bedpans and urinals. Room deodorizers help remove many unpleasant odors. Always empty and rinse bedpans or urinals promptly. Thorough hygiene measures are the best way to control body or breath odors. Most health care institutions now prohibit smoking. Before using room deodorizers, determine that the patient is not allergic to or sensitive to the deodorizer itself.

## OUTCOME EVALUATION

**TABLE 27-7**

| Nursing Action | Patient Response/Finding | Achievement of Outcome |
|---|---|---|
| Turned Mrs. Foster every 90 minutes. | Mrs. Foster did not report sensations of pressure, burning, or tingling over bony areas or other areas of the skin. Mrs. Foster was able to assist with position change. | Mrs. Foster's skin remains intact without erythema. |
| Gave hygiene and perineal care following each episode of incontinence. | Mrs. Foster stated that skin felt clean. Mrs. Foster did not report sensations of wetness, burning, pain, or tingling in perineal region. | Mrs. Foster's skin remains dry and intact. Perineal skin is free of odor, redness, and swelling. |

## EVALUATION

James provides Mrs. Foster with a shower and modifies her plan of care to include a shower every other day. He includes a teaching plan on oral hygiene. Mrs. Foster tells James that she really appreciates having more frequent showers and that they really help her feel and do her best. Although Mrs. Foster is very tired and needs a rest period after the shower, she feels it is worth it. Mrs. Foster was also able to demonstrate proper oral hygiene. Mrs. Foster knows that James provides the extra effort to her care and the subsequent modification of the care plan, and she is happy and feels somewhat in control of her care.

**Documentation Note**
"Assisted patient in shower. Nursing care plan modified to include shower every other day followed by a 30-minute rest period. Moved physical and occupational therapy times to accommodate shower and rest periods. Patient went to dining room for lunch. Included oral hygiene (brushing teeth twice a day [AM and PM] and flossing at least once daily) in care plan modification."

**BOX 27-11** PATIENT TEACHING

Mrs. Foster tells James that she is concerned about needing more dental care. She has just had three root canals. Although the care she received controlled the pain and discomfort that she experienced, her insurance did not cover the total expense. Consequently, her family is paying the balance of the bill. She asks him what she can do to help prevent or minimize the need for dental services outside of routine maintenance.

James develops the following teaching plan for Mrs. Foster:

**Outcome**
- At the end of the teaching session Mrs. Foster will demonstrate or verbalize strategies for good dental hygiene.

**Teaching Strategies**
- Inspect Mrs. Foster's current dental supplies.
- Provide a basic background about course of dental disease.
- Demonstrate how to brush teeth and gums.
- Explain that she needs to brush teeth twice a day with an American Dental Association–accepted fluoride toothpaste.
- Explain how to floss teeth; explore dental flossing devices as well as floss string.

- Explain that flossing at least once a day removes any bacteria trapped between teeth.
- Provide information on foods that contribute to decay or prevent it. Examples of foods that promote tooth decay include soda, juices, and candy that contain sugar. Those that promote healthy teeth include fruits and vegetables.
- Identify and explain that she needs to report symptoms such as reddened, painful, or bleeding gums or teeth with a white or darkened spot to nursing staff and physician or health care provider.
- Summarize the lesson.

**Evaluation Strategies**
- Use open-ended questions.
- Ask Mrs. Foster to verbalize when to perform dental hygiene.
- Ask Mrs. Foster to demonstrate proper brushing and flossing of her teeth.
- Have Mrs. Foster identify what dietary items to avoid.
- Have Mrs. Foster describe what signs and symptoms she needs to report.

Ill patients seem to be more sensitive to common facility noises. Until the patient is familiar with facility noises, try to control the noise level. You also need to explain the source of any unfamiliar noises.

Proper lighting is necessary for everyone's safety and comfort. A brightly lit room is usually stimulating, but a darkened room is best for rest and sleep. Adjust room lighting by closing or opening drapes, regulating over-bed and floor lights, and closing or opening room doors.

### Room Equipment

A typical room contains certain basic pieces of furniture. The over-bed table rolls on wheels and adjusts to various heights over the bed or a chair. Usually two storage areas are under the tabletop. The table provides ideal working space for performing procedures. It also provides a surface on which to place meal trays, toiletry items, and objects the patient frequently uses. Make sure to clean the top of the bed table with an antiseptic cleaner before using the table for meals. Do not place the bedpan and urinal on the overbed table. Use the bedside stand to store the patient's personal possessions and hygiene equipment. Most patients use the bedside stand for the telephone, water pitcher, and drinking cup.

Most rooms contain an armless straight-backed chair and an upholstered lounge chair with arms. Patients and visitors use the lounge chair, which is usually placed at the foot of the bed or beside it. Straight-backed chairs are convenient when temporarily transferring the patient from the bed, such as during bed making.

Each room usually has an over-bed light. Position moveable lights that extend over the bed from the wall for easy reach, but move then aside when not in use. Gooseneck or special examination lights are portable standing lights used to provide extra light during bedside procedures.

Other equipment usually found in a patient's room includes a call light, a television set or radio, a blood pressure gauge, oxygen and vacuum wall outlets, and personal care items. Special equipment designed for comfort or positioning patients include footboards and foot boots (Figure 27-2), special mattresses, and bed boards.

**BEDS.** Seriously ill patients sometimes remain in bed for a long time. Because a bed is the piece of equipment patients use most, it is designed for comfort, safety, and adaptability for changing positions.

The typical hospital bed has a firm mattress on a metal frame that you and the patient can raise and lower horizontally. You will use different bed positions to promote patients' lung expansion and for procedures such as postural drainage (Table 27-8).

You change the position of a bed by electrical controls on the side or foot of the bed or on a bedside table. Patients thus raise or lower sections of the bed without expending much energy. Instruct patients in the proper use of controls, and caution them against raising the bed to a position that causes harm. It is generally recommended to keep a bed at a height that is appropriate for easy patient transfer.

Beds contain safety features such as locks on the wheels or casters. Make sure wheels are locked when the bed is sta-

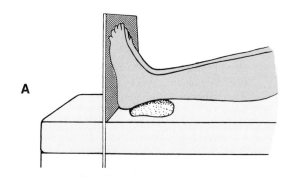

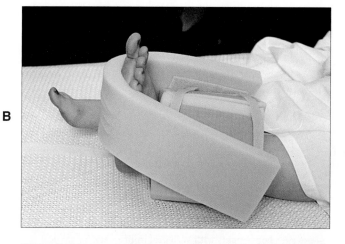

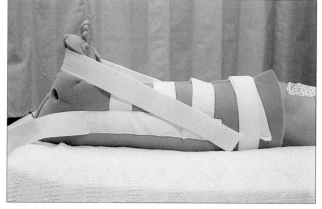

FIGURE **27-2 A,** Footboard. **B,** Foot boot. **C,** Foot boot with lower leg extension.

tionary to prevent accidental movement. Side rails allow patients to move more efficiently in bed and prevent accidents. Do not use side rails to restrict a patient from moving in bed. When using side rails as a restraint, you need a physician's or health care provider's order (see Chapter 26). The headboard is removable from most beds. This is important when the medical team needs to have easy access to the head, such as during cardiopulmonary resuscitation.

**Bed Making.** Keep a patient's bed as clean and comfortable as possible. This requires frequent inspections to be sure linen is clean, dry, and free of wrinkles.

Usually make a bed in the morning after the patients' bath or while the patient is bathing, in a shower, sitting in a chair eating, or out of the room for procedures or tests. Throughout the day straighten linen that becomes loose or wrinkled. Also, check the bed linen for food particles after meals and for wetness or soiling. Change linen that becomes soiled or wet.

When changing the bed linen, follow basic principles of asepsis by keeping soiled linen away from the uniform. Place soiled linen in special linen containers before discarding it in the linen hamper. To avoid air currents, which spread microorganisms, you never fan linen. To avoid transmitting infection, do not place soiled linen on the floor. Immediately discard any clean linen that touches the floor.

During bed making, use proper body mechanics (see Chapter 25). Make sure you raise the bed to its highest position before changing linen so you do not have to bend or stretch over the mattress.

The patients' privacy, comfort, and safety are important when making a bed. Using side rails, keeping call lights within the patient's reach, and maintaining the proper bed position help promote comfort and safety. After making a bed you always return it to the lowest horizontal position to prevent accidental falls.

When possible, make the bed while it is unoccupied (Box 27-12). If the patient is confined to bed, organize bed-making activities to conserve time and energy (Skill 27-5). When making an unoccupied bed follow the same basic principles as for bed making. The surgical, recovery, or postoperative bed is a modified version of the unoccupied bed. Fold the top covers of the surgical bed to one side or fanfold them to the bottom third of the bed. This allows for easy transfer of patient into the bed. After a patient is discharged, send all bed linen to the laundry. Housekeeping personnel clean the mattress and bed and apply new bed linen.

**Linens.** Before bed making, it is important to collect not only bed linens but also the patient's personal linens. Linens come pressed and folded to prevent the spread of microorganisms and to make bed making easier. Bed linens have a center crease that you place in the center of the bed from the head to the foot. The linens unfold easily to the sides, with creases often fitting over the mattress edge. Apply new linens whenever there is soiling.

*Text continued on p. 765*

| TABLE 27-8 | Common Bed Positions | |
|---|---|---|

| Position | Description | Uses |
|---|---|---|
| Fowler's | Head of bed raised to angle of 45 degrees or more; semisitting position. | Preferred while patient eats; used during nasogastric tube insertion and nasotracheal suction; promotes lung expansion. |
| Semi-Fowler's | Head of bed raised approximately 30 degrees; incline is less than Fowler's position. | Promotes lung expansion. |
| Trendelenburg's | Entire bed tilted downward with head of bed down. | For postural drainage; facilitates venous return in patients with poor peripheral perfusion. |
| Reverse Trendelenburg's | Entire bed frame tilted downward with foot of bed down. | Used infrequently; promotes gastric emptying and prevents esophageal reflux. |
| Flat | Entire bed frame parallel with floor. | For patients with vertebral injuries and in cervical traction; used by hypotensive patients; generally preferred by patients for sleeping. |

---

| BOX 27-12 | PROCEDURAL GUIDELINES FOR |
|---|---|

### Making an Unoccupied Bed

**Delegation:** You can delegate making an unoccupied bed to assistive personnel.

**Equipment:** linen bag, mattress pad (optional depending on facility's practice), bottom sheet (flat or fitted), drawsheet (optional), top sheet, blanket, bedspread, waterproof pads (optional), pillowcases, bedside chair or table, disposable gloves (if linen is soiled), washcloth, and antiseptic cleanser

1. Perform hand hygiene.
2. Determine if patient has been incontinent or if excess drainage is on linen. Gloves will be necessary.
3. Assess activity orders or restrictions in mobility in planning if patient can get out of bed for procedure. Assist to bedside chair or recliner.
4. Lower side rails on both sides of bed, and raise bed to comfortable working position.
5. Remove soiled linen, and place in laundry bag. Avoid shaking or fanning linen.
6. Reposition mattress, and wipe off any moisture using a washcloth moistened in antiseptic solution. Dry thoroughly.
7. Apply all bottom linen on one side of bed before moving to opposite side. Apply bottom sheet, flat or fitted.
8. Be sure to place fitted sheet smoothly over mattress. To apply a flat unfitted sheet, allow about 25 cm (10 inches) to hang over mattress edge. Lower hem of sheet lies seam down, even with bottom edge of mattress. Pull remaining top portion of sheet over top edge of mattress.
9. While standing at head of bed, miter top corner of bottom flat sheet (see Skill 27-5, step 14).
10. Tuck remaining portion of unfitted sheet under mattress.
11. Optional: Apply drawsheet, laying center fold along middle of bed lengthwise. Smooth drawsheet over mattress and tuck excess edge under mattress, keeping palms down.
12. Move to opposite side of bed, and spread bottom sheet smoothly over edge of mattress from head to foot of bed.
13. Apply fitted sheet smoothly over each mattress corner. For an unfitted sheet, miter top corner of bottom sheet (see step 9), making sure corner is stretched tight.

**BOX 27-12** PROCEDURAL GUIDELINES FOR

## Making an Unoccupied Bed—cont'd

14. Grasp remaining edge of unfitted bottom sheet, and tuck tightly under mattress while moving from head to foot of bed. Smooth folded drawsheet over bottom sheet, and tuck under mattress, first at middle, then at top, and then at bottom.
15. If needed, apply waterproof pad over bottom sheet or drawsheet.
16. Place top sheet over bed with vertical center fold lengthwise down middle of bed. Open sheet out from head to foot, being sure top edge of sheet is even with top edge of mattress.
17. Make horizontal toe pleat: stand at foot of bed and fanfold top sheet 5 to 10 cm (2 to 4 inches) across bed. Pull sheet up from bottom to make fold approximately 15 cm (6 inches) from bottom edge of mattress.
18. Tuck in remaining portion of sheet under foot of mattress. Then place blanket over bed with top edge parallel to top edge of sheet and 15 to 20 cm (6 to 8 inches) down from edge of sheet. (Optional: Apply additional spread over bed.)
19. Make cuff by turning edge of top sheet down over top edge of blanket and spread.
20. Standing on one side at foot of bed, lift mattress corner slightly with one hand, and with other hand tuck top sheet, blanket, and spread under mattress. Be sure toe pleats are not pulled out.

21. Make modified mitered corner with top sheet, blanket, and spread. After making triangular fold, do not tuck tip of triangle (see illustration).
22. Go to other side of bed. Spread sheet, blanket, and spread out evenly. Make cuff with top sheet and blanket. Make modified corner at foot of bed.
23. Apply clean pillowcase.
24. Place call light within patient's reach on bed rail or pillow, and return bed to height allowing for patient transfer. Assist patient to bed.
25. Arrange patient's room. Remove and discard supplies. Perform hand hygiene.

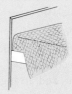

STEP **21** Modified mitered corner.

---

**SKILL 27-5** ┆ Making an Occupied Bed

### Delegation Considerations

You can delegate making an occupied bed to assistive personnel. Before delegating this skill, instruct the assistive personnel about:

- Any precautions or activity restrictions for the patient
- What to do if wound drainage, dressing material, drainage tubes, or IV tubing becomes dislodged or if assistive personnel find it in the linens
- What to do if patient becomes fatigued

### Equipment (Figure 27-3)

- Linen bag(s)
- Mattress pad (optional depending on facility practice)
- Bottom sheet (flat or fitted)
- Drawsheet
- Top sheet
- Blanket
- Bedspread

- Waterproof pads and/or bath blankets (optional)
- Pillowcases
- Bedside chair or table
- Disposable gloves (optional)
- Towel
- Disinfectant

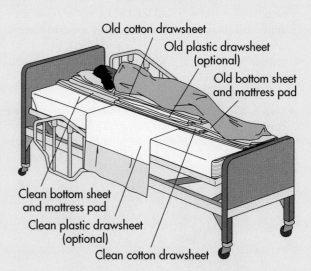

Old cotton drawsheet
Old plastic drawsheet (optional)
Old bottom sheet and mattress pad
Clean bottom sheet and mattress pad
Clean plastic drawsheet (optional)
Clean cotton drawsheet

FIGURE **27-3** Equipment for making an occupied bed.

## SKILL 27-5 | Making an Occupied Bed

| STEP | RATIONALE |
|---|---|
| **ASSESSMENT** | |
| 1. Assess potential for patient incontinence or for excess drainage on bed linen. | Determines need for protective waterproof pads or extra bath blankets on bed. |
| 2. Check chart for orders or specific precautions concerning movement and positioning. | Ensures patient safety and use of proper body mechanics. |
| **PLANNING** | |
| 1. Explain procedure to the patient, noting that the patient will be asked to turn on side and roll over linen. | Minimizes anxiety and promotes cooperation. |
| **IMPLEMENTATION** | |
| 1. Perform hand hygiene, and apply disposable gloves (wear gloves only if linen is soiled or there is risk for contact with body secretions). | Reduces transmission of microorganisms. |
| 2. Assemble equipment, and arrange on bedside chair or table. Remove unnecessary equipment such as a dietary tray or items used for hygiene. | Assembling all equipment provides for smooth procedure and assists in increasing patient's comfort. Placing linen on clean surface minimizes spread of infection. |
| 3. Draw room curtain around bed or close door. | Maintains patient's privacy. |
| 4. Adjust bed height to comfortable working position. Lower any raised side rail on one side of bed. Remove call light. | Minimizes strain on back. It is easier to remove and apply linen evenly to bed in flat position. Provides easy access to bed and linen. |
| 5. Loosen top linen at foot of bed. | Makes linen easier to remove. |
| 6. Remove bedspread and blanket separately. If spread and blanket are soiled, place them in linen bag. Keep soiled linen away from uniform. | Reduces transmission of microorganisms. |
| 7. If you reuse blanket and spread, fold them by bringing the top and bottom edges together. Fold farthest side over onto nearer bottom edge. Bring top and bottom edges together again. Place folded linen over back of chair. | Folding method facilitates replacement and prevents wrinkles. |
| 8. Cover patient with bath blanket placed over top sheet. If patient is able to help, have him or her hold top edge of bath blanket. If patient is unable to help, tuck top of bath blanket under shoulder. Grasp top edge of sheet under bath blanket, and remove sheet. Discard sheet in linen bag. | Bath blanket provides warmth and keeps body parts covered during linen removal. |
| 9. With assistance from another nurse, slide mattress toward head of bed. | If mattress slides toward foot of bed when head of bed is raised, it is difficult to tuck in linen. In addition, it is uncomfortable for the patient because the patient's feet will press against or hang over the foot of the bed. |
| 10. Position patient on the far side of the bed, turned onto side and facing away from you. Be sure side rail in front of patient is up. Adjust pillow under patient's head. | Turning patient onto side provides space for placement of clean linen. Side rail ensures patient's safety by preventing forward falls from the bed surface and helps patient in moving. |

| STEP | RATIONALE |
|---|---|

11. Loosen bottom linens, moving from head to foot. With seam side down (facing the mattress), fanfold bottom sheet and drawsheet toward patient—first drawsheet, then bottom sheet. Tuck edges of linen just under buttocks, back, and shoulders. Do not fanfold mattress pad if it is to be reused (see illustration).

Prepares for removal of all bottom linen simultaneously.

12. Wipe off any moisture on exposed mattress with towel and appropriate disinfectant.

Provides maximum work space for placing clean linen. Later, when patient turns to other side, you can remove soiled linen easily.

Reduces transmission of microorganisms.

13. Apply clean linen to exposed half of bed:

Applying linen over bed in successive layers minimizes energy and time used in bed making.

  a. Place clean mattress pad on bed by folding it lengthwise with center crease in middle of bed. Fanfold top layer over mattress. (If you reuse pad, simply smooth out any wrinkles.)

  b. Unfold clean bottom sheet lengthwise so that center crease is situated lengthwise along center of bed. Fanfold sheet's top layer toward center of bed alongside the patient (see illustration). Smooth bottom layer of sheet over mattress, and bring edge over closest side of mattress. Pull fitted sheet smoothly over mattress ends. Allow edge of flat unfitted sheet to hang about 25 cm (10 inches) over mattress edge. Lower hem of bottom flat sheet lies seam down and even with bottom edge of mattress.

Proper positioning of linen on one side ensures that adequate linen will be available to cover opposite side of bed. Keeping seam edges down eliminates irritation to patient's skin.

14. Miter bottom flat sheet at head of bed:

Ensures secure flat sheet will not loosen easily.

  a. Face head of bed diagonally. Place hand away from head of bed under top corner of mattress, near mattress edge, and lift.

  b. With other hand, tuck top edge of bottom sheet smoothly under mattress so that side edges of sheet above and below mattress meet if brought together.

  c. Face side of bed and pick up top edge of sheet at approximately 45 cm (18 inches) from top of mattress (see illustration).

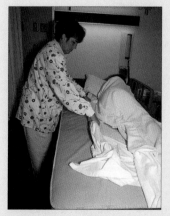

STEP **11** Old linen tucked under patient.

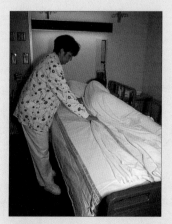

STEP **13b** Clean linen applied to bed.

SKILL 27-5 | Making an Occupied Bed—cont'd

| STEP | RATIONALE |
|---|---|
| d. Lift sheet, and lay it on top of mattress to form a neat triangular fold, with lower base of triangle even with mattress side edge (see illustration). | |
| e. Tuck lower edge of sheet, which is hanging free below the mattress, under mattress. Tuck with palms down, without pulling triangular fold (see illustration). | |
| f. Hold portion of sheet covering side of mattress in place with one hand. With the other hand, pick up top of triangular linen fold and bring it down over side of mattress (see illustrations). Tuck this portion under mattress (see illustration). | Mitered corner is not easy to loosen even if patient moves frequently in bed. |
| 15. Tuck remaining portion of sheet under mattress, moving toward foot of bed. Keep linen smooth. | Folds of linen are source of irritation. |
| 16. *(Optional)* Open clean drawsheet so that it unfolds in half. Lay centerfold along middle of bed lengthwise, and position sheet so that it will be under the patient's buttocks and torso (see illustration). Fanfold top layer toward patient, with edge along patient's back. Smooth bottom layer out over mattress, and tuck excess edge under mattress (keep palms down). | You will use drawsheet to lift and reposition patient. Placement under patient's torso distributes most of patient's body weight over sheet. |
| 17. Place waterproof pad over drawsheet, with centerfold against patient's side. Fanfold top layer toward patient. | Protects bed linen from being soiled. |
| 18. Have patient roll slowly toward you, over the layers of linen. Raise side rail on working side, and go to other side. | Positions patient for removal of old linen and placement of new linens. Maintains patient's safety and body alignment during turning. |

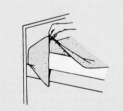

STEP **14c** Top edge of sheet picked up.

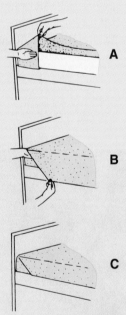

A

B

C

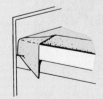

STEP **14d** Sheet on top of mattress in a triangular fold.

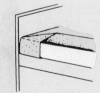

STEP **14e** Lower edge of sheet tucked under mattress.

STEP **14f** **A** and **B**, Triangular fold placed over side of mattress. **C,** Linen tucked under mattress.

| STEP | RATIONALE |
|------|-----------|
| 19. Lower side rail. Assist patient in positioning on other side, over folds of linen. Loosen edges of soiled linen from under mattress (see illustration). | Exposes opposite side of bed for removal of soiled linen and placement of clean linen. Makes linen easier to remove. |
| 20. Remove soiled linen by folding it into a bundle or square, with soiled side turned in. Discard in linen bag. If necessary, wipe mattress with antiseptic solution, and dry mattress surface before applying new linen. | Reduces transmission of microorganisms. |
| 21. Pull clean, fanfolded linen smoothly over edge of mattress from head to foot of bed. | Smooth linen will not irritate patient's skin. |
| 22. Assist patient in rolling back into supine position. Reposition pillow. | Maintains patient's comfort. |
| 23. Pull fitted sheet smoothly over mattress ends. Miter top corner of bottom sheet (see step 14). When tucking corner, be sure that sheet is smooth and free of wrinkles. | Wrinkles and folds cause irritation to skin. |
| 24. Facing side of bed, grasp remaining edge of bottom flat sheet. Lean back; keep back straight; and pull while tucking excess linen under mattress. Proceed from head to foot of bed. (Avoid lifting mattress during tucking to ensure fit.) | Proper use of body mechanics while tucking linen prevents injury. |
| 25. Smooth fanfolded drawsheet out over bottom sheet. Grasp edge of sheet with palms down; lean back; and tuck sheet under mattress. Tuck from middle to top and then to bottom. | Tucking first at top or bottom pulls sheet sideways, causing poor fit. |
| 26. Place top sheet over patient with centerfold lengthwise down middle of bed. Open sheet from head to foot, and unfold over patient. | Correctly positioning centerfold distributes sheet equally over bed. |
| 27. Ask patient to hold clean top sheet, or tuck sheet around patient's shoulders. Remove bath blanket and discard in linen bag. | Sheet prevents exposure of body parts. Having patient hold sheet encourages patient participation in care. |
| 28. Place blanket on bed, unfolding it so that crease runs lengthwise along middle of bed. Unfold blanket to cover patient. Make sure top edge is parallel with edge of top sheet and 15 to 20 cm (6 to 8 inches) from top sheet's edge. | Place blanket to cover patient completely and provide adequate warmth. |

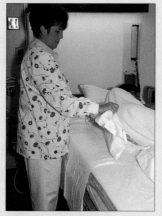

STEP **16** Optional drawsheet.

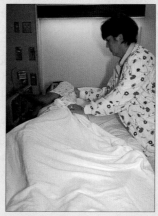

STEP **19** Assisting patient to roll over folds of linen.

SKILL 27-5 | Making an Occupied Bed—cont'd

| STEP | RATIONALE |
|---|---|
| 29. Place spread over bed according to step 28. Be sure that top edge of spread extends about 2.5 cm (1 inch) above blanket's edge. Tuck top edge of spread over and under top edge of blanket. | Gives bed neat appearance and provides extra warmth. |
| 30. Make cuff by turning edge of top sheet down over top edge of blanket and spread. | Protect patient's face from rubbing against blanket or spread. |
| 31. Standing on one side at foot of bed, lift mattress corner slightly with one hand and tuck linens under mattress. Tuck top sheet and blanket under together. Be sure that linens are loose enough to allow movement of patient's feet. Making a horizontal toe pleat is an option. | Makes neat-appearing bed. Pressure ulcers develop on patient's toes and heels from feet rubbing against tight-fitting bed sheets. |
| 32. Make modified mitered corner with top sheet, blanket, and spread (see illustration in Box 27-12 ) | Ensures top covers will not loosen easily. |
|    a. Pick up side edge of top sheet, blanket, and spread approximately 45 cm (18 inches) from foot of mattress. Lift linen to form triangular fold, and lay it on bed. | |
|    b. Tuck lower edge of sheet, which is hanging free below mattress, under mattress. Do not pull triangular fold. | |
|    c. Pick up triangular fold, and bring it down over mattress while holding linen in place along side of mattress. Do not tuck tip of triangle. | Secures top linen but keeps even edge of blanket and top sheet draped over mattress. |
| 33. Raise side rail. Make other side of bed; spread sheet, blanket, and bedspread out evenly. Fold top edge of spread over blanket and make cuff with top sheet (see step 30); make modified mitered corner at foot of bed (see step 32). | Side rail protects patient from accidental falls. |
| 34. Change pillowcase: | |
|    a. Have patient raise head. While supporting neck with one hand, remove pillow. Allow patient to lower head. | Support of neck muscles prevents injury during flexion and extension of neck. |
|    b. Remove soiled case by grasping pillow at open end with one hand and pulling case back over pillow with the other hand. Discard case in linen bag. | Pillows slide out easily, thus minimizing contact with soiled linen. |
|    c. Grasp clean pillowcase at center of closed end. Gather case, turning it inside out over the hand holding it. With the same hand, pick up middle of one end of the pillow. Pull pillowcase down over pillow with the other hand. | Eases sliding of pillowcase over pillow. |
|    d. Be sure pillow corners fit evenly into corners of pillowcase. Place pillow under patient's head. | Poorly fitting case constricts fluffing and expansion of pillow and interferes with patient comfort. |
| 35. Place call light within patient's reach, and return bed to comfortable position. | Ensures patient safety and comfort. |
| 36. Open room curtains, and rearrange furniture. Place personal items within easy reach on over-bed table or bedside stand. Return bed to a comfortable height. | Promotes sense of well-being. |
| 37. Discard dirty linen in hamper or chute, and perform hand hygiene. | Prevents transmission of microorganisms. |
| 38. Ask if patient feels comfortable. | Ensures bed linens are clean and smooth. |

| STEP | RATIONALE |
|---|---|
| **EVALUATION** | |
| 1. Inspect skin for areas of irritation. | Folds in linen cause pressure on skin. |
| 2. Observe patient for signs of fatigue, dyspnea, pain, or discomfort. | Provides you with data about patient's level of activity tolerance and ability to participate in other procedures. |

**RECORDING AND REPORTING**

■ It is not necessary to record the making of an occupied bed.

■ Patient's skin shows signs of breakdown.
  • Institute skin care measures to reduce risk of pressure ulcer (see Chapter 35).
  • Change patient's position frequently.

**UNEXPECTED OUTCOMES AND RELATED INTERVENTIONS**

■ Patient feels discomfort from linen fold.
  • Tighten sheets.
  • Change patient's position frequently.

## KEY CONCEPTS

- Provide patients' daily hygiene needs if they are unable to care for themselves adequately.
- Providing hygiene care gives you the chance to assess external body surfaces and the patient's emotional state.
- While providing daily hygiene needs, use teaching and communication skills to develop a relationship with the patient.
- Always consider the patient's personal preferences when you plan daily hygiene care.
- Maintain privacy and comfort when providing the patient's daily care.
- The absence of saliva movement and production in the unconscious or orally intubated (artificial airway) patient has the potential for the development of gram-negative bacteria in the oral mucosa.
- During assessment of the skin and oral mucosa, observe characteristics influenced by hygiene.

- Patients who are immobilized and poorly nourished and who have reduced sensation or peripheral circulation are at risk for altered skin integrity.
- Wear gloves during hygiene care when the risk of contacting body fluids is high, and always wear gloves during perineal care.
- Patients with diabetes or poor peripheral circulation need special nail and foot care.
- Because hygiene is a personal matter, patients from different cultures will vary in the perceptions of who can assist in their care.
- When administering oral care to unconscious patients, take measures to prevent aspiration.
- Base evaluation of hygiene care on the patient's sense of comfort, relaxation, well-being, and understanding of hygiene techniques.

## CRITICAL THINKING IN PRACTICE

*Mr. Roberts, an 80-year-old widower who lives alone, is admitted to the intensive care unit. He was admitted with a diagnosis of chest pain 24 hours ago. Past medical history includes a myocardial infarction 2 years ago, type 2 diabetes controlled by a 1200-calorie, low-fat, low-sugar diet. He is allergic to penicillin. He is obese and has poor hygiene. His skin is rough and dry with some areas of excoriation. Mr. Roberts has his own teeth, which are in poor condition. Your report this morning included the following information. Vital signs are blood pressure, 134/84; pulse, 84; respirations, 20; and afebrile. Continuous use of 2 L of oxygen per nasal cannula. Oxygen saturation is 99%. Normal sinus rhythm, and respirations are regular. Patient denies chest pain. Orders given to transfer to the step-down unit, awaiting*

*bed placement. Activity includes up at bedside with assistance. Patient requires at least one person to assist with transfer to chair. Gait is unsteady, and patient complains of being tired after activity. Patient has just completed breakfast.*

– – – – – – – – – – – – – – – – – – –

1. Based on your assessment of the patient's activity level, he will probably require a:
   a. Shower
   b. Tub bath
   c. Partial bed bath
   d. Complete bed bath
2. While assisting Mr. Roberts with his bath, your assessment reveals that his heels are cracked and bleeding and

that his toenails are long and curved. What action do you take as a result of your assessment?
a. Complete the bath, and document information.
b. Apply lotion to the heels and cut patient's nails, using a straight-line cut across the nail.
c. Complete the bath, document your assessments, and notify the charge nurse of your findings.
c. Contact a podiatrist.

3. In addition to bathing, all of the following interventions will assist in promoting patient comfort except:
a. Keeping linen free from wrinkles
b. Making the bed with tight-fitting top sheet
c. Shampooing patient's hair
d. Assisting with oral care

*Mrs. John, a 30-year-old woman, is admitted to the neurological unit following a spinal cord injury. She is 2 weeks post admission, and she is now a quadriplegic. Mrs. John is alert and oriented and has spontaneous respirations and intact gag reflex. She was transferred from trauma ICU 2 days ago. Patient has a percutaneous endoscopic gastrostomy (PEG) tube in place for supplemental enteral feedings and is still experiencing diarrhea from the tube feedings. Mrs. John needs to be catheterized with a straight catheter every 4 to 6 hours. A stage I pressure ulcer is present on her left heel. Plan of care includes the following nursing diagnoses: diarrhea, impaired physical mobility, impaired*
skin integrity, bathing/hygiene and dressing/grooming self-care deficits, latex allergy response, and powerlessness.

– – – – – – – – – – – – – – – – – – – – –

4. Your assessment reveals the following information. Mrs. John will not open her eyes and responds to your questions with one-syllable answers or not at all. Vital signs are stable, and she is afebrile; enteral feedings are running at 50 ml/hour, and 200 ml remains in the bag. Patient is incontinent of a large amount of liquid stool. She is scheduled to be catheterized with a straight catheter in 10 minutes. How would you prioritize your activities?

5. Mrs. John requires complete assistance with her oral care. List the following steps in order of how you would proceed with providing her oral care. Note that you have already explained the procedure to patient, gathered your equipment, raised the bed to a comfortable working level, and lowered the side rail.
a. Inspect oral cavity by having patient open mouth.
b. Brush teeth holding bristles at a 45-degree angle to gum line.
c. Floss teeth.
d. Clean biting surfaces of teeth.
e. Wash hands, and apply nonlatex disposable gloves.
f. Have patient rinse mouth (suction if needed).
g. Elevate head of bed.
h. Clean inner and outer surfaces of upper and lower teeth.

## NCLEX® REVIEW

1. Mr. Houseff has been hospitalized following an auto accident. He has suffered multiple traumatic injuries and requires complete assistance with bathing. The patient is a Muslim. When providing a bath you should know that:
1. Muslims consider the top parts of the body cleaner than the lower parts
2. Touching is taboo between related males and females
3. For a Muslim the left hand is used for cleaning
4. When bathing a male you should avoid uncovering the lower torso and exposing the arms

2. While assessing a patient's skin, you notice a flaky, rough texture on exposed areas of the hands, face, and legs. Good skin care for this patient includes:
1. Bathing the patient more frequently
2. Increasing fluid intake
3. Lessening the amount of rinsing of the skin
4. Avoiding cleansing over areas of dryness

3. Which of the following patients is at greatest risk for having oral hygiene problems?
1. Mr. Garcia, who is 84 years old, has cataracts, and is receiving antibiotic therapy for pneumonia
2. Ms. Louiza, who is 56 years old, drinks seven glasses of fluids daily, and has been hospitalized for diagnostic tests because of liver disease
3. Mr. Simon, who is 72 years old and has thyroid disease and diabetes mellitus

4. Ms. Hornbeck, who is 62 years old, has been NPO for 3 days following a colon resection, and has a nasogastric (NG) tube

4. As a nurse caring for four different patients, you plan to organize your morning care so that the patient most in need of a bath can be attended to first. You would likely provide hygiene care to which of the following patients first?
1. A patient who has just completed physical therapy and reports feeling very fatigued.
2. A patient who has returned to the nursing unit following hip surgery and reports pain at a level of 6 on a scale of 0 to 10
3. A patient who has an intestinal infection and is experiencing diaphoresis and fecal incontinence
4. A patient who experienced a stroke 2 days ago and has reduced function of his right arm

5. An older adult who has practiced poor oral hygiene and has an impaired gag reflex is at risk for developing pneumonia for which of the following reasons?
1. Acquiring mouth ulcerations
2. Aspirating bacteria that accumulate in the oral cavity
3. Acquiring an increased incidence of dental caries
4. Developing a resistance to antibiotics effective against dental plaque organisms

**6.** Which of the following patients should not soak his or her feet before nail care?

**1.** A cancer patient undergoing chemotherapy

**2.** A patient with a neurological disorder causing decreased sensation in the lower extremities

**3.** A patient who has excessively dry, flaky skin

**4.** A patient with diabetes mellitus

## REFERENCES

Agency for Health Care Policy and Research: *Pressure ulcers in adults: prediction and prevention,* Pub Nos 92-0047, 92-0050, Rockville, Md, 1992, Public Health Service, U.S. Department of Health and Human Services.

American Dental Association: *Oral heath topics A-Z,* http://www. ada.org/public/topics/cleaning.asp.

American Diabetes Association: *Foot complications,* 2005, http://www.diabetes.org/type-1-diabetes-foot-complications.jsp.

Armstrong DG, Lavery LA: Diabetic foot ulcers: prevention, diagnosis and classification, *Am Fam Physician* 57(6):1325, 1998.

Bauroth K and others: The efficacy of an essential oil antiseptic mouthwash vs. dental flossing in controlling interproximal gingivitis: a comparative study, *J Am Dent Assoc* 144(3):359, 2003.

Bennett MA: Report of the task force on the implications for darkly pigmented intact skin in the prediction and prevention of pressure ulcers, *Adv Wound Care* 8(6):34, 1995.

British Dental Health Foundation: *Frequently asked questions,* 2002, http://www.dental health org.

Champion VL: Instrument development for health belief model constructs, *Adv Nurs Sci* 6(3):73, 1984.

Cooppan R, Habershaw G: Preventing leg and foot complications, *Patient Care* 29(3):35, 1995.

Dochterman JM, Bulechek GM, editors: *Nursing interventions classification (NIC),* ed 4, St. Louis, 2004, Mosby.

Dunn JC and others: Bathing: pleasure or pain? *J Gerontol Nurs* 28(11):6, 2002

El-Solh A and others: Colonization of dental plaques: a reservoir of respiratory pathogens for hospital-acquired pneumonia in institutionalized elders, *Chest* 126(5):1575, 2004.

Family Gentle Dental Care: *Gum disease linked to heart disease,* 2004, http://www.dentalgentlecare.com.

Fitch JA and others: Oral care in the adult intensive care unit, *Am J Crit Care* 8(2):314, 1999.

Grap MJ and others: Oral care interventions in critical care: frequency and documentation, *Am J Crit Care* 12(2):114, 2003.

*How to care for contact lenses,* 2005, http://www.com/research/ HowtoCareforContactLenses.htm.

Labyak SE, Metzger BL: The effects of effleurage backrub on the physiological components of relaxation: a meta analysis, *Nurs Res* 46:59, 1997.

Mahoney DF: Cerumen impaction: prevalence and detection in nursing homes, *J Gerontol Nurs* 54(12):56, 1993.

Maklebust J: Pressure ulcer update, *RN* 41(12):56, 1991.

Marsh P, Martin M: *Oral Microbiology,* ed 3, London, Chapman Hall, 1992.

McNally M, Kenney N: Ethics in an aging society: challenge for oral health care, *J Can Dent Assoc* 65(11):623, 1999.

Meiner SE, Lueckenotte AG: *Gerontologic nursing,* ed 3, St. Louis, 2006, Mosby.

Moorhead S, Johnson M, Maas M: *Nursing outcomes classification (NOC),* ed 3, St. Louis, 1004, Mosby.

National Pediculosis Association: *Child care provider's guide to controlling head lice,* 2001, http://www.headlice.org.

Neil JA: Assessing foot care knowledge in a rural population with diabetes, *Ostomy Wound Manage* 48(1):50, 2002.

Ney DF: Cerumen impaction, ear hygiene practices, and hearing acuity, *Geriatr Nurs* 14(2):70, 1993.

Osterman HM, Struck KM: The aging foot, *Orthop Nurs* 9:43, 1990.

Panel for the Prediction and Prevention of Pressure Ulcers in Adults: Assessing risk and preventing pressure ulcers, *Patient Care* 27(7):36, 1993.

Poland JM: Comparing Moi-Stir to lemon glycerin swabs, *Am J Nurs* 87:422, 1987.

Scully C and others: Oral mucositis: a challenging complication of radiotherapy, chemotherapy, and radiochemotherapy. II. Diagnosis and management of mucositis, *Head Neck* 26(1):77, 2004.

Sheppard CM, Brenner PS: The effects of bathing and skin care practices on skin quality and satisfaction with an innovative product, *J Gerontol Nurs* 26(10):36, 2000.

Skewes SM: No more bed baths! *RN* 57:34, 1994.

Stiefel KA and others. Improving oral hygiene for the seriously ill patient: implementing research-based practice, *Medsurg Nurs* 9(1):40, 2000.

Strauss MB and others: Preventive foot care: a user friendly system for patients and physicians, *Postgrad Med* 103(5):233, 1998.

# CHAPTER 28

# Oxygenation

## MEDIA RESOURCES

**CD COMPANION** *evolve* **WEBSITE**

http://evolve.elsevier.com/Potter/basic

- **NCLEX® Review**
- **Audio Glossary**
- **English/Spanish Audio Glossary**
- **Video Clips**

## OBJECTIVES

- Describe the structure and function of the cardiopulmonary system.
- Identify the physiological processes of cardiac output, myocardial blood flow, coronary artery circulation, and respiratory gas exchange.
- Describe the relationship of cardiac output, preload, afterload, contractility, and heart rate.
- Diagram the electrical conduction system of the heart.
- Identify the physiological processes involved in ventilation, perfusion, and exchange of respiratory gases.
- Describe the impact of the patient's health status, age, lifestyle, and environment on tissue oxygenation.

- Identify and describe clinical outcomes as a result of disturbances in conduction, altered cardiac output, impaired valvular function, myocardial ischemia, and impaired tissue perfusion.
- Identify nursing interventions for promotion, maintenance, and restoration of cardiopulmonary function in the primary care, acute care, and restorative and continuing care settings.
- Identify and describe clinical outcomes for hyperventilation, hypoventilation, and hypoxemia.

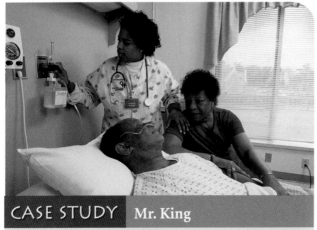

## CASE STUDY    Mr. King

Mr. King, a 74-year-old man, came to the emergency department with a 6-day history of chest pain, shortness of breath, cough, and generalized malaise. His wife and son are with him. Mr. King is a retired bookbinder who lives with his wife. Both have preexisting health conditions that put them at risk for pneumonia. Mrs. King is diabetic and takes insulin twice daily. Mr. King has a history of alcohol abuse but at present is not drinking. Both individuals have been heavy smokers for more than 50 years. Mrs. King performs most of the household duties. Mrs. King grocery shops weekly with the help of her daughter-in-law. Mr. King used to help out with the housework and loves to tinker in the garden; however, lately he has been unable to participate in any of the activities. His wife states, "All he seems to be able to do is sit in his chair and watch TV."

Mary Brown is a junior nursing student assigned to her first hospital-based clinical experience. Mary has had some experience in health assessment and patient teaching related to health promotion activities from her recent clinical rotation in a clinic. In the previous clinical experience, patients were motivated to

adjust their at-risk health behaviors, such as smoking or poor diet. Mary feels confident when she arrives in the clinical area this morning because Mr. King has similar health needs to the clinical experiences she has had. However, when Mary goes to meet Mr. King and performs her morning assessment, she is overwhelmed. This patient is in a great deal of respiratory distress. It seems that every breath is a struggle for him. Everything that Mary has planned to do seem less important. The patient is extremely anxious. His wife is at his side, anticipating Mary's every move and demanding some action.

## KEY TERMS

accessory muscles, p. 773
afterload, p. 771
atelectasis, p. 773
atrioventricular (AV) node, p. 771
bundle of His, p. 771
cardiac index, p. 771
cardiac output (CO), p. 770
cardiopulmonary rehabilitation, p. 811
cardiopulmonary resuscitation (CPR), p. 811
chest percussion, p. 799
chest physiotherapy (CPT), p. 798

chest tube, p. 799
cough, p. 781
cyanosis, p. 782
diaphragmatic breathing, p. 812
diffusion, p. 772
dyspnea, p. 778
dysrhythmias, p. 774
electrocardiogram (ECG), p. 771
hemoptysis, p. 781
hemothorax, p. 801
humidification, p. 798
hypercapnia, p. 773
hyperventilation, p. 772
hypoventilation, p. 772

*Continued*

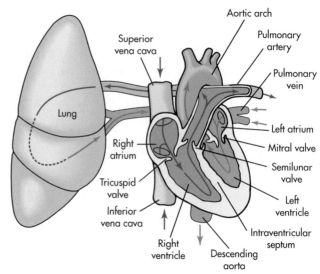

FIGURE **28-1** Schematic representation of blood flow through the heart. Arrows indicate direction of flow. (From Lewis SM and others: *Medical surgical nursing: assessment and management of clinical problems,* ed 6, St. Louis, 2004, Mosby.)

## Scientific Knowledge Base

Oxygen is a basic human need and is required for life. You will frequently meet patients who are unable to meet their oxygenation needs, which is often the result of an ineffective pump (heart disease) or ineffective gas exchange (lung disease).

### Cardiopulmonary Physiology

The function of the cardiopulmonary system is to provide oxygen to the tissues and remove carbon dioxide and waste products from the body.

### Structure and Function

The heart delivers oxygenated blood from the lungs to the body. Once the body receives oxygenated blood, the tissues of the body are able to carry out selected metabolic activities and waste products, such as carbon dioxide. The cardiovascular system then delivers carbon dioxide and other waste products to the lung and kidney for elimination. The pumping action of the heart is essential, and the four heart valves (tricuspid, pulmonic, mitral, and aortic) ensure the one-way flow of blood through the heart (Figure 28-1).

**REGULATION OF BLOOD FLOW.** There are multiple regulators of blood flow (Table 28-1). Heart rate affects blood flow because of the interaction between rate and diastolic filling time. Diastolic filling time affects the amount of blood in the ventricle at the end of diastole (**preload**). With a sustained heart rate greater than 160 beats per minute, diastolic filling time decreases, causing **stroke volume (SV)** and **cardiac output (CO)** to decrease. In some situations you will also care for patients with long-term cardiovascular disease whose SV and CO decrease with heart rates greater than 120 beats per minute. Patients with decreased myocardial reserve experience decreased SV and CO with a heart rate less than 160 beats per minute. The heart rate of the older adult is slow to increase under stress. To compensate for this, the SV increases in order to increase the CO and blood pressure.

**CONDUCTION SYSTEM.** The rhythmic relaxation and contraction of the atria and ventricles depend on continuous, organized transmission of electrical impulses to the muscle. The conduction system generates controls and transmits these impulses (Figure 28-2).

The conduction system generates the impulses that initiate the electrical mechanical chain of events. The autonomic nervous system influences the rate of impulse generation, the transmission speed through the conductive pathway, and the strength of contractions through sympathetic and parasympathetic (vagus nerve) nerve fibers in the atria and ventricles. The vagus nerve (parasympathetic) also innervates sinoatrial and atrioventricular nodes and is able to reduce the rate of impulse generation.

The conduction system originates with the **sinoatrial (SA) node,** the "pacemaker" of the heart. The SA node is in the right atrium next to the entrance of the superior vena cava. Impulses begin at the SA node at an intrinsic rate of 60 to 100 beats per minute. The resting adult rate ranges from 60 to 80 beats per minute. The older adult has a wide range from the 40s to more than 100 beats per minute (Seidel and others, 2003).

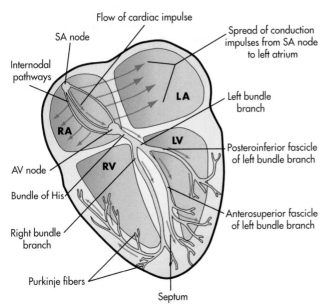

FIGURE **28-2** Conduction system of the heart. *AV*, Atrio-ventricular; *LA*, left atrium; *LV*, left ventricle; *RA*, right atrium; *RV*, right ventricle; *SA*, sinoatrial. (From Lewis SM and others: *Medical surgical nursing: assessment and management of clinical problems,* ed 6, St. Louis, 2004, Mosby.)

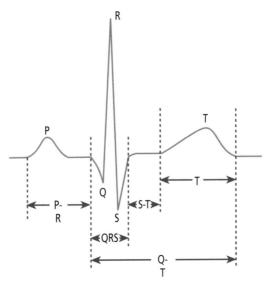

FIGURE **28-3** Normal ECG waveform. (Modified from Canobbio MM: *Cardiovascular disorders,* St. Louis, 1990, Mosby.)

| TABLE 28-1 | **Regulation of Blood Flow** |
|---|---|
| **Regulator** | **Definition** |
| Cardiac output | Amount of blood ejected from the left ventricle per minute |
| | Normal range (adult): 4-6 L/min |
| **Cardiac index** | Measure of adequacy of the cardiac output; cardiac index equals cardiac output divided by the patient's body surface area |
| | Normal range (adult): 2.5-4 L/min/m3 |
| Stroke volume | Amount of blood ejected from the ventricle with each contraction Normal range (adult): 50-75 ml per contraction |
| Preload | Amount of blood in the ventricles at end diastole |
| **Afterload** | Resistance of the ejection of blood from the left ventricle |
| **Myocardial contractility** | Ability of the heart to squeeze blood from the ventricles and prepare for the next contraction |

The electrical impulses are then transmitted along intra-atrial pathways to the **atrioventricular (AV) node.** The AV node mediates impulse transmission between the atria and the ventricles. Delaying the impulse at the AV node before transmitting it through the **bundle of His** and ventricular **Purkinje network** assists atrial emptying.

An **electrocardiogram (ECG)** records the electrical activity of the conduction system as waves and complexes. An ECG monitors the regularity and path of the electrical impulse through the conduction system; however, it does not reflect the muscular work of the heart. The normal sequence of electrical impulses on the ECG is called **normal sinus rhythm (NSR)** (Figure 28-3). A normal ECG waveform consists of a P wave (atrial depolarizing), QRS complex (ventricular depolarization), and T wave (ventricular repolarization).

Care providers can interpret the size, appearance, and sequence of waves to identify dysrhythmias.

## Gas Exchange

For the exchange of respiratory gases to occur, the organs, nerves, and muscles of respiration must be intact and the central nervous system must regulate the respiratory cycle (Figure 28-4).

**STRUCTURE AND FUNCTION.** Diseases that change the structure and function of the lung also alter respiration, or breathing. The respiratory muscles, pleural space, lungs, and alveoli (see Figure 28-4) are essential for ventilation, perfusion, and exchange of respiratory gases. There are two lungs, a right and left lung. The right lung is made up of three lobes, the right upper, middle, and lower lobes. The left

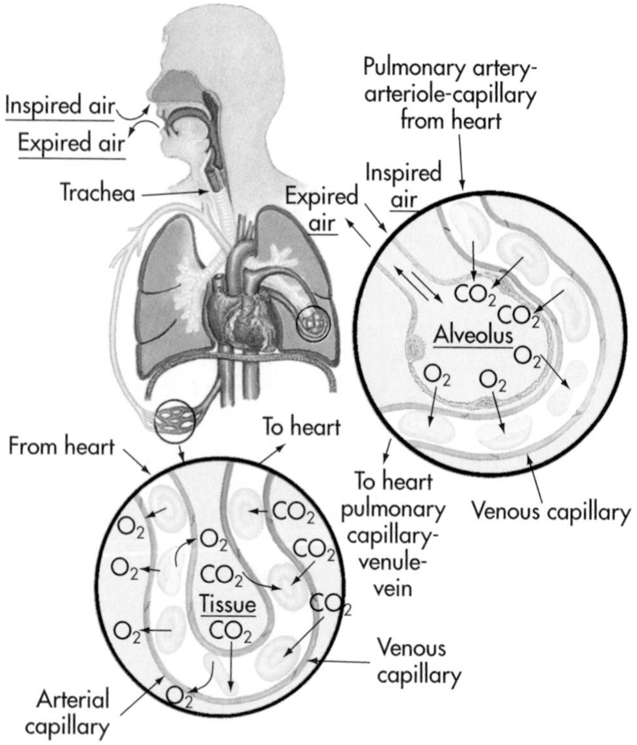

FIGURE **28-4** Structures of the pulmonary system. The circles denotes the alveoli. (Modified from Wilson SF, Thompson JM: *Mosby's clinical nursing series: respiratory disorders,* St. Louis, 1990, Mosby.)

---

**BOX 28-1** **Neural and Chemical Regulation of Respiration**

**Neural Regulation**

Neural regulation maintains rhythm and depth of respiration, as well as the balance between inspiration and expiration.

**Cerebral Cortex**

Voluntary control of respiration delivers impulses to the respiratory motor neurons by way of the spinal cord. Voluntary control of respiration accommodates speaking, eating, and swimming.

**Medulla Oblongata**

Automatic control of respiration occurs continuously.

**Chemical Regulation**

Chemical regulation maintains appropriate rate and depth of respirations based on changes in the blood's carbon dioxide ($CO_2$), oxygen ($O_2$), and hydrogen ion ($H^+$) concentration.

**Chemoreceptors**

Chemoreceptors are located in the medulla, aortic body, and carotid body. Changes in chemical content of $O_2$, $CO_2$, and $H^+$ stimulate chemoreceptors, which in turn stimulate neural regulators to adjust the rate and depth of ventilation to maintain normal arterial blood gas levels. Chemical regulation occurs during physical exercise and in some illnesses. It is a short-term adaptive mechanism.

---

lung has two lobes, the upper and middle lobes. The trachea enters the thorax and bifurcates, or branches out, into the right and left mainstem bronchus. The bronchi branch into smaller and smaller bronchioles, similar to a tree. The last branch of the airways ends at the exchanging unit of the lung, the alveoli.

**REGULATION OF RESPIRATION.** Respiratory regulation provides for adequate oxygen to meet the metabolic demand, such as during exercise, infection, or pregnancy. Respiratory regulation promotes exhalation of metabolically produced carbon dioxide, which is a determinant of acid-base status (see Chapter 15).

Neural and chemical regulators control respiration (Box 28-1). Neural regulation involves the central nervous system control of respiratory rate, depth, and rhythm. Chemical regulation involves the influence of chemicals, such as carbon dioxide and hydrogen ions, on the rate and depth of respiration.

**OXYGEN TRANSPORT.** The delivery of oxygen depends on the amount of oxygen entering the lungs (oxygenation), blood flow to the lungs and tissues (perfusion), the oxygen-carrying capacity of the blood (rate of **diffusion**), and the amount of carbon dioxide excreted by the lungs (**ventilation**). The amount of dissolved oxygen in the plasma, the amount of hemoglobin, and the tendency of hemoglobin to bind with oxygen all influence the capacity of

the blood to carry oxygen. Only a relatively small amount of oxygen, about 3%, is dissolved in the plasma. Hemoglobin transports most oxygen and serves as a carrier for both oxygen and carbon dioxide. The hemoglobin molecule combines with oxygen to form oxyhemoglobin. The formation of oxyhemoglobin is easily reversible, allowing hemoglobin and oxygen to dissociate, which frees oxygen to enter tissues.

**CARBON DIOXIDE TRANSPORT.** Carbon dioxide diffuses into red blood cells and is rapidly hydrated into carbonic acid ($H_2CO_3$). The carbonic acid then dissociates (breaks apart) into hydrogen ($H^+$) and bicarbonate ($HCO_3^-$) ions. Hemoglobin buffers the hydrogen ion, and the $HCO_3^-$ diffuses into the plasma (see Chapter 15). Reduced hemoglobin (deoxyhemoglobin) combines with carbon dioxide more easily than oxyhemoglobin, and therefore venous blood transports most of the carbon dioxide back to the lungs for excretion in expired air.

## Factors Affecting Oxygenation

Any condition that affects cardiopulmonary functioning directly affects the body's ability to meet oxygen demands. The general classifications of cardiac disorders include disturbances in conduction, impaired valvular function, myocardial ischemia, cardiomyopathic conditions, and peripheral tissue hypoxia. Respiratory disorders include **hyperventilation, hypoventilation,** and **hypoxia.**

Other pathophysiological processes affect a patient's oxygenation. These include alterations that affect the oxygen-carrying capacity of blood (e.g., anemia), increases in the body's metabolic demands (e.g., fever, infection), and alterations that affect the patient's chest wall movement or the central nervous system.

**DECREASED OXYGEN-CARRYING CAPACITY.** Ninety-seven percent of oxygen is carried on the hemoglobin molecule. Any process that decreases or alters hemoglobin, such as anemia or inhalation of toxic substances, decreases the oxygen-carrying capacity of blood. Carbon monoxide is the most common toxic inhalant decreasing the oxygen-carrying capacity of blood. Hemoglobin tends to bind with carbon monoxide 210 times more readily than with oxygen, creating a functional hypoxemia (Thibodeau and Patton, 2004). Because of the bond's strength, it is not easy for carbon monoxide to dissociate from hemoglobin, making the hemoglobin unavailable for oxygen transport.

**DECREASED INSPIRED OXYGEN CONCENTRATION.** When the concentration of inspired oxygen declines, the oxygen-carrying capacity of the blood decreases. An upper or lower airway obstruction limiting delivery of inspired oxygen to alveoli causes a decrease in the fraction of inspired oxygen ($F_IO_2$) concentration. Decreased environmental oxygen (as occurs at high altitudes) or decreased delivery of inspired oxygen, as the result of an incorrect oxygen concentration setting on respiratory therapy equipment, also results in a decreased $F_IO_2$.

**HYPOVOLEMIA.** Hypovolemia is a reduced circulating blood volume resulting from extracellular fluid losses that occurs in conditions such as shock and severe dehydration. If the fluid loss is significant, the body tries to adapt by increasing the heart rate and constricting peripheral vessels to increase the volume of blood returned to the heart and increase the cardiac output.

**INCREASED METABOLIC RATE.** Increases in metabolic activity of the body result in an increased oxygen demand. When the body is unable to meet the increased oxygen demand, the oxygen level falls. An increased metabolic rate is a normal response of the body to pregnancy, wound healing, and exercise because the body is building tissue. Most people are able to meet the increased oxygen demand and do not display signs of oxygen deprivation.

Fever increases the tissues' need for oxygen. As a result, carbon dioxide production also increases. If the fever lasts for a period of time, the metabolic rate remains high and the body begins to break down protein stores, resulting in muscle wasting and decreased muscle mass. Respiratory muscles, such as the diaphragm and intercostals, are also wasted. The body attempts to adapt to the increased carbon dioxide (**hypercapnia**) levels by increasing the rate and depth of respiration to eliminate the excess carbon dioxide. The patient's work of breathing increases, and the patient will eventually display signs and symptoms of **hypoxemia,** a decreased arterial oxygen level in the blood. Early clinical signs and symptoms of hypoxemia include:

- Anxiety
- Restlessness
- Inability to concentrate
- Increases in heart rate
- Increased respiratory rate and blood pressure
- Cardiac dysrhythmias, such as premature ventricular contractions, premature atrial contractions, and sinus tachycardia

As the hypoxemia worsens, some patients lose consciousness. Patients with pulmonary diseases, such as chronic obstructive pulmonary disease (COPD), are at greater risk for hypoxemia and hypercapnia, an elevated arterial carbon dioxide level. Patient assessments often show an increased rate and depth of respiration and use of pursed-lip breathing and **accessory muscles** of respiration.

**CONDITIONS AFFECTING CHEST WALL MOVEMENT.** Any condition that reduces chest wall movement will decrease ventilation. If the diaphragm is unable to fully descend with breathing, the volume of inspired air decreases, delivering less oxygen to the alveoli and subsequently to tissues.

**Musculoskeletal Abnormalities.** Abnormalities in the thoracic region such as abnormal structural shapes and muscle disease contribute to decreased oxygenation and ventilation. Abnormal structural shapes impairing oxygenation include those that affect the rib cage, such as pectus excavatum, and those that affect the spinal column, such as kyphosis. The angle of curvature in kyphosis can progress with time, resulting in severe hypoventilation and hypoxemia.

Muscle diseases, such as muscular dystrophy, affect oxygenation by decreasing the patient's ability to expand and contract the chest. This impairs ventilation, and **atelectasis,** hypercapnia, and hypoxemia occur.

**Nervous System Diseases.** Myasthenia gravis, Guillain-Barré syndrome, and poliomyelitis are examples of nervous system diseases that result in hypoventilation. These diseases impair nervous and muscular control, causing reduced ventilation (hypoventilation) occurs.

Disease or trauma involving the medulla oblongata and spinal cord of the central nervous system has the ability to impair respiration. When the medulla oblongata is affected, neural regulation of respiration is damaged and abnormal breathing patterns develop. Damage to the spinal cord affects respiration in two ways. If the phrenic nerve is damaged, the diaphragm does not descend, thus reducing inspiratory lung volumes and causing hypoxemia. Cervical trauma at C3 to C5 level results in paralysis of the phrenic nerve. Spinal cord trauma below the fifth cervical vertebra usually leaves the phrenic nerve intact but damages nerves that innervate the intercostal muscles, preventing anteroposterior chest expansion.

**Trauma.** Trauma to the chest wall also impairs inspiration. The person with multiple rib fractures sometimes develops a flail chest, a condition in which fractures cause instability in part of the chest wall. This causes paradoxical breathing in which the lung underlying the injured area contracts on inspiration and expands on expiration.

Chest wall or upper abdominal incisions also decrease chest wall movement because incisional pain causes the patient to inhale shallowly, which decreases chest wall movement.

**Chronic Disease.** Oxygenation decreases either as a direct consequence of chronic disease or decreases as a secondary effect, as with anemia. The physiological response to chronic hypoxemia is the development of a secondary polycythemia, which is an increase in red blood cells. This is an adaptive response of the body to increase the amount of circulating hemoglobin to improve oxygen transport; as a result the patient's oxygenation improves.

## Alterations in Cardiac Functioning

Illnesses and conditions that affect cardiac rate, rhythm, strength of contraction, blood flow through the chambers, myocardial blood flow, and peripheral circulation alter cardiac functioning.

**DISTURBANCES IN CONDUCTION.** Some disturbances in conduction are the result of electrical impulses that do not originate from the SA node. These rhythm disturbances are called **dysrhythmias,** meaning a deviation from the normal sinus rhythm (Table 28-2). Dysrhythmias occur as primary conduction disturbances; as a response to ischemia, valvular abnormality, anxiety, and drug toxicity; as a result of caffeine, alcohol, or tobacco use; or as a complication of acid-base or electrolyte imbalance (see Chapter 15).

In addition to the site of impulse origin, cardiac response is used to classify dysrhythmias. The response can be an increase in heart rate or tachycardia (a rate greater than 100 beats per minute), a decrease in rate, or bradycardia (a rate less than 60 beats per minute), premature (early beat) atrial or ventricular beats, or blocked (delayed or absent beat) atrial or ventricular beats.

**DECREASED CARDIAC OUTPUT.** Failure of the myocardium to eject sufficient blood volume to the systemic and pulmonary circulations results in heart failure. Failure of the myocardial pump results from primary coronary artery disease (CAD), cardiomyopathic conditions, valvular disorders, and pulmonary disease.

**MYOCARDIAL ISCHEMIA. Myocardial ischemia** happens when the coronary artery does not supply sufficient blood to the heart (myocardium). Decreased perfusion to the myocardium results in chest pain, especially with activity. Angina or angina pectoris is the result of decreased blood flow to the myocardium as a result of coronary artery spasms or temporary constriction. When decreased myocardial blood perfusion is extensive or completely blocked, the tissue becomes necrotic and a **myocardial infarction** occurs. Myocardial infarction presents clinically as severe chest pain, breathlessness, diaphoresis, and hypotension (a fall in blood pressure).

**LEFT-SIDED HEART FAILURE. Left-sided heart failure** is an abnormal condition characterized by impaired functioning of the left ventricle, usually caused by chronically elevated arterial pressures and pulmonary congestion. If left ventricular failure is significant, the amount of blood ejected from the left ventricle drops greatly, resulting in decreased cardiac output.

**RIGHT-SIDED HEART FAILURE. Right-sided heart failure** results from impaired functioning of the right ventricle. Venous congestion in the systemic circulation is characteristic of this. Signs of this are distended jugular veins and peripheral edema. Right-sided heart failure more commonly results from pulmonary diseases or as an outcome of left-sided heart failure.

**IMPAIRED VALVULAR FUNCTION. Valvular heart disease** is an acquired or congenital disorder of a cardiac valve characterized by stenosis and obstructed blood flow or valvular degeneration and regurgitation (backflow) of blood. When stenosis occurs in the aortic and pulmonic valves the adjacent ventricles work harder to move the ventricular volume beyond the stenotic valve. When regurgitation occurs, there is a backflow of blood into an adjacent chamber.

## Alterations in Respiratory Functioning

Illnesses and conditions that affect ventilation or oxygen transport cause alterations in respiratory functioning. The three primary alterations are hyperventilation, hypoventilation, and hypoxia.

**HYPERVENTILATION.** Hyperventilation is an increase in respiratory rate resulting in excess amounts of carbon dioxide elimination. Anxiety, fever, infection, exercise, drugs, or acid-base imbalance cause hyperventilation. Hypoxia associated with pulmonary embolus or shock also results in hyperventilation. Acute anxiety and an increased respiratory rate cause loss of consciousness from excess carbon dioxide exhalation. In fever an increase of 1° F causes a 7% increase in the metabolic rate, thereby increasing carbon dioxide production. The clinical response is increased rate and depth of respiration.

Hyperventilation produces signs and symptoms including tachycardia, shortness of breath, chest pain, dizziness, light-headedness, decreased concentration, paresthesia, circumoral and/or extremity numbness, tinnitus, blurred vision, disorientation, and tetany (carpopedal spasm).

**HYPOVENTILATION.** Hypoventilation occurs when ventilation is inadequate to meet the body's oxygen demand or to eliminate carbon dioxide. As ventilation decreases, arterial carbon dioxide ($PaCO_2$) is elevated. Severe atelectasis, a collapse of the alveoli, produces hypoventilation. When alveoli collapse, less of the lung is ventilated and hypoventilation occurs. Clinical signs and symptoms include dizziness, occipital headache upon awakening, lethargy, disorientation, decreased ability to follow instructions, cardiac dysrhythmias, electrolyte imbalances, convulsions, and possible coma or cardiac arrest.

When caring for patients with COPD and chronically elevated $PaCO_2$ levels, remember that inappropriate administration of excessive oxygen will result in hypoventilation. Patients with COPD and hypercapnia (high $CO_2$ level) have adapted to the higher carbon dioxide level. The carbon dioxide–sensitive chemoreceptors are essentially not functioning, and the stimulus to breathe is a decreased partial pressure of oxygen ($PaO_2$).

| TABLE 28-2 | Common Basic Cardiac Dysrhythmias |
|---|---|

| Rhythm Characteristics | Etiology | Clinical Significance | Management |
|---|---|---|---|

**Sinus Tachycardia**

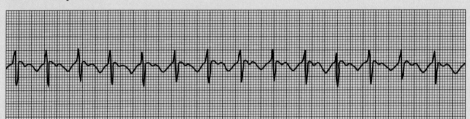

| Regular rhythm, rate 100-180 beats/min (higher in infants), normal P wave, normal QRS complex | Rate increase is a normal response to exercise, emotion, or stressors, such as pain, fever, pump failure, hyperthyroidism, and certain drugs (e.g., caffeine, nitrates, nicotine) | Patient with damaged heart may be unable to sustain increased workloads (increased myocardial oxygen consumption) brought on by persistent increases in heart rate | Correct underlying factors; remove offending drugs |

**Sinus Bradycardia**

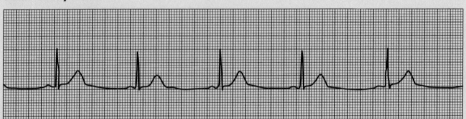

| Regular rhythm, rate <60 beats/min, normal P wave, normal PR interval, normal QRS complex | Rate decrease is a normal response to sleep or in well-conditioned athlete; abnormal drops in rate caused by diminished blood flow to SA node, vagal stimulation, hypothyroidism, increased intracranial pressure, or certain drugs (e.g., digoxin, propranolol, procainamide) | Has clinical significance when associated with signs of impaired cardiac output and symptoms of dizziness, syncope, chest pain | Correct underlying causes; administer atropine, 0.5-1.0 mg IV; may need to implant transvenous pacemaker |

**Sinus Dysrhythmia**

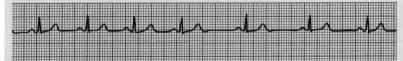

| Irregular rhythm; often associated with respiration, slowing during inspiration and increasing with expiration; rate of 60-100 beats/min; normal P wave, PR interval, and QRS complex | Sinus rhythm with cyclical variation caused by vagal impulses that influence rhythm during respiration; occurs commonly in children, young adults, and older adults; usually disappears as heart rate increases | No clinical significance unless heart rate decreases and symptoms of dizziness occur with decreased rate | None indicated unless heart rate decreases and symptoms occur |

*Continued*

| TABLE 28-2 | **Common Basic Cardiac Dysrhythmias—cont'd** |
|---|---|

| Rhythm Characteristics | Etiology | Clinical Significance | Management |
|---|---|---|---|
| **Atrial Fibrillation (A-Fib)** | | | |

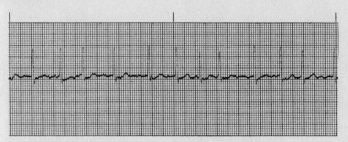

| Rhythm Characteristics | Etiology | Clinical Significance | Management |
|---|---|---|---|
| Irregular atrial activity resulting in an irregular ventricular response with resultant irregular cardiac rate and rhythm. No identifiable P wave. Rate is determined by the conduction of the multiple atrial impulses across the AV node | Caused by aging, calcification of the SA node, or changes in myocardial blood supply | Loss of the atrial kick (portion of the cardiac output squeezed in the ventricles with a coordinated atrial contraction), pooling of blood in the atria, and development of microemboli. Patients complain of fatigue, a fluttering in the chest, and shortness of breath if ventricular response is rapid | Managed with blood thinners such as warfarin (Coumadin) or if the patient is experiencing cardiopulmonary compromise, carotid sinus massage or elective synchronized cardioversion |
| **Supraventricular Tachycardia (SVT)** | | | |

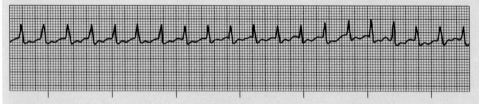

| | | | |
|---|---|---|---|
| Sudden, rapid onset of tachycardia with stimulus originating above AV node; regular rhythm; rate 150-250 beats/min; P wave often hidden; normal QRS complex | Begins and ends spontaneously or is precipitated by excitement, fatigue, or caffeine, smoking, or alcohol use | Usually no significant impairment; patient complains of palpitations and shortness of breath; if persistent or occurring in patient with preexisting heart disease, causes decrease in cardiac output and/or blood pressure, resulting in heart failure or shock | Experienced clinicians perform vagal stimulation with carotid sinus massage. Decrease ventricular response with medications to block AV conduction: verapamil, IV push; propranolol slowly IV (contraindicated in patients with heart failure); edrophonium, test dose initially. If resistant to preceding measures, properly trained health care provider will perform synchronized cardioversion |

## TABLE 28-2 Common Basic Cardiac Dysrhythmias—cont'd

| Rhythm Characteristics | Etiology | Clinical Significance | Management |
|---|---|---|---|
| **Premature Ventricular Contractions (PVCs)** | | | |

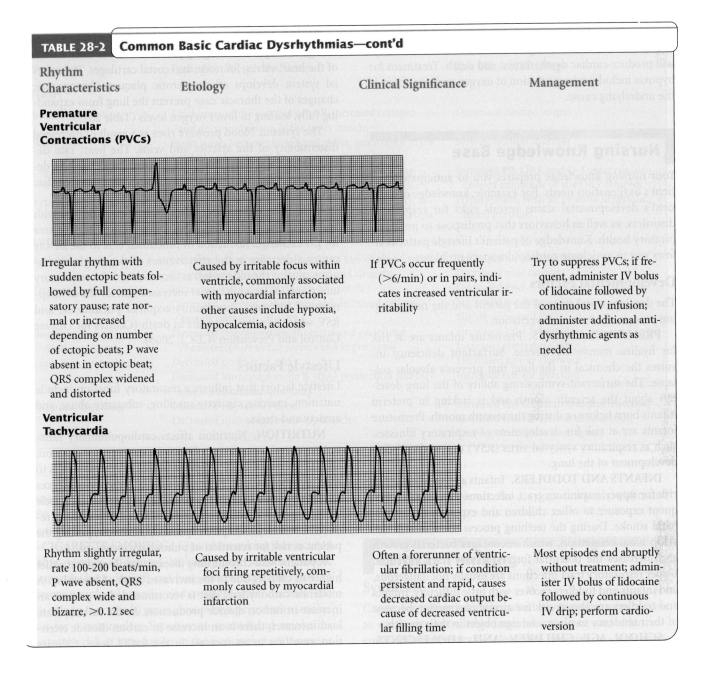

| | | | |
|---|---|---|---|
| Irregular rhythm with sudden ectopic beats followed by full compensatory pause; rate normal or increased depending on number of ectopic beats; P wave absent in ectopic beat; QRS complex widened and distorted | Caused by irritable focus within ventricle, commonly associated with myocardial infarction; other causes include hypoxia, hypocalcemia, acidosis | If PVCs occur frequently (>6/min) or in pairs, indicates increased ventricular irritability | Try to suppress PVCs; if frequent, administer IV bolus of lidocaine followed by continuous IV infusion; administer additional antidysrhythmic agents as needed |
| **Ventricular Tachycardia** | | | |
| Rhythm slightly irregular, rate 100-200 beats/min, P wave absent, QRS complex wide and bizarre, >0.12 sec | Caused by irritable ventricular foci firing repetitively, commonly caused by myocardial infarction | Often a forerunner of ventricular fibrillation; if condition persistent and rapid, causes decreased cardiac output because of decreased ventricular filling time | Most episodes end abruptly without treatment; administer IV bolus of lidocaine followed by continuous IV drip; perform cardioversion |

When you administer excessive oxygen, this satisfies the body's oxygen requirement and negates the stimulus to breathe. High concentrations of oxygen (e.g., greater than 24% to 28% [1 to 3 L/min]) prevent the $PaO_2$ from falling. As a result, this destroys the stimulus to breathe, resulting in hypoventilation. The excessive retention of carbon dioxide leads to respiratory arrest. If untreated, your patient's status will rapidly decline and death is possible.

Treatment for hyperventilation and hypoventilation involves treating underlying cause, improving tissue oxygenation, restoring ventilation, and achieving acid-base balance.

**HYPOXIA.** Hypoxia is inadequate tissue oxygenation with a deficiency in oxygen delivery or oxygen utilization at the cellular level. Causes of hypoxia include:

- A lowered oxygen-carrying capacity, as in anemia or carbon monoxide poisoning
- Diminished concentrations of inspired oxygen, as in high altitudes and airway obstruction
- The inability of the tissues to extract oxygen from the blood, as in septic shock and cyanide poisoning
- Decreased diffusion of oxygen from the lung (alveoli) into the blood, as in pneumonia or atelectasis
- Poor tissue perfusion with oxygenated blood as in hypovolemic shock, cardiogenic shock, or cardiomyopathy
- Impaired ventilation from multiple rib fractures, chest trauma, spinal cord injury, or head trauma

When the $PaO_2$ level is low (hypoxemia; less than 60 mm Hg), your patient is at risk for developing hypoxia. Some pa-

chair or completing personal hygiene. Ask patients what they want to accomplish. If they are diaphoretic, they will appreciate clean sheets and a bath after being medicated for pain.

Base your decision to delegate responsibility to an assistive person on your assessment of the patient and the type of care the patient will receive. Consider what tasks are safe to delegate, within the skill set of the assistive personnel, and how the patient will feel about the care that you have delegated. The priority is to maintain or improve the patient's oxygenation and meet the patient's needs. You are ultimately responsible for all the total patient care.

**CONTINUITY OF CARE.** Impaired levels of oxygenation affect all aspects of your patient's life, not just the physical component. Designing collaborative nursing interventions with physical and occupational therapy and social services will improve your patient's level of functioning. Respiratory therapy assists in designing measures to improve breathing and cough control. Social services can recommend support groups. When planning care for patients with impaired oxygenation, be sensitive to the needs of the patient as well as the family. Chronic illness changes the dynamics of family relationships. Sometimes roles need to change, and the patient and family have difficulty coping. You will need to provide an empathic ear to the family as well as the patient. Help them develop solutions that maintain the dignity of both parties and continue to support the family unit.

### ✹ Implementation

Nursing interventions for patients with oxygenation alterations are diverse. Health promotion activities improve healthier lifestyle habits. Symptom management aids in reducing the severity of cardiopulmonary problems. Interventions aimed at improving respiration and ventilation make it easier for patients to breathe.

**HEALTH PROMOTION.** Maintaining the patient's optimal level of health is important in reducing the number and severity of respiratory symptoms. Prevention of respiratory infections maintains optimal health. You provide health education to help patients make choices for improving health practices (Box 28-4). Some patient education topics to consider include regular blood pressure checkups and taking blood pressure medication as prescribed; low-fat, low-salt, proper caloric diet; importance and benefits of pneumococcal vaccine and annual influenza vaccine; smoking cessation and avoiding secondhand smoke exposure. Be sure to individualize the patient teaching to meet the needs of the patient. Older adults have differing needs with educational material and respond differently than younger patients (Box 28-5).

**Influenza and Pneumococcal Vaccine.** The Centers for Disease Control and Prevention (CDC) recommends annual influenza vaccines for older patients age 65 years and older and patients with chronic illness, regardless of age (CDC, 2004). The value of vaccination for immunocompromised patients is unclear. HIV-positive patients may receive the flu vaccine. Persons with a known hypersensitivity to eggs, chickens,

---

| BOX 28-4 | PATIENT TEACHING |
|---|---|

**Cardiopulmonary Health Promotion**

Mr. and Mrs. King are both interested in how to prevent hospitalizations in the future and what they can do to maintain their health. Mary has developed the following teaching plan to help the Kings meet their goals.

**Outcome**
- Upon completion of the teaching session Mr. and Mrs. King will be able to verbalize the steps they need to take to improve their health maintenance and reduce the risk of future hospitalizations.

**Teaching Strategies**
- Establish rapport with the Kings, and maintain eye contact during the teaching session.
- Use words the Kings will understand; avoid medical jargon when possible.
- Provide an overview of the material.
- Provide a written copy of the material taught for reinforcement and reference.
- Demonstrate how to monitor the pulse and check the blood pressure.
- Have Mr. King purchase the blood pressure monitor and cuff they will use at home to practice within the hospital.
- Allow Mrs. King time to become familiar with the blood pressure cuff and manometer.
- Provide written abnormal lab/test results that they need to review with their primary care physician or health care provider.
- Allow time for questions and answer honestly.
- Summarize the material.

**Evaluation Strategies**
- Ask Mr. and Mrs. King to verbalize what they learned.
- Ask Mrs. King to return demonstrate taking a pulse and blood pressure.
- Ask Mr. King to verbalize which pulse and blood pressure readings they need to report to the physician or health care provider.
- Ask the Kings to list the signs and symptoms they need to report to the physician or health care provider.
- Ask Mr. and Mrs. King if they have any questions or need any additional information.

---

or feathers should not receive the vaccine. If the patient has fever, delay the influenza vaccine until the patient is afebrile.

Give the pneumococcal vaccine every 10 years for low-risk patients and every 5 years for those with multiple underlying conditions. You can give both the influenza vaccine and pneumococcal vaccine to pregnant women after the first trimester. However, in all cases consult the patient's obstetrician before administering either vaccine.

**Environmental Modifications.** Avoiding exposure to secondhand smoke is important for patients with cardiopulmonary illnesses. Most public places and businesses have now adopted a no-smoking policy or offer separate smoking areas. When a patient lives with secondhand smoke in the

BOX 28-5 CARE OF THE OLDER ADULT

### Care of the Older Adult

- Risk factor modification is important, including smoking cessation, weight reduction, a low-cholesterol diet, management of hypertension, and exercise.
- Coronary artery disease is the leading cause of death and disability in women older than 40 years of age.
- Older adults have more atypical signs and symptoms of coronary artery disease.
- The incidence of atrial fibrillation increases with age and is the leading contributing factor for stroke in the older adult.
- Healthy behavior changes sometimes slow or halt the progression of the older adult's disease. However, it is often more difficult to get older adults to change long-term unhealthy habits.
- Mental status changes are often the first sign of respiratory problems in the older adult and include subtle increases in forgetfulness and irritability.
- The older adult often does not complain of dyspnea until it impacts activities of daily living, and then only if the activities are important to the older adult.
- Use cough suppressants with caution because of changes in the older patient's cough mechanism. Cough suppression leads to retention of pulmonary secretions, plugged airways, and atelectasis.
- Chronic illness in the older adult sometimes results in unacceptable behavior patterns because of loss of control experienced with a chronic illness.

home, you will need to provide counseling and support to help the smoker understand the effects of secondhand smoke on the patient. The patient, smoker, and you will need to develop a plan that takes into account the patient's and smoker's needs.

**ACUTE CARE.** Patients with acute pulmonary illnesses require nursing interventions directed toward halting the pathological process, such as a respiratory tract infection; shortening the duration and severity of the illness, such as hospitalization with pneumonia; and preventing complications from illness or treatments, such as nosocomial infection resulting from invasive procedures.

**Dyspnea Management.** Dyspnea is difficult to measure and treat, thus requiring individualized treatments for each patient. You will usually need to implement more than one therapy. Initially you will treat and stabilize the underlying processes that cause or worsen dyspnea, and then administer four additional therapies:

1. Medications (e.g., bronchodilators, steroids, mucolytics, antianxiety drugs)
2. Oxygen therapy as indicated
3. Physical techniques (e.g., cardiopulmonary reconditioning, breathing techniques, cough control)
4. Psychosocial techniques (e.g., relaxation techniques, biofeedback, meditation) to lessen the sensation of dyspnea

**Maintenance of a Patent Airway.** The airway is patent when the trachea, bronchi, and large airways are free from obstructions. You use three types of interventions to maintain a patent airway: coughing techniques, suctioning, and insertion of an artificial airway.

*Coughing Techniques.* Coughing maintains a patent airway by removing secretions from both the upper and lower airways. You evaluate cough effectiveness by sputum expectoration, the patient's report of swallowed sputum, or clearing of adventitious lung sounds. Encourage patients with chronic pulmonary diseases, upper respiratory tract infections, and lower respiratory tract infections to deep breathe and cough at least every 2 hours while awake. Encourage patients with a large amount of sputum to cough every hour while awake and to awaken to cough every 2 to 3 hours while asleep until the acute phase of sputum production has ended.

CASCADE COUGH. With the cascade cough, the patient takes a slow, deep breath and holds it for 2 seconds while contracting expiratory muscles. Then the patient opens the mouth and performs a series of coughs throughout exhalation, thereby coughing at progressively lowered lung volumes. This technique promotes airway clearance and a patent airway in patients with large volumes of sputum.

HUFF COUGH. The huff cough stimulates a natural cough reflex and is generally effective only for clearing central airways. While exhaling, the patient opens the glottis by saying the word *huff*. With practice the patient inhales more air and is able to progress to the cascade cough.

QUAD COUGH. The quad cough technique is for patients without abdominal muscle control, such as those with spinal cord injuries. While the patient breathes out with a maximal expiratory effort, the patient or you push inward and upward on the abdominal muscles toward the diaphragm, causing the cough.

*Suctioning Techniques.* When a patient is unable to effectively clear respiratory tract secretions with coughing, suctioning clears the airways. The primary suctioning techniques are oropharyngeal and nasopharyngeal suctioning, orotracheal and nasotracheal suctioning, and tracheal suctioning through an artificial airway (Skill 28-1).

These techniques are based on common principles. Because the nasotrachea and trachea are considered sterile, sterile technique is required for orotracheal and nasotracheal suctioning. The mouth is considered clean, and therefore the suctioning of oral and nasopharyngeal secretions requires only clean technique. Always suction oral secretions after suctioning of the nasotrachea and trachea when combining suction techniques. Suctioning requires the use of a round-tipped, multihole catheter. Frequency of suctioning is determined by clinical assessment. When secretions are identified by inspection or auscultation techniques, suctioning is required. Sputum is produced as a response to a pathological condition. There is no rationale for routine suctioning every 1 to 2 hours.

Although suctioning is a frequent procedure, there is ongoing research to determine best practices to promote airway clearance without causing complications. The practice

*Text continued on p. 796*

---

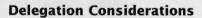

## SKILL 28-1 Suctioning

### Delegation Considerations

The skills of nasotracheal and artificial airway suctioning are not routinely delegated to assistive personnel. However, when the patient is assessed by the nurse to be stable oral and tracheostomy tube suctioning can be delegated. These situations include patients with permanent tracheostomy tubes. Before delegation the nurse instructs assistive personnel about:

- Any individualized aspects of care that pertain to suctioning, such as position, duration of suction, and pressure settings
- Signs and symptoms of hypoxemia or respiratory distress, such as change in patient's respiratory status, confusion, and restlessness, and to immediately report these signs to the nurse
- Reporting changes in patient's secretion quality, quantity, and color

### Equipment

- Appropriate-size suction catheter or closed-suction catheter (smallest diameter that will remove secretions effectively) or Yankauer catheter (oral suction)
- Nasal or oral airway (if indicated)
- Sterile gloves
- Clean gloves
- Clean towel or paper drape
- Portable or wall suction
- Mask or face shield
- Connecting tube (6 feet)

*If Not Using Closed-Suction Catheter*

- Small Y-adapter (if catheter does not have a suction control port)
- Water-soluble lubricant
- Sterile basin
- Sterile normal saline solution or water (about 100 ml)

| STEP | RATIONALE |
|---|---|

## ASSESSMENT

1. Assess signs and symptoms of upper and lower airway obstruction, including wheezes, crackles, or gurgling on inspiration or expiration; restlessness; ineffective coughing; unilateral, segmental, or lobar absent or diminished breath sounds (in absence of pneumonectomy or lobectomy); tachycardia; hypertension or hypotension; cyanosis; decreased level of consciousness, especially acute; or excess nasal secretions, drooling, or gastric secretions or vomitus in the mouth (Moore, 2003).

Physical signs and symptoms result from decreased oxygen to tissues, as well as pooling of secretions in upper and lower airways. Complete assessment before and following the suction procedure (Moore, 2003).

2. Determine the presence of apprehension, anxiety, decreased ability to concentrate, lethargy, decreased level of consciousness (especially acute), increased fatigue, dizziness, behavioral changes (especially irritability), decreased oxygen saturation (from pulse oximetry), increased pulse rate, increased rate of breathing, decreased depth of breathing, elevated blood pressure, cardiac dysrhythmias, pallor, cyanosis, and dyspnea or use of accessory muscles.

Signs and symptoms associated with hypoxia (low oxygen at the cellular or tissue level), hypoxemia (low oxygen tension in the blood), or hypercapnia (elevated carbon dioxide tension in the blood). Patients report sensations of pain and discomfort with the suctioning procedure; as a result, this increases their anxiety before suctioning. Anxiety and pain consume oxygen and in turn worsen the signs of hypoxia (Puntillo and others, 2002).

3. Assess for risk factors for upper or lower airway obstruction, including obstructive lung disease; pulmonary infections; impaired mobility; sedation; decreased level of consciousness; seizures; presence of feeding tube; anatomy of nasopharynx and oral pharynx; decreased gag or cough reflex; decreased swallowing ability; allergies; sinus drainage; and head, neck, or chest trauma.

Presence of these risk factors impairs the patient's ability to clear secretions from the airway and necessitates nasopharyngeal or nasotracheal suctioning.

| STEP | RATIONALE |
|------|-----------|
| 4. Determine additional factors that normally influence upper or lower airway function: recent surgery, ineffective or absent cough, chemical neuromuscular blockade, neuromuscular diseases, congestive heart failure, pulmonary edema, adult respiratory distress syndrome, hyaline membrane disease, or diaphragmatic weakness or paralysis (Moore, 2003). | Allows nurse to identify patients at risk for airway obstruction needing endotracheal tube (ET) or tracheostomy tube suctioning. |
| 5. Assess the following factors that influence character of secretions: | |
|    a. Fluid status | Fluid overload increases amount of secretions. Dehydration promotes thicker secretions. |
|    b. Lack of humidity | The environment influences secretion formation and gas exchange, necessitating airway suctioning when the patient cannot clear secretions effectively. |
|    c. Infection (e.g., pneumonia) | Patients with respiratory infections are likely to have increased secretions that are thicker and sometimes more difficult to expectorate. |
| 6. Identify contraindications to nasotracheal suctioning:<br>   a. Facial traumas/surgery<br>   b. Bleeding disorders<br>   c. Nasal bleeding<br>   d. Epiglottitis or croup<br>   e. Laryngospasm<br>   f. Irritable airway | The passage of a catheter though the nasal route will cause additional trauma, increase nasal bleeding, or cause severe bleeding in the presence of bleeding disorders. In the presence of epiglottitis, croup, laryngospasm, or irritable airway, the entrance of a suction catheter via the nasal route causes intractable coughing, hypoxemia, and severe bronchospasm, necessitating emergency **intubation** or tracheostomy (Moore, 2003). |
| 7. Examine sputum microbiology data. | Certain bacteria are easy to transmit or require isolation because of virulence or antibiotic resistance. |
| 8. Obtain patient's vital signs and oxygen saturation via pulse oximetry. Keep oximeter probe on during procedure. | Establishes physiological baseline. |
| 9. Assess patient's understanding of procedure. | Reveals need for patient instruction and encourages cooperation. |

## PLANNING

| | |
|------|-----------|
| 1. Explain to patient how procedure will help clear airway and relieve breathing problems. Explain that temporary coughing, sneezing, gagging, or shortness of breath is normal during the procedure. Encourage patient to cough out secretions. Practice coughing, if able. Splint surgical incisions, if necessary. | Encourages cooperation and minimizes risks, anxiety, and pain of procedure. |
| 2. Explain importance of coughing during procedure. | Facilitates secretion removal and may reduce frequency and duration of future suctioning. |
| 3. Assist patient with assuming position comfortable for nurse and patient (usually semi-Fowler's or sitting upright with head hyperextended, unless contraindicated). | Reduces stimulation of gag reflex, promotes patient comfort and secretion drainage, and prevents aspiration and nurse strain. |
| 4. Place towel across patient's chest, if needed. | Reduces transmission of microorganisms by protecting gown from secretions. |

## SKILL 28-1 | Suctioning—cont'd

| STEP | RATIONALE |
|---|---|

### IMPLEMENTATION

**1.** Perform hand hygiene, and apply face shield if splashing is likely.

Reduces transmission of microorganisms.

**2.** Connect one end of connecting tubing to suction machine, and place other end in convenient location near patient. Turn suction device on, and set vacuum regulator to appropriate negative pressure.

Excessive negative pressure damages nasal pharyngeal and tracheal mucosa and will induce greater hypoxia.

**3.** If indicated, increase supplemental oxygen therapy to 100% or as ordered by physician or health care provider. Encourage patient to breathe deeply.

Hyperoxygenation provides some protection from suction-induced decline in oxygenation. Hyperoxygenation is most effective in the presence of hyperinflation, such as encouraging the patient to deep breathe or increasing ventilator tidal volume (Moore, 2003).

---

• **Critical Decision Point:** You must readjust oxygen as ordered by physician or health care provider after procedure to avoid increased risk of oxygen toxicity and absorption, atelectasis from prolonged administration of high concentrations of oxygen, and increased carbon dioxide retention in patients with chronic obstructive lung diseases.

---

**4.** Prepare suction catheter.
   a. One-time-use catheter
      (1) Open suction kit or catheter using aseptic technique. If sterile drape is available, place it across patient's chest or on the over-bed table. Do not allow the suction catheter to touch any nonsterile surfaces.

Maintains asepsis and reduces transmission of microorganisms.

      (2) Unwrap or open sterile basin, and place on bedside table. Be careful not to touch inside of basin. Fill with about 100 ml sterile normal saline solution or water (see illustration).

Use saline or water to clean tubing after each suction pass.

      (3) Open lubricant. Squeeze small amount onto open sterile catheter package without touching package. NOTE: Lubricant is not necessary for artificial airway suctioning.

Prepares lubricant while maintaining sterility. Use water-soluble lubricant to avoid lipoid aspiration pneumonia. Excessive lubricant occludes catheter.

   b. Closed (in-line) suction catheter (see Box 28-7)

**5.** Turn on suction device, and set regulator to appropriate pressure.

Excessive negative pressure results in damage to the nasal pharyngeal and tracheal mucosa and increases suction-induced hypoxia.

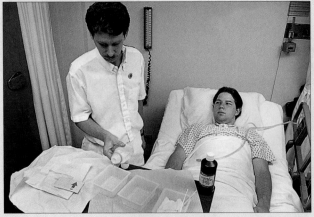

STEP **4a(2)** Pouring sterile saline into tray.

| STEP | RATIONALE |
|------|-----------|

6. Apply a pair of clean gloves for oropharyngeal suction. Apply sterile glove to each hand or clean glove to nondominant hand and sterile glove to dominant hand for all other suction techniques.

7. Pick up suction catheter with dominant hand without touching nonsterile surfaces. Pick up connecting tubing with nondominant hand. Secure catheter to tubing (see illustration).

    Maintains catheter sterility. Connects catheter to suction.

8. Check that the equipment is functioning properly by suctioning small amount of normal saline solution from basin.

    Ensures equipment function. Lubricates internal catheter and tubing.

9. Suction airway.

  **a. Oropharyngeal suctioning**

    (1) Remove oxygen mask if present. Nasal cannula may remain in place. Keep oxygen mask near patient's face. Insert Yankauer catheter along gum line to pharynx. With suction applied, move catheter around mouth until you clear the secretions. Encourage patient to cough. Replace oxygen mask, as appropriate.

      Intermittent suction prevents invagination of oral mucosa into suction catheter. Invagination of mucosa causes trauma to the mucous membranes.
      Coughing moves secretions from lower to upper airways into mouth.

    (2) Rinse catheter with water in basin until catheter and connecting tube are cleared of secretions.

      Clearing secretions before they dry reduces probability of transmission of microorganisms and enhances delivery of preset suction pressures.

    (3) Place catheter or Yankauer in a clean, dry area for reuse with suction turned off. If patient able to suction self, place within patient's reach with suction on.

      Facilitates prompt removal of airway secretions for future suctioning.

  **b. Nasopharyngeal and nasotracheal suctioning**

    (1) Lightly coat distal 6 to 8 cm (2 to 3 inches) of catheter tip with water-soluble lubricant.

      Lubricates catheter for easier insertion.

    (2) Remove oxygen delivery device, if applicable, with nondominant hand. Without applying suction and using dominant thumb and forefinger, gently but quickly insert catheter into naris during inhalation. Following the natural course of the naris, slightly slant the catheter downward or through mouth. Do not force through naris (see illustration).

      Application of suction pressure while introducing catheter into trachea increases risk of damage to mucosa and increases risk of hypoxia because of removal of entrained oxygen present in airways.

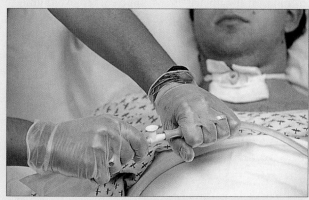

STEP **7** Attaching catheter to suction

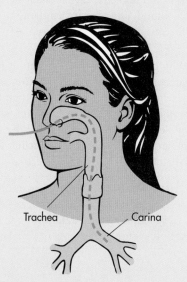

STEP **9b(2)** Pathway for nasotracheal catheter progression.

Trachea      Carina

SKILL 28-1 | Suctioning—cont'd

| STEP | RATIONALE |
|---|---|

• *Critical Decision Point:* Be sure to insert catheter during patient inhalation, especially if inserting catheter into trachea, because epiglottis is open. Do not insert during swallowing or catheter will most likely enter esophagus. Never apply suction during insertion. Make sure patient coughs. If patient gags or becomes nauseated, catheter is most likely in esophagus and you must remove it.

| STEP | RATIONALE |
|---|---|
| (a) *Nasopharyngeal suctioning:* In adults, insert catheter about 16 cm (6 inches); in older children, 8 to 12 cm (3 to 5 inches); in infants and young children, 4 to 8 cm (2 to 3 inches). Rule of thumb is to insert catheter distance from tip of nose (or mouth) to base of earlobe. | Ensures that you position catheter tip correctly in pharynx or trachea for suctioning. |
| (b) *Nasotracheal suctioning:* In adults, insert catheter about 20 cm (8 inches); in older children, 14 to 20 cm ($5\frac{1}{2}$ to 8 inches); and in young children and infants, 8 to 14 cm (3 to $5\frac{1}{2}$ inches) (see step 9b(2)). | |

• *Critical Decision Point:* When there is difficulty passing the catheter, ask patient to cough or say "ahh," or try to advance the catheter during inspiration. Both these measures assist in opening the glottis to permit passage of the catheter into the trachea.

| STEP | RATIONALE |
|---|---|
| [1] *Positioning for nasotracheal suctioning:* In some instances turning patient's head to right helps nurse suction left mainstem bronchus; turning head to left helps nurse suction right mainstem bronchus. If you feel resistance after insertion of catheter for maximum recommended distance, catheter has probably hit carina. Pull catheter back 1 to 2 cm before applying suction. | Turning the patient's head to the side elevates the bronchial passage on the opposite side. |

• *Critical Decision Point:* Use the nasal approach, and perform tracheal suctioning before pharyngeal suctioning whenever possible. The mouth and pharynx contain more bacteria than the trachea does. If there is an abundance of oral secretions present before beginning the procedure, suction mouth with oral suction device.

| STEP | RATIONALE |
|---|---|
| (3) With catheter tip in position, apply intermittent suction for up to 10 seconds (Moore, 2003) by placing and releasing nondominant thumb over vent of catheter and slowly withdrawing catheter while rotating it back and forth between dominant thumb and forefinger. Encourage patient to cough. Replace oxygen device, if applicable. | Intermittent suction and rotation of catheter prevent injury to mucosa. If catheter "grabs" mucosa, remove thumb to release suction. Suctioning longer than 10 seconds causes cardiopulmonary compromise, usually from hypoxemia or vagal overload. |

• *Critical Decision Point:* Monitor vital signs and oxygen saturation throughout suction procedure. If the pulse drops more than 20 beats per minute or increases more than 40 beats per minute, or if pulse oximetry falls below 90% or 5% from baseline, cease suctioning. Any deteriorating change in the patient's physiological status during suctioning requires termination of the procedure, hyperoxygenation, and other appropriate interventions (e.g., position change) (Moore, 2003).

| STEP | RATIONALE |
|---|---|
| (4) Rinse catheter and connecting tubing with normal saline or water until cleared. | Secretions that remain in suction catheter or connecting tubing decrease suctioning efficiency. |
| (5) Assess for need to repeat suctioning procedure. Observe for alterations in cardiopulmonary status. When possible, allow adequate time (1 to 2 minutes) between suction passes for ventilation and oxygenation. Assist patient with deep breathing and coughing. | Suctioning sometimes induces hypoxemia, dysrhythmias, laryngospasm, and bronchospasm. Deep breathing reventilates and reoxygenates alveoli. Repeated passes clear the airway of excessive secretions but also remove oxygen and induce **laryngospasm.** |

**c. Artificial airway suctioning**

| STEP | RATIONALE |
|---|---|
| (1) Hyperinflate and/or hyperoxygenate patient before suctioning, using manual resuscitation bag-valve mask connected to oxygen source or sigh mechanism on mechanical ventilator. Some mechanical ventilators have a button that when pushed delivers 100% oxygen for a few minutes and then resets to the previous value. | Hyperinflation decreases the risk for atelectasis caused by negative pressure of suctioning. Preoxygenation converts large proportion of resident lung gas to 100% oxygen to offset amount used in metabolic consumption while interrupting ventilator or oxygenation, as well as to offset volume lost during suction procedure (Day and others, 2002). |

---

· *Critical Decision Point:* Use caution when suctioning patients with a head injury. The suction procedure causes elevations in intracranial pressure (ICP). You reduce this risk by presuctioning hyperventilation, which results in hypocarbia that in turn induces vasoconstriction. It is the vasoconstriction that reduces the potential increase in ICP. It is recommended that you limit the introduction of a catheter to two times with each suctioning procedure (Moore, 2003).

---

| STEP | RATIONALE |
|---|---|
| (2) If patient is receiving mechanical ventilation, open swivel adapter, or if necessary remove oxygen or humidity delivery device with nondominant hand. | Exposes artificial airway. |
| (3) Without applying suction, gently but quickly insert catheter using dominant thumb and forefinger into artificial airway (it is best to try to insert catheter into the artificial airway while patient is inhaling) until you meet resistance or until patient coughs, then pull back 1 cm (½ inch) (see illustration). | Application of suction pressure while introducing catheter into trachea increases risk of damage to tracheal mucosa, as well as increased hypoxia related to removal of entrained oxygen present in airways. Pulling back stimulates cough and removes catheter from mucosal wall so that catheter is not resting against tracheal mucosa during suctioning. |

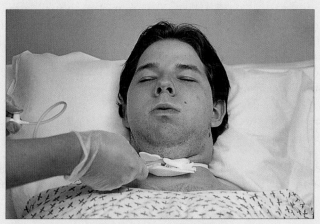

STEP **9c(3)** Suctioning tracheostomy.

**SKILL 28-1** | **Suctioning—cont'd**

| STEP | RATIONALE |
|---|---|

• *Critical Decision Point:* If you are unable to insert catheter past the end of the ET tube, the catheter is probably caught in the Murphy eye (i.e., side hole at the distal end of the ET tube that allows for collateral airflow in the event of tracheal mainstem intubation). If so, rotate the catheter to reposition it away from the Murphy eye, or withdraw it slightly and reinsert with the next inhalation. Usually the catheter meets resistance at the carina. One indication that the catheter is at the carina is acute onset of coughing, because the carina contains many cough receptors. Pull the catheter back 1 cm (½ inch).

| | |
|---|---|
| (4) Apply intermittent suction by placing and releasing nondominant thumb over vent of catheter; slowly withdraw catheter while rotating it back and forth between dominant thumb and forefinger. Encourage patient to cough. Watch for respiratory distress. | Intermittent suction and rotation of catheter prevent injury to tracheal mucosal lining. If catheter "grabs" mucosa, remove thumb to release suction. |

• *Critical Decision Point:* If patient develops respiratory distress during the suction procedure, immediately withdraw catheter, and supply additional oxygen and breaths as needed. In an emergency, you can administer oxygen directly though the catheter. Disconnect suction, and attach oxygen at prescribed flow rate through the catheter.

| | |
|---|---|
| (5) If patient is receiving mechanical ventilation, close swivel adapter, or replace oxygen delivery device. | Reestablishes artificial airway. |
| (6) Encourage patient to deep breathe, if able. Some patients respond well to several manual breaths from the mechanical ventilator or bag-valve-mask. | Reoxygenates and reexpands alveoli. Suctioning sometimes causes hypoxemia and atelectasis. |
| (7) Rinse catheter and connecting tubing with normal saline until clear. Use continuous suction. | Removes catheter secretions, which can decrease suctioning efficiency and provide environment for microorganism growth. |
| (8) Assess patient's cardiopulmonary status for secretion clearance. Repeat steps (1) through (7) once or twice more to clear secretions. Allow at least 1 full minute between suction passes. | Suctioning induces dysrhythmias, hypoxia, and bronchospasm and impairs cerebral circulation or adversely affects hemodynamic stability (Akgul and Akyolcu, 2002; Moore, 2003). Repeated passes with suction catheter clear airway of excessive secretions and promote improved oxygenation. |
| (9) When you have cleared pharynx and trachea sufficiently of secretions, perform oropharyngeal suctioning to clear mouth of secretions. Do not suction nose again after suctioning mouth. | Removes upper airway secretions. More microorganisms are generally present in mouth. Upper airway is considered "clean" and lower airway is considered "sterile." Use the same catheter to suction from sterile to clean areas, but not from clean to sterile areas. |
| 10. When you have completed suctioning, disconnect catheter from connecting tubing. Roll catheter around fingers of dominant hand. Pull glove off inside out so that catheter remains coiled in glove. Pull off other glove over first glove in same way to seal in contaminants. Discard in appropriate receptacle. Turn off suction device. | Reduces transmission of microorganisms. |
| 11. Remove towel, place in laundry or appropriate receptacle, and reposition patient. (You will need to wear clean gloves for personal care.) | Reduces transmission of microorganisms. Promotes comfort. |
| 12. If indicated, readjust oxygen to original level because patient's blood oxygen level should have returned to baseline. | Prevents absorption atelectasis and oxygen toxicity while allowing patient time to reoxygenate blood. |

| STEP | RATIONALE |
|---|---|
| 13. Discard remainder of normal saline into appropriate receptacle. If basin is disposable, discard into appropriate receptacle. If basin is reusable, rinse it out and place it in soiled utility room. | Reduces transmission of microorganisms. |
| 14. Remove face shield, and discard into appropriate receptacle. Perform hand hygiene. | Reduces transmission of microorganisms. |
| 15. Place unopened suction kit on suction machine table or at head of bed. | Provides immediate access to suction catheter for next procedure. |
| 16. Assist patient to a comfortable position, and provide oral hygiene as needed. | |

## EVALUATION

1. Compare patient's respiratory assessment before and after suctioning.

2. Observe airway secretions.

3. Ask patient if breathing is easier and if there is less congestion.

Provides subjective confirmation that you relieved airway obstruction during suctioning procedure.
Provides data to document presence or absence of respiratory tract infection.
Provides data to determine if you met patient expectations.

## RECORDING AND REPORTING

■ Record the amount, consistency, color, and odor of secretions.
■ Record the patient's response to the suction procedure.
■ Record and report the presuctioning and postsuctioning cardiopulmonary status.

## UNEXPECTED OUTCOMES AND RELATED INTERVENTIONS

■ Worsening cardiopulmonary status
  • Limit length of time suctioning.
  • Determine need for presuctioning hyperoxygenation and hyperinflation.
  • Determine need for more frequent, shorter-duration suctioning.
  • Notify physician or health care provider of changes.
■ Return of bloody secretions
  • Determine amount of suction pressure used, and adjust accordingly.
  • Evaluate frequency of suctioning, and reduce if appropriate.
  • Determine other factors that lead to blood secretions (e.g., prolonged bleeding time).
  • Provide more frequent oral hygiene.

■ Unable to pass suction catheter through first naris attempted
  • Try other naris or oral route.
  • Insert nasal airway, especially if suctioning through patient's naris frequently.
  • Guide catheter along naris floor to avoid turbinates.
  • If obstruction is mucus, apply suction to relieve obstruction, but do not apply suction to mucosa. If you think the obstruction is a blood clot, consult physician or health care provider.
■ Paroxysms of coughing
  • Administer supplemental oxygen.
  • Allow patient to rest between passes of suction catheter.
  • Consult physician or health care provider regarding need for inhaled bronchodilators or topical anesthetics.
■ Unable to obtain secretions
  • Determine adequacy of humidification of oxygen delivery device.
  • Evaluate patient's fluid status.
  • Determine need for chest physiotherapy.
  • Assess for signs of infection.

**Research Summary**

The practice of normal saline instillation (NSI) into artificial airways before suctioning has the potential for causing detrimental effects, such as decreased heart rate and hypotension, which in turn have an adverse effect on the patient's oxygen status. In addition, newer research is identifying a link between NSI and nosocomial infections. NSI in conjunction with artificial airway suctioning may lead to the dispersion of microorganisms into the lower respiratory tract and subsequent pulmonary infection.

**Application to Nursing Practice**

- Use noninvasive techniques, such as chest physiotherapy or coughing, to improve airway clearance and optimize the suctioning procedure.
- Maintain adequate hydration so that the patient's secretions remain thin.
- Encourage activity and position change to prevent secretions from accumulating in the dependent region of the lung.
- Maintain sterile asepsis when suctioning a patient's airway.

Data from Freytag CC and others: Prolonged application of closed in-line suction catheters increase microbial colonization of lower respiratory tract bacterial growth on catheter surface, *Infection* 31(1):31, 2003.

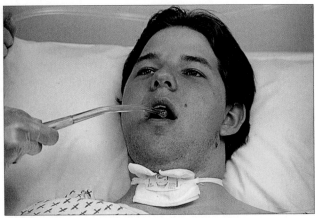

FIGURE **28-5** Oropharyngeal suctioning. (From Perry AG, Potter PA: *Clinical nursing skills and techniques,* ed 6, St. Louis, 2006, Mosby.)

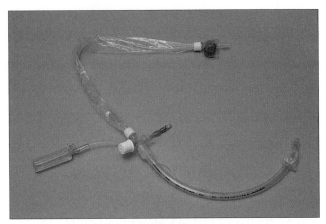

FIGURE **28-6** Ballard tracheal care closed suction.

of normal saline instillation into artificial airways to improve secretion clearance is inconclusive and may in fact cause further complications (Box 28-6).

*OROPHARYNGEAL AND NASOPHARYNGEAL SUCTIONING.* You use oropharyngeal or nasopharyngeal suctioning to assist the patient who is able to cough effectively but is unable to clear secretions by expectorating or swallowing. Use a Yankauer or tonsillar tip suction device for oropharyngeal suctioning (Figure 28-5). A Yankauer suction catheter is a rigid plastic catheter with one large and several small eyelets through which mucus is removed. The catheter is angled to facilitate removal of secretions from the mouth. Use the Yankauer suction catheter when oral secretions are thick and plentiful. Do not use the Yankauer suction catheter in the nares because of its size.

*OROTRACHEAL AND NASOTRACHEAL SUCTIONING.* Orotracheal or nasotracheal suctioning is necessary when the patient is unable to cough and does not have an artificial airway (see Skill 28-1). You pass a catheter through the mouth or nose into the trachea. The nose is the preferred route because stimulation of the gag reflex is minimal. The procedure is similar to nasopharyngeal suctioning, but the catheter tip is in the trachea.

*TRACHEAL SUCTIONING.* You perform tracheal suctioning through an artificial airway, such as a tracheostomy tube or endotracheal tube. Two methods of suctioning currently used include use of a single catheter for one-time use and closed suctioning, including a multiple-use catheter. The suction catheter in closed suctioning is encased in a plastic sheath and used for 24 to 48 hours. You will use closed suctioning most often for patients who require mechanical ventilation because it continuously delivers oxygen during suctioning (Box 28-7).

*Artificial Airways.* An artificial airway is for a patient with decreased level of consciousness, airway obstruction, mechanical ventilation, and removal of tracheobronchial secretions (see Skill 28-1).

*ORAL AIRWAY.* The oral airway (Figure 28-7), the simplest type of artificial airway, prevents obstruction of the trachea by displacement of the tongue into the oropharynx. The oral airway extends from the teeth to the oropharynx, maintaining the tongue in the normal position. You determine proper oral airway size by measuring the distance from the corner of the mouth to the angle of the jaw just below the ear. The length is equal to the distance from the flange of the airway to the tip. You need to use the correct-size airway. If the airway is too small, the tongue will not stay in the anterior portion of the mouth; if too large, it will force the tongue toward the epiglottis and obstruct the airway.

| BOX 28-7 | PROCEDURAL GUIDELINES FOR |

## Closed (In-Line) Suctioning

**Delegation Considerations:** The airway suctioning with a closed (in-line) suction catheter is not routinely delegated to assistive personnel. In some situations, such as suctioning a patient with a permanent tracheostomy tube, this procedure may be delegated. The nurse is responsible for assessing the patient's cardiopulmonary status, and before delegation the nurse must instruct assistive personnel about:

- Any individualized aspect of care that pertain to suctioning, such as position, duration of suction, and pressure settings
- Signs and symptoms of hypoxemia or respiratory distress, such as change in patient's respiratory status, confusion, and restlessness, and to immediately report these signs to the nurse
- Reporting changes in patient's secretion quality, quantity, and color

**Equipment:** closed system or in-line suction catheter (Figure 28-6); suction machine; 6 feet of connecting tubing; two clean gloves (optional), face shield

1. Perform assessment as in Skill 28-1.
2. Explain the procedure to the patient and the importance of coughing during the suctioning procedure.
3. Assist patient with assuming a position of comfort for both patient and nurse, usually semi-Fowler's or high Fowler's position. Place towel across the patient's chest.
4. Perform hand hygiene, and attach suction.
   a. In many institutions the catheter is attached to the mechanical ventilator circuit by a respiratory therapist. If catheter is not already in place, open suction catheter package using aseptic technique, attach closed suction catheter to ventilator circuit by removing swivel adapter and placing closed suction catheter apparatus on ET or tracheostomy tube, and connect Y on mechanical ventilator circuit to closed suction catheter with flex tubing (see illustration).

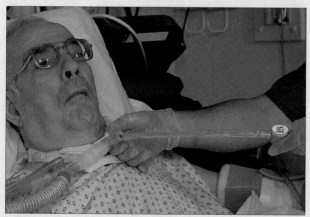

STEP **4a** Suctioning tracheostomy with closed system suction catheter.

b. Connect one end of connecting tubing to suction machine, and connect other to the end of a closed system or in-line suction catheter, if not already done. Turn suction device on, and set vacuum regulator to appropriate negative pressure (see manufacturer's directions). Many closed system suction catheters require slightly higher suction; consult manufacturer's guidelines.
5. Hyperinflate and/or hyperoxygenate patient with bag-valve-mask or manual breathing mechanism on mechanical ventilator according to institution protocol and clinical status (usually 100% oxygen).
6. Unlock suction control mechanism if required by manufacturer. Open saline port, and attach saline syringe or vial.
7. Pick up suction catheter enclosed in plastic sleeve with dominant hand.

---

- *Critical Decision Point:* The use of normal saline instillation with closed in-line suction catheters is not appropriate for all patients and needs further investigation. Normal saline instillation in conjunction with endotracheal suction leads to the dispersion of microorganisms into the lower respiratory tract (Freytag and others, 2003; Sole and others, 2003).

---

8. Insert catheter; use a repeating maneuver of pushing catheter and sliding (or pulling) plastic sleeve back between thumb and forefinger until you feel resistance or patient coughs.
9. Encourage patient to cough, and apply suction by squeezing on suction control mechanism while withdrawing catheter. It is difficult to apply intermittent pulses of suction and nearly impossible to rotate the catheter compared with a standard catheter. Be sure to withdraw catheter completely into plastic sheath so it does not obstruct airflow.
10. Reassess cardiopulmonary status, including pulse oximetry, to determine need for subsequent suctioning or complications. Repeat steps 5 through 9 one to two more times to clear secretions. Allow adequate time (at least 1 full minute) between suction passes for ventilation and reoxygenation.
11. When airway is clear, withdraw catheter completely into sheath. Be sure that colored indicator line on catheter is visible in the sheath. Squeeze vial or push saline syringe while applying suction to rinse inner lumen of catheter. Use at least 5 to 10 ml of saline to rinse the catheter until you clear it of retained secretions, which cause bacterial growth and increase the risk of infection (Freytag and others, 2003). Lock suction mechanism, if applicable, and turn off suction.
12. If patient requires oral or nasal suctioning, perform Skill 28-1 with separate standard suction catheter.
13. Reposition patient.
14. Remove gloves and discard them, and perform hand hygiene.
15. Compare patient's cardiopulmonary assessments before and after suctioning, and observe airway secretions.

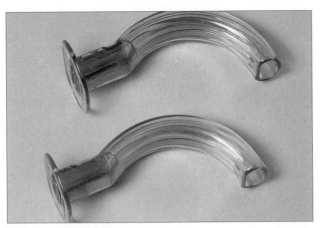

FIGURE **28-7** Artificial oral airways.

Turning the curve of the airway toward the cheek and placing it over the tongue, insert the airway. When the airway is in the oropharynx, turn it so the opening points downward. Correctly placed, the airway moves the tongue forward, away from the oropharynx, and the flange, the flat portion of the airway, rests against the patient's teeth. Incorrect insertion merely forces the tongue back into the oropharynx.

*TRACHEAL AIRWAY.* Tracheal airways include endotracheal, nasotracheal, and tracheal tubes. These allow easy access to the trachea for deep tracheal suctioning. Because of the artificial airway, the patient no longer has normal humidification of the tracheal mucosa. Ensure that nebulization or the oxygen delivery system is supplying humidity to the airway. This humidification is protective and helps reduce the risk of airway plugging.

**Mobilization of Pulmonary Secretions.** The ability of a patient to mobilize pulmonary secretions makes the difference between a short-term illness and a long recovery involving complications.

*Hydration.* Maintenance of adequate hydration promotes mucociliary clearance, the body's natural mechanism for removing mucus and cellular debris from the respiratory tract. In patients with adequate hydration, pulmonary secretions are thin, white, watery, and easily removable with minimal coughing. A fluid intake of 1500 to 2000 ml per day will help keep pulmonary secretions thin and easy to expectorate, unless contraindicated by cardiac condition.

*Humidification.* Humidification is necessary for patients receiving oxygen therapy at more than 4 L/min. You humidify a nasal catheter, nasal cannula, or face mask by bubbling it through water. When using humidity, make sure to use sterile saline for inhalation. Also, make sure to change the solution according to agency procedures. Humidification is a source for nosocomial infections because the moist environment supports the growth of pathogens.

*Nebulization.* Nebulization uses the aerosol principle to suspend a maximum number of water drops or particles of the desired size in inspired air. The moisture added to the respiratory system through nebulization improves clearance and is often used for administration of bronchodilators and mucolytic agents.

**Maintenance or Promotion of Lung Expansion.** Nursing interventions to maintain or promote lung expansion include positioning, incentive spirometry, chest physiotherapy, and chest tube management.

*Positioning.* Healthy people maintain adequate ventilation and oxygenation by frequent position changes. When a person has restricted mobility, this increases his or her risk for respiratory impairment. Frequent position changes are a simple and cost-effective method for reducing the patient's risk for pooled airway secretions and decreased chest wall expansion.

The most effective position for patients with cardiopulmonary diseases is the 45-degree semi-Fowler's position, using gravity to assist in lung expansion and reduce pressure from the abdomen on the diaphragm. Ensure that the patient does not slide down in bed, causing reduced lung expansion. Position patients with unilateral lung disease, such as a pneumothorax or atelectasis, with the healthy lung down. This promotes better perfusion of the healthy lung, improving oxygenation. In the presence of pulmonary abscess or hemorrhage, place the affected lung down to prevent drainage toward the healthy lung.

*Incentive Spirometry.* Incentive spirometry (**IS**) is a method of encouraging voluntary deep breathing by providing visual feedback to patients about inspiratory volume. IS promotes deep breathing to prevent or treat atelectasis in the postoperative patient. It encourages patients to breathe to their normal inspiratory capacities. A postoperative inspiratory capacity one half to three fourths of the preoperative volume is acceptable because of postoperative pain. Administration of pain medications before IS will help the patient achieve deep breathing by reducing pain and splinting. There is no clinical benefit to using IS in place of early ambulation. Encourage your postoperative patients to ambulate as soon as possible.

Flow-oriented incentive spirometers consist of one or more plastic chambers that contain freely moving colored balls. The patient inhales slowly with an even flow to elevate the balls and keep them floating as long as possible. This will allow a maximally sustained inhalation.

Volume-oriented IS devices have a bellows that raises to a predetermined volume by an inhaled breath. An achievement light or counter is used to provide feedback. Some devices will not turn the light on unless the bellows is at a minimum desired volume for a specified period of time.

*Chest Physiotherapy.* Chest physiotherapy (**CPT**) is used to mobilize pulmonary secretions (Box 28-8). CPT includes postural drainage, chest percussion, and vibration, followed by productive coughing or suctioning. CPT is for patients who produce more than 30 ml of sputum per day or have evidence of atelectasis by chest x-ray film.

| BOX 28-8 | **Assessment Criteria for Chest Physiotherapy** |

Nursing care and selection of CPT skills are based on specific assessment findings. The following guidelines help you with physical assessment and subsequent decision making:

- Know the patient's normal range of vital signs. Conditions requiring CPT, such as atelectasis and pneumonia, affect vital signs. The degree of change is related to the level of hypoxia, overall cardiopulmonary status, and tolerance to activity.
- Know the patient's medications. Certain medications, particularly diuretics and antihypertensives, cause fluid and hemodynamic changes. These decrease the patient's tolerance to positional changes and postural drainage. Long-term steroid use increases the patient's risk of pathological rib fractures and often contraindicates vibration.
- Know the patient's medical history. Certain conditions, such as increased intracranial pressure, spinal cord injuries, and abdominal aneurysm resection, contraindicate the positional changes of postural drainage. Thoracic trauma or surgery also contraindicates percussion, and vibration.
- Know the patient's level of cognitive function. Participation in controlled cough techniques requires the patient to follow instructions. Congenital or acquired cognitive limitations alter the patient's ability to learn and participate in these techniques.
- Be aware of the patient's exercise tolerance. CPT maneuvers are fatiguing. When the patient is not used to physical activity, usually the patient will have little tolerance for the maneuvers. However, with gradual increases in activity and planned CPT, patient tolerance to the procedure improves.

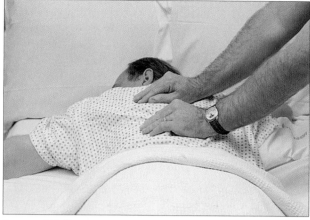

FIGURE 28-8 Hand position for chest wall percussion during physiotherapy.

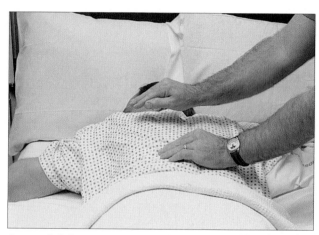

FIGURE 28-9 Chest wall percussion, alternating hand motion against the patient's chest wall.

*CHEST PERCUSSION.* **Chest percussion** involves striking the chest wall over the area being drained. You position the hand so that the fingers and thumb touch, cupping the hand (Figure 28-8). Percussion on the surface of the chest wall sends waves of varying amplitude and frequency through the chest, changing the consistency and location of the sputum. You perform chest percussion by alternating hand motion against the chest wall (Figure 28-9). Perform percussion over a single layer of clothing, not over buttons, snaps, or zippers. The single layer of clothing prevents slapping the patient's skin. Thicker or multiple layers of material dampen the vibrations.

Be cautious when percussing the lung fields not to percuss the scapular area, or trauma will occur to the skin and underlying musculoskeletal structures. Percussion is contraindicated in patients with bleeding disorders, osteoporosis, or fractured ribs.

*VIBRATION.* **Vibration** is a fine, shaking pressure applied to the chest wall only during exhalation. This technique increases the velocity and turbulence of exhaled air, facilitating secretion removal. Vibration increases the exhalation of trapped air, shakes mucus loose, and induces a cough. You will use vibration most often used with pa-

tients with cystic fibrosis. It is not recommended for infants and young children.

*POSTURAL DRAINAGE.* **Postural drainage** is the use of positioning techniques that drain secretions from specific segments of the lungs and bronchi into the trachea. The procedure for postural drainage includes most lung segments (Table 28-8). Because some patients do not require postural drainage of all lung segments, you base the procedure on clinical assessment findings. For example, some patients with left lower lobe atelectasis will require postural drainage of only the affected region, whereas a child with cystic fibrosis requires postural drainage of all segments.

*Chest Tubes.* **A chest tube** is a catheter inserted through the thorax to remove air and fluids from the pleural space and to reestablish normal intrapleural and intrapulmonic pressures. Chest tubes are used after chest surgery and chest

## TABLE 28-8    Positions for Postural Drainage

| Lung Segment | Position of Patient | Lung Segment | Position of Patient |
|---|---|---|---|
| **Adult** | | Right middle lobe— posterior segment | Prone with thorax and abdomen elevated |
| Bilateral | High Fowler's | | |
| Apical segments Right upper lobe— anterior segment | Sitting on side of bed Supine with head elevated | Both lower lobes— anterior segments | Supine in Trendelenburg's position |
| Left upper lobe— anterior segment | Supine with head elevated | Left lower lobe— lateral segment | Right side-lying in Trendelenburg's position |
| Right upper lobe— posterior segment | Side-lying with right side of chest elevated on pillows | | |
| Left upper lobe— posterior segment | Side-lying with left side of chest elevated on pillows | Right lower lobe— lateral segment | Left side-lying in Trendelenburg's position |
| Right middle lobe— anterior segment | Three-fourths supine position with dependent lung in Trendelenburg's position | Right lower lobe— posterior segment | Prone with right side of chest elevated in Trendelenburg's position |
| | | Both lower lobes— posterior segment | Prone in Trendelenburg's position |

| TABLE 28-8 | Positions for Postural Drainage—cont'd | | |
|---|---|---|---|
| **Lung Segment** | **Position of Patient** | **Lung Segment** | **Position of Patient** |
| **Child** | | Bilateral lobes— anterior segments | Lying supine on nurse's lap, back supported with pillow |
| Bilateral—apical segments | Sitting on nurse's lap, leaning slightly forward flexed over pillow | | |
| Bilateral—middle anterior segments | Sitting on nurse's lap, leaning against nurse | | |

trauma and for pneumothorax or hemothorax to promote lung expansion (Skill 28-2).

A **pneumothorax** is a collection of air or other gas in the pleural space. The gas causes the lung to collapse because it obliterates the negative intrapleural pressure and exerts a counterpressure against the lung making it unable to expand. There are a variety of mechanisms for a pneumothorax. It occurs spontaneously or from chest trauma.

A patient with a pneumothorax usually feels pain as atmospheric air irritates the parietal pleura. The pain is sharp and pleuritic. Dyspnea is common and worsens as the size of the pneumothorax increases.

**Hemothorax** is an accumulation of blood and fluid in the pleural cavity between the parietal and visceral pleurae, usually as the result of trauma. It produces a counterpressure and prevents the lung from full expansion. In addition to pain and dyspnea, signs and symptoms of shock will develop if blood loss is severe.

Disposable chest drainage systems, such as Thora-Seal III or Pleur-Evac chest drainage system (DeKental), are one-piece molded plastic units that you use to evaluate any volume of air or fluid with controlled suction (see Figure 28-10). The first chamber provides a water seal to prevent air from being drawn back into the pleural space. The second chamber collects fluid or blood. The third chamber is for suction, to facilitate removal of chest drainage. The suction pressure causes gentle, continuous bubbling in the third chamber. Suction pressure is measured in centimeters of water. You will usually set suction at $-15$ to $-20$ cm $H_2O$ for adults. Children require lesser amounts of suction pressure.

The disposable units appear to be the system of choice because they are cost-effective and some facilitate autotransfusion, a common practice in open heart surgeries. Knowledge of the basics of chest tube management and troubleshooting maneuvers reduces the patient's risk of complications.

The one-bottle system, used for smaller amounts of drainage, is the simplest closed drainage system. The single bottle serves as a collector and a water seal. The long glass drainage tube submerged in water establishes a level of suction to remove fluid and air from the chest cavity. Most health care settings rarely use this system, except for the drainage of exudates from an empyema. During normal respiration the fluid ascends with inspiration and descends with expiration.

*SPECIAL CONSIDERATIONS.* Clamping chest tubes is contraindicated when the patient is ambulating or being transported. Handle the chest drainage unit carefully, and maintain the drainage device below the patient's chest. If the tubing disconnects from the unit, instruct the patient to exhale as much as possible and to cough. This maneuver rids the pleural space of as much air as possible. Then cleanse the tip of the tubing, and reconnect the tubing to the unit quickly. Clamping the chest tube is not recommended, because it results in a tension pneumothorax, which is a life-threatening event.

*CHEST TUBE REMOVAL.* Removal of a chest tube requires patient preparation. An analgesic administered before removal helps to minimize discomfort and anxiety. Generally the physician or health care provider removes the tube and places an occlusive petrolatum gauze dressing over the wound. You will monitor the patient's vital signs and $SpO_2$.

*Text continued on p. 807*

## SKILL 28-2 | Care of Patients With Chest Tubes

### Delegation Considerations

Do not delegate this skill. However, the nurse should inform assistive personnel about:
- Proper positioning of the patient with chest tubes to facilitate chest tube drainage and optimal functioning of the system
- How to ambulate and transfer the patient with chest drainage
- Reporting any changes in vital signs, level of comfort, $SpO_2$, or excessive bubbling in water-seal chamber
- Immediately notifying the nurse if there is a disconnection of the system, change in type and amount of drainage, bleeding, or sudden cessation of bubbling

### Equipment

- Disposable chest drainage system (Figure 28-10)
- Suction source and setup (wall canister or portable)
  - Water suction system: add sterile water or normal saline (NS) solution to cover the lower 2.5 cm (1 inch) of water-seal U tube, sterile water or NS to put into the suction control chamber if suction is to be used (see manufacturer's directions)
  - Waterless system: add vial of 30 ml injectable sodium chloride or water, 20-ml syringe, 21-gauge needle, and antiseptic swab
- Nonsterile gloves

- 2-inch tape
- Sterile gauze sponges
- Two shodded hemostats

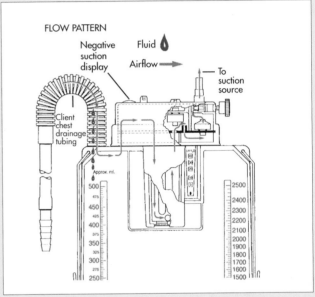

FIGURE **28-10** Disposable waterless chest drainage system with suction.

| STEP | RATIONALE |
| --- | --- |

### ASSESSMENT

1. Perform hand hygiene.
2. Assess pulmonary status:
   a. Assess for respiratory distress and chest pain, and breath sounds over affected lung area (see Chapters 12 and 13).
   b. Signs and symptoms of increased respiratory distress and/or chest pain are decreased breath sounds over the affected and nonaffected lungs, marked cyanosis, asymmetrical chest movements, presence of subcutaneous emphysema around tube insertion site or neck, hypotension, and tachycardia (Carroll, 2002).
   c. Chest pain on inspiration.
3. Obtain vital signs, oxygen saturation ($SpO_2$), and level of cognition.
4. If possible, ask patient to rate level of comfort on a visual analog scale of 0 to 10.

5. Observe:
   a. Chest tube dressing and site surrounding tube insertion.

Signs and symptoms reflect improvement in respiratory distress and chest pain after insertion of chest tube. If respiratory distress is not relieved or worsens or if there is sharp stabbing chest pain with or without decreased blood pressure and increased heart rate, notify physician or health care provider immediately. These symptoms indicate a pneumothorax (Woodruff, 1999).

Changes in pulse and blood pressure indicate infection, respiratory distress, or pain.

Chest tubes are often painful and interfere with patient's mobility, coughing and deep breathing, and rehabilitation (Puntillo, 2003).

Ensures that dressing is intact, without air or fluid leaks and that area surrounding insertion site is free of drainage or skin irritation (Carroll, 2002).

| STEP | RATIONALE |
|---|---|
| b. Tubing for kinks, dependent loops, or clots. | Maintains a patent, freely draining system, preventing fluid accumulation in chest cavity. The presence of kinks, dependent loops, or clotted drainage increases the patient's risk for infection, atelectasis, and tension pneumothorax (Allibone, 2003). |
| c. Chest drainage system, to ensure it is upright and below level of tube insertion. | Facilitates drainage. Ensures system is in position to function properly. |

## PLANNING

1. Provide two shodded hemostats for each chest tube, attached to top of patient's bed with adhesive tape. Chest tubes are only clamped under specific circumstances per physician's or health care provider's order or nursing policy and procedure:
   a. To assess air leak (Table 28-9).
   b. To quickly empty or change disposable drainage system; performed by a nurse who has received education in the procedure.
   c. To assess if patient is ready to have chest tube removed (which is done by physician's or health care provider's order); monitor the patient for recurrent pneumothorax.

Shodded hemostats have a covering to prevent hemostat from penetrating chest tube once changed. The use of these shodded hemostats or other clamp prevents air from reentering the pleural space (Allibone, 2003).

| TABLE 28-9 | Problem Solving With Chest Tubes |
|---|---|

| Assessment | Intervention |
|---|---|
| Air leak can occur at insertion site, connection between tube and drainage, or within drainage device itself. Continuous bubbling is noted in water-seal chamber and water seal. | Locate leak by clamping tube at different intervals along the tube. Leaks are corrected when constant bubbling stops. |
| Assess for location of leak by clamping chest tube with two rubber-shodded or toothless clamps close to the chest wall. If bubbling stops, air leak is inside patient's thorax or at chest insertion site. | Unclamp tube, reinforce chest dressing, and notify physician or health care provider immediately. Leaving chest tube clamped can cause collapse of lung, mediastinal shift, and eventual collapse of other lung from buildup of air pressure within the pleural cavity. |
| If bubbling continues with the clamps near the chest wall, gradually move one clamp at a time down drainage tubing away from patient and toward suction control chamber. When bubbling stops, leak is in section of tubing or connection between the clamps. | Replace tubing or secure connection, and release clamps. |
| If bubbling still continues, this indicates the leak is in the drainage system. Notify physician or health care provider immediately, and prepare for another chest tube insertion. | Change the drainage system. Make sure chest tubes are patent: remove clamps, eliminate kinks, or eliminate occlusion. |
| Assess for tension pneumothorax, as indicated by:<br>• Severe respiratory distress<br>• Low oxygen saturation<br>• Chest pain<br>• Absence of breath sounds on affected side<br>• Tracheal shift to unaffected side<br>• Hypotension and signs of shock<br>• Tachycardia | Obstructed chest tubes trap air in intrapleural space when air leak originates within the thorax.<br>A flutter (Heimlich) valve or large-gauge needle may be used for short-term emergency release of pressure in the intrapleural space. Have emergency equipment, oxygen, and code cart available because condition is life-threatening. |
| Water seal tube is no longer submerged in sterile fluid due to evaporation. | Add sterile water to water-seal chamber until distal tip is 2 cm under surface level. |

SKILL 28-2 | Care of Patients With Chest Tubes—cont'd

| STEP | RATIONALE |
|---|---|
| 2. Position the patient. | Permits optimal drainage of fluid and/or air. |
| a. Semi-Fowler's position to evacuate air (pneumothorax). | Air rises to highest point in chest. Pneumothorax tubes are usually placed on the anterior aspect at midclavicular line, second or third intercostal space. |
| b. High Fowler's position to drain fluid (hemothorax). | Permits optimal drainage of fluid. Posterior tubes are placed on midaxillary line, eighth or ninth intercostal space. |

## IMPLEMENTATION

| | |
|---|---|
| 1. Be sure tube connection between chest and drainage tube is intact and taped. | Secures chest tube to drainage system and reduces risk of air leak causing breaks in airtight system. |
| a. Make sure water-seal vent is not occluded. | Permits displaced air to pass into atmosphere. |
| b. Make sure suction control chamber vent is not occluded when using suction. Waterless systems have relief valves without caps. | Provides safety factor of releasing excess negative pressure into atmosphere. |
| 2. Coil excess tubing on mattress next to patient. Secure with rubber band, safety pin, or plastic clamp. | Prevents excess tubing from hanging over edge of mattress in dependent loop. It is possible for drainage to collect in loop and occlude drainage system (Allibone, 2003). |
| 3. Adjust tubing to hang in straight line from top of mattress to drainage chamber. | Promotes drainage and prevents fluid or blood from accumulating in pleural cavity. |
| 4. If chest tube is draining fluid, indicate time (e.g., 0900) that you began drainage on drainage bottle's adhesive tape or on write-on surface of disposable commercial system. | Provides a baseline for continuous assessment of type and quality of drainage. |
| 5. Strip or milk chest tube only if indicated (this means compressing the tube to encourage clots to press through the tube): | Stripping causes complications because it creates excessive negative intrapleural pressure (over –100 cm $H_2O$). Milking causes less of a pressure change. |
| *Stripping*—compression along length of the tubing beginning at patient and continuing until reaching the drainage unit. | |
| *Milking*—compressing and releasing the tube sequentially. | |

• *Critical Decision Point:* Check your institutional policy before stripping or milking chest tubes. Most institutions have stopped this practice because stripping the tube greatly increases intrapleural pressure, which possibly damages the pleural tissue and will cause or worsen an existing pneumothorax. However, even though the literature is contradictory, you will perform stripping or milking in selected patients (e.g., fresh postoperative thoracic surgery or chest traumas). The rationale for selective use of stripping or milking is that the presence of clotted tube drainage decreases reexpansion and increases risk of tension pneumothorax (Allibone, 2003). Thus the benefits of stripping or milking outweigh the risks.

| | |
|---|---|
| a. You manipulate postoperative mediastinal chest tubes if nursing assessment indicates an obstruction or decreased drainage from clots or debris in the tubing. | Stripping is controversial and performed only if hospital policy permits and there is a physician's or health care provider's order. Stripping creates a high degree of negative pressure and has potential of pulling lung tissue or pleura into drainage hole of the chest tube (Carroll, 1991). |
| 6. Perform hand hygiene. | Reduces transmission of microorganisms. |

| STEP | RATIONALE |
|---|---|

## EVALUATION

1. Monitor vital signs, pulse oximetry as ordered.

Provides ongoing data regarding patient level of oxygenation.

2. Observe:

a. Chest tube dressing. Check the dressing carefully; it can come loose from the skin, although this is not always readily apparent.

Appearance of drainage is sometimes due to an occluded tube, causing drainage to exit around tube.

b. Make sure tubing is free of kinks and dependent loops.

Straight and coiled drainage tube positions are optimal for pleural drainage. However, when dependent loop is unavoidable, periodic lifting and draining of the tube will also promote pleural drainage.

c. Make sure the chest drainage system is upright and below level of tube insertion. Note presence of clots or debris in tubing. Monitor the position of the system relative to the chest tube carefully, especially during patient transport.

Ensures system is in position to function.

d. Water seal for fluctuations with patient's inspiration and expiration.

(1) Waterless system: diagnostic indicator for fluctuations with patient's inspirations and expirations.

In the non–mechanically ventilated patient, fluid rises in the water seal or diagnostic indicator with inspiration and falls with expiration. The opposite occurs in the patient who is mechanically ventilated. This indicates that the system is functioning properly (Lewis and others, 2004).

(2) Water-seal system: bubbling in the water-seal chamber.

When you initially connect system to the patient, expect bubbles from the chamber. These are from air that was present in the system and in the patient's intrapleural space. After a short time, the bubbling stops. Fluid continues to fluctuate in the water seal on inspiration and expiration until the lung reexpands or the system becomes occluded.

(3) Water-seal system: bubbling is in the suction control chamber (when suction is being used).

Suction control chamber has constant gentle bubbling. Tubing should be free of obstruction, and the suction source should be turned to the appropriate setting.

e. Waterless system: bubbling is diagnostic indicator.

Mechanism serves for presence of tidaling.

f. Type and amount of fluid drainage: Note color and amount of drainage, patient's vital signs, and skin color. What is the normal amount of drainage?

(1) In the adult, less than 50 to 200 ml/hr immediately after surgery in a mediastinal chest tube; approximately 500 ml in the first 24 hours.

Dark-red drainage is normal only in the postoperative period, turning serous with time (Lewis and others, 2004).

(2) Between 100 and 300 ml of fluid drains in a pleural chest tube in an adult during the first 2 hours after insertion. This rate decreases after 2 hours; expect 500 to 1000 ml in the first 24 hours. Drainage is grossly bloody during the first several hours after surgery and then changes to serous (Lewis and others, 2004). A sudden gush of drainage is often retained blood and not active bleeding and is usually the result of patient repositioning.

Reexpansion of lungs forces drainage into the tube. Coughing also causes large gushes of drainage or air. Report excessive amounts and/or the continued presence of frank bloody drainage the first several hours after surgery to the physician or health care provider, along with patient's vital signs and respiratory status.

---

- *Critical Decision Point:* If drainage suddenly increases or if there is more than 100 ml/hour of blood drainage (except for the first 3 hours postoperative), inform the physician or health care provider and remain with the patient and assess vital signs, oxygen saturation by pulse oximetry, and cardiopulmonary status (Allibone, 2003).

## SKILL 28-2 ¦ Care of Patients With Chest Tubes—cont'd

| STEP | RATIONALE |
|---|---|
| g. Waterless system: The suction control (float ball) indicates the amount of suction the patient's intrapleural space is receiving. | The suction float ball dictates the amount of suction in the system. The float ball allows no more suction than dictated by its setting. If the suction source is set too low, the suction float ball cannot reach the prescribed setting. In this case, increase the suction for the float ball to reach the prescribed setting. |
| 3. Evaluate patient for decreased respiratory distress and chest pain, breath sounds over affected lung area, and $SpO_2$. | Increase in respiratory distress, decrease in breath sounds, marked cyanosis, asymmetrical chest wall movements, presence of subcutaneous emphysema around insertion site or neck, hypotension, tachycardia, and/or mediastinal shift are critical and indicate a severe change in patient status, such as excessive blood loss or tension pneumothorax. Notify physician or health care provider immediately. |
| 4. Ask patient to rate level of comfort on a scale of 0 to 10. | Indicates need for analgesia. Patient with chest tube discomfort hesitates to take deep breaths and as a result is at risk for pneumonia and atelectasis. |

## RECORDING AND REPORTING

■ Record and report patency of chest tubes; presence, type, and amount of drainage; presence of fluctuations; patient's vital signs; chest dressing status; amount of suction and/or water seal; patient's level of comfort.

## UNEXPECTED OUTCOMES AND RELATED INTERVENTIONS

■ Air leak unrelated to patient respirations
  • Locate source (see Table 28-10, p. 812).
  • Notify physician or health care provider.
  • Drain tubing contents into drainage bottle. Coil excess tubing on mattress and secure in place, or place in a straight line down the length of the bed.
■ Tension pneumothorax is present.
  • Determine that chest tubes are not clamped, kinked, or occluded. Obstructed chest tubes trap air in intrapleural space when air leak originates within patient.
  • Notify physician or health care provider immediately.
  • Prepare immediately for another chest tube insertion. Obtain a flutter (Heimlich) valve or large-gauge needle for short-term emergency release of air in intrapleural space. Have emergency equipment (e.g., oxygen, code cart) near patient.

■ Continuous bubbling is in water-seal chamber, indicating that leak is between patient and water seal.
  • Tighten loose connections between patient and water seal.
  • Cross-clamp the chest tube closest to patient's chest. If bubbling stops, the air leak is inside patient's thorax or at chest tube insertion site. Unclamp tube, and notify physician or health care provider immediately. Reinforce chest dressing. Leaving chest tube clamped causes a tension pneumothorax and mediastinal shift.
  • Gradually move clamps down drainage tubing away from patient and toward drainage chamber, moving one clamp at a time. When bubbling stops, leak is in section of tubing or connection distal to the clamp. Replace tubing, or secure connection and release clamp.

The most frequent sensations reported during removal of a chest tube include burning, pain, and a pulling sensation.

***Noninvasive Ventilation.*** Noninvasive ventilation (NIV) maintains positive airway pressure and improves alveolar ventilation without the need for an artificial airway. In addition, this mechanical ventilator alternative reduces and reverses atelectasis, improves oxygenation, reduces pulmonary edema, and improves cardiac function (Woodrow, 2003a). Continuous positive airway pressure keeps the terminal airways (alveoli) partially inflated, reducing the risk for atelectasis. If atelectasis has occurred, positive pressure assists in reinflation. Because the alveoli remain partially inflated, there is a continuous exchange of respiratory gases, and as a result the patient's oxygenation improves. In the cardiac patient, NIV reduces pulmonary edema because the increased alveolar pressure forces interstitial fluid out of the lungs and back into the pulmonary circulation. In patients with altered cardiac function secondary to sleep apnea, NIV provides improved myocardial oxygenation and improved function.

In selected patients, such as those with postpolio syndrome and other neuromuscular diseases, congestive heart failure, sleep disorders, and pulmonary diseases, this is often the treatment of choice in supporting ventilation without the hazards associated with endotracheal intubation (Preston, 2001, Woodrow, 2003b). In addition, when using NIV there is a reduced risk for pneumonia, gastric aspiration, and ventilator dependency (Perkins and Shortall, 2000).

Continuous positive airway pressure (CPAP) has been available for many years and maintains a set positive airway pressure throughout the patient's breathing cycle (Figure 28-11). Therefore a CPAP of 5 cm $H_2O$ provides 5 cm of pressure during inspiration and expiration. It is very beneficial to the patient with sleep apnea. During sleep the upper airway collapses and prevents normal airflow. When the airflow is interrupted, there is a drop in the patient's oxygen saturation and frequent awakenings occur. CPAP uses continuous positive pressure to keep the airway open and prevent upper airway collapse. As a result the patient breathes more normally, sleeps better, and has markedly reduced snoring. The usual CPAP pressure is 5 to 20 cm of water (Perkins and Shortall, 2000). However, there are disadvantages to this device (Box 28-9).

Bilevel positive airway pressure (BiPAP) works by providing assistance during inspiration and preventing airway closure during expiration. During inspiration BiPAP generates a preset positive pressure support, which increases the patient's tidal volume and ultimately alveolar ventilation. This pressure support ends when the patient begins the exhaling; however, a CPAP is maintained within the airways throughout the expiratory phase (Preston, 2001). As a result there is an increase in the functional residual capacity (the amount of air remaining in the lungs at the end of expiration), reduced airway closure, reexpansion of atelectatic area, and improved oxygenation. BiPAP is delivered via a large face mask, so patients may find it uncomfortable and noisy as well.

The goals of NIV include improved ventilation and sleep, enhanced quality of life, reduction of morbidity, improvement of physical and physiological function, and cost-effectiveness

*Text continued on p. 810*

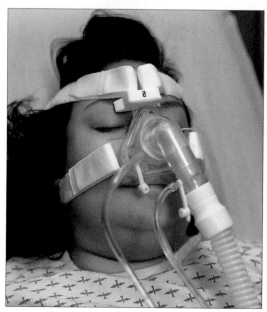

FIGURE **28-11** Mask suitable for either continuous positive airway pressure (CPAP) or bilevel positive airway pressure (BiPAP) device.

### BOX 28-9 Problems Associated With CPAP

| Problem | Cause |
|---|---|
| Discomfort | Large tight-fitting mask that fits over patient's nose.<br>Oxygen flow rate causes dry mucous membranes. |
| Risks to skin integrity | Tight fit of the mask causes pressure and diaphoresis. Patients need to remove the mask to relieve pressure. |
| Hypercapnia | Although CPAP improves alveolar function, which increases carbon dioxide clearance from the blood, it also causes air trapping. In some patients this causes a rise in carbon dioxide levels. |
| Gastric distention | CPAP forces more air into the stomach, which causes distention and discomfort in some patients. In addition, severe gastric distention impedes diaphragmatic motion and reduces lung volumes. |
| Noise | Some patients find the machine very noisy. It interferes not only with sleep, but also with leisure activities. |

Data from Perkins L, Shortall SP: Ventilation without intubation, *RN* 63(1):34, 2000; Woodrow P: Using non-invasive ventilation in acute wards: part I, *Nurs Stand* 18(1):39, 2003.

## SKILL 28-3 | Care of the Patient With Noninvasive Ventilation

### Delegation Considerations

Do not delegate this skill. The nurse is responsible for assessment and evaluation of the patient receiving noninvasive ventilation, as well as determining the safe functioning of the equipment. The nurse must instruct assistive personnel:

- To report any changes in patient's vital signs or $SpO_2$, mental status, or change in skin color
- To notify nurse of a change in patient's level of comfort
- To notify nurse of any difficulty in awakening patient

### Equipment

(NOTE: When device is used in the home, the home care equipment vendor provides the equipment.)
- Nasal mask/full face mask (with quick-release straps) or nasal pillows
- Oxygen source and tubing
- CPAP/BiPAP per physician's or health care provider's order
- Humidification source, if needed
- Pressure generator (in institutional health care settings, the patient's room may have a pressure source)
- Delivery tubing
- Pulse oximetry
- Gloves
- Goggles (if splash risk exists)

| STEP | RATIONALE |
|---|---|
| **ASSESSMENT** | |
| 1. Assess patient's respiratory status, including symmetry of chest wall expansion, respiratory rate and depth, $SpO_2$, sputum production, and lung sounds (see Chapter 13); when possible ask patient about dyspnea, and observe for signs and symptoms associated with hypoxia. | Decreased chest wall movement, crackles or decreased lung sounds, increased respiratory rate, increased sputum production, or hypoxia can indicate the need for noninvasive ventilation to improve oxygenation. |

- *Critical Decision Point:* Patients with sudden changes in their vital signs, level of consciousness, or behavior are possibly experiencing profound hypoxia. Patients who demonstrate subtle changes over time have worsening of a chronic or existing condition or a new medical condition (Jevon and Evans, 2001).

| | |
|---|---|
| 2. Observe patient's ability to clear and remove airway secretions. | Secretions plug the airway, decreasing the amount of oxygen that is available for gas exchange in the lung. |
| 3. If available, note patient's most recent arterial blood gas (ABG) results or arterial oxygen saturation. | Objectively documents the patient's pH, arterial oxygen, arterial $CO_2$, or arterial oxygen saturation. |

- *Critical Decision Point:* If the patient is currently on NIV, evaluate if the therapy is meeting the patient's oxygenation and ventilation needs. Determine what factors have changed, resulting in the new assessment findings.

| | |
|---|---|
| 4. Obtain vital signs before initiation of therapy. | Provides baseline data to compare desired or problematic vital sign changes resulting from the therapy. |
| 5. Review patient's medical record for the medical order for CPAP/BiPAP and appropriate settings. | Physician's or health care provider's order is necessary for this therapy. |

| PLANNING | |
|---|---|
| 1. Explain to patient and family the purpose and reasons for CPAP/BiPAP. | Helps reduce the sense of claustrophobia from the mask. In addition, information reduces anxiety and increases cooperation and compliance with the therapy (Woodrow, 2003a). |

| STEP | RATIONALE |
|---|---|

## IMPLEMENTATION

1. Perform hand hygiene; apply gloves and goggles. Apply barrier gown if secretions are projectile.

2. Determine correct mask size. Use supplied masking charts to determine the correct size (S, M, L, and XL) (see illustration).

3. Connect CPAP/BiPAP device delivery tubing to pressure generator.

Reduces transmission of microorganisms and exposure to pulmonary secretions.

Make sure the mask fits snugly over patient's nose (CPAP) or nose and mouth (BiPAP) because a tight seal is necessary to deliver the positive pressure. It is essential that the mask has quick-release straps so in the case of an emergency (e.g., vomiting, respiratory arrest) you can quickly remove the mask. This quick-release system also allows the patient to remove the mask quickly when needed (Preston, 2001).

Ensures patient is receiving proper noninvasive ventilation as ordered.

---

• **Critical Decision Point:** In some patients it is also necessary to connect oxygen delivery source; however, you will frequently use this equipment without oxygen.

---

4. Connect patient to pulse oximetry.

5. Set CPAP/BiPAP initial settings:
   a. CPAP: 4 to 8 cm $H_2O$
   b. BiPAP:
      (1) Inspiratory usually set at 8 cm $H_2O$
      (2) Expiratory usually set at 4 cm $H_2O$ (Preston, 2001)

6. Perform frequent skin assessment to determine the presence of pressure, skin irritation, or skin breakdown.

7. Dispose of supplies as appropriate, and perform hand hygiene.

It is important to continually monitor the patient's level of oxygenation when beginning NIV (Perkins and Shortall, 2000).

These settings allow the health care team to determine initial patient response. CPAP provides single positive pressure at the end of exhalation, which helps to keep the alveoli open at end-expiration.

BiPAP supplies pressures at both inhalation and exhalation. The inhalation pressure prevents airway closure and the expiratory pressure helps to keep the alveoli open at end-expiration (Preston, 2001).

A mask that is too tight increases the risk for skin breakdown over the bridge of the nose.

Reduces transmission of microorganisms.

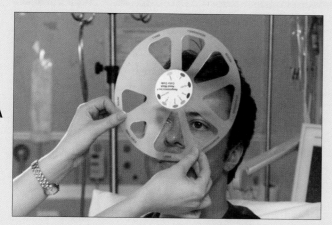

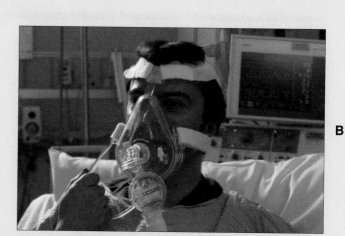

STEP 2 **A,** Mask sizing. **B,** Full face mask with quick-release restraining straps.

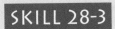

## SKILL 28-3 | Care of the Patient With Noninvasive Ventilation—cont'd

| STEP | RATIONALE |
|---|---|

### EVALUATION

1. Evaluate patient's response to noninvasive ventilation. Observe for decreased anxiety; improved level of consciousness and cognitive abilities; decreased fatigue; absence of dizziness; decreased pulse, regular rhythm; decreased respiratory rate and work of breathing; return to normal blood pressure; improved color.

As hypoxia and hypercapnia are reduced or corrected, the patient's physical assessment parameters will improve.

2. Monitor ABG levels—observe pulse oximetry.

Documents patient's level of oxygenation. When first initiating NIV, especially in patients with underlying COPD, it is important to obtain ABGs after the first hour and every 2 to 6 hours during the first day. These patients often retain carbon dioxide (Perkins and Shortall, 2000).

3. Observe skin integrity over the bridge of the patient's nose.

A mask that is too tight causes skin breakdown, and frequent skin assessment is necessary.

4. Monitor patient's and family's ability to manipulate device and face mask.

Determines patient's ability to perform self-care and to follow CPAP/BiPAP plan.

### RECORDING AND REPORTING

■ Record respiratory assessment findings, CPAP/BiPAP settings, SpO₂, and the patient's response to the noninvasive ventilation.

■ Report any sudden change in patient's respiratory status or worsening ABGs or pulse oximetry.

### UNEXPECTED OUTCOMES AND RELATED INTERVENTIONS

■ Patient experiences hypoxia.
  • Notify physician or health care provider.
  • Reassess patient.
  • Determine correct settings and integrity of noninvasive ventilation system.

■ Patient experiences hypercapnia.
  • Notify physician or health care provider.
  • Reassess patient.
  • Determine correct settings and integrity of noninvasive ventilation system.

■ Patient states a sense of smothering or claustrophobia.
  • Reexplain system to patient.
  • Demonstrate use of quick-release straps.
  • Have patient demonstrate use of quick-release straps.

---

(Perkins and Shortall, 2000; Woodrow, 2003b). You prepare patients and families who are candidates for noninvasive ventilation for discharge by using a multidisciplinary team.

**Maintenance and Promotion of Oxygenation.** Some patients require oxygen therapy to keep a healthy level of tissue oxygenation. The goal of **oxygen therapy** is to prevent or relieve hypoxia. Any patient with impaired tissue oxygenation will benefit from controlled oxygen administration. Oxygen is not a substitute for other treatments. Use it only when indicated. Oxygen is a drug. It is expensive and has dangerous side effects. As with any drug, you continuously monitor the dosage or concentration of oxygen. Routinely

check the physician's or health care provider's orders to verify that the patient is receiving the prescribed oxygen concentration. The six rights of medication administration also apply to oxygen administration (see Chapter 14).

*Safety Precautions With Oxygen Therapy.* Oxygen is a highly combustible gas and fuels fire readily. Although it will not spontaneously burn or cause an explosion, it can easily cause a fire to ignite in a patient's room if it contacts a spark from a cigarette or electrical equipment.

With increasing use of home oxygen therapy, patients and health care professionals need to be aware of these dangers of combustion. Promote safety by using the following measures:

- Place "No smoking" signs on the patient's room door and over the bed. Inform the patient, visitors, roommates, and all personnel that smoking is not permitted in areas where oxygen is in use.
- Determine that all electrical equipment in the room is functioning correctly and is properly grounded (see Chapter 26).
- Know the fire procedures and the location of the closest fire extinguisher.
- Check the oxygen level of portable tanks before transporting to ensure there is enough oxygen in the tank.

***Oxygen Supply.*** Oxygen tanks or a permanent wall-piped system supplies oxygen to the patient's bedside. Oxygen tanks are transported on wide-based carriers that allow the tank to be upright at the patient's bedside. Regulators control the amount of oxygen delivered. One common type of oxygen tank is an upright flow meter with a flow-adjustment valve at the top. A second type is a cylinder indicator with a flow-adjustment handle.

***Methods of Oxygen Delivery.*** Nasal cannula, nasal catheter, face mask, and the mechanical ventilator are all ways to deliver oxygen to the patient (Table 28-10).

HOME OXYGEN. Indications for home oxygen therapy include $PaO_2$ of 55 mm Hg or less or $SaO_2$ of 88% or less on room air at rest, on exertion, or with exercise.

When home oxygen is necessary, it is usually delivered by nasal cannula. If your patient has a permanent tracheostomy, a T tube or tracheostomy collar is necessary to provide humidification to the airway.

Three types of oxygen systems are used: compressed oxygen, liquid oxygen, and oxygen concentrators. You assess the advantages and disadvantages of each type, along with the patient's needs and community resources, before placing a certain delivery system in the home. In the home the major consideration is the oxygen delivery source.

Patients requiring home oxygen need extensive teaching to be able to continue oxygen therapy at home efficiently and safely. This includes oxygen safety, regulation of the amount of oxygen, and how to use the prescribed home oxygen delivery system. You will need to coordinate the efforts of the patient and the family, home care nurse, home respiratory therapist, and home oxygen equipment vendor. The social worker usually assists with arranging the home care nurse and oxygen vendor.

**Restoration of Cardiopulmonary Functioning.** When hypoxia is severe and prolonged, cardiac arrest results. A cardiac arrest is a sudden cessation of cardiac output and circulation. When this occurs, the tissues do not receive oxygen, carbon dioxide is not transported from tissues, tissue metabolism becomes anaerobic, and metabolic and respiratory acidosis occurs. Permanent heart, brain, and other tissue damage occur within 4 to 6 minutes.

***Cardiopulmonary Resuscitation.*** An absence of pulse and respiration characterizes cardiac arrest. If you determine that the patient has experienced a cardiac arrest, begin **cardiopulmonary resuscitation (CPR)**. CPR is a basic emergency procedure of artificial respiration and manual external cardiac

massage. The "ABCs" of CPR are to establish an airway, initiate breathing, and maintain circulation. When you cannot establish an airway, reassess proper head position and assess for airway obstruction. The 2005 guidelines for CPR do not recommend that lay rescuers perform blind sweeps of the mouth or abdominal thrusts (American Heart Association, 2005). The recommendation is to begin standard CPR after calling 9-1-1 for adult victims, unless they have been involved in a drowning, drug overdose, or trauma. The rate of compression for an adult, child, or infant is more than 100 compressions per minute. The ratio of compressions to breaths in one- and two-rescuer CPR for persons 8 years or older and for one-rescuer child or infant is 30 compressions to 2 ventilations. A ratio of 15 compressions to 2 ventilations is used in infant and child 2-rescuer CPR (American Heart Association, 2005).

Defibrillation is recommended within 5 minutes for an out-of-hospital sudden cardiac arrest and within 3 minutes for an in-hospital victim. The recommendation further states that in addition to health care providers, specific lay individuals, police, firefighters, security personnel, ski patrol members, ferryboat crews, and airline flight attendants need training in CPR and the use of an automated external defibrillator (AED) (American Heart Association, 2005) (Box 28-10).

When a 12-lead ECG finds an acute myocardial infarction (AMI), this indicates the administration of clot-busting medications, usually administered in the prehospital setting. You must give the medication within a few hours of the myocardial infarction or stroke (American Heart Association, 2005).

**RESTORATIVE AND CONTINUING CARE.** Restorative and continuing care emphasize cardiopulmonary reconditioning as a structured rehabilitation program. **Cardiopulmonary rehabilitation** is actively assisting the patient to achieve and maintain an optimal level of health through controlled physical exercise, nutrition counseling, relaxation and stress management techniques, prescribed medications, and oxygen administration. As physical reconditioning occurs, the patient's physical symptoms, anxiety, depression, or somatic concerns decrease. The patient and the rehabilitation team define the goals of rehabilitation.

**Respiratory Muscle Training.** Respiratory muscle training improves strength and endurance, resulting in improved activity tolerance. Respiratory muscle training will possibly prevent respiratory failure in patients with COPD.

***Breathing Exercises.*** Breathing exercises include techniques to improve ventilation and oxygenation. The three basic techniques are deep breathing and coughing exercises, pursed-lip breathing, and diaphragmatic breathing. Review coughing techniques on p. 787.

**Pursed-lip breathing** involves deep inspiration and prolonged expiration through pursed lips to prevent alveolar collapse. While sitting up, instruct the patient to take a deep breath and to exhale slowly through pursed lips. Patients need to gain control of the exhalation phase so that exhalation is longer than inhalation. The patient is usually able to perfect this technique by counting inhalation time and gradually increasing the count during exhalation.

| TABLE 28-10 | **Oxygen Delivery Systems** | | |
|---|---|---|---|
| **Delivery System** | **Indications** | **O₂ Concentration (Flow Rate)** | **Considerations** |
| Nasal cannula | Simple, comfortable device to deliver low-concentration $O_2$ (<6 L/min) | 24% (1 L/min)<br>28% (2 L/min)<br>32% (3 L/min)<br>36% (4 L/min)<br>40% (5 L/min)<br>44% (6 L/min) | Flow rates more than 4 L/min often cause drying effect on mucosa; humidify oxygen; be alert for skin breakdown over ears and in nares; questionable efficiency in mouth breathers |
| Transtracheal $O_2$ (TTO) | For chronic lung diseases; small, IV-size catheter inserted directly into trachea | Flow requirements may be reduced to 60%-80%, which greatly increases amount of time available from portable source of $O_2$ | No $O_2$ lost to atmosphere; patients achieve adequate oxygenation at lower rates (more efficient, less expensive, and produces fewer side effects); patients more likely to use $O_2$ because of mobility, comfort, and cosmetic improvement |
| **Oxygen masks** | Administer $O_2$, humidity, or heated humidity | | Be alert for skin breakdown around face and ears |
| Simple face mask | Short-term $O_2$ therapy | 30%-60% (6-8 L/min) | Contraindicated for patients with carbon dioxide retention; effective for mouth breathers (see illustration) |
| Plastic face mask with a reservoir bag | Delivers high concentrations of $O_2$ | 80%-90% (10 L/min) | Frequently inspect the bag to make sure it is inflated (see illustration) |
| Venturi mask | Can deliver precise, high-flow rates of $O_2$; adapters can be applied to increase humidification | 24% (2 L/min)<br>28% (3 L/min)<br>30% (4 L/min)<br>35% (6 L/min)<br>40% (8 L/min)<br>45% (10 L/min)<br>55% (14 L/min) | Mask must be removed when patient eats (see illustration) |

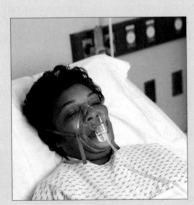

Simple face mask.

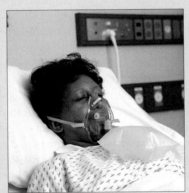

Plastic face mask with inflated reservoir bag.

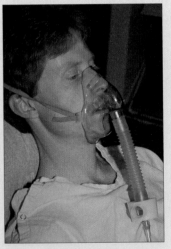

Venturi mask.

**Diaphragmatic breathing** is more difficult and requires the patient to relax intercostal and accessory respiratory muscles while taking deep inspirations. The patient concentrates on expanding the diaphragm during controlled inspiration. Teach the patient to place one hand flat below the breastbone above the waist and the other hand 2 to 3 cm below the first hand. Then ask the patient to inhale while the lower hand moves outward during inspiration. The patient observes for inward movement as the diaphragm ascends. You initially teach these exercises with the patient in the supine position and then practice while the patient sits and stands. The exercise is often used with the pursed-lip breathing technique.

- Is a device used to administer an electrical shock through the chest wall to the heart.
- Has built-in computers that assess the victim's heart rhythm and determine if defibrillation is needed.
- Delivers a shock to the victim after announcing "Everyone stand back."

- Can be used by nonmedical personnel.
- Is used to strengthen the chain of survival. Every minute of a sudden cardiac death without defibrillation decreases the survival rate by 7% to 10% (American Heart Association, 2003).

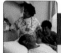

## EVALUATION

Mary cares for Mr. King throughout his hospital stay. He is able to go home with improved activities of daily living. He is now able to walk to the mailbox to get the mail, bathe himself, and accompany his wife to the grocery store. He does not require supplemental oxygen use at home. Because he now practices pursed-lip breathing, his breathing is more controlled, relieving his subsequent anxiety.

Mr. King is afebrile, his white blood cells are within normal limits, and his sputum cultures are negative at discharge. He is able to describe ways to prevent respiratory infections, because they aggravate airways and precipitate an episode of acute respiratory failure.

While Mary is observing Mr. King preparing for discharge, it is quite evident that Mr. King is using the various breathing techniques that they have worked on together. His wife even appears less anxious and states she feels as though for the first time they have taken a step (even though small) to improve the quality of their lives.

**Documentation Note**

"Mr. King discharged to home. Able to state the purpose of breathing exercises and each medication, able to list causes and symptoms of respiratory tract infection. Has an appointment in 1 week with a community-based rehabilitation program. Scheduled to see his physician or health care provider in 2 weeks. Prescriptions explained and given to patient. Accompanied to the exit. Left with wife and son."

## OUTCOME EVALUATION

TABLE 28-11

| Nursing Action | Patient Response/Finding | Achievement of Outcome |
|---|---|---|
| Ask Mr. King to keep track of his fluid intake. | Mr. King has completed accurate intake list daily, averaging 2400 ml/hr. Coughing thin secretions. | Good daily fluid intake. Secretions are thin, white, and watery. Outcome met. |
| Ask Mr. King to ambulate for 10 minutes every 4 hours. | Mr. King ambulates once every 8 hours. | Mr. King has met the goal half of the time. Outcome not completely achieved. |
| Auscultate the chest. | Lung sounds are clear. | Outcome met. |
| Ask Mr. King to keep track of deep breathing every 2 hours while awake. | Diary completed for each day. Mr. King has documented deep breathing every 2 hours while awake 85% of the time. | Secretions are thin, the lung is clear, and there is no evidence of infection. Outcome met. |

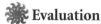 **Evaluation**

**PATIENT CARE.** You evaluate nursing interventions and therapies by comparing the patient's progress to the goals and desired outcomes of the nursing care plan. When nursing measures directed to improve oxygenation are unsuccessful, modify the care plan by revising existing interventions or introducing new interventions. Do not hesitate to notify the physician or health care provider about a patient's deteriorating oxygenation status. Prompt notification will help to avoid an emergency situation or even the need for CPR.

Management of the patient with COPD depends on achieving three major goals: reduction of airflow obstruction, prevention or management of complications, and improvement in the patient's quality of life.

Patients with chronic cardiopulmonary disease present a nursing challenge. They require frequent nursing interventions when they are acutely ill. Because this is a chronic disease, do not think in terms of recovery, but rather health maintenance. You are caring for patients with a debilitating disease. You will not see a dramatic cure. You will be assisting patients to improve the quality of their lives in small but significant ways.

**PATIENT EXPECTATIONS.** Individualize the goals that you set for the patient, and make sure they are realistic. Patients need to know how to cope with this chronic disease. Before any teaching program is effective, the patient must want to learn. Ask the patient if he or she would like to know more about COPD and how to control it. Inform the patient that it is possible to gain greater independence, improve mobility, decrease dyspnea, and decrease the frequency of acute respiratory infections. Presenting an individualized education program, based on assessment data, helps to ensure the patient will comprehend, learn, use, and ultimately benefit from the education (Table 28-11).

## KEY CONCEPTS

- The primary function of the heart is to deliver deoxygenated blood to the lungs for oxygenation and to deliver oxygen and nutrients to the tissues.
- Cardiac dysrhythmias are classified by cardiac activity and site of impulse origin.
- The primary function of the lungs is to transfer oxygen from the atmosphere into the alveoli and carbon dioxide out of the body as a waste product.
- Ventilation is the process of providing adequate oxygenation from the alveoli to the blood.
- The process of inspiration (active process) and expiration (passive process) is achieved with lung changes in pressures and volumes.
- The central nervous system and chemicals within the blood control respiration.
- Decreased hemoglobin levels alter the patient's ability to transport oxygen.
- Impaired chest wall movement reduces the level of tissue oxygenation.
- Hyperventilation is a respiratory rate greater than that required to maintain normal levels of carbon dioxide.
- Hypoventilation causes carbon dioxide retention.
- Hypoxia occurs if the amount of oxygen delivered to tissues is too low.
- The nursing assessment includes information about the patient's cough, dyspnea, fatigue, wheezing, chest pain, environmental exposures, respiratory infection, cardiopulmonary risk factors, use of medications, and physical functioning.
- Pursed-lip breathing is an effective intervention to control breathing and increase oxygenation.
- Breathing exercises improve ventilation, oxygenation, and sensations of dyspnea.
- Nebulization delivers small drops of water or particles of medication to the airways.
- Chest physiotherapy includes postural drainage, percussion, and vibration to mobilize pulmonary secretions.
- Coughing and suctioning techniques maintain a patent airway.
- Oxygen therapy improves levels of tissue oxygenation and is delivered by nasal cannula, nasal catheter, or oxygen mask.

## CRITICAL THINKING IN PRACTICE

*You are assigned to care for Mrs. Schwartz, a 63-year-old retired executive. She has a history of COPD and has been complaining of upper respiratory symptoms, including increasing shortness of breath, fever, nonproductive cough, nausea, and malaise.*

- - - - - - - - - - - - - - - - - - - -

1. Mrs. Schwartz complains that she is unable to expectorate her sputum. She is able to cough up the pulmonary secretions, but the secretions remain in her mouth, causing her nausea. What nursing intervention is appropriate to help with her oral secretions?
   a. Nasotracheal suctioning
   b. Oropharyngeal suctioning
   c. Yankauer suctioning
   d. Closed inline suctioning
2. During your rounds you assess Mrs. Schwartz. You observe she has labored breathing and is using the accessory muscles of respiration. Her lungs have bibasilar crackles and diminished breath sounds. She is complaining of increasing shortness of breath and right-sided chest pain.

Her temperature is 102.8° F, and she is diaphoretic. Your next actions would include:
   a. Notifying the charge nurse and physician or health care provider of a change in condition
   b. Checking a pulse oximeter and blood pressure
   c. Forcing fluids and changing her position frequently
   d. Arranging for a chest x-ray examination
3. The physician or health care provider has examined the patient and ordered ABGs, chest x-ray examination, continuous pulse oximetry, vital signs every 2 hours, and oxygen via face mask at 40%. What signs do you need to observe for in this patient?
   a. Worsening respiratory failure
   b. Increased sputum production
   c. Respiratory rate and pattern
   d. Fatigue
   e. All of the above
4. What preparations do you make in anticipation of acute respiratory failure? List possible nursing interventions.

## NCLEX® REVIEW

1. Assessment of your patient with tachycardia should include:
   1. Risk factors for CAD
   2. Consumption of caffeine and herbal substances
   3. Heart rate, blood pressure, and respiratory rate
   4. Nutritional assessment for high-fat foods and poor nutrition

2. When assessing the patient's oxygenation you would include:
   1. Complete blood count (CBC) and chest x-ray examination
   2. Heart rate and respiratory rate
   3. ABG levels and pulse oximetry
   4. Chest x-ray examination, heart rate, respiratory rate, and ABG levels

**3.** A normal-appearing ECG tracing with a heart rate of 125 beats per minute would be considered:
 **1.** Sinus rhythm
 **2.** Sinus bradycardia
 **3.** Sinus tachycardia
 **4.** Ventricular tachycardia

**4.** Incentive spirometry is used to:
 **1.** Promote coughing
 **2.** Replace the need for early ambulation
 **3.** Promote deep breathing and prevent atelectasis
 **4.** Decrease the need for analgesia

**5.** More precise oxygen concentrations can be achieved using a:
 **1.** Nasal cannula
 **2.** Simple face mask without inflated reservoir bag
 **3.** Venturi mask system
 **4.** Plastic face mask with inflated reservoir bag

**6.** When caring for a patient with a decreased hemoglobin level, it is important to remember that:
 **1.** The patient is at risk for bleeding
 **2.** The patient has altered oxygen transport
 **3.** The patient is at risk for elevated carbon dioxide levels
 **4.** The patient has alterations in the chemical regulators of respiration

**7.** A patient is a candidate for chest physiotherapy if:
 **1.** The patient is receiving long-term steroids
 **2.** The patient has had abdominal surgery
 **3.** The patient has increased intracranial pressure
 **4.** The patient has good exercise tolerance and can follow instructions

## REFERENCES

Akgul S, Akyolcu N: Effects of normal saline on endotracheal suction, *J Clin Nurs* 11(6):826, 2002.

Allibone L: Nursing management of chest drains, *Nurs Stand* 17(22):45, 2003.

American Heart Association: *CPR and AEDs,* 2003, http://www.AHA.org.

American Heart Association: *CPR,* 2005, http://www.Americanheart.org.

American Heart Association: Part 3 Overview of CPR, *Circulation,* 112: IV-12: 2005.

Canobbio MM: *Cardiovascular disorders,* St. Louis, 1990, Mosby.

Carroll P: A guide to mobile chest drains, *RN* 65(5):56, 2002.

Carroll PF: What's new in chest-tube management, *RN* 54(5):34, 1991.

Centers for Disease Control and Prevention: Recommended adult immunization schedule—United States, October 2004-September 2005, *MMWR* 53(45):Q1, 2004.

Centers for Disease Control and Prevention: *Respiratory syncytial virus,* 2005, http://www.cdc.gov/neidod/dyra/revb/resp/rsvfeat.htm.

Day T and others: Tracheal suctioning: an exploration of nurses' knowledge and competence in acute and high dependency ward areas, *J Adv Nurs* 39(1):35, 2002.

Dochterman JM, Bulechek GM, editors: *Nursing interventions classification (NIC),* ed 4, St. Louis, 2004, Mosby.

Freytag CC and others: Prolonged application of closed in-line suction catheters increase microbial colonization of lower respiratory tract bacterial growth on catheter surface, *Infection* 31(1):31, 2003.

Jevon P, Ewens B: Assessment of a breathless patient, *Nurs Stand* 15(16):48, 2001.

Lewis SL and others: *Medical surgical nursing: assessment and management of clinical problems,* ed 6, St. Louis, 2004, Mosby.

Moore T: Suctioning techniques for the removal of respiratory secretions, *Nurs Stand* 18(9):47, 2003.

Moorhead S, Johnson M, Maas M: *Nursing outcomes classification (NOC),* ed 3, St. Louis, 2004, Mosby.

Perkins L, Shortall SP: Ventilation without intubation, *RN* 63(1):34, 2000.

Perry AG, Potter PA: *Clinical nursing skills and techniques,* ed 6, St. Louis, 2006, Mosby.

Preston R: Introducing non-invasive positive pressure ventilation, *Nurs Stand* 15(26):42, 2001.

Puntillo KA and others: Pain assessment and management in the critically ill: wizardry or science? *Am J Crit Care* 12(4):10, 2003.

Seidel HM and others: *Mosby's guide to physical examination,* ed 5, St. Louis, 2003, Mosby.

Sole ML and others: A multisite survey of suction techniques and airway management practices, *Am J Crit Care* 12(30):220, 2003.

Thibodeau GA, Patton KT: *Structure and function of the body,* ed 12, St. Louis, Mosby, 2004.

Wilson SF, Thompson JM: *Mosby's clinical nursing series: respiratory disorders,* St. Louis, 1990, Mosby.

Woodrow P: Using non-invasive ventilation in acute wards: part I, *Nurs Stand* 18(1):39, 2003a.

Woodrow P: Using non-invasive ventilation in acute wards: part II, *Nurs Stand* 18(1):41, 2003b.

Woodruff DW: Pneumothorax, *RN* 62(9):62, 1999.

# CHAPTER 29

# Sleep

## MEDIA RESOURCES

**CD COMPANION** **evolve** **WEBSITE**

http://evolve.elsevier.com/Potter/basic

- **NCLEX® Review**
- **Audio Glossary**
- **English/Spanish Audio Glossary**

## OBJECTIVES

- Compare the characteristics of rest and sleep.
- Explain the effect the 24-hour sleep-wake cycle has on biological function.
- Discuss mechanisms that regulate sleep.
- Describe the normal stages of sleep.
- Explain the functions of sleep.
- Compare and contrast the characteristics of sleep for different age-groups.
- Identify factors that normally promote and disrupt sleep.

- Discuss characteristics of common sleep disorders.
- Gather a sleep history for a patient.
- Describe interventions appropriate in promoting sleep for patients with various sleep disorders.
- Discuss differences in sleep interventions used for patients of different age-groups.
- Develop a teaching plan to improve a patient's sleep hygiene.
- Describe ways to evaluate sleep therapies.

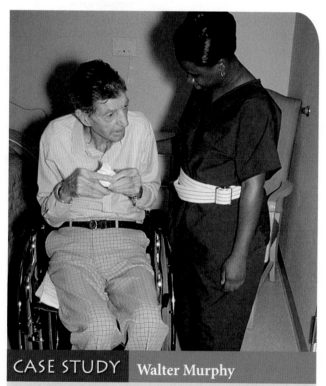

## CASE STUDY  Walter Murphy

Walter Murphy is an 82-year-old patient who has resided in the local nursing home for the last 3 months. His wife, Mary, still lives at home but visits Walter on a daily basis. Walter is confined to a wheelchair as a result of osteoarthritis and a mild stroke he experienced just 1 year ago. Even though he has physical limitations, he is alert and oriented. Over the last several weeks, Mary has found her husband to be very sleepy when she visits him just before lunchtime. Walter tells Mary that he has trouble falling asleep at night, and once he does fall asleep, he reawakens frequently during the night. Mary is concerned because her husband does not seem as alert or interested during her visit.

Anna is a 23-year-old junior student assigned to the nursing home for her second semester in nursing school. She has had experience in nursing homes, having worked in one center as a nurse assistant during the last two summers. Anna's assignment is to care for Mr. Murphy over the next 4 weeks.

### KEY TERMS

Advanced sleep phase syndrome, p. 820
Biological clock, p. 818
Cataplexy, p. 824
Circadian rhythm, p. 818
Excessive daytime sleepiness, p. 820
Hypnotics, p. 832
Insomnia, p. 822

Narcolepsy, p. 824
Nocturia, p. 831
Nonrapid eye movement (NREM) sleep, p. 818
Rapid eye movement (REM) sleep, p. 818
Sedatives, p. 832
Sleep, p. 818
Sleep apnea, p. 822
Sleep deprivation, p. 824

Physical and emotional health depend on adequate sleep and rest. Without proper amounts of rest and sleep, the ability to concentrate, make judgments, promote healing, and participate in daily activities decreases. To help a patient gain needed rest and sleep, you need to understand the nature of sleep, the factors influencing it, and the patient's sleep habits. Nurses care for patients who often have preexisting sleep disturbances and for patients who develop sleep problems as a result of illness or being in the health care environment. You will learn to use an individualized approach based on patients' personal sleep habits and pattern of sleep to provide effective sleep therapies.

## Scientific Knowledge Base

### Sleep and Rest

When people are at rest, they usually feel mentally relaxed, free from anxiety, and physically calm. They are in a state of mental and physical activity that leaves them feeling refreshed, rejuvenated, and ready to resume the activities of the day. Rest does not imply inactivity, although everyone often thinks of it as settling down in a comfortable chair or taking a brief nap. All persons have their own habits for obtaining rest. For example, reading a book, practicing a relaxation exercise (see Chapter 30), or taking long walks are all restful habits.

**Sleep** is a recurrent, altered state of consciousness that occurs for sustained periods. When persons get proper sleep, they feel that their energy has been restored. Some experts believe that these feelings of energy restoration imply that sleep provides time for the repair and recovery of body systems for the next period of wakefulness.

## Physiology of Sleep

Sleep is a cyclical physiological process that alternates with longer periods of wakefulness. The sleep-wake cycle influences and regulates body functions and behavioral responses.

**CIRCADIAN RHYTHMS.** People experience cyclical rhythms as part of their everyday life. The most familiar rhythm is the 24-hour, day-night cycle known as the diurnal or **circadian rhythm.** Light and temperature affect all circadian rhythms, including the sleep-wake cycle. External factors such as social activities and environmental stressors also affect circadian rhythms. The natural secretion of melatonin supports circadian rhythm in the sleep-wake cycle by helping to ensure a smooth transition from wakefulness to sleep (Hilton, 2002). Every person has a **biological clock** that is normally synchronized by exposure to light and activity. Some people fall asleep at 8 PM, whereas others go to bed at midnight or early in the morning. Different people also function best at different times of the day.

The normal rhythm of sleep is synchronized with other body functions. Normal variations in body temperature, for example, correlate with sleep-wake patterns (see Chapter 12). When the sleep-wake cycle becomes disrupted (e.g., by working rotating shifts), other physiological functions change as well. For example, a person sometimes experiences a decreased appetite and loses weight. Failure to obtain sufficient sleep adversely affects a person's overall health. For example, a change in sleep patterns may lead to overeating or loss of appetite.

**SLEEP-WAKE REGULATION.** Sleep-wake is a dual process that has two distinct states (Jones, 2005). It involves a sequence of physiological states maintained by highly integrated central nervous system (CNS) activity that is associated with changes in the peripheral nervous, endocrine, cardiovascular, respiratory, and muscular systems (McCance and Heuther, 2002). Each sequence is identified by specific physiological responses and patterns of brain activity. The control and regulation of the sleep-wake state depends on the interrelationship between two cerebral mechanisms that intermittently activate and suppress the brain's higher centers to control sleep and wakefulness (Figure 29-1). The neurons in the brain stem reticular formation maintain a state of wakefulness, whereas the neurons in the parasympathetic control centers maintain a state of sleep.

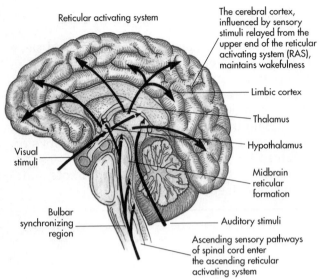

FIGURE **29-1** The RAS and BSR control sensory input, intermittently activating and suppressing the brain's higher centers to control sleep and wakefulness.

When you try to fall asleep, you close your eyes, assume a relaxed position, and have the room dark, quiet, and at a comfortable temperature. Stimuli to the reticular activating system (RAS) in the upper brain stem decline. Gradually the bulbar synchronizing region (BSR) takes over, causing sleep. You will generally not reawaken until you finish your usual sleep cycle or stimuli in the environment (e.g., traffic outside or chirping of birds) stimulate the RAS to awaken.

**Stages of Sleep.** Normal sleep involves two phases: **nonrapid eye movement (NREM) sleep** and **rapid eye movement (REM) sleep** (Box 29-1). During NREM an individual progresses through four stages during a typical 90-minute sleep cycle. The quality of sleep from stage 1 through stage 4 becomes increasingly deep. Lighter sleep is characteristic of stages 1 and 2, when a person is more easily arousable. Stages 3 and 4 involve a deeper sleep called slow-wave sleep from which a person is more difficult to arouse. REM sleep is the phase at the end of each 90-minute sleep cycle. During REM sleep there is increased brain activity associated with rapid eye movements and muscle atonia. REM sleep is not divided into stages.

**Sleep Cycle.** Normally an adult's routine sleep pattern begins with a presleep period during which the person is aware only of a gradually developing sleepiness. This period normally lasts 10 to 30 minutes. Individuals experiencing difficulty falling asleep often remain in this stage for an hour or more.

Once asleep, the person usually passes through four to six complete sleep cycles, each consisting of four stages of NREM sleep and a period of REM sleep. The cyclical pattern usually progresses from stage 1 through stage 4 of NREM, followed by a reversal from stage 4 to 3 to 2, ending with a period of REM sleep (Figure 29-2).

With each successive cycle, stages 3 and 4 of NREM sleep shorten and the period of REM lengthens. REM sleep lasts

---

**BOX 29-1  Stages of the Sleep Cycle**

**NREM Stage 1**

Stage includes lightest level of sleep.

Stage lasts a few minutes.

Decreased physiological activity begins with gradual fall in vital signs and metabolism.

Sensory stimuli, such as noise, easily arouse sleeper.

If awakened, person feels as though daydreaming has occurred.

**NREM Stage 2**

Stage is period of sound sleep.

Relaxation progresses.

Arousal is still relatively easy.

Stage lasts 10 to 20 minutes.

Body functions continue to slow.

**NREM Stage 3**

It involves initial stages of deep sleep.

Sleeper is difficult to arouse and rarely moves.

Muscles are completely relaxed.

Vital signs decline but remain regular.

Stage lasts 15 to 30 minutes.

**NREM Stage 4**

It is deepest stage of sleep.

It is very difficult to arouse sleeper.

If sleep loss has occurred, sleeper will spend considerable portion of night in this stage.

Vital signs are significantly lower than during waking hours.

Stage lasts approximately 15 to 30 minutes.

Sleepwalking and enuresis sometimes occur.

**REM Sleep**

Vivid, full-color dreaming occurs.

Stage usually begins about 90 minutes after sleep has begun.

Stage typified by autonomic response of rapidly moving eyes, fluctuating heart and respiratory rates, and increased or fluctuating blood pressure.

Loss of skeletal muscle tone occurs.

Gastric secretions increase.

It is very difficult to arouse sleeper.

Duration of REM sleep increases with each cycle and averages 20 minutes.

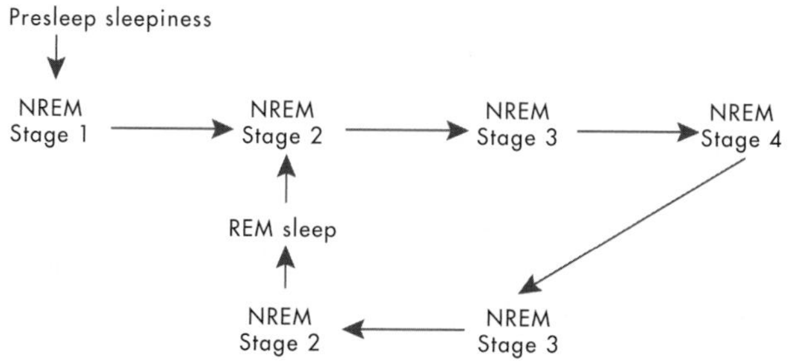

---

FIGURE 29-2 The stages of the adult sleep cycle.

up to 60 minutes during the last sleep cycle. Not all people progress consistently through the usual stages of sleep. For example, a sleeper fluctuates back and forth for short intervals between NREM stages 2, 3, and 4 before entering REM sleep. The amount of time spent in each stage varies. The number of sleep cycles depends on the total amount of time that the person spends sleeping.

## Functions of Sleep

The purpose of sleep is still unclear. One theory suggests that sleep is a time of restoration and preparation for the next period of wakefulness (McCance and Huether, 2002). During NREM sleep, biological functions slow. A healthy adult's normal heart rate throughout the day averages 70 to 80 beats per minute. However, during sleep the heart rate normally falls to 60 beats per minute or less, thus preserving cardiac function.

Sleep is also a part of maintaining normal biological processes and optimal immune performance (Davis, Parker, and Montgomery, 2004). During NREM stage 4 sleep, the body

releases human growth hormone for the repair and renewal of epithelial and specialized cells such as brain cells (Jones, 2005; McCance and Huether, 2002). Protein synthesis and cell division for the renewal of tissues also occur during rest and sleep.

REM sleep appears to be important for cognitive restoration. Researchers associate REM sleep with changes in cerebral blood flow, increased cortical activity, increased oxygen consumption, and epinephrine release. This association assists with memory storage and learning.

The benefits of sleep often go unnoticed until a person develops a problem resulting from sleep deprivation. A loss of REM sleep leads to feelings of confusion. Various body functions (e.g., motor performance, memory, and immune function) alter when prolonged sleep loss occurs.

**DREAMS.** The dreams of REM sleep are more vivid and elaborate than those of NREM sleep, and researchers believe them to be functionally important to the consolidation of long-term memory and emotional healing (Honkus, 2003). REM dreams progress in content throughout the night from dreams about current events to emotional dreams of childhood or the past. Personality influences the quality of dreams; for example, a creative person may have very vivid, unusual dreams, whereas a depressed person may have dreams of helplessness.

Dreams help people sort out immediate concerns or erase certain fantasies or nonsensical memories. Because most dreams are forgotten, many people have little dream recall and do not believe they dream at all. To remember a dream, a person must consciously think about it on awakening. People who recall dreams vividly usually awaken just after a period of REM sleep.

## Nursing Knowledge Base

### Normal Sleep Requirements and Patterns

Sleep duration and quality vary among persons of all age-groups. The neonate and infant up to the age of 3 months average about 16 hours of sleep a day. Approximately 50% of this sleep is REM sleep, which stimulates the higher brain centers (Hockenberry and others, 2003). Infants usually develop a nighttime pattern of sleep by 3 months of age. Infants sometimes take several naps during the day but usually sleep an average of 9 to 11 hours during the night. Infants spend about 30% of sleep time in the REM cycle. Awakening commonly occurs early in the morning, although infants sometimes wake during the night.

By the age of 2 years, children usually sleep through the night and take daily naps. Total sleep averages 12 hours a day. Some children stop taking naps altogether at age 3. It is common for toddlers to awaken during the night. The percentage of REM sleep continues to fall. Toddlers are often unwilling to go to bed at night. A preschooler sleeps an average of 12 hours a night (about 20% is REM). By the age of 5, the preschooler rarely takes daytime naps (Hockenberry and others, 2003) except in cultures where a siesta is the custom. The preschooler usually has difficulty relaxing or quieting down after long, active days. A preschooler also has problems with bedtime fears, waking during the night, and nightmares.

The school-age child usually does not require a nap. A 6-year-old averages 11 to 12 hours of sleep nightly, whereas an 11-year-old sleeps about 9 to 10 hours (Hockenberry and others, 2003). Encouraging quiet activities usually persuades the 6- or 7-year-old to go to bed. The older child often resists sleeping because of an unawareness of fatigue or a need to be independent. Adolescents need between $8\frac{1}{2}$ and $9\frac{1}{2}$ hours of sleep. At a time when sleep needs actually increase, the typical adolescent is subject to a number of changes that often reduce the time spent sleeping (Carno and others, 2003). The typical teenager gets about $7\frac{1}{2}$ hours of sleep per night. Usually parents no longer set a specific bedtime. School demands, after-school social activities, and part-time jobs lessen time available for sleep. Teens go to bed later and rise earlier during the high school years. Because of lifestyle demands that shorten the time available for sleep and physiological needs, teens often experience **excessive daytime sleepiness (EDS)**. Poor school performance, vulnerability to accidents, behavioral problems, and increased use of alcohol and stimulants are the result of EDS due to insufficient sleep (Walsh and others, 2005).

Most young adults average 6 to $8\frac{1}{2}$ hours of sleep a night, but this varies. Young adults rarely take regular naps. Young adults spend approximately 20% of sleep time in REM sleep, which remains consistent throughout the remainder of life. Healthy young adults require adequate sleep to participate in the day's busy activities. However, lifestyle demands often interrupt usual sleep patterns, which results in insomnia. During middle adulthood the total time spent sleeping at night begins to decline. The amount of stage 4 sleep begins to fall, a decline that continues with advancing age. Health care workers often initially diagnose sleep disturbances among people in this age range even when the symptoms of a disorder have been present for several years. Members of this age-group sometimes rely on sleeping medications.

Complaints of sleeping difficulties increase with age. More than 50% of persons age 65 and older report regular problems with sleep (Hoffman, 2003). Older adults spend more time in stage 1 and have less stage 3 and stage 4 NREM sleep; some older adults have almost no NREM stage 4, or deep sleep. Episodes of REM sleep tend to shorten. Older adults awaken more often during the night, and it takes more time for them to fall asleep. Their sleep efficiency (the amount of time asleep given the amount of time in bed) is reduced, and they increase the number of naps taken during the day (Kryger and others, 2004). Often older adults do not feel refreshed after sleeping (Hoffman, 2003). Tests show that older adults do not have an increased need for sleep, but have a reduction in the ability to sleep.

As people age, their circadian clock advances, causing **advanced sleep phase syndrome.** The syndrome is common in older adults and often is the reason behind the complaint of waking early in the morning and being unable to get back to sleep (Shneerson, 2000). People with the syndrome get sleepy early in the evening (e.g., 8 or 9 PM). If they go to bed at that time, they will sleep for about 8 hours and wake up around 4 or 5 AM. However, when people with advanced sleep phase syndrome stay up until their customary 10 or 11 PM, their bodies still awaken at 4 or 5 AM. Consequently, they receive only 5 to 6 hours of sleep, the amount of time they are in bed before their advanced sleep-wake cycle wakes them up.

### Factors Affecting Sleep

A number of factors (physical, psychological, and environmental) affect the quantity and quality of sleep. Often more than one factor combine to cause a sleep problem.

**PHYSICAL ILLNESS.** Any illness or condition that causes pain, difficulty breathing, nausea, or mood problems such as anxiety or depression can result in sleep problems. Individuals with such alterations have trouble falling or staying asleep. Illnesses also force patients to sleep in positions to which they are unaccustomed. Table 29-1 summarizes illnesses and conditions that have the potential for causing sleep alterations.

**DRUGS AND SUBSTANCES.** A considerable number of drugs cause either sleepiness, insomnia, or fatigue as a side effect (Box 29-2). Medications prescribed for sleep often cause more problems than benefits. L-Tryptophan is a natural protein found in foods such as milk, cheese, and meats and sometimes helps a person sleep. It is a precursor, or forerunner, to the neurotransmitter serotonin, which has a role in the sleep-wake cycle.

**LIFESTYLE.** A persons' daily routine influences sleep patterns. For example, an individual who alternately works

| TABLE 29-1 | **Illnesses and Conditions That Can Alter Sleep** |

| Illness/Condition | Nature of Sleep Alteration |
|---|---|
| Respiratory disease (e.g., emphysema, asthma, bronchitis, allergic rhinitis, common cold) | Shortness of breath requires use of two to three pillows to raise head. Altered rhythm of breathing. Nasal congestion and sore throat impair breathing and ability to relax. |
| Coronary heart disease with episodes of chest pain and irregular heart rates | Frequent awakenings and sleep stage changes during sleep and significant alterations in all stages of sleep. |
| Hypertension | Reduced length and depth of NREM sleep and a shortened REM latency period cause arousals and early morning awakening resulting in fatigue. |
| Hypothyroidism | Decreases slow-wave sleep and REM sleep and increased movements during sleep contribute to daytime sleepiness. |
| Hyperthyroidism | Increase in metabolism causes insomnia due to increased time needed to fall asleep. |
| Nocturia (reduced bladder tone, diabetes, urethritis, prostate disease) | Awakenings at night to urinate; difficulty returning to sleep. |
| Gastric reflux | Burning pain in lower esophagus; increases when lying flat in bed. |
| Depression | Awakenings in early morning with inability to return to sleep; worsened by anxiety or agitation. |
| Pain | Delay in sleep onset, increased sleep awakenings, and decreased slow-wave activity during sleep result in poor sleep quality. Worsened by increased sympathetic activity resulting in high cardiac heart rate. |

| BOX 29-2 | **Effect of Medications and Other Substances on Sleep** |

**Hypnotics**

Interfere with reaching deeper sleep stages
Provide only temporary (1 week) increase in quantity of sleep
Eventually cause "hangover" feeling during day
In some cases, sleep apnea worsens in older adults

**Diuretics (Administered Late in the Day)**

Cause nocturia

**Antidepressants and Stimulants**

Suppress REM sleep
Decrease total sleep time

**Alcohol**

Speeds onset of sleep and disrupts REM sleep
Awakens person during night and causes difficulty returning to sleep

**Caffeine**

Stimulant prevents person from falling asleep
Causes person to awaken during night

**Beta-Adrenergic Blockers**

Cause nightmares and insomnia
Cause awakening from sleep

**Benzodiazepines**

Increase sleep time
Increase daytime sleepiness

**Narcotics (Opiates)**

Suppress REM sleep
Cause increased daytime drowsiness

**Antihistamines**

Cause drowsiness
Excess amounts cause insomnia

**Nasal Decongestants**

Cause daytime sleepiness

day and night shifts often has difficulty adjusting to the altered sleep schedule. Other alterations in routine that disrupt sleep patterns include performing unaccustomed heavy work or exercise, engaging in late-night social activities, and changing evening mealtime.

**USUAL SLEEP PATTERNS AND EXCESSIVE DAYTIME SLEEPINESS.** On average, adults sleep 7 to 7.5 hours per nights on weeknights and 8 or more hours per night on weekends (National Sleep Foundation, 2002). Many Americans suffer from sleep deprivation and experience EDS during the day. EDS often results in impairment of waking function, poor work or school performance, accidents while driving or using equipment, and behavioral or emotional problems. Feelings of sleepiness are usually most intense upon awakening from sleep or right before going to sleep and about 12 hours after the midsleep period.

Sleepiness becomes pathological when it occurs at times when persons need or want to be awake. Persons who temporarily experience sleep deprivation as a result of an active social evening or lengthened work schedule usually feel sleepy the next day. However, they are sometimes able to overcome these feelings even though they have difficulty performing tasks and remaining attentive. Chronic lack of sleep is much more serious than temporary sleep deprivation and causes serious alterations in the ability to perform daily activities. EDS is most difficult to overcome during sedentary tasks (e.g., driving).

**EMOTIONAL STRESS.** Worry over personal problems or situations interfere with sleep. Emotional stress causes tension and often leads to frustration when sleep does not come. Stress also causes a person to try too hard to fall asleep, to awaken frequently during the sleep cycle, or to oversleep. Continued stress causes poor sleep habits in some cases.

**ENVIRONMENT.** The physical environment in which a person sleeps has a significant influence on the ability to fall and remain asleep. Good ventilation, a comfortable temperature, and a darkened or softly lit room are essential for restful sleep. The size, firmness, and position of a bed also affect sleep quality. Hospital beds are often harder than those at home. If a person usually sleeps with another individual, sleeping alone during times of illness causes wakefulness. However, sleeping with a restless or snoring bed partner also disrupts sleep.

**SOUND.** Noise affects sleep activity by decreasing REM activity (Honkus, 2003). Noise easily disturbs older adults' sleep because most of their sleep is in lighter sleep stages. Some persons require silence to fall asleep, whereas others prefer background noise such as soft music or television.

In health care facilities, noise created by caregivers, equipment, and other patients causes a problem for patients. Noise in health care settings is usually new or strange to the patient. This problem is greatest the first night a patient stays in a hospital or other facility, when patients often experience increased total wake time, increased awakening, and decreased REM sleep and total sleep time. Nursing activities are a source of increased sound levels. The intensive care setting is one of the loudest, where close proximity of patients, noise from confused and ill patients, and ringing of alarm systems and telephones make the environment very disruptive.

**EXERCISE AND FATIGUE.** A person who is moderately fatigued usually achieves restful sleep, especially if the fatigue results from enjoyable work or exercise. Completing vigorous exercise within 2 hours or more before bedtime allows the body to cool down and maintains a state of fatigue that promotes relaxation. Vigorous exercise before bedtime interferes with sleep onset due to increased body temperature. Also, excess fatigue resulting from exhausting or stressful work makes falling asleep difficult.

**FOOD AND CALORIC INTAKE.** Following good eating habits is important for proper health, including sleep. Eating a large, heavy, and/or spicy meal within 3 to 4 hours of bedtime sometimes results in indigestion that interferes with sleep. Alcohol consumed in the evening has insomnia-producing and diuretic effects. Coffee, tea, cola, and chocolate contain caffeine and xanthines that cause sleeplessness as a result of CNS stimulation.

Weight loss or weight gain influences sleep patterns. Weight gain contributes to obstructive sleep apnea due to increased size of the soft tissue structures in the upper airway (Schwab and others, 2005). Weight loss causes insomnia and decreased amounts of sleep (Benca and Schenck, 2005). Certain sleep disorders are the result of the semistarvation diets popular in a weight-conscious society.

## Sleep Disorders

Sleep disorders are conditions that, if untreated, cause disturbed nighttime sleep that results in one of three problems: insomnia; abnormal movements or sensation during sleep or when awakening at night; or excessive daytime sleepiness (Malow, 2005). The occurrence of sleep disorders is becoming a significant health problem, especially for persons living in stressful environments. The American Academy of Sleep Medicine developed the International Classification of Sleep Disorders version 2 (ICSD-2), which classifies sleep disorders into eight major categories (Box 29-3).

In sleep-related movement disorders the person experiences simple stereotyped movements that disturb sleep. The isolated symptoms, apparently normal variants, and unresolved issues category includes sleep-related symptoms that fall between normal and abnormal sleep. Other sleep disorders contain sleep problems that do not fit into other categories.

**INSOMNIA.** Insomnia is a symptom experienced by patients who have chronic difficulty falling asleep, frequent awakenings from sleep, and/or a short sleep or nonrestorative sleep (Edinger and Means, 2005). The person with insomnia complains of EDS, as well as insufficient quantity and quality of sleep. Frequently, however, the patient gets more sleep than he or she realizes. Insomnia sometimes signals an underlying physical or psychological disorder.

Often people experience transient or temporary insomnia as a result of situational stresses such as work or family problems. Insomnia sometimes recurs, but between episodes the patient is able to sleep well. However, a temporary case of insomnia caused by a stressful event has the ability to lead to chronic difficulty in obtaining sufficient sleep. Insomnia is often associated with poor sleep habits. If the condition continues, the fear of not being able to sleep is enough to cause wakefulness. During the day a person with chronic insomnia feels sleepy, fatigued, depressed, and anxious.

Direct treatments, such as improved sleep hygiene measures, biofeedback, and relaxation techniques, at the symptoms. It is important to treat underlying emotional or medical problems that cause the insomnia.

**SLEEP APNEA.** Sleep apnea is a disorder in which the individual is unable to breathe and sleep at the same time. There is a lack of airflow through the nose and mouth for periods from 10 seconds to 1 to 2 minutes in length. There can be 10 or 15 to more than 100 respiratory events per hour of sleep (Dobbin and Strollo, 2002). There are three types of sleep apnea: obstructive, central, and mixed apnea, which has both an obstructive and a central component.

---

### BOX 29-3 Classification of Select Sleep Disorders

**Insomnias**

Adjustment sleep disorder (acute insomnia)
Inadequate sleep hygiene
Paradoxical insomnia
Insomnia due to mental disorder
Behavioral insomnia of childhood
Idiopathic insomnia
Insomnia due to medical condition

**Sleep-Related Breathing Disorder**

**Central Sleep Apnea Syndromes**

Primary central sleep apnea
Central sleep apnea due to a drug or substance
Central sleep apnea due to a medical condition

**Obstructive Sleep Apnea Syndromes**

Obstructive sleep apnea, adult
Obstructive sleep apnea, child

**Hypersomnias Not Due To a Sleep-Related Breathing Disorder**

Narcolepsy (four specified types)
Menstrual-related hypersomnia
Idiopathic hypersomnia with long sleep time
Behaviorally induced insufficient sleep syndrome
Hypersomnia due to a medical condition

**Parasomnias**

**Disorders of Arousal**

Sleepwalking
Sleep terrors

**Parasomnias Usually Associated With REM Sleep**

Nightmare disorder
REM sleep behavior disorder
Sleep paralysis

**Other Parasomnias**

Sleep-related groaning
Sleep-related hallucinations
Sleep-related eating disorder
Sleep-related enuresis (bed-wetting)

**Circadian Rhythm Sleep Disorders**

**Primary Circadian Rhythm Sleep Disorders**

Delayed sleep phase type
Advanced sleep phase type

**Behaviorally Induced Circadian Rhythm Sleep Disorders**

Jet lag type
Shift work type
Delayed sleep phase type
Due to a drug or substance

**Sleep-Related Movement Disorders**

Restless leg syndrome
Periodic limb movements
Sleep-related leg cramps
Sleep-related bruxism (teeth grinding)

**Isolated Symptoms, Apparently Normal Variants, and Unresolved Issues**

Long sleeper
Short sleeper
Snoring
Sleep talking
Benign sleep myoclonus of infancy

**Other Sleep Disorders**

Physiological (organic) sleep disorders
Environmental sleep disorder
Sleep disorder not due to a substance or physiological condition

Data from American Sleep Disorders Association, Diagnostics Classification Steering Committee: International Classification of Sleep Disorders. In Kryger M and others, editors: *Principles and practice of sleep medicine,* ed 4, Philadelphia, 2005, WB Saunders.

---

The most common form, obstructive sleep apnea (OSA), is a cessation or stopping of airflow despite the effort to breathe. It occurs when muscles or soft structures of the oral cavity or throat relax during sleep. The upper airway becomes partially or completely blocked and nasal airflow diminishes (hypopnea) or stops (apnea). The person tries to breathe because chest and abdominal movement continues, which often results in loud snoring sounds. When breathing is partially or completely diminished, the person becomes sufficiently hypoxic that he or she must awaken to breathe. Structural abnormalities such as a deviated septum, nasal polyps, narrow lower jaw, or enlarged tonsils sometimes predispose a patient to obstructive apnea.

Cessation of diaphragmatic and intercostal respiratory effort causes central sleep apnea. This cessation is a result of dysfunction of the brain's respiratory control center. The impulse to breathe temporarily fails. Nasal airflow and chest wall movement cease, with oxygen saturation of the blood also falling. You will see central sleep apnea in patients with congestive heart failure, brain stem injury, muscular dystrophy, and encephalitis, as well as in people who breathe normally during the day. It is the least common sleep apnea.

EDS is the most common complaint of people with obstructive sleep apnea. Patients with OSA are at risk for cardiac dysrhythmias, right heart failure, pulmonary hypertension, angina attacks, stroke, and hypertension. A serious decline in the arterial oxygen and cardiac arrhythmias occur (see Chapter 28).

Treatment for sleep apnea includes therapy for underlying cardiac, respiratory, or emotional problems. The treatment of choice is use of a nasal continuous positive airway pressure (CPAP) device at night. The CPAP machine pushes positive air pressure into the airway in an attempt to reduce the apnea periods the patient experiences during sleep by serving as a splint for the airway. Improved sleep hygiene and a weight loss program are also helpful to treat OSA.

**NARCOLEPSY. Narcolepsy** is a CNS dysfunction of mechanisms that regulate sleep and wake states. EDS is the most common complaint associated with narcolepsy. During the day a person suddenly feels an overwhelming wave of sleepiness and falls asleep. It is possible for REM sleep to occur within 15 minutes of falling asleep. There are two narcolepsy states: with or without cataplexy. **Cataplexy** is a sudden muscle weakness during intense emotions such as anger or laughter that occurs at any time during the day. If the cataplectic attack is severe, the patient loses voluntary muscle control and falls to the floor.

A person with narcolepsy often falls asleep uncontrollably at inappropriate times. Unless you recognize this disorder, you will mistake a sleep attack for laziness, lack of interest in activities, or drunkenness. Typically symptoms first occur in adolescence and are sometimes confused with EDS. You treat narcoleptics with stimulants that sometimes only partially increase wakefulness and reduce sleep attacks. Medications that suppress cataplexy and the other REM-related symptoms are also effective.

**SLEEP DEPRIVATION. Sleep deprivation** is a problem many patients have as a result of a sleep disorder. Causes include illness (e.g., fever, difficulty breathing, or pain), emotional stress, medications, environmental disturbances (e.g., frequent interruptions in sleep during nursing care), and variability in the timing of sleep as a result of shift work. Sleep deprivation occurs from insufficient sleep or disrupted sleep.

Hospitalization, especially in intensive care units, makes patients vulnerable to the circadian sleep disorders (Honkus, 2003). Sleep deprivation involves decreases in the quantity and quality of sleep, as well as inconsistency in the timing of sleep. When sleep becomes interrupted or fragmented, changes in the normal sequencing of the sleep cycles occur. A cumulative sleep deprivation develops over time.

Individuals respond to sleep deprivation differently. Some patients experience a variety of physiological and psychological symptoms such as blurred vision, decreased reflexes, slow response time, cardiac arrhythmias, confusion, and irritability. The severity of symptoms is often related to the duration of sleep deprivation. The most effective treatment for sleep deprivation is elimination or correction of factors that disrupt the sleep pattern. Nurses play an important role in identifying treatable sleep deprivation problems.

**PARASOMNIAS.** The parasomnias are sleep disorders that produce abnormal sleep movements, behaviors, emotions, perceptions, and dreaming as a result of autonomic nervous system changes and skeletal muscle activity during sleep (Thorpy, 2005). Disorders of arousal, partial arousal, and sleep transition are more common in children than in adults. An individual often experiences more than one parasomnia. Specific treatment for these disorders varies based on the underlying cause. However, in all cases it is important to support patients experiencing a disorder and to maintain their safety.

## Critical Thinking

### Synthesis

It is not uncommon for almost any patient to experience some type of sleep disorder. However, it is important not to overlook such a problem or consider it as normal. Use of a critical thinking approach helps you to correctly identify the nature of a sleep problem and then to initiate appropriate nursing care. Apply your knowledge, experience, and appropriate critical thinking attitudes and standards to make the correct clinical judgments for patients.

**KNOWLEDGE.** To make decisions about the nature and cause of a patient's sleep problems, it is important for you to synthesize knowledge regarding the physiology and functions of sleep and factors that affect sleep. Knowledge of the pathophysiology of select disease processes further helps in understanding the mechanisms for certain sleep problems. In addition, a good knowledge of pharmacological information is important because many of the medications patients receive may contribute to sleeping difficulties.

Another important area of knowledge to synthesize is the patient's personal routine and cultural orientation. Infant care practices such as co-sleeping and the practice of regular siestas or naps are examples of cultural variations influencing sleep. Anticipate how such cultural factors ultimately influence an individual patient's ability to sleep.

**EXPERIENCE.** You know of factors that have either disrupted or promoted your own ability to sleep. This personal experience is valuable when assessing patients' sleep problems or in selecting therapies for sleep promotion. Previous clinical experience with patients helps you to appreciate that environmental and lifestyle variations significantly affect the quality and quantity of sleep a patient receives.

**ATTITUDES.** When dealing with sleep problems, it sometimes takes a long time to find effective therapies. For example, it is not easy to eliminate chronic insomnia in a short period. Perseverance is an important critical thinking attitude to use if you are to help find effective solutions for the patient. The problems that result from sleep disturbances also often require creative approaches. Sometimes an original idea is necessary to minimize or control environmental stressors in the patient's sleep environment.

**STANDARDS.** When learning about a patient's sleep problem, you will use numerous intellectual standards in conducting the nursing assessment. Always conduct a detailed sleep assessment to understand the nature of the sleep problem and potential causes and solutions. A clear, precise, specific, and accurate assessment is very important so that you establish an appropriate plan of care. One acceptable standard for gathering a complete history of the quality of sleep over time is the use of a sleep diary.

# Nursing Process

## Assessment

Assess a patient's sleep pattern to gather information about factors that usually influence sleep. Because sleep is a subjective experience, only the patient is able to report whether it is sufficient and restful. If a patient admits to or you suspect a sleep problem, you will need a more detailed history. Aim your assessment at understanding the characteristics of any sleep problem and the patient's usual sleep habits so that you incorporate ways for promoting sleep into nursing care.

**SOURCES FOR SLEEP ASSESSMENT.** Patients are your best resource for describing a sleep problem and any change from their usual sleep and waking patterns. Parents or bed partners offer information on patients' sleep patterns that reveal the nature of certain disorders.

Obtain a child's sleep history from the parents. Older children often are able to relate their fears or worries that prevent them from falling asleep. If a child frequently awakens in the middle of bad dreams, parents are usually able to identify the problem without necessarily knowing the meanings of the dreams. Parents can also describe typical behavior patterns that encourage or impair sleep. With chronic sleep problems, parents relate the duration of the problem, its progression, and the child's responses. It is a good idea for parents of an infant to keep a 24-hour log of their infant's waking and sleeping behavior over a period of several days.

**SLEEP HISTORY.** Obtain a brief sleep history from patients who report they enjoy adequate sleep. Determine usual bedtime, normal bedtime rituals, preferred environment for sleeping, and what time the patient usually rises to plan care to support the patient's positive sleep habits and patterns. You need to assess the quality and characteristics of sleep in greater depth when you suspect a sleep problem.

**Sleep Pattern.** Begin the sleep history with the patient's self-report of his or her sleep pattern. Most patients will give a reasonably accurate estimate of their sleep patterns, particularly if any changes have occurred. An effective, subjective method for you to use for assessing sleep quality is the visual analog scale (Lashley, 2004). Draw a straight horizontal line about 100 mm (4 inches) long. Opposing statements such as "best night's sleep" and "worst night's sleep" are at each end of the line. Patients are asked to place a mark along the horizontal line at the point that best matches their perception of the previous night's sleep. The distance of the mark along the line in millimeters offers a numerical value for satisfaction with sleep. Use the scale repeatedly to show change in sleep over time. Do not use the scale to compare the quality of sleep for different patients.

It is important to have patients describe their usual sleep pattern in case there are significant changes created by a sleep disorder. To assess the patient's sleep pattern, ask the following questions:

1. What time do you usually get in bed?
2. What time do you usually fall asleep? Do you do anything special to help you fall asleep?
3. How many times do you awaken during sleep? Why do you think you awaken? What do you do about awakening?
4. What time do you typically wake up?
5. What time do you get out of bed, and how long do you stay up once you have awakened?
6. What is the average number of hours you sleep?

Compare the assessment data with the pattern usually found for other patients of the same age, and look for patterns that suggest problems. Sometimes patients with sleep problems show patterns very different from their usual one, and sometimes the change is relatively minor. Hospitalized patients usually need or want more sleep as a result of illness. However, some will require less sleep because they are less active. Some patients who are ill think that it is important to try to sleep more than what is usual for them, eventually making sleeping difficult.

**Description of Sleeping Problems.** When a patient admits to or you suspect a sleep problem, ask open-ended questions to help a patient describe the problem more fully. A general description of the problem followed by more focused questions usually reveals specific sleep characteristics (Table 29-2).

You need to understand the nature of the sleep problem, its signs and symptoms, its onset and duration, its severity, predisposing factors or causes, and the overall effect on the patient. Assessment questions include the following:

1. *Nature of the problem:* Tell me what type of problem you have with your sleep. Tell me why you think you are not getting enough sleep. Describe for me a recent typical night's sleep. How is this sleep different from what you are used to?
2. *Signs and symptoms:* Have you been told that you snore loudly? Do you have headaches when awakening? Does your child awaken from nightmares? Ask bed partner or parents whether patient has restful sleep or problems such as going to the bathroom frequently.
3. *Onset and duration:* When did you notice the problem? How long has this problem lasted?
4. *Severity:* How long does it take you to fall asleep? How often during the week do you have trouble falling asleep or staying asleep?
5. *Predisposing factors:* Tell me what you do just before going to bed. Have you recently had any changes at work, school, or home? How would you describe your current mood, and have you noticed any recent changes? What medications or recreational drugs do you take regularly? Do you eat foods (e.g., spicy or greasy foods) or drink liquids (e.g., alcohol, caffeinated beverages) that disrupt your sleep? If so, how much do you eat or drink daily?

## FOCUSED PATIENT ASSESSMENT

TABLE 29-2

| Factors to Assess | Questions and Approaches | Physical Assessment Strategies |
|---|---|---|
| Bedtime routines | Determine what the patient does to prepare for sleep. | Observe for dark circles under patient's eyes and excessive daytime sleepiness. |
| Bedtime environment | Ask the patient to describe the bedroom sleeping condition (e.g., level of light, noise, temperature). | Observe the number of times the patient yawns. |
| Current life events | Ask patient about normal hours worked. Determine if changes in job or home responsibilities have occurred. Ask patient about social activities outside of work. | Ask patient or sleeping partner about multiple patient position changes during sleep. Observe the patient's ability to concentrate on the conversation. |

6. *Effect on patient:* How has the loss of sleep affected you? Do you feel excessively sleepy or irritable or have trouble concentrating? Do you have trouble staying awake? Have you fallen asleep at inappropriate times? Ask a family member or friend: Have you noticed any changes in the patient's behavior since the sleep problem started?

**Sleep Log.** In addition to the sleep history, ask a patient and bed partner to keep a sleep-wake log for 1 to 2 weeks (Lashley, 2004). Have them complete the log daily to provide information on day-to-day variations in sleep-wake patterns over time. Entries in the log often include 24-hour information on waking and sleeping activities such as exercise, work activities, mealtimes, and alcohol and caffeine intake. They should also include time and length of daytime naps, evening and bed routines, the time the patient tries to fall asleep, time and number of awakenings, and the time of morning awakening. If necessary, have the partner help to complete the sleep-wake log. The log is most helpful if the patient is motivated to complete it thoroughly. Use of a tape recorder is a helpful option for patients with visual impairment or who have difficulty writing. Do not use the log with acutely ill patients who have short hospital stays.

**Physical Illness.** Assess for any physical or psychological problems that affect a patient's sleep. Review of known medical conditions will reveal symptoms (e.g., pain, shortness of breath, or fear) that interfere with the patient's normal sleep pattern. Assess the patient's medication history, including over-the-counter and prescribed drugs. If a patient takes medications for sleep, gather information about the type and amount of medication the person uses. If a patient is scheduled for surgery, be sure to ask about a history of sleep apnea. Patients with sleep apnea who receive general anesthesia and pain medications after surgery have increased risk for developing airway obstruction during recovery (Cullen, 2001). If the patient has recently undergone surgery, expect the patient to experience some disturbance in sleep. The effect on sleep depends on the severity of pain experienced after surgery and the amount of care received during the night (Tranmer and others, 2003).

**Current Life Events.** Changes in lifestyle disrupt a patient's sleep. A person's family situation or occupation offers clues to the nature of a sleep problem. Changes in job responsibilities, rotating shifts, or the recent birth of a child or loss of a family member sometimes contribute to a sleep disturbance. Questions about social activities, recent travel, or mealtime schedules also help clarify the sleep assessment.

**Emotional and Mental Status.** If a patient is anxious, fearful, or angry, mental preoccupations seriously disrupt sleep. In this situation the patient experiences emotional stress related to illness or situational crises. Ask patients to explore feelings about family relationships, job, or other meaningful situations. When a sleep disturbance is related to an emotional problem, the key is to treat the primary problem, and its resolution will improve sleep (Schneider, 2002).

**Bedtime Routines.** Ask how the patient prepares for sleep. Assess habits that are beneficial compared with those that disturb sleep. You will need to point out that a particular habit is interfering with sleep and help patients find ways to change or eliminate their habits that disrupt sleep. A patient's activity or exercise pattern before bedtime offers additional information about sleep quality. Does the patient perform strenuous exercise within 2 hours of going to sleep? Does the patient usually spend 1 to 2 hours cooling down or relaxing before sleep?

**Bedtime Environment.** Ask the patient to describe preferred bedroom conditions. For example, ask if the patient keeps the bedroom dark or softly lit and closes the door. Some patients listen to a radio or watch TV or prefer a quiet environment if noise prevents the patient from falling asleep. Also ask about room temperature and ventilation.

Assess the type of bed in which the person sleeps. Does the patient sleep in the same bed every night? Is the mattress comfortable? Does the patient need several pillows or cushions in bed to sit up during sleep? Does the patient use a lounge chair to sleep? Information about the sleeping environment helps you design better sleeping conditions.

**Behaviors of Sleep Deprivation.** Some patients are unaware of how their sleep problems are affecting their behavior. Observe for behaviors such as irritability, disorientation (similar to a drunken state), and slurred speech. If sleep deprivation has lasted a long time, psychotic behavior such as delusions and paranoia develop. For example, a patient reports seeing strange objects or colors in the room or the patient acts afraid when you or other health personnel enter the room suddenly or without warning.

## SYNTHESIS IN PRACTICE

As Anna prepares to conduct an assessment of Mr. Murphy, she knows it is important to consider how sleep is altered in older adults. Because they typically have less deep sleep and more awakenings to begin with, it will be important to consider what factors in the nursing home environment disrupt sleep. In addition, she has learned that the pain of Mr. Murphy's osteoarthritis is a contributing factor to any possible sleep disturbance. His immobility resulting from the stroke adds discomfort. Anna also plans to assess Mr. Murphy's medications carefully to determine if any drugs are adding to a sleep alteration.

From Anna's experience in a nursing home, she knows that a resident's sleep is often fragmented. Furthermore, she has read in a journal article that multiple factors affect sleep in the nursing home patient, including physical illness, dementia, depression, high prevalence of sleep-disordered breathing, chronic bed rest, circadian rhythm disturbances, and the noise and lighting of the nursing home environment (Kryger and others, 2004). She wants to be sure that her assessment considers all potential factors influencing Mr. Murphy's sleep pattern. Anna plans to include Mr. Murphy's wife in the assessment to learn more about Mrs. Murphy's perceptions of changes in Mr. Murphy's behavior. A complete assessment needs to be clear and precise; thus Anna plans to talk with Mr. Murphy more than one time to gather the necessary information and to keep her patient from becoming fatigued.

In the health care setting, determine whether environmental stimuli are disrupting the patient's sleep. A roommate who stays up late or has multiple visitors, the presence of electrical equipment at a patient's bedside, and the likelihood of noise coming from an outside hallway are examples of factors to consider that you are able to reduce or control.

**PATIENT EXPECTATIONS.** After assessing the patient's sleep history, determine the patient's expectations regarding nursing care. Use a caring and skilled approach to assess the patient's sleep needs. For example, ask, "Now that I understand more about your sleep habits and the recent problems you have had, what is it that you expect from us regarding your care?" or "In order to improve your sleep, what do you feel is most important that we do for you?" The patient sometimes has a different view on the relationship of sleep and health from your own. Examining patient expectations helps to clarify any misconceptions you have. In the hospital setting some patients are more concerned about being sure you are checking their condition routinely than about whether you wake them and disturb sleep.

### Nursing Diagnosis

Your assessment will reveal clusters of data that include defining characteristics for a sleep problem or other nursing diagnoses that result from disturbed sleep. If you identify a sleep pattern disturbance, it is helpful for you to specify the exact condition. By determining the nature of a sleep disturbance, you will design more effective interventions. The following is a list of potential nursing diagnoses that you may apply after identifying a sleep problem:

- Anxiety
- Ineffective breathing pattern
- Acute confusion
- Ineffective coping
- Compromised family coping
- Fatigue
- Ineffective protection
- Disturbed sensory perception
- Sleep deprivation
- Disturbed sleep pattern

Your assessment also needs to identify the probable cause or related factor for the sleep disturbance, such as a noisy environment, a high intake of caffeine, or stress involving work. The cause becomes the focus of interventions for minimizing or eliminating the problem. For example, a hospitalized patient who experiences insomnia as a result of a noisy sleeping environment will benefit from a reduction in hospital equipment noise or minimizing interruptions. If the insomnia is related to worry over a threatened marital separation, your interventions involve introducing coping strategies. If you define the probable cause or related factors incorrectly, the patient will not benefit from your care.

### Planning

**GOALS AND OUTCOMES.** After identifying all relevant nursing diagnoses for a patient, you develop a plan of care (see care plan). You will develop an individualized care plan only after you understand how the nursing diagnosis relates to the patient's normal and current sleep pattern, the patient's perception of the sleep problem, and the factors disrupting sleep. Together you and the patient develop realistic goals and outcomes. For example, the goal of "Patient establishes a healthy sleep pattern" will include outcomes such as "Patient will fall asleep within ½ hour of planned time" and "Patient will have less than two awakenings during the night." This will be realistic if you know from your assessment that it now takes the patient an hour to fall asleep and that awakenings occur 3 to 4 times a night. The outcomes will serve as measurable guidelines to determine goal achievement. An effective plan includes outcomes established over a realistic time frame that focus on the goal of improving the quality of sleep. This type of plan requires many weeks to accomplish.

**SETTING PRIORITIES.** Using the data you gathered about the nature of the patient's problem, you need to identify priority strategies and interventions to promote sleep. Together, you and the patient identify and select the strategies and interventions that are most likely to be beneficial in the home or health care setting. The plan of care includes priority strategies that support positive sleep habits and patterns that fit the patient's living environment, cultural orientation, and lifestyle. For example, the patient decides that purchasing a new mattress to increase comfort is the first step toward improving sleep. In a health care setting, you will plan treatments or routines to give the patient more time to rest. For example, you turn and reposition a patient at the same time you give him or her medication or perform a

CARE PLAN Disturbed Sleep Pattern

### ASSESSMENT

Anna learns that Mr. Murphy usually slept from 10:30 PM to 6:00 AM when he was at home, usually awakening once or twice during the night to urinate. He rarely had difficulty falling asleep, but according to his wife, listening to music helped him relax. Since being in the nursing home, he now reports, **"I have so much trouble falling asleep; it probably takes over an hour."** When asked if he awakens during the night, Mr. Murphy responds, "Are you kidding? No one can sleep here; something is always going on." Mr. Murphy admits to **awakening as many as 3 or 4 times during the night.** The patient estimates he received maybe **4 hours of sleep the previous night.** He denies that he is having discomfort from the osteoarthritis but is **having difficulty** changing positions and **getting comfortable.** While Mr. Murphy describes his situation, he **yawns frequently** and states, **"I really feel tired."** Anna asks him to rate the quality of the previous night's sleep, and he places a **mark on the analog scale near "worst night's sleep."** Anna notices during the assessment that Mr. Murphy's roommate is frequently calling out to anyone who passes the room door. The roommate's television is also on.

*Defining characteristics are shown in bold type.

### NURSING DIAGNOSIS Disturbed sleep pattern related to excessive environmental stimuli.

### PLANNING

**GOAL**

• Patient will obtain a sense of restfulness following sleep within 1 month.

**EXPECTED OUTCOMES\***
*Sleep*

• Patient will have fewer than two self-reported awakenings during the night within 2 weeks.
• Patient will report being able to fall asleep within ½ hour of going to bed within 2 weeks.
• Patient will obtain an average of 7 hours of sleep per night within 4 weeks.

*Outcomes classification label from Moorhead S, Johnson M, Maas M: *Nursing outcomes classification (NOC),* ed 3, St. Louis, 2004, Mosby.

### INTERVENTIONS†

**Sleep Enhancement**

• Have Mr. Murphy sit in the sunroom near the window for 30 to 60 minutes in the morning each day.
• Discourage frequent daytime napping or naps longer than 30 minutes.
• Have an egg-crate–mattress placed over bed mattress. Have staff position patient with extra pillows.
• Encourage Mr. Murphy to decrease his fluids 2 to 4 hours before sleep.

**Simple Relaxation Therapy**

• Arrange for patient to have a CD player with earphones to play music of his choice when first going to sleep.
• Arrange for Mr. Murphy to have some of his favorite reading material at his bedside.

**Exercise Promotion**

• Have patient get regular exercise (e.g., have Mr. Murphy propel down hallways in wheelchair for 5 minutes, 4 times a day before dinner).

### RATIONALE

Bright light increases melatonin levels and improves the average time older adults sleep (Hoffman, 2003).
Daytime napping interferes with sleeping.

Increases comfort of sleeping position, enhancing relaxation, which will promote a sleep state.
Decreases number of times patient awakens to urinate (Ebersole, Hess, and Luggen, 2004).

Soothing music blocks out sounds from the environment, promotes relaxation, and decreases the time to sleep onset (Johnson, 2003).
Reading before bedtime is a rest-promoting pre-bedtime activity.

Regular exercise improves sleep quality by slightly increasing the amount of stage 3 and stage 4 sleep (Hoffman, 2003).

†Intervention classification labels from Dochterman JM, Bulechek GM, editors: *Nursing interventions classification (NIC),* ed 4, St. Louis, 2004, Mosby.

### EVALUATION

• Ask Mr. Murphy to use a visual analog scale to rate the quality of his sleep at the end of each week.
• Ask Mrs. Murphy to evaluate her perceptions of Mr. Murphy's level of fatigue.

• Have Mr. Murphy report on the time he estimates falling asleep and the number of awakenings at night.
• Ask Mr. Murphy at the end of 4 weeks to keep a record for a week of the length of time he estimates sleeping.

**BOX 29-4** CARE OF THE OLDER ADULT

**Sleep-Wake Pattern**
- Maintain a regular rising time and bedtime.
- Eliminate naps unless they are a routine part of the schedule.
- If patient takes naps, limit to 20 minutes or less twice a day.
- Avoid extremes of sleep, that is, becoming excessively sleepy on the weekends.
- Go to bed when sleepy.
- Use relaxation techniques and a regular bedtime routine to promote sleep.
- If unable to sleep in 15 to 30 minutes, get out of bed.

**Environment**
- Expose to bright light for 30 minutes to 2 hours daily, preferably soon after waking.
- Sleep where you sleep best.
- Keep noise to a minimum; use soft music to mask noise if necessary.
- Use night-light and keep path to bathroom free of obstacles.
- Set room temperature to preference; use blankets and socks to promote warmth.

**Medications**
- Use sedatives and hypnotics as last resort and then only short term if needed.
- Adjust medications being taken for other conditions, and look for drug interactions that cause insomnia or EDS.

**Diet**
- Limit alcohol, caffeine, and nicotine in late afternoon and evening.
- Drink warm milk as a light snack before bedtime.
- Decrease fluids 2 to 4 hours before sleep.

**Physiological/Illness Factors**
- Elevate head of bed and provide extra pillows as preferred.
- Use analgesics 30 minutes before bed to ease aches and pains.
- Use prescribed medications to control symptoms of chronic conditions.

---

treatment such as suctioning, to limit the number of nurse-patient contacts. All staff caring for the patient need to know the plan so that they will cluster activities at times to reduce awakenings. In a nursing home some plan rest periods around the activities of other residents.

**CONTINUITY OF CARE.** The nature of a sleep disturbance determines whether referrals to additional health care providers are necessary. For example, if a sleep problem is related to a situational crisis or emotional problem, refer the patient to a psychiatric clinical nurse specialist, pastoral care professional, or clinical psychologist for counseling. This helps to ensure that you attend to the patient's problems not only in the health care setting but in the home as well. When chronic insomnia is the problem, a medical referral or referral to a sleep center is beneficial.

## Implementation

Your nursing interventions for improving the quality of a person's sleep will largely focus on health promotion. In an acute care setting, your focus becomes managing the environment in a way that supports the patient's normal sleep habits and keeps the patient safe. When patients enter long-term care or nursing home environments, you will need to make special considerations to promote adequate sleep and rest.

**HEALTH PROMOTION.** Patients need adequate sleep and rest to maintain active and productive lifestyles. Your specific interventions will promote a person's normal sleep and rest pattern.

**Environmental Controls.** All patients require a sleeping environment with a comfortable room temperature and proper ventilation, minimal noise, a comfortable bed, and proper lighting. Infants sleep best when the room tempera-

ture is 18° to 21° C (64° to 70° F) and covered with a light, warm blanket. Place healthy infants on their sides or backs when being put to sleep (American Academy of Pediatrics, 2000). The national "Back to Sleep" campaign has been very successful in teaching parents and infant caregivers to place infants on their backs for sleeping to reduce the incidence of sudden infant death syndrome (SIDS) (National Institute of Child Health and Human Development, 2005). Children and adults vary more in regard to comfortable room temperature but usually sleep best in cooler environments. Some prefer to sleep without covers. Older adults sometimes require extra blankets or covers or sleep wearing socks (Box 29-4).

Eliminate or reduce distracting noise so that the bedroom is as quiet as possible. In the home the TV or the ringing of the telephone disrupts a patient's sleep. The family members become important participants in care when each has a different schedule for going to sleep. It often requires the cooperation of several people living with the patient to reduce noise. Some patients sleep better with familiar inside noises, such as the hum of a ceiling fan.

Make sure the bed and mattress provide support and comfortable firmness. Place a bed board under the mattress to add support. Sometimes extra pillows help a person to position more comfortably in bed. The position of the bed in the room also makes a difference for some patients.

For any patient prone to confusion or falls, safety is critical. In the home a small night-light assists the patient in becoming oriented to the room environment before arising to go to the bathroom. Beds set lower to the floor will reduce the risk of falls when a person stands. Remove clutter from the path a patient uses to walk from the bed to the bath-

---

**PATIENT TEACHING**

On one of her visits to the nursing home, Mary Murphy tells Anna, the nurse, that she is having trouble sleeping and does not feel rested. Anna asks Mrs. Murphy to describe her current sleep habits. Using what she knows about sleep hygiene measures, Anna then develops a teaching plan to help Mrs. Murphy improve her sleeping.

**Outcome**

At the end of the teaching session, Mrs. Murphy will develop a plan that includes good sleep hygiene practices.

**Teaching Strategies**

- Discuss with Mrs. Murphy the need to practice good sleep hygiene habits regularly.
- Caution Mrs. Murphy against delaying bedtime or sleeping long hours during weekends or holidays to maintain her normal sleep-wake cycle.
- Explain to her not to use the bedroom for watching television, snacking, or other nonsleep activity, besides sex.

- Encourage Mrs. Murphy to take a warm bath before bedtime.
- Encourage Mrs. Murphy to walk for 30 minutes every morning.
- Instruct Mrs. Murphy to play soft relaxing music at bedtime to help her fall asleep.
- Demonstrate relaxation techniques to Mrs. Murphy.
- Advise Mrs. Murphy if that she does not fall asleep within 20 minutes, she needs to get out of bed and do some quiet activity until feeling sleepy enough to go back to bed.
- Instruct Mrs. Murphy to avoid heavy meals for 3 hours before bedtime; a light snack helps.
- Answer questions that Mrs. Murphy has about sleep problems.

**Evaluation Strategies**

- Ask Mrs. Murphy to describe three good sleep hygiene habits.
- Have Mrs. Murphy demonstrate a relaxation technique to use to promote sleep.
- Ask Mrs. Murphy to identify an appropriate bedtime snack.
- Ask Mrs. Murphy to identify soothing music to use at bedtime to help her relax.

---

room. If a patient needs help in ambulating from the bed to the bathroom, have a small bell at the bedside to call family members.

Patients vary in regard to the amount of light that they prefer at night. Infants and older adults sleep best in softly lit rooms. Do not have light shining directly on their eyes. Small table lamps or night-lights prevent total darkness. For older adults this reduces the chance of confusion when arising from bed. If streetlights shine through windows or when patients nap during the day, heavy shades, drapes, or slatted blinds are helpful.

**Promoting Bedtime Routines.** Bedtime routines and sleep hygiene measures relax patients in preparation for sleep. It is important for persons to go to sleep when they feel fatigued or sleepy. To develop good sleep hygiene at home, patients and their bed partners need to learn techniques that promote sleep and conditions that interfere with sleep (Box 29-5).

Newborns and infants benefit from quiet activities such as holding them snugly in blankets, talking or singing softly, and gently rocking. A bedtime routine (e.g., same hour for bedtime or quiet activity) used consistently helps toddlers and preschool children avoid delaying sleep. Parents need to reinforce patterns of preparing for bedtime. Reading stories, allowing children to sit in a parent's lap while listening to music or prayer, and coloring are routines associated with preparing for bed.

Adults need to avoid excessive mental stimulation just before bedtime. Reading a light novel, watching a relaxing television program, or listening to music helps a person relax (Box 29-6). Relaxation exercises and praying induce calm (see Chapter 30).

**Promoting Comfort.** People fall asleep only after feeling comfortable and relaxed. You will recommend and use sev-

eral measures to promote comfort, such as encouraging the patient to wear loose-fitting nightwear and to void before bedtime. Have family members give a relaxing back rub. Minor irritants keep persons awake. Change diapers before placing infants in bed. An extra blanket prevents chilling when trying to fall asleep.

Have patients who suffer painful illnesses try a variety of measures at home to promote comfort. Application of dry or moist heat, use of supportive dressings or splints (see Chapter 35), and proper positioning with the use of extra pillows for support are very helpful. For patients with temporary acute pain (e.g., following surgery), it is sometimes advantageous to the patient and bed partner to let the patient sleep alone until the pain subsides.

You will help patients with physical illness learn ways to control symptoms that disrupt sleep. For example, a patient with respiratory abnormalities needs to sleep with two pillows or in a semisitting position to ease the effort to breathe. The patient will often benefit from taking prescribed bronchodilators before sleep to prevent airway obstruction.

**Promoting Activity.** In the home encourage patients to stay physically active during the day so that they are more likely to sleep at night. Increasing daytime activity lessens problems with falling asleep. Always plan rigorous exercise at least several hours before bedtime.

Research indicates that exercise is beneficial to older adults because it improves nighttime sleep. However, individuals with chronic diseases that influence their functional abilities are likely to have limited activity (Ebersole and others, 2004). Recommend activities that are safe for older patients to perform. Walking, swimming, and cycling on a stationary bike are excellent for those patients with limited physical impairment. Repetitions of sit-to-stand or transferring and up to 5 minutes of walking or wheelchair propulsion are excellent for

**BOX 29-6** USING EVIDENCE IN PRACTICE

**Research Summary**

Sleep problems, especially insomnia, are common in persons over 65. This affects more women than men. Researchers found music to have a relaxing effect. One research study examined the effect of using an individualized music program on persons with sleep problems. The study participants were 52 women over the age of 70 who self-reported sleep problems. The women selected their own music. Researchers collected data on sleep patterns for 10 days before the participants used music and for 10 days of music use.

The researchers found that the majority of the women selected classical music. The results of the study showed that the use of music decreased the amount of time that it took the women to fall asleep and decreased the number of times the women reawakened during the night. As a result, the women reported increased satisfaction with sleep.

**Application to Nursing Practice**

The results from this study will help nurses promote sleep for patients, especially older patients experiencing sleep problems such as insomnia. The nurse first performs an assessment of the patients' patterns of sleep. Early recognition of a problem allows the nurse to intervene promptly. Nurses help patients select music that is pleasant and soothing for them. They instruct patients to begin listening to the softly played selected music when they get into bed. The nurse further instructs patients to turn out the lights and close their eyes. Music will vary according to the patient's preference. Use music as an intervention for at least 5 nights in order to see a benefit. These nursing interventions will help patients obtain improved sleep.

Data from Johnson JE: The use of music to promote sleep in older women, *J Community Health Nurs* 20(1):27, 2003.

**BOX 29-7** CULTURAL FOCUS

Co-sleeping is a culturally preferred habit. Co-sleeping is more common in nonindustrialized countries. This practice is also common in the United States with Asian-American and African-American families. Health care personnel in the United States discourage this practice because of safety issues even though research does not show that the practice is unsafe. American culture promotes independence in childhood. Co-sleeping does not promote this independence, and thus health care workers discourage it. As a nurse you need to be culturally sensitive when discussing co-sleeping practices with parents and developing sleeping plans for children.

**Implications for Practice**

- Complete a thorough sleep assessment of the child and family.
- Discuss the risks of co-sleeping with parents. During the discussion remain culturally sensitive and respectful of the parents' views.
- Co-sleeping affects the infant's normal sleep pattern by decreasing slow wave sleep and increasing the number of nighttime arousals.
- Co-sleeping has been linked to increased risk of sudden infant death syndrome (SIDS) under certain conditions such as parental smoking, alcohol or drug use.
- Instruct parents that co-sleep to avoid using alcohol or drugs that impair arousal. Decreased arousal prevents the parents from awakening if the child is having problems.
- Co-sleeping should only occur with parents and not another adult or child.
- Avoid soft bedding surfaces. Infants and children will become entangled or have their head covered if the bed contains loose coverings, pillows, or stuffed toys.
- Encourage the parents to use light sleeping clothes, keep the room temperature comfortable, and to not bundle the child tightly or in too many clothes.

From Davis KF, Parker KP, Montgomery GL: Sleep in infants and young children. I. Normal sleep, *J Pediatr Health Care* 18(2):65, 2004.

those with physical limitations (Alessi and others, 1995). Weight lifting using light weights (e.g., 2 to 5 lb) is also excellent to build upper body strength and endurance.

**Stress Reduction.** When patients feel emotionally upset, urge them to try not to force sleep. Otherwise, insomnia often develops, and soon they will associate bedtime with the inability to relax. Encourage a patient who has difficulty falling asleep to get up and pursue a relaxing activity rather than staying in bed and thinking about sleep. When the emotional problem is ongoing and the patient finds little relief, encourage referral to an appropriate counselor.

Children often have problems going to bed and falling asleep. After nightmares, have parents enter children's rooms immediately and talk to them briefly about their fears to provide a cooling-down period. Comforting children while they lie in their own bed is reassuring. Keeping a light on in the room also helps. Usually experts do not recommend that a child be allowed to sleep with parents; however, cultural traditions cause families to approach sleep practices differently. For example, Hispanic and Asian families often practice co-sleeping, in which parents allow children to sleep with them or siblings to lessen the child's anxiety and promote a sense of security (Box 29-7).

**Bedtime Snacks.** Some persons enjoy bedtime snacks, whereas others cannot sleep after eating. A dairy product snack such as warm milk, which contains L-tryptophan, helps to promote sleep. A full meal before bedtime often causes gastrointestinal upset and interferes with the ability to fall asleep.

Make sure patients avoid drinking excess fluids or ingesting caffeine before bedtime. Coffee, tea, cola, and chocolate will cause a person to stay awake or awaken throughout the night. Alcohol interrupts sleep cycles and reduces the amount of deep sleep. Coffee, tea, colas, and alcohol act as diuretics, which cause **nocturia**.

**Pharmacological Approaches to Promoting Sleep.** Many of the drugs patients take to manage symptoms can cause insomnia. Make sure patients use CNS stimulants such as amphetamines, nicotine, terbutaline, theophylline, and pemoline sparingly and under medical management (McKenry and Salerno, 2003). Withdrawal from CNS depressants such as alcohol, barbiturates, and tricyclic antidepressants also causes insomnia and must be managed carefully.

Sleep medications help a patient if used correctly. **Sedatives** and **hypnotics** are groups of drugs used to induce and/or maintain sleep. However, long-term use of these drugs disrupts sleep and leads to more serious problems. One group of drugs considered to be relatively safe is the benzodiazepines. These medications do not cause general CNS depression as sedatives or hypnotics do. Experts recommend a low dose of a short-acting benzodiazepine such as zolpidem (Ambien) for short-term use (no longer than 2 to 3 weeks) (Nagel and others, 2003).

The use of benzodiazepines in the older adult population is potentially dangerous because of the drug's tendency to remain active in the body for a longer time. This means the drugs can potentially interact with other agents (Hoffman, 2003). Short-acting benzodiazepines (e.g., oxazepam, lorazepam, or temazepam) at the lowest possible dose are recommended. Initial doses should be small, and increments are added gradually, based on patient response, for a limited time.

Melatonin is a hormone produced in the brain that helps control circadian rhythms. It is a popular nutritional supplement in the United States used to aid sleep. Melatonin is usually sold in 3-mg tablets, but the body produces less than 0.5 mg. Because of the lack of large-scale studies on its safety, caution patients about the regular use of melatonin as a sleep aid (Hoffman, 2003).

The use of nonprescription sleeping medications is not advisable. Over the long term, these drugs lead to further sleep disruption even when they initially seem effective. Caution older adults about using over-the-counter antihistamines because of their long duration of action that causes confusion, constipation, and urinary retention (Nagel and others, 2003). Help patients with interventions that do not require the use of drugs.

Regular use of any sleep medication leads to tolerance, and withdrawal then causes rebound insomnia. Make sure all patients understand the possible side effects of sleep medications. Routine monitoring of patient response to sleeping medications is important.

**Managing Specific Sleep Disturbances.** Patients who suffer specific sleep disturbances will likely benefit from the health promotion strategies discussed so far. Weight loss can be effective for the patient with obstructive sleep apnea. It is important for the patient to follow an appropriate weight reduction plan (see Chapter 31). In milder cases of obstructive sleep apnea, body position during sleep is effective. One suggestion is to elevate the head of the bed (Ebersole and others, 2004).

**ACUTE CARE.** The nursing interventions described for health promotion are applicable to a patient requiring acute care. The nature of the acute care setting requires you to be creative in finding ways to maintain the patient's normal sleep pattern.

**Managing Environmental Stimuli.** A challenge for you in the hospital is controlling noise. Because many patients spend only a short time in hospitals, it is easy to forget the importance of establishing good sleep conditions.

In the hospital setting, plan care to avoid awakening patients. Try to schedule assessments, treatments, procedures, and routines for times when patients are awake. Perform nursing activities before the patient receives sleeping medication or begins to fall asleep. For example, you have a patient who has had surgery. Before the patient retires for the night, change the surgical dressing, reposition the patient, administer pain medication, and check vital signs. Give medications and draw blood during waking hours when possible. Plan with other departments and services to schedule therapies at intervals that give patients time to rest. Whenever it becomes necessary to awaken a patient, do it as quickly as possible so that the patient can fall back to sleep as soon as possible.

**Safety.** Safety precautions are important for patients who awaken during the night to use the bathroom and for those with excessive daytime sleepiness. Set beds lower to the floor to lessen the chance of the patient's falling when first standing. Remove clutter, and move equipment from the path a patient uses to walk from the bed to the bathroom. If a patient needs assistance in ambulating from the bed to the bathroom, make sure the call light is within the patient's reach. Be sure the patient knows how to turn the light on correctly.

If patients normally use a CPAP machine at home because of sleep apnea, it is important that they bring their home equipment with them to the hospital and use it every night. This is even more important for patients with sleep apnea who have surgery and receive general anesthesia. In these patients the anesthesia in combination with pain medications used after surgery reduces the patient's defenses against airway obstruction. After surgery, the patient achieves very deep levels of REM sleep that leads to muscle relaxation and airway obstruction (Cullen, 2001). These patients need ventilatory support in the postoperative period to prevent respiratory complications. Make sure that the patients use their home CPAP equipment. Use pain medication carefully in these patients. Monitor the patient's breathing and oxygen levels regularly. Notify the physician or health care provider right away if the patient is difficult to arouse or is having trouble breathing.

Patients who experience daytime sleepiness can fall asleep while sitting up in a chair or wheelchair. Position patients so that they will not fall out of the chair when sleeping. Elevating the patient's feet on an ottoman or small bench may assist in positioning the patient safely. A pillow placed in the patient's lap offers some support. If a patient enjoys leaning over an over-bed table while sitting in a chair, be sure the table is locked and secure. Avoid using safety belts because they are considered restraints (see Chapter 26).

**Comfort Measures.** You will make the patient more comfortable in an acute care setting by providing personal hygiene before bedtime. A warm bath or shower is very relaxing. Offer patients restricted to bed the opportunity to wash their face and hands. Toothbrushing and care of dentures also help to prepare the patient for sleep. Have patients void before retiring so they are not kept awake by a full bladder. While a patient prepares for bed, help to position the patient off any potential pressure sites. Offering a back rub or massage helps relax the patient.

Removal of irritating stimuli is another way to improve the patient's comfort for a restful sleep. Changing or removal of moist dressings, repositioning drainage tubing, reapplying wrinkled thromboembolic hose, and changing tape on nasogastric tubes eliminate constant irritants to the patient's skin. When an intravenous (IV) site becomes irritated and painful, reinsertion of the IV is usually recommended (see Chapter 15). Cleanse the perineal or anal area thoroughly for patients who are incontinent. Diaphoretic patients will benefit from a cool sponging.

**RESTORATIVE AND CONTINUING CARE.** The quality of sleep in a long-term care or nursing home environment is often fragmented. Residents of a nursing home often suffer chronic disease, incontinence, and dementia and take multiple medications, all of which can disrupt sleep. Patients commonly use psychotropic medications in nursing homes, with some evidence of a change in normal diurnal variation in sleep (Alessi and others, 1995). Noise, light, and repositioning of nursing home residents during linen changes are factors that cause patients to awaken. Besides care activities, nursing home residents themselves are very disruptive when they call out loudly to roommates or nursing staff.

In the long-term care environment many patients require rehabilitation or supportive care. The nature of their illnesses and treatment requirements disrupt sleep. For example, patients who are ventilator dependent will likely get brief periods of sleep throughout the day rather than prolonged sleep because of disruptions from ventilator alarm sounds and the need for occasional suctioning.

**Maintaining Activity.** General recommendations to improve sleep in older adults have often suggested increasing daytime activity or exercise (Hoffman, 2003). The general benefits of activity and exercise—improved activity endurance, improved mobility, and improved sense of well-being—may prove to be beneficial to those older adults who

are not institutionalized and thus not exposed to repetitive environmental distractions.

In the restorative care setting try to limit the time patients spend in bed. In the nursing home serve meals in the resident dining area. Otherwise patients should be up in a chair for meals and for personal hygiene activities. It is also important to keep the residents involved in social activities planned at the nursing home (e.g., card playing or arts and crafts). Regular exercise keeps the patients active and stimulated. It is also ideal to limit naps to once a day for 30 minutes or less (Elliott, 2001).

Patients with dementia often have disrupted sleep-wake cycles. They often become easily fatigued and experience periods of insomnia (Ebersole and others, 2004). In this situation activities and visits need to be shortened to allow the patient to maintain an adequate energy level. If the patient awakens during the night, keeping the lights at a low level and using soothing techniques such as quiet music or a back rub will promote sleep.

**Reducing Sleep Disruption.** Knowing the many factors that disrupt sleep in restorative care settings, you will find ways to make the environment more favorable to sleep. Noise control is critical. Often staff within a nursing home naturally speak louder because of residents' difficulties with hearing. Walking up close to a patient and talking in a normal but clear voice will likely improve the patient's hearing and reduce the chance of awakening a nearby roommate. Teaching assistive personnel to be more sensitive to the sources of noise that disrupt patients' sleep is very useful.

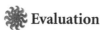 **Evaluation**

**PATIENT CARE.** Evaluation of therapies designed to promote sleep and rest must be individualized. Patients in relatively good health often do not need as much sleep as patients whose physical conditions are poor.

If you have established realistic goals of care, the expected outcomes become guidelines for evaluating the patient's progress and response to interventions (Table 29-3). Use evaluative measures shortly after trying a therapy. Use other evaluative measures after a patient awakens from

---

 **OUTCOME EVALUATION**　　　　　　　　　　　　　　　　　　　　　　　　**TABLE 29-3**

| Nursing Action | Patient Response/Finding | Achievement of Outcome |
| --- | --- | --- |
| Encourage Mr. Murphy to decrease fluid intake 2 to 4 hours before sleep. | Did not consume further fluids after dinner. | Mr. Murphy is obtaining an average of 6 hours of uninterrupted sleep per night. |
| Have an egg-crate–style mattress placed over bed mattress. Have staff position Mr. Murphy with extra pillows. | Mr. Murphy feels more comfortable lying on his side with pillows behind his back. | Mr. Murphy reports two or three awakenings during the night. |
| Arrange for Mr. Murphy to have a CD player with earphones to play music of his choice when first going to bed. | Within 20 minutes, Mr. Murphy's eyes are closed and his breathing is deep and even, at a rate of 12 breaths per minute. | Mr. Murphy is falling asleep within ½ hour of going to bed. |

## EVALUATION

After 4 weeks at the nursing home, Anna has been able to have Mr. Murphy transferred to a new room and has been monitoring his progress. He has been in the new room for 2 weeks. Anna asks Mr. Murphy, "Tell me how our plan to improve your sleep has been working. Have the music and headphones been helpful?" Mr. Murphy replies, "Well, it has helped to be down here at the end of the hall. It still is a bit noisy, especially if the nurses are working with people across the way. I have used the headphones the last 2 weeks, and they have helped me relax and fall asleep in about 20 or 30 minutes." Anna questions Mr. Murphy further and learns that he is awakening 2 or 3 times during the night. However, during the last week he estimated getting about 6 hours of sleep, an improvement from a month ago. Mr. Murphy also reports that the staff has usually been good about reminding him to do his daily exercises with the wheelchair. He dislikes staying in his room and has tried to exercise as much as possible.

Anna decides to revise the care plan, adding an intervention for placing a sign on the patient's door at night asking staff to keep the door closed. Mr. Murphy's sleep is improving, and Anna selects an additional measure aimed at reducing awakenings.

Anna wants to know Mr. Murphy's level of satisfaction with her care. She asks, "Have I met your expectations so far? If not, tell me how I can better help you." Mr. Murphy replies, "You've been great. I know you can't make this place like home. There is so much to think about when you are here. I think about my wife a lot." Anna responds, "Tell me more. What do you mean there is so much to think about?" Anna recognizes that psychological and physical stressors alter sleep. She decides to reassess Mr. Murphy to determine if additional nursing interventions will be appropriate.

**Documentation Note**

"Reports some improvement in overall sleep quality. Able to fall asleep within 20 to 30 minutes using headphones with music. Reports sleeping approximately 6 hours per night. Continues to experience reawakenings, resulting from noise in outside hallway. Recommend closing room door at night to reduce noise further. Admits to thinking about his wife and possibly other concerns. Will explore further with him."

sleep (e.g., asking a patient to describe the number of awakenings during the night). Together the patient and bed partner can usually provide accurate information. If the patient lives or sleeps alone, reliability of evaluation can be questioned.

When the patient does not meet expected outcomes, revise the nursing measures based on the patient's needs or preferences. Document the patient's response to sleep therapies so that a continuum of care can be maintained.

**PATIENT EXPECTATIONS.** Review the progress in the plan of care with the patient, and determine if the patient's expectations were met. Does the patient believe your interventions were helpful and useful? Did you incorporate the patient's typical sleep routine into the plan of care? For the hospitalized patient, did staff avoid unnecessary interruptions, giving the patient a chance to rest? The patient's perceptions are valuable sources of information regarding the overall success in improving the quality of the patient's sleep.

## KEY CONCEPTS

- Researchers believe sleep provides physiological and psychological restoration.
- The 24-hour sleep-wake cycle is a circadian rhythm that influences physiological function and behavior.
- The control and regulation of sleep depends on a balance between CNS regulators.
- During a typical night's sleep a person fluctuates between NREM stages 2, 3, and 4 before entering REM sleep. The amount of time in each stage varies.
- The number of hours of sleep needed by each person to feel rested is variable.
- Long-term use of sleeping pills leads to difficulty in initiating and maintaining sleep.
- The hectic pace of a person's lifestyle, emotional and psychological stress, and drug and alcohol ingestion disrupt the sleep pattern.
- An environment with a darkened room, reduced noise, comfortable bed, appropriate temperature, and good ventilation promotes sleep.

- The most common type of sleep disorder is insomnia. Characteristics of insomnia are the inability to fall asleep, to remain asleep during the night, or to go back to sleep after awakening earlier than is desired.
- Only a patient can report whether sleep is restful.
- When using environmental controls to promote sleep, consider the usual characteristics of the patient's home environment and normal lifestyle.
- Noise can disrupt sleep and enhance pain perception.
- A bedtime routine of relaxing activities prepares a person physically and mentally for sleep.
- Pain or other symptom control is essential to promote the ability to sleep.
- One of the most important nursing interventions for promoting sleep is establishing periods for uninterrupted sleep.

## CRITICAL THINKING IN PRACTICE

*Edward Pena is a 34-year-old businessman who comes to the physician's office complaining of being very sleepy during the day. He has noticed the problem for about 3 months. He states, "If I'm lucky, I get about 4 or 5 hours of sleep each night." He spends most of the workweek flying to various cities across the country as part of his sales job.*

1. To help Mr. Pena with his problem, what data do you gather first?
   a. A description of a recent typical night's sleep
   b. A detailed medication history
   c. History of current health problems and past surgeries
   d. Description of job responsibilities

*Mr. Pena goes on to tell you that his day begins at 5 AM and often does not end until 7 PM or later. He admits that his eating habits are irregular; sometimes he does not have a meal until 8 or 9 at night. He drinks coffee during the day for energy. Mr. Pena likes to play golf on weekends but exercises little during the week. Last month his boss had a long talk with Mr. Pena after hearing that he had fallen asleep during a business meeting.*

2. Which signs and symptoms that you assessed in Mr. Pena correlate with his documented sleep problems? (Mark all that apply.)
   a. Dark circles under his eyes
   b. Multiple changes in position
   c. Complaints of leg cramps
   d. Frequent yawning
   e. Increasing frequency of headaches
   f. Dry oral mucous membranes

3. What recommendations will you make to Mr. Pena to help him sleep? (Mark all that apply.)
   a. Go to bed at the same time each night.
   b. Drink a glass of wine at bedtime to relax.
   c. Increase your amount of sleep to at least 7 hours each night.
   d. Work out after dinner to make yourself tired.
   e. Turn on quiet, soothing music when you get in bed.
   f. Get up and do a relaxing activity if you do not fall asleep within 20 minutes.

4. Mr. Pena returns for a follow-up visit in 1 month. Which statement made by him indicates that the interventions for sleep are working?
   a. I am getting 7 to 8 hours of sleep after I take the sleeping pill.
   b. I fell more refreshed and rested in the morning.
   c. It only takes me about 45 minutes to fall asleep now.
   d. I only get sleepy during the afternoon meetings now.

## NCLEX® REVIEW

1. Which complaint by a patient is indicative of obstructive sleep apnea?
   1. Headache
   2. Early wakening
   3. Memory loss
   4. Excessive daytime sleepiness

2. The nurse recognizes that a problem with using benzodiazepines in older adults is that:
   1. Increasingly larger doses are required to initiate sleep
   2. The liver metabolizes the drug rapidly
   3. The drug remains active in the body for an extended time period
   4. The drugs are very expensive for older persons with a fixed income

3. A priority nursing intervention to promote sleep in the hospitalized patient is to:
   1. Encourage patient to continue to follow regular bedtime routines
   2. Coordinate laboratory draws for blood to be completed at 5:00 AM
   3. Give patient his or her prescribed sleeping medication by 11:00 PM
   4. Turn television on low to late night programming

4. An older patient complains about difficulty falling asleep. A priority nursing goal for the patient is to:
   1. Sleep for 7 hours each night
   2. Limit napping during the day to three or four naps
   3. Decrease awakenings to two or three a night
   4. Fall asleep within 20 minutes of getting in bed

5. Mrs. Riley, 68 years old, tells you that she is having problems sleeping and does not feel rested in the morning. What is the **first** action you will take with the patient?
   1. Instruct her to start keeping a sleep diary.
   2. Ask her to describe a recent typical night's sleep.
   3. Discuss her sleep patterns with her husband.
   4. Talk to her about increasing her daytime activity.

6. You teach a patient to limit caffeine intake in the evening because it interferes with normal sleep patterns by:
   1. Causing nocturia
   2. Increasing daytime sleepiness
   3. Causing awakenings during the night
   4. Increasing dreaming time

7. You are developing a care plan for an older patient who is having difficulty sleeping. An intervention to include on the plan is to:
   1. Encourage the patient to decrease fluids 2 to 4 hours before going to bed
   2. Have the patient exercise in the evening to increase fatigue
   3. Allow the patient to sleep as late as possible
   4. Encourage the patient to nap during the day to make up lost sleep

8. A mother tells the nurse that her 4-year-old is having sleep problems. When gathering assessment data related

to this problem, an important issue you will question the mother about is:

1. The age of other siblings in the home
2. Usual bedtime practices for the child
3. Growth and development patterns for the child
4. The type of preschool the child attends during the day

9. A patient in the community clinic becomes upset after learning he has narcolepsy. He asks you what this means. Your best response is that narcolepsy is:

1. A sudden muscle weakness during periods of stress
2. Stopping breathing for very short periods while sleeping

3. Frequent awakenings during the night with difficulty falling back asleep
4. A dysfunction in which the patient falls asleep uncontrollably at inappropriate times

10. A nursing measure to promote sleep in young children is to:

1. Make sure the room is dark and quiet
2. Encourage reading a story just before bedtime
3. Increase evening activities to promote fatigue
4. Allow children to fall asleep in parents' bed

## References

Alessi CA and others: Does physical activity improve sleep in impaired nursing home residents? *J Am Geriatr Soc* 43:1098, 1995.

American Academy of Pediatrics: Changing concepts of sudden infant death syndrome: implications for infant sleeping environment and sleep position, *Pediatrics* 105:650, 2000.

American Sleep Disorders Association, Diagnostic Classification Steering Committee; International Classification of Sleep Disorders. In Thorpy M: Classification of sleep disorders. In Kryger M and others, editors: *Principles and practice of sleep medicine*, ed 4, Philadelphia, 2005, WB Saunders.

Benca RM, Schenck CH: Sleep and eating disorders. In Kryger M and others, editors: *Principles and practice of sleep medicine*, ed 4, Philadelphia, 2005, WB Saunders.

Carno MA and others: Developmental stages of sleep from birth to adolescence, common childhood disorders: overview and nursing implications, *J Pediatr Nurs* 18(4):274, 2003.

Cullen DJ: Obstructive sleep apnea and postoperative analgesia: a potentially dangerous combination, *J Clin Anesth* 13:83, 2001.

Davis KF, Parker KP, Montgomery GL: Sleep in infants and young children. I. Normal sleep, *J Pediatr Health Care* 18(2):65, 2004.

Dobbin KR, Strollo PJ: Obstructive sleep apnea: recognition and management considerations for the aged patient, *AACN Clin Issues* 13(1):103, 2002.

Dochterman JM, Bulechek GM, editors: *Nursing interventions classification (NIC)*, ed 4, St. Louis, 2004, Mosby.

Ebersole P, Hess P, Luggen AS: *Toward healthy aging: human needs and nursing response*, ed 6, St. Louis, 2004, Mosby.

Edinger JD, Means MK: Overview of insomnia: definitions, epidemiology, differential diagnosis, and assessment. In Kryger MH and others: *Principles and practice of sleep medicine*, ed 4, St. Louis, 2005, WB Saunders.

Elliott AC: Primary care assessment and management of sleep disorders, *J Am Acad Nurse Pract* 13(9):409, 2001.

Hilton G: Melatonin and the pineal gland, *J Neurosci Nurs* 34(2):74, 2002.

Hockenberry MJ and others: *Wong's nursing care of infants and children*, ed 7, St. Louis, 2003, Mosby.

Hoffman S: Sleep in the older adult: implications for nurses, *Geriatr Nurs* 24(4):210, 2003.

Honkus VL: Sleep deprivation in critical care units, *Crit Care Nurs* 26(3):179, 2003.

Johnson JE: The use of music to promote sleep in older women, *J Community Health Nurs* 20(1):27, 2003.

Jones B: Basic mechanisms of sleep-wake states. In Kryger M and others, editors: *Principles and practice of sleep medicine*, ed 4, Philadelphia, 2005, WB Saunders.

Kryger M and others: Bridging the gap between science and clinical practice, *Geriatrics* 59(1):24, 2004.

Lashley F: Measuring sleep. In Frank-Stromborg M, Olsen SJ, editors: *Instruments for clinical health-care research*, ed 3, Boston, 2004, Jones & Bartlett Publishers.

Malow BA: Approach to the patient with disordered sleep. In Kryger M and others, editors: *Principles and practice of sleep medicine*, ed 4, Philadelphia, 2005, WB Saunders.

McCance K, Huether S: *Pathophysiology: the biologic basis for disease in adults and children*, ed 4, St. Louis, 2002, Mosby.

McKenry LM, Salerno E: *Mosby's pharmacology in nursing*, ed 21, St. Louis, 2003, Mosby.

Moorhead S, Johnson J, Maas M: *Nursing outcomes classification (NOC)*, ed 3, St. Louis, 2004, Mosby.

Nagel CL and others: Sleep promotion in hospitalized elders, *MedSurg Nurs* 12(5):279, 2003.

National Institute of Child Health and Human Development: *SIDS: "Back to Sleep" campaign*, http://www.nichd.nih.gov/sids/sids.cfm.

National Sleep Foundation: *2002 Sleep in America poll*, http://www.sleepfoundation.org/2005poll.html.

Schneider DL: Insomnia: safe and effective therapy for sleep problems in the older adult, *Geriatrics* 57(5):24, 2002.

Shneerson J: *2000 Handbook of sleep medicine*, Cambridge, UK, 2000, Blackwell Science.

Schwab RJ and others: Anatomy and physiology of upper airway obstruction. In Kryger MH and others: *Principles and practice of sleep medicine*, ed 4, St. Louis, 2005, WB Saunders.

Thorpy M: Classification of sleep disorders. In Kryger M and others, editors: *Principles and practice of sleep medicine*, ed 4, Philadelphia, 2005, WB Saunders.

Tranmer JE and others: The sleep experience of medical and surgical patients, *Clin Nurs Res* 12(2):159, 2003.

Walsh JK and others: Sleep medicine, public policy, and public health. In Kryger MH and others: *Principles and practice of sleep medicine*, ed 4, St. Louis, 2005, WB Saunders.

# CHAPTER 30

# Promoting Comfort

## MEDIA RESOURCES

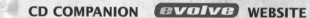

**CD COMPANION** *evolve* **WEBSITE**

http://evolve.elsevier.com/Potter/basic

- **NCLEX® Review**
- **Audio Glossary**
- **English/Spanish Audio Glossary**

## OBJECTIVES

- Discuss common misconceptions about pain.
- Describe the physiology of pain.
- Identify components of the pain experience.
- Explain how the gate control theory relates to selecting nursing therapies for pain relief.
- Assess a patient experiencing pain.
- Develop appropriate nursing diagnoses for a patient in pain.
- Describe guidelines for selecting and individualizing pain therapies.
- Describe applications for use of nonpharmacological pain therapies.

- Discuss nursing implications for administering analgesics.
- Differentiate the nursing implications associated with managing cancer pain versus non-cancer pain.
- Describe interventions for the relief of acute pain following operative or medical procedures.
- Describe the sequence of treatments recommended in pain management for cancer patients.
- Evaluate a patient's response to pain therapies.

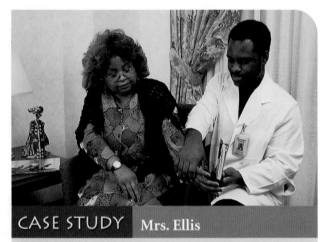

**CASE STUDY**   Mrs. Ellis

Mrs. Ellis is a 70-year-old African-American woman with hypertension, diabetes, and rheumatoid arthritis. She is receiving home visits following a recent hospitalization for the control of her diabetes. Her current health priority is the discomfort and disability associated with her rheumatoid arthritis. Arthritis has severely deformed her hands and feet. The pain in her feet is so severe that Mrs. Ellis often only walks short distances. The pain interferes with sleep and reduces her energy both physically and emotionally; as a result, she does not leave her home often. She has lived alone since her husband's death 6 years ago.

Jim is a 26-year-old sophomore nursing student assigned to do home visits with the community health nurse. Jim conducts assessments, performs procedures, and teaches health promotion to a variety of patients with various illnesses. This is Jim's first experience caring for a patient with severe chronic pain.

## KEY TERMS

analgesics, p. 855
cutaneous stimulation,
 p. 854
endorphins, p. 841
epidural infusion,
 p. 859
exacerbations, p. 842
guided imagery, p. 855
local anesthesia,
 p. 858
neurotransmitters,
 p. 840
nociceptors, p. 839
opioid, p. 856
pain, p. 838
patient-controlled
 analgesia (PCA),
 p. 844

perception, p. 839
placebos, p. 858
prostaglandins,
 p. 855
reaction, p. 845
reception, p. 839
relaxation, p. 854
remissions, p. 842
synapse, p. 841
threshold, p. 839
tolerance, p. 843
transcutaneous
 electrical nerve
 stimulation (TENS),
 p. 854

influence how they interpret and experience comfort. An understanding of comfort gives you, as a nurse, a larger range of choices when selecting pain therapies. Pain management is more than administering analgesics. First you need to understand how the pain experience affects a patient's ability to function and then use therapies that meet the unique needs of patients (Pasero and McCaffery, 2004).

### Nature of Pain

**Pain** is more than a single physiological sensation caused by a specific stimulus. It is subjective and highly individualized. The person experiencing pain is the only authority on it. According to McCaffery (1979), "Pain is whatever the experiencing person says it is, existing whenever he says it does." Acute pain is a physiological mechanism that protects the in-

## Scientific Knowledge Base

### Comfort

The provision of comfort is a concept central to the art of nursing. All patients bring physiological, sociocultural, spiritual, psychological, and environmental characteristics that

| BOX 30-1 | Common Biases and Misconceptions About Pain |

Patients who are knowledgeable about opioids and who make regular efforts to obtain them are drug seeking (addicted).

There is no reason for patients to hurt when you cannot find a physical cause for pain.

Administering analgesics regularly leads to patients' tolerance and drug dependence.

The amount of tissue damage in an injury accurately indicates pain intensity.

Health care personnel are the best judge of the existence and severity of pain.

The pain **threshold** and tolerance is the same for everyone.

Illness and its associated suffering are an inevitable part of aging.

You use physical or behavioral signs of pain to verify the existence and severity of pain.

Patients who fall asleep really do not have pain.

dividual from a harmful stimulus. For example, a patient with a sprained ankle avoids bearing full weight on the foot to prevent further injury. Acute pain warns of tissue damage and alerts the body to protect itself (McCaffery and Pasero, 1999). However, if patients are unable to express their pain (e.g., patients with aphasia, who are intubated, or who have mental status changes), this does not necessarily mean that they do not experience pain. Careful pain assessment is crucial. On the other hand, some patients (e.g., some with spinal cord injuries) are unable to experience pain. If patients cannot sense painful stimuli, you take special precautions to protect them from additional injury.

Health care providers often have prejudices about patients in pain. Unless patients have objective signs of pain, nurses do not always believe all their patients are experiencing pain. The extent to which you make uneducated assumptions about patients in pain influences your nursing assessment and seriously limits your ability to offer pain relief (Simpson and others, 2002). Too often, nurses allow misconceptions about pain (Box 30-1) to affect their willingness to provide pain relief (McCaffery and Pasero, 1999). Many nurses avoid acknowledging a patient's pain because of their own fear of contributing to addiction. In addition, nurses do not always accept the patient's report of pain. These fears and beliefs lead to mistrust between the nurse and patient, increased patient recovery time, increased complications and mortality, increased psychological problems, and increased cost (Letizia and others, 2004).

The failure of health care providers to assess pain accurately and consistently results in poor pain management and increased patient suffering. National and international organizations have made efforts to correct this problem (Agency for Health Care Policy and Research [AHCPR], 1992; American Pain Society [APS], 2003). The Joint Commission on Accreditation of Health Care Organizations (JCAHO) (2000) introduced a pain standard that requires that health

care workers assess all patients for pain on a regular basis. Many health care institutions have adopted this standard by recommending that staff include pain as a "fifth vital sign." It is important that you develop a "pain conscience" when you care for patients. Learn to assess for pain in every patient, select proper pain therapies, and evaluate the effects of your actions in relieving patients' pain.

## Physiology of Pain

**TRANSDUCTION.** Cellular damage from thermal (e.g., exposure to high or low temperatures), mechanical (e.g., edema distending body tissues), chemical (e.g., leakage of hydrochloric acid out of the stomach), or electrical (e.g., electrical burn) stimuli releases pain-producing substances such as histamine, bradykinin, and potassium. This stimulation causes an action potential on **nociceptors** (receptors that respond to harmful stimuli), thus converting the original stimuli into a pain impulse (McCaffery and Pasero, 1999). This conversion is known as transduction.

**TRANSMISSION.** Painful stimuli produce nerve impulses that travel along afferent peripheral nerve fibers. There are primarily two types of peripheral nerve fibers that conduct painful stimuli: the fast, myelinated A-delta fibers and the small, slow unmyelinated C fibers. The A fibers send sharp, localized, and distinct sensations. The small C fibers relay slower impulses that are poorly localized, visceral, and persistent (Menefee and Katz, 2003). For example, after stepping on a nail, a person initially feels a sharp localized pain, which is the result of A-fiber transmission. Within a few seconds, the whole foot aches from C-fiber stimulation.

A-delta and C fibers transmit impulses from the periphery to the dorsal horn of the spinal cord, where an excitatory neurotransmitter, substance P, is released. This causes a synaptic transmission from the afferent (sensory) peripheral nerve to spinothalamic tract nerves. Pain stimuli travel through nerve fibers in the spinothalamic tracts, cross to the opposite side of the spinal cord, and then travel up the spinal cord. Figure 30-1 shows the normal pain **reception** pathway. After the pain impulse ascends the spinal cord, information is sent quickly to higher centers in the brain.

**PERCEPTION.** As the pain impulse ascends to the brain, the central nervous system extracts information, such as location, duration, and quality of the pain impulse. The thalamus is the first structure in the brain to process the impulse. It sends the impulse to many areas in the brain, including the cerebral cortex, hypothalamus, and limbic system. Thus the patient becomes aware of the experience of pain. There is no one "pain center" in the brain that supports the complex nature of pain. Any factor that interrupts or influences normal pain **perception**, such as normal fatigue, depression, or pain therapies affects the patient's awareness and response to pain.

**MODULATION.** When a person perceives a harmful impulse, the brain stimulates descending neurons. The neurons then inhibit nociceptive and interneurons in the ascending pathway. In addition, endogenous opioids and other

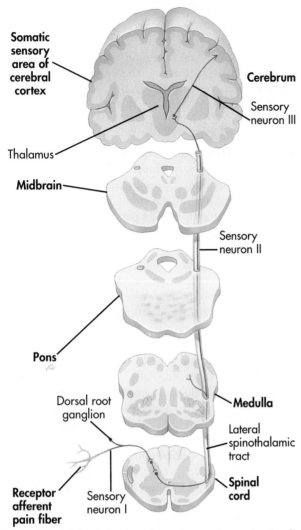

FIGURE 30-1 Spinothalamic pathway that conducts pain stimuli to the brain.

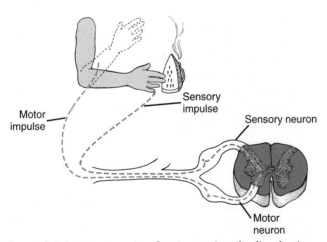

FIGURE 30-2 Protective pain reflex. Sensory impulse directly stimulates motor nerves, bypassing the brain, causing withdrawal from pain stimulus.

**BOX 30-2** **Neurophysiology of Pain: Neurotransmitters**

**Excitatory Neurotransmitters**

**Substance P**

Found in the pain neurons of the dorsal horn (excitatory peptide)

Needed to transmit pain impulses from the periphery to higher brain centers

Causes vasodilation and edema

**Bradykinin**

Released from the brain stem and dorsal horn to inhibit pain transmission

**Prostaglandins**

Increase sensitivity to pain

**Inhibitory Neurotransmitters**

**Endorphins, Enkephalins, and Dynorphins**

Body's natural supply of morphinelike substances

Activated by stress and pain

Located within the brain, spinal cord, and gastrointestinal tract

Cause analgesia when they attach to opiate receptors in the brain

**Serotonin**

Released from plasma that leaks from surrounding blood vessels at the site of tissue injury

Binds to receptors on peripheral nerves, increasing pain stimuli

neurotransmitters (serotonin and norepinephrine) further inhibit the transmission of the painful stimuli to the brain (Menefee and Katz, 2003).

A protective reflex response also occurs with pain (Figure 30-2). When a person is injured, a noxious stimulus from the skin travels along sensory neurons to the dorsal horn of the spinal cord where it synapses with spinal motor neurons. The impulse continues to travel along the spinal nerve to the skeletal muscle, causing the person to withdraw from the source of the pain.

Pain reception requires an intact peripheral nervous system and spinal cord. Common factors that disrupt pain reception include trauma, drugs, tumor growth, and metabolic disorders.

After a patient gains some pain relief, plan other therapies such as patient education, use of relaxation exercises, or the application of heat to enhance the effect of analgesics.

**Neurotransmitters.** **Neurotransmitters** are substances that affect the sending of nerve stimuli (Box 30-2). They either excite or inhibit nerve transmission. Excitatory neurotransmitters, such as substance P, send electrical impulses across the synaptic cleft between two nerve fibers enhancing the transmission of the painful impulse. Inhibitory neurotransmitters

| TABLE 30-1 | Physiological Reactions to Acute Pain |
|---|---|
| **Response** | **Cause or Effect** |
| **Sympathetic Stimulation*** | |
| Dilation of bronchial tubes and increased respiratory rate | Provides increased oxygen intake |
| Increased heart rate | Provides increased oxygen transport |
| Peripheral vasoconstriction (pallor, elevation in blood pressure) | Elevates blood pressure with shift of blood supply from periphery and viscera to skeletal muscles and brain |
| Increased blood glucose level | Provides additional energy |
| Diaphoresis | Controls body temperature during stress |
| Increased muscle tension | Prepares muscles for action |
| Dilation of pupils | Affords better vision |
| Decreased gastrointestinal motility | Frees energy for more immediate activity |
| **Parasympathetic Stimulation†** | |
| Pallor | Causes blood supply to shift away from periphery |
| Muscle tension | Results from fatigue |
| Decreased heart rate and blood pressure | Results from vagal stimulation |
| Rapid, irregular breathing | Causes body defenses to fail under prolonged stress of pain |
| Nausea and vomiting | Causes return of gastrointestinal function |
| Weakness or exhaustion | Results from expenditure of physical energy |

*Pain of low to moderate intensity and superficial pain.
†Severe or deep pain.

such as **endorphins** decrease neuron activity without directly transferring a nerve signal through a **synapse**. Researchers believe endorphins act indirectly by increasing or decreasing the effects of neurotransmitters. Pain perception is influenced by balancing neurotransmitters and by the descending pain-control fibers originating from the cerebral cortex.

**Gate Control Theory of Pain.** The gate control theory gives you a way to understand pain-relief measures. The gate control theory of Melzack and Wall (1996) suggests that pain impulses can be regulated or even blocked by gating mechanisms along the central nervous system. The gating mechanism occurs within the spinal cord, thalamus, reticular formation, and limbic system (Melzack and Wall, 1996). The brain determines whether the gate will be opened or closed, either increasing or decreasing the intensity of the ascending pain impulse (Menefee and Katz, 2003). The theory suggests that pain impulses pass through when the gate is open and not while it is closed. The gate control theory suggested the importance of psychological variables (thoughts and feelings), as well as physiological sensations, in the perception of pain. Thus pain intensity can be lowered by using psychological, physiological, and/or pharmacological interventions to close the gate (Dalton and Coyne, 2003). For example, therapies such as exercise, heat, cold, massage, and transcutaneous electrical nerve stimulation (TENS) are thought to release endorphins, which close the gate (Rakel and Barr, 2003). This prevents or reduces the patient's perception of pain.

**Physiological Responses.** When acute pain impulses travel up the spinal cord toward the brain stem and thalamus, the autonomic nervous system is stimulated as part of the stress response. Acute pain of low-to-moderate intensity

and superficial pain cause the fight-or-flight response of the general adaptation syndrome. Acute stimulation of the sympathetic branch of the autonomic nervous system results in transient physiological responses summarized in Table 30-1. If pain is unrelenting, severe, or deep, typically involving visceral organs, the parasympathetic nervous system goes into action. Most patients quickly adapt, with physical signs, such as vital signs, returning to normal. Thus a patient in pain, especially persistent pain, will not always have physical signs (McCaffery and Pasero, 1999).

It is important to understand that patients with chronic pain do not have the same physiological responses as acute pain. They do not demonstrate autonomic or sympathetic nervous system reactions. In addition, if you do not treat acute pain adequately, it can progress to chronic pain. It appears that unrelieved pain sensitizes and changes nerves (neuroplasticity), resulting in enhanced intensity, duration, and distribution of pain (Arnstein, 2003). These permanent neuroplastic changes contribute to the development of chronic pain syndromes. Chronic pain is not simply acute pain that lasts a long time.

**Behavioral Responses.** The response to pain is complex and variable. Responses integrate biological, social and psychological characteristics of the individual. Whether the pain is acute or chronic also influences the behavioral response. Clenching the teeth, facial grimacing, holding or guarding the painful part, and bent posture are all indications of acute pain. Chronic pain affects the patient's activity (eating, sleeping, working, hygiene, social interactions), thinking (confusion, forgetfulness, helplessness, catastrophizing), or emotions (anger, depression, irritability, frustration) (Arnstein,

2003). Recognizing the patient's unique response to pain is important in assessing the success of the pain management plan. Improvement in the negative effects of chronic pain suggests successful pain relief because comfort usually results in improved function. However, lack of pain expression does not mean a patient is not having pain. Unless a patient openly reacts to pain, it is difficult to assess the nature and extent of the discomfort. You need to help a patient communicate the pain response effectively.

## Nursing Knowledge Base

### Acute and Chronic Pain

As a result of the physical, psychological, and financial toll of inadequate pain management, President Clinton declared 2001 to 2010 as the Decade of Pain Control and Research (Loeser, 2003). Chronic pain is emerging as a common and expensive twenty-first century health care problem. An estimated 10% of Americans are unable to work or perform activities of daily living independently because of severe pain (Arnstein, 2003). The most common types of pain you will observe in patients include acute/transient and chronic/persistent that includes cancer and noncancer pain.

**ACUTE PAIN.** Acute pain usually has an identifiable cause following acute injury, disease, or surgery. It begins rapidly, varies in intensity (mild to severe), and lasts briefly. Acute pain warns people of impending injury or disease; thus it is protective. It eventually resolves after a damaged area heals. Patients in acute pain are frightened, anxious, and expect relief quickly. Acute pain is self-limiting, and the patient therefore knows an end is in sight. Because acute pain usually has an identifiable cause and is usually of short duration, health team members are willing to treat it aggressively. However, conflict between you and the patient will arise if you do not provide quick relief.

Acute pain seriously threatens a patient's recovery by hampering the patient's ability to become active and involved in self-care. It causes complications such as physical and emotional exhaustion, immobility, sleep deprivation, delayed wound healing, and pulmonary complications (McCaffery and Pasero, 1999). If you are unable to control acute pain, it is likely that patient education and rehabilitation will be delayed and hospitalization will be prolonged. If not adequately controlled, acute pain progresses to chronic pain. When you relieve acute pain, the patient is able to direct full attention toward recovery.

**CHRONIC PAIN.** Chronic pain is prolonged, varies in intensity, and usually lasts longer than is typically expected or predicted (Arnstein, 2003; McCaffery and Pasero, 1999). In chronic pain, endorphins either cease to function or are reduced. For example, chronic pain from cancer is sometimes a result of the tumor itself, the treatment (chemotherapy, radiation therapy, or surgery), or complications of the disease (fistulas).

Chronic noncancer pain such as low back pain often results from nonprogressive or healed tissue injury. Frequently there are no identifiable causes. The pain is ongoing and often does not respond to treatment. Health care workers are usually less willing to treat chronic pain as aggressively as acute pain. The Agency for Health Care Policy and Research (AHCPR) reported that up to 90% of the 8 million Americans who have cancer can have their pain managed effectively (Jacox and others, 1994). Too often health care workers undertreat these patients' pain.

Patients with chronic pain often have periods of **remissions** (partial or complete disappearance of symptoms) and **exacerbations** (increases in severity). This unpredictability frustrates the patient, often leading to depression. Chronic pain is a major cause of psychological and physical disability, leading to problems such as job loss, inability to perform simple daily activities, sexual dysfunction, and social isolation. The patient with chronic pain often does not show overt symptoms and does not adapt to the pain. But the patient seems to suffer more with time because of physical and mental exhaustion. Symptoms of chronic pain include fatigue, insomnia, anorexia, weight loss, withdrawal, depression, hopelessness, and anger.

Caring for the patient with chronic pain is a challenge. Do not become frustrated or offer false hope for a cure. Instead, help the patient identify ways to cope and to minimize the perception of pain.

Providing care to the primary family caregiver is also important. The stress of caring for a loved one with persistent pain causes physical and emotional problems (da Cruz and others, 2004). In addition, a family caregiver needs to understand and accept the pain plan in order to successfully implement it.

### Factors Influencing Pain

To accurately assess and then treat a patient's pain, you need to understand the various factors that influence the pain experience.

**AGE.** Developmental differences influence how infants, children, and older adults react to pain. Infants demonstrate pain through crying, changes in vital signs, facial expression, and extremity movement (Schechter and others, 2003). Children have trouble understanding pain and nursing or medical care that causes pain. Children without full vocabularies have difficulty verbally describing and expressing pain to parents or caregivers. Children's temperaments affect how they cope with pain. Children often describe treatments and procedures as the most difficult part of being sick or in the hospital.

Children are grossly undermedicated for pain. When comparing children with adults having the same medical diagnoses, children received fewer medication doses. In addition, analgesic doses are often too small or given too infrequently to be effective (Schechter and others, 2003). It is necessary for you to understand a child's response to pain. If a child is too young to speak, observe behavioral changes such as irritability, loss of appetite, unusual quietness, disturbed sleep patterns, restlessness, and rigid posturing as signs of pain (Jacox and others, 1994; Schechter and others, 2003). If a behavior such as crying changes after a child receives an analgesic, pain was probably the cause of the behavior.

Pain is not a natural part of aging. Likewise, pain perception does not decrease with age. However, older adults often suffer from acute and chronic painful diseases, which the person, the family, and health care providers frequently take for granted or underestimate. They use words such as *hurting* or *aching* instead of using the word *pain* to describe their pain. Older adults sometimes also have more than one painful site. They often hesitate to discuss their pain because of concerns of bothering their physician or health care provider. These barriers contribute to the inadequate pain management of older adults (Ardery and others, 2003). Older adults suffer serious loss of functional status as a result of pain. Pain reduces mobility, self-care activities, socialization, and activity tolerance (McCaffery and Pasero, 1999). A patient with cognitive impairment or who is nonverbal (aphasic, mental status changes, or not fluent in English) will have trouble communicating pain and providing a detailed description (Closs and others, 2004). Yet you will be able to assess pain accurately in most patients using physical and behavioral cues (American Geriatrics Society [AGS], 2002; Fuchs-Lacelle and Hadjistavropoulos, 2004).

The ability of older adults to interpret pain is sometimes complicated by multiple diseases and vague symptoms affecting similar parts of the body. When older patients have more than one source of pain, you gather detailed assessments. Different diseases cause similar symptoms. For example, a patient who has had a below-knee amputation continues to perceive pain from the foot that has been amputated (phantom pain) and has suture-line pain from the surgery. A patient who has had a stroke sometimes experiences pain in the paralyzed arm and in areas of the body unaffected by the stroke (Widar and others, 2004).

**GENDER.** Previously researchers did not believe gender influenced pain perception or response. Recent research (Logan and Gedney, 2004; Rustoen and others, 2004) on pain in men and women demonstrate a difference in responses to pain due to gender. Women appear to be more sensitive to pain, requiring less stimulation to evoke a pain response than men (Robinson and others, 2003). However, this topic needs further research.

**CULTURE.** Culture influences how people perceive the causes of and learn to react to and express pain. Italian, Jewish, African-American, and Spanish-speaking persons smile readily and use facial expressions and gestures to communicate pain or displeasure (Taylor and Herr, 2003). In contrast, Irish, English, and Northern European persons tend to have less facial expression and are less responsive, especially to strangers such as professional caregivers. Understanding cultural background and personal characteristics will help you to more accurately assess pain and its meaning for patients (Taylor and Herr, 2003) (Box 30-3). Even more important is recognizing how your own culture influences your attitude about pain (Weissman and others, 2002). Understanding your values, personal biases, and assumptions will help you become culturally sensitive to others who are different from you.

**MEANING OF PAIN.** The meaning a patient attributes to pain affects the pain experience. Patients perceive pain differently if it suggests a threat, loss, punishment, or challenge. The degree and quality of pain perceived by a patient are related to the meaning of pain (Feinberg, 2004).

**ATTENTION.** The degree to which a patient focuses on pain influences pain perception. Increased attention has been associated with increased pain, whereas distraction has been associated with decreased pain. You will apply this concept when you use pain-relief therapies such as listening to music and rhythmical breathing. By focusing a patient's attention and concentration on other stimuli, you help turn the patient's focus away from the pain. Usually, increased **tolerance** for pain lasts only during the time of distraction (McCaffery and Pasero, 1999).

**ANXIETY.** High anxiety levels increase pain perception. In addition, pain also causes anxiety. Autonomic arousal patterns are similar in pain and anxiety. Health anxiety negatively influenced the response of patients with chronic pain to pain and treatment (Hadjistavropoulos and others, 2002). Nurses act to reduce health anxiety levels to lower the perception of pain.

**DEPRESSION.** The incidence of depression is very high in patients with chronic pain. They experience many losses, such as their ability to enjoy life, to be in control, to work, to socialize and to be independent (Bair, 2003). Suicidal thoughts are relatively common in patients with chronic pain. Therefore you need to routinely assess for suicidal tendencies (Menefee and Katz, 2003). As a nurse, be aware of the possibility of depression in patients with persistent pain and suggest a referral if symptoms of major depression emerge.

**FATIGUE.** Fatigue heightens pain perception. This intensifies pain and decreases coping abilities (Block, 2002). Patients are more likely to experience pain at the end of a tiring day than after restful sleep.

**PREVIOUS EXPERIENCE.** Previous experience of pain includes pain the patient has experienced personally and pain the patient has heard about from someone else. Previous pain experience does not necessarily mean a patient will accept pain more easily in the future. Frequent episodes of pain without relief or bouts of severe pain produce anxiety or fear. In contrast, when the patient has experiences with the same type of pain that has successfully been relieved, it is easier for the patient to interpret the pain sensation. As a result, the patient is better prepared to take steps to relieve the pain. A patient who has had no experience with a particular type of pain sometimes has an impaired ability to cope with it. You prepare such a patient with a clear explanation of the type of pain that he or she will experience and the methods to reduce it (Wells, 2003).

**COPING STYLE.** Pain can be lonely for some. Frequently patients feel a loss of control over their environments or the outcome of events. Coping style thus influences the ability to cope with pain. Patients with internal loci of control perceive themselves as having personal control over their environments and the outcome of events. They ask questions, desire

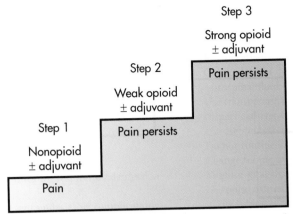

FIGURE **30-10** WHO analgesic ladder is a three-step approach to using drugs in cancer pain management. ± *adjuvant,* With or without adjuvant medications. (From World Health Organization: *Cancer pain relief and palliative care,* Report of a WHO expert committee, WHO Technical Report Series No. 804, Geneva, Switzerland, 1990, WHO.)

acute pain. WHO (1990) recommends a three-step approach to managing cancer pain (Figure 30-10). Therapy begins with NSAIDs and/or adjuvants and then progresses to strong opioids if pain persists. When a patient with cancer first has pain, it is best to begin with a higher dosage than what will be routinely needed. This provides the patient with immediate pain relief. The physician or health care provider then slowly decreases the dosage to the amount that successfully controls pain. The physician or health care provider treats side effects of analgesia aggressively so the patient is able to continue using analgesia. Patients receiving long-term opioids often develop a drug tolerance. Therefore they require higher dosages to attain pain relief. Higher dosages are not lethal, because most patients also develop tolerance to life-threatening side effects (McCaffery and Pasero, 1999). However, tolerance does not prevent the side effect of constipation. Unless contraindicated, patients receiving long-term ATC opioids also receive ATC stimulant laxatives and not just stool softeners.

For patients with cancer the aim of drug therapy is to anticipate and prevent or minimize pain. Therefore it is necessary to give required analgesic dosages regularly, even when pain subsides. Regular administration maintains blood levels for ongoing pain control. However, patients still have flares of pain or "breakthrough pain" that requires additional bolus doses of medication (rescue doses). A decrease in the duration of pain relief or an increase in the intensity of pain relief provided by the regular analgesia therapy and the need for an increased number of rescue doses are indications that the patient needs a higher opioid dose (McCaffery and Pasero, 1999).

Transdermal drug systems administer drugs (e.g., fentanyl) via a patch placed on the skin. This is useful when patients are unable to take drugs orally. Self-adhesive patches deposit the opioid into the subcutaneous tissue. The subcutaneous tissue releases the drug slowly over time at predetermined rates for 48 to 72 hours. This results in effective analgesia throughout the day and night. Inform patients

that it sometimes takes 12 to 16 hours for analgesia to take effect when they first begin to use an analgesic patch (Asburn and others, 2003). Therefore it is important for you to obtain an order for an immediate-release opioid to be used for breakthrough pain. Heat causes more rapid drug absorption. For this reason, warn patients to avoid external heat such as heating pads, hot showers, and prolonged exposure to the sun while using a patch. Only patients who have chronic stable pain and who have routinely received 40 mg or more of morphine (or its equivalent) daily on an ATC basis for a week or more are candidates for a fentanyl patch.

Another measure to treat severe persistent cancer pain is morphine given by continuous intravenous drip or intermittently by a PCA pump. Continuous infusions provide uniform pain control at lower dosages. Thus there are fewer side effects. Continuous-drip morphine is given in acute care settings and the home. An infusion control pump delivers morphine intravenously to ensure safe and accurate administration. Each agency has guidelines for morphine dose and infusion rates.

When a patient receives continuous-drip morphine, assess the intravenous site to ensure it is patent and without complications (e.g., no redness, swelling, or drainage). When a patient starts on continuous IV morphine, you need to prevent overdose and central nervous system depression. Record baseline blood pressure and respiratory rates before the infusion begins. After the infusion starts, monitor vital signs as often as every 15 to 30 minutes for the first few hours until the patient gains relief at a constant dosage. If the patient's blood pressure or respirations decrease, the infusion rate is reduced according to the physician's or health care provider's order or agency policy. For severe respiratory depression, administer small doses of the opioid antagonist naloxone (Narcan) intravenously, according to policy, to increase respiratory rate and depth, but not reverse the pain relief (Sargent, 2002).

**RESTORATIVE AND CONTINUING CARE.** Patients in need of restorative care for pain usually are suffering chronic persistent pain that is unrelenting. You will continue to use nonpharmacological measures that are effective for individual patients. However, additional pharmacological measures designed to give a patient better long-term pain control are required. The focus in restorative care is to use a comprehensive approach in supporting the patient and family.

**Opioid Infusions.** In the home or extended care settings, patients will use ambulatory infusion pumps for opioid infusions. The pumps are lightweight, compact, and allow free movement. The pump is battery powered and worn in a pouch attached to a belt or harness. The bag of medication and parenteral fluid fits inside the pump. A dose of opioid, delivered continuously over 24 hours, is usually slowly infused intravenously through a peripherally inserted central catheter (PICC) or a subclavian placed catheter (see Chapter 15). Both catheters are left in place for an extended period of time. Sometimes pain medication is infused subcutaneously (sub-Q) using a small catheter that the patient inserts into sub-Q tissue and replaces every 72 hours. The ambulatory pumps differ from PCA devices, which deliver only small, preset

## BOX 30-12 PATIENT TEACHING

### Ambulatory Infusion Pumps

If your patient is discharged home with an opioid infusion pump, develop a teaching plan that will ensure adequate pain management with minimal adverse effects from the analgesic.

### Outcome

- At the end of the teaching session, the patient and/or family member will verbalize possible analgesic adverse effects and demonstrate proper pump management, correct catheter maintenance, and administration of naloxone.

### Teaching Strategies

- Plan teaching session in a quiet environment.
- Determine a time that is convenient for patient and family.
- Avoid teaching during times of moderate to severe pain.
- Teach patient and family the most frequent adverse effects associated with analgesic.
- Instruct family on administration of naloxone (Narcan) intramuscularly to reverse respiratory depression.
- Demonstrate how to assess the central venous catheter (CVC), PICC line, or sub-Q catheter insertion site and maintain or change pump flow rate. If the patient has a CVC or PICC, teach how to maintain the patency of the catheter by routinely flushing the catheter with saline or heparin (see agency policy or prescriber's orders to determine type, amount, and frequency of flush).
- Show how to prevent air from entering catheter and how to clamp catheter when infusion has stopped.
- Explain how to change medication bag and tubing, how to prevent infection at catheter site, and how to change the dressing per agency policy. Teach patients how frequently to change the medication bag and tubing and the catheter dressing, and teach those with sub-Q catheters how to change the catheter site and how frequently to change the site.
- Describe a preventive bowel routine using stool softeners, laxatives, dietary fiber, hydration, and routine exercise.
- Warn patient against wearing pump in shower or submerging in bathtub. Temporarily disconnect pump during shower or place in a plastic bag hung outside shower or tub.
- Suggest keeping the pump on the bed or on a nightstand when sleeping. During lovemaking, set pump to the side so it does not interfere with closeness and intimacy.
- Instruct the patient and family on the purpose of the pump alarms and what to do when they sound.
- Provide a 24-hour emergency telephone number.
- Answer questions honestly.
- Summarize what you taught, and clarify questions or concerns.

### Evaluation Strategies

- Use open-ended questions (e.g., "Tell me some of the adverse effects that could occur that you would let the physician or health care provider or nurse know about.")
- Have patient/family demonstrate how to assess catheter insertion site and verify pump flow rate.
- If the patient has a CVC or PICC, have patient/family demonstrate how to flush the catheter.
- Have patient/family demonstrate cleaning/care of the catheter site and insertion of new sub-Q catheter (if appropriate).
- Ask patient to explain what to do with the pump during bathing, sleeping, and lovemaking.
- Have patient verbalize what to do if the pump alarm sounds and the number to call for emergencies.

---

doses of medication. The patient and family learn to manage the pump, observe for drug side effects, and maintain function of the catheter that delivers the medication (Box 30-12). Because the patient is initially managed on the opioid in the hospital before going home, the risk of side effects is not as great. A home care nurse makes routine visits to be sure the patient or family members manage the pump correctly.

**Palliative Care.** End-of-life or hospice pain management is not the same as palliative care. Palliative care offers treatments to help patients live, perhaps years, with a variety of incurable conditions, including persistent pain. The goal of palliative care is to relieve suffering and to support the best possible quality of life for patients with chronic and life-threatening conditions and their family members (National Consensus Project, 2004). Patients with chronic pain require a different approach to pain management than patients with acute pain. Unfortunately, physicians, nurses, and other health care providers cannot eliminate all pain, and learning to live with daily pain is not easy. Therefore it is important for patients with chronic pain to gain control of their pain versus allowing the pain to control them.

Consider making a referral to a palliative care team when you care for patients diagnosed with incurable conditions that have persistent pain as a symptom. These teams are composed of a variety of health care professionals who help patients achieve a level of pain control that allows patients to function and enjoy life (National Consensus Project, 2004). The patient is an active participant in the management of the pain. Without patient involvement, adequate pain control will not be possible.

**Hospice.** Hospices are programs to care for the terminally ill. The programs help terminally ill patients continue to live at home in comfort and privacy with the help of a health care team. Pain control is a priority. Families learn to monitor the patient's symptoms and become primary caregivers. Chapter 23 discusses hospice in more detail.

**End-of-Life Care.** You will need to teach and reassure family members and patients about the use of analgesics at the end of life (EOL). Emphasize the need to provide maximum pain relief by increasing (titrating) the dosage of medication to meet the patient's pain-control needs (Ersek and others, 2004). It is acceptable to increase opioids by 25% to 100% depending on the patient's response and pain intensity (Curtiss, 2004). Titrating is based on percent change of a drug dose because the body does not recognize milligram or microgram changes. It is the concentration of the drug in the blood, not

## OUTCOME EVALUATION

TABLE 30-6

| Nursing Action | Patient Response/Finding | Achievement of Outcome |
|---|---|---|
| Have Mrs. Ellis tell you, on a scale of 0 to 10, how her pain feels when it is most severe. | Mrs. Ellis rates pain at a 5. | Most severe level of pain has reduced from a 9 to a 5. Improved pain relief. |
| Ask Mrs. Ellis to describe how the pain is affecting her ability to perform daily chores such as bathing and dressing and washing the dishes. | Mrs. Ellis reports less stiffness in hands; able to wash dishes and says warm water is soothing. States she still has some difficulty putting on clothes, "My hands really hurt when I have to reach behind my back to pull a zipper." She reports that getting up to walk to bathroom and kitchen still creates discomfort in knees and hips, although she has less pain while she walks through her home. | She is able to perform limited activities of daily living (ADLs), showing some improvement by being able to wash dishes. Joint pain continues to affect ability to dress self. Pain persists during standing but has less of an effect during walking. Continue plan of care, suggest use of heat compresses before dressing. Also suggest use of Velcro closures on clothes. |

## EVALUATION

After 2 weeks, Jim returns to evaluate Mrs. Ellis's progress. Mrs. Ellis reports that she has seen her nurse practitioner and has been referred to physical therapy for supportive hand splints. In addition, the nurse practitioner has prescribed NSAIDs for pain control and to reduce gastrointestinal irritation caused by her aspirin. Mrs. Ellis reports that she falls asleep more easily if she takes her medication 30 minutes before going to bed. Jim gets the chance to observe Mrs. Ellis use a warm compress on her hands and wrist. Afterward, he asks her to rate her pain on a scale of 0 to 10. Mrs. Ellis rates it as a 3. During the visit, Mrs. Ellis gets up to walk to the kitchen. Jim notes that although it takes her time to stand, her gait is steadier. She is ambulating with a walker that the physical therapist recommended. Jim asks if Mrs. Ellis has found someone she can call when she needs assistance. The patient mentions that she has talked with her neighbor, who has offered to help her with shopping and to take her to church.

**Documentation Note**
"Patient reports improved satisfaction with pain control, able to fall asleep more easily. After using warm compress, rates pain at 3 on a scale of 0 to 10. Appears less fatigued and is ambulating with steadier gait, using walker. Has initiated social contact with neighbor as support system. Will evaluate effectiveness of supportive devices and ongoing NSAID effectiveness at next visit."

the number of milligrams or micrograms, that causes an effect. If the maximum dose ordered by the physician or health care provider is ineffective, you are responsible for notifying the physician or health care provider (ASPMN, 2003). The dosage needed to relieve the patient's pain sometimes exceeds the normal dosage range published in printed drug information. It is important to emphasize that the opioid will *not* hasten the loved-one's death. In fact, appropriately dosed opioids will alleviate suffering and improve the quality of life as the end approaches (Arnold and others, 2004). You use the fastest route of medication administration until pain is under control. Once pain is controlled, use the least invasive route possible including oral, rectal, transdermal, or sublingual routes. Remember, you will often need to use a combination of opioid, nonopioid, adjunct, and/or nonpharmacological therapies to provide adequate pain relief.

### Evaluation

**PATIENT CARE.** With regard to pain management, the patient is the source for evaluating outcomes. The patient is the only one who will know if the severity of pain has lessened

and which therapies bring most relief. To evaluate the effectiveness of nursing interventions, compare baseline pain assessments before treatments with ongoing assessment findings after treatment. Similarly, evaluate whether the patient's response to pain (e.g., positioning and body movements or ability to socialize or perform self-care) has changed. Compare actual outcomes with expected outcomes (Table 30-6) to determine if your patient met his or her goal (McCaffery and Pasero, 1999). Is the patient able to perform those activities that pain had prevented? Continuous evaluation allows you to determine whether the patient needs new or revised therapies and if new nursing problems have developed. It is important to discuss the patient's ongoing pain management needs with family members and health care providers who will be involved in the patient's care upon discharge or transfer.

Part of the evaluation of the success of treatment involves consideration of abuse or misuse of the opioid. Although addiction to opioids used to manage pain is rare, it is a concern that you need to evaluate (Compton and Athanasos, 2003; Passik and Kirsh, 2004). You will reassess patients receiving long-term opioids for indicators of addiction such as worsening psychological well-being and social and vocational function despite aggressive attempts at pain management (Compton and Athanasos, 2003). If addiction is suspected, recommend a referral to a clinician who specializes in chemical dependency to facilitate a thorough evaluation and an appropriate treatment plan.

**PATIENT EXPECTATIONS.** Subtle behaviors such as a gentle smile or a sigh of relief indicate the level of a patient's satisfaction with pain relief. However, it is important for you to *ask* patients if you have met their expectations. Do not ask patients if they are satisfied with their pain management, because patients often answer "yes" even when their pain is severe (Whelan and others, 2004). If a patient's expectations have not been met, then you need to spend more time understanding the patient's desires. Working closely with the patient will enable you to help the patient set realistic expectations that will be met within the limits of the patient's condition and treatment. It is also important to review the current pain management plan and suggest changes as appropriate.

## KEY CONCEPTS

- Acute pain, a protective mechanism that warns a person of tissue injury, is completely subjective.
- Misconceptions about pain lead to undertreatment.
- A patient's age, gender, anxiety, culture, previous experience and meaning of pain influence the pain experience.
- A patient's pain tolerance influences your perceptions of the seriousness of the discomfort.
- The difference between acute and chronic pain involves the duration of discomfort, physical signs and symptoms, and the patient's perceptions regarding relief.
- Pain scales attempt to communicate the severity of pain and the effectiveness of pain therapies.
- The patient's family and friends are a key resource in pain assessment.
- You individualize pain therapy by collaborating closely with the patient, using assessment findings, trying a variety of therapies, and maintaining the patient's well-being.
- Eliminating sources of painful stimuli is a basic nursing measure for promoting comfort.

- Nonpharmacological therapies are effective in altering patient perception of pain, promoting muscle relaxation, and giving the patient control over pain experienced.
- Using a regular schedule for analgesic administration is more effective than an as-needed schedule.
- A PCA device gives patients pain control with a low risk of overdose.
- Your primary role in caring for a patient who receives local anesthesia is protecting the patient from injury.
- The aim of therapy for patients with chronic pain is to anticipate and prevent pain rather than to treat it.
- A serious but rare side effect of morphine infusions is respiratory depression, which you reverse with intravenous Narcan.
- Evaluation of pain therapy requires consideration of the changing character of pain, response to therapy, ability to function, and the patient's perceptions of a therapy's effectiveness.

## CRITICAL THINKING IN PRACTICE

*The nurse arrives for a follow-up visit at the home of Mrs. Menendez, who is 84 years old and has inoperable breast cancer. Gloria, Mrs. Menendez's daughter, has been caring for her mother by herself for the past 3 weeks. She is concerned because her mother's pain seems worse and she does not know what to do. Upon physical assessment, you note that the breast tumor remains dry; however, the tumor mass has increased in size. Mrs. Menendez describes the pain as a constant, intense, burning sensation at the site of the tumor. In addition, she reports shooting, stabbing pain in her lower back that is worse when she tries to move. This pain has made it difficult to lie in bed or to move. She is unable to give you a pain intensity number (on the 0 to 10 scale). She has been unable to sleep at night for the past week and has started losing weight. In addition, she refuses to go to church as she has been doing for the past few years. She has been taking two Darvocet capsules by mouth every 4 hours as needed, although yesterday Gloria reports that out of desperation she gave her mother two Darvocet capsules every 2 hours until Mrs. Menendez became nauseated. The nurse recalls that morphine (4 mg orally [PO] every 4 hours as needed [prn]) was also ordered for the patient in anticipation of increased pain not controlled with*

*Darvocet. When questioned, Gloria states that she did not want to give her mother this "dope" for fear of addiction. Plus, she is "saving" the morphine for when her mother "really needs it." Gloria also reports that her mother's bowels are "locked up" even though she tried an over-the-counter medication to alleviate the constipation. Mrs. Menendez appears very stoic with minimal nonverbal expression of pain. Her major concern is that she is too weak to have her grandchildren, relatives, and friends visit. She tells you that she thinks that the pain is worse because the cancer is spreading, but that God would only give her pain that she could "put up with."*

- - - - - - - - - - - - - - - - - - -

1. Using the PQRSTU model of pain assessment, describe the pain you would assess in this case.
2. What kind of pain is Mrs. Menendez describing?
   a. Neuropathic
   b. Somatic
   c. Visceral
3. What major patient and caregiver barrier(s) are Mrs. Menendez and Gloria demonstrating? (Mark all that apply.)
   a. Concern about overreporting pain
   b. Fear of addiction

c. Unfounded reliance on God to relieve the pain
d. Worries about side effects of medications
e. Anxiety about inadequate pain control as disease progresses

4. What pain medication plan would you recommend?
   a. Continue using the Darvocet for another week to give it a fair trial.
   b. Stop the Darvocet, and call the physician or health care provider for a different opioid order.
   c. Stop the Darvocet, begin the morphine every 4 hours ATC, and consult with physician about an adjuvant drug for the neuropathic pain.
   d. Continue the Darvocet, but add an over-the-counter (OTC) NSAID to help treat the somatic pain.

5. Mrs. Menendez is experiencing _____, an adverse effect of opioids. Thus the nurse should consider calling the physician or health care provider for an order for a(n) _____ _____.

6. Given Mrs. Menendez's history and culture, which non-pharmacological nursing intervention would the nurse recommend she use to help alleviate the pain?
   a. Guided imagery
   b. Massage
   c. Prayer
   d. Progressive relaxation

## NCLEX® REVIEW

1. The following are common physiological responses to chronic pain (mark all that apply):
   1. Increased blood glucose level
   2. Increased heart rate and blood pressure
   3. Diaphoresis
   4. Dilation of pupils
   5. All the above
   6. None of the above

2. A patient who describes burning or electric-like pain is most likely experiencing _____ pain.

3. After receiving report, which of the following patients should you see first? A patient:
   1. Who is waking up from IV moderate sedation and has a physician in attendance
   2. With a pain intensity of 8 out of 10 after receiving morphine 4 mg IV 45 minutes ago
   3. Who received two Percocet tablets for pain 30 minutes ago
   4. With a PCA that the previous nurse neglected to clear at the end of the shift

4. A patient who is confused and has a history of aphasia just returned from having a gastrointestinal tube inserted. The physician or health care provider ordered acetaminophen 650 mg per tube every 6 hours prn. The best nursing intervention at this time is to:
   1. Administer the Tylenol every 6 hours
   2. Wait for the patient to experience pain
   3. Ask the physician or health care provider for an around-the-clock dosing schedule of Tylenol
   4. Ask the family member to rate the patient's pain and act accordingly

5. A patient with cancer was receiving 20 mg of immediate-release oxycodone every 4 hours around-the-clock for pain for the past 2 months. The patient has been allowed nothing by mouth (NPO) for the past 10 hours because of uncontrolled nausea. He begins to sweat and report abdominal pains. These are symptoms of:
   1. Addiction
   2. Drug tolerance
   3. Physical dependence
   4. Pseudotolerance

6. When applying a fentanyl patch for the first time to a patient, you consult with the physician or health care provider to be sure that the following is available:
   1. An immediate-release opioid for breakthrough pain
   2. A stool softener ordered around-the-clock
   3. A heating pad to place over the patch
   4. Acetaminophen 650 mg PO every 6 hours prn

7. When you assess the patient with pain, the most accurate assessment of the pain comes from the:
   1. Patient
   2. Family member
   3. Primary health care provider
   4. Significant other

8. A good indicator of the effectiveness of the patient's pain plan is:
   1. What the family members believe about the patient's pain intensity
   2. How well the patient is functioning
   3. How much pain medication the patient is using
   4. How satisfied the patient is with the pain plan

## REFERENCES

Agency for Health Care Policy and Research, Acute Pain Management Guideline Panel: *Acute pain management in infants, children and adolescents: operative or medical procedures and trauma.* Clinical practice guideline, AHCPR Pub No. 92-0032, Rockville, Md, February 1992, Agency for Health Care Policy and Research, Public Health Service, U.S. Department of Health and Human Services.

American Geriatrics Society: The management of persistent pain in older persons, *J Am Geriatr Soc* 50(6):S205, 2002.

American Pain Society: *Principles of analgesic use in the treatment of acute and cancer pain,* ed 5, Glenview, Ill, 2003, The Society.

American Pain Society: *Guidelines for the management of cancer pain in adults and children,* Glenview, Ill, 2005, The Society.

American Society for Pain Management Nursing: *Pain management in patients with addictive disease,* 2002, http://www.aspmn.org/html/PSaddiction.htm.

American Society for Pain Management Nursing: *On end of life care,* 2003, http://www.aspmn.org/html/endoflifecare.pdf.

American Society for Pain Management Nursing: *Use of placebos for pain management,* 2005, http://www.aspmn.org/html/Placebos%20revised_2005.pdf.

Arnold E and others: Consideration of hastening death among hospice patients and their families, *J Pain Symptom Manage* 27(6):523, 2004.

Arnstein P: Comprehensive analysis and management of chronic pain, *Nurs Clin North Am* 38(3):403, 2003.

Arnstein P: Personal communication, April 2005.

Arthritis Foundation: *Pain center: take medications wisely,* 2004, http://www.arthritis.org/conditions/pain_center/medications.asp.

Asburn M and others: The pharmacokinetics of transdermal fentanyl delivered with and without heat, *J Pain* 4(6):301, 2003.

Bair M: Depression and pain comorbidity: a literature review, *Arch Intern Med* 163(20):2433, 2003.

Baird C, Sands L: Pilot study of the effectiveness of guided imagery with progressive muscle relaxation to reduce chronic pain and mobility difficulties of osteoarthritis, *Pain Manag Nurs* 5(3):7, 2004.

Beaule P and others: Meperidine-induced seizure after revision hip arthroplasty, *J Arthroplasty* 19(4):516, 2004.

Beyer J and others: The creation, validation, and continuing development of the Oucher: a measure of pain intensity in children, *J Pediatr Nurs* 7(5):335, 1992.

Block K: Pain, depression, and fatigue in cancer, *Integr Cancer Ther* 1(4):323, 2002.

Byers J, Thornley K: Cueing into infant pain, *MCN Am J Matern Child Nurs* 30(2):84, 2004.

Closs S and others: A comparison of five pain assessment scales for nursing home residents with varying degrees of cognitive impairment, *J Pain Symptom Manage* 27(3):196, 2004.

Compton P, Athanasos P: Chronic pain, substance abuse and addiction, *Nurs Clin North Am* 38(3):525, 2003.

Curtiss C: Consensus statements, positions, standards, and guidelines for pain and care at the end of life, *Semin Oncol Nurs* 20(2):121, 2004.

da Cruz Dde A and others: Caregivers of patients with chronic pain: responses to care, *Int J Nurs Terminol Classif* 15(1):5, 2004.

Dalton J, Coyne P: Cognitive-behavioral therapy: tailored to the individual, *Nurs Clin North Am* 38(3):465, 2003.

Davidhizar R, Giger J: A review of the literature on care of patients in pain who are culturally diverse, *Int Nurs Rev* 51:47, 2004.

Dochterman JM, Bulecheck GM, editors: *Nursing interventions classification (NIC),* ed 4, St. Louis, 2004, Mosby.

Ersek M and others: HPNA position paper: providing opioids at the end of life, *J Hospice Palliat Nurs* 6(4):244, 2004.

Feinberg S: Race, ethnicity, cultural factors and chronic pain, *Am Chronic Pain Assoc Chronicle* 21(2):6, 2004.

Feldt K: The Checklist of Nonverbal Pain Indicators (CNIP), *Pain Manag Nurs* 1(1):13, 2000.

Ferrell B and others: Analysis of pain content in nursing textbooks, *J Pain Symptom Manage* 19(3):216, 2000.

Fisher S and others: Pain assessment and management in cognitively impaired nursing home residents: association of certified nursing assistant pain report, minimum data set pain report, and analgesic medication use, *J Am Geriatr Soc* 50(1):152, 2002.

Fuchs-Lacelle S, Hadjistavropoulos T: Development and preliminary validation of the pain assessment checklists for seniors with limited ability to communicate (PACSLAC), *Pain Manag Nurs* 5(1):37, 2004.

Gelinas G and others: Assessment in nonverbal populations (infants, mentally impaired, etc.): development of a critical care pain observation tool (CCPOT), *J Pain* 5(3, suppl 1):S106, 2004.

Gordon D: Nonopioid and adjuvant analgesics in chronic pain management: strategies for effective use, *Nurs Clin North Am* 38(3):447, 2003.

Green C and others: The unequal burden: confronting racial and ethnic disparities in pain, *Pain Med* 4(3):277, 2003.

Gunnarsdottir S and others: Interventions to overcome clinician- and patient-related barriers to pain management, *Nurs Clin North Am* 38(3):419, 2003.

Hadjistavropoulos H and others: The role of health anxiety among patients with chronic pain in determining response to therapy, *Pain Res Manag* 7(3):127, 2002.

Jacox A and others: *Management of cancer pain,* Clinical Practice Guideline No. 9, AHCPR Pub No. 94-0592, Rockville, Md, March 1994, Agency for Health Care Policy and Research, U.S. Department of Health and Human Services, Public Health Service.

Joint Commission on Accreditation of Healthcare Organizations: *Comprehensive accreditation manual for hospital standards: the official handbook,* Oak Brook, Ill, 2000, The Commission.

Kwekkeboom K and others: A pilot study to predict success with guided imagery for cancer pain, *Pain Manag Nurs* 4(3):112, 2003.

Leavitt S: *Using patient-controlled analgesia (PCA) for acute pain management,* 2003. http://www.baxter.com/doctors/iv_therapies/education/iv_therapy_ce/pca/pca.html.

Letizia M and others: Barriers to caregiver administration of pain medication in hospice care, *J Pain Symptom Manage* 27(2):114, 2004.

Loeser J: The decade of pain control and research, *Am Pain Soc Bull* 13(3):13, 2003.

Logan H, Gedney J: Sex differences in the long-term stability of forehead cold pressor pain, *J Pain* 5(7):406, 2004.

Mayer D and others: Speaking the language of pain, *Am J Nurs* 101(2):44, 2001.

McCaffery M: *Nursing management of the patient with pain,* ed 2, Philadelphia, 1979, Lippincott.

McCaffery M, Pasero C: *Pain: clinical manual,* ed 2, St. Louis, 1999, Mosby.

Melzack R, Wall P: *The challenge of pain,* ed 2, London, 1996, Penguin.

Menefee L, Katz N: *The pain EDU.org manual: a clinical companion,* Newton, Mass, 2003, Inflexxion.

Merkel S: Pain assessment in infants and young children: the finger span scale, *Am J Nurs* 102(11):55, 2002.

Merkel S and others: Pain assessment in infants and young children: the FLACC scale, *Am J Nurs* 102(10):55, 2002.

Moorhead S, Johnson M, Maas M: *Nursing outcomes classification (NOC),* ed 3, St. Louis, 2004, Mosby.

National Consensus Project: *Clinical practice guidelines for quality palliative care,* 2004, http://www.nationalconsensusproject.org.

Palos G and others: Perceptions of analgesic use and side effects: what the public values in pain management, *J Pain Symptom Manage* 28(5):460, 2004.

Pasero C: Pain assessment in infants and young children: neonates, *Am J Nurs* 102(8):61, 2002.

Pasero C: *Epidural analgesia for acute pain management in adults,* 2003a, http://www.baxter.com/doctors/iv_therapies/eduction/iv_therapy_ce/epidural/epidural.html.

Pasero C: Epidural analgesia for postoperative pain, *Am J Nurs* 103(10):62, 2003b.

Pasero C: Epidural analgesia for postoperative pain, part II, *Am J Nurs* 103(11):43, 2003c.

Pasero C: *Intravenous patient-controlled analgesia for acute pain management,* Pensacola, Fla, 2003d, American Society for Pain Management Nursing.

Pasero C, McCaffery M: Comfort-function goals, *Am J Nurs* 104(9):77, 2004.

Passik S, Kirsh K: Opioid therapy in patients with a history of substance abuse, *CNS Drugs* 18(1):13, 2004.

Pulido P and others: The efficacy of continuous bupivacaine infiltration for pain management following orthopaedic knee surgery: anterior cruciate ligament reconstruction and total knee arthroplasty, *Orthop Nurs* 21(1):31, 2002.

Rakel B, Barr J: Physical modalities in chronic pain management, *Nurs Clin North Am* 38(3):477, 2003.

Redinbaugh E and others: Factors associated with the accuracy of family caregiver estimates of patient pain, *J Pain Symptom Manage* 23(5):31, 2003.

Robinson M and others: Altering gender role expectations: effects on pain tolerance, pain threshold, and pain ratings, *J Pain* 4(6):284, 2003.

Rushton P and others: Knowledge and attitudes about cancer pain management: a comparison of oncology and nononcology nurses, *Oncol Nurse Forum* 30(5):849, 2003.

Rustoen T and others: Gender differences in chronic pain: findings from a population-based study of Norwegian adults, *Pain Manag Nurs* 5(3):105, 2004.

St. Marie B: The complex pain patient: interventional treatment and nursing issues, *Nurs Clin North Am* 38(3):539, 2003.

Sargent C: Naloxone: How well do you know this drug? *Clin J Oncol Nurs* 6(1):17, 2002.

Schechter N, Berde C, Yaster M: *Pain in infants, children, and adolescents,* ed 2, Philadelphia, 2003, Lippincott Williams & Wilkins.

Silka P and others: Pain scores improve analgesic administration patterns for trauma patients in the emergency department, *Acad Emerg Med* 11(3):264, 2004.

Simpson K and others: The effects of a pain management education program on the knowledge level and attitudes of clinical staff, *Pain Manag Nurs* 3(3):87, 2002.

Snyder M, Wieland J: Complementary and alternative therapies: what is their place in the management of chronic pain? *Nurs Clin North Am* 38(3):495, 2003.

Taylor L, Herr K: Pain intensity assessment: a comparison of selected pain intensity scales for use in cognitively intact and cognitively impaired African American older adults, *Pain Manag Nurs* 4(2):87, 2003.

Thomas S and others: Effects of morphine analgesia on diagnostic accuracy in emergency department patients with abdominal pain: a prospective, randomized trial, *J Am Coll Surg* 196(1):18, 2003.

Turner J: *The importance of placebo effects in pain treatment and research,* 2003, http://www.hsc.missouri-edu/shrp/ptwww/courses/assign/turner.html.

Vallerand A: The use of long-acting opioids in chronic pain management, *Nurs Clin North Am* 38(3):435, 2003.

Weisse C and others: The influence of gender and race on physician's pain management decisions, *J Pain* 4(9):505, 2003.

Weissman D and others: *Cultural aspects of pain management,* 2002, http://www.eperc.mcw.edu/fastFact/ff_78.htm.

Wells N: Improving cancer pain management through patient and family education, *J Pain Symptom Manage* 23(5):344, 2003.

Wheeler M and others: Adverse events associated with postoperative opioid analgesia: a systemic review, *J Pain* 3(3):159, 2002.

Whelan C and others: Pain and satisfaction with pain control in hospitalized medical patients, *Arch Intern Med* 164:175, 2004.

White P and others: Use of a continuous local anesthetic infusion for pain management after median sternotomy, *Anesthesiology* 99(4):918, 2003.

Widar M and others: Coping with long-term pain after stroke, *J Pain Symptom Manage* 27(3):215, 2004.

Wong DL, Baker CM: Pain in children: comparison of assessment scales, *Pediatr Nurs* 14(1):9, 1988.

World Health Organization: *Cancer pain relief and palliative care,* Report of a WHO expert committee, WHO Technical Report Series No. 804, Geneva, Switzerland, 1990, WHO.

# CHAPTER 31

# Nutrition

## MEDIA RESOURCES

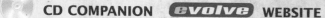

**CD COMPANION** *evolve* **WEBSITE**

http://evolve.elsevier.com/Potter/basic

- **NCLEX® Review**
- **Audio Glossary**
- **English/Spanish Audio Glossary**
- **Video Clips**

## OBJECTIVES

- Explain the importance of a balance between energy intake and output.
- List the end products of carbohydrate, protein, and lipid metabolism.
- Explain the significance of saturated, unsaturated, and polyunsaturated lipids in nutrition.
- Describe the basic food groups (using the food guide pyramid) and their value in planning meals for good nutrition.
- Explain dietary guidelines.

- Discuss the major areas of nutritional assessment.
- Identify nutritional problems, and describe a patient at risk for these problems.
- Establish a plan of care to meet the nutritional needs of the patient.
- Discuss methods for feeding patients.
- Describe the procedure for initiating and maintaining tube feedings.
- Describe the procedure for initiating and maintaining total parenteral nutrition.

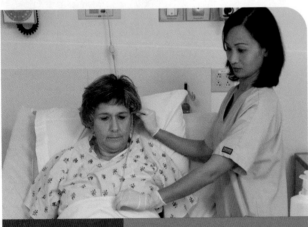

## CASE STUDY  Mrs. Gonzalez

Mrs. Gonzalez is a 65-year-old Hispanic woman who comes to the emergency department with slurred speech, right facial droop, and weakness in her upper and lower right side extremities. She has a history of hypertension and coronary artery disease. She lives alone in a senior apartment complex and works part-time at the Salvation Army providing meals to the homeless. Mrs. Gonzalez has a daughter and two small grandchildren that live in another state. She is admitted to the hospital with acute stroke.

Mrs. Gonzalez is awake and alert in her hospital room but is drooling from the right side of her mouth. When she tries to drink water, she starts to cough and she is unable to swallow her pills. The physician has ordered Mrs. Gonzalez be allowed nothing by mouth (NPO) until the speech language pathologist (SLP) is able to evaluate her.

The SLP performs a bedside swallowing evaluation and a modified barium swallow, which indicates inadequate clearance of food and liquid from the vocal folds and aspiration of thickened liquids. Mrs. Gonzalez is unable to swallow and is diagnosed with oropharyngeal dysphagia. The speech language pathologist recommends nasogastric (NG) tube feedings and speech and swallowing therapy.

Sarah Lee is a senior nursing student assigned to Mrs. Gonzalez. As Sarah prepares to assess Mrs. Gonzalez, she recalls information about the effect of dysphagia on nutrition and rehabilitation. She will assess Mrs. Gonzalez's weight and weight history, diet history, and cultural customs. Sarah knows that

consulting with a registered dietitian (RD) to assess Mrs. Gonzalez's nutritional status and to assist with nutrition interventions is necessary. The RD will make recommendations regarding the tube feeding type, rate, and schedule. Sarah and the RD will work as a team with the SLP to assist Mrs. Gonzalez in the rehabilitation of her speech and swallowing.

It is Sarah's responsibility to insert Mrs. Gonzalez's NG tube and start her tube feedings. The RD has recommended a continuous tube feeding for 12 hours during the day to reduce the risk of aspiration.

## KEY TERMS

absorption, p. 872
amino acids, p. 871
anabolism, p. 873
anthropometry, p. 879
carbohydrates, p. 871
catabolism, p. 873
dietary reference intakes (DRIs), p. 873
digestion, p. 872
dysphagia, p. 889
enteral nutrition (EN), p. 890
gluconeogenesis, p. 873
glucose, p. 873
glycogen, p. 873
glycogenesis, p. 873
jejunostomy tube, p. 892

lipid, p. 871
lipogenesis, p. 873
metabolism, p. 873
minerals, p. 872
monosaturated fatty acid, p. 871
nutrients, p. 871
obesity, p. 885
parenteral nutrition (PN), p. 892
polyunsaturated fatty acid, p. 871
proteins, p. 871
saturated fatty acid, p. 871
unsaturated fatty acid, p. 871
vitamins, p. 872

Nutrition is a basic component of health and is essential for normal growth and development, tissue maintenance and repair, cellular metabolism, and organ function. The human body needs an adequate supply of nutrients for essential functions of cells.

Scientific principles regarding nutrition and the role of various nutrients in metabolism and health form a basis for the nutritional plan of care that you develop with your patients. Disease processes, age, gender, and activity all affect utilization of nutrients and nutritional requirements. Pharmaceutical agents prescribed to treat disease also interact with nutrients and foods.

## Scientific Knowledge Base

### Principles of Nutrition

The body requires food to provide energy for movement, maintenance of body temperature, growth and development, cellular metabolism, synthesis and repair of tissues, and organ function. The gastrointestinal system is made up of a number of organs and structures that enable the body to nourish itself through the ingestion of food. Each organ or structure in the gastrointestinal (GI) tract has a specific function aimed toward preparing food for the digestion and absorption of its nutrients.

NUTRIENTS. A **nutrient** is a chemical substance that provides nourishment and affects metabolic and nutritive processes. The essential nutrients include carbohydrates, proteins, lipids, vitamins, minerals, and water. Only carbohydrates, proteins, and lipids provide energy. Vitamins and minerals are catalysts for the use of nutrients for energy. Minerals and water regulate body processes.

**Carbohydrates.** **Carbohydrates** are composed of carbon, hydrogen, and oxygen. They are starches and sugars obtained mainly from plant foods, with the exception of lactose, which is found in milk (milk sugar). Carbohydrates contribute as much as 90% of the total caloric intake in parts of the world where grains are a major food source. Carbohydrates are a source of energy, providing 4 kilocalories per gram (kcal/g).

Another type of carbohydrate is fiber. Fiber provides the structural part of plants and is sometimes called nonstarch polysaccharides. Fiber also includes some nonpolysaccharides such as lignins and tannins. Human digestive enzymes cannot break down fiber. Therefore they do not contribute calorically to the diet. Each fiber has a different structure. Most contain monosaccharides; however, they differ in types of monosaccharides and types of bonds. Fiber is either soluble or insoluble. Soluble fiber becomes a gel in water and delays gastrointestinal transit time; because of this, soluble fiber helps prevent diarrhea in tube-fed patients. Insoluble fiber does not change in water and accelerates intestinal transit; this is helpful in preventing constipation in patients taking pain medication.

**Proteins.** Amino acids are the building blocks of **proteins** and are made of hydrogen, oxygen, carbon, and nitrogen.

**Amino acids** are the most important components of proteins in the human body, and they are essential for synthesis of body tissue in growth, maintenance, and repair. The body is unable to synthesize some amino acids, such as essential amino acids. These can be obtained only from daily food sources. Proteins are a source of energy, providing 4 kcal/g.

The required daily intake of protein varies according to age. For example, infants under 6 months of age require 2.2 g/kg daily. Adolescents require 1 g/kg daily. Most healthy adults require only about 0.8 g/kg of body weight per day. In disease, protein requirements will double or triple, such as for major burns. Pregnant women require an additional 30 g and lactating women an additional 20 g above the usual daily need.

Nutrition experts believe that the intake of protein in America is generally greater than required. Protein foods are expensive to buy and produce, and fatty cuts of meat, whole milk, cheese, and eggs contain significant amounts of saturated fatty acids and cholesterol. The 2005 Dietary Guidelines for Americans recommend Americans change their diet by increasing daily intake of fruits and vegetables, whole grains, and nonfat or low-fat milk and milk products; choosing fats and carbohydrates wisely for good health (Dietary Guidelines Advisory Committee, 2004).

**Lipids.** **Lipid** is a comprehensive term applied to compounds that are insoluble in water but soluble in organic solvents such as ethanol and acetone. At room temperature these include solid fats and liquid oils. Lipids are composed of carbon, hydrogen, and oxygen. Lipids are a source of energy, providing 9 kcal/g.

Approximately 98% of the lipids in foods and 90% of the lipids in the human body are in the form of triglycerides. Triglycerides contribute to high blood levels of certain lipoproteins linked to cardiovascular diseases.

A **saturated fatty acid** contains as much hydrogen as it is able to hold. A **monounsaturated fatty acid** is able to take up another hydrogen atom, and a **polyunsaturated fatty acid** is able to take up many more hydrogen atoms and become hydrogenated or saturated fat. Ingestion of saturated fatty acids appears to increase blood cholesterol levels. Ingestion of **unsaturated fatty acids** has a minimal effect on blood cholesterol. Monounsaturated fatty acids appear to lower blood cholesterol levels. Fatty acids are usually not purely saturated, unsaturated, or polyunsaturated. Most animal fats have high proportions of saturated fatty acids; most vegetable fats have higher amounts of unsaturated and polyunsaturated fatty acids (e.g., safflower oil is about 75% polyunsaturated, olive oil about 25%).

There are also essential fatty acids (EFA.) The two primary EFA are linoleic acid (an omega-6 fatty acid) and linolenic acid (an omega-3 fatty acid). EFA have many roles in the body, including the production of cell membranes and hormones, among others. The metabolism of EFA has effects on the regulation of blood pressure, blood clot formation, and immune response.

Adipose is the body's form of energy stored as fat. The metabolism of 1 g of lipid yields 9 kcal (38 J), more than twice the energy provided by carbohydrates or proteins. Lipids account for 35% to 45% of the American diet. The American Heart Association (AHA) recommends limiting total fat intake to 30% or less of calories and saturated fats to less than10% of total energy intake for the total population, with more severe restrictions in individuals with hypercholesterolemia or cardiovascular disease (Krauss and others, 2000). In addition to restrictions in saturated fat intake, the AHA recommends increasing intake of dietary omega-3 fatty acids to assist in the treatment of hypertriglyceridemia (Kris-Etherton and others, 2002).

**Vitamins.** **Vitamins** are organic substances present in small amounts in foods and are essential for normal metabolism. They serve as coenzymes in cellular enzyme reactions. The body is unable to synthesize vitamins in the required amounts and depends on dietary intake. The exception to this is vitamin K, which the body synthesizes by bacteria in the intestine. The Food and Nutrition Board of the Institute of Medicine (1998) reviews ongoing research and periodically revises the recommended allowances for vitamins and other nutrients. Although vitamins are contained in many foods, processing, storage, and preparation all affect them. Vitamin content is usually highest in foods that are fresh and used quickly after minimal exposure to heat, air, or water. Vitamins are water-soluble and fat-soluble.

Water-soluble vitamins are stored in limited amounts for short periods of time, necessitating daily consumption. It was once assumed that water-soluble vitamins were not toxic, due to limited storage capacity. However, continuous high doses of niacin, vitamin $B_6$, choline, and vitamin C result in toxicity. Vitamins are catalysts in biochemical reactions. When there is enough of a vitamin to meet the catalyst demands, the remaining serum level of the vitamin supply acts as a free chemical and is sometimes toxic to the body.

Fat-soluble vitamins are able to be stored in the body for longer periods; however, dietary intake is still necessary, with some exceptions. Vitamin K is in dark leafy green vegetables, but the body also produces it within the large intestine. In addition, the body produces vitamin D as a response to sunlight exposure. Toxicity to all of the fat-soluble vitamins is possible, usually related to intake of synthetic vitamins.

It has been suggested that all adults consume a standard multivitamin supplement daily to prevent chronic disease. The reasoning behind this suggestion is the proposed link between supplemental folate and vitamins $B_{12}$, $B_6$, and D and prevention of cardiovascular disease, cancer, and osteoporosis (Fletcher and Fairfield, 2002). Although this is a good concept, there are risks associated with widespread supplementation. Multivitamin supplementation needs to be individualized.

**Minerals.** **Minerals** are inorganic elements that act as catalysts in biochemical reactions. Minerals are classified as macrominerals when the daily requirement is 100 mg or more and microminerals when the body needs less than 100 mg daily. Macrominerals play a role in balancing the pH of the body, and specific amounts are necessary in the blood and cells to promote acid-base balance. Microminerals are also called trace elements because the required amount is usually very small or a trace. Trace mineral content of food is variable and often depends upon the content of those minerals in soil and water. Interactions occur among trace minerals. Excess of one trace mineral sometimes causes the deficiency of another. The deficiency of one allows for toxicity of another, and the deficiency of a trace mineral will sometimes worsen the deficiency of another.

**Water.** Water is an important nutrient because the function of cells depends on an aqueous environment. The roles of water in the body include transportation of nutrients and waste products; providing structure to large molecules (protein, glycogen); participation in metabolic reactions; serving as solvent, lubricant, and cushion; regulating body temperature; and maintaining blood volume.

A lean person's body contains a higher percentage of water than an obese person's body. Infants have the greatest percentage of total body weight as water; older adults have the least. Infants and older adults are most vulnerable to water deprivation or water loss.

The human body requires 1.5 ml of water for every kilocalorie of energy used. The ingestion of liquids and solid foods, such as fresh fruits and vegetables, aids the body in meeting fluid needs. The body also produces water when food is oxidized during digestion.

Thirst is a protective mechanism that alerts the oriented person to the need for fluids. Thirst is a less reliable guide for infants and confused patients. These patients are usually unable to communicate that they are thirsty.

**DIGESTION.** The process of **digestion** begins in the mouth, where mastication, or chewing, breaks down food into smaller particles, and amylase in saliva begins to break down starches. Mucus lubricates food particles for their passage through the esophagus into the stomach. Churning movements of the stomach mix food particles with hydrochloric acid. The most significant absorption of nutrients occurs in the small intestine. Digestive proteins, or enzymes, in the gastrointestinal system break food particles into a simpler form. The small intestine digests and absorbs most nutrients; the large intestine absorbs electrolytes and water, thus helping to maintain the body's electrolyte balance (see Chapter 15).

**ABSORPTION.** The small intestine is the primary site of **absorption** of simple nutrients. It is lined with villi, which project into the lumen and greatly increase the surface area available for absorption. The upper duodenum absorbs cholesterol, vitamins E and K, folic acid, riboflavin, and thiamin. The lower duodenum and upper jejunum absorb glucose, amino acids, minerals, and fats, and the lower jejunum and ileum absorb sucrose, lactose, and maltose. Understanding sites of absorption explains the nature of diseases that might affect intestinal function.

Intestinal contents move by peristaltic action into the large intestine. Water and electrolytes are absorbed from the large intestine. The body excretes other nutrients remaining in the intestinal contents when they reach the large intestine as waste products. When intestinal motility is increased, such as in diarrhea, the body loses nutrients that move through the small intestine too quickly for complete absorption.

**METABOLISM.** Nutrients are transported through the circulatory system to body tissues. Through **metabolism,** nutrients are converted into necessary substances for cell function. Metabolism refers to all of the biochemical and physiological processes by which the body maintains itself.

Carbohydrates, protein, and fat produce chemical energy and maintain a dynamic balance of tissue buildup and breakdown. The chemical energy produced by metabolism is converted to other types of energy by different tissues. Muscle contraction involves mechanical energy, the nervous system involves electrical energy, and the mechanisms of heat production involve thermal energy. These forms of energy all begin in metabolism.

Absorbed nutrients are carried to the liver, where major metabolic processes occur. The liver also regulates energy through its control of glucose metabolism. **Glucose** is the primary fuel for the body. The liver and muscles store glucose in the form of **glycogen** via a process called **glycogenesis. Lipogenesis** converts glucose to fat for storage. Insulin and glucagon act as regulatory hormones to promote glucose storage or use. Insulin promotes glucose use, and glucagon promotes glucose storage. During states where energy needs exceed glycogen storage, the body breaks down fat and amino acids for conversion to glucose via a process called **gluconeogenesis.**

The basal metabolic rate (BMR) represents the energy needs of a person at rest after awakening. Energy needs are based on BMR along with activity level, energy required to break down food, and energy required for healing during illness. Energy balance occurs when energy requirements equal energy intake. In general, when a person exceeds his or her energy needs or his or her needs are insufficient, the person gains weight or loses weight, respectively.

The two basic types of metabolism are anabolism and catabolism. **Anabolism** is the production of more-complex chemical substances by synthesis of nutrients. **Catabolism** is the breakdown of body tissues into simpler substances. Although catabolism produces some energy, both processes require energy, which comes from food or stored sources.

**STORAGE.** The body stores energy as adipose tissue. Glycogen is stored in small reserves in liver and muscle tissue, and protein is stored in muscle mass. When the body's energy demands exceed dietary sources, the body uses stored (fat) energy. When the body has unused energy, it is stored principally in fat.

Fat-soluble vitamins are also stored in limited reserves (6 to 8 months), and the body releases them to meet the needs when dietary intake is insufficient. Most water-soluble vitamins are stored for a minimal amount of time (3 to 5 days).

**ELIMINATION.** The intestinal contents move through the large intestine by peristalsis (see Chapter 33). As the material moves toward the rectum, water is reabsorbed through the mucosa. The end products of digestion include cellulose and similar fibrous substances the body is unable to digest. The body also eliminates sloughed cells from the intestinal walls, mucus, digestive secretions, water, and microorganisms.

## Foundations of Nutrition

A number of agencies and organizations in the United States regularly publish and update dietary guidelines. The guidelines change as nutritional researchers discover new knowledge.

**U.S. DEPARTMENT OF AGRICULTURE FOOD GUIDE PYRAMID.** The food guide pyramid revised in 2005 is designed as a part of the Food Guidance System of the U.S. Department of Agriculture (USDA). It is designed to be used as part of a system intended to educate the American public on healthy eating for weight maintenance and health promotion (Center for Nutrition Policy and Promotion, 2005). The 2005 version of the food guide pyramid (Figure 31-1) reflects the revisions to the Dietary Guidelines for Americans. In addition to the pyramid, the USDA also developed interactive educational tools that are accessible through CD-ROM, the Internet, and other venues. The specific goals of the revisions are to:

- Balance energy expenditure and caloric intake to prevent weight gain
- Promote weight loss and/or maintain a healthy weight
- Increase the intake of vitamins, minerals, fiber, and other key nutrients
- Lower chronic disease risks by lowering intake of saturated fats, trans fats, cholesterol, sodium, and other food components (Hentges, 2004)

**DIETARY GUIDELINES FOR AMERICANS.** The dietary guidelines are designed to provide advice for the public based on a review of the science. The goal of these guidelines is to promote health and to reduce risk for major chronic diseases through diet and physical activity (Dietary Guidelines Advisory Committee, 2004). They were most recently updated in 2005 (Box 31-1).

**DIETARY REFERENCE INTAKES.** The Food and Nutrition Board of the National Academy of Sciences has published recommended daily allowances (RDAs) since 1943. In 1997 these recommendations were renamed **dietary reference intakes (DRIs)** in response to the increased public use of nutritional supplements. The DRIs define the recommended amounts of nutrients based on scientific evidence with the goal of chronic disease prevention. There are four components to the DRIs: estimated average requirement (EAR), recommended dietary allowances (RDAs), adequate intakes (AIs), and tolerable upper intake levels (ULs). The EAR is the amount of a nutrient that appears sufficient to maintain a specific body function for 50% of the population, and it is recommended based on age and gender. The RDA represents the average needs of 98% of the population, not the exact needs of an individual. The AI is the suggested intake for individuals based on observed or experimentally deter-

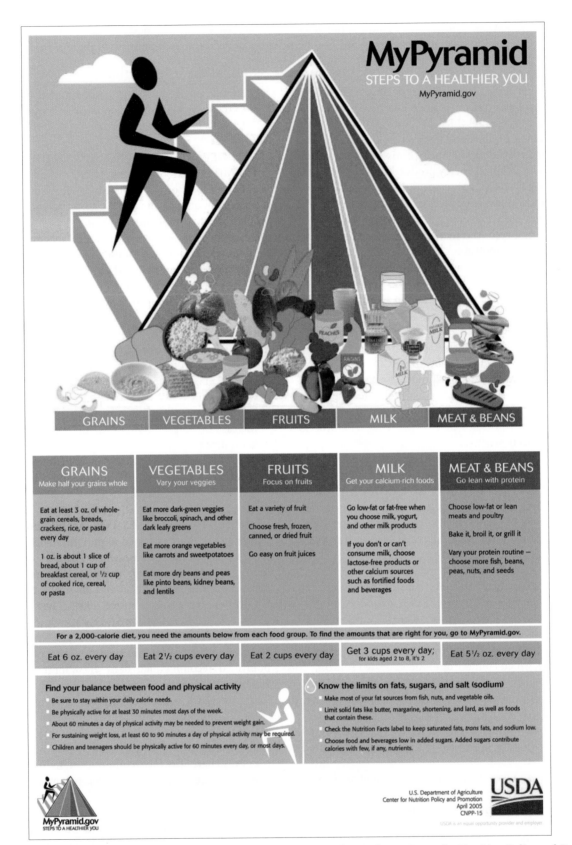

FIGURE 31-1 Sample food guide pyramid for adults. (From U.S. Department of Agriculture: Center for Nutrition Policy and Promotion, April 2005, http://www.MyPyramid.gov.)

---

**BOX 31-1    Dietary Guidelines for Americans**

Adequate Nutrients Within Calorie Needs
Weight Management
Physical Activity
Food Groups to Encourage in Moderation
  Fats
  Carbohydrates
  Sodium and Potassium
  Alcoholic Beverages
  Food Safety

---

Modified from U.S. Department of Health and Human Services and
U.S Department of Agriculture: *Executive summary: Dietary Guidelines
for Americans 2005*, 2005, http://www.health.gov/dietaryguidelines/
dga2005/document/html/executivesummary.htm.

---

**BOX 31-2    Examples of Nutrition Objectives from Healthy People 2010**

Increase the proportion of adults who are at a healthy weight
  (BMI 18.5 to 24.9)
Reduction of obesity in children and adolescents to 5% and
  adults to 15%
Decrease in growth retardation to 5% in low-income children
  <5 years
Decrease in fat intake to <30% and saturated fat intake to
  <10% of total calories daily
Decrease in saturated fat intake to <10% of total calories daily
Vegetable and fruit intake of five daily servings in 75% of people
Increase intake of grain products to six daily servings in 50% of
  people
Calcium DRI met in 75% of people
Sodium daily intake no more than 2400 mg in 65% of people
Reduction of prevalence of anemia in pregnant women to 20%
Nutrient-dense meals and snacks at school for children and
  adolescents
Nutritional education and counseling services for diabetics at
  primary care sites
Increase in prevalence of food security to 94% of households

---

Data from Food and Drug Administration, National Institutes of
Health: Nutrition and overweight. In U.S. Department of Health
and Human Services, Public Health Service: *Healthy People 2010*, ed 2,
Washington, DC, 2000, U.S. Government Printing Office.

---

mined estimates of nutrient intakes by groups and is provided when there is insufficient evidence to set RDA. The UL is the highest level that likely poses no risk of adverse health events. It is not a recommended level of intake (Food and Nutrition Board 1998).

**OTHER DIETARY GUIDELINES.** Other professional organizations have published dietary guidelines. Examples of this are the American Cancer Society Guidelines for Cancer Prevention and the American Heart Association Guidelines for Heart Healthy Eating. These guidelines are similar to the Dietary Guidelines for Americans.

In 1997 the U.S. Department of Health and Human Services (USDHHS) and the Public Health Service (PHS) began a consensus process that resulted in the updated publication of *Healthy People 2010: Understanding and Improving Health* (see Chapter 1). The report defines national goals or objectives to be met in this decade to increase the proportion of Americans who live long, healthy lives. Nutrition-related goals for the year 2010 include increasing intake of fruits, vegetables, and grain products and reducing fat and sodium consumption. There continues to be an effort to integrate these goals with the food guide pyramid, the nutrition facts label, and the healthy index recommended by the USDA (Food and Drug Administration and National Institutes of Health, 2000) (Box 31-2).

## Nursing Knowledge Base

There are social, cultural, and emotional aspects in eating and drinking in all societies (Negus 1994; Shaw and Power, 1999). We celebrate holidays and events with food, bring food to those who are grieving, and use food for medicinal purposes. We also recognize cultural food differences, incorporate food into family traditions and rituals, and associate appearance with eating behaviors. Some abstain from or recognize foods in religious beliefs and practices and as-

sociate certain foods and dining practices with socioeconomic status.

For most people, food has sociological and psychological significance, which varies with each individual. In attempting to affect eating patterns, understand patients' values, beliefs, and attitudes about food and how those values affect food purchase, preparation, and intake.

Nutritional requirements depend upon many factors. Individual caloric and nutrient requirements vary by stage of development, body composition, activity levels, conditions such as pregnancy and lactation, and the presence of disease. Culture and religion also influence dietary patterns and needs (Box 31-3). Registered dietitians (RD) use predictive equations that take into account some of those factors to estimate patient's nutrition requirements.

### Alternative Food Patterns

Individuals follow special patterns of food intake based on religion, cultural background, ethics, health beliefs, personal preference, or concern about the environment. Such special diets do not necessarily provide more or less nutritional benefit than diets based on the food guide pyramid or other nutritional guidelines. Adequate nutritional intake depends on balanced consumption of all required nutrients. The vegetarian diet is an example of a dietary pattern that is commonly consumed because of religious or personal beliefs. The vegetarian diet is primarily plant based and includes the elimination of many animal-based foods.

| BOX 31-3 | **Culture and Religious Factors Influencing Dietary Patterns** |

**Culture**

- Acceptability of food
- Healing properties of some foods
- Place of birth and upbringing
- Geography and climate
- Customs and traditions
- Fasting practices

**Religion**

- Acceptability of foods in accordance with religious customs (e.g., kosher, halal)
- Ethical conviction (e.g., the use of genetically modified organisms, avoidance of animal products)

Modified from Brown A: *Understanding food: principles and preparation*, ed 2, Belmont, Calif, 2004, Wadsworth Publishing.

Vegetarians are grouped into several categories. Ovolactovegetarians avoid meat, fish, and poultry but eat eggs and milk. Lactovegetarians drink milk but avoid eggs and other animal-based foods. Vegans eat only foods of plant origin. Individuals consuming the vegan diet are susceptible to vitamin $B_{12}$ and protein deficiency. Vegans need to supplement their diets with vitamin $B_{12}$ and carefully choose foods to ensure ingestion of essential amino acids. Knowledge of high biological value protein versus low biological value protein sources is necessary to ensure intake of all of the essential amino acids.

## Developmental Needs

Stage of life also affects energy and protein needs. As an individual matures into an adult, the energy required per kilogram of body weight for adequate growth decreases (see Chapter 19).

In addition, when rapid growth periods end, as with the young and middle adult, the energy needs decline and the risk of weight gain increases. If unchecked, this weight gain will result in obesity. Increased physical exercise, a healthy dietary intake that is low in fat and high in fresh fruits and vegetables, and moderate use of convenience foods all help to reduce the risk of weight gain.

## ▌Critical Thinking

### Synthesis

Critical thinking enables you to synthesize information gathered from knowledge, experience, attitudes, and standards to provide appropriate nutritional care. The end result of critical thinking will be your clinical judgment of the patient's nutritional problems and subsequent nursing interventions.

**KNOWLEDGE.** Application of knowledge from nutritional principles and the basic and social sciences form your knowledge base related to nutritional care. Information that comes from interviewing and observing the patient and the responses you obtain during nursing interventions will guide you toward application of knowledge. For example, your patient reports a dietary pattern of avoiding cabbage. This pattern could arise from physiological discomfort (gas-forming food), psychological issues (forced to eat cabbage as a child), sociological reasons (associated with lower socioeconomic class), ethnicity (not readily available in the country of origin), teaching- or learning-related reasons (never taught how to prepare cabbage), or mythology (a food that contains harmful chemicals). A nurse will consider these factors in planning a nutritious diet.

**EXPERIENCE.** Just as multiple factors influence your patients' choices of dietary practices, multiple factors also influence your dietary patterns. Individuals who have nutritional or health problems change their long-standing dietary practices to enhance health. In assisting a patient in changing dietary patterns, draw on examples from your own experience. Perhaps you attempted to change a dietary practice or have a family member who requires a special diet. Previous experiences with therapeutic diets or behavioral changes will assist in the identification of nursing interventions that will be successful for the patient.

**ATTITUDES.** Integrity and discipline are critical thinking skills that are beneficial during nutritional assessment and counseling. Although you will encounter patients whose dietary practices are dramatically different from yours, you assist those patients in attaining a nutritionally balanced diet. In addition, you will encounter patients whose dietary patterns are not healthful. Changes in dietary practices often occur over time. Perseverence will be necessary in educating patients to understand the impact of unhealthful food choices.

**STANDARDS.** Standards established by the DRIs, AHA, American Society of Parenteral and Enteral Nutrition (AS-PEN), American Dietetic Association (ADA), or other professional organizations help to structure nutrition interventions. ASPEN and ADA provide recommendations for aggressive nutrition intervention, as well as intervention in end-of-life care. Ethical issues in health care have arisen around the withdrawal or withholding of specialized feeding (Burck, 1996). Food symbolizes love and care to many individuals (Schwarte, 2001). Patients and families with advanced disease view nutrition support as life sustaining and sometimes use this to elicit some control in their final days. Some patients and family members request enteral nutrition or parenteral nutrition when patients are eating poorly (Whitworth and others, 2004). The use of this aggressive nutrition intervention in terminal patients is usually unnecessary and produces little benefit (ASPEN, 2002). You can avoid these issues partially with the use of advance directives and intensive education. As part of an advance directive, patients are asked if they wish to have nutrition or hydration as a

## SYNTHESIS IN PRACTICE

As Sarah prepares to assess Mrs. Gonzalez, she recalls information about nutrition and its effect on rehabilitation, especially the importance of adequate caloric protein intake in patients who have had a stroke. She will focus assessment on Mrs. Gonzalez's weight, need for enteral nutrition, elimination patterns, and rehabilitation efforts. Sarah knows that it is important to assess for tolerance of feeding as well.

Sarah knows that consulting with a dietitian to further assess Mrs. Gonzalez's nutritional status and assist with nutritional in-

terventions will be beneficial. The dietitian will use data from Sarah's initial nursing assessment and assist Sarah in collecting further nutrition-related information.

Experience has taught Sarah that economic and cultural preferences will also affect the acceptance of tube feeding. She is aware that Mrs. Gonzalez may perceive the initiation of enteral feedings as a loss of independence. Sarah will reassure the patient that the tube feeding is necessary for her safety and explains that the goal will be to restart oral feedings as soon as it is safe to do so.

means of life support. Advance directives make the patients' wishes known and have become a standard area of assessment for patients in the hospital and in the home care setting.

## Nursing Process

### Assessment

**SCREENING.** Nutritional screening is part of your initial assessment of the patient. The nutrition screening is a quick method of identifying malnutrition or risk of malnutrition (ASPEN, 2002). Nutritional screenng tools commonly include objective measures such as height, weight, weight change, primary diagnosis, and the presence of comorbidities (ASPEN, 2002). Single objective measures alone are ineffective predictors of nutrition risk (Sarhill and others, 2003). You combine multiple objective measures with subjective measures related to nutrition to screen for nutrition risk (Council on Practice [COP], 1994).

There are several standardized nutrition screening tools for you to use in the outpatient setting. The Mini Nutritional Assessment (MNA) (Figure 31-2) was developed for the older adult population. This 18-item tool has two sections: screening and assessment. The screening contains 6 questions related to decline in food intake, weight loss, mobility, stress, and body mass index (BMI). The health care practitioner completes the assessment portion if the patient scores 11 or less (Guigoz and others, 1996). The 12-item assessment includes specific medical history and eating habits, as well as some anthropometric measurements. A score of less than 17 points indicates protein-energy malnutrition (PEM) (Guigoz and others, 1996; Guigoz and Vellas, 1999).

Acute care institutions commonly use the initial nursing assessment as a nutrition screening. Certain nutrition risk factors, such as unintentional weight loss, the presence of a modified diet, or the presence of nutrition impact symptoms (i.e., nausea, vomiting, diarrhea, constipation), are triggers for nutritional consultation.

**NUTRITION ASSESSMENT.** If you find a patient is at risk for nutritional problems, the next step is a more in-depth nutritional assessment by an RD, if possible. Nutrition assessment is different from nutrition screening. Nutrition assessment is

an in-depth exploration of medical history, dietary history, physical examination, anthropometric measurements, and laboratory data (Table 31-1) (COP, 1994). This process leads to the identification and diagnosis of nutritional issues (Lacey and Pritchett, 2003). Nutrition assessment includes the determination of nutrient and protein needs. In an acute care setting the RD is available to make these calculations. In an outpatient setting, there is not always an RD to complete the nutrition assessment. Tools such as the MNA can help nurses perform nutrition assessment.

**Diet History.** The diet history focuses on habitual intake of food and liquids and information about preferences, allergies, and digestive problems (Box 31-4). Open-ended questions encourage the patient to elaborate on food intake during the interview. For example, ask a patient who reports that she avoids dairy products, "Tell me what led you to avoid dairy products?" The patient's answer to this question will lead to physiological, psychological, sociological, religious, cultural, or food preference factors that you will further explore.

Ask a patient to keep a detailed record of food intake over 3 days, representing a typical eating pattern. Have the patient include a weekend day. This record allows you to calculate the patient's nutritional intake and to compare it with the DRIs. Instruct your patients to record the specific type of foods and the exact amounts ingested. This requires the use of measuring cups and scales. Information on patient's activity level and presence of disease will be necessary to estimate energy needs. For example, a patient who has a fever or has suffered severe trauma has high caloric demands even though the activity level is limited. You compare estimated energy need, as calculated through prediction equations, to actual caloric intake, through calorie counts. Calorie counts use records of exact amounts of food trays consumed as documented by the nursing or nutrition staff to calculate total calories and protein consumed daily. You will need to consult with an RD to determine an exact calorie count or requirements.

**Medication History.** Prescribed and over-the-counter medications have the potential for drug-nutrient interactions. Knowing what medications your patients take is important when meeting nutritional needs. Consultation with a pharmacist will determine the specific risks for nutrient/drug interactions for your patients.

**Nestlé**

# Mini Nutritional Assessment
## MNA®

Last name:      First name:      Sex:      Date:

Age:      Weight, kg:      Height, cm:      I.D. Number:

*Complete the screen by filling in the boxes with the appropriate numbers.*
*Add the numbers for the screen. If score is 11 or less, continue with the assessment to gain a Malnutrition Indicator Score.*

## Screening

**A** Has food intake declined over the past 3 months due to loss of appetite, digestive problems, chewing or swallowing difficulties?
0 = severe loss of appetite
1 = moderate loss of appetite
2 = no loss of appetite

**B** Weight loss during the last 3 months
0 = weight loss greater than 3 kg (6.6 lbs)
1 = does not know
2 = weight loss between 1 and 3 kg (2.2 and 6.6 lbs)
3 = no weight loss

**C** Mobility
0 = bed or chair bound
1 = able to get out of bed/chair but does not go out
2 = goes out

**D** Has suffered psychological stress or acute disease in the past 3 months
0 = yes      2 = no

**E** Neuropsychological problems
0 = severe dementia or depression
1 = mild dementia
2 = no psychological problems

**F** Body Mass Index (BMI) (weight in kg) / (height in m)$^2$
0 = BMI less than 19
1 = BMI 19 to less than 21
2 = BMI 21 to less than 23
3 = BMI 23 or greater

**Screening score** (subtotal max. 14 points)
12 points or greater   Normal – not at risk – no need to complete assessment
11 points or below   Possible malnutrition – continue assessment

## Assessment

**G** Lives independently (not in a nursing home or hospital)
0 = no      1 = yes

**H** Takes more than 3 prescription drugs per day
0 = yes      1 = no

**I** Pressure sores or skin ulcers
0 = yes      1 = no

**J** How many full meals does the patient eat daily?
0 = 1 meal
1 = 2 meals
2 = 3 meals

**K** Selected consumption markers for protein intake
• At least one serving of dairy products (milk, cheese, yogurt) per day?   yes ☐   no ☐
• Two or more servings of legumes or eggs per week?   yes ☐   no ☐
• Meat, fish or poultry every day   yes ☐   no ☐
0.0 = if 0 or 1 yes
0.5 = if 2 yes
1.0 = if 3 yes

**L** Consumes two or more servings of fruits or vegetables per day?
0 = no      1 = yes

**M** How much fluid (water, juice, coffee, tea, milk…) is consumed per day?
0.0 = less than 3 cups
0.5 = 3 to 5 cups
1.0 = more than 5 cups

**N** Mode of feeding
0 = unable to eat without assistance
1 = self-fed with some difficulty
2 = self-fed without any problem

**O** Self view of nutritional status
0 = views self as being malnourished
1 = is uncertain of nutritional state
2 = views self as having no nutritional problem

**P** In comparison with other people of the same age, how does the patient consider his/her health status?
0.0 = not as good
0.5 = does not know
1.0 = as good
2.0 = better

**Q** Mid-arm circumference (MAC) in cm
0.0 = MAC less than 21
0.5 = MAC 21 to 22
1.0 = MAC 22 or greater

**R** Calf circumference (CC) in cm
0 = CC less than 31      1 = CC 31 or greater

**Assessment** (max. 16 points)

**Screening score**

**Total Assessment** (max. 30 points)

## Malnutrition Indicator Score
17 to 23.5 points      at risk of malnutrition

Less than 17 points      malnourished

Ref.: Guigoz Y, Vellas B and Garry P.J. 1994. Mini Nutritional Assessment: A practical assessment tool for grading the nutritional state of elderly patients. *Facts and Research in Gerontology.* Supplement #2:15-59.
Rubenstein LZ, Harker J, Guigoz Y and Vellas B. Comprehensive Geriatric Assessment (CGA) and the MNA: An Overview of CGA, Nutritional Assessment, and Development of a Shortened Version of the MNA. In: "Mini Nutritional Assessment (MNA): Research and Practice in the Elderly". Vellas B, Garry P.J and Guigoz Y, editors. Nestlé Nutrition Workshop Series. Clinical & Performance Programme, vol. 1. Karger, Bâle, in press.

FIGURE **31-2** Mini Nutritional Assessment (MNA). (Reprinted with permission by Nestle Nutrition.)

## FOCUSED PATIENT ASSESSMENT

TABLE 31-1

| Factors to Assess | Questions and Approaches | Physical Assessment Strategies |
|---|---|---|
| Food and nutrient intake<br>Patterns and dietary history | Ask patient or family for a 24-hour diet recall<br>Ask patient or family about food preferences, allergies, dislikes | Inspect oral cavity for physical barriers to eating, (e.g., tooth decay, poor fitting dentures)<br>Observe patient swallowing<br>Observe percentage of food consumed from meal tray |
| Changes in weight | Ask patient about any recent change in weight<br>Determine if weight change was desired<br>Determine presence of medications that alter taste or appetite | Weigh patient<br>Observe patient's muscle tone<br>Assess skin turgor<br>Inspect oral cavity for signs of malnutrition, such as cheilosis, stomatitis, and dry lesions at corners of mouth (see Table 31-2) |
| Skin | Ask patient if there is a change in skin, for example, acne, or bruising | Observe skin for color, moisture, changes in pigment, or bruising (see Table 31-2) |

Modified from Council on Practice (COP) Quality Management Committee: Identifying patients at risk: ADA's definitions for nutrition screening and nutrition assessment, *J Am Diet Assoc* 94(8):838, 1994.

---

### BOX 31-4 | Information Contained in a Diet History

Twenty-four-hour diet recall of the day
- Use of enteral or parenteral nutrition
- Food consumed for breakfast, lunch, dinner, and snacks
- Number of meals and snacks a day
- Timing of meals and snacks
- Use of nutritional supplements

Dietary restrictions
- Medically prescribed diets
- Modified-consistency diets

Food preferences, allergies, and aversions
- Foods that cause indigestion, diarrhea, or gas

Chewing or swallowing difficulties (examine the mouth)
- Use of dentures (have patient remove dentures to examine the mouth)
- Presence of tooth decay
- Presence of xerostomia, mucositis, or mouth sores

Usual bowel movements
- Presence of constipation or diarrhea
- Duration of constipation or diarrhea

Meal procurement and preparation responsibility

Appetite changes

Modified from Whitney E, Rolfes S, editors: *Understanding Nutrition*, ed 9, Stamford, 2002, Wadsworth Publishing.

---

**PATIENTS AT RISK FOR NUTRITIONAL PROBLEMS.** A patient with a condition that interferes with the ability to ingest, digest, or absorb adequate nutrients needs to be assessed for malnutrition (Figure 31-3). Congenital anomalies and surgical revisions of the gastrointestinal tract interfere with normal function. Patients fed only by intravenous infusion of 5% to 10% dextrose are at risk for nutritional defi-

ciencies. Older adults, infants, or the malnourished are at greatest risk. Box 31-5 summarizes common conditions and pathophysiology that place patients at nutritional risk.

**PHYSICAL EXAMINATION.** Examine the patient for signs of actual or potential nutritional alterations (Table 31-2). The skin and hair are primary areas that reflect nutrient deficiencies. Be alert for rashes, dry scaly skin, poor skin turgor, skin lesions, hair loss, easily pluckable hair, hair without luster, and an unhealthy scalp.

**ANTHROPOMETRY. Anthropometry** is a systematic measurement of the size and makeup of the body using height and weight as the principle measures. You typically obtain height and weight measurements during a patient's admission to any health care setting. If the patient is unable to stand, you estimate height by measuring the patient's length with a tape measure while lying supine. Weight can be assessed with bed scales. You then compare height and weight with usual measurements, called usual body weight (UBW) and standard norms for normal height-weight relationships, called ideal body weight (IBW). Serial measures of weight over time provide more useful information than one measurement. When collecting serial measurements of weight, you weigh the patient about the same time each day, on the same scale, and with the same amount of clothing. In some patients, weight changes of 2 lb in 24 hours is significant because 1 lb is roughly equivalent to 500 ml of fluid.

BMI is an indicator of the relationship of height to weight. You calculate it by dividing weight in kilograms (kg) by height in meters squared ($m^2$). A BMI range of 18.5 to 24.9 is recommended for optimal health. BMI is commonly used to describe disease risk with respect to adiposity. BMI underestimates body fat in those who have lost muscle mass, such as older adults or those with chronic disease (National Heart Lung and Blood Institute, 2000). Body builders and patients with large amounts of edema or ascites also experience false

## Nutrition Risk Assessment

Name _____ Adm date _____ Rm _____ Assess type _____

DOB _____ Age _____ Sex: M  F  Advance directive _____ Physician _____

Diagnosis _____

Ht (in) _____ Wt (lb) _____ Wt (kg) _____ Usual body wt range _____ BMI _____

BEE _____ Activity factor _____ Injury factor _____ Total cal _____ Total protein _____ g ( _____ g/kg)

Total fluids _____ cc ( _____ cc/kg) Fluid restriction _____

Diet order _____ Food allergies/sensitivities _____

Supplement/snacks _____ Cultural/religious preferences _____

| Risk Factor | No/Low Risk (0 pts) | Moderate Risk (1 pt) | High Risk (3 pts) | MDS Ref | Pts | Comments |
|---|---|---|---|---|---|---|
| Weight status; loss or gain | BMI 19-27 No weight change | <5% wt change in 30 days; <7.5% within 90 days; or <10% within 6 mo | BMI <19 or >27 ≥5% wt change in 30 days; ≥7.5% in 90 days; or ≥10% within 6 mo | J, K, E | | |
| Oral/nutrition intake; food | Intake meets 76-100% of estimated needs | Intake meets 26-75% of estimated needs | Intake meets ≤25% of estimated needs | AC, J, K | | |
| Oral/nutrition intake; fluids | Consumes 1,500-2,000 cc/day | Consumes 1,000-1,499 cc/day | Consumes < 1,000 cc/day | AC, J, K | | |
| Medications; nutrition-related | 0-1 drugs/day | 2-4 drugs/day | 5 or more drugs/day | O | | |
| Relevant conditions and diagnoses | HTN, DM, heart disease, or other controlled diseases/conditions | Anemia, infection, CVA (recent), fracture, UTI, alcohol abuse, drug abuse, COPD, edema, surgery (recent), osteoporosis, hx of GI bleed, food intolerances and allergies, poor circulation, constipation, diarrhea, GERD, anorexia, Parkinson's | Cancer (advanced), septicemia, liver failure, dialysis, ESRD, Alzheimer's, dementia, depression, dehydration, dysphagia, radiation/chemo, active GI bleed, chronic nausea, vomiting, ostomy, gastrectomy, fecal impaction, uncontrolled diseases or conditions | E, H, I, J, M, P | | |
| Physical and mental functioning | Ambulatory, alert, able to feed self, no chewing or swallowing problems | Out of bed w/assistance, motor agitation (tremors, wandering), limited feeding assistance, supervision while eating, chewing or swallowing problems, teeth in poor repair, ill-fitting dentures or refusal to wear dentures, edentulous, taste and sensory changes, unable to communicate needs | Bedridden, inactive, total dependence, extensive or total assistance or dependence while eating, aspirates, tube feeding, TPN, mouth pain | A, B, E, G, L, P | | |
| Lab values | Albumin and other nutrition-related lab values WNL | Albumin 3.0-3.4 g/dL, 1-2 other nutrition-related labs abnormal | Albumin less than 3.0 g/dL, 3-5 other nutrition-related labs abnormal | P | | |
| Skin conditions | Skin intact | Stage I/II pressure ulcers or skin tears not healing, hx of pressure ulcers, stasis ulcer, fecal incontinence | Stage III/IV pressure ulcers or multiple impaired areas | M | | |

**Overall Risk Category:**   0-2 points: NO/LOW RISK     3-7 points: MODERATE RISK   ≥8 points: HIGH RISK

**Total Points:** _____         **Overall Risk Category:** _____

Signature: _____ Date: _____

FIGURE **31-3** Nutrition Risk Assessment (NRA). (Reprinted with permission by Consultant Dietitians in Health Care Facilities Practice Group of the American Dietetic Association.)

| BOX 31-5 | **Indicators of Risk for Malnutrition in Adults** |
|---|---|

Involuntary loss or gain of
- ≥10% of usual body weight within 6 months
- ≥5% of usual body weight in 1 month

Current weight 20% over or under ideal body weight (as determined by a prediction equation)

Presence of chronic disease or increased metabolic requirements
Inadequate nutrient intake
- Altered diets or diet schedules
- Inability to ingest or absorb food

Modified from ASPEN Board of Directors and Clinical Guidelines Task Force: Guidelines for the use of parenteral and enteral nutrition in adult and pediatric patients, *JPEN J Parenter Enteral Nutr* 26(1 Suppl):1SA, 2002.

| TABLE 31-2 | **Physical Signs of Nutritional Status** |
|---|---|

| Body Area | Normal Appearance | Indicators of Malnutrition |
|---|---|---|
| General appearance | Alert, responsive | Listless, apathetic, cachectic |
| Weight | Normal for height, age, body build | Overweight or underweight (special concern for underweight) |
| Posture | Erect, arms and legs straight | Sagging shoulders, sunken chest, humped back |
| Muscles | Well-developed, firm, good tone, some fat under skin | Flaccid, poor tone, undeveloped, tender, "wasted" appearance, impaired ability to walk |
| Nervous control | Good attention span, not irritable or restless, normal reflexes, psychological stability | Inattentive, irritable, confused, burning and tingling of hands and feet (paresthesia), loss of position and vibratory sense, weakness and tenderness of muscles (may result in inability to walk), decrease or loss of ankle and knee reflexes |
| Gastrointestinal function | Good appetite and digestion, normal regular elimination, no palpable (perceptible to touch) organs or masses | Anorexia, indigestion, constipation or diarrhea, liver or spleen enlargement |
| Cardiovascular function | Normal heart rate and rhythm, no murmurs, normal blood pressure for age | Rapid heart rate (above 100 beats per minute, tachycardia), enlarged heart, abnormal rhythm, elevated blood pressure |
| General vitality | Endurance, energetic, sleeps well, vigorous | Easily fatigued, no energy, falls asleep easily, looks tired, apathetic |
| Hair | Shiny, lustrous, firm, not easily plucked, healthy scalp | Stringy, dull, brittle, dry, thin and sparse, depigmented, easily plucked |
| Skin (general) | Smooth, slightly moist, good color | Rough, dry, scaly, pale, pigmented, irritated, bruises, petechiae |
| Face and neck | Skin color uniform, smooth, healthy appearance, not swollen | Greasy, discolored, scaly, swollen, skin dark over cheeks and under eyes, lumpiness or flakiness of skin around nose and mouth |
| Lips | Smooth, good color, moist, not chapped or swollen | Dry, scaly, swollen, redness and swelling (cheilosis), or angular lesions at corners of the mouth or fissures or scars (stomatitis) |
| Mouth, oral mucous membranes | Reddish pink mucous membranes in oral cavity | Swollen, deep red or magenta oral mucous membranes, oral lesions |
| Gums | Good pink color, healthy, red, no swelling or bleeding | Spongy, bleed easily, marginal redness, inflamed, receding |
| Tongue | Good pink color or deep reddish in appearance, not swollen or smooth, surface papillae present, no lesions | Swelling, scarlet and raw, magenta color, beefy (glossitis), hyperemic and hypertrophic papillae, atrophic papillae |
| Teeth | No pain, no sensitivity | Missing teeth, broken teeth |
| Eyes | Bright, clear, shiny, no sores at corner of eyelids, membranes moist and healthy pink color, no prominent blood vessels or mound of tissue or sclera, no fatigue circles beneath | Eye membranes pale (pale conjunctivae), redness of membrane (conjunctival injection), dryness of infection, Bitot's spots, redness and fissuring of eyelid corners (angular palpebritis), dryness of eye membrane (conjunctival xerosis), dull appearance of cornea (corneal xerosis), soft cornea (keratomalacia) |
| Neck (glands) | No enlargement | Thyroid or lymph nodes enlarged |
| Nails | Firm, pink | Spoon-shaped (koilonychia), brittle, ridged |
| Legs and feet | No tenderness, weakness, or swelling; good color | Edema, tender calf, tingling, weakness, lesions |
| Skeleton | No malformations | Bowlegs, knock-knees, chest deformity at diaphragm, beaded ribs, prominent scapulas |

Data from Nix S: *Williams' basic nutrition and diet therapy,* ed 12, St. Louis, 2005, Mosby.

---

**BOX 31-6** **Causes of Dysphagia**

| Myogenic | Neurogenic | Obstructive | Other |
|---|---|---|---|
| Myasthenia gravis | Stroke | Benign peptic stricture | Gastrointestinal or esophageal resection |
| Aging | Cerebral palsy | Lower esophageal ring | Rheumatologic disorders |
| Muscular dystrophy | Guillain-Barré syndrome | Candidiasis | Connective tissue disorders |
| Polymyositis | Multiple sclerosis | Head and neck cancer | Vagotomy |
| | Amyotrophic lateral sclerosis (Lou Gehrig disease) | Inflammatory masses | |
| | Diabetic neuropathy | Trauma/surgical resection | |
| | Parkinson's disease | Anterior mediastinal masses | |
| | | Cervical spondylosis | |

---

overestimation of the degree of fatness, so use clinical judgment when evaluating the BMI of these individuals (Expert Panel on the Identification, Evaluation and Treatment of Overweight and Obesity in Adults, 2000).

**DYSPHAGIA.** **Dysphagia** refers to swallowing dysfunction. It occurs as a result of neurogenic, myogenic, and obstructive causes (Box 31-6). The complications of dysphagia are diverse, including increased length of stay, pulmonary infections, disability/decreased functional status, decreased nutrition status, increased likelihood of discharge to institutionalized care, and increased mortality (Elmstahl and others, 1999; Perry and Love, 2001).

There are several indicators that warn you that your patient has dysphagia. Cough; change in voice tone or quality after swallowing; abnormal movements of the mouth, tongue, or lips; and slow, weak, imprecise or uncoordinated speech are all signs of dysphagia. Some other signs are abnormal gag, delayed swallowing, incomplete oral clearance or pocketing, regurgitation, pharyngeal pooling, delayed or absent trigger of swallow, and inability to speak consistently (Groher, 1997). Patients with dysphagia do not usually exhibit overt signs such as coughing when food enters the airway. "Silent aspiration," or aspiration that occurs without a cough, is a common cause of complications (Hammond and others, 2001). Silent aspiration accounts for 40% to 70% of aspiration in patients with dysphagia (Daniels and others, 2000).

Dysphagia includes two primary types: oropharyngeal and esophageal. Oropharyngeal dysphagia is further subdivided into the voluntary oral phase of swallowing and the pharyngeal phase. Causes of oropharyngeal dysphagia include neurogenic disorders, decreased salivation, oropharyngeal lesions, weakness of lips, decreased oral sensitivity, Sjögren's syndrome (dry mouth), or cognitive disorders. Esophageal dysphagia affects the involuntary phase of swallowing and is related to obstructive disorders, motility disorders, or motor dysfunction (Spieker, 2000).

Dysphagia cause decreases in food intake, which subsequently results in malnutrition. Patients that experience dysphagia illustrate changes in skinfold thickness and albumin, indicating malnutrition. This malnutrition commonly occurs secondary to inability to consume an adequate volume of food. Frustrations with the process of feeding and swallowing impede adequate ingestion of food. The period of adjustment to new dietary restrictions and the rehabilitation period affect intake for long periods of time. Malnutrition due to inadequate protein, calorie, and micronutrient intake will significantly slow down recovery (Bending, 2001; Elmstahl and others, 1999; Perry and Love, 2001). Early screening and treatment of dysphagia lead to more cost-effective treatment and improved quality of care (Elmstahl and others, 1999; Hinds and Wiles, 1998).

**Dysphagia Screening.** Similar to nutrition screening, the purpose of dysphagia screening is to quickly identify problems with swallowing and to refer at-risk patients for a more in-depth assessment (Skill 31-1). There are many dysphagia screening tools. The Registered Dietitian Dysphagia Screening Tool includes medical record review, observation of a patient at a meal for change in voice quality, posture and head control, percentage of meal consumed, eating time, drooling of liquids and solids, cough during/after a swallow, facial or tongue weakness, difficulty with secretions, pocketing, and presence of voluntary and dry cough (Brody and others, 2000). Screening tools such as the Burke Dysphagia Screening Test and the Standardized Swallowing Assessment have also been validated in patients with dysphagia (Perry and Love, 2001). All of these tools look at holding, leakage, coughing, choking, breathlessness, and quality of voice. Each also contains a component with or without the administration of water (Perry, 2001; Wood and Emick-Herring, 1997). These tools are designed for multidisciplinary use by RNs, RDs, physicians, or SLPs (Brody and others, 2000; Daniels and others, 2000; Perry and Love, 2001).

**LABORATORY VALUES.** Laboratory values useful in nutritional assessment include complete blood count (CBC), albumin, prealbumin (transferrin), electrolytes, blood urea nitrogen, creatinine, glucose, cholesterol, and triglycerides. A low red blood cell count and depressed hemoglobin value indicates anemia. The hemoglobin, hematocrit, electrolyte, and blood urea nitrogen values also help to reflect the state of hydration. Researchers have linked decreased serum levels of albumin and prealbumin with malnutrition; however, disease state and metabolic stress highly affect these values (Fuhrman and others, 2004). Individual laboratory measures alone are not specific enough to indicate nutrition risk (Sarhill and oth-

*Text continued on p. 885*

# SKILL 31-1 Aspiration Precautions

## Delegation Considerations

The assessment of a patient's risk for aspiration and determination of positioning should not be delegated. However, assistive personnel may feed patients after receiving instruction in aspiration precautions. The nurse must instruct assistive personnel to:

- Report to the nurse in charge, as soon as possible, any onset of coughing, gagging, or pocketing of food

## Equipment

- Chair or electric bed (to allow patient to sit upright)
- Thickening agents as needed (rice, cereal, yogurt, gelatin, commercial thickening agent)
- Tongue blade
- Penlight

| STEP | RATIONALE |
|---|---|
| **ASSESSMENT** | |
| 1. Perform nutritional screening. | Patients at risk for aspiration from dysphagia may alter their eating patterns or choose foods that do not provide adequate nutrition (Perry and McLaren, 2003). |
| 2. Assess patients who are at increased risk of aspiration (Box 31-6) for signs and symptoms of dysphagia (e.g., cough, pharyngeal pooling, change in voice after swallowing). | Patient may exhibit symptoms or demonstrate poor lip and tongue control. Patients at risk include those who have neurological or neuromuscular diseases and those who have had trauma to or surgical procedures of the oral cavity or throat. |
| 3. Observe patient during mealtime for signs of dysphagia, and allow patient to attempt to feed self. Observe patient consume various consistencies of foods and liquids. Note at end of meal if patient fatigues. | Can detect abnormal eating patterns such as frequent clearing of throat or prolonged eating time. Fatigue increases risk of aspiration. |
| 4. Ask patient about any difficulties with chewing or swallowing various textures of food. | Select foods may be more easily aspirated than others. |
| 5. Report signs and symptoms of dysphagia to the physician or health care provider. | Patient may need to have an evaluation performed by a radiologist or speech language pathologist (Perry, 2001). |
| 6. Place identification on patient's chart or Kardex indicating that dysphagia is present. | Identifying patient as having dysphagia reduces risk of his or her receiving oral nutrients without supervision (Dangerfield and Sullivan, 1999). |
| **PLANNING** | |
| 1. Instruct patient about what you are going to do and why. | Increases patient cooperation. |
| 2. Explain to patient why you are observing him or her while he or she eats. | Signs or symptoms associated with aspiration may indicate the need for further evaluation of swallowing, such as a fluoroscopic swallow study (Perry, 2001). |
| **IMPLEMENTATION** | |
| 1. Perform hand hygiene. | Reduces transmission of microorganisms. |
| 2. Using penlight and tongue blade, gently inspect mouth for pockets of food. | Pockets of food in the mouth can indicate difficulty swallowing. |
| 3. Elevate head of patient's bed so that hips are flexed at a 90-degree angle and head is flexed slightly forward, or help patient to same position in a chair. | Reduces risk of aspiration. |
| 4. Observe patient consume various consistencies of foods and liquids. | Referral to a dietitian is appropriate if a patient has difficulty with a particular consistency. |
| 5. Add thickener to thin liquids to create the consistency of mashed potatoes, or serve client pureed foods. | Thin liquids such as water and fruit juice are difficult to control in the mouth and are more easily aspirated (Goulding and Bakheit, 2000). |
| 6. Place ½ to 1 teaspoon of food on unaffected side of the mouth, allowing utensil to touch the mouth or tongue. | |

SKILL 31-1 ¦ Aspiration Precautions—cont'd

| STEP | RATIONALE |
|---|---|
| 7. Place hand on throat to gently palapte swallowing event as it occurs. Swallowing twice is often necessary to clear the pharynx. | |
| 8. Provide verbal coaching while feeding client and positive reinforcement to client.<br>a. Open your mouth.<br>b. Feel the food in your mouth.<br>c. Chew and taste the food.<br>d. Raise your tongue to the roof of your mouth.<br>e. Think about swallowing.<br>f. Close your mouth and swallow.<br>g. Swallow again.<br>h. Cough to clear airway. | Verbal cueing keeps client focused on swallowing. Positive reinforcement enhances client's confidence in ability to swallow. |
| 9. Observe for coughing, choking, gagging, and drooling of food; suction airway as necessary. | These are indications that suggest dysphagia and risk for aspiration. |
| 10. Provide rest periods as necessary during meal. | Avoiding fatigue decreases the risk of aspiration. |
| 11. Ask patient to remain sitting upright for at least 30 minutes after the meal. | Reduces the risk of gastroesophageal reflux, which can cause aspiration. |
| 12. Help patient to perform hand hygiene and perform mouth care. | Mouth care after meals helps prevent dental caries. |
| 13. Return patient's tray to appropriate place, and perform hand hygiene. | Reduces spread of microorganisms. |

## EVALUATION

| | |
|---|---|
| 1. Observe patient's ability to ingest foods of various textures and thickness. | Indicates whether aspiration risk is increased with thin liquids. |
| 2. Monitor patient's food and fluid intake. | Patient may avoid certain types and textures of food that are difficult to swallow. |
| 3. Weigh patient weekly. | Determines if weight is stable and reflects adequate caloric level. |
| 4. Observe patient's oral cavity after meal to detect pockets of food. | Determines presence of pockets of food when meal has included foods of various textures. |

## RECORDING AND REPORTING

■ Document the following in patient's chart: patient's tolerance of various food textures, amount of assistance required, position during meal, absence or presence of any symptoms of dysphagia, and amount eaten.

■ Report any coughing, gagging, choking, or swallowing difficulties to nurse in charge or physician or health care provider.

## UNEXPECTED OUTCOMES AND RELATED INTERVENTIONS

■ Patient coughs, gags, complains of food "stuck in throat," or has pockets of food in mouth.
  • Patient may require a swallowing evaluation (see Box 31-6).

• Consider consultation with a speech therapist for swallowing exercises and techniques to improve swallowing and reduce risk of aspiration.
• Notify physician or health care provider of any symptoms that occurred during meal and which foods caused the symptoms.

■ Patient avoids certain textures of food.
  • Change consistency and texture of food.

■ Patient experiences weight loss.
  • Discuss findings with physician or health care provider and/or dietitian.

ers, 2003), so they are combined with multiple objective measures determine malnutrition (COP, 1994).

**PATIENT EXPECTATIONS.** Patients who require assistance with nutritional problems have a variety of expectations. Patients with impairments in upper arm mobility expect assistance with activities such as preparing the meal, setting up the meal tray or plate, or being fed. Other patients expect information on the availability and use of assistive devices, used to increase one's independence with meals. A consultation with occupational therapy will help patients obtain these assistive devices and provide education on their proper use. You need to teach patients who have impaired vision how to feed themselves. It is also important for you to learn what the patient expects in terms of resuming a normal diet or learning to adjust to a therapeutic diet.

## Nursing Diagnosis

Following nursing assessment, cluster relevant defining characteristics to determine whether actual or potential nutritional problems exist. An alteration occurs when the body does not ingest a nutrient in sufficient quantity, poorly digests or does not completely absorb nutrients, or when total daily caloric needs are deficient or excessive. The following are examples of nursing diagnoses appropriate for patients with nutritional alterations:

- Risk for aspiration
- Disturbed body image
- Diarrhea
- Fatigue
- Deficient fluid volume
- Excess fluid volume
- Imbalanced nutrition: less than body requirements
- Imbalanced nutrition: more than body requirements
- Risk for imbalanced nutrition: more than body requirements
- Feeding self-care deficit
- Ineffective tissue perfusion: gastrointestinal

The overweight patient also has nutrient deficiencies and sometimes requires supplements or specialized nutritional support during episodes of acute illness. The nursing assessment identifies dietary patterns that have contributed to **obesity.** An assessment is needed that focuses on adequacy of all food groups. Patterns such as intake of high-fat foods and inadequate fruit and vegetable intake are examples of food habits that lead to nutrient deficiencies. Make sure the nursing diagnosis is as precise as possible. Related factors need to be accurate so that you select the appropriate interventions. For example, a diagnosis of *deficient fluid volume related to vomiting* will require different interventions than *deficient fluid volume related to anorexia.*

## Planning

During planning you will select nursing interventions intended to improve nutrition status and the monitoring and evaluation to assess the effectiveness of those interventions (Lacey and Pritchett, 2003). The input of all disciplines involved in patient care is necessary for the planning of the nutrition interventions. Reflect on the causes of malnutrition or risk for malnutrition (COP, 1994). You will individualize the intervention to the patient and take into consideration the patient's comfort and wishes. Although there are variables between and among patients, common nutritional goals include symptom management, weight maintenance, and preservation of functional status (Luthringer and Kulakowski, 2000). The use of modified diets, the addition of oral nutritional supplements, or the initiation of enteral or parenteral nutrition is sometimes required to improve nutrition status. Consider the cost of these modifications, as well as patient and caregiver burden, before beginning an intervention. The services of financial planners and social workers are very beneficial in situations where patients are not able to afford the intervention.

**GOALS AND OUTCOMES.** The goal in caring for patients with nutritional alterations is to improve the patient's nutritional status. If the nutritional diagnosis is *imbalanced nutrition: less than body requirements,* the outcome will be for the patient to gain weight or to ingest adequate nutrients in a certain category. If a patient is obese, a goal of care will be to safely achieve weight reduction. You determine specific, individualized goals by identifying patient behaviors that have led to the nutritional alteration (see care plan). You achieve the goals through a prescribed diet, patient education, and assisting the patient in developing new behaviors that will enable the patient to achieve an adequate nutritional status. Professionals who assist in providing care include the registered dietitian, nutritional support clinical nurse specialist, pharmacists, and physicians or health care providers

Weight gain or loss of $\frac{1}{2}$ to 1 lb/wk is a realistic level for patients who are underweight or overweight. Patients often have unrealistic expectations about nutritional repletion or dieting in reference to weight gain or loss. Assist patients in understanding this concept by asking them to reflect on their rate of weight gain or loss. Changes in weight usually occur over months or years unless an acute illness has occurred. When patients do not see rapid achievement of weight goals, they become discouraged. Remember that correction of poor dietary patterns is a long-term rather than a short-term goal. Short-term goals usually involve achieving calorie or nutrient targets on a daily or weekly basis.

**SETTING PRIORITIES.** Patients at risk for nutritional problems will have a plan of care aimed at improving nutritional status. However, many factors can influence how you set priorities so that a patient receives proper nourishment. For example, if a patient is on oral intake, your priority may involve symptom control (e.g., nausea or pain) before a patient feels comfortable to eat. Physiological factors such as fear or depression may influence a person's willingness to eat. In such a situation, discussing a patient's concerns may take precedence over starting mealtime. Food is important for all persons, but when illness dis-

## CARE PLAN  Nutrition

### ASSESSMENT

Mrs. Gonzalez's diet history reveals that she ate balanced meals three times daily, including at least three servings of fruits and vegetables. However, now that she has had a stroke, she is **unable to swallow** and **aspirates pills and thickened liquids.** The speech language pathologist has diagnosed her with **oropharyngeal dysphagia.** Mrs. Gonzalez states, "I just don't know about this NG tube. I wish my doctor would just let me eat."

*Defining characteristics are shown in bold type.

### NURSING DIAGNOSIS Risk for aspiration.

### PLANNING

#### GOAL

- Patient will receive adequate nutrients safely through enteral tube feeding.

- Patient will participate in speech therapy daily with the SLP.

#### EXPECTED OUTCOMES*
#### Nutritional Status: Nutrient Intake

- Patient will maintain weight.
- Patient will not exhibit signs of aspiration.
- Patient's albumin and prealbumin levels will remain normal.
- Patient will progress to an oral diet before discharge to restorative care facility.

*Outcomes classification label from Moorhead S, Johnson M, Maas M: *Nursing outcomes classification (NOC)*, ed 3, St. Louis, 2004, Mosby.

### INTERVENTIONS†
#### Nutritional Management
- Insert NG tube.


- Initiate enteral feeding as prescribed.


- Advance tube feeding as tolerated; monitor for tolerance.


#### Aspiration Precautions
- Continue with speech therapy.

### RATIONALE

Enteral tube feeding will allow for safe provision of nutrients while swallowing is rehabilitated with the assistance of the speech language pathologist (SLP) (Brody and others, 2000).
The tube feeding is initiated at a low rate of infusion and increased slowly to allow for maximum tolerance.
Abdominal pain, large volume of gastric residuals, and diarrhea, are signs of feeding intolerance and need to be evaluated promptly.


Speech therapy will assist the patient in regaining the ability to swallow foods and liquids. The SLP provides this on a regular basis (Elmstahl and others, 1999; Perry, 2001).
Speech therapy includes trials of various consistencies of foods and liquids. Make sure the patient is properly positioned and supervised during these trials. Aspiration of food and liquids lead to chest congestion and pneumonia (National Dysphagia Diet Task Force [NDDTF], 2002).

†Intervention classification labels from Dochterman JM, Bulechek GM, editors: *Nursing interventions classification (NIC)*, ed 4, St. Louis, 2004, Mosby.

### EVALUATION
- Weigh Mrs. Gonzalez on a weekly basis.
- Review Mrs. Gonzalez's tolerance of enteral formula.
- Measure laboratory values at 2-week intervals.

---

rupts appetite or the ability to eat, you must anticipate what is most important to help your patient achieve good nutrition.

The development of the care plan requires collaboration of the health, care team, the patient and the caretakers. Family and caretakers are often involved in food purchase and preparation. The nutritional plan of care will not succeed without their commitment to, involvement in, and understanding of nutritional goals. Table 31-3 describes commonly prescribed diets for hospitalized patients.

**CONTINUITY OF CARE.** Patient nutritional needs extend beyond the acute, hospital setting and into the home or rehabilitation care setting. Some patients with physiological conditions causing more severe cases of malnutrition require enteral tube feeding or parenteral nutrition to meet fluid, electrolyte, and nutritional needs.

| TABLE 31-3 | **Hospital Therapeutic Diets** |
|---|---|
| **Diet** | **Description** |
| Clear liquid | Clear fluids that you can see through |
| | Clear fluids, sodas, pulp-free juices, broth, gelatin, popsicles (without pieces of fruit), hard candy |
| | Uses: Bowel surgery or examination, as a transition to oral diet after a period of NPO, in acute GI distress |
| Full liquid | Fluids, foods blenderized to a liquid form |
| | All fluids, pureed food mixed with liquid to thin consistency, cream soup, milk and yogurt drinks, ice cream |
| | Uses: Patients who are unable to chew swallow, or tolerate solid food |
| National Dysphagia Diet (NDD)— dysphagia puree (National Dysphagia Diet Task Force [NDDTF], 2002) | Uniform, pureed, cohesive, "puddinglike" texture |
| | Smooth hot cereals cooked to a "pudding" consistency, mashed potatoes, pureed meat, pureed pasta or rice, pureed vegetable, yogurt |
| NDD—dysphagia mechanically altered (NDDTF, 2002) | Moist, soft-textured, easily forms a bolus |
| | Cooked cereals, dry cereals moistened with milk, canned fruit (excluding pineapple), moist ground meat, well-cooked noodles in sauce/gravy, well-cooked diced vegetables |
| NDD—dysphagia advanced (NDDTF, 2002) | Regular foods (with the exception of very hard, sticky, or crunchy foods) |
| | Moist breads (with butter, jelly, etc.), well-moistened cereals, peeled soft fruits (peach, plum, kiwi), tender, thin-sliced meats, baked potato (without skin), tender cooked vegetables |
| Regular (NDDTF, 2002) | All foods |
| | No restrictions |
| High fiber | Fresh fruits and vegetables, whole grains, bran, oatmeal, seeds, nuts, beans, and dried fruits |
| | Uses: Increase fecal bulk, normalize serum lipids, control postprandial blood glucose, remissions of diverticulosis, irritable bowel syndrome, or ulcerative colitis |
| Low sodium | 4-g (no added salt), 2-g, 1-g, or 500-mg sodium diets |
| | Allow all foods except those high in sodium, such as processed food products, tomato juice, salad dressing, smoked or cured meats, pickles, commercial pasta, and rice mixes or soups |
| | Uses: Limit amount of sodium to prevent fluid accumulation or loss of excess body water, congestive heart failure, renal, liver dysfunction, or hypertension |
| Low cholesterol | 300 mg/day cholesterol, also commonly includes 30% of calories from fat, <10% of calories from saturated fat, focusing on monounsaturated fat as a preferred fat choice |
| | Allow all foods except those high in saturated fat and cholesterol such as whole fat milk, ice cream, egg yolk, untrimmed meat, fried foods, pastries, donuts, and bacon |
| | Uses: AHA guidelines for serum lipid reduction with coronary artery disease |
| Diabetic | Based on calorie level; restricts carbohydrate to 45%-55% of calories; <30% of calories from fat; 25-30 g of fiber |
| | Includes all foods with restricted portion sizes |
| | Uses: Patients with diabetes |

Modified from Chicago Dietetic Association and others: *Manual of Clinical Dietetics,* ed 6, Chicago, 2000, American Dietetic Association.

Patients and family members need to learn the skills to administer these therapies safely and effectively. Home health care nurses play an important role in initially establishing enteral and parenteral nutrition routes and then assisting patients and families with monitoring and supplement delivery. Long-term nutritional management is a challenge that requires collaboration between the patient, family, and health care team.

### Implementation

**HEALTH PROMOTION.** You play a major role in promoting healthy dietary practices. Using tools such as the food guide pyramid, assists patients with food choices, menu planning, and dietary patterns. You will also educate patients about food labels and their meanings. An area of particular importance is education about product claims that are misleading: some "reduced fat" foods still have significant amounts of fat, some "lite" foods still contain considerable calories, and "low cholesterol" does not always mean low fat.

Obesity is an epidemic in the United States. One out of two Americans is obese or overweight (Ruser and others, 2005). Proposed contributing factors are sedentary lifestyle, work schedules, and poor meal choices. More patients are acknowledging their weight and seeking weight loss strategies (Lee and others, 2004).

| TABLE 31-4 | Food-Borne Illness | | |
|---|---|---|---|
| **Food-Borne Illness** | **Organisms** | **Food Source** | **Symptoms** |
| Botulism | *Clostridium botulinum* | Spores widespread; toxin produced only in anaerobic conditions<br>Improperly home-canned foods, smoked and salted fish, ham, sausage, shellfish | Onset: 4-36 hours post consumption<br>Symptoms vary from mild discomfort to death in 24 hours, initially dizziness, progressing to motor (respiratory) paralysis<br>Duration: Variable; average 10 days with administration of antitoxin within 24 hours; 41 days with administration after 24 hours (Frattarelli and Abdel-Haq, 2004) |
| *E. coli* | *Escherichia coli* 0157:H7 | Bacteria found on animals that graze<br>Undercooked meat (ground beef) and poultry, unpasteurized milk | Onset: 2-5 days post consumption<br>Severe cramps, diarrhea (may be bloody), renal failure<br>Duration: 7-10 days |
| Listeriosis | *Listeria monocytogenes* | Bacteria resist heat, salt, nitrate, acid, and survive at low temperatures<br>Soft cheese, meat (hot dogs, pate, lunch meats), unpasteurized milk, shellfish, seafood | Onset: 2-30 days post consumption<br>Nausea, vomiting, fever, headache, pneumonia, meningitis, spontaneous abortion, death in elderly and infants*<br>Duration: 5-10 days |
| Perfringens enteritis | *C. perfringens* | Caused by prolonged periods of temperatures >40° F and <150° F<br>Cooked meats, meat dishes held at room or warm temperature | Onset: 8-12 hours<br>Diarrhea, abdominal pain, nausea, vomiting*<br>Duration: <24 hours |
| Salmonellosis | *Salmonella typhi*<br>*S. paratyphi* | Milk, custards, egg dishes, salad dressings, sandwich fillings, raw meats, polluted shellfish | Onset: 8-72 hours<br>Diarrhea, cramps, vomiting<br>Duration: 4-7 days (U.S. Food and Drug Administration and Center for Food Safety, 2001) |
| Shigellosis | *Shigella dysenteriae* | Usually secondary to cross contamination with uncooked foods<br>Milk, milk products, potato salads | Onset: 1-7 days<br>Mild diarrhea to fatal dysentery<br>Duration: 5-7 days (U.S. Food and Drug Administration and Center for Food Safety, 2001) |
| *Staphylococcus* | *Staphylococcus aureus* | Toxin produced at room temperature<br>Custards, cream fillings, processed meats, ham, cheese, ice cream, potato salad, sauces, casseroles | Onset: 30 minutes-8 hours<br>Severe abdominal cramps, pain, vomiting, diarrhea, perspiration, headache, fever, prostration<br>Duration: 1-2 days |

Modified from Partnership for Food Safety Education: *Organisms that can bug you,* 2005, http://www.fightbac.org/sources.cfm.
*Symptoms are generally most severe for youngest and oldest age-groups.

A high percentage of those who attempt to lose weight are unsuccessful, regaining lost weight over time. Diet and exercise compliance affects success with weight loss. Many individuals are willing to pay for weight loss programs if the program meets individual needs (Roux and others, 2004). Information on weight loss diets is available everywhere, from the bookstore to the Internet. However, there is a lack of good evidence evaluating the effectiveness of commercial weight loss programs. Scientifically controlled studies, which assess safety and efficacy, are necessary before making recommendations to use a specific diet (Hamilton and Greenway, 2004).

Food safety is a commonly overlooked aspect of health promotion. Contaminated and undercooked food products,

especially eggs and meats, will result in severe debilitating and even fatal illnesses (Table 31-4). Patient education is one method of improving safe food practices for patients and their families (Box 31-7).

**ACUTE CARE.** It is common for oral intake to decrease during periods of stress. This occurs as a result of the anorexic effects of stress-induced hormones (Takeda and others, 2004). It is important that you monitor the patient's nutrient intake, identify influences that reduce appetite, and plan interventions to increase intake.

One of the most disruptive influences on intake in acute care is diagnostic testing (McClave and others, 1999). Some blood and radiographic studies require the patient to fast.

BOX 31-7 PATIENT TEACHING

Through her studies Sarah learns that food safety is an important public health issue. The very young, older adults, patients with chronic illness, and those patients who are immunosuppressed are at risk for food-borne illnesses (see Table 31-4). As Mrs. Gonzalez improves and tolerates more food, Sarah consults with the dietitian and together they develop a teaching plan regarding food safety for the foods that her patient's family will be preparing.

**Outcome**
- At the end of the teaching session the patient's family will be able to state measures to reduce food-borne illnesses.

**Teaching Strategies**
- Describe precautionary measures to avoid food-borne illnesses:
  ◦ Wash hands, food preparation surfaces, and utensils with hot, soapy water.
  ◦ Cook meat, poultry, fish, eggs until well done (180° F).
  ◦ Wash fresh fruits and vegetables thoroughly.
  ◦ Do not eat raw meat or unpasteurized milk or juices.
  ◦ Do not use food past expiration date.
  ◦ Refrigerate foods at 40° F within 2 hours of cooking.
  ◦ Keep foods properly refrigerated.
  ◦ Thaw frozen foods in the refrigerator.
  ◦ Discard food that you suspect is spoiled.
  ◦ Do not use wooden cutting boards. Instead use plastic laminate or solid surface cutting boards that can be disinfected.
  ◦ Wash dishrags, dishtowels, sponges regularly with bleach, or use paper towels.
  ◦ Clean inside of refrigerator and microwave regularly with bleach or soap.

Modified from Partnership for Food Safety Education: *Tools You Can Use*, 2005, http://portal.fightbac.org/pfse/toolsyoucanuse/.

Therefore the patient's food is withheld until the patient returns from the test or the testing is completed. This disrupts mealtimes, and sometimes patients are too fatigued to eat or experience discomfort related to the test. Emotional stress also influences intake. Patients who are worried about their families, finances, employment, or illness are not always able to eat or eat enough to compensate for the effect of stress on metabolism.

Medications also affect intake and in some cases the use of nutrients. The use of certain medications is associated with anorexia, malabsorption, and increased metabolism. Medication-induced nausea, vomiting, and diarrhea also greatly affect intake (Moriguti and others, 2001). Taste changes occur with the use of medications such as chemotherapy and diuretics and mineral preparations such as zinc (Whitman, 2000). Keep these factors in mind when designing measures to promote nutrition.

Symptoms associated with illness can have a major effect on appetite. Pain, nausea, and shortness of breath make it difficult for patients to chew, swallow, and tolerate stomach filling. Often patients refuse to eat to avoid the associated discomfort.

Food presentation is a factor in appetite. Hot foods that are cold or cold foods that are warm are not appetizing. Overcooked or undercooked foods are unappealing. A meal tray precariously balanced on a crowded, soiled over-bed table does not enhance the meal. Removal of the tray lid outside of the patient's room will help to decrease distress in those patients sensitive to odors, such as patients with nausea. Attention to details in food presentation, meal scheduling, and the patient's difficulties with food will enhance a patient's intake. You help to stimulate a patient's appetite through environmental adaptations, consultation with an RD, attention to food preferences, and patient and family counseling.

The use of therapeutic diets has also been associated with the development of protein-energy malnutrition (Moriguti and others, 2001). The unpalatability of diets that are low in sodium and fat affect dietary intake. In this situation you need to weigh the benefits associated with the therapeutic diet against the detrimental effects of weight loss and malnutrition (Huffman, 2002).

**Providing a Comfortable Environment.** In the acute setting provide an environment conducive to eating. Make sure the patient's room is free of reminders of treatments and odors. Provide mouth care when necessary to remove unpleasant tastes. Plan to administer analgesics or antiemetics early enough so that patients are more comfortable to eat at mealtime. Position the patient comfortably so that the meal is more enjoyable. If a patient refuses a portion of the meal, make every effort to replace it with a suitable alternative.

**Assisting Patients With Feeding.** Hospitalized patients may be unable to feed themselves adequately because of the severity of their illness or the fatigue and debilitation of the condition. You will improve patient feeding by carefully protecting patients' dignity and actively involving them. When assisting patients with feeding, encourage the patient to ingest and adequate volume of food at a comfortable pace. Provide independence through use of adaptive devices (see Figure 31-4) or finger foods. Always position a patient in a chair or high Fowler's position (if possible) to improve swallowing and digestion. Allow the patient time to empty the mouth after every spoonful, attempting to match the speed of feeding to the patient's readiness. Encourage patients to direct the order in which they wish to eat food items. Mealtime is a good time to instruct patients and their families about the selection of appropriate foods and the importance of a balanced diet.

**Dysphagia.** A certified SLP identifies patients at risk for **dysphagia** and provides recommendations for dysphagia therapy (Perry and Love, 2001). The assessment focuses on oral-motor and oral-sensory function, protective reflexes, respiratory status, level of arousal, cognitive-linguistic status, and perception. The SLP administers trials of several consistencies of foods and fluids to obtain a comprehensive description of the phases of swallowing. This is usually accompanied by judgment of degree of dysfunction and aspiration risk (Perry and Love, 2001). The SLP then makes treatment recommendations focusing on consistencies of foods and fluids and the use of swallowing therapies based on the assessment (Elmstahl and others, 1999).

*Dysphagia Treatment.* Treatment of dysphagia commences immediately after diagnosis. The patient care plan includes the promotion of good nutrition status, weight maintenance, diminution of the risk of aspiration, promotion of eating independence, and enjoyment of mealtime (Dorner, 2002). Treatment including a combination of oral motor exercises, swallowing techniques, positioning during feeding, and diet modification will lead to a reduced degree of oral and pharyngeal dysfunction, in turn leading to improved nutrition status (Elmstahl and others, 1999).

*Diet Management.* The safe initiation of oral nutrition and hydration is a priority for patients with dysphagia (Wood and Emick-Herring, 1997). The most common dietary modifications for patients with dysphagia includes the thickening of liquids, modification of food texture, and the replacement of oral feeding with enteral tube feeding. Patients experiencing dysphagia because of mechanical disorders or obstruction tend to tolerate liquid or pureed foods. On the other hand, it is necessary for patients with oropharyngeal dysphagia to avoid these foods and to use semisolid consistencies that are easy to chew (Groher, 1997). Liquids often have to be thickened with a commercial thickener to decrease transit time and to allow for protection of the airway (Dorner, 2002; Groher, 1997). If aspiration is present, maintain NPO status with enteral tube feeding.

The American Dietetic Association published the National Dysphagia Diet Task Force's (NDDTF's) National Dysphagia Diet in 2002 to provide uniformity to diets provided by all facilities to patients with dysphagia (NDDTF, 2002). The diet is made of four levels: dysphagia puree, dysphagia mechanically altered, dysphagia advanced, and regular. There are also four levels of liquid consistencies: thin liquids (low viscosity), nectarlike liquids (medium viscosity), honeylike liquids (viscosity of honey), and spoon-thick liquids (viscosity of pudding) (NDDTF, 2002).

The puree diet is unappetizing to patients previously eating solid foods. This can lead to noncompliance, especially if using commercial baby food (Dorner, 2002; Groher, 1997; Shaw and Power, 1999). Institutional food service companies have used this as an opportunity to develop flavorful pureed alternatives, molded into appetizing forms. Unfortunately these items are often very expensive, preventing their widespread use.

*Patient Positioning.* You position patients with dysphagia properly before eating to prevent misdirection of food. Have the patient sit upright to correctly align the anatomy of the pharynx and esophagus. Make sure the body is well supported in a bed or chair, and do not leave the patient unsupervised.

**Disabled Patients.** Allow patients with disabilities that interfere with independent food intake to do as much as possible for themselves. When necessary, prepare the tray, cutting food into bite-size pieces, buttering bread, and pouring liquids. Use special eating utensils if necessary or as recommended by occupational therapy. Some patients become fatigued during the course of the meal, leading to suboptimal intake. Provide assistance at the end of meals as needed. Evaluate the results of self-feeding on the basis of food intake. Recognize and commend any success the patient has.

**Enteral Tube Feedings.** **Enteral nutrition (EN)** refers to nutrients given into the stomach or intestinal tract via a feeding tube. Nasogastric feedings are delivered through a feeding tube introduced through the nose and into the stomach. Nasointestinal feedings are delivered through a feeding tube inserted through the nose and into the jejunum. When patients have obstructions or are not candidates for nasal feeding tubes, physicians surgically insert tubes directly into the stomach (gastrostomy) or jejunum (jejunostomy). The most desirable and appropriate method of providing nutrition is the oral route; unfortunately, this is not always possible. When oral feedings are not possible, yet the stomach or intestine is able to digest nutrients, enteral tube feeding is an alternative. Enteral feeding is preferred over parenteral nutrition (intravenous nutrition) because it improves utilization of nutrients, is generally safer for patients, maintains structure and function of the gut, and is less expensive (ASPEN, 2002). A variety of enteral feeding formulas are available in whole protein or partially digested form. Special enteral formulas for renal disease, hepatic disease, pulmonary disease, or diabetes are also available, as well as adult and pediatric formulas. The skills presented in this chapter focus on the administration of nutritional feedings directly into the gastrointestinal tract with the goal of restoring the patient's nutritional status.

Research has demonstrated a beneficial effect of EN over parenteral routes in patients with a functional GI tract (Box 31-8). Postoperative feeding by the enteral route is associated with earlier return of bowel function and decreased incidence of infection (Braunschweig and others, 2001) and postoperative stay (Bozzetti and others, 2001). EN is also associated with improved protein balance (Harrison and others, 1997) and reduced incidence of hypoglycemia and electrolyte abnormalities when compared to PN (Braga and others, 2001).

Skill 31-2 describes insertion of a feeding tube. Feeding tubes are referred to as being nasally placed because that is the route most frequently used, primarily because the nose provides a natural stability for tubes. However, in the event of trauma to the nose, or in the event that the patient already has an endotracheal tube placed in the mouth, feeding tubes are sometimes placed orally. Avoid large-bore NG tubes for primary use as a feeding tube because they carry an increased risk of aspiration and are more irritating to the nasopharyngeal and esophageal mucosa (ASPEN, 2002). Occasionally you will use large-bore tubes inserted for gastric decompression to initiate enteral feeding because they are already in place. If the feeding continues for more than a

| BOX 31-8 | USING EVIDENCE IN PRACTICE |
|---|---|

**Research Summary**

Indications for EN generally fall into one of three categories: impaired swallowing or gag reflex (which is usually related to a neurological problem); nutritional deficit due to reduced food ingestion or hypermetabolic state even when the patient is able to eat; or an inability to eat related to surgery, injury, or disease process. This last category is often associated with altered or decreased level of consciousness. According to a recent study, complications of enteral nutrition include displacement of the tube, electrolyte alterations, hyperglycemia, constipation, diarrhea, clogging of the tube, vomiting, and pulmonary aspiration (Pancorbo-Hidalgo and others, 2001). Complications of prolonged intubation also include nasal erosion, nasopharyngeal ulcers, sinusitis, otitis, esophagitis, and vocal cord paralysis (ASPEN, 2002).

One of the most dreaded complications associated with tube feedings is pulmonary aspiration, potentially leading to pneumonia. Two traditional bedside methods used to assess for pulmonary aspiration of enteral feeding into the respiratory tract included the glucose method and the dye method. The premise of the glucose method was that normal tracheal secretions contain minimal levels of glucose. Therefore, if glucose-rich enteral formula is aspirated into the airway, glucose levels of tracheal secretions increase. However, researchers have shown that the glucose levels of tracheal secretions vary widely (Metheny, St. John and Clouse, 1998).

Another common practice was the addition of food coloring to enteral tube feeding. Food coloring, typically blue, added to enteral feeding caused suctioned tracheal secretions to turn blue if the patient aspirated the tube feeding into the respiratory tract. However, the dye is able to be systemically absorbed, interferes with hemocult testing of stool, and has questionable safety (Maloney and Metheny, 2002; Metheny and others, 2002a). There is even an association between death and the use of dye in enteral feedings (Maloney and Metheny, 2002). The most recent recommendations from members of the North American Summit on Aspiration in the Critically Ill Patient indicate not to use the dye method and the glucose method of testing for aspiration at all (McClave and others, 2002). Researchers are currently trying to develop new bedside methods for assessing for pulmonary aspiration, such as assessing for the presence of pepsin, a substance produced in the stomach, in tracheal secretions (Metheny and others, 2002b).

Routine assessment for placement of feeding tubes is primarily a nursing responsibility. Traditionally nurses used the auscultatory method of assessing placement. Since the late 1980s there have been several studies showing that the auscultatory method to detect gastric or intestinal feeding tube placement is unreliable. This method does not detect when a feeding tube has inadvertently been placed into the respiratory tract (Dobranowski and others, 1992; Roubenoff and Ravich, 1989) and does not distinguish between placement in the stomach versus the intestine (Metheny and others, 1990).

Tube feeding has been associated with inadequate delivery of nutrients, potentially leading to malnutrition or electrolyte disturbances, because of interruptions in feeding (McClave and others, 1992). Previously, health care providers have often delayed beginning administration of enteral nutrition until they auscultate bowel sounds in the patient.

**Application to Nursing Practice**

The most important nursing intervention to decrease the risk of aspiration is to keep the head of the bed elevated at least 30 degrees (ASPEN, 2002; Metheny and others, 2002b). If the patient has the bed in a flat position, it is possible to keep the bed flat yet elevate the head by placing the bed in reverse Trendelenburg's position (Metheny and others, 2002b).

Initially use x-ray to verify that a feeding tube is positioned in the desired site, and verify the tube position every 4 to 12 hours and as needed. Certain characteristics of fluid aspirated from feeding tubes are helpful in assessing placement of the tube. Color differentiates gastric from intestinal placement. Because most intestinal aspirates are stained by bile to a distinct yellow color, and most gastric aspirates are not, the difference often distinguishes the sites (Metheny and others, 1998b). The pH of an aspirate offers valuable data as well in assessing placement of a feeding tube (Metheny and others, 1999). Bedside testing of pH using pH paper covering a range from 0 to 14 is sufficient for this purpose (Metheny and others, 1994) and is standard protocol to aid in the assessment of feeding tube placement.

Research has suggested that when compared to total PN, initiation of EN within the first 24 hours in critically ill patients helps to lower infection rates and decrease length of intensive care unit admission (Kudsk and others, 1992). In addition, early EN helps to maintain bowel mucosal integrity, improve wound healing, and reduce rates of septic morbidity. Furthermore, it is not necessary to wait for the presence of bowel sounds to begin tube feeding.

Data from: ASPEN Board of Directors and the Clinical Guidelines Task Force: Guidelines for the use of parenteral and enteral nutrition in adult and pediatric patients, *JPEN J Parenter Enteral Nutr* 26(1 Suppl):1SA, 2002; Kudsk KA and others: Enteral versus parenteral feeding: effects on septic morbidity after blunt and penetrating abdominal trauma, *Ann Surg* 215:503, 1992; Metheny NA and others: Pepsin as a marker for pulmonary aspiration, *Am J Crit Care* 11:150, 2002b; Metheny NA and others: pH testing of feeding-tube aspirates to determine placement, *Nutr Clin Pract* 9:185, 1994; Metheny and others: pH, color, and feeding tubes, *RN* 61:25, 1998; Metheny NA and others: pH and concentration of bilirubin in feeding tube aspirates as predictors of tube placement, *Nurs Res* 48(4):189, 1999.

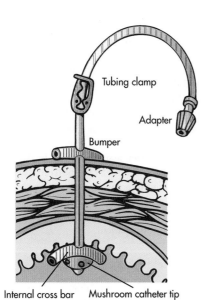

FIGURE **31-4** Percutaneous endoscopic gastrostomy tube.

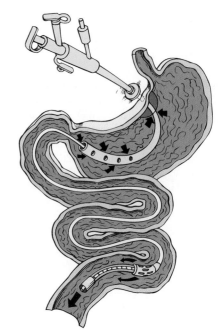

FIGURE **31-5** Endoscopic insertion of jejunostomy tube.

few days, or if the patient is at high risk for aspiration, consult with the health care provider about placement of a small-bore feeding tube.

*Feeding Tube Insertion.* When the patient cannot ingest, chew, or swallow food but can digest and absorb nutrients, a feeding tube is placed nasally, laparoscopically, or surgically into the stomach or small intestine (Skills 31-2 and 31-3). When making the decision regarding enteral access, the physician or health care provider considers rate of gastric emptying, GI anatomy, aspiration risk, and anticipated duration of requirement for enteral access (Directors, 2002). Nasal tubes are associated with sinusitis, otitis, vocal cord paralysis, and ulcers of the nose and sinuses. For this reason they are not used as long-term enteral access. Intestinal feedings require an infusion pump to allow for controlled slow administration and do not measure residual volume (RV). The ideal choice for long-term EN access is a gastrostomy (ASPEN, 2002).

Intestinal tubes do not reduce the risk of aspiration of formula into the lungs during enteral feeding because formula refluxes into the stomach (Pearce and Duncan, 2002). You decrease the risk of aspiration by elevating the head of the bed 30 degrees, avoiding bolus feedings, and using isosmotic feedings to avoid delaying intestinal emptying (ASPEN, 2002; Pearce and Duncan, 2002). Aspiration of enteral formula into the lungs irritates the bronchial mucosa, resulting in decreased blood supply to affected pulmonary tissue. This leads to pneumonia. The glucose content of formula serves as a medium for bacterial growth, promoting infection.

Traditional bedside methods of testing placement of feeding tubes, such as injection of air, are ineffective. The "gold standard" is radiographic confirmation of feeding tube location (ASPEN, 2002), but this is costly. pH testing is now recommended to confirm the placement.

*Gastrostomy/Jejunostomy Tube Feedings.* When patients cannot tolerate nasally or orally placed tubes, there are other options. One is a gastrostomy tube (G-tube), surgically placed in the stomach and exiting through an incision in the upper left quadrant of the abdomen, where it is sutured in place. An alternative is a percutaneous endoscopic gastrostomy (PEG) tube. This tube also exits through a puncture wound in the upper left quadrant of the abdomen, but it is held securely in place by virtue of its design (Figure 31-4). When patients who cannot tolerate a nasal or oral tube have gastric ileus, delayed gastric emptying, gastric resections, or neurological impairments that place them at greater risk of aspiration, enteral nutrition is delivered via a **jejunostomy tube** (Box 31-10). Jejunostomy feeding tubes, like gastrostomy tubes, are inserted during surgery (J-tube) or endoscopy (PEJ). Endoscopic insertion of a jejunostomy tube is also done through a PEG tube. After insertion of the large-bore PEG tube, the PEJ tube passes through the PEG and advances into the jejunum (Figure 31-5). A Y connector attached to the jejunostomy tube caps the PEG tube and closes the system. This Y connector labels the gastrostomy tube and designates the jejunostomy tube for feeding. You need to know which port is gastric and which port is jejunal.

**Providing PN.** **Parenteral nutrition (PN)** is the administration of a solution consisting of glucose, amino acids, lipids, minerals, electrolytes, trace elements, and vitamins provided through an indwelling peripheral or central venous catheter. Administration of PN is only for use when the GI tract is not functioning. PN is not appropriate for patients who are able to absorb adequate nutrients via EN or oral feeding. PN use is associated with increased risk of infection and cost (Heyland and Dhaliwal, 2005; Koretz and others,

*Text continued on p. 905*

## SKILL 31-2 ¦ Intubating the Patient With a Nasogastric or Nasointestinal Feeding Tube

### Delegation Considerations

Intubating a patient with a feeding tube should not be delegated to assistive personnel. However, assistive personnel may assist with patient positioning during tube insertion.

### Equipment

- NG tube or nasointestinal (NI) tube (8 to 12 Fr) with guide wire or stylet
- 60-ml or larger Luer-lok or catheter-tip syringe
- Stethoscope
- Hypoallergenic tape and tincture of benzoin or tube fixation device

- pH indicator strip (scale 0.0 to 14.0)
- Glass of water and straw for patients able to swallow
- Emesis basin
- Towel
- Facial tissues
- Clean gloves
- Suction equipment in case of aspiration
- Penlight to check placement in nasopharynx
- Tongue blade

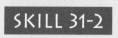

| STEP | RATIONALE |
|---|---|

### ASSESSMENT

1. Verify patient's need for enteral tube feedings: impaired swallowing, deccreased level of consciousness, surgeries of the upper alimentary tract, need for long-term enteral nutrition. Also assess patient's height, weight, hydration status, electrolyte balance, and organ function.

Identifying patients who need tube feedings before they become nutritionally depleted is essential. Up to 40% of hospitalized patients are malnourished (Pearce and Duncan, 2002).

2. Assess patency of nares. Have patient close each nostril alternately and breathe. Examine each naris for patency and skin breakdown.

Nares are sometimes obstructed or irritated, or septal defect or facial fractures are present.

3. Assess patient's medical history: nosebleeds, facial trauma, nasal surgery, deviated septum, anticoagulant therapy, coagulopathy.

Conditions may contraindicate nasal insertion of a tube.

4. Assess patient for gag reflex. Place tongue blade in patient's mouth, touching uvula.

Identifies patient's ability to swallow and determines if a greater risk of aspiration exists.

• ***Critical Decision Point:*** You insert NG or NI feeding tubes in patients with altered or decreased level of consciousness, but risk of inadvertent respiratory placement increases if there is an impaired gag reflex (Wendell and others, 1991).

5. Assess patient's mental status.

Alert patient is better able to cooperate with procedure. If vomiting occurs, an alert patient will usually expectorate vomitus, which will help to reduce the risk of aspiration.

6. Assess for bowel sounds.

Absence of bowel sounds indicates decreased or absent peristalsis and increased risk of aspiration.

7. Determine if the health care provider wants a prokinetic agent administered before the placement of a NI tube.

Prokinetic agents, such as metoclopramide, given *before* NI tube placement help advance the tube into the intestine (Kittinger, Sandler, and Heizer, 1987).

### PLANNING

1. Explain procedure to patient.
2. Explain to patient how to communicate during intubation by raising index finger to indicate gagging or discomfort.

Increases patient's cooperation with intubation procedure.

It is important for patient to have a way of communicating to alleviate stress. Pause to decrease gagging.

SKILL 31-2 | **Intubating the Patient With a Nasogastric or Nasointestinal Feeding Tube—cont'd**

| STEP | RATIONALE |
| --- | --- |

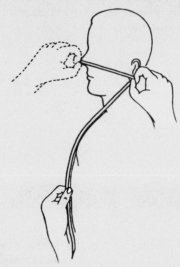

STEP **5** Determine length of tube you will insert.

| STEP | RATIONALE |
| --- | --- |
| 3. Position patient in sitting or high-Fowler's position. If patient is comatose, place in semi-Fowler's position with head propped forward using a pillow. An assistant is often necessary to help with positioning of confused or comatose patients. | Reduces risk of pulmonary aspiration if patient vomits. Assists with closure of airway and passage of the tube into the esophagus. The natural response to an object being inserted into the nose is to tip the head backward; avoid this because it opens the airway. |
| 4. Examine feeding tube for flaws: rough or sharp edges on distal end and closed or clogged outlet holes. | Flaws in feeding tube hamper tube intubation and will injure patient. Clogged outlets do not allow passage of feeding. |
| 5. Determine length of tube you will insert, and mark with tape or indelible ink (see illustration). | Being aware of proper length to intubate determines approximate depth of insertion. |

---

• *Critical Decision Point:* Tip of tube must reach stomach. Measure distance from tip of nose to earlobe to xyphoid process of sternum. Add additional 20 to 30 cm (8 to 12 inches) for NI tube (Hanson, 1979; Lord and others, 1993; Welch, 1996).

---

| STEP | RATIONALE |
| --- | --- |
| 6. Prepare NG or NI tube for intubation: | |
|   a. Perform hand hygiene. | Reduces spread of microorganisms. |
|   b. If the tube has a guide wire or stylet, inject 10 ml of water from 60-ml Luer-Lok or catheter-tip syringe into the tube. | Aids in guide wire or stylet insertion. |
|   c. Make certain that you position guide wire securely against weighted tip and that both Luer-Lok connections are snugly fitted together. | Promotes smooth passage of tube into GI tract. Improperly positioned stylet will induce serious trauma. |
| 7. Cut adhesive tape 10 cm (4 inches) long, or prepare tube fixation device. | |

---

## IMPLEMENTATION

| STEP | RATIONALE |
| --- | --- |
| 1. Put on clean gloves. | Reduces transmission of microorganisms. |
| 2. Dip tube with surface lubricant into glass of room temperature water, or apply water-soluble lubricant. Do not place plastic tubes in cold water or ice water. | Activates lubricant to facilitate passage of tube. Tubes will become stiff and inflexible, causing trauma to mucous membranes. |
| 3. Hand the alert patient a glass of water with straw or glass with crushed ice (if able to swallow). | Asking patient to swallow water will facilitate tube passage. |

| STEP | RATIONALE |
|---|---|
| 4. Gently insert tube through nostril to back of throat (posterior nasopharynx). May cause patient to gag. Aim back and down toward ear (see illustration). | Natural contours ease passage of tube into GI tract. |
| 5. Check for position of tube in back of throat with penlight and tongue blade. | Checking ensures tube is not coiled, kinked, or entering trachea. |

• *Critical Decision Point:* Encourage patient to swallow by giving small sips of water or ice chips. Advance tube as patient swallows. Rotate tube 180 degrees while inserting. Swallowing facilitates passage of tube past oropharynx. Rotating decreases friction.

| STEP | RATIONALE |
|---|---|
| 6. Have patient flex head toward chest after tube has passed through nasopharynx. | Closes off glottis and reduces risk of tube entering trachea. |
| 7. Emphasize need to mouth breathe and swallow during insertion. | Helps facilitate passage of tube and alleviates patient's fears during the procedure. |
| 8. When you insert the tube approximately 10 inches (in the adult), stop and listen for air exchange from the distal portion of the tube. | If air is heard, tube is in respiratory tract; remove tube and start over (Metheny and Titler, 2001). |
| 9. Advance tube each time patient swallows until it has passed the desired length. | Reduces discomfort and trauma to patient. |

• *Critical Decision Point:* Do not force tube. If you meet resistance or if patient starts to cough, choke, or become cyanotic, stop advancing the tube and pull tube back and start over.

| STEP | RATIONALE |
|---|---|
| 10. Check for position of tube in back of throat with penlight and tongue blade. | |
| 11. Temporarily anchor tube to the nose with a small piece of tape, and check placement of tube (see Skill 31-3). | Movement of the tube stimulates gagging. Assesses general position before anchoring tube more securely. |
| 12. After you obtain gastric aspirates, anchor tube to nose to avoid pressure on nares. Mark exit site with indelible ink. Use one of following options for anchoring: | A properly secured tube allows the patient more mobility and prevents trauma to nasal mucosa. |
| a. **Apply tape:** | |
| (1) Apply tincture of benzoin or other skin adhesive on tip of patient's nose and allow it to become "tacky." | Helps tape adhere better. Protects skin. |

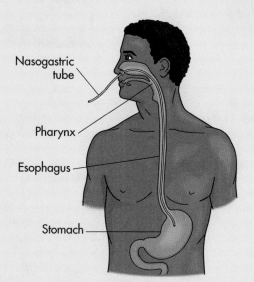

STEP **4** NG tube inserted through nose and esophagus into stomach.

| SKILL 31-2 | Intubating the Patient With a Nasogastric or Nasointestinal Feeding Tube—cont'd |
| --- | --- |

| STEP | RATIONALE |
| --- | --- |

     (2) Split one end of the adhesive tape strip lengthwise 5 cm (2 inches).

     (3) Wrap each of the 5-cm strips in opposite directions around tube as it exits nose (see illustration).

  b. Apply tube fixation device using shaped adhesive patch:

     (1) Apply wide end of patch to bridge of nose (see illustration).

     (2) Slip connector around feeding tube as it exits nose (see illustration).

**13.** Fasten end of NG tube to patient's gown using a piece of tape. Do not use safety pins to pin the tube to the patient's gown (see illustration).

Reduces traction on the nares if tube moves.
Safety pins become unfastened and cause injury to the patient.

**14.** Assist patient to a comfortable position. Some previously believed that positioning the patient on right side facilitated intestinal tube placement.

Promote patient comfort. Researchers indicate that placing the patient on the right side does not promote passage of the tube into the small intestine (Kittinger and others, 1987).

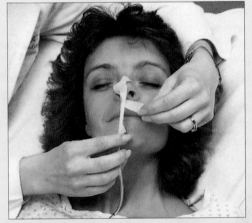

STEP **12a(3)** Wrapping tape to anchor nasoenteral tube.

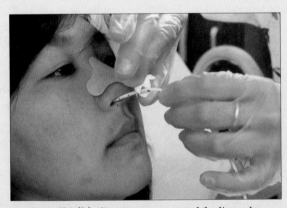

STEP **12b(2)** Slip connector around feeding tube.

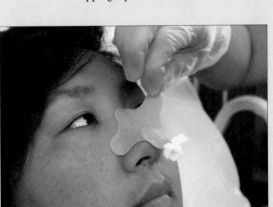

STEP **12b(1)** Applying tube fixation patch to bridge of nose.

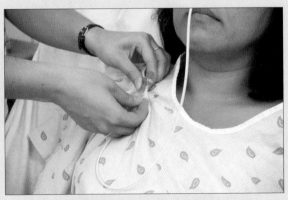

STEP **13** Fastening feeding tube to patient's gown.

| STEP | RATIONALE |
|---|---|

• *Critical Decision Point:* Leave guide wire or stylet in place until you ensure correct position by x-ray film. Never attempt to reinsert a partially or fully removed guide wire or stylet while feeding tube is in place. This will cause perforation of the tube and injure the patient.

| | |
|---|---|
| 15. Obtain x-ray film of chest/abdomen. | X-ray examination is currently the most accurate method to determine feeding tube placement. |
| 16. Change gloves, and administer oral hygiene (see Chapter 27). Cleanse tubing at nostril with washcloth dampened in mild soap and water. | Promotes patient comfort and integrity of oral mucous membranes. |
| 17. Remove gloves, dispose of equipment, and perform hand hygiene. | Reduces transmission of microorganisms. |

## EVALUATION

| | |
|---|---|
| 1. Observe patient to determine response to NG or NI tube intubation. Have the patient speak. Check vital signs and oxygen saturation. | A patient who is comfortable, is able to speak without difficulty, and has normal oxygen saturation is likely to have a correctly placed tube. |
| 2. Confirm x-ray film results. | Proper position is essential before initiating feedings. |
| 3. Remove the guide wire or stylet after x-ray verification of correct placement. | |
| 4. Routinely assess location of external exit site marking on the tube, as well as color and pH of fluid withdrawn from the NG or NI tube. | Will reveal if end of tube has changed position. However, it is possible that the tube changed position inside the gastrointestinal tract with no external evidence of the change. |

## RECORDING AND REPORTING

■ Record and report type and size of tube placed, location of distal tip of tube, patient's tolerance of procedure, and confirmation of tube position by x-ray examination. Documentation of nonrespiratory placement by x-ray examination is standard practice when you initially insert a small-bore tube. Record and report any type of unexpected outcome and the interventions performed.

## UNEXPECTED OUTCOMES AND RELATED INTERVENTIONS

■ Tube placed in the respiratory tract. Usually seen on x-ray.
  • Remove the tube, and report the incident to the physician or health care provider; obtain order for reinsertion.
■ Aspiration of stomach contents into respiratory tract (immediate response) in the alert patient, evidenced by coughing, dyspnea, cyanosis, or decreases in oxygen saturation values during the procedure.

  • Position the patient on side to facilitate drainage of oral secretions.
  • Suction the patient nasotracheally or orotracheally to try to remove aspirated substance.
  • Report the event immediately to the physician or health care provider.
■ Aspiration of stomach contents into respiratory tract (delayed response or small-volume aspiration), evidenced by auscultation of crackles or wheezes, dyspnea, or fever.
  • Report change in patient condition to the physician or health care provider; if there has not been a recent chest x-ray examination, suggest one be ordered.
  • Prepare for possible initiation of antibiotics.
■ Nasal mucosa becomes inflamed, tender, and/or eroded.
  • Retape the tube in a different position to relieve pressure on mucosa.
  • If the tube has been in the same site for an extended period, consider reinsertion of the tube in the opposite nares (health care provider's order required).

# SKILL 31-3 | Verifying Feeding Tube Placement

## Delegation Considerations

This skill cannot be delegated to assistive personnel. The nurse must instruct assistive personnel to immediately inform the nurse if:

- The patient's respirations change or the patient complains of being short of breath, coughing, or choking
- The patient vomits or assistive personnel notices vomitus in patient's mouth during oral hygiene
- Nasal irritation is present
- Displacement of the feeding tube occurs

## Equipment

- 60 ml Luer-Lok or catheter-tip syringe
- Clean gloves
- Medicine cup
- pH indicator strip (scale 0.0 to 14.0)
- Normal saline or tap water

| STEP | RATIONALE |
|---|---|
| **ASSESSMENT** | |
| 1. Know the policy and procedures for frequency and method of checking tube placement in your facility. | Verifies agency procedure for checking placement of feeding tube. Regardless of the method, make sure you obtain x-ray confirmation at the time of placement. |
| 2. Identify signs and symptoms of coughing, choking, or cyanosis. | Indicates accidental migration of feeding tube into the airway. However, their absence does not ensure that respiratory migration has not occurred, especially in the patient with altered level of consciousness and/or altered gag and cough reflexes. |
| 3. Identify conditions that increase the risk for spontaneous tube dislocation from the intended position:<br>  a. Retching/vomiting<br>  b. Nasotracheal suctioning<br>  c. Severe bouts of coughing. | Increased intraabdominal pressure dislocates tube (e.g., stomach to esophagus, intestine to stomach). |
| 4. Observe the external portion of the tube for movement of the ink mark away from the mouth or nares (see Skill 31-2). | Increased external length of a tube indicates that the distal tip is no longer in the correct position. |
| 5. Review patient's medication record: is patient receiving a gastric acid inhibitor (e.g., cimetidine, ranitidine, famotidine, nizatidine) or a proton pump inhibitor (e.g., omeprazole)? | $H_2$ receptor antagonists reduce volume of gastric acid secretion and the acid content of secretions, thus causing the pH value to be higher, that is, more basic (Metheny and Stewart, 2002). |
| 6. Review patient's record for history of prior tube displacement. | Patients who have a history of tube displacement are at increased risk. |
| **PLANNING** | |
| 1. Explain procedure to patient. | Improves patient cooperation. |
| **IMPLEMENTATION** | |
| 1. Perform hand hygiene, and apply gloves. | Reduces transmission of microorganisms. |
| 2. Measures to verify placement of tube should be conducted at the following times:<br>  a. For intermittently tube-fed patients, test placement immediately before each feeding and before medications.<br>  b. For continuously tube-fed patients, test placement at least once every 12 hours and before medication administration.<br>  c. Wait at least 1 hour after medication administration by tube or mouth. | Premature aspiration of contents will remove unabsorbed medication, reducing dose delivered to patient. Medication also interferes with pH testing and appearance of aspirate (Metheny and others, 1994). |

| STEP | RATIONALE |
|------|-----------|
| **3.** Unplug end of feeding tube. Draw up 10 to 30 ml of air into a 60-ml syringe, then attach to end of feeding tube. Flush tube with 30 ml of air before attempting to aspirate fluid. Repositioning the patient from side to side is helpful. More than one bolus of air through the tube is necessary in some cases. | Burst of air aids in aspirating fluid more easily (Metheny and others, 1993b). Smaller syringes generate unnecessarily high pressures inside the tube.<br>It is sometimes more difficult to aspirate fluid from the small intestine than from the stomach. |
| **4.** Draw back on syringe slowly, and obtain 5 to 10 ml of gastric aspirate (see illustration *A*). Observe appearance of aspirate to help assess the position of the tube (see illustration *B*). | Drawing back quickly, or with a smaller syringe, increases intratubular pressure and causes the tube to collapse.<br>Aspirates from NG tubes of continuously tube-fed patients often have appearance of curdled enteral formula. Aspirates from NI tubes are often stained yellow from bile. Gastric aspirates from intermittent tube-fed patients are not typically bile stained (unless intestinal fluid has refluxed into the stomach). |
| **5.** Gently mix aspirate in syringe and expel into medicine cup. Dip the pH strip into the fluid or by applying a few drops of the fluid to the strip. Compare the color of the strip with the color on the chart provided by the manufacturer (see illustration) (Metheny and others, 1998a). | Mixing ensures equal distribution of contents for testing. pH paper covering a range from 0 to 11 provides most accurate readings of gastric pH levels (Metheny and others, 1994). |
|    a. Gastric fluid from patient who has fasted for at least 4 hours usually has pH range of 1 to 4. | Range of 1 to 4 is a reliable indicator of stomach placement, especially when a gastric acid inhibitor is *not* being used. |
|    b. Fluid from NI tube of fasting patient usually has pH greater than 6. | Intestinal contents are less acidic than stomach contents (Metheny and others, 1999). |

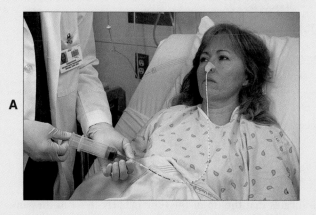

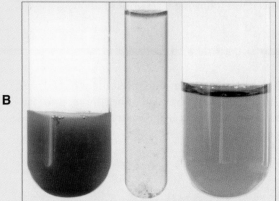

STEP **4 A,** Obtaining gastric aspirate. **B,** Typical color of aspirates from stomach, intestine, and airway. (Used with permission from Metheny NA and others: pH, color, and feeding tubes, *RN* 61(1):25, 1998.)

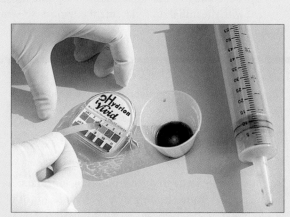

STEP **5** Compare color on test strip with color on pH chart.

## SKILL 31-3 | Verifying Feeding Tube Placement—cont'd

| STEP | RATIONALE |
|---|---|
| c. Patient with continuous tube feeding may have pH of 5 or higher. | Formulas contain solutions that are basic. |
| d. pH of pleural fluid from the tracheobronchial tree is generally greater than 6. | The pH of pleural fluid makes it difficult to differentiate between respiratory and intestinal placement (Metheny and others, 1999). |
| e. Patient who takes acid inhibitor medication will usually have an acidic pH (4 to 6). | |

• *Critical Decision Point:* Do not use auscultation of an air bolus to assess tube position. See Box 31-8.

| | |
|---|---|
| 6. If after repeated attempts, it is not possible to aspirate fluid from a tube that you originally established by x-ray examination to be in desired position, and (a) there are no risk factors for tube dislocation, (b) tube has remained in original taped position, and (c) patient is not experiencing respiratory distress, assume tube is correctly placed (Metheny and others, 1993a). | It is reasonable to assume you correctly placed the tube. When you obtain abdominal x-ray films for clinical reasons, take advantage of the reports to monitor tube location. |
| 7. Irrigate tube. | Keeps tube patent. |
|   a. Draw up 30 ml normal saline or tap water in syringe. | Will flush full length of tube. |
|   b. Kink feeding tube and then insert tip of syringe into end of feeding tube. | Prevents leakage of gastric secretions. |
|   c. Release kink and slowly instill irrigation solution. | Irrigant clears tubing. |
|   d. If unable to irrigate, reposition patient on left side, then try again. | Tip of tubing may be against stomach wall. Repositioning moves tip. |
|   e. When irrigant is instilled remove syringe. Reinstitute continuous tube feeding or replug end of tube. | Tube is clear and patent. |
| 8. Remove and dispose of gloves. Perform hand hygiene. | Reduces transmission of microorganisms. |

## EVALUATION

| | |
|---|---|
| 1. Observe patient for respiratory distress: | Feeding entered airway |
|   a. persistent gagging | |
|   b. Paroxysms of coughing | |
|   c. Respiratory patterns (e.g., rate and depth) that are inconsistent with patient's baseline measures | |
| 2. Verify that color, pH, and appearance of aspirate is consistent with the initial tube placement according to x-ray results. | Indicates that the tip of the tube is likely to be in the same place as it was following x-ray confirmation. |

## RECORDING AND REPORTING

■ Record and report pH and appearance of aspirate.

## UNEXPECTED OUTCOMES AND RELATED INTERVENTIONS

■ Red or brown coloring (coffee grounds in appearance) of fluid aspirated from a feeding tube is an indicator of new or old blood, respectively, in the gastrointestinal tract.

• If the color is not related to medications recently administered, notify the physician or health care provider. Red or brown coloring is an indicator of new or old blood, respectively.

# Administering Enteral Nutrition via a Feeding Tube

## Delegation Considerations

Administration of enteral tube feeding may be delegated to assistive personnel. However, the nurse must first verify tube placement and patency. Instruct assistive personnel to:
• Infuse feeding slowly.
• Report any difficulty infusing the feeding or any discomfort voiced by the patient

## Equipment

• Disposable feeding bag and tubing or ready-to-hang system
• 60-ml Luer-lok or catheter-tip syringe
• Stethoscope
• Infusion pump (required for continuous or intestinal feedings): Use pump designed for tube feedings
• Prescribed enteral feeding
• Normal saline or tap water
• Gloves
• Equipment to obtain blood glucose by finger stick

| STEP | RATIONALE |
|---|---|

## ASSESSMENT

1. Assess patient's need for enteral tube feedings (see Skill 31-2).

   Identify patients who need tube feedings before they become nutritionally depleted.

2. Assess patient for food allergies.

   Prevents patient from developing localized or systemic allergic responses.

3. Auscultate for bowel sounds.

   Absent bowel sounds indicate decreased ability of GI tract to digest or absorb nutrients.

4. Obtain baseline weight and review laboratory values. Assess patient for fluid volume excess or deficit, electrolyte abnormalities, and metabolic abnormalities such as hyperglycemia.

   Provides objective data to measure effectiveness of feedings.

5. Verify health care provider's order for formula, rate, route, and frequency.

   Ensures you will administer correct formula in appropriate volume.

6. For feeding tubes placed through the abdominal wall, assess stoma site for breakdown, irritation, or drainage.

   Infection, pressure from gastrostomy tube, or drainage of gastric secretions cause skin breakdown.

## PLANNING

1. Explain procedure to patient.

   Decreases patient anxiety.

2. Perform hand hygiene.

   Reduces transmission of microorganisms.

3. Prepare feeding container to administer formula continuously:

   a. Check expiration date on formula and integrity of container.

   Ensures GI tolerance of formula. Prevents leakage of tube feeding.

   b. Have tube feeding at room temperature.

   Cold formula causes gastric cramping and discomfort because the mouth and esophagus did not warm the liquid.

   c. Connect tubing to container or prepare ready-to-hang container. Use aseptic technique, and avoid handling the feeding system. If you need to handle the system, perform hand hygiene and wear gloves.

   Ensures the feeding system, including the bag, connections, and tubing, is free of contamination to prevent bacterial growth (Padula and others, 2004).

   d. Shake formula container well, and fill container with formula (see illustration). Open stopcock on tubing, and fill tubing with formula to remove air (prime tubing). Hang on pole.

   Filling the tubing with formula prevents excess air from entering gastrointestinal tract once infusion begins.

4. For intermittent feeding, measure formula in container and have syringe ready. Be sure formula is at room temperature.

   Cold formula causes gastric cramping.

5. Place patient in high-Fowler's position, or elevate head of bed at least 30 degrees.

   Elevated head helps prevent aspiration.

# Administering Enteral Nutrition via a Feeding Tube—cont'd

| STEP | RATIONALE |
|---|---|

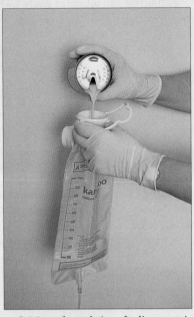

STEP **3d** Pour formula into feeding container.

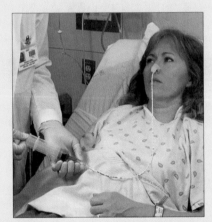

STEP **3** Check for gastric residual (small-bore tube).

## IMPLEMENTATION

1. Apply gloves.

Reduces transmission of microorganisms.

2. Determine tube placement (see Skill 31-3).

Feedings instilled into a misplaced tube sometimes cause serious injury or death.

3. Check gastric residual volume (see illustration).

For adults, a volume in excess of 200 ml for NG tubes and 100 ml for gastrostomy tubes raises concern about intolerance; however, have feedings continue while conducting further examinations (ASPEN, 2002; McClave and others, 1992; McClave and others, 1999; Murphy and Bickford, 1999). Fluids aspirated from the stomach contain electrolytes that, if withheld, will cause electrolyte imbalances. Notify the health care provider if residual volume is excessive, and request an order regarding whether or not to return the residual fluid to the patient.

   a. Draw up 10 to 30 ml of air and connect syringe to end of feeding tube. Flush tube with air. Pull back slowly, and aspirate the total amount of gastric contents that may possibly be aspirated.

   b. Return aspirated contents to stomach unless volume is excessive.

   c. Assess residual volume before each feeding for intermittent feedings. Researcher recommendations for continuous feeding range from every 4 to every 12 hours.

4. Irrigate tube (see Skill 31-3).

5. Initiate feeding:

---

• *Critical Decision Point:* Do not add food coloring or dye to enteral nutrition (see Box 31-8).

---

   a. Syringe or intermittent feeding

      (1) Pinch proximal end of feeding tube.

Prevents air from entering patient's stomach.

      (2) Remove plunger from syringe, and attach barrel of syringe to end of tube.

Barrel receives formula for instillation.

      (3) Fill syringe with measured amount of formula (see illustration). Release tube, elevate syringe to no more than 18 inches (45 cm) above insertion site, and allow it to empty gradually by gravity. Repeat steps 1 to 3 until you have delivered prescribed amount to patient.

Height of syringe allows for safe, slow, gravity drainage of formula. Total delivery of bolus feedings take several minutes, depending on the amount of the bolus. Administering the feeding too quickly will cause abdominal discomfort to the patient or increase the risk for aspiration.

| STEP | RATIONALE |
|------|-----------|

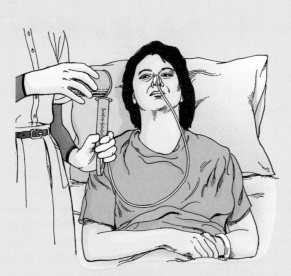

STEP **5a(3)** Fill syringe with formula.

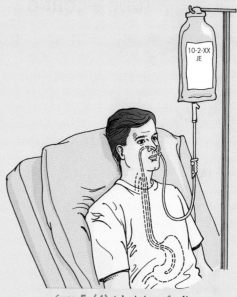

STEP **5a(4)** Administer feeding.

(4) If using a feeding bag, prime tubing and attach gavage tubing to end of feeding tube. Set rate by adjusting roller clamp on tubing or placing on a feeding pump. Allow bag to empty gradually over 30 to 60 minutes (see illustration). Label bag with tube-feeding type, strength, and amount. Include date, time, and initials. Change bag every 24 hours.

Gradual emptying of tube feeding by gravity from syringe or feeding bag reduces risk of abdominal discomfort, vomiting, or diarrhea induced by bolus or too-rapid infusion of tube feedings. Helps decrease bacterial colonization.

b. Continuous-drip method

(1) Prime and hang feeding bag and tubing on feeding pump pole.

(2) Connect distal end of tubing to proximal end of feeding tube.

Continuous-feeding method delivers prescribed hourly rate of feeding with less risk of abdominal discomfort.

(3) Connect tubing through infusion pump, and set rate (see illustration).

Delivers continuous feeding at a steady rate and pressure. Alarms for increased resistance.

---

• *Critical Decision Point:* Maximum hang time for formula is 8 hours in an open system, 24 hours in closed, ready-to-hang system (if it remains closed). Refer to manufacturer's guidelines.

---

6. Advance rate of concentration of tube feeding gradually (Box 31-9).

Helps to prevent diarrhea and gastric intolerance to formula.

7. Following intermittent infusion or at end of infusion, irrigate feeding tube per hospital policy. Have registered dietitian recommend total free water requirement per day, and obtain a physician's or health care provider's order.

Provides patient with source of water to help maintain fluid and electrolyte balance. Clears tubing of formula.

8. When you are not administering tube feedings, cap or clamp the proximal end of the feeding tube.

Prevents air from entering stomach between feedings.

9. Rinse bag and tubing with warm water whenever feedings are interrupted. Use a new administration set every 24 hours.

Rinsing bag and tubing with warm water clears old tube feedings and reduces bacterial growth.

10. For tubes placed through the abdominal wall, the exit site of the tube is usually left open to air.

# Administering Enteral Nutrition via a Feeding Tube—cont'd

## STEP

## RATIONALE

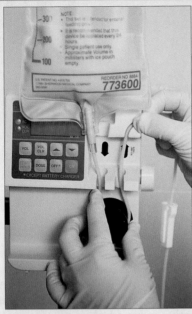

STEP **5b(3)** Connect tubing through infusion pump.

---

**BOX 31-9** | **Advancing the Rate of Tube Feeding**

Protocols for advancing tube feedings are commonly facility specific. Most of these protocols are untested for validity. There does not appear to be a benefit to slow initiation of EN over days. Most patients can tolerate feedings 2 to 3 days post initiation (ASPEN, 2002; Parrish and McCray, 2003).

**Intermittent**

1. Start formula at full strength. Do not dilute formulas with water; this increases the risk of bacterial contamination (ASPEN, 2002).
2. Infuse bolus of formula over at least 20 to 30 minutes via syringe or feeding container.
3. Begin feedings with no more than 150 to 250 ml at one time. Increase by 30 to 60 ml per feeding per 8 to 12 hours to achieve needed volume and calories in four to six feedings (Parrish and McCray, 2003).

**Continuous**

1. Start formula at full strength. Do not dilute formulas with water; this increases the risk of bacterial contamination (ASPEN, 2002).
2. Begin infusion rate at designated initiation rate.
3. Advance rate slowly (e.g., 30 to 60 ml/hr per 8 to 12 hours) (Parrish and McCray, 2003) to target rate if tolerated (tolerance indicated by absence of nausea and diarrhea, and low gastric residuals).

---

## EVALUATION

1. Measure residual volume per policy.
2. Monitor finger-stick blood glucose (usually at least every 6 hours until maximum administration rate is reached and maintained for 24 hours).

3. Monitor intake and output at least every 8 hours.

4. Weigh patient daily until patient reaches and maintains maximum administration rate for 24 hours, then weigh patient 3 times per week.

5. Monitor laboratory values (e.g., albumin, transferrin, and prealbumin).
6. Observe patient's respiratory status.

7. Observe patient's level of comfort.
8. Auscultate bowel sounds.
9. For tubes placed through the abdominal wall, observe stoma site for skin integrity.

Evaluates tolerance of tube feeding.

Requires a physician or health care provider order. Alerts nurse to patient's tolerance of enteral nutrition. Changes in blood glucose levels require physician or health care provider to revise type of formula administered.

Intake and output are indications of fluid balance or fluid volume excess or deficit.

Weight gain is indicator of improved nutritional status; however, sudden gain of more than 2 lb in 24 hours usually indicates fluid retention.

Laboratory values are indicators of patient nutritional status.

Change in respiratory status may indicate aspiration of tube feeding.

Reduced gastric emptying will lead to abdominal discomfort.

Assess gastric peristalsis.

Gastric or intestinal secretions cause injury and necrosis at stoma site.

| STEP | RATIONALE |
|------|-----------|

## RECORDING AND REPORTING

- Record amount and type of feeding, patient's response to tube feeding, patency of tube.
- Record volume of formula and any additional water on intake and output form.
- Report type of feeding, status of feeding tube, patient's tolerance, and adverse effects.

## UNEXPECTED OUTCOMES AND RELATED INTERVENTIONS

- The feeding tube becomes clogged.
  - To avoid this problem, flush the tube with water after checking the residual volume (Edwards and Metheny, 2000). Do not use cranberry juice to unclog feeding tubes; water works better than cranberry juice (Metheny and others, 1988).
- There is excessive gastric residual volume.
  - Notify physician or health care provider to determine if you need to hold feedings. If feedings are held, reassess residual volume 1 hour after you stop the feeding to determine if volume has lessened or increased. If it has increased, make sure the physician or health care provider is aware.
  - Maintain patient in semi-Fowler's position; have head of bed elevated at least 30 degrees.
- Patient aspirates formula.
  - (See interventions following Skill 30-2.)

- The patient develops diarrhea three times or more in 24 hours; indicates intolerance.
  - Notify physician or health care provider, and confer with dietitian to determine need to modify type of formula, concentration, or rate of infusion.
  - Consider other causes (e.g., bacterial contamination of the feeding, patient infection) (Eisenberg, 2002).
  - Determine if patient is receiving antibiotics or medications (e.g., those containing sorbitol), which will induce diarrhea (Benya and others, 1991; Guenter and others, 1991).
- Patient develops nausea and vomiting.
  - Indicates gastric ileus. Withhold tube feeding, and notify physician or health care provider.
  - Be sure tubing is patent; aspirate for residual.
- Drainage (signs of hemorrhage, infection, or obstruction) from the abdominal insertion site of a gastrostomy or jejunostomy (ASPEN, 2002).
  - Notify the physician or health care provider; describe and document the type of drainage.
  - For purulent drainage anticipate the need for cultures.
  - Place a dry drain-gauze around the site, and change every shift and prn.
- There is a foul odor or unusual appearance of the aspirated fluid.
  - Notify the physician or health care provider, and document the findings. Do not return aspirated material of unusual odor or appearance without first consulting the physician or health care provider.

2001). Parenteral nutrition is a specialized nutrition support that provides a specific amount of micronutrients and macronutrients intravenously. PN is selected when the gastrointestinal tract cannot be used or cannot absorb nutrients in sufficient amounts to provide adequate nutrition. A physician or health care provider reevaluates the patient daily for continued need for PN. The goal is to move toward the use of the gastrointestinal tract for enteral nutrition and eventual normal oral intake (ASPEN, 2002).

You will reduce the complications of PN by meticulous aseptic care of the central venous access device (ASPEN, 2002), a gradual increase in the nutrient provision over several days, careful monitoring of laboratory results for metabolic or electrolyte abnormalities, and assessment of fluid balance.

PN solutions that contain 10% dextrose or greater are hyperosmolar (i.e., highly concentrated) and irritate small peripheral veins. As a result, you infuse PN at this concentration through central venous lines. This is called central

PN. You administer solutions less than 900 mOsm through peripheral veins. This is referred to as peripheral PN (Gottschlich, 2001). Each day the physician or health care provider will prescribe PN, and it is mixed in the pharmacy. This prescribed solution reflects the patient's most recent laboratory values and metabolic and nutritional status. The solution itself is made for the patient's specific nutritional needs, containing amino acids, dextrose, vitamins, minerals (electrolytes), and water. The solution may or may not contain lipid. Some patients receive no lipids or receive lipids only 2 to 3 times per week.

If the PN prescription includes lipid, it is sometimes combined with the other nutrients (total nutrient admixture [TNA]) or provided in a separate bag. Do not use TNA if you observe oil droplets or an oily or creamy layer on the surface of the solution. You co-infuse lipid emulsion peripherally or centrally using a Y connector, below an in-line filter. Infusion rate is 0.5 to 1.0 ml/min for the first 30 minutes. Reactions to lipid infusion include dyspnea, cyanosis, vomiting, headache,

| BOX 31-10 | PROCEDURAL GUIDELINES FOR |
|---|---|

## Administering Enteral Feedings via Gastrostomy or Jejunostomy Tube

**Delegation Considerations:** Administration of gastrostomy feedings may be delegated to assistive personnel. However, the nurse must first verify tube placement and patency. The nurse should instruct assistive personnel about:
- The prescribed rate to infuse the feeding
- Reporting any difficulty infusing the feeding or any discomfort by the patient
- Reporting any gagging, paroxysms of coughing, or choking

**Equipment:** disposable feeding container or ready-to-hang bag, 30-ml or larger Luer-Lok or catheter-tip syringe, stethoscope, infusion pump designed for tube feedings (required for continuous or intestinal feedings): Use pump designed for tube feedings, pH indicator strip, prescribed enteral feeding, normal saline or tap water, gloves, equipment to obtain blood glucose by finger stick, if needed.

1. Assess appropriateness of initiation of EN (see Skill 31-2).
2. Auscultate for bowel sounds before feeding. Consult physician or health care provider if bowel sounds are absent.
3. Obtain baseline weight and laboratory values.
4. Verify physician's or health care provider's order for formula, rate, route, and frequency.
5. Assess skin around gastrostomy/jejunostomy site for breakdown, irritation, or drainage.
6. Explain procedure to patient and perform hand hygiene.
7. Prepare feeding container to administer formula continuously:
   a. Check expiration date on formula and integrity of container.
   b. Have tube feeding at room temperature.
   c. Connect tubing to container as needed or prepare ready-to-hang container.
   d. Shake formula well. Fill container and tubing with formula.
8. For intermittent feeding, measure feeding in container and have syringe ready. Be sure formula is at room temperature.
9. Place patient in high-Fowler's position, or elevate head of bed at least 30 degrees.
10. Apply gloves, and verify tube placement (see Skill 31-3).
11. Check gastric residual volume (RV).
    a. *Gastrostomy tube:* Attach syringe, and aspirate gastric secretions. Return aspirated contents to stomach unless the RV exceeds 100 ml. If the RV is 100 ml on several occasions, hold feeding and notify physician or health care provider.
    b. *Jejunostomy tube:* Aspirate intestinal secretions, observe volume, and return contents as above.
12. Irrigate tube with 30 ml water (see Skill 31-3).
13. Initiate feedings:

- *Critical Decision Point:* Do not add food coloring or dye to enteral nutrition.

- *Critical Decision Point:* Jejunostomy feedings are given continuously to ensure proper absorption. Do not bolus these feedings because there is no reservoir in which the feeding can collect. Bolusing into a jejunostomy will lead to intolerance and diarrhea.

   A. **Syringe or Intermittent Feeding**
      (1) Pinch proximal end of the gastrostomy/jejunostomy tube.

      (2) Remove plunger from syringe, and attach barrel of syringe to end of tube.
      (3) Fill syringe with measured amount of formula. Release tube, and elevate syringe. Allow syringe to empty gradually by gravity, refilling until you have delivered the prescribed amount to the patient.
      (4) If feeding bag is used, prime tubing and attach gavage tubing to end of feeding tube. Set rate by adjusting roller clamp on tubing or placing on a feeding pump. Allow bag to empty gradually over 30 to 60 minutes. Label bag with tube feeding type, strength, and amount. Include date, time, and initials. Change bag every 24 hours.
   B. **Continuous-Drip Method**
      (1) Connect distal end of tubing to proximal end of feeding tube.
      (2) Connect tubing through feeding pump according to manufacturer's directions, and set rate (see Skill 31-4).
14. Advance rate or concentration of tube feeding gradually (see Box 31-9).
15. Administer water via feeding tube as ordered with or between feedings.
16. Flush tube with 30 ml of water or normal saline every 4 to 6 hours around the clock and before and after administering medications via the tube.
17. When patient is not receiving tube feedings, cap or clamp the proximal end of the gastrostomy/jejunostomy tube.
18. Rinse container and tubing with warm water after all intermittent feedings.
19. The gastrostomy/jejunostomy exit site is usually left open to air. However, if patient needs a dressing because of drainage, change dressing daily or as needed and report the drainage to the physician or health care provider; inspect exit site every shift.
20. Dispose of supplies, and perform hand hygiene.
21. Evaluate patient's tolerance of tube feeding. Check amount of gastric RV every 8 to 12 hours.
22. Monitor finger-stick blood glucose level every 6 hours until patient reaches and maintains maximum rate of administration for 24 hours.
23. Monitor intake and output every 8 hours.
24. Weigh patient daily until maximum administration rate is reached and maintained for 24 hours, then weigh patient 3 times per week.
25. Monitor laboratory values.
26. Observe stoma site for skin integrity.
27. Observe patient's level of comfort.
28. Auscultate bowel sounds.
29. Record amount and type of feeding, patient's response to feeding, patency of tube, any untoward effects, and condition of gastrostomy/jejunostomy site in nurses' notes.
30. Record amount of feeding on intake and output form.
31. Report type of feeding, status of gastrostomy tube, patient's tolerance, and adverse effects.

and/or chest pain (Gottschlich, 2001). If reactions occur stop the infusion, and notify the physician or health care provider. If the patient tolerates the slow lipid infusion, advance the rate as ordered by the physician or health care provider.

*Initiating PN.* PN therapy requires a central venous catheter (CVC) inserted into the jugular or subclavian vein (ASPEN, 2002). Nurses assist with this procedure for inserting a central venous catheter. Specially trained nurses insert peripherally inserted central catheters (PICCs) (see Chapter 15). A chest x-ray film will confirm the location of the central venous catheter. Alternately, some patients have a long-term central venous access device, such as a tunneled catheter or an implanted port.

Before beginning an infusion, verify the physician's or health care provider's order. You always use an infusion pump. The solution is provided at a specified rate over the course of the day. Patients receiving PN at home frequently administer the entire daily solution over 12 hours at night. This allows the patient to disconnect from the infusion each morning, flush the central line, and have independent mobility during the day.

*Caring for the Patient Receiving PN.* Nursing care for the patient receiving PN is based on four major nursing goals: (1) preventing infection; (2) maintaining the PN system; (3) preventing metabolic, electrolyte, or fluid balance complications; and (4) assessing the patient's readiness for EN or discharge planning for home PN.

Primary methods to prevent infection include asepsis during insertion and care of the central venous catheter and dressing, use of an in-line intravenous filter, and maintaining secure, uncontaminated tubing connections. Make sure PN solutions do not exceed their 24-hour infusion limit.

Patients receiving PN have laboratory measurements monitored regularly. Capillary blood glucose testing or urine glucose testing occurs during the initiation of PN to assess for metabolic tolerance. Be alert for changes in vital signs or fluid balance and abnormal laboratory results that indicate infection, **hyperglycemia,** glucosuria, or electrolyte imbalance (Andris and Krzywda, 1999; Souba, 1997). Report any unusual symptoms to the physician or health care provider. An increased temperature is an early sign of infection. Report this to the physician or health care provider.

## RESTORATIVE AND CONTINUING CARE

**Diet Therapy in Disease Management.** Patients discharged from a hospital with diet prescriptions often need dietary education to plan meals that meet specific therapeutic requirements. Restorative care includes immediate post-surgical care, posthospitalization care, and routine medical care. Therefore integrate preparation for the restorative aspect of patient care within the acute care setting.

Patients with specific diseases often need modified dietary intake patterns in order to achieve good nutrition. These include gastrointestinal diseases, such as irritable bowel syndrome and malabsorption syndromes; metabolic disorders, such as diabetes mellitus and hypoglycemia; cardiovascular diseases; renal diseases; and cancers. Diet modifications are necessary to correspond with the body's ability to metabolize certain nutrients, to correct nutritional deficiencies, and to eliminate harmful foods from the diet. In all cases, work with the physician or health care provider and RD when planning and implementing modified diets.

**Home Care.** Sometimes specialized nutrition therapies, such as EN and PN, need to be continued beyond the hospital setting to the home care setting. In home care you are often the only care provider who sees the patient on a regular basis. As a home care nurse you teach patients or caregivers how to administer PN or EN, assess the patient for tolerance of the nutrition prescription, and evaluate the patient's progress toward nutritional goals.

##  Evaluation

**PATIENT CARE.** An ongoing evaluation will measure the value of your activities in meeting the patient's nutritional needs. Allow enough time to test a nursing approach to a problem.

Evaluation of clinical progress includes objective data, such as weight gain or improved laboratory parameters, or subjective data, such as the patient's reporting improvement in food choices or in self-reporting improved intake (Table 31-5). When clinical progress does not occur, determine whether the interventions were not effective, were not done or accepted by the patient, were not realistic or appropriate, or were affected by unanticipated or unidentified factors.

## OUTCOME EVALUATION

TABLE 31-5

| Nursing Action | Patient Response/Finding | Achievement of Outcome |
|---|---|---|
| Ask Mrs. Gonzalez if she is experiencing any gastrointestinal discomfort. | Mrs. Gonzalez admits she has occasional constipation. | Mrs. Gonzalez is not experiencing diarrhea, but bowel movements need to be regular. |
| Weight patient weekly. | Patient is weighed. | Weight is maintained. |
| Monitor the laboratory values. | Prealbumin remains 20 and albumin is 4.0. | Prealbumin and albumin values are maintained within normal limits. |
| Ask SLP about Mrs. Gonzalez's swallowing rehabilitation. | Patient is able to tolerate ground diet and nectar-thickened liquids. | Calorie count indicates oral intake does not currently meets anticipated needs. |

## EVALUATION

Sarah sees Mrs. Gonzalez before discharge to a restorative care facility. Mrs. Gonzalez is now able to consume all of her required nutrients with a ground diet and nectar-thickened liquids. Sarah removes her NG tube in preparation for her transport to the new facility. Before Mrs. Gonzalez regained her ability to orally consume adequate nutrients, her physician changed her EN formula to a fiber-containing formula. This relieved her constipation and promoted daily bowel movements.

Sarah advises Mrs. Gonzalez to continue the current plan of care and emphasizes that it is important to continue speech therapy. She discusses the importance of compliance with diet modifications until swallowing function returns completely.

### Documentation Note
"Swallows without aspirating. Daily regular bowel movements post initiation of fiber-containing formula. Oral intake of mechanically altered diet meets 100% of estimated needs. To be followed by restorative care facility."

If outcomes are not met, reassess the patient to determine if you missed any important data. Some patients need reeducation if they have forgotten or misunderstood essential skills or knowledge. Also, attempt to validate that the patient is in agreement with the goals and is willing and able to follow the nutritional plan of care.

**PATIENT EXPECTATIONS.** Nutritional interventions often depend on the patient's willingness and ability to change behavior patterns and learn new patterns. If the patient is not fully committed to the expected changes, the interventions will not always be successful. Some patients also find it difficult to change behavior and are less motivated with the passage of time. It is important to remember to individualize the nutrition care plan and focus on the patient.

Most patients respond well to the opportunity to make informed choices. Your explanations of the reasons for the behavioral change and providing the patient options for how to achieve the change will assist the patient in making the change. Provide education in several brief sessions, if necessary, to maximize the retention of information.

## KEY CONCEPTS

- Nutrients needed by the body to carry out vital functions are water, carbohydrates, protein, lipids, vitamins, microminerals, and macrominerals.
- You maintain body weight when energy intake as food or fluids equals energy requirements.
- Protein is essential for growth, maintenance, and repair.
- Digestion is the mechanical and chemical process by which food is broken down into its simplest form for absorption. Digestion and absorption occur mainly in the small intestine.
- Dietary reference intakes (DRIs), another basis for diet selection, were formulated for population groups, not individuals.
- Guidelines for dietary change advocate reduced intake of fat, saturated fat, salt, refined sugar, and cholesterol and increased intake of complex carbohydrates and fiber.
- Age affects the requirements for essential nutrients. Periods of rapid growth increase the need for protein, vitamins, and minerals.

- Because improper nutrition affects all body systems, nutritional assessment includes a review of the total physical assessment.
- Proper feeding techniques protect the dependent patient from loss of dignity and self-esteem.
- Special hospital diets alter the composition, texture, digestibility, and residue of foods to suit the patient's particular needs.
- Enteral nutrition is for patients who are unable to ingest food but are able to digest and absorb foods.
- Enteral nutrition protects intestinal structure and function and enhances immunity.
- Evaluation of the outcomes of nursing intervention in the area of nutritional support is essential to revise, update, or continue nursing activities.

## CRITICAL THINKING IN PRACTICE

*You are completing a nursing history for a 24-year-old patient who has diabetes. The patient is slightly underweight and tells you that he is vegetarian and eats no animal products, including fish, eggs, and milk.*

- - - - - - - - - - - - - - - - - -

1. a. What information about his diet do you need to determine whether it is adequate in calories and protein?
   b. What laboratory tests would reflect protein status?
   c. What physical assessment findings might suggest inadequate protein intake?
2. Mrs. Evans is 75 years of age and lives alone. She receives a Social Security check, which pays for her rent and utili-

ties with about $100 a month left over. She has arthritis, takes aspirin, and has difficulty ambulating more than about 50 feet at a time. How does Mrs. Evans's situation affect her nutritional status?
3. While giving Mr. Orzo a bath, you notice that his PN solution looks odd. There is a small yellow layer at the top of the bag. Mr. Orzo is receiving lipids, amino acids, and dextrose in a single solution. What does this layer indicate, and what do you do first?

## NCLEX® REVIEW

1. The nutrient that provides the body's most preferred energy source is:
    1. Fat
    2. Protein
    3. Vitamin
    4. Carbohydrate
2. The nutrient that is preferred to repair tissue is:
    1. Fat
    2. Protein
    3. Vitamin
    4. Carbohydrate
3. When feeding tubes are first positioned, verification is done by:
    1. Auscultation
    2. X-ray confirmation
    3. pH testing of gastric contents
    4. Confirmation of distal mark on feeding tube
4. The most accurate method for bedside confirmation of feeding tube placement is:
    1. Auscultation
    2. X-ray confirmation
    3. pH testing for gastric contents
    4. Confirmation of distal mark on feeding tube
5. Parenteral nutrition is used when the patient is:
    1. NPO
    2. Critically ill
    3. Recovering from abdominal surgery
    4. Experiencing a condition resulting in gastrointestinal dysfunction
6. Assessment of glucose balance in a patient receiving parenteral nutrition is most accurate with:
    1. Fasting blood glucose
    2. Urine testing for ketones
    3. Urine testing for glucose
    4. Serum glucose monitoring
7. You have been working with an overweight patient to achieve weight reduction. The patient is adhering to his diet but wants faster results. You tell the patient that he is having a steady weight loss progression. Ideal weight loss is:
    1. 0.5 lb/wk
    2. 1 to 2 lb/wk
    3. 2 to 3 lb/wk
    4. More than 3 lb/wk

## REFERENCES

Andris DA, Krzywda EA: Central venous catheter occlusion: successful management strategies, *Medsurg Nurs* 8(4):229, 1999.

ASPEN Board of Directors and the Clinical Guidelines Task Force: Guidelines for the use of parenteral and enteral nutrition in adult and pediatric patients, *JPEN J Parenter Enteral Nutr* 26(1 Suppl):1SA, 2002.

Bending A.: Meeting the challenges of managing dysphagia, *Community Nurse* 7(1):13, 2001.

Benya R, Layden TJ, Mobarhan S: Diarrhea associated with tube feeding: the importance of using objective criteria, *J Clin Gastroenterol* 13:167, 1991.

Bozzetti F and others: Postoperative enteral versus parenteral nutrition in malnourished patients with gastrointestinal cancer: a randomized multicentre trial, *Lancet* 358(9292):1487, 2001.

Braga ML and others: Early postoperative enteral nutrition improves gut oxygenation and reduces costs compared with total parenteral nutrition, *Crit Care Med* 29(2):242, 2001.

Braunschweig CL and others: Enteral compared with parenteral nutrition: a meta-analysis, *Am J Clin Nutr* 74(4):534, 2001.

Brody RR and others: Role of registered dietitians in dysphagia screening, *J Am Diet Assoc* 100(9):1029, 2000.

Brown A: *Understanding food: principles and preparation*, ed 2, Belmont, Calif, 2004, Wadsworth Publishing.

Burck R: Feeding, withdrawing, and withholding: ethical perspectives, *Nutr Clin Pract* 11(6):243, 1996.

Center for Nutrition Policy and Promotion: *Backgrounder: revision of the Food Guidance System,* Washington, DC, 2004, U.S. Department of Agriculture.

Chicago Dietetic Association and others: *Manual of clinical dietetics,* ed 6, Chicago, 2000, American Dietetic Association.

Council on Practice (COP) Quality Management Committee: Identifying patients at risk: ADA's definitions for nutrition screening and nutrition assessment, *J Am Diet Assoc* 94(8):838, 1994.

Dangerfield L, Sullivan R: Screening for and managing dysphagia after stroke, *Nurs Times* 95(19): 44, 1999.

Daniels S and others: Clinical predictors of dysphagia and aspiration risk: outcome measures in acute stroke patients, *Arch Phys Med Rehabil* 81:1030, 2000.

Dietary Guidelines Advisory Committee: *Report of the Dietary Guidelines Advisory Committee on the Dietary Guidelines for Americans, 2005,* Washington, DC, 2004, U.S. Department of Agriculture.

Dobranowski J and others: Incorrect positioning of nasogastric feeding tubes and the development of pneumothorax, *Can Assoc Radiol J* 43:35, 1992.

Dochterman JM, Bulechek GM, editors: *Nursing interventions classification (NIC),* ed 4, St. Louis, 2004, Mosby.

Dorner B: Tough to swallow, *Today's Dietitian* 2002(August):28, 2002.

Edwards SJ, Metheny NA: Measurement of gastric residual volume: state of the science, *Medsurg Nurs* 9(3):125, 2000.

Eisenberg P: An overview of diarrhea in the patient receiving enteral nutrition, *Gastroenterol Nurs* 25:95, 2002.

Elmstahl S and others: Treatment of dysphagia improves nutritional conditions in stroke patients, *Dysphagia* 14:61, 1999.

Expert Panel on the Identification, Evaluation, and Treatment of Overweight and Obesity in Adults: *The practical guide to identification, evaluation, and treatment of overweight and obesity in adults,* Bethesda, Md, 2000, National Institutes of Health.

Fletcher RH, Fairfield KM: Vitamins for chronic disease prevention in adults: clinical applications, *JAMA* 287(23):3127, 2002.

Food and Drug Administration and National Institutes of Health: Nutrition and overweight. In U.S. Department of Health and Human Services, Public Health Service: *Healthy People 2010*, Washington, DC, 2000, U.S. Government Printing Office.

Food and Nutrition Board, Institute of Medicine: *Dietary reference intakes: a risk assessment model for establishing upper intake levels for nutrients*, Washington, DC, 1998, National Academy Press.

Frattarelli D, Abdel-Haq N: *Botulism*, 2004, http://www.emedicine.com/ped/topic273.htm.

Fuhrman MP P and others: Hepatic proteins and nutrition assessment, *J Am Diet Assoc* 104(8):1258, 2004.

Goulding R, Bakheit AMO: Evaluation of the benefits of monitoring fluid thickness in the dietary management of dysphagic stroke patients, *Clin Rehab* 14(2):119, 2000.

Gottschlich M, editor: *The science and practice of nutrition support*, Dubuque, Iowa, 2001, Kendall Hunt Publishing.

Groher M: *Dysphagia: diagnosis and management*, ed 3, Boston, Mass, 1997, Butterworth-Heinemann.

Guenter PA and others: Tube feeding-related diarrhea in acutely ill patients, *JPEN J Parenter Enteral Nutr* 15:277, 1991.

Guigoz Y, Vellas B: The Mini Nutritional Assessment (MNA) for grading the nutritional state of elderly patients: presentation of the MNA, history and validation, *Nestle Nutr Workshop Ser Clin Perform Programme* 1:3, 1999.

Guigoz YB and others: Assessing the nutritional status of the elderly: The Mini Nutritional Assessment as part of the geriatric evaluation, *Nutr Rev* 54(1 pt 2):S59, 1996.

Hamilton M, Greenway F: Evaluating commercial weight loss programmes: an evolution in outcomes research, *Obes Rev* 5(4):217, 2004.

Hammond CL and others: Assessment of aspiration risk in stroke patients with quantification of voluntary cough, *Neurology* 56:502, 2001.

Hanson RL: Predictive criteria for length of nasogastric tube insertion for tube feeding, *JPEN J Parenter Enteral Nutr* 3(3):160, 1979.

Harrison LE and others: Early postoperative enteral nutrition improves peripheral protein kinetics in upper gastrointestinal cancer patients undergoing complete resection: a randomized trial, *JPEN J Parenter Enteral Nutr* 21(4):202, 1997.

Hentges E: Center for Nutrition Policy and Promotion: Notice of proposal for food guide graphic presentation and consumer education materials: opportunity for public comment, *Federal Register* 69(133):42030, 2004.

Hinds N, Wiles C: Assessment of swallowing and referral to speech and language therapists in acute stroke, *Q J Med* 919(12):829, 1998.

Huffman GB: Evaluating and treating unintentional weight loss in the elderly, *Am Fam Physician* 65(4):640, 2002.

Kittinger JW, Sandler RS, Heizer WD: Efficacy of metoclopramide as an adjunct to duodenal placement of small-bore feeding tubes: a randomized, placebo-controlled, double-blind study, *JPEN J Parenter Enteral Nutr* 11:33, 1987.

Koretz RL and others: AGA technical review on parenteral nutrition, *Gastroenterology* 121(4):970, 2001.

Krauss RM and others: AHA dietary guidelines: revision 2000—a statement for healthcare professionals from the Nutrition Committee of the American Heart Association, *Circulation* 102(18):2284, 2000.

Kris-Etherton PM and others: Fish consumption, fish oil, omega-3 fatty acids, and cardiovascular disease, *Circulation* 106(21):2747, 2002.

Kudsk KA and others: Enteral versus parenteral feeding: effects on septic morbidity after blunt and penetrating abdominal trauma, *Ann Surg* 215:503, 1992.

Lacey K, Pritchett E: Nutrition care process and model: ADA adopts road map to quality care and outcomes management, *J Am Diet Assoc* 103(8):1061, 2003.

Lee JS and others: Weight-loss intention in the well-functioning, community-dwelling elderly: associations with diet quality, physical activity, and weight change, *Am J Clin Nutr* 80(2):466, 2004.

Lord LM and others: Comparison of weighted vs unweighted enteral feeding tubes for efficacy of transpyloric intubation, *JPEN J Parenter Enteral Nutr* 17:271, 1993.

Luthringer S, Kulakowski K: Medical nutrition therapy protocols. In McCallum P, Polisena C: *The clinical guide to oncology nutrition*, Chicago, 2000, American Dietetic Association.

Maloney J, Metheny N: Controversy in using blue dye in enteral tube feeding as a method of detecting pulmonary aspiration, *Crit Care Nurse* 22:84, 2002.

McClave SA and others: Use of residual volume as a marker for enteral feeding intolerance: prospective blinded comparison with physical examination and radiographic findings, *JPEN J Parenter Enteral Nutr* 16:99, 1992.

McClave SA and others: Enteral tube feeding in the intensive care unit: factors impeding adequate delivery, *Crit Care Med* 27(7):1252, 1999.

McClave SA and others: North American Summit on Aspiration in the Critically Ill Patient: consensus statement, *JPEN J Parenter Enteral Nutr* 26:S80, 2002.

Metheny N and others: Effect of feeding tube properties and three irrigants on clogging rates, *Nurs Res* 37:165, 1988.

Metheny N, St. John RE, Clouse RE: Measurement of glucose in tracheobronchial secretions to detect aspiration of enteral feedings, *Heart Lung* 27:285, 1998.

Metheny N and others: Effectiveness of pH measurements in predicting feeding tube placement, *Nurs Res* 38(5):280, 1989.

Metheny N and others: Effectiveness of the auscultatory method in predicting feeding tube location, *Nurs Res* 39:262, 1990.

Metheny N and others: How to aspirate fluid from small-bore feeding tubes, *Am J Nurs* 93(5):86, 1993b.

Metheny NA, Stewart BJ: Testing feeding tube placement during continuous tube feedings, *Appl Nurs Res* 15:254, 2002.

Metheny NA, Titler MG: Assessing placement of feeding tubes, *Am J Nurs* 101:36, 2001.

Metheny NA and others: pH testing of feeding-tube aspirates to determine placement, *Nutr Clin Pract* 9:185, 1994.

Metheny NA and others: Detection of improperly positioned feeding tubes, *J Healthc Risk Manage* 18(3):37, 1998a.

Metheny NA and others: pH, color, and feeding tubes, *RN* 61(1):25, 1998b.

Metheny NA and others: pH and concentration of bilirubin in feeding tube aspirates as predictors of tube placement, *Nurs Res* 48(4):189, 1999.

Metheny NA and others: Efficacy of dye-stained enteral formula in detecting pulmonary aspiration, *Chest* 122:276, 2002a.

Metheny NA and others: Pepsin as a marker for pulmonary aspiration, *Am J Crit Care* 11:150, 2002b.

Moorhead S, Johnson M, Maas M: *Nursing outcomes classification (NOC)*, ed 3, St. Louis, 2004, Mosby.

Moriguti JC and others: Involuntary weight loss in elderly individuals: assessment and treatment, *Sao Paulo Med J* 119(2):72, 2001.

Murphy LM, Bickford V: Gastric residuals in tube feeding: how much is too much? *Nutr Clin Pract* 14:304, 1999.

National Dysphagia Diet Task Force: *National Dysphagia Diet: standardization for optimal care*, Chicago, 2002, American Dietetic Association.

Negus E: Stroke induced dysphagia in the hospital: the nutritional perspective, *Br J Nurs* 3(6):263, 1994.

Nix S: *Williams' basic nutrition and diet therapy*, ed 12, St. Louis, 2005, Mosby.

Padula CA and others: Enteral feedings: what the evidence says, *Am J Nurs* 104:62, 2004.

Pancorbo-Hidalgo PL, Garcia-Fernandez FP, Ramirez-Perez C: Complications associated with enteral nutrition by nasogastric tube in an internal medicine unit, *J Clin Nurs* 10:482, 2001.

Parrish C, McCray S: Enteral feeding: dispelling myths, *Pract Gastroenterol* 9:33, 2003.

Partnership for Food Safety Education: *Organisms that can bug you*, 2004, http://www.fightbac.org/sources.cfm.

Partnership for Food Safety Education: *Tools You Can Use*, 2005, http://portal.fightbac.org/pfse/toolsyoucanuse/.

Pearce CB, Duncan HD: Enteral feeding: nasogastric, nasojejunal, percutaneous endoscopic gastrostomy, or jejunostomy—its indications and limitations, *Postgrad Med J* 78(918):198, 2002.

Perry L: Screening swallowing function of patients with acute stroke. II. Detailed evaluation of the tool used by nurses, *J Clin Nurs* 10:474, 2001.

Perry L, Love C: Screening for dysphagia and aspiration in acute stroke: a systematic review, *Dysphagia* 16:7, 2001.

Perry L, McLaren S: Eating difficulties after stroke, *J Adv Nurs* 43(4):360, 2003.

Roubenoff R, Ravich WJ: Pneumothorax due to nasogastric feeding tubes: report of four cases, review of the literature, and recommendations for prevention, *Arch Intern Med* 149:184, 1989.

Roux L and others: Valuing the benefits of weight loss programs: an application of the discrete choice experiment, *Obes Res* 12(8):1342, 2004.

Ruser CB and others: Whittling away at obesity and overweight: small lifestyle changes can have the biggest impact, *Postgrad Med* 117(1):31, 2005.

Sarhill N and others: Evaluation of nutritional status in advanced metastatic cancer, *Support Care Cancer* 11(10):652, 2003.

Schwarte A.: Ethical decisions regarding nutrition and the terminally ill, *Gastroenterol Nurs* 24(1):29, 2001.

Shaw C, Power J: Nutritional management of patients with dysphagia, *Br J Community Nurs* 4(7):338, 1999.

Souba WW: Nutritional support, *N Engl J Med* 336(1):41, 1997.

Spieker M: Evaluating dysphagia, *Am Fam Physician* 61:3639, 2000.

Takeda EJ and others: Stress control and human nutrition, *J Med Invest* 51(3-4):139, 2004.

U.S. Department of Agriculture: *Steps to a healthier you*, 2005, http://www.mypyramid.gov/downloads/MiniPoster.pdf.

U.S. Department of Health and Human Services and U.S. Department of Agriculture: *Executive summary: Dietary Guidelines for Americans 2005*, 2005, http://www.health.gov/dietaryguidelines/dga2005/document/html/executivesummary.htm.

U.S. Food and Drug Administration and Center for Food Safety and Applied Nutrition: *Science and our food supply*, 2001, http://www.cfsan.fda.gov/dms/a2z-term.html.

Welch SK: Certification of staff nurses to insert enteral feeding tubes using a research-based procedure, *Nutr Clin Pract* 11(1):21, 1996.

Wendell GD, Lenchner GS, Promisloff RA: Pneumothorax complicating small bore feeding tube placement, *Arch Intern Med* 151:599, 1991.

Whitman MM: The starving patient: supportive care for people with cancer, *Clin J Oncol Nurs* 4(3):121, 2000.

Whitney E, Rolfes S, editors: *Understanding nutrition*, ed 9, Stamford, Conn, 2002, Wadsworth Publishing.

Whitworth MK and others: Doctor, does this mean I'm going to starve to death? *J Clin Oncol* 22(1):199, 2004.

Wood P, Emick-Herring B: Dysphagia: a screening tool for stroke patients, *J Neurosci Nurs* 29(5):325, 1997.

# CHAPTER 32

# Urinary Elimination

## MEDIA RESOURCES

**CD COMPANION** *evolve* **WEBSITE**

http://evolve.elsevier.com/Potter/basic

- **NCLEX® Review**
- **Audio Glossary**
- **English/Spanish Audio Glossary**
- **Video Clips**

# OBJECTIVES

- Explain the function of each organ in the urinary system.
- Describe the process of urination.
- Identify factors that commonly influence urination.
- Compare and contrast common alterations in urination.
- Obtain a nursing history from a patient with an alteration in urination.
- Describe physical assessment techniques used to assess urinary elimination.
- Describe characteristics of normal and abnormal urine.

- Describe nursing implications of common diagnostic tests of the urinary system.
- Identify nursing diagnoses relevant to the urinary system.
- Discuss nursing measures to assist the patient with urinary elimination.
- Describe nursing measures to control incontinence.
- Discuss nursing measures to reduce urinary tract infections.
- Apply or insert an external or indwelling catheter.

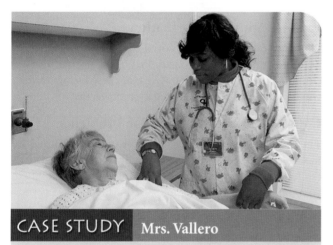

## CASE STUDY — Mrs. Vallero

Mrs. Vallero is an 85-year-old woman. She has been in the hospital for 4 days for congestive heart failure with pulmonary edema. At the 3 PM report Phyllis learns her indwelling urinary catheter and intravenous (IV) line were removed at 8 AM today. Her total input since that time has been 1400 ml orally. It is now 4:30 PM. Mrs. Vallero was incontinent of a small amount of urine and was complaining of lower abdominal pain. She has no recorded urine output for the day. She was catheterized at 6 PM for 600 ml of pale, clear yellow urine after the physician or health care provider was called. The physician or health care provider ordered "single catheterization now and times one."

Mrs. Phyllis Stone is a 43-year-old divorced mother of two daughters. Phyllis is a sophomore nursing student in her sixth week of clinical rotation at a community hospital. She was in the hospital as a patient at the birth of her daughters. At the birth of her second child a year ago she had a cesarean section and had a urinary catheter in for 2 days.

### KEY TERMS

bacteriuria, p. 916
catheterization, p. 931
continent urinary diversion (CUR), p. 921
dysuria, p. 916
glomerulus, p. 914
graduated measuring container, p. 922
hematuria, p. 923
micturition, p. 914
nephrons, p. 914
nosocomial, p. 916
proteinuria, p. 914
residual urine, p. 916

suprapubic catheter, p. 942
ureterostomy, p. 917
urinal, p. 928
urinary diversion, p. 914
urinary incontinence, p. 916
urinary reflux, p. 944
urinary retention, p. 914
urine hat, p. 922
urometer, p. 922
urosepsis, p. 916
voiding, p. 914

Normal elimination of urinary wastes is a function most people take for granted. When the urinary system fails to function properly, it affects virtually all body systems. Patients with alterations in urinary elimination may also have body image problems as a result.

## Scientific Knowledge Base

Knowledge from the biological and social sciences helps you to identify actual and potential urinary tract problems that patients encounter. A thorough understanding of related information helps you to provide complete and competent care to the patient with altered elimination.

## Urinary Elimination

Urinary elimination depends on the function of the kidneys, ureters, bladder, and urethra. The kidneys remove wastes from the blood and urine. The ureters transport urine from the kidneys to the bladder. The bladder holds urine until the urge to urinate develops and urine leaves the body through the urethra. All these organs must be intact and functional for the successful removal of urinary wastes. The normal range of urine production is 1 to 2 L/day (Huether and McCance, 2004). Fluid intake and body temperature affect urine production. Urine is usually 95% water and 5% solutes. These solutes include electrolytes and organic solutes such as urea, uric acid, creatinine, and ammonia.

**KIDNEYS.** The kidneys are reddish brown, bean-shaped organs that lie on either side of the vertebral column behind the abdominal peritoneum and against the deep muscles of the back. The kidneys are level with the twelfth thoracic and third lumbar vertebrae. The functional units, **nephrons,** remove waste products from the blood and regulate water and electrolyte concentrations in body fluids. The kidneys efficiently filter the blood of waste products in part because of their high blood flow, which represents approximately 25% of the cardiac output.

A cluster of capillaries forms the **glomerulus,** which is the initial site of urine formation. These capillaries filter water and glucose, amino acids, urea, uric acid, creatinine, and major electrolytes. Protein does not normally filter through the glomerulus. Therefore protein in the urine, **proteinuria,** is a sign of glomerular injury.

However, not all glomerular filtrate is excreted as urine. The body reabsorbs approximately 99% of the filtrate into the plasma. When the filtrate leaves the glomerulus, it passes through a system of tubules in which water and glucose, amino acids, uric acid, sodium, potassium, and bicarbonate ions are selectively reabsorbed into plasma. Hydrogen and potassium ions and ammonia are secreted into the tubules and become a part of the urine.

**URETERS.** A ureter is attached to each kidney pelvis and carries urinary wastes into the bladder. Urine draining from the ureters to the bladder is sterile. Peristaltic waves cause the urine to enter the bladder in spurts rather than steadily. To prevent urine from returning to the ureters, a small flaplike fold of mucous membrane acts as a valve and covers the juncture of the ureters and bladder.

**BLADDER.** The urinary bladder is a hollow, distensible, muscular organ that is a reservoir for urine. When empty, the bladder lies in the pelvic cavity behind the symphysis pubis. In the male the bladder rests against the rectum posteriorly, and in the female it rests against the anterior wall of the uterus and vagina.

The bladder's shape changes as it fills with urine. When the bladder is full, its superior surface expands up into a dome and pushes above the symphysis pubis. A greatly distended bladder may reach the umbilicus. In a pregnant woman the fetus pushes against the bladder, causing a feeling of fullness and reducing its capacity.

**URETHRA.** Urine travels from the bladder through the urethra and passes to the outside of the body through the urethral meatus. Mucous membrane lines the urethra, and urethral glands secrete mucus into the urethral canal. The external urethral sphincter, located about halfway down the urethra, permits voluntary flow of urine.

## Act of Urination

Urination, **micturition,** and **voiding** are all terms for expelling urine from the urinary bladder. You sense a desire to urinate when the bladder contains only a small amount of urine (150 to 200 ml in an adult and 50 to 100 ml in a child). As the volume of urine increases, the bladder wall stretches. Normally a person is conscious of the need to urinate. If the person chooses not to void, the external urinary sphincter remains contracted, inhibiting the reflex. However, when a person is ready to void, the external sphincter relaxes, the micturition reflex stimulates the detrusor muscle to contract, and urination occurs.

## Factors Influencing Urination

Physiological factors, psychosocial conditions, and diagnostic or treatment-induced factors all affect normal urinary elimination (Box 32-1). Knowledge of these factors enables you to anticipate possible elimination problems.

## Common Urinary Elimination Problems

The most common urinary problems involve disturbances in urination. These disturbances result from impaired bladder function, obstruction to urine outflow, or an inability to voluntarily control micturition. Some patients have permanent or temporary changes in the normal pathway of urination. For example, the patient with a **urinary diversion** has special problems because urine drains through an artificial opening (stoma) on the abdominal wall.

**URINARY RETENTION. Urinary retention** is an accumulation of urine in the bladder because the bladder is unable to partially or completely empty. The patient who retains at least 25% of total bladder capacity is experiencing urinary retention. Urine collects in the bladder, stretching its walls and causing feelings of pressure, discomfort, tenderness over the symphysis pubis, restlessness, and diaphoresis. These findings along with an absence of urinary output over several hours and a distended bladder may indicate urinary retention. In urinary retention the bladder sometimes holds more than 1000 ml of urine.

Eventually retention with overflow will develop. Pressure in the bladder builds so that the external urethral sphincter is unable to hold back urine. The sphincter opens to allow a small volume of urine (25 to 60 ml) to escape, after which the bladder pressure falls enough to allow the sphincter to close. The patient may void or be incontinent of small amounts of urine 2 or 3 times an hour with no relief of distention or discomfort. This symptom of retention incontinence is called overflow urinary incontinence (Milne, 2004).

| BOX 32-1 | Factors Influencing Urinary Elimination |
| --- | --- |

### Growth and Development

Infants and young children are unable to concentrate urine and reabsorb water effectively.

Children cannot control urination voluntarily until 18 to 24 months.

A child must be able to recognize the feeling of bladder fullness, to hold urine for 1 to 2 hours, and to communicate the sense of urgency to a parent.

With age, the ability to concentrate urine declines and the frequency of urination increases.

The process of aging impairs micturition by interfering with mobility, sometimes making it difficult for older adults to reach the toilet or bedside commode in time (Figure 32-1).

### Sociocultural Factors

Cultural and gender norms vary on the privacy or publicness of urination. North Americans expect toilet facilities to be private, whereas some European cultures accept communal toilet facilities. Religious or cultural norms dictate who is acceptable to assist in elimination practices.

Social expectations (e.g., school recesses) influence the time of urination.

### Psychological Factors

Anxiety and stress do not affect the characteristics of urine but sometimes affect a sense of urgency and increase the frequency of urination.

Anxiety prevents complete urination because tension makes it difficult to relax abdominal muscles.

### Personal Habits

Privacy and adequate time to urinate are usually important to most people. Some people need distractions to relax.

### Muscle Tone

Weak abdominal and pelvic floor muscles impair bladder contraction and control of the external sphincter.

Immobility, childbirth, or trauma sometimes cause decreased muscle tone.

Continuous drainage of urine through an indwelling catheter often causes loss of the bladder's muscle tone.

### Fluid Intake

Foods with high fluid content, such as fruits and vegetables, increase urine production.

If fluids, electrolytes, and solutes are balanced, increased fluid intake increases urine production.

Alcohol stops the release of antidiuretic hormones, thus promoting urine production.

Fluids containing caffeine increase urinary output frequency and urgency.

### Pathological Conditions

Diabetes mellitus and multiple sclerosis cause neuropathies that alter bladder function.

Rheumatoid arthritis, degenerative joint disease, and parkinsonism slow or hinder physical activity and interfere with urination.

Chronic diseases, such as stroke, alter urinary patterns by interfering with mobility or bladder sensation.

Acute renal disease reduces urine volume; chronic renal disease initially increases volume of poorly concentrated urine.

Febrile conditions reduce the amount of urine but increase the concentration.

Spinal cord injuries interrupt voluntary bladder emptying.

### Surgical Procedures

The stress response to surgery reduces the amount of urinary output to increase circulatory fluid volume.

Anesthetics and pain-killing drugs slow the filtration rate and reduce urinary output.

Local trauma during lower abdominal and pelvic surgery sometimes obstructs urine flow, making indwelling catheters necessary.

### Medications

Diuretics prevent reabsorption of water and certain electrolytes, and urinary output increases.

Some drugs also change the color of urine (e.g., amitriptyline turns it blue-green, methyldopa turns it red, warfarin sodium turns it orange, indomethacin turns it green).

Some medications affect the ability to relax and empty the bladder.

### Diagnostic Examinations

Following intravenous pyelograms, monitor patient for complications such as hypersensitivity reactions and acute renal failure.

Cystoscopy causes localized edema of the urethral passageway and bladder sphincter spasm, resulting in urinary retention and the passing of red or pink urine.

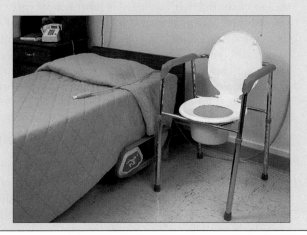

FIGURE **32-1** Bedside commode. (From Sorrentino S: *Mosby's textbook for nursing assistants*, St. Louis, 2004, Mosby.)

| TABLE 32-1 | Urinary Disorders | |
|---|---|---|
| **Disorder** | **Causes** | |
| **Urinary Retention** | | |
| Urine flow is obstructed; urine accumulates in bladder. Low fluid intake leads to retention. | Prostate gland enlargement, fecal impaction, pregnancy in third trimester, urethral stricture or edema after childbirth, and urethral edema after surgery or diagnostic examination obstruct urine flow. | |
| | Spinal cord and peripheral nerve trauma and degeneration of peripheral nerves (e.g., diabetic neuropathy) alter sensory and motor innervation. | |
| | Emotional anxiety and muscle tension alter ability to relax sphincters. | |
| | Medications (anesthetics and narcotics) dull bladder sensations. | |
| **Lower Urinary Tract Infection** | | |
| Microorganisms enter urethra resulting in bacterial spread, causing inflammation of bladder muscle. | Kinked or blocked urethral catheter and urinary retention cause obstruction of urine flow. | |
| | Poor perineal hygiene, frequent sexual intercourse, ingredients in bubble baths, improperly handled diagnostic instruments, improperly sterilized instruments, and contaminated urine receptacles cause spread of bacteria. | |
| **Urinary Incontinence** | | |
| Incontinence involves incompetent or weakened sphincter and loss of control of voiding. | Multiple childbirths, pelvic organ surgery, and removal of prostate gland weaken sphincter. | |
| | Mental confusion, sedatives or analgesics, spinal cord injury, bladder spasm, and bladder atrophy cause loss of voiding control. | |

Decreased urine production causes retention by filling the bladder gradually, thus preventing activation of the stretch receptors. After distending beyond a certain point, the bladder cannot contract. Retention also occurs because of many other factors (Table 32-1).

**URINARY TRACT INFECTIONS.** Urinary tract infections account for 36% to 40% of hospital-acquired (**nosocomial**) infections in the United States. Most of these infections are directly due to catheterization. **Bacteriuria** (bacteria in the urine) is often inevitable once a retention catheter is inserted (Foxman, 2002). The catheter is a source of injury to the mucosa, thus allowing bacterial invasion. It is important to keep catheterization at a minimum because bacteriuria leads to the spread of organisms into the bloodstream (**urosepsis**) and kidneys, especially in the severely ill patient.

Microorganisms are able to enter the urinary tract through the urethral meatus or the bloodstream. However, the ascending route through the urethra is more common. Bacteria inhabit the vagina in women and the distal urethra and external genitalia in men and women. Organisms enter the urethral meatus easily and travel up the inner mucosal lining to the bladder. Women are more susceptible to urinary tract infection because of the proximity of the anus to the urethral meatus and because of a short urethra. In the male the length of the urethra and the antibacterial substance in prostatic secretions reduce the risk of urinary tract infection.

Normally the body flushes out organisms during voiding. However, bladder distention reduces blood flow to the mucosal and submucosal layer, and tissues become more susceptible to bacteria. **Residual urine,** urine that remains in the bladder after urination, is an ideal site for microorganism growth. Table 32-1 summarizes the causes of lower urinary tract infection.

Patients with urinary tract infections often have pain or burning during urination (**dysuria**) and urgency. An irritated bladder also causes a frequent and urgent sensation of the need to void. Fever, chills, nausea and vomiting, and malaise sometimes develop. Irritation to bladder and urethral mucosa results in blood-tinged urine (hematuria). The urine appears concentrated and cloudy because of bacteria. If infection spreads to the kidneys (pyelonephritis), fever, flank pain, tenderness, and chills are common symptoms. The older adult with urinary tract infection with an accompanying fever also exhibits an alteration in mental status such as acute confusion (Lewis, Heitkemper, and Dirksen, 2004).

**URINARY INCONTINENCE.** Urinary incontinence is the loss of control over voiding. It is either temporary or permanent. The patient is unable to control the external urethral sphincter. Leakage is continuous or intermittent. In some cases, you will be the first or only professional to whom patients will reveal their incontinence. Therefore be sensitive to this problem, which researchers believe occurs in more than a third of nursing home residents and in 13% to 56% of nonhospitalized adults (Mason and others, 2003). There are five types of incontinence (Table 32-2). The causes of incontinence vary by type.

Incontinence is a common problem that develops in people of every age. It is a myth that incontinence is part of the aging process. The annual cost of incontinence for patients in the community and in nursing homes is over $16 billion annually (Sampselle, 2003). Urinary incontinence has an impact on body image and social interaction. Clothing be-

| TABLE 32-2 | Types of Urinary Incontinence | |
|---|---|---|
| **Description** | **Causes** | **Symptoms** |
| **Total** | | |
| Total uncontrollable and continuous loss of urine | Neuropathy of sensory nerves<br>Trauma or disease of spinal nerves or urethral sphincter | Constant flow of urine at unpredictable times<br>Nocturia<br>Lack of awareness of bladder filling or incontinence |
| **Functional** | | |
| Involuntary unpredictable passage of urine in patient with intact urinary and nervous systems | Fistula between bladder and vagina<br>Change in environment<br>Sensory, cognitive, or mobility deficits | Strong urge to void with loss of urine before reaching appropriate receptacle |
| **Stress** | | |
| Increased intraabdominal pressure causing leakage of small amount of urine | Coughing, laughing, vomiting, or lifting with full bladder<br>Obesity<br>Full uterus pressing against bladder during third trimester of pregnancy<br>Incompetent bladder outlet<br>Weak pelvic musculature | Dribbling of urine with increased intraabdominal pressure<br>Urinary urgency<br>Frequency |
| **Urge** | | |
| Involuntary passage of urine after strong sense of urgency to void | Decreased bladder capacity<br>Irritation of bladder stretch receptors<br>Alcohol or caffeine ingestion<br>Increased fluid intake | Urinary urgency<br>Abnormal frequency (more often than every 2 hours)<br>Bladder contracture or spasm<br>Nocturia<br>Voiding in small (less than 100 ml) or in large (more than 550 ml) amounts |
| **Reflex** | | |
| Involuntary loss of urine occurring at somewhat predictable intervals when patient reaches specific bladder volume. | Upper spinal cord injury or disease involving area above reflex arc, blocking cerebral awareness<br>Lower spinal cord injury blocking impulses to reflex arc | Lack of awareness of bladder filling<br>No urge to void<br>Uninhibited bladder contraction or spasm at regular intervals |

comes wet with urine, and the accompanying odor adds to embarrassment. Patients with this problem often avoid physical and social activities (Wyman, 2003).

Older adults are more susceptible to incontinence because of functional limitations and the environment in which they live. An older person with restricted mobility has a greater chance of being incontinent because of the inability to reach toilet facilities in time. Low-set chairs and high beds are additional obstacles for the older adult who needs to get up to reach a toilet. An older adult who has difficulty undoing buttons or manipulating zippers faces another obstacle. Some older adults with chronic health problems lack the energy to walk very far at one time, and if there is only one toilet in the home, the distance is sometimes too far for the patient with urge incontinence (Lekan-Rutledge and Colling, 2003). Continued episodes of incontinence create skin breakdown. Acidic urine is irritating to the skin. The patient who has frequent incontinence is especially at risk for pressure ulcers (see Chapter 35).

## Urinary Diversions

With surgery it is possible to divert the drainage of urine from a diseased or dysfunctional bladder. There are two classifications for urinary diversions: continent and incontinent (Figure 32-2). A **ureterostomy** (an incontinent diversion) is any surgical procedure that creates stomas on the outer abdominal wall for continuous urine drainage. Typically the patient with a ureterostomy has had the bladder removed surgically because of a malignant growth, birth defects, or a spinal cord injury. A ureterostomy is often the preferred treatment for chronic incontinence. The ileal loop or conduit, commonly used for the last 40 years, involves separating a loop of intestinal ileum with its blood supply intact. A ureterostomy involves bringing the end of one or both

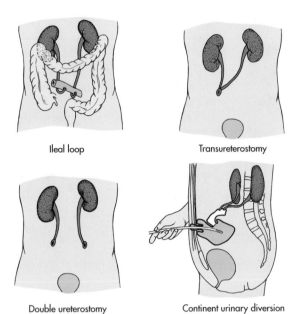

Ileal loop

Transureterostomy

Double ureterostomy

Continent urinary diversion

FIGURE **32-2** Types of incontinent and continent urinary diversions.

ureters to the abdominal surface. To avoid the need for two collecting devices, a transureterostomy connects the ureters and brings one out through the abdominal wall.

Surgery for continent diversion creates an internal pouch to store urine. Patients do not need to wear an external ostomy pouch over the urinary stoma. Instead they learn to insert a catheter into their stoma to drain urine periodically throughout the day. A urinary diversion poses threats to body image. Some patients with an incontinent diversion wear an artificial device to collect urine and learn to manage it. The patient with a urinary diversion is able to wear normal clothing, engage in any physical activity, travel, and have sexual relations.

## Nursing Knowledge Base

Urinary elimination is a natural and often private process that requires physiological and psychological health. Therefore providing nursing care for a patient with potential or actual urinary problems requires an understanding beyond anatomy and physiology. Be knowledgeable about concepts such as infection control, hygiene measures, growth, and development, and also be sensitive to the patient's psychosocial needs when a urinary problem develops.

### Infection Control and Hygiene

The urinary tract is a common site for infection, and therefore you will follow the principles of infection control to prevent the onset and spread of urinary tract infections and to promote the treatment of infections that do occur (see Chapter 11). *Escherichia coli* often causes urinary tract infections, and the infections occur anywhere along the urinary tract from the urethra to the kidneys. Urinary tract infec-

tions that occur after admission to a health care facility are called nosocomial infections and are sometimes the result of procedures such as urinary catheterization. The major reason for most nosocomial infections is a lack of hand washing (Lewis and others, 2004).

You will need to follow the principles of medical and surgical asepsis meticulously when carrying out procedures involving the urinary tract or external genitalia. Any instrumentation used on the urinary tract, such as catheterization, requires the use of sterile technique. Procedures that involve manipulation of the perineum, such as perineal care or examination of the genitalia, require the use of medical asepsis.

### Developmental Considerations

Throughout the life span, normal growth and development processes affect a person's ability to void. Normally, neonates void within 24 hours after birth. In the neonate and infant, urination is a voiding response and produced by a full bladder. As the child reaches the age of 2 or 3 years, the neuromuscular and cognitive functions develop to the point where the child begins to control voiding (see Chapter 19).

As we age, changes occur in both the male and female that contribute to the development of voiding problems. In the male it is possible for prostate enlargement to start after age 40 and continue until the 80s, causing partial obstruction of the urethra and resulting in inadequate emptying of the bladder. This change produces increased urinary frequency. In the female, childbearing and hormonal levels influence urination. Changes associated with pregnancy often produce urinary frequency and urgency. With repeated deliveries or hormone changes after menopause, temporary or permanent changes can occur that result in decreased perineal muscle tone. These changes may lead to urgency and stress incontinence (see Table 32-2). Hormonal changes may also contribute to an increased susceptibility to infection. Decreased levels of estrogen tend to cause the urethral mucosa to become thinner and more fragile and consequently more easily traumatized and infected (Huether and McCance, 2004).

### Psychosocial Implications

Self-concept, culture, and sexuality are all closely related concepts that are affected when a patient has elimination problems. Self-concept changes over our life span and includes one's body image, self-esteem, roles, and identity (see Chapter 20). When children begin to achieve bladder control and learn the appropriate skills, they sometimes resist urinating on the toilet. Children often associate their urine and feces as extensions of self, and they do not want to flush part of themselves away.

Gender influences the position we use to urinate. Males tend to stand to urinate, and females assume a sitting position. Culture influences how people talk about urination and how much privacy a person needs. It is considered improper in some cultures for a male to ask a female patient about private matters such as urination (Box 32-2).

CULTURAL FOCUS

- Accommodate need for gender-congruent care among cultures emphasizing separate gender roles and female modesty such as African, Hispanic, Asian, Islamic, Arabic, Hindu, Jewish Orthodox, and Amish cultures.
  - Explain the procedure you will perform, and ask the patient how he or she wants this done.
  - Assign female caregivers to catheterize females and male caregivers for male patients.
  - Allow presence of a family member at the bedside if requested by the patient.
  - Provide privacy through adequate draping and use of bedside screens.
  - Prevent entrance of the opposite sex during the procedure.
  - Avoid prolonged exposure of the patient.
    - Assign a skilled practitioner to perform urinary procedures.
- Control verbal and nonverbal communication when performing catheterization of a circumcised female.
  - Avoid judgmental comments, and assess for landmarks in a professional manner.
  - Use a smaller catheter when scarring constricts the area.
  - Explain the procedure you will perform.
- Promote understanding of patients of the procedure to be done.
  - Use an interpreter as needed.
  - Repeat explanations because patient's anxiety about the loss of privacy creates distraction.
  - Explain measures to protect the patient's privacy.
- Provide patients' hygiene needs.
  - Certain cultures, such as Hindus and Muslims, observe meticulous hygiene practices that designate the left hand to perform unclean procedures such as catheterization.
    - Wash your hands before touching the patient, and use your right hand.
    - Use the left hand to handle the urinal and/or urinary secretions.
    - Change the bed linens and gown of the patient promptly if contaminated with urine.
    - Do not place the urinal or soiled bed linens on top of the bedside table or surface used for praying or eating.
    - Provide the patient with the equipment and supplies for cleansing after elimination (Lawrence and Rozmus, 2001).

## Critical Thinking

### Synthesis

In caring for patients with altered patterns of elimination, you need to synthesize knowledge, draw from experience, apply critical thinking attitudes, and be knowledgeable about the standards of practice. Practical experience and knowledge from science and nursing will assist you in providing individualized nursing care for these patients.

**KNOWLEDGE.** In order to properly care for patients with elimination problems it is important that you understand changes in normal urinary elimination caused by pathological conditions and changes associated with age,

gender, and improper hygiene practices. This knowledge and a comprehensive view of your patient's situation allow you to make the most accurate decisions about patient care. Information regarding a patient's fluid balance and knowledge of medication will further complement your knowledge base. When patients have changes in their fluid balance, this affects elimination patterns. In addition, these changes increase the patients' risks for problems in urination related to infection, incontinence, or retention.

**EXPERIENCE.** Previous and personal experience provide a basis for determining elimination needs. Perhaps you have cared for a previous patient who was incontinent. Perhaps you or a close friend has had the experience of an indwelling catheter or a urinary tract infection and experienced frequency, burning, urgency, and hesitancy. Maybe you have learned, when caring for previous patients, that voiding patterns are individual. To find out about voiding patterns, you ask patients about their usual patterns of elimination.

**ATTITUDES.** Patients have individual and very personal elimination needs. Be flexible, and use different positioning techniques to meet patients' unique elimination needs. Always consider the patient's preferences in planning elimination practices and setting priorities. Curiosity is another critical thinking attitude that enables you to learn more about patients so you will make the best clinical decision with them.

**STANDARDS.** Because urination is often a private matter, you will protect the patient's privacy. In addition, it is important that you adhere to the standards of medical and surgical asepsis. Some of the interventions you select to restore urinary elimination will be invasive. Follow the standards of asepsis to reduce the risk of infection (see Chapter 11).

## Nursing Process

### Assessment

You need to complete a nursing history, perform a physical assessment, assess the patient's urine, and review information from laboratory and diagnostic tests to identify a urinary elimination problem.

**NURSING HISTORY.** Information from the scientific and the nursing knowledge base assist you in completing a nursing history. The nursing history includes a review of the patient's elimination patterns, symptoms of urinary alterations, and assessment of factors that are affecting the ability to urinate normally.

**Pattern of Urination.** Ask the patient about daily voiding patterns, including frequency and times of day, normal volume at each voiding, and history of recent changes. Frequency varies among individuals. Most people void an average of 5 or more times a day. The patient who voids frequently during the night often has renal or cardiovascular disease. Information about the pattern of urination is necessary to establish a baseline for comparison.

**Symptoms of Urinary Alterations.** Certain symptoms of alterations occur in more than one type of urinary disor-

| TABLE 32-3 | Common Symptoms of Urinary Alterations |
|---|---|

| Description | Causes or Associated Factors |
|---|---|
| **Urgency**<br><br>Feeling of the need to void immediately | Full bladder<br>Inflammation or irritation to bladder mucosa from infection<br>Incompetent urethral sphincter<br>Psychological stress |
| **Dysuria**<br><br>Painful or difficult urination | Bladder inflammation<br>Trauma or inflammation of urethra |
| **Frequency**<br><br>Voiding at frequent intervals | Increased fluid intake<br>Bladder inflammation<br>Increased pressure on bladder (e.g., pregnancy, psychological stress) |
| **Hesitancy**<br><br>Difficulty in initiating urination | Prostate enlargement<br>Anxiety<br>Urethral edema |
| **Polyuria**<br><br>Voiding large amount of urine | Excess fluid intake<br>Diabetes mellitus or insipidus<br>Use of diuretics |
| **Oliguria**<br><br>Diminished urinary output in relation to fluid intake | Dehydration<br>Renal failure<br>Urinary tract obstruction<br>Increased secretion of antidiuretic hormone (ADH) |
| **Nocturia**<br><br>Urination, particularly excessive, at night | Excess intake of fluids (especially coffee or alcohol before bedtime)<br>Renal disease<br>Cardiovascular disease |
| **Dribbling**<br><br>Leakage of urine despite voluntary control of micturition | Urine retention from incomplete bladder emptying<br>Stress incontinence |
| **Hematuria**<br><br>Presence of blood in urine | Neoplasms of kidney, certain glomerular diseases, infections of kidneys or bladder, traumatic injury to urinary structure, calculi, blood dyscrasia |
| **Retention**<br><br>Accumulation of urine in bladder, with inability of bladder to empty | Urethral obstruction, bladder inflammation, decreases in sensory activity, neurogenic bladder, prostate enlargement after anesthesia, side effects of certain medications (e.g., anticholinergics, antispasmodics, antidepressants) |
| **Residual Urine**<br><br>Volume of urine remaining in bladder after voiding (volumes of 100 ml or more) | Inflammation or irritation of bladder mucosa from infection, neurogenic bladder, prostatic enlargement, trauma, or inflammation of urethra |

## FOCUSED PATIENT ASSESSMENT

**TABLE 32-4**

| Factors to Assess | Questions and Approaches | Physical Assessment Strategies |
|---|---|---|
| Fluid intake | Determine if patient has any fluid restrictions.<br>Ask if patient is able to obtain fluids independently.<br>Ask what patient's usual 24-hour intake equals. | Observe skin and mucous membranes.<br>Obtain intake and output. |
| Urinary elimination | In ambulatory patients:<br>  Ask patient about ability to use toileting facilities.<br>For patients with restricted mobility:<br>  Determine patient's frequency and need for assistance in using toileting facilities.<br>  Ask patient what type of assistance he or she uses at home. | Observe patient's ability to use toileting facilities.<br>Observe if assistance needed with transfer and ambulation to and from the toilet area. |
| Bladder function | Ask or determine when patient last voided, noting amount of urine.<br>Ask patient about perception of urge to void.<br>Ask patient if bladder feels empty after voiding. | Palpate bladder. |

der. During assessment ask the patient about the presence of symptoms listed in Table 32-3. Also determine whether the patient is aware of conditions or factors that precipitate or aggravate the symptoms.

**Factors Affecting Urination.** Focused assessment enables you to gather data relevant to your patient's elimination pattern (Table 32-4). In addition, there are important factors in the patient's history that normally affect urination. These factors include the following:

1. *Medication usage:* You need to ask about prescription, over-the-counter, and herbal supplements because they sometimes affect fluid and electrolyte balance. Diuretics are successfully used to regulate fluid balance; however, side effects cause fluid and electrolyte imbalances. Narcotic analgesics cause urinary retention. Some anesthetics temporarily depress renal or bladder function.

2. *Mobility status:* Assess patients' use of walking aids, the ability to remove clothing, or the ability to get in and out of the bathroom or up and down from the toilet.

3. *Environmental barriers:* Assess both home and health care setting for barriers that prevent the patient from accessing the toilet. Some patients need an elevated toilet seat, grab bars, or a portable commode. Also consider the lack of lighting and distance to the toilet (Lekan-Rutledge and Colling, 2003).

4. *Sensory restrictions:* Assess for those sensory changes that obstruct self-toileting (e.g., patients with visual problems who have trouble reaching toilet facilities safely). If the patient has difficulty with hand coordination, assess the type of clothing and the patient's ease in using clothing fasteners.

5. *Past illness:* Assess for history of urinary tract infection or bladder surgery that may increase the risk for recur-

rent problems. Chronic diseases (e.g., multiple sclerosis) that impair bladder function require you to consider preventive care measures. Patients returning from surgery often have difficulty voiding the first few hours until the effects of anesthesia diminish.

6. *Major surgery:* Patients recovering from major surgery and suffering critical illness or disability often have an indwelling catheter to aid urinary drainage and provide a measurement of urinary output. A catheter places a patient at risk for infection.

7. *Urinary diversion:* If the patient has a urinary diversion, assess its type, location, and function. Also assess the condition of surrounding skin and usual methods for management (presence of appliance or pouch, type of skin care products and application). If the patient has an incontinent diversion, assess the methods and frequency of appliance changes and the type of nighttime drainage system. In addition, in the patient with a **continent urinary diversion (CUR)**, determine the frequency and type of catheters used to drain urine.

8. *Personal habits:* Some personal habits may inhibit urination or put the patient at risk for infection (i.e., poor hand or perineal hygiene). If a patient is hospitalized, assess how this alters his or her personal habits. Privacy is often difficult to accomplish in a health care setting, particularly if a patient uses a bedpan (see Chapter 33) or a urinal. Determine the patient's knowledge and practices of perineal hygiene.

9. *Fluid intake:* A patient's physical condition affects the frequency with which you monitor fluid intake (see Chapter 15). Regular intake and output (I&O) measurements help to assess a patient's overall fluid balance. Patients who have urinary tract infections and are experiencing urgency, burning, and frequency often mistakenly decrease their fluid intake to try to fix the symptoms.

10. *Age:* Toilet training and enuresis are concerns that arise in the toddler and preschooler. In the adult, increasing age sometimes brings disease and physiological changes that predispose to incontinence.

**PATIENT EXPECTATIONS.** Note the patient's responses to questions about urination. Does the patient seem hesitant or embarrassed? Psychosocial factors such as culture or sexuality sometimes influence the patient's response. In addition, ask the patient what he or she expects from care. Does the patient expect the infection to be resolved? Does the woman who has stress incontinence expect this condition to be relieved?

Because urination is often considered a private matter, some patients find it difficult to talk about their voiding habits. Postoperative patients or patients taking medications that affect urination become concerned that something is wrong when you ask them every couple of hours if they have voided. Also, patients receiving intravenous (IV) fluids do not always realize that they have an increased need for urination. Urinary catheters indicate to some that the patient is very ill; they do not know that urinary catheters are used for diagnosis and monitoring for a variety of patients.

**PHYSICAL ASSESSMENT**

**Skin and Mucosa.** Assess the skin's hydration status by noting texture and turgor. Observe the skin around periurethral tissues and stomas for excoriation, drainage, and tenderness. Urinary incontinence, fluid imbalance, and electrolyte disturbances increase the risk for skin breakdown. Observation of the oral mucosa also reveals whether hydration is adequate.

**Kidneys.** If the kidneys become infected or inflamed, flank pain typically develops. You assess for tenderness early in the disease by gently percussing the costovertebral angle (the angle formed by the spine and twelfth rib). Inflammation of the kidney results in pain on percussion.

**Bladder.** Normally the bladder rests below the symphysis pubis and you are unable to palpate it. When distended, the bladder rises above the symphysis pubis at the midline of the abdomen and just below the umbilicus. Then, when you apply light pressure to the bladder, the patient feels tenderness or even pain. Palpation also causes the urge to urinate.

**Urethral Meatus.** The female patient assumes a dorsal recumbent position to provide full exposure of the genitalia. Using the gloved nondominant hand, retract the labial folds to observe the urethral meatus. Look for drainage and lesions, and ask the patient if there is discomfort. There is normally no discharge from the meatus. Drainage indicates infection. Be sure you note the color and consistency of drainage.

The male's urethral meatus is normally a small opening at the tip of the penis. To inspect the meatus for discharge, lesions, and inflammation, it is necessary for you to retract the foreskin in uncircumcised males. Following inspection of the meatus, return foreskin over the meatus.

**Assessment of Urine.** The assessment of urine involves measuring the patient's fluid intake and urinary output and observing the characteristics of the urine.

*Intake and Output.* When patients have altered or impaired urinary elimination, you measure their I&O to help monitor fluid and electrolyte balance. Although often written as part of a physician's or health care provider's order, placing a patient on I&O is often a nursing judgment. Placing a patient on I&O measurement requires cooperation and assistance from the patient and family. Intake measurements must include all oral liquids and semiliquids; all enteral feedings through nasogastric, gastrostomy, or jejunostomy tubes; and all parenteral fluids such as intravenous solutions, blood components, and parenteral nutrition (see Chapter 15).

You are responsible for accurate recording. Measurements are kept throughout the day and totaled every 8 hours, but sometimes you will decide that you need more frequent measurements. Recording I&O when the patient has voided or eaten is often a task that you delegate. Before delegating this task, inform the care provider what the metric conversions are for common liquid-holding containers such as a coffee cup or milk carton and ensure that the care provider knows aseptic principles relating to body fluids. In addition, caution the care provider to be sensitive to the privacy needs of the patients and clarify what he or she needs to report to you about I&O, such as changes in color, amount, or odor of urine or presence and frequency of incontinence. If the patient needs assistance, inform the care provider about the amount of assistance the patient requires. Also inform the care provider if the patient needs to use a urinal or bedpan or if the patient has bathroom privileges.

Urinary output is a key indicator of kidney function. A change in urine volume is a significant indicator of fluid imbalance, kidney dysfunction, or decreased blood volume. For example, in a catheterized postoperative patient, hourly urinary output provides an indirect measure of circulating blood volume. If the urinary output falls below 30 ml/hour, notify the physician or health care provider and assess for other signs of blood loss.

Assess urine volume by measuring with a **graduated measuring container** (receptacle for volume measurement) the output collected in a bedpan, urinal, **urine hat** (a receptacle that fits inside the commode) (Figure 32-3), or catheter bag. It is critical that each patient have an individual measuring container with name and room number marked on it and that you use only one graduate for each patient. Transmission of microorganisms occurs when you use equipment that belongs to other patients.

Special **urometers** attach to catheter drainage tubing and are a convenient means of measuring small urine volume on a regular basis (Figure 32-4). A urometer holds 100 to 200 ml of urine. After measuring urine from a urometer, drain the cylinder into the urinary drainage bag or into a receptacle for disposal.

If you need a precise measurement of fluid intake from a patient who is at home, you need to ask the patient to show a commonly used glass or cup on which the intake estimate is based.

*Characteristics.* Inspect the patient's urine for color, clarity, and odor. Monitor and document any changes. You

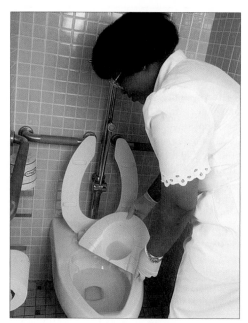

FIGURE **32-3** Urine hat.

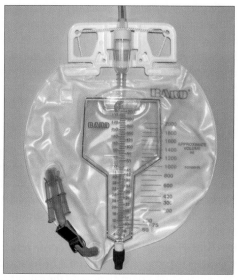

FIGURE **32-4** Urometer. (Courtesy Michael Gallager, RN, BSN, MSN, OSF Saint Francis Medical Center, Peoria, Ill.)

monitor and record unusual characteristics, such as sediment in the urine, for improvement.

*COLOR.* Normal urine ranges in color from a pale straw color to amber, depending on its concentration. Urine is usually more concentrated in the morning. As the person drinks more fluids, it becomes less concentrated.

Unexpected changes such as the appearance of blood in the urine (**hematuria**) alert you to assess for associated signs and symptoms and report the information to the physician or health care provider. Bleeding from the kidneys or ureters usually causes urine to become dark red; bleeding from the bladder or urethra usually causes bright red urine.

Drugs also change the urine's color. For example, patients taking metronidazole or docusate sodium will notice a darkening of their urine to a reddish brown. Beets, rhubarb, and blackberries cause red urine. The kidneys excrete special dyes used in intravenous diagnostic studies, and this discolors the urine. Dark amber urine is the result of high concentrations of bilirubin (urobilinogen) in patients with liver disease. Report unexpected color changes to the physician or health care provider.

*CLARITY.* Normal urine appears transparent at the time of voiding. Urine that stands several minutes in a container becomes cloudy. In patients with renal disease, freshly voided urine appears cloudy because of protein concentration. Urine also appears thick and cloudy as a result of bacteria.

*ODOR.* Urine has a characteristic ammonia odor. The more concentrated the urine, the stronger the odor. As urine remains standing (e.g., in a collection device), more ammonia breakdown occurs, and the odor becomes stronger.

**LABORATORY AND DIAGNOSTIC TESTING.** You are responsible for collecting urine specimens for laboratory testing. The type of test determines the method of collection. Label all specimens with the patient's name, date, and time of collection. Table 32-5 lists routine urinary analysis values and specific nursing interpretations for each type of measurement.

**Specimen Collection.** You will sometimes collect several types of urine specimens for testing. Always collect specimens in appropriate containers, at the correct time, and in the correct manner. Also, you need to properly label all specimens with the patient's identification and complete the laboratory requisition with the necessary information. Urine specimens need to reach the laboratory within 1 hour of collection or be refrigerated. Urine that stands in a container at room temperature will grow bacteria.

*Urinalysis Sample.* A simple urinalysis does not require a sterile urine specimen, or sample. The laboratory performs urinalysis on a routine or clean-voided specimen or on a specimen obtained from a catheter. The urinalysis is a screening test for renal disease, metabolic disorders, lower urinary tract alterations, and fluid imbalances (see Table 32-5). For a quick screening, you perform certain portions of the urinalysis with special reagent strips. Dip the strip into the urine, and watch for a color change, which indicates the presence of protein, blood, sugar, ketones, and other solutes. You will also perform a specific gravity test in the clinic or hospital unit.

The patient voids into a clean urine cup, a urinal, or a bedpan. The patient needs to void before defecating so feces do not contaminate the specimen. If a woman is menstruating, make note of this on the specimen requisition in case red blood cells appear. Transfer the urine to the proper container, and send it to the laboratory. Do not allow a specimen to sit unrefrigerated.

*Clean-Voided or Midstream Specimen.* To obtain a specimen relatively free of the microorganisms growing in the lower urethra, you need to instruct the patient on the method for obtaining a clean-voided specimen. Give pa-

| TABLE 32-5 | Routine Urinalysis Values |
|---|---|
| **Measurement (Normal Value)** | **Interpretation** |
| pH (4.6 to 8.0) | pH level helps to indicate acid-base balance. Urine that stands for several hours becomes alkaline from bacterial growth. |
| Protein (up to 8 mg/100 ml) | Protein is normally not present in urine. It is seen in renal disease because damage to glomerular membrane allows protein to enter urine. However, temporary presence of protein occurs after strenuous exercise, exposure to cold, or psychological stress. |
| Glucose (not normally present) | Diabetic patients have glucose in urine because of inability of tubules to reabsorb high serum glucose concentrations (over 180 mg/100 ml). Ingestion of high concentrations of glucose causes some to appear in urine of healthy persons. |
| Ketones (not normally present) | With poor control of diabetes, patients experience breakdown of fatty acids. End product of fatty acid metabolism is ketones. Patients with dehydration, starvation, or excessive aspirin ingestion also have ketonuria. |
| Blood (up to two red blood cells) | Damage to glomerulus or tubules causes blood cells to enter urine. Trauma or disease of lower urinary tract also causes hematuria. |
| Specific gravity (1.01 to 1.03) | Specific gravity tests measure concentration of particles in urine. High specific gravity reflects concentrated urine, and low specific gravity reflects diluted urine. Dehydration, reduced renal blood flow, and increase in ADH secretion elevate specific gravity. Overhydration and inadequate ADH secretion reduce it. |

tients a sterile urine cup, sterile disinfectant wipes, and clean gloves. The cup and disinfectant wipes are often prepackaged together. The package usually contains instructions, but instruct the patient in how to wash and how to collect the specimen. Anxiety, difficulty or inability to read, or language barriers will prevent the patient from fully comprehending the instructions independently.

Instruct female patients to use the disinfectant wipes to clean from the meatus toward the rectum. Instruct men to clean the meatus in a circular motion moving from the center of the meatus to the outside. Caution the patient against wiping repeatedly with the contaminated cloth. The patient then opens a sterile urine cup. Tell your patient to start and discard the initial stream into a toilet or bedpan. This cleans or flushes the urethral orifice and meatus of resident bacteria. During the midstream, or middle portion of voiding, collect the specimen. Immediately after obtaining the specimen, place a sterile top securely over the container and send it to the laboratory for testing.

*Sterile Specimen.* Another method for collecting a sterile urine specimen for culture is by catheterizing a patient or by obtaining the specimen from an existing indwelling catheter. Do not collect urine specimens for culture from urine drainage bags unless it is the first urine drained into a new sterile bag. Bacteria grow rapidly in drainage bags, giving the specimen a false measurement of bacteria.

During catheterization collect the specimen as soon as urine flows from the catheter's end. After filling the sample container, you withdraw the straight catheter or connect the newly inserted indwelling catheter to a drainage tube (Skill 32-1).

If a patient already has an indwelling catheter, use a sterile syringe to withdraw urine. Most urine drainage tubes have special ports referred to as sampling ports to withdraw specimens. Some companies have catheters with a sampling port that ac-

cepts most plastic or blunt cannulas (needleless) to reduce the risk of needle stick. Read the manufacturer's instructions to determine if the catheter tubing in use accepts blunt cannulas.

First, clamp the tubing about 3 inches below the sampling port, allowing fresh sterile urine to collect in the tube. Then wipe the port with a disinfectant swab. Using the agency-recommended procedure, withdraw 3 ml for a culture. While aspirating urine, be careful not to raise the tubing, which causes urine to return (backflow) to the bladder.

After obtaining the specimen, transfer the urine into a sterile container using sterile aseptic technique, and place it in a plastic pouch or bag per agency policy for transportation to the laboratory. The laboratory requisition will indicate the way you collected the specimen. Inspect the site from which you obtained the specimen periodically to check that the catheter is not leaking.

*Twenty-Four-Hour Urine Specimen.* Some tests of renal function and urine composition require a 24-hour collection of urine. You indicate the starting time on the gallon container and on the laboratory requisition. **Always discard the first sample.** The 24-hour collection period begins after you throw away the first specimen. The patient then collects all urine voided in 24 hours. Any missed specimens make the results inaccurate and require you to restart the test. You remind the patient to void before defecating so feces do not contaminate urine. If there is fecal contamination, consult the laboratory for instructions. The patient needs to void the last specimen as close as possible to the end of the 24-hour period.

*Common Urine Tests.* In addition to urinalysis, other tests that you will perform are measurement of specific gravity, urine culture, and glucose and ketone levels. Your role in collecting specimens is that of teaching. You explain the purpose of all tests, identify what preparation (if any) the patient needs before the test, what you expect of the patient during the test, and any posttest care.

SPECIFIC GRAVITY. To measure specific gravity use a urinometer and cylinder. The urinometer has a specific gravity scale at the top and a weighted mercury bulb at the bottom. Pour a urine specimen into a clean dry cylinder, and suspend the weighted urinometer in it. The concentration of dissolved substances in the urine determines the depth at which the urinometer will float. The point the level of urine reaches on the urinometer scale is the specific gravity measurement.

URINE CULTURE. A urine culture simply requires a sterile sample of urine. It takes approximately 72 hours before the laboratory is able to report significant findings of bacterial growth. If bacteria are present, an additional test for sensitivity determines the antibiotics that will be effective or ineffective.

**Diagnostic Examinations.** The urinary system is one of the few organ systems accessible to accurate diagnostic study by radiographic techniques. The two approaches for visualizing urinary structures, namely direct and indirect techniques, are either quite simple or very complex, requiring extensive nursing interventions. These procedures are further subdivided into invasive and noninvasive categories.

### Noninvasive Procedures

ABDOMINAL ROENTGENOGRAM. An abdominal roentgenogram, also referred to as a plain film, KUB, or flat plate of the abdomen, assesses the gross structures of the urinary tract for abnormalities. Physicians or health care providers use the x-ray film to determine the size, shape, and location of the kidneys, ureters, and bladder structures. It is also useful in visualizing calculi (stones) or tumors in these organs.

INTRAVENOUS PYELOGRAM. The physician or health care provider performs an excretory urogram or intravenous pyelogram (IVP) to view the entire urinary system and to assess some renal functions. Although these procedures are noninvasive, the IVP does require that the patient receive an intravenous injection of a radiopaque dye. Because the kidneys and ureters lie behind the intestines, it is necessary that the patient receive a bowel preparation before the procedure.

Nursing implications before the test include recognizing patients at risk for complications caused by the contrast material. The contrast material becomes toxic to the kidney tissue if the patient is dehydrated. Any patient with preexisting renal insufficiency is at risk. Older adults in particular are prone to problems because of their risk for volume depletion during bowel preparation. It is important to appropriately assess fluid volume status before this procedure (see Chapter 15).

Additional nursing implications before the test are as follows:

1. Assess the patient for allergy: intravenous contrast materials; shellfish or iodine allergy, which sometimes predicts allergies to the IVP dye.
2. If ordered, have the patient complete bowel preparation the evening before the test.
3. Explain that the patient is allowed nothing by mouth (NPO) after midnight.

4. Explain that you start an intravenous infusion for dye injection before the test.
5. Explain that facial flushing is normal during dye injection and that the patient may feel dizzy, warm, or nauseous.
6. Explain that the test involves x-ray studies taken at several intervals and that the patient will void near the end of the test.

Nursing implications after the test are as follows:

1. Ensure that the patient resumes a normal diet.
2. Encourage fluid intake to minimize dehydration caused by fasting and to avoid the potential nephrotoxic effects of the contrast material.
3. Remind the patient to report itching, rash, or hives, which indicate delayed hypersensitivity to IVP dye.
4. Monitor I&O, or explain to the patient to report decreased or absent urination.

RENAL SCAN. Renal scans allow indirect visualization of urinary tract structures after an intravenous injection of radioactive isotopes. Except for the venipuncture, the procedure is painless. The scanning procedure takes approximately 1 hour. You obtain information about renal blood flow, anatomical structures, and their excretory function from this procedure. This procedure is used for patients who are unable to receive IVP dyes.

Nursing implications before the test include the following:

1. Explain that the radiologist will inject the radioisotope intravenously through an existing IV line or needle.
2. Explain that the patient will feel no discomfort but needs to lie still.
3. Explain that there is no risk of radioactive exposure.

COMPUTERIZED AXIAL TOMOGRAPHY. Computerized axial tomography is used to visualize abnormal pathological conditions such as tumors, obstructions, retroperitoneal masses, and lymph node enlargement. The computer allows enhancement of the x-ray to show "slices" of the body part. Although this procedure is noninvasive, in some examinations oral and/or intravenous contrast material is used to enhance the areas under study.

RENAL ULTRASOUND. Ultrasonography is a painless, noninvasive diagnostic tool in the assessment of urinary disorders. Sound waves are bounced off the underlying body structures, and the resulting picture is used to identify gross renal anatomy and structural abnormalities of the kidneys or lower urinary tract.

### Invasive Procedures

ENDOSCOPY. Endoscopy is the visualization of organs with the aid of a telescope or fiber-optic imaging. To view the interior of the bladder and urethra, the physician or health care provider performs a cystoscopy. The cytoscope looks like a urinary catheter, although it is not as flexible. It is inserted through the urethra. The procedure is painful during instrument insertion. Unless the patient lies still, the bladder may be perforated. Cystoscopy is performed under general or local anesthesia with sedation. A patient's age, general health, and expected duration of the procedure affect the choice of anesthesia. Because the test requires insertion of a foreign object into a sterile cavity, the patient receives large amounts of fluids (intravenously or orally) before and during the procedure to maintain a continuous urine flow and to flush out bacteria. Antibiotics are often administered intravenously. During the test, some urine and tissue specimens are collected.

Nursing implications before the test include the following:

1. Verify that the patient signed an informed consent form.
2. Perform a bowel preparation or enema, or administer a cathartic on the evening before the test.
3. If local anesthetic will be used, encourage intake of oral fluids.
4. If general anesthetic will be used, ensure that the patient is NPO after midnight.
5. Because this procedure is considered a minor surgical procedure, you will need to complete a preoperative checklist in some cases (see Chapter 37).
6. Explain that insertion of the cystoscope is similar to insertion of a urethral catheter.
7. Explain the importance of lying still during the test, if local anesthesia is used.
8. Explain that an intravenous line will be started to give fluids during the test.
9. Administer a sedative or analgesic per the physician's or health care provider's orders.

Nursing implications after the test include the following:

1. Instruct the patient to remain in bed as ordered.
2. Assess for signs of urinary retention and first voiding.
3. Observe characteristics of urine, noting bloody or cloudy urine.
4. Encourage increased fluid intake, and monitor I&O.
5. Observe for fever, dysuria, or a change in blood pressure.
6. Administer medications to calm bladder spasms and/or lower back pain.

In addition to complete visual inspection of the bladder and urethra through the cystoscope, the radiologist sometimes performs a retrograde pyelography. During this procedure the radiologist passes a small catheter through the cystoscope into the bladder that allows catheterizing of the ureters and renal pelvis. Urine specimens are then collected separately from each ureter. Radiopaque dye is instilled into the renal pelvis while taking serial x-ray films to examine the filling of the renal collecting system.

Invasive examinations to visualize the bladder and urethra include retrograde cystograms, voiding cystourethrogram, and cystourethrogram. All of these studies involve the instillation of a radiopaque fluid into the bladder via a catheter (urethral or suprapubic). Serial x-ray films taken during this procedure will provide information regarding

## SYNTHESIS IN PRACTICE

As Phyllis prepares to assess Mrs. Vallero again, she remembers that urinary problems are common in older adults but that age alone does not cause incontinence. She recalls that patients with urinary retention sometimes leak urine and are therefore misdiagnosed as incontinent. She knows patients generally void at least every 6 to 8 hours and that Mrs. Vallero's recent catheterization and her decreased mobility since hospitalization make her more prone to urinary retention or incontinence. In addition, she knows she will need to assess if Mrs. Vallero feels the urge to urinate. She determines that no one has taken Mrs. Vallero to the bathroom recently. Phyllis also needs to find out more about her patient's urination patterns at home.

Previous clinical experience has taught Phyllis that palpation of the abdomen over a distended bladder causes some discomfort. Mrs. Vallero grimaces slightly when her abdomen is palpated and says she's only got a little *dolor* (pain).

Because congestive heart failure and bed rest have left Mrs. Vallero in a weakened state, Phyllis is flexible and creative in designing a plan of care to meet the patient's elimination needs. This plan needs to incorporate scheduled voiding, oral fluids, and increased physical activity.

abnormalities. Nursing implications for this procedure are the same as those for the cystoscopy procedure.

*ARTERIOGRAM (ANGIOGRAM).* The renal angiogram is an invasive radiographic procedure with radiopaque contrast material that outlines the vascular supply to the kidneys. Most frequently this procedure evaluates the arterial system; however, techniques to investigate the venous system (venogram) are available. Pretest nursing implications are similar to those for the IVP except in some cases you will need a signed consent form. Patients are often given a narcotic or antianxiety agent for relaxation before the examination.

Nursing implications after the angiogram include the following:

1. Monitor the patient's vital signs hourly until you verify the patient is stable, and then advance the intervals to every 2 hours, then every 4 hours.
2. Ensure that the patient maintains bed rest for 4 to 8 hours.
3. Check pulses and assess circulation in the extremity used.
4. Observe for bleeding, increased tenderness, or hematoma formation at the catheter insertion site for 24 hours.
5. Maintain a pressure dressing over the site for 24 hours.
6. Observe the patient for possible delayed allergic reactions to the contrast material.
7. Monitor the patient's I&O, and report abnormalities in urine volume to the physician or health care provider.

*URODYNAMIC TESTING.* Urodynamic testing is a group of tests that measure transport, elimination, and storage of urine in the lower urinary tract. The tests do not cause much pain, but they do require catheterization. A contraindication to testing is a urinary tract infection. Care after the procedures includes teaching the patient the signs and symptoms of infection and to report to the physician or health care provider if any of those signs and symptoms appears.

### Nursing Diagnosis

Thorough assessment of the patient's urinary function identifies defining characteristics that support actual or at-risk elimination problems. Identification of the defining characteristics leads you to select an appropriate NANDA International nursing diagnostic label. It is very helpful to read the definition of the diagnosis and to examine whether there is a match between the data you collected and the defining characteristics (see Chapter 7).

For example, there are five recognized diagnoses for incontinence, and it is not easy for a beginning student to make a decision without looking for a match between data and defining characteristics. The differentiation between stress and urge incontinence is a common problem. In both, the patient has an involuntary loss of urine, but the accuracy of data collection helps to identify the correct diagnosis. If the patient loses urine after sneezing or coughing, then the diagnosis is stress incontinence. If the patient reports that there was a strong urge to urinate just before the incontinence occurred, then the diagnosis is urge incontinence. Other nursing diagnoses are appropriate when the urinary problem affects other patient functions. A selected list of possible nursing diagnoses include:

- Disturbed body image
- Functional urinary incontinence
- Reflex urinary incontinence
- Stress urinary incontinence
- Total urinary incontinence
- Urge urinary incontinence
- Risk for infection
- Deficient knowledge
- Toileting self-care deficit
- Impaired skin integrity
- Impaired urinary elimination
- Urinary retention

Associated problems require interventions that often have no direct effect on urinary elimination. For example, when the patient has the diagnosis *toileting self-care deficit related to limited lower extremity mobility,* appropriate nursing interventions provide the patient a means of easy access to toileting facilities. Selection of an appropriate related factor ensures that you select the relevant interventions. If you identify the related factor in the example as a loss of voluntary control of micturition, you would select interventions to prevent incontinence. It is important to identify the correct related factors for a given nursing diagnosis; otherwise, your nursing interventions will be ineffective.

### Planning

**GOALS AND OUTCOMES.** Establish patient-centered goals and outcomes in collaboration with the patient and family. For example, a realistic patient goal is that the pa-

tient has normal micturition with complete bladder emptying within 1 month. To achieve this goal you identify a number of outcomes; for example, the patient will ingest at least 2000 ml of fluids per day, empty the bladder within 2 hours of drinking, and have less than 50 ml of residual urine. Problems develop when you make goals and outcomes without adequate assessment and collaboration with the patient.

You and the patient work together to maintain patient involvement in care and to maintain normal elimination patterns when possible (see care plan). If you reinforce good health habits that the patient already follows, the patient will be more likely to comply with the plan of care. Determine the patient's educational needs. Return demonstrations of psychomotor and self-care skills by the patient verify learning of procedures and accuracy in their performance.

**SETTING PRIORITIES.** It is important to establish priorities of care based on the patient's immediate physical and safety needs, patient expectations, and readiness to perform some self-care activities. For example, a patient with a long-term continent urinary diversion admitted with a severe urinary tract infection expects to resume his or her self-care routine. However, due to the severity of the infection, you perform all care for the patient's urinary diversion with sterile technique. In this case the priorities are to treat the infection, prevent reinfection, and teach the patient how to perform sterile techniques.

**CONTINUITY OF CARE.** In the hospital, planning for care also includes preparations for discharge. You need to explore the need for home care services and make appropriate referrals. Planning includes consideration of the patient's home environment and normal elimination routines. Determine if there is a need to collaborate with other disciplines in this planning process (e.g., social services) to explore family financial resources or other influences that may affect the discharge process. Use community resources as well, such as ostomy support groups for patients with incontinent diversions.

Significant others are also included in discharge planning and in teaching sessions. Identify who will be involved with the care of the patient at home. Your active and thoughtful role in planning these interventions will result in the patient's progress toward improved urinary elimination.

### Implementation

Your care of patients with elimination alterations is focused in three general areas: health promotion, acute care, and restorative and continuing care. The specific interventions include patient education, promoting normal micturition and complete bladder emptying, prevention of infection, skin integrity, and comfort. As part of their education, patients need to know the basic mechanisms for urine production and voiding.

**HEALTH PROMOTION.** Success of therapies aimed at optimizing normal urinary elimination depends in part on successful patient education (Box 32-3). Instruct patients about their specific elimination problems. For example, a

# CARE PLAN  Urinary Retention

### ASSESSMENT

Mrs. Vallero was **unable to void 6 hours after catheter removal.** She was catheterized at that time and 700 ml of urine obtained. It is now 4 hours since the catheterization. She has been drinking fluids, including hot tea and tomato juice, to increase her chances of urinating on her own. She now complains of **dribbling** and being unable to urinate even though **she feels the urge.** She was also **incontinent** on the last shift of a **small amount of urine several times.** She complains of a feeling of pressure over her lower abdomen. The nursing assessment reveals a **distended bladder.**

*Defining characteristics are shown in bold type.

---

### NURSING DIAGNOSIS Urinary retention related to detrusor inadequacy secondary to catheterization.

---

### PLANNING

| GOAL | EXPECTED OUTCOMES* |
|---|---|
| | **Urinary Continence** |
| • Patient will have normal micturition with complete bladder emptying in 1 month | • Patient will void greater than 150 ml each time.<br>• Patient will empty bladder completely.<br>• Patient will be free of irritative symptoms. |

*Outcomes classification label from Moorhead S, Johnson M, Maas M: *Nursing outcomes classification (NOC),* ed 3, St. Louis, 2004, Mosby.

---

### INTERVENTIONS†

**URINARY RETENTION CARE**

• Provide privacy for elimination.

• Use the power of suggestion by running water or flushing the toilet.

• Use double voiding technique—have patient void and then rest on the toilet for 3 to 5 minutes before voiding again.

### RATIONALE

Urination is generally a private matter, and the presence of another person may prevent relaxation of the urinary sphincter. The sound of running water often causes the urge to void.

Double voiding promotes more efficient bladder emptying by allowing detrusor muscle to contract, rest, and contract again (Gray, 2000).

†Intervention classification labels from Dochterman JM, Bulechek GM, editors: *Nursing interventions classification (NIC),* ed 4, St. Louis, 2004, Mosby.

---

### EVALUATION

• Ask Mrs. Vallero about her urge to void, sensation of bladder fullness, and dribbling episodes.

• Have Mrs. Vallero report her pattern of urinary elimination, including dribbling (if any), nocturia, and types and volumes of fluid ingested during the 1-month period.

• If interventions are unsuccessful, she will need a referral to a continence specialist.

---

patient who practices poor hygiene will benefit from learning about normal sterility of the urinary tract and ways to prevent bacterial invasion of the urinary tract. It is also useful to discuss the basic mechanism for urine production and voiding for patients with elimination alterations. Knowledge of factors that promote normal urine production and voiding will also help. Health promotion skills are always the initial focal point of teaching.

It will be easy for you to incorporate teaching during delivery of care (Box 32-4). For example, if you are attempting to increase the patient's fluid intake, a good time to discuss benefits is while giving fluids with medications or meals. You will possibly be more successful in teaching about perineal hygiene during a bath or while giving catheter care. When possible, include family members in these discussions.

### Normal Micturition

*Stimulating the Micturition Reflex.* The patient's ability to void depends on feeling the urge to urinate, on being able to control the urethral sphincter, and on being able to relax.

You promote relaxation and stimulate the reflex to void by helping patients to assume the normal position for voiding.

Females are better able to void in a squatting position. This position promotes contraction of the pelvic and intraabdominal muscles that assist in sphincter control and bladder contraction. If the patient cannot use a toilet, position her on a bedpan or bedside commode (see Chapter 33).

The male patient voids more easily in the standing position. At times it is necessary for one or more nurses to assist the male patient to stand. If the patient is unable to reach a toilet, have him stand at the bedside and void into a **urinal** (a plastic or metal receptacle for urine) (Figure 32-5). Always determine mobility status before having a patient stand to void.

If the patient is unable to stand at the bedside, you will need to assist him to use the urinal in bed. When possible, the patient holds the urinal and positions the penis in the urinal. If the patient needs assistance, position the penis completely within the urinal and hold the urinal in place or

---

**BOX 32-3** | **Urinary Elimination Health Promotion/Restoration Activities**

### Adequate Hydration

A patient with normal renal function who does not have heart disease or alterations requiring fluid restriction should drink six to eight glasses of fluid daily (Huether and McCance, 2004).

### Micturition Habits

Ensure patient comfort and privacy.

Allow sufficient time to void (at least 15 minutes).

Integrating the patient's habits into the care plan fosters a more normal voiding pattern.

Offer the patient use of toilet facilities if possible, avoiding bedpans.

Ensure access to toilet facilities.

Assist the patient in the appropriate position for voiding (i.e., females—sitting, males—standing).

### Personal Hygiene

Instruct female patients to cleanse the perineum and urethra from front to back after each voiding and bowel movement.

Encourage patients prone to urinary tract infections to shower instead of bathing.

### Complete Bladder Emptying

Patients who have difficulty starting or stopping the urine stream benefit from exercises to strengthen pelvic muscles (Milne, 2004).

Credé's method of manual bladder compression helps to stimulate urination and manually expels urine when bladder tone is reduced.

Drug therapy alone or in conjunction with other therapies is useful for treating problems of incontinence and retention (Thompson and Smith, 2002).

### Infection Prevention

Ensure adequate fluid intake.

Encourage good hand washing.

Prevent breaks in closed catheter drainage systems.

Follow tips for preventing infection in catheterized patients.

Teach patient how to keep urine acidic. Acid urine tends to inhibit growth of microorganisms. Meats, eggs, whole-grain breads, cranberries, and prunes increase urine acidity (Gray, 2002).

### Skin Integrity

The skin is the first barrier of defense.

The normal acidity of urine is irritating to the skin.

Washing with mild soap and warm water is the best way to remove urine from the skin.

After performing hygiene, apply dry clothing immediately on incontinent patient.

Patients with external urinary devices need to receive assistance in selecting appliances that fit appropriately. Also, teach them preventive skin care measures.

---

**BOX 32-4** | PATIENT TEACHING

Mrs. Vallero is concerned about regaining her urinary function. Phyllis develops the following teaching plan for her:

### Outcome

At the end of the teaching session Mrs. Vallero will be able to tell Phyllis the activities that she will do to help in her own recovery.

### Teaching Strategies

- Establish rapport with Mrs. Vallero.
- Find out what Mrs. Vallero already knows about good practices for urinary health.
- Use the correct terms for the anatomy that you will discuss, but explain them so Mrs. Vallero knows what they are.
- Provide appropriate visual diagrams and written materials for Mrs. Vallero.
- Instruct her about observations to make regarding urinary output.

- Instruct her about adequate fluid intake, incorporating her fluid preferences.
- Discuss how to do intake and output measurement at home.
- Reinforce correct perineal hygiene measures to reduce the risk of urinary tract infection.
- Provide Mrs. Vallero with pertinent signs and symptoms of infection to report to her physician or health care provider.

### Evaluation Strategies

- Use open-ended questions to determine level of learning.
- Ask Mrs. Vallero to verbalize her understanding of normal urinary function.
- Ask Mrs. Vallero to verbalize the abnormal signs and symptoms to report to her physician or health care provider.
- Have Mrs. Vallero measure water in a container to simulate intake and output measures.

---

assist the patient in holding the urinal. Make sure you place the penis completely within the urinal to avoid urine spills.

Once the patient has finished voiding, remove the urinal and wash and dry the penis to prevent growth of microorganisms and to aid in preventing skin breakdown.

Other measures to promote normal micturition include the use of sensory stimuli (e.g., turning on running water, putting a patient's hand in a pan of warm water, or stroking the female patient's inner thigh). Each tends to promote relaxation and the reflex to void.

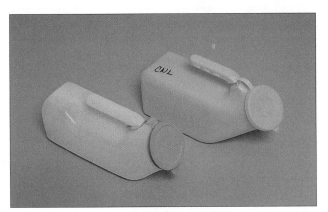

FIGURE **32-5** Types of male urinals.

***Maintaining Elimination Habits.*** Many patients follow set routines of normal voiding. In a hospital or long-term care facility, routines often conflict with those of the patient. Integrating the patient's habits into the care plan fosters a more normal voiding pattern.

Make sure you give the patient privacy, and do not rush him or her. Privacy is essential for normal voiding. If the patient is unable to reach the bathroom, make sure the bedside area is private. In the home, some debilitated patients may prefer using a bedside commode enclosed behind a partition or room divider. Some patients are embarrassed by the sound of voiding. Running water or flushing the toilet masks the sound effectively. Young children are often unable to void in the presence of persons other than parents.

Assess the times when a patient normally voids, and offer the opportunity to use a toilet at those times. Respond in a timely manner to the patient's urge to urinate. Delay in assisting the patient to the bathroom may interfere with normal micturition. Research has shown that promptly assisting patients to toileting facilities reduces incontinence when the patients were able to perceive the urge to void (Palmer and Newman, 2004). Older adults may also require other special interventions owing to the aging process (Box 32-5).

Comfort is an important factor in facilitating voiding. Therefore activities that increase patient comfort will aid urination. If the patient typically uses special measures to void (e.g., reading or listening to music), encourage continued use at home and, when possible, in the health care setting. Use toilet seat extenders for patients with arthritis or after a total hip replacement to aid the patient in sitting and in rising off the toilet.

Encourage and provide appropriate personal hygiene, including hand washing and perineal care (see Chapter 27) as needed. Nosocomial genitourinary infections are second only to respiratory infections (see Chapter 11). Bacteria are the most common cause of these infections, and *E. coli* invasion through the urethra is the most frequent organism and route (O'Donnell and Hofman, 2002).

***Maintaining Adequate Fluid Intake.*** A simple method of promoting normal micturition is maintenance of a good

---

**BOX 32-5** CARE OF THE OLDER ADULT

- The older patient sometimes experiences urinary elimination problems as a result of mobility problems or neurological impairments. Be aware of these problems, and arrange scheduled toileting and promote access to toileting facilities.
- Older patients are prone to physiological urinary retention as a result of diminished bladder muscle tone, capacity, and contractility. This increases their risk for large postvoid residuals with an associated risk of frequent infections. Teaching sessions include techniques to stimulate the voiding reflex and to provide for complete bladder emptying and prevention of infections (Wyman, 2003).
- Older patients also experience delayed sensations to void, resulting in urgency. Educate the patient regarding any factor that interferes with the patient's perceptions of sensation to void (e.g., medications, emotional disturbances, decreased fluid intake).
- Older adults experience the following physiological changes that make them more prone to incontinence. During teaching sessions, consider these normal physiological changes to plan appropriate interventions:
  ○ Decreased renal blood flow secondary to decreased cardiac output (*make sure patient takes ordered medications that increase cardiac output, such as digoxin and diuretics*)
  ○ Decreased ability to concentrate urine secondary to decrease in nephron mass (*unless patient is fluid restricted, ensure adequate intake to prevent dehydration*)
  ○ Decreased tone of the pelvic floor muscles (Huether and McCance, 2004) (*encourage strengthening of pelvic floor muscles by teaching Kegel exercises*)
- Older adults in institutionalized settings (e.g., hospitals, nursing homes) are at the greatest risk for experiencing incontinence problems because of sensory and physical mobility losses (Lekan-Rutledge and Colling, 2003).
- Older adults also experience sensory alterations, such as diminished vision, which delay attempts to locate toilet facilities. In care settings, orient patients to their environment with special emphasis on the location of toileting facilities, bedpans or urinals, and assistive devices (e.g., walkers, call light).

---

fluid intake. A patient with normal renal function who does not have heart disease or alterations requiring fluid restriction needs to drink six to eight glasses of fluid daily. When a person increases fluid intake, excreted urine flushes out solutes or particles that collect in the urinary system. Because a patient probably is not accustomed to drinking eight glasses of water daily, offer fluids the patient prefers. At home it helps to set a schedule for drinking fluids (e.g., with meals or medications). A simple trick is to encourage the patient to drink a cup of water after voiding. Voiding becomes a natural cue to drinking fluids. The patient will not need a rigid schedule. To prevent nocturia, suggest that the patient avoid drinking fluids 2 hours before bedtime.

**Promotion of Bladder Emptying.** Patients with urinary retention and incontinence are frequently unable to empty

**TABLE 32-6** | Treatment Options for Incontinence

| Type | Treatments to Attain Continence |
|---|---|
| Functional | Toileting programs/bladder training |
| | Environmental alterations |
| Stress | Conditioning (Kegel) exercises |
| | Estrogen replacement |
| | Alpha-adrenergic agonists |
| | Intravaginal electrical stimulation |
| | Bladder neck suspension surgery |
| | Artificial sphincter |
| | Penile clamp |
| Urge | Anticholinergic drug therapy |
| | Biofeedback |
| | Treatment of associated urinary tract infection |
| | Treatment of associated vaginitis |
| | Diet modification to minimize bladder irritants |
| Reflex (upper motoneuron lesion) | Intermittent self-catheterization |
| | Bladder training |
| | Electrical stimulation |
| | Credés's method |

the bladder. Incontinence is a major nursing challenge. Choosing from a variety of treatment options, you and the patient will work together to design interventions that promote continence (Table 32-6). The use of indwelling catheters is a last resort because infection is always a threat. Encourage use of protective absorbent materials to control wetness when other treatments fail, but do not recommend these instead of treatment (Thompson and Smith, 2002).

***Strengthening Pelvic Floor Muscles.*** Patients who have difficulty starting and stopping the urine stream benefit from exercises to strengthen pelvic muscles (Sampselle, 2003). This technique is helpful for both men and women with urinary problems. The patient is able to practice the Kegel exercises anytime and anywhere. No one will be aware that the patient is doing this exercise. Simple steps will show gradual improvement in urinary control. The patient follows these instructions:

1. Squeeze and hold the muscles around the vagina and /or anus for 10 seconds without tensing leg, buttock, or abdominal muscles. Then relax the muscles for 10 seconds. This maneuver allows the patient to identify the posterior muscles of the pelvic floor.
2. Do this exercise 15 times in the morning; 15 times in the afternoon, and 20 times at night. Work up to 25 times each time period. If done consistently the patient will see improvement in urinary control (Wyman, 2003).

***Manual Bladder Compression.*** By manually compressing the walls of the bladder, a person improves bladder emptying. Credé's method helps to stimulate micturition and manually expels urine when bladder tone is reduced. Instruct the patient to place both hands flat on the abdomen below the umbilicus and above the symphysis pubis with the fingers pointed down toward the bladder's dome. The patient compresses the hands downward against the bladder's walls while tightening the perineum, contracting the abdominal wall, and holding the breath. When urine is in the bladder, Credé's compression causes the sensation of bladder fullness. The maneuver also promotes bladder emptying by relaxing the urethral sphincter.

***Drug Therapy.*** Drug therapy alone or along with other therapies is useful for treating problems of incontinence and retention. Drugs are used to increase bladder emptying (e.g., retention), bladder capacity (e.g., urge incontinence), and sphincter tone (e.g., stress incontinence).

When the bladder empties, the detrusor muscle contracts in response to stimulation. Incomplete bladder emptying results from impaired innervation or weakness of the detrusor muscle. As a result, the patient experiences retention and overflow incontinence. Therapy with cholinergic drugs increases bladder contraction and improves emptying. Bethanechol (Urecholine) stimulates nerves to increase bladder wall contraction and relax the sphincter. You administer this drug subcutaneously or orally. Alpha-adrenergic agents such as phenoxybenzamine are also used to improve bladder emptying. Using Credé's method or other measures for stimulating micturition increases the effect of the drug.

If urine is in the bladder, urge incontinence sometimes occurs as a result of hyperactivity of the bladder muscle that suddenly increases pressure. Local irritants such as stones or infection cause uncontrolled bladder contractions. The elimination of caffeine, carbonated drinks, and alcohol is useful in reducing urge incontinence (Thompson and Smith, 2002). Anticholinergic drugs (e.g., propantheline) reduce incontinence by blocking contractility of the bladder. Patients with heart disease, glaucoma, high blood pressure, kidney and liver disease, and urinary retention must use these drugs with caution. Direct smooth-muscle relaxants (e.g., oxybutynin) are also used. These drugs work by decreasing the contractility of the bladder. Patient instructions are similar to those for propantheline (McKenry and Salerno, 2003).

To treat stress incontinence, alpha-adrenergic drugs are often used. Many patients commonly use phenylpropanolamine. This medication along with pelvic strengthening exercises works in some women. Some have used estrogen therapy to decrease stress incontinence (McKenry and Salerno, 2003).

**ACUTE CARE.** Often patients need care in hospitals, clinics, or their homes for urinary conditions of sudden onset. One of the most frequent treatments is urinary catheterization.

**Catheterization. Catheterization** of the bladder involves introducing a rubber or plastic tube through the urethra and into the bladder. The catheter provides a continuous flow of urine in patients unable to control micturition or in patients with obstructions. Because bladder catheterization carries a high risk of urinary tract infection, first try other interventions to empty the bladder. Gray (2004b) has

## BOX 32-6 USING EVIDENCE IN PRACTICE

**Research Summary**

Although urinary catheters are not used as frequently or for as long as in the past, it is important to be aware of the risk for urinary tract infection whenever catheters are used. One researcher studied nursing interventions to discover if those interventions really made a difference in the development of urinary tract infection in persons with indwelling catheters. Infections in a person with a long-term indwelling catheter (longer than 2 weeks) are complicated because they are often caused by multiple or resistant microorganisms.

The researcher did a literature search to find published studies to answer his questions. The findings were startling. The intervention that had the strongest risk reduction was the use of silver-containing catheters. Those catheters were more likely to prevent bacteruria. The maintenance of a sterile, closed drainage system, especially in the short term, was also an important intervention. Over the long term the evidence was not as strong. Contrary to popular opinion, sterile insertion technique did not reduce urinary tract infection risk. The use of special antiseptic solutions to perform catheter/perineal care was less effective than mild soap and water.

**Application to Nursing Practice**

Although most hospital facilities will not abandon the practice of using sterile technique for catheter insertion, it is clear that the type of catheter material and the maintenance of a closed system have a greater effect on risk reduction. Be aware that breaking the closed system to irrigate with any saline or antiseptic solution actually raises the risk of infection. If a catheter is blocked, it is safer to remove it and insert another one. Hand hygiene remains a very important factor in minimizing the spread of catheter-related infection from patient to patient. Perineal care is more effective using mild soap and water than using potentially harmful or ineffective commercial solutions.

Data from Gray M: What nursing interventions reduce the risk of symptomatic urinary tract infection in the patient with an indwelling catheter, *J Wound Ostomy Continence Nurs* 31(1):3, 2004.

reported new evidence regarding factors most likely to contribute to infection from catheterization (Box 32-6).

*Types of Catheterization.* Intermittent catheterizations and indwelling catheterization are the two types of catheter insertion. With the intermittent technique, the patient has a single-use straight catheter introduced for a short period to drain the bladder (5 to 10 minutes). When the bladder is empty, the catheter is removed. Intermittent catheterization is repeated as necessary. An indwelling or Foley catheter remains in place until a patient is able to void completely and voluntarily. It is sometimes necessary to change indwelling catheters periodically.

The single-use straight catheter has a single lumen with a small opening approximately 1.3 cm (½ inch) from the tip. Urine drains from the tip, through the lumen, and to a receptacle. An indwelling Foley catheter has a small inflatable balloon that encircles the catheter just below the tip. When inflated, the balloon rests against the bladder outlet to anchor the catheter in place. The indwelling catheter also has as many as two or three separate lumens within the body of the catheter. One lumen drains urine through the catheter to a collecting tube. A second lumen carries sterile water to and from the balloon when it is inflated or deflated. A third (optional) lumen is used to instill fluids or drugs into the bladder. You insert a three-lumen catheter when you anticipate irrigations of the catheter. Usually you use three-way catheters with male patients who have had a transurethral resection of the prostate.

*Indications for Use.* Intermittent catheterization is preferred for short-term use or to minimize infection in patients who are chronically unable to void. Intermittent catheterization is indicated in the following situations:

1. For immediate relief of acute bladder distention
2. For long-term management of patients with incompetent bladders
3. To obtain a sterile urine specimen
4. To assess for residual urine after voiding
5. To instill a medication

Done correctly, intermittent catheterization has a lower risk of infection than indwelling catheterization. However, if a patient requires frequent intermittent catheterization, an indwelling catheter is preferable. Indwelling catheterization is indicated in the following situations:

1. Obstruction to urine outflow
2. Patients undergoing surgical procedures involving the urinary tract or surrounding structures
3. To prevent urethral obstruction from blood clots
4. To accurately record output in critically ill or comatose patients
5. To prevent skin breakdown in incontinent comatose patients
6. To provide continuous or intermittent bladder irrigations

*Catheter Insertion.* Urethral catheterization requires a physician's or health care provider's order. Insert the catheter using strict sterile technique. The steps for inserting an indwelling and a single-use straight catheter are the same. The difference lies in the procedure taken to inflate the indwelling catheter balloon and secure the catheter. You collect needed specimens while inserting either catheter. Skill 32-1 lists steps for performing female and male urethral catheterization.

*CLOSED DRAINAGE SYSTEMS.* After you insert an indwelling catheter it is necessary to maintain a closed urinary drainage system to minimize the risk of infection. Urinary drainage bags are plastic and hold approximately 2000 ml of urine. The bag hangs on the lower bed frame without touching the floor. Some urinary drainage bags have special urometers between the collection tubing and bag. When the patient ambulates, instruct patient or caregiver to carry the bag below the level of

*Text continued on p. 942*

## SKILL 32-1 ¦ Inserting a Straight or Indwelling Catheter

### Delegation Considerations

Usually you do not delegate this skill to assistive personnel. The use of assistive personnel for inserting urinary catheters occurs in some settings (e.g., emergency department), but it has not become routine practice. However, assistive personnel assist with positioning the patient, focusing lighting for the procedure, and aiding in the patient's comfort during the procedure by measures such as holding the patient's hand or keeping the patient warm.

### Equipment

- Disposable gloves
- Warm water for perineal care
- Cleansing soap or solution
- Waterproof, absorbent pads
- Catheterization kit containing the following sterile items:
  - Gloves (extra pair optional)
  - Drapes, one fenestrated
  - Water-soluble lubricant
  - Antiseptic cleansing solution
  - Cotton balls
  - Forceps
  - Sterile specimen cup

- Prefilled syringe with sterile water to inflate balloon of indwelling catheter
- Catheter of correct size and type for procedure (i.e., intermittent or indwelling) (Figure 32-6)
- Sterile drainage tubing with collection bag and multipurpose tube holder or tape, safety pin, and elastic band for securing tubing to bed if patient is bed-bound (for indwelling catheter)
- Receptacle or basin (usually bottom of catheterization tray)
- Bath blanket

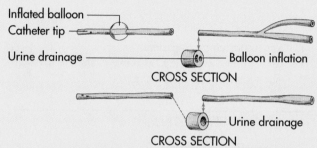

FIGURE **32-6** Indwelling and straight urinary catheters

| STEP | RATIONALE |
| --- | --- |

### ASSESSMENT

**1.** Assess status of patient:
   a. Ask patient time of last urination. Check I&O flow sheet, or palpate the bladder.

   b. Level of awareness or developmental stage.

   c. Mobility and physical limitations of patient.
   d. Patient's gender and age.

   e. Distended bladder.

   f. Perform hand hygiene and put on clean, disposable gloves. Assess perineum for erythema, drainage, and odor.
   g. Assess for any pathological condition that will impair passage of catheter (e.g., enlarged prostate gland in men).
   h. Allergies to antiseptic (e.g., povidone-iodine [Betadine]), tape, latex, lubricant, and shellfish.

**2.** Review patient's medical record, including physician's or health care provider's order, medical history, and nurses' notes. Review data on preparation for surgery, urinary irrigations, collection of sterile urine specimen, or measurement of residual urine.

Bladder fullness may be detected with deep palpation above the symphysis pubis.

Reveals patient's ability to cooperate and level of explanation needed.

Will determine how you position the patient.

Determines catheter size: 8 to 10 Fr for children, 14 to 16 Fr for women, 12 Fr for young girls, and 16 to 18 Fr for male patients unless the physician or health care provider orders a larger size (Daneshgari and others, 2002).

Causes pain. Indicates need to insert catheter if patient is unable to void independently.

Determines condition of perineum.

Obstruction prevents passage of catheter through urethra into bladder.

Betadine allergies are common. Exposure to agents cause local reaction at urinary meatus or even anaphylaxis (McKenry and Salerno, 2003).

Determines purpose for inserting catheter.

## SKILL 32-1 ¦ Inserting a Straight or Indwelling Catheter—cont'd

| STEP | RATIONALE |
|---|---|
| 3. Assess for previous catheterization, including catheter size, response of patient, and time of last catheterization. | Offers useful data in selecting catheter for this procedure and in approach needed to prepare patient. |
| 4. Identify any pathological condition that may impair passage of catheter (e.g., enlarged prostate in men). | Obstruction prevents passage of catheter through urethra into bladder. |

- *Critical Decision Point:* Determine allergy to antiseptic, tape, latex, and lubricant. Povidone-iodine (Betadine) allergies are common; if the client is unaware of allergy, ask if allergic to shellfish.

| STEP | RATIONALE |
|---|---|
| 5. Assess patient's knowledge of the purpose for catheterization. | Reveals need for patient instruction. |

### PLANNING

| | |
|---|---|
| 1. Explain procedure to patient. | Promotes cooperation. |
| 2. Arrange for extra nursing personnel to assist as necessary. | Patient may be unable to assume positioning for procedure. |
| 3. Collect appropriate equipment. | |

### IMPLEMENTATION

| | |
|---|---|
| 1. Perform hand hygiene. | Reduces transmission of microorganisms. Infection is common after catheterization. Bacteria often colonize Foley catheter systems within 48 hours of catheterization (Griffiths, Fernandez, and Murie, 2004). |
| 2. Close curtain or door. | Offers privacy, reduces embarrassment, and aids in relaxation during procedure. |
| 3. Raise bed to appropriate working height. | Promotes use of proper body mechanics. |
| 4. Facing patient, stand on left side of bed if right-handed (on right side if left-handed). Clear bedside table, and arrange equipment. | Successful catheter insertion requires nurse to assume comfortable position with all equipment easily accessible. |
| 5. Raise side rail on opposite side of bed, and put side rail down on working side. | Promotes patient safety. |
| 6. Place waterproof pad under patient. | Prevents soiling of bed linen. |
| 7. Position patient: | Provides good visualization of perineal structures. |
|   **A. Female Patient** | |
|     (1) Assist to dorsal recumbent position (supine with knees flexed). Ask patient to relax thighs so she is able to externally rotate the hip joints. | Most natural position for catheter insertion. Support legs with pillows to reduce muscle tension and promote comfort. |
|     (2) Position female patient in side-lying (Sims') position with upper leg flexed at knee and hip if unable to be supine. If you use this position, take extra precautions to cover rectal area with drape during procedure to reduce chance of cross contamination. | This alternate position is for patients unable to move or abduct the leg at the hip joint (e.g., if patient has arthritic joints). Also, this position is more comfortable for patient. Support patient with pillows if necessary to maintain position. |
|   **B. Male Patient** | |
|     (1) Assist to supine position with thighs slightly abducted. | Comfortable position for patient that aids in visualization. |
| 8. Drape patient: | Avoids unnecessary exposure of body parts and maintains patient's comfort. |
|   **A. Female Patient** | |
|     (1) Drape with bath blanket (see illustration). Place blanket diamond fashion over patient, with one corner at patient's neck, side corners over each arm and side, and last corner over perineum. | |

| STEP | RATIONALE |
|---|---|
| **B. Male Patient** | |
| (1) Drape upper trunk with bath blanket, and cover lower extremities with bed sheets, exposing only genitalia (see illustration). | |
| 9. Wearing disposable gloves, wash perineal area with soap and water as needed; dry and dispose of gloves (see Chapter 27). | Reduces microorganisms near urethral meatus and allows further opportunity to visualize perineum and landmarks. |
| 10. Position lamp to illuminate perineal area. (When using flashlight, have assistant hold it.) | Permits accurate identification and good visualization of urethral meatus. |
| 11. Perform hand hygiene. When inserting an indwelling catheter, open package containing drainage system (unless it comes preattached to catheter); place drainage bag over edge of bottom bed frame, and bring drainage tube up between side rail and mattress. | Prepares bag for attachment to catheter. (Most newer catheters are preattached to a drainage bag, eliminating the connection site). |

---

• *Critical Decision Point:* This step is necessary only if indwelling catheter is to be inserted and drainage system is not part of the catheterization kit.

---

| STEP | RATIONALE |
|---|---|
| 12. Open catheterization kit according to directions, keeping bottom of container sterile. | Prevents transmission of microorganisms from table or work area to sterile supplies. The materials in the kit are ordered in sequence of use. |
| 13. Place plastic bag that contains kit within reach of work area to use as waterproof bag to dispose of used supplies. | |
| 14. Apply sterile gloves (see Chapter 11). | Allows nurse to handle sterile supplies without contamination. |

---

• *Critical Decision Point:* If underpad is first item in kit, place the pad plastic side down under the patient, touching only the edges so as to maintain sterility. Then apply sterile gloves (see Chapter 11, Sterile Fields).

---

| STEP | RATIONALE |
|---|---|
| 15. Organize supplies on sterile field. Open inner sterile package containing catheter. Pour sterile antiseptic solution into correct compartment containing sterile cotton balls. Open lubricant packet. Remove specimen container (place lid loosely on top). An indwelling catheter kit includes a syringe. Take the prefilled syringe from collection compartment of tray, and set it aside on sterile field if needed. | Maintains principles of surgical asepsis and organizes work area. |

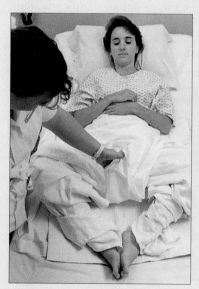

STEP **8A(1)** Draping female for catheterization.

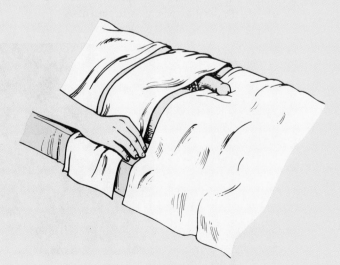

STEP **8B(1)** Draping male for catheterization.

SKILL 32-1 | Inserting a Straight or Indwelling Catheter—cont'd

| STEP | RATIONALE |
|---|---|
| 16. Before inserting an indwelling catheter, a common practice is to test the balloon by injecting fluid from prefilled syringe into balloon port (see illustration). | Checks integrity of balloon. Do not use the catheter if the balloon does not inflate, inflates unevenly, or leaks. This is a controversial step. **Follow manufacturer's recommendations. Checking the balloon in this way sometimes stretches the balloon and causes increased trauma on insertion.** |
| 17. Lubricate catheter 2.5 to 5 cm (1 to 2 inches) for women and 12.5 to 17.5 cm (5 to 7 inches) of men. NOTE: Some catheter kits will have a plastic sheath over the catheter that you need to remove before lubrication. (Optional: Physician or health care provider sometimes orders use of lubricant containing local anesthetic.) | Eases insertion of catheter through urethral canal. Length of urethra determines how much of the catheter needs lubrication. |
| 18. Apply sterile drape, keeping gloves sterile: | |
| **A. Female Patient** | |
| (1) Allow top edge of drape to form cuff over both hands. Place drape down on bed between patient's thighs. Slip cuffed edge just under buttocks, taking care not to touch contaminated surface with gloves. | Outer surface of drape covering hands remains sterile. Sterile drape against sterile gloves is sterile. |
| (2) Pick up fenestrated sterile drape, and allow it to unfold without touching an unsterile object. Apply drape over perineum, exposing labia and being sure not to touch contaminated surface. | Maintains sterility of work surface. |
| **B. Male Patient:** You will use one of two methods for draping, depending on preference. | Maintains sterility of work surface. |
| (1) First method: Apply drape over thighs, and carefully slip under penis without contaminating drape or completely opening fenestrated drape. | |
| (2) Second method: Apply drape over thighs and just below penis. Pick up fenestrated sterile drape, allow it to unfold, and drape it over penis with fenestrated slit resting over penis. | |
| 19. Place sterile tray and contents on sterile drape between legs. Open specimen container. NOTE: Patient's size and positioning will dictate exact placement. This method works best with flexible, average-size patients. | Provides easy access to supplies during catheter insertion. Maintains aseptic technique during procedure. |

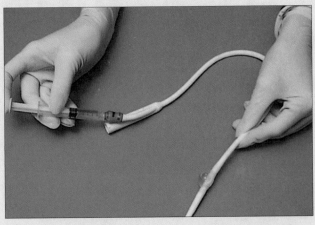

STEP **16** Inserting fluid to test catheter balloon.

| STEP | RATIONALE |
|---|---|

**20.** Cleanse urethral meatus.

   **A. Female Patient**

      (1) With nondominant hand, carefully retract labia to fully expose urethral meatus. **Maintain position of nondominant hand throughout procedure.** Use sterile fenestrated drape to protect sterile field.

Provides full visualization of urethral meatus. Full retraction prevents contamination of urethral meatus during cleansing.

---

• *Critical Decision Point:* Closure of labia during cleansing requires that you repeat the procedure because the area has become contaminated.

---

      (2) Using forceps in sterile dominant hand, pick up cotton ball saturated with antiseptic solution and clean perineal area, wiping front to back from clitoris toward anus. Using a new cotton ball for each area, wipe along the far labial fold, near labial fold, and directly over center of urethral meatus (see illustration).

Cleansing reduces number of microorganisms at urethral meatus. Use of single cotton ball for each wipe prevents transfer of microorganisms. Cleansing moves from areas of least contamination to that of most contamination (see Chapter 11). Dominant hand remains sterile.

   **B. Male Patient**

      (1) If patient is not circumcised, retract foreskin with nondominant hand. Grasp penis at shaft just below glans. Retract urethral meatus between thumb and forefinger. **Maintain nondominant hand in this position throughout procedure.** Use the sterile fenestrated drape as your sterile field.

Accidental release of foreskin or dropping of penis during cleansing requires you to restart procedure because area has become contaminated.

---

• *Critical Decision Point:* If the foreskin does not remain retracted during insertion, then repeat the cleansing procedure because the area has become contaminated.

---

      (2) With dominant hand, pick up cotton ball with forceps and clean penis. Move it in circular motion from urethral meatus down to base of glans. Repeat cleansing three more times, using clean cotton ball each time (see illustration).

Reduces number of microorganisms at urethral meatus and moves from areas of least to most contamination. Dominant hand remains sterile.

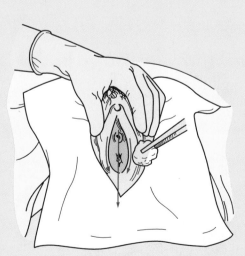

STEP **20A(2)** Cleansing technique (female).

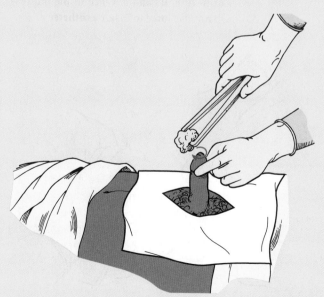

STEP **20 B(2)** Cleansing technique (male).

## SKILL 32-1 ⌐ Inserting a Straight or Indwelling Catheter—cont'd

| STEP | RATIONALE |
|---|---|
| 21. Pick up catheter with gloved dominant hand 7.5 to 10 cm (3 to 4 inches) from catheter tip. Hold end of catheter loosely coiled in palm of dominant hand. (Optional: Grasp catheter with forceps.) Place distal end of catheter in urine tray receptacle if performing a straight catheterization. | Having control of catheter tip allows for less traumatic insertion. Controlling distal end prevents accidental contamination. |
| 22. Insert catheter:<br>  **A. Female Patient**<br>    (1) Ask patient to bear down gently as if to void, and slowly insert catheter through urethral meatus (see illustration). | Relaxation of external sphincter aids in insertion of catheter. |
|     (2) Advance catheter a total of 5 to 7.5 cm (2 to 3 inches) in adult **or until urine flows out catheter's end.** When urine appears, advance catheter another 2.5 to 5 cm (1 to 2 inches). Do not force against resistance. Place end of catheter in urine tray receptacle. | Female urethra is short. Appearance of urine indicates that catheter tip is in bladder or lower urethra. Advancement of catheter ensures bladder placement. |

• *Critical Decision Point:* If no urine appears, check if catheter is in vagina. If misplaced, leave catheter in vagina as landmark indicating where not to insert, and insert another sterile catheter.

| | |
|---|---|
|     (3) Release labia, and hold catheter securely with nondominant hand. | Bladder or sphincter contraction sometimes causes accidental expulsion of catheter. |
|   **B. Male Patient**<br>    (1) Lift penis to position perpendicular to patient's body, and apply light traction (see illustration). | Straightens urethral canal to ease catheter insertion. |
|     (2) Ask patient to bear down as if to void, and slowly insert catheter through urethral meatus. | Relaxation of external sphincter aids in insertion of catheter. |
|     (3) Advance catheter 17.5 to 22.5 cm (7 to 9 inches) to the bifurcation of the injection port and catheter end in an adult male. If you initially feel resistance, withdraw catheter slightly and wait; do not force it through urethra. As you advance the catheter, note when urine appears and advance to the bifurcation. **Do not use force to insert a catheter.** | The adult male urethra is long. It is normal to meet resistance at the prostatic sphincter. When you meet resistance, hold catheter firmly against sphincter without forcing catheter. After a few seconds, the sphincter usually relaxes and you are able to advance the catheter. Appearance of urine indicates catheter tip is in bladder or urethra. Advancement of catheter to the bifurcation ensures proper placement (Daneshgari and others, 2002). |

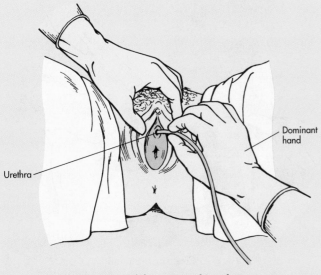

STEP **22A(1)** Inserting the catheter.

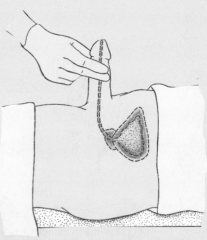

STEP **22B(1)** Position of penis perpendicular to body for catheter insertion.

| STEP | RATIONALE |
|---|---|
| (4) Lower penis, and hold catheter securely in non-dominant hand. Place end of catheter in urine tray receptacle. | Bladder or urethral contraction accidentally expels catheter. Collection of urine prevents soiling and provides output measurement. |
| (5) Reduce (or reposition) the foreskin. | Paraphimosis (retraction and constriction of the foreskin behind the glans penis) secondary to catheterization will occur if you do not reduce the foreskin. |
| 23. Collect urine specimen as needed. Fill sterile specimen cup to desired level (20 to 30 ml) by holding end of catheter in dominant hand over cup. | Allows you to obtain sterile specimen for culture analysis. |
| 24. Allow bladder to empty fully unless institution policy restricts maximal volume of urine drained with each catheterization (about 800 to 1000 ml). | Retained urine serves as reservoir for growth of microorganisms. |

• *Critical Decision Point:* If you inserted a straight, single-use catheter, wait until urine has drained, then withdraw catheter slowly but smoothly until removed.

| | |
|---|---|
| 25. Inflate balloon of indwelling catheter fully per manufacturer's recommendations (see illustrations).<br> a. With free dominant hand, attach syringe to injection port at end of catheter.<br> b. While holding catheter with nondominant hand at urethral meatus, take end of catheter and place it between first two free fingers of nondominant hand.<br> c. Slowly inject total amount of solution. If patient complains of sudden pain, aspirate solution and advance catheter farther.<br> d. After inflating balloon, release catheter with nondominant hand and pull gently to feel resistance. Then move catheter slightly back into bladder. | Inflation of balloon anchors catheter tip in place above bladder outlet to prevent removal of catheter. Note the size of balloon on the catheter. Most commonly you will use a 5-ml balloon, but a 30-ml balloon is sometimes ordered. A prefilled syringe is often included with the kit; use only the amount included. Do not overinflate or underinflate the balloon. |

• *Critical Decision Point:* If you notice resistance to inflation or if the patient complains of pain, the balloon is probably not entirely within the bladder. Stop inflation; aspirate any fluid injected into the balloon, and advance the catheter a little more before reattempting to inflate.

| | |
|---|---|
| 26. Newer catheters are usually preattached to drainage system. If not, attach end of catheter to collecting tube of drainage system. Drainage bag needs to be below level of bladder; do not place bag on side rails of bed (see illustration). | Establishes closed system for urine drainage. Raising bag on side rail will cause backflow of urine into bladder. |

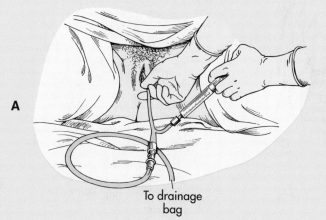

To drainage bag

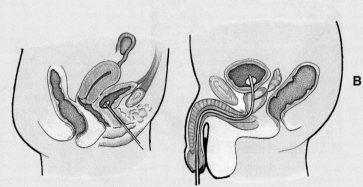

STEP 25 **A,** Inflating the balloon (indwelling catheter) **B,** Position of balloon in bladder.

## SKILL 32-1 | Inserting a Straight or Indwelling Catheter—cont'd

| STEP | RATIONALE |
|---|---|

**27.** Anchor catheter:

   **A. Female Patient**

     (1) Secure catheter tubing to inner thigh with strip of nonallergenic tape (commercial multipurpose tube holders with a Velcro strap or adhesive patches are available). Allow for slack so movement of thigh does not create tension on catheter (see illustration).

   *Anchoring catheter to inner thigh reduces pressure on urethra, thus reducing possibility of tissue injury in this area. In addition, anchoring the catheter assists in prevention of accidental dislodgement (Hanchett, 2002).*

   **B. Male Patient**

     (1) Secure catheter tubing to top of thigh or lower abdomen (with penis directed toward chest). Allow slack in catheter so movement does not create tension on catheter (see illustration).

   *Anchoring catheter to lower abdomen reduces pressure on urethra at junction of penis and scrotum, thus reducing possibility of tissue injury in this area (Hanchett, 2002). This method is impractical for ambulatory patients especially in the home.*

---

• *Critical Decision Point:* Be sure there are no obstructions in tubing. Coil excess tubing on bed, and fasten it to bottom sheet with clip from kit or with rubber band and safety pin.

---

**28.** Assist patient to comfortable position. Wash and dry perineal area as needed.

   Maintains comfort and security.

**29.** Remove gloves, and dispose of equipment, drapes, and urine in proper receptacles.

   Reduces transmission of microorganisms.

**30.** Perform hand hygiene.

   Reduces spread of microorganisms.

**31.** Palpate bladder.

   Determines if distention is relieved.

***Removal of indwelling catheter***

**32.** Before removing an indwelling catheter, check the patient's medical orders to determine if you need a sterile urine specimen.

   Allows for you to obtain a sterile specimen without another catheterization.

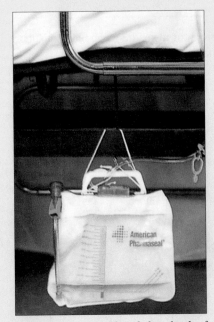

STEP **26** Drainage bag below level of bladder.

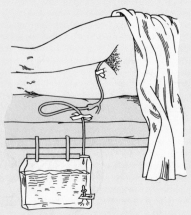

STEP **27A(1)** Securing the female indwelling catheter.

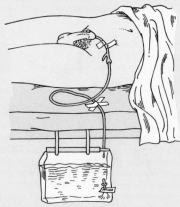

STEP **27B(1)** Securing the male indwelling catheter.

| STEP | RATIONALE |
|---|---|
| 33. Explain the procedure to patient. | Patient will have realistic expectations of the removal process and be able to cooperate more fully. |
| 34. Place an absorbent, waterproof pad between thighs (female patient) or over thighs (male patient). | Provides for decreased soiling of bed linens in case urine drips from the catheter as it is removed. |
| 35. Perform hand hygiene. | Reduces spread of microorganisms. |
| 36. Put on clean disposable gloves. | Reduces spread of microorganisms. |
| 37. Remove adhesive tape or Velcro tube holder used to pressure and anchor catheter. | Allow for positioning of catheter for removal. |
| 38. Using a sterile syringe fitted with a tip that matches the catheter inflation valve, aspirate all the instilled fluid used to inflate the balloon. | Ensure total deflation of the balloon to decrease trauma to urethra and urinary meatus. The catheter will have a label stating the balloon volume. |
| 39. After removing the instilled fluid, gently and smoothly pull out the catheter while asking the patient to breathe slowly with an open mouth. | By removing the catheter slowly you will reduce potential trauma. If patient experiences discomfort or the catheter is not coming out, attempt to remove more fluid from the balloon before retrying. |
| 40. After removal of catheter, wrap in absorbent pad and dispose of properly. | Reduces transmission of microorganisms. |
| 41. Remove any tape residue from abdomen or inner thigh. | Removes source of skin irritation. |
| 42. Instruct to save urine after removal of catheter and provide measuring device. | Allows for assessment for urinary retention following catheter removal. |

## EVALUATION

| | |
|---|---|
| 1. Ask about patient's comfort. | Determines if patient's sensation of discomfort or fullness has been relieved. |
| 2. Observe character and amount of urine in drainage system. | Determines if urine is flowing adequately. |
| 3. Determine that there is no urine leaking from catheter or tubing connections. | Prevents injury to patient's skin and ensures a closed sterile system. |
| 4. Determine patient's ability to void after catheter removal and measure urine output from first void. | Patient should be able to void within 6 to 8 hours of catheter removal. Normal symptoms during first void after catheter removal include hesitancy and dysuria. |

## RECORDING AND REPORTING

■ Report and record type and size of catheter inserted, amount of fluid used to inflate balloon, characteristics of urine, amount of urine, reason for catheterization, specimen collection, and patient's response to procedure.

■ Ensure that times for catheter care are set in the care plan. Patients with indwelling catheters receive perineal and catheter care every 8 hours and after bowel movements.

■ Record in nurses' notes when catheter care was given and condition of urethral meatus.

■ Record removal of catheter, assessment of urethral meatus, and character and amount of urine in drainage bag. Record patient's next voiding.

## UNEXPECTED OUTCOMES AND RELATED INTERVENTIONS

■ Urethral or perineal irritation is present.
  • Observe for leaking, and replace catheter if necessary.
  • If catheter is present, ensure that indwelling catheter is anchored.

  • If securing catheter does not help or if catheter has been removed after several days, notify physician or health care provider of urethral irritation.

■ Patient has fever and/or odor is present, or patient experiences small, frequent voidings or any burning or bleeding.
  • Monitor vital signs and urine, but report findings to physician or health care provider because any of these symptoms/signs may indicate a urinary tract infection.

■ Patient experiences urinary retention and is unable to void after catheter removal.
  • Ensure adequate intake and privacy, and facilitate urination by relaxation.
  • If patient unable to void within 6 to 8 hours of catheter removal, notify physician or health care provider and anticipate order for straight catheterization.

the patient's bladder. Never raise a drainage bag and tubing above the level of the patient's bladder. Urine in the bag and tubing is a medium for bacteria, and infection will develop if urine is allowed to reflux (return to the bladder).

Most drainage bags contain an antireflux valve to prevent urine from reentering the drainage tubing and contaminating the bladder. A spigot at the base of the bag provides a means to empty the bag. Make sure the spigot is always clamped, except during emptying, and tucked into the protective pouch at the bag's side.

To keep the drainage system patent, check for kinks or bends in the tubing, avoid positioning the patient on drainage tubing, prevent tubing from becoming dependent, and observe for clots or sediment that block the tubing.

***Routine Catheter Care.*** Patients with indwelling catheters require specific perineal hygiene care to reduce the risk of urinary tract infection. In most institutions, patients receive catheter care every 8 hours as the minimal standard of care. In addition, provide catheter care each time the patient defecates or has bowel incontinence. Proper care involves removal of any secretions or encrustation at the catheter insertion site and cleansing of the first 4 inches of the catheter.

Provide thorough perineal care (see Chapter 27), and observe the urethral meatus and surrounding tissues for inflammation, swelling, and discharge. Note the amount, color, odor, and consistency of discharge to determine local infection and status of hygiene. Use soap and water to cleanse along the length of the catheter for 4 inches (10 cm) (Figure 32-7). Hold the catheter firmly as you cleanse from the urethra up toward the end of the catheter. Cleansing away from the urethra reduces microorganisms around the meatus. The use of powders or lotions on the perineum is contraindicated because of the risk of growth of microorganisms, which travel up the urinary tract.

Replace, as necessary, the adhesive tape or multipurpose tube holder that anchors the catheter to the patient's leg or abdomen, and remove adhesive residue from the skin. Secure the catheter, thus reducing the risk of the catheter being pulled on and exposing the portion that was in the urethra. This also prevents drag on the catheter and avoids pressure from the balloon on the bladder neck. Replace the urinary tubing and collection bag if necessary, adhering to principles of surgical asepsis. Change the urinary tubing and collection bag if there are signs of leakage, odor, or sediment buildup. Check the drainage tubing and bag to ensure that no tubing loops hang below the level of the bladder. Make sure that the tube is coiled and secured onto the bed linen, the tube is not kinked or clamped, and the drainage bag is positioned on the bed frame.

**Alternatives to Urethral Catheterization.** To avoid the risks associated with catheters inserted through the urethra, alternatives for urinary drainage exist. A **suprapubic catheter** is inserted surgically into the bladder through the lower abdomen above the symphysis pubis (Figure 32-8). Although most successfully used for short periods with patients who have had gynecological and bladder surgery, the suprapubic catheter is sometimes used in older adult males who require

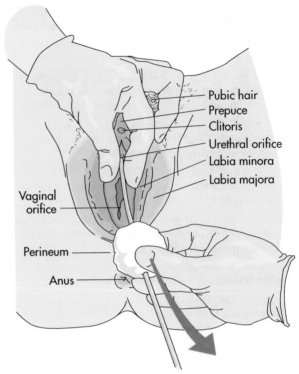

FIGURE **32-7** Cleansing the catheter during catheter care. (From Sorrentino S: *Mosby's textbook for nursing assistants*, St. Louis, 2004, Mosby.)

a long-term alternative to urinary catheterization. As with indwelling urinary catheters, the suprapubic catheter predisposes the patient to urinary tract infections, but the incidence is lower. Spread of infection to the kidneys requires removing the catheter. The advantages of a suprapubic catheter for patients are that they void naturally when the catheter is clamped and it is more comfortable. Daily care will depend on policy, but the cleaning and dressing of the site are similar to care of any surgical drain (see Chapter 37).

The condom catheter is suitable for incontinent or comatose male patients who still have complete and spontaneous bladder emptying (Box 32-7). The condom catheter poses little risk of infection. Local infections, however, result from buildup of secretions around the urethra, trauma to the urethral meatus, or buildup of pressure in the outflow tubing.

It is necessary to remove the condom catheter daily to check for skin irritation. Clean the urethral meatus and penis thoroughly with each condom catheter change. Twisting of the condom at the drainage tube attachment irritates the skin and obstructs urine outflow. Check the drainage tubing frequently for patency. For a man with a retracted foreskin, maintaining the intactness of a conventional condom catheter is difficult. Special devices are available to help with the problem. Review manufacturer's guidelines for product application.

There is a lack of a full spectrum of devices and appliances for incontinent adults, particularly women (Mason and others, 2003). Some women wear the newer absorbent

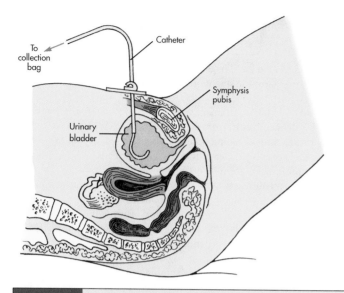

FIGURE 32-8 Placement of suprapubic catheter above the symphysis pubis.

---

### BOX 32-7  PROCEDURAL GUIDELINES FOR

## Applying a Condom Catheter

**Delegation Considerations:** You can delegate the skill of applying a condom catheter to assistive personnel.

- Instruct assistive personnel to ask whether patient has a latex allergy.
- Caution caregiver to be sensitive to privacy needs of patients.
- Clarify that skin of penile shaft is intact and free from swelling, redness, or open lesions before applying the condom catheter.
- Clarify the caregiver's understanding of how to apply the adhesive strip that secures the condom catheter.

**Equipment:** Condom catheter (sometimes comes with self-adhesive or an elastic adhesive), collection bag, basin with warm water, towel and washcloth, clean gloves, scissors

1. Check physician's or health care provider's order.
2. Perform hand hygiene.
3. Assess urinary elimination patterns, patient's ability to voluntarily urinate, and continence.
4. Assess mental status of patient and explain procedure.
5. Raise bed to working height, and raise far upper side rail.
6. Assist patient to a supine position. Using sheet, drape patient, only exposing the genitalia.
7. Apply disposable gloves; provide perineal care and dry thoroughly.

8. Prepare condom catheter and drainage bag (see manufacturer's directions).
9. Assess condition of penis and scrotum. Provide perineal care.
   a. If needed, clip hair at base of penile shaft.
10. Apply skin prep to penile shaft, and allow to dry.
11. Holding penis in nondominant hand, apply condom by rolling smoothly onto penis. NOTE: Leave a 2.5- to 5-cm (1- to 2-inch) space between tip of penis and end of catheter (see illustration).
12. Secure condom catheter:
    a. If using elastic adhesive, wrap the strip of adhesive over the condom to secure it in place by using a spiral technique (see illustration). **NOTE: Never use adhesive tape.**
    b. For self-adhesive catheter, follow manufacturer's directions.
13. Attach catheter to large-volume drainage bag or leg bag. Attach large-volume drainage bag to lower bed frame.
14. Make patient comfortable.
15. Observe urinary drainage, drainage tube patency, condition of penis, and tape placement.

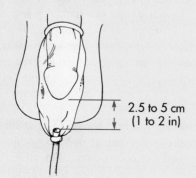

STEP 10 Distance between end of penis and tip of condom.

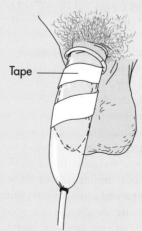

STEP 11 Apply elastic tape in a spiral fashion to secure the condom catheter to the penis.

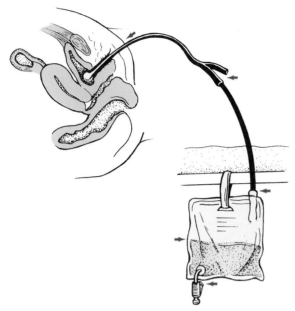

FIGURE **32-9** Potential sites for introduction of infection.

**BOX 32-8** **Tips for Preventing Infection in Catheterized Patients**

Follow good hand hygiene techniques.

Do not allow the spigot on the drainage bag to touch a contaminated surface.

Do not open the drainage system at connection points to obtain specimens or measure urine.

If the drainage tubing becomes disconnected, do not touch the ends of the catheter or tubing. Wipe the ends of the tube with antiseptic solution before reconnecting.

Each patient needs to have a separate receptacle for measuring urine to prevent cross contamination.

Prevent pooling of urine and reflux of urine into the bladder. Avoid raising the drainage bag above the level of the bladder.

Avoid allowing any dependent loops of tubing.

If it is necessary to raise the bag during transfer of the patient to a bed or stretcher, clamp the tubing.

Before patient exercises or ambulates, drain all urine from tubing into bag.

Avoid prolonged clamping or kinking of the tubing (except during bladder conditioning).

Empty the drainage bag at least every 8 hours.

Remove the catheter as soon as possible after conferring with physician or health care provider.

Secure the catheter in place, noting specific guidelines regarding the male patient's taping procedure.

Perform routine perineal hygiene every 8-hour shift and after defecation.

pads and adult disposable undergarments. However, wearers of these disposable undergarments report skin irritation, odor, and increased infection rate. For the active incontinent woman, behavioral treatment options such as pelvic floor exercises and diet management will promote more independence (Macaulay and others, 2004).

**RESTORATIVE AND CONTINUING CARE.** Returning to normal micturition often means preventing complications from treatment. Many restorative functions are related to preventing infection after catheterization, promoting comfort, and preventing skin breakdown if the patient is incontinent.

**Preventing Infection.** Maintaining a closed urinary drainage system is important in infection control. A break in the system leads to introduction of microorganisms. Sites at risk are at the place of catheter insertion, drainage bag, spigot, tube junction, and junction of tube and bag (Figure 32-9). In addition, monitor the patency of the system to prevent pooling of urine. Urine in the drainage bag is an excellent medium for microorganism growth. Bacteria are able to travel up drainage tubing to grow in pools of urine. Therefore it is important to prevent the abnormal backward flow of urine (**urinary reflux**). If this urine flows back into the bladder, an infection will probably develop. Box 32-8 gives suggestions for ways to prevent infections in catheterized patients.

**Promotion of Comfort.** Patients with urinary alterations are often uncomfortable as a result of the symptoms of urinary problems. Frequent or unpredictable voiding, dysuria, and painful distention are sources of discomfort.

The incontinent patient gains comfort from having clean, dry clothing. When incontinence is the problem, a protective pad or sanitary belt offers protection against soiling. Wet clothing adheres to the skin and can cause rubbing and irritation. Check pads frequently, and change them as needed.

Giving urinary analgesics that act on the urethral and bladder mucosa sometimes relieve dysuria. Phenazopyridine

(Pyridium) helps to relieve dysuria, burning, and itching. It is available in combination with sulfonamide antibiotics in preparations such as Azo Gantanol and Azo Gantrisin. The sulfonamide provides additional antibacterial action. Make patients taking drugs with phenazopyridine aware that their urine will appear orange and possibly stain their clothing. They need to drink large amounts of fluids to prevent toxicity from the sulfonamides and to maintain optimal flow through the urinary system. Always ask patients about allergies to sulfa before giving these drugs (McKenry and Salerno, 2003).

If the patient has local discomfort from an inflamed urethra, a warm sitz bath will provide pain relief (see Chapter 35). The warm water soothes inflamed tissues near the urethral meatus by improving blood supply. The patient is often relaxed after a sitz bath, so voiding occurs easily.

The pain of distention cannot be relieved unless the patient is able to empty the bladder. Methods for stimulating micturition or intermittent catheterization are often the only sources of pain relief.

**Maintenance of Skin Integrity.** The acidity of urine is irritating to the skin. When urine becomes alkaline, encrustation or precipitate collects on the skin, causing breakdown. Continuous exposure of the skin to urine leads to gradual maceration and excoriation. Washing with mild soap and warm water is the best way to remove urine from the skin. Special no-rinse cleansers are particularly useful. They avoid the problem of skin irritation that results from incomplete

## OUTCOME EVALUATION

| Nursing Action | Patient Response/Finding | Achievement of Outcome |
|---|---|---|
| Measure and time each voiding. Compare with fluid intake.<br>Palpate bladder. | Mrs. Vallero's fluid intake was 800 ml in 6 hours.<br>Mrs. Vallero voided twice in 6 hours and voided 200-400 ml with each void.<br>Bladder nondistended upon palpation following voiding.<br>Mrs. Vallero did not perceive increased urge to void during palpation. | Mrs. Vallero is ingesting and voiding fluid appropriately, indicating normal micturition.<br>She voids >150 ml each time.<br>Complete bladder emptying achieved. |

removal of cleansers from the skin (Gray, 2004a). Body lotion keeps the skin moisturized and provides a barrier to the urine. Patients who wet their clothing need a clean set of clothes after each voiding.

When the skin becomes irritated or inflamed, the physician or health care provider often prescribes a cream or spray containing steroids to reduce inflammation (e.g., triamcinolone [Kenalog]). If fungal growth develops, the antifungal drug nystatin (Mycostatin), available in cream or powder form, is effective (McKenry and Salerno, 2003; Wound, Ostomy, and Continence Nurses Society [WOCN], 2004).

The patient with a ureterostomy has a special hygiene problem because urine drains from the ostomy site continuously. The drainage pouch or appliance frequently becomes moist and slips from the skin (WOCN, 2005). Continual oozing of urine around the stoma causes skin breakdown. Skin barriers provide a layer of protection between the skin and ostomy pouch. When urine leaks, it frequently covers the outer skin barrier. An enterostomal therapist helps the patient select an ostomy appliance that fits snugly against the skin's surface around the stoma (see Chapter 33).

## Evaluation

**PATIENT CARE.** To evaluate the care plan use the expected outcomes developed during planning to determine whether interventions were effective (Table 32-7) This evaluation process is a dynamic one. You use this information to monitor the patient's progress and to direct future interventions. The optimal goal is the patient's ability to urinate voluntarily without dysuria, urgency, or frequency. The patient's urine needs to be an amber color, clear, without abnormal constituents, and within the normal range of pH and specific gravity.

You also evaluate specific outcomes designed to demonstrate normal urinary function and prevent complications of urinary alterations. Has the patient's intake been at least 2000 ml? Is the bladder distended? Is there less than 50 ml of residual urine on the second voiding? Is urinary output in proportion to fluid intake? Are there a reduced number of incontinent episodes? Is the urine culture showing negative bacterial growth? Does the patient use correct hand hygiene? Are there any areas of skin breakdown around the perineum, stoma, or condom?

Be systematic in evaluating the patient's response to care. Nursing research is being conducted to validate the effec-

## EVALUATION

Phyllis and her instructor talk with Mrs. Vallero and explain that she probably needs a catheterization again. She asks to try to "go" and nods to the bathroom. Phyllis suggests that she sit for at least 15 minutes and leave the water running in the sink. Phyllis also shows Mrs. Vallero how to push on her abdomen after she is sitting in the bathroom. Mrs. Vallero was able to void after 5 minutes.

**Documentation Note**

"Moved slowly to the bathroom. Gait was steady, slow, and slightly stooped. Breathing was even and nonlabored, and while sitting on the toilet, stated, 'I'm ready.' Used manual bladder compression and turned the water on in the sink. Voided 400 ml of clear, pale yellow urine. Stated 'I don't feel so full now.' Returned to bed. No evidence of residual urine in bladder using portable ultrasound."

tiveness of nursing interventions. Evidence-based practice will improve the quality of care you provide.

**PATIENT EXPECTATIONS.** Many take control over urination for granted until it is lost. Patients report that it is degrading and they feel like a baby when they lose control over voiding. Therefore evaluation of care from the incontinent patient's standpoint centers around maintaining a level of dryness that is personally satisfactory. Patients want to have control, and to achieve that outcome they need to have confidence in utilizing triggering mechanisms to initiate voiding.

Patients who have a urinary tract infection find that pain, urgency, and frequency rule their lives. Patients who have an infection will be satisfied with their care if they are able to report an absence or decrease in their symptoms. Does the patient void without dysuria? Does the patient sleep and carry out activities of daily living with lessened or no discomfort?

For all patients with urinary problems, lack of privacy is a potential issue. Did they feel that staff were considerate, and did the staff protect their privacy? Patients will also evaluate whether you include them in the planning of their care. Were they able to tell you the important information about their habits? Did you consider that information when you suggested a plan of care or implemented an intervention?

# KEY CONCEPTS

- Voluntary control from higher brain centers and involuntary control from the spinal cord influence micturition or voiding.
- Symptoms common to urinary disturbances include urgency, dysuria, polyuria, oliguria, and difficulty in starting the urinary stream.
- When collected properly, a clean-voided urine specimen does not contain bacteria picked up from the urethral meatus.
- A patient will better understand the importance of perineal hygiene by knowing that the urinary tract is normally sterile.
- Methods of promoting the micturition reflex assist patients in sensing the urge to urinate and controlling urethral sphincter relaxation.
- An increased fluid intake results in urine formation that flushes particles and solutes from the urinary system.

- Incontinence is classified as total, urge, stress, reflex, or functional. Each type of incontinence has specific nursing interventions.
- An indwelling urinary catheter remains in the bladder for an extended period, making the risk of infection greater than with intermittent catheterization.
- Closed drainage systems deliver sterile solutions and medication to the bladder. Strict asepsis is necessary when caring for a patient with a closed bladder drainage system.
- Because urine drains almost continuously from a ureterostomy, there is risk of skin breakdown around a stoma site.
- A primary function of the elimination process is fluid balance.

# CRITICAL THINKING IN PRACTICE

*Ms. Miller is an 18-year-old college student who has symptoms of a lower urinary tract infection (cystitis). She has made an appointment with the nurse practitioner at the student health service at her college.*

1. What additional information is needed before planning care and treatment?
2. A female has a higher risk of urinary tract infection than a male does because of:
   a. Inadequate fluid intake
   b. Poor hygiene
   c. Length of urethra
   d. Continuity of mucous membrane
Explain your choice:

3. When assessing her urine you should observe each specimen for:
   a. Clarity
   b. Viscosity

   c. Specific gravity
   d. Sugar and acetone
Explain your choice:

*After discussion with Ms. Miller, she tells you she has become sexually active since coming to college. You discuss her choice from a health-related viewpoint. You talk with her about sexually transmitted infections and give her some related literature to read. You also discuss the importance of preventing future episodes of cystitis.*

4. The major result of recurrent cystitis is potential for:
   a. Scarring of bladder lining
   b. Fluid and electrolyte imbalance
   c. Ascending infection to the kidney
Explain your choice:

# NCLEX® REVIEW

1. An adult patient has not voided in 8 hours and complains about a continued perception of the urge to urinate. Your initial action is to:
   1. Notify the physician or health care provider
   2. Insert a straight catheter
   3. Palpate the patient's bladder
   4. Increase patient's fluid intake
2. Identification of a "2 + hematuria" in your female patient with a urinary tract infection indicates:
   1. A response to the antibiotic therapy
   2. A ruptured vessel within the bladder

   3. Irritation of the bladder mucosa from the pathogen
   4. The result of a straight catheter used to obtain a sterile specimen
3. When applying a condom catheter, it is important to secure the catheter to the penile shaft in such a manner that the _____ circulation is not impaired and urine is able to flow out.
4. When a patient with an indwelling catheter complains of discomfort in the bladder, you first:
   1. Notify the physician or health care provider
   2. Milk the tube gently
   3. Check the patency of the tube
   4. Irrigate the catheter with antiseptic solution

5. Maintaining a Foley catheter drainage bag in the dependent position prevents:
   1. Urinary reflux
   2. Urinary retention
   3. Reflex incontinence
   4. Urinary incontinence
6. The purpose of instructing the patient to begin and discard the initial stream of urine when obtaining a midstream urine specimen is to:
   1. Allow for patient comfort
   2. Allow sufficient urine to be obtained for the culture specimen
   3. Allow the initial urine to wash bacteria from the external genitalia
   4. Allow the initial urine to drain from the bladder to avoid inaccurate urine cultures
7. Which of the following statements by the patient indicates that she is at risk for a recurrence of cystitis (inflammation of the bladder)?
   1. "I can go 8 to 10 hours without needing to urinate."
   2. "I take a shower every morning."

3. "I wipe from front to back after urinating."
4. "I drink a lot of water during the day."
8. When collecting a 24-hour urine specimen, you:
   1. Discard the first voided specimen of the 24-hour period.
   2. Weigh the patient before the collection begins
   3. Discard the last voided specimen of the 24-hour period
   4. Check the intake and output of the previous day
9. A routine urinalysis is ordered for a patient. If you cannot send the specimen to the laboratory immediately, you:
   1. Take no special action
   2. Refrigerate the specimen
   3. Place the specimen in "dirty" utility until you can send it
   4. Discard the specimen and collect it later

## REFERENCES

Daneshgari F and others: Evidence-based multidisciplinary practice: improving the safety and standards of male bladder catheterization, *MedSurg Nurs* 11(5):236, 2002.

Dochterman JM, Bulechek GM, editors: *Nursing interventions classification (NIC)*, ed 4, St. Louis, 2004, Mosby.

Foxman B: Epidemiology of urinary tract infections: incidence, morbidity, and economic costs, *Am J Med* 113(1A):5S, 2002.

Gray M: Urinary retention: management in the acute care setting, part II , *Am J Nurs* 100(8):36, 2000.

Gray M: Are cranberry juice or cranberry products effective in the prevention or management of urinary tract infection? *J Wound Ostomy Continence Nurs* 29(3):122, 2002.

Gray M: Preventing and managing perineal dermatitis: a shared goal of wound and continence care, *J Wound Ostomy Continence Nurs* 31(suppl 1):S2, 2004a.

Gray M: What nursing interventions reduce the risk of symptomatic urinary tract infection in the patient with an indwelling catheter, *J Wound Ostomy Continence Nurs* 31(1):3, 2004b.

Griffiths RD, Fernandez RS, Murie P: Removal of short-term indwelling urethral catheters: the evidence, *J Wound Ostomy Continence Nurs* 31(5):299, 2004.

Hanchett M: Techniques for stabilizing urinary catheters, *Am J Nurs* 102(3):44, 2002.

Huether SE, McCance KL: *Understanding pathophysiology*, ed 3, St. Louis, 2004, Mosby.

Lawrence P, Rozmus C: Culturally sensitive care of the Muslim patient, *J Transcult Nurs* 12(3):228, 2001.

Lekan-Rutledge D, Colling J: Urinary incontinence in the frail elderly, *Am J Nurs* 103(suppl 3):36S, 2003.

Lewis SM, Heitkemper MM, Dirksen SR: *Medical-surgical nursing*, ed 6, St. Louis, 2004, Mosby.

Macaulay M and others: A pilot study to evaluate reusable absorbent body-worn products for adults with moderate/heavy urinary incontinence, *J Wound Ostomy Continence Nurs* 31(6):357, 2004.

Mason DJ, Newman DK, Palmer MH: Changing UI practice, *Am J Nurs* 103(suppl 3):2S, 2003.

McKenry LM, Salerno E: *Mosby's pharmacology in nursing*, ed 21, St. Louis, 2003, Mosby.

Milne JL: Behavioral therapies at the primary care level: the current state of knowledge, *J Wound Ostomy Continence Nurs* 31(6):367, 2004.

Moorhead S, Johnson M, Maas M: *Nursing outcomes classification (NOC)*, ed 3, St. Louis, 2004, Mosby.

O'Donnell JA, Hofman MT: Urinary tract infection: how to manage nursing home patients with or without chronic catheterization, *Geriatrics* 57(5):45, 2002.

Palmer MH, Newman DK: Bladder matters: urinary incontinence in nursing homes, *Am J Nurs* 104(11):57, 2004.

Sampselle CM: Behavioral interventions in young and middle-aged women, *Am J Nurs* 103(suppl 3):9S, 2003.

Sorrentino S: *Mosby's textbook for nursing assistants*, St. Louis, 2004, Mosby.

Thompson DL, Smith DA: Continence nursing: a whole person approach, *Holist Nurs Pract* 16(2):14, 2002.

Wound, Ostomy, and Continence Nurses Society: *Peristomal skin complications: best practice for clinicians*, Glenview, Ill, 2004, The Society.

Wound, Ostomy, and Continence Nurses Society: *Stoma complications: best practice for clinicians*, Glenview, Ill, 2005, The Society.

Wyman JF: Treatment of urinary incontinence in men and older women, *Am J Nurs* 103(suppl 3):26S, 2003.

# CHAPTER 33

# Bowel Elimination

## MEDIA RESOURCES

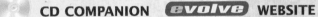

**CD COMPANION** *evolve* **WEBSITE**

http://evolve.elsevier.com/Potter/basic

- NCLEX® Review
- Audio Glossary
- English/Spanish Audio Glossary
- Video Clips

## OBJECTIVES

- Explain the physiology of digestion, absorption, and bowel elimination.
- Discuss physiological and psychological factors that influence bowel elimination.
- Describe common physiological alterations in bowel elimination.
- Assess a patient's bowel elimination pattern.
- Perform a fecal occult blood test.
- List nursing diagnoses related to alterations in bowel elimination.

- Describe nursing implications for common diagnostic examinations of the gastrointestinal tract.
- Administer an enema.
- List nursing measures aimed at promoting normal elimination and defecation.
- Describe nursing care required to maintain structure and function of a bowel diversion.

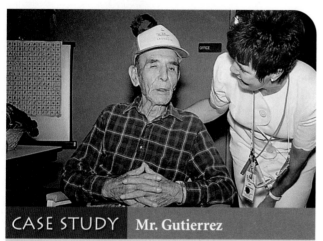

### CASE STUDY  Mr. Gutierrez

Mr. Gutierrez resides in an assisted living apartment of a long-term care center. He busies himself in his small garden plot and enjoys other activities of the center, such as nightly card/bingo games and outings to major league baseball and local museums. He is 82 years old, widowed, and has lived in this particular area of the care center for over 3 years. His family, with whom he is quite close, is scattered across the country. He has one niece who lives in the same town. Mr. Gutierrez feels he is in good health. He believes as long as he eats green chili peppers every day, he will remain healthy. Because he has a small kitchen in his apartment, he is able to make some of his favorite foods. His diet consists of flour and corn tortillas, beans, and rice. He likes most meats, but he prefers chicken and asado (pork). For breakfast he usually has huevos rancheros. He has been hospitalized only twice, once for the flu and once for placement of a pacemaker. He presently takes only three medications: digoxin, Zestril, and Metamucil.

This afternoon Mr. Gutierrez has telephoned his niece for the fourth time. The complaint is always the same: Mr. Gutierrez reports, " My bowels are locked up and haven't moved in the last 2 days." He ate a big meal the previous evening and now reports feeling "all gassed up." His niece tried to explain about eating foods containing fiber and more vegetables but in exasperation reminded Mr. Gutierrez that the nursing student was coming later this afternoon and he could talk to the student about his problem.

Vickie, a 45-year-old married mother of two sons, is Mr. Gutierrez's nursing student. Vickie's oldest son is a freshman at the same college she is attending; the other is a sophomore in high school. Her husband, Roger, is very supportive of her being in school. Vickie has been seeing Mr. Gutierrez once a week for 5 weeks as a portion of a home care clinical experience. They have developed a good rapport. Mr. Gutierrez's self-identified problems with his bowels are a frequent topic of conversation.

### KEY TERMS

cathartics, p. 966
colon, p. 950
constipation, p. 952
defecation, p. 951
diarrhea, p. 953
enema, p. 967
fecal impaction, p. 953
fecal incontinence, p. 953
fecal occult blood test (FOBT), p. 961

feces, p. 951
flatus, p. 950
hemorrhoids, p. 953
laxatives, p. 966
melena, p. 961
ostomy, p. 954
peristalsis, p. 950
segmentation, p. 950
stoma, p. 954
Valsalva maneuver, p. 951

Regular bowel elimination is essential for the maintenance of a healthy body state. Alterations in bowel elimination are often early signs or symptoms of problems within either the gastrointestinal or other body systems. Because bowel function depends on the balance of several factors, elimination patterns and habits vary among individuals.

Although often considered a common and expected occurrence in the older adult, individuals of any age experience changes in intestinal elimination. These changes are sometimes the result of illness, diagnostic testing, the aging process, or surgical intervention. Alterations in intestinal elimination respond to both preventive and supportive nursing care.

## Scientific Knowledge Base

### Anatomy and Physiology of the Gastrointestinal Tract

The gastrointestinal (GI) tract is a series of hollow mucous membrane–lined muscular organs that begin at the mouth and end at the anal orifice. The functions of the GI tract are to break down ingested food for use by the body's cells and to promote the absorption of fluid and nutrients. The GI tract is a complex system, and changes in any one area alter total body functioning.

**MOUTH.** The mouth mechanically and chemically breaks down nutrients into usable size and form. The teeth masticate food, breaking it down into a size suitable for swallowing. Saliva, produced by the salivary glands in the mouth, dilutes and softens the food in the mouth for easier swallowing. Digestion begins in the mouth and ends in the small intestine.

**ESOPHAGUS.** As food enters the upper esophagus, it passes through the upper esophageal sphincter, a circular muscle that prevents air from entering the esophagus and food from refluxing into the throat. The bolus of food travels down the esophagus and **peristalsis,** contractions that propel food through the length of the GI tract, pushes the food.

The food moves down the esophagus and reaches the cardiac sphincter, which lies between the esophagus and the upper end of the stomach. The sphincter prevents reflux of stomach contents back into the esophagus.

**STOMACH.** The stomach performs three tasks: the storage of the swallowed food and liquid; the mixing of food, liquid, and digestive juices; and the emptying of its contents into the small intestine. The stomach produces and secretes hydrochloric acid (HCl), mucus, the enzyme pepsin, and intrinsic factor. Pepsin and HCl facilitate the digestion of protein. Mucus protects the stomach mucosa from acidity and enzyme activity. The intrinsic factor is essential in the absorption of vitamin $B_{12}$.

**SMALL INTESTINE.** Movement within the small intestine, occurring by both **segmentation** and peristalsis (Figure 33-1), facilitates both digestion and absorption. Approximately 7 to 10 L of liquid chyme moves through on an average day. Reabsorption in the small intestine is so efficient that by the time the chyme reaches the end of the small intestine, it is pastelike in consistency, with a volume of 600 to 800 ml (McCance and Huether, 2002). The small intestine is divided into three sections: the duodenum, the jejunum, and the ileum.

The duodenum is approximately 2 feet long and continues to process the chyme from the stomach. The second section, the jejunum, is approximately 9 feet long and has the primary function of absorption of carbohydrates and proteins. The ileum, which is approximately 12 feet long, specializes in the absorption of water, fats, and bile salts. The duodenum and jejunum absorb most nutrients and electrolytes in the small intestine. The ileum absorbs certain vitamins, iron, and bile salts.

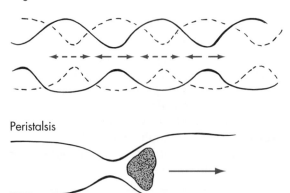

FIGURE **33-1** Segmented and peristaltic waves.

When small intestine function is impaired, this greatly alters the digestive process. Conditions such as inflammation, surgical resection, or obstruction disrupt peristalsis, reduce the area of absorption, or block the passage of chyme. Electrolyte and nutrient deficiencies then develop.

**LARGE INTESTINE.** The lower GI tract is called the large intestine **(colon)** because it is larger in diameter than the small intestine. However, its length (1.5 to 1.8 m [5 to 6 feet]) is much shorter. The large intestine is divided into the cecum, colon, and rectum (Figure 33-2). The large intestine is the primary organ of bowel elimination.

Chyme enters the large intestine by waves of peristalsis through the ileocecal valve, a circular muscle layer that prevents regurgitation. The colon is divided into the ascending, transverse, descending, and sigmoid colons. The colon's muscular tissue allows it to accommodate and eliminate large quantities of waste and gas **(flatus).** The colon has three functions: absorption, secretion, and elimination. The colon absorbs a large volume of water (up to 1.5 L) and significant amounts of sodium and chloride daily (Doughty, 2006). The amount of water absorbed from chyme depends on the speed at which colonic contents move. Chyme is normally a soft, formed mass. If peristalsis is abnormally fast, there is less time for water to be absorbed and the stool will be watery. If peristaltic contractions slow down, water continues to be absorbed and a hard mass of stool forms, resulting in constipation.

The secretory function of the colon aids in electrolyte balance. Bicarbonate is secreted in exchange for chloride. About 4 to 9 mEq of potassium is also excreted daily. Serious alterations in colon function (e.g., diarrhea) cause severe electrolyte disturbances.

Slow peristaltic contractions move contents through the colon. Intestinal content is the main stimulus for contraction. Mass peristalsis pushes undigested food toward the rectum. These mass movements occur only three or four times daily, with the strongest during the hour after mealtime.

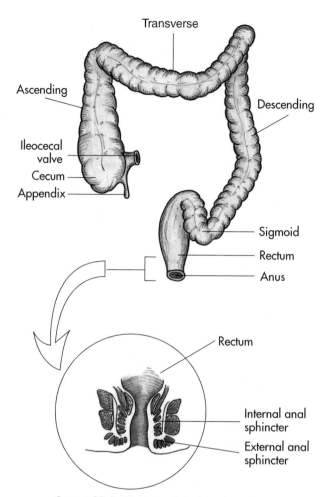

Transverse

Ascending

Descending

Ileocecal
valve

Cecum

Appendix

Sigmoid

Rectum

Anus

Rectum

Internal anal
sphincter

External anal
sphincter

FIGURE **33-2** Divisions of the large intestine.

The rectum is the final portion of the large intestine. Normally, the rectum is empty of waste products (**feces**) until just before defecation. The rectum contains vertical and transverse folds of tissue that help to temporarily hold fecal contents during **defecation.** Each fold contains an artery and veins that can become distended from pressure during straining. This distention results in hemorrhoid formation.

**ANUS.** Feces and flatus (gas) are expelled from the rectum through the anal canal and anus. Contraction and relaxation of the internal and external sphincters, innervated by sympathetic and parasympathetic stimuli, aid in the control of defecation. The anal canal contains a rich supply of sensory nerves that help to control continence.

**DEFECATION.** The physiological factors critical to bowel function and defecation include normal GI tract function, sensory awareness of rectal distention and rectal contents, voluntary sphincter control, and adequate rectal capacity and compliance (Doughty, 2000). Normal defecation begins with movement in the left colon, moving stool toward the anus. When stool reaches the rectum, the distention causes relaxation of the internal sphincter and an awareness of the need to defecate. At the time of defecation,

the external sphincter relaxes and abdominal muscles contract, increasing intrarectal pressure and forcing the stool out (Doughty, 2000). Pressure can be exerted to expel feces through voluntary contractions of the abdominal muscles while maintaining forced expiration against a closed airway. This is termed the **Valsalva maneuver,** and it assists in stool passage. Patients with cardiovascular disease, such as hypertension or abnormal cardiac rhythm, glaucoma, increased intracranial pressure, or a new surgical wound are at risk with this maneuver. Caution them against straining at stool. Normal defecation is painless, resulting in passage of soft, formed stool.

## Nursing Knowledge Base

To manage your patient's elimination problems, you need to understand normal elimination and factors that promote, impede, or cause alterations in elimination, such as constipation, diarrhea, and fecal incontinence (Box 33-1). Supportive nursing care respects the patient's privacy and emotional needs. In addition, interventions designed to promote normal bowel elimination will also minimize discomfort.

Any alteration in bowel elimination is embarrassing for a patient. Because of the sensitivity many patients experience regarding elimination of the bowel with its associated sounds and odors, be very sensitive to communication techniques, especially nonverbal. The patient may perceive changes in facial expression as disgust. Be aware of the patient's need for privacy during elimination.

Patients with chronic diseases of the GI system often have numerous hospitalizations, perhaps multiple surgeries, and significant changes in eating habits and lifestyles. They are often on complicated medication schedules that are taxing both physically and financially. Their desire for wellness sometimes leads them to consider alternative forms of medical treatment, such as vitamin or herbal supplements. It is important for you to remain accepting of patient's health care choices.

Some patients with chronic gastrointestinal diseases require an ostomy, which results in body image changes, with patients losing control over a very basic body function. Even though clothing conceals the ostomy, the patient feels different. The idea of being different or not a whole person affects the patient's social interaction with others, resulting in isolation. Some patients experience difficulty in maintaining or initiating normal sexual relations. One important factor in the patient's acceptance of this change in body functioning is the ability to control fecal secretions. Foul odors, spillage, leakage of liquid stools, and the inability to regulate bowel movements further place the patient at risk for loss of self-esteem.

### Common Bowel Elimination Problems

Alteration in bowel elimination results from a variety of factors. Below is a discussion of some of the more common alterations.

| BOX 33-1 | Factors Influencing Bowel Elimination |

### Age

Infants have a smaller stomach capacity, less secretion of digestive enzymes, and more rapid intestinal peristalsis. The ability to control defecation does not occur until 2 to 3 years of age.

Adolescents experience rapid growth and increased metabolic rate. There is also rapid growth of the large intestine. There is also increased secretion of gastric acids to dissolve food fibers and act as a bactericide against swallowed organisms (McCance and Huether, 2002).

Older adults have decreased chewing ability. Partially chewed food is not digested as easily. Peristalsis declines, and esophageal emptying slows. This impairs absorption by the intestinal mucosa. Muscle tone in the perineal floor and anal sphincter weakens, causing difficulty in controlling defecation (see Box 33-2).

### Diet

Regular daily food intake promotes peristalsis.

High-fiber foods such as raw fruits, cooked fruits, greens, raw vegetables, and whole grains (cereals and breads) promote peristalsis and defecation by creating bulk.

Low-fiber foods (e.g., pasta, lean meats, milk) slow peristalsis.

Gas-producing foods (e.g., broccoli, cauliflower, onions, dried beans) stimulate peristalsis.

Persons with lactose intolerance lack the enzyme lactose, which is needed to digest the simple sugars in milk. Such intolerance leads to diarrhea and cramping.

### Position During Defecation

Squatting allows a person to lean forward, exert intraabdominal pressure, and contract thigh muscles to normally defecate.

Older adults or those with arthritis are sometimes unable to rise from a toilet seat.

Immobilized patients, required to use a bedpan while lying, cannot contract muscles to defecate.

### Pregnancy

As pregnancy advances and the fetus enlarges, this exerts pressure on the rectum. Constipation commonly occurs.

### Diagnostic Tests

Certain examinations involving visualization of GI structures require the emptying of bowel contents. Patients receive nothing by mouth (NPO), bowel evacuants, and enema administration to cleanse the bowel before a test. These factors interfere with normal elimination.

Barium examinations require ingestion of barium, a mixture that hardens and causes serious constipation unless eliminated soon after a test.

### Fluid Intake

The body absorbs fluid into the fecal mass and increases bulk for easier passage.

Hot beverages and fruit juices soften stool and increase peristalsis.

Large quantities of milk slow peristalsis and cause constipation.

### Activity

Immobilization depresses colon motility.

Regular physical exercise promotes peristalsis.

### Psychological Factors

Stress, anxiety, or fear initiates parasympathetic impulses, causing the acceleration of digestion and peristalsis. Diarrhea and gaseous distention will result.

Emotional depression decreases peristalsis and leads to constipation.

### Personal Habits

Personal habits such as failing to respond to the need to defecate and lack of privacy interfere with normal elimination patterns and lead to constipation.

Hospitalized patients often share toilet facilities or use bedpans or bedside commodes. The resulting embarrassment causes them to ignore the urge to defecate.

### Pain

Hemorrhoids, rectal surgery, and abdominal surgery cause a patient to suppress defecation because of pain; constipation develops.

### Medications

Laxatives and cathartics soften stool and promote peristalsis.

Antidiarrheal agents inhibit peristalsis.

Narcotic analgesics, opiates, and anticholinergic drugs depress peristalsis and cause constipation.

Antibiotics alter normal bowel flora and produce diarrhea.

Drugs that contain iron sometimes turn the stool black. Antacids cause a white discoloration. Anticoagulants result in frank or occult blood in the stool.

### Surgery and Anesthesia

General anesthetics cause slowing or halting of peristalsis.

Surgery involving bowel manipulation temporarily stops peristalsis (paralytic ileus) for 24 to 48 hours.

---

**CONSTIPATION. Constipation** is a symptom and usually includes infrequent bowel movements, difficult passage of feces, inability to defecate at will, and hard feces (Dosh, 2002). Common causes of constipation include changes in diet, medications, inflammation, environmental factors (e.g., unavailability of toilet facilities or lack of privacy), and lack of knowledge about regular bowel habits (Box 33-2). In the older adult, constipation is usually diet related, most commonly a lack of fiber (Thompson and others, 2003). Regardless of etiology, intestinal motility slows, causing prolonged exposure of the fecal mass to the intestinal walls. Fecal water continues to be absorbed, leaving the stool hard

## BOX 33-2 Common Causes of Constipation

- Irregular bowel habits and ignoring the urge to defecate.
- Chronic illnesses (e.g., Parkinson's disease, multiple sclerosis, rheumatoid arthritis, chronic bowel diseases, depression, eating disorders) (Annells and Koch, 2002; Richmond, 2003).
- Low-fiber diet high in animal fats (e.g., meats, dairy products, eggs) and refined sugars (rich desserts). Also, low fluid intake slows peristalsis (Bliss and others, 2001).
- Situational stress (e.g., illness of a family member, death of a loved one, divorce) (Dosh, 2002).
- Lengthy bed rest or physical inactivity (Thompson and others, 2003).
- Heavy laxative use causes loss of normal defecation reflex. In addition, the lower colon is completely emptied, requiring time to refill with bulk (Annells and Koch, 2002).
- Older adults experience slowed peristalsis, loss of abdominal muscle elasticity, and reduced intestinal mucus secretion. Older adults often eat low-fiber foods (Dosh, 2002).
- Neurological conditions that block nerve impulses to the colon (e.g., spinal cord injury, tumor).
- Organic illnesses such as hypothyroidism, hypocalcemia, or hypokalemia (Richmond, 2003).

and underlubricated. Constipation causes abdominal distension, loss of appetite, nausea/vomiting, and bad breath (Thompson and others, 2003).

Constipation is a significant threat to a patient's well-being. Straining during defecation is contraindicated for patients with cardiovascular problems or for those who have had recent abdominal or rectal surgery. Patients who exert effort to pass a stool experience Valsalva maneuver. When a person strains, this maneuver causes blood to be trapped in veins within the chest, and upon relaxing the venous blood rushes to the heart. Because of an increased venous return the heart is overloaded, which results in an increased cardiac workload, leading to possible cardiac dysrhythmias or angina. The Valsalva maneuver also traps blood in the veins of the abdomen, causing increases in intraabdominal pressure, which leads to stress on suture lines.

**IMPACTION. Fecal impaction** results from unrelieved constipation. It is a collection of hardened feces wedged in the rectum that the patient is unable to expel. In severe impaction the hardened fecal mass extends up into the sigmoid colon. Patients at greatest risk for impaction include those who are confused or unconscious, badly constipated, or those who have experienced an interruption in nerve supply to the bowel.

An obvious sign of impaction is the inability to pass a stool for several days, despite a repeated urge to defecate. When a continuous oozing of diarrhea stool develops, this indicates impaction. This diarrhea is liquid stool seeping around the fecal mass. Anorexia, abdominal distention and cramping, nausea and/or vomiting, and rectal pain also occur.

**DIARRHEA. Diarrhea** is an increased frequency in the passage of loose stools (Table 33-1). Fluid and electrolyte

imbalances result from diarrhea. Older adults and the very young are at the greatest risk for electrolyte imbalance. Because of the irritating effects of the intestinal contents, persistent diarrhea readily leads to skin breakdown in the perianal region.

The aim of treatment is first to maintain adequate hydration. Parenteral replacement of fluids is necessary when the patient is at risk for fluid and electrolyte imbalance. You will aim interventions at identifying and correcting causative factors. Depending on the cause, you use antispasmodic or antidiarrheal medications to slow peristalsis.

**INCONTINENCE. Fecal incontinence** is the inability to control the passage of feces and gas from the anus. Any condition that impairs function or control of the anal sphincter causes fecal incontinence. Conditions creating frequent, loose, large-volume, watery stools also predispose a patient to incontinence. Some of these conditions may be from nosocomial infections, such as *Clostridium difficile*, or iatrogenic effects of treatment, such as tube feedings or antibiotic therapy (Bliss and others, 2000).

Management of fecal incontinence requires a complete understanding of the causes. The presence of diarrhea is frequently associated with the incontinence episodes. In some situations this diarrhea is due to diet, antibiotic use, or a combination of both. Antibiotics alter the normal flora in the gastrointestinal tract, causing diarrhea to occur. Diets with inadequate fiber affect the bulk of the stool and absorption of water into the fecal mass.

In many situations the patient is mentally alert but physically unable to avoid defecation. Some patients may have little or no warning before the incontinence episode of loose, watery diarrhea presents itself.

Incontinence affects patients in many ways. Because of the associated embarrassment, incontinence leads to social isolation, changes in body image, sexuality (see Chapter 20), and feelings of inadequacy or guilt. Like diarrhea, incontinence predisposes the patient to skin breakdown.

**FLATULENCE. Flatulence** (gas) is one of the most common GI disorders. It refers to a sensation of bloating and abdominal distention accompanied by excess gas. As gas accumulates in the lumen of the intestines, the bowel wall stretches and distends. Normally, intestinal gas escapes through the mouth (belching) or the anus. However, when there is a reduction in the intestinal motility resulting from analgesics (usually opiates), general anesthetic, abdominal surgery, or immobilization, flatulence becomes severe, causing abdominal distention and severe sharp pain (Gong, 2004).

**HEMORRHOIDS. Hemorrhoids** are made up of a mass of dilated blood vessels that lie beneath the lining of the skin in the anal mucosa. Increased venous pressure resulting from straining at defecation, pregnancy, and chronic illnesses, such as congestive heart failure and chronic liver disease, lead to hemorrhoids. Passage of hard stool causes hemorrhoid tissue to stretch and bleed. Hemorrhoid tissue becomes inflamed and tender, and patients complain of itching, and burning. Because pain worsens during defecation,

| TABLE 33-1 | Conditions That Cause Diarrhea |
|---|---|
| **Condition** | **Physiological Effects** |
| Emotional stress (anxiety) | Increased intestinal motility |
| Intestinal infection (streptococcal or staphylococcal enteritis) | Inflammation of intestinal mucosa, increased mucus secretion in colon |
| Food allergies | Reduced digestion of food elements |
| Food intolerance (greasy foods, coffee, alcohol, spicy foods) | Increased intestinal motility, increased mucus secretion in colon |
| Tube feedings | Hyperosmolarity of some enteral solutions results in diarrhea, because hyperosmolar fluids draw fluids into the gastrointestinal tract |
| Medications | |
| Iron | Irritation of intestinal mucosa |
| Antibiotics | Suprainfection allowing overgrowth of normal flora, inflammation and irritation of mucosa |
| Laxatives (short term) | Increased intestinal motility |
| Inflammatory bowel disease (colitis, Crohn's disease) | Inflammation and ulceration of intestinal walls, reduced absorption of fluids, increased intestinal motility |
| Surgical alterations | |
| Gastrectomy | Loss of reservoir function of stomach, improper absorption because food moves into duodenum too quickly |
| Colon resection | Reduced size of colon, reduced amount of absorptive surface |

the patient sometimes ignores the urge to defecate, resulting in constipation.

**BOWEL DIVERSIONS.** Certain diseases prevent the normal passage of intestinal contents throughout the small and large bowel. The treatment for these disorders results in the need for a temporary or permanent artificial opening (**stoma**) in the abdominal wall. Surgical openings are made in the ileum (ileostomy) or colon (colostomy) by bringing the end of the intestine through the abdominal wall to create the stoma.

The standard bowel diversion creates a stoma, or the patient has reconstructive surgery that uses the native sphincter. The reconstructive surgery includes either a continent stoma procedure (rarely done anymore) or reconstructive surgery, the ileoanal pouch anastomosis, which is described in a later section (Colwell and others, 2001).

**Ostomies.** The location of the **ostomy** determines stool consistency. The more intestine remaining, the more formed and normal the stool. For example, an ileostomy bypasses the entire large intestine, creating frequent, liquid stools. The sigmoid colostomy emits near-normal stool. The location of an ostomy depends on the patient's medical problem and general condition.

Loop colostomies are frequently done on an emergency basis and are temporary large stomas constructed in the transverse colon (Figure 33-3). The surgeon pulls a loop of bowel onto the abdomen and places a plastic rod, bridge, or rubber catheter temporarily under the bowel loop to keep it from slipping back. The surgeon then opens the bowel and sutures it to the skin of the abdomen. The loop ostomy has two openings through the stoma. The proximal end drains stool, and the distal portion drains mucus.

The end colostomy consists of one stoma formed from the proximal end of the bowel with the distal portion of the

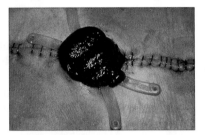

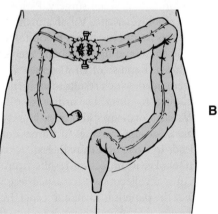

FIGURE **33-3 A**, A temporary transverse loop colostomy supported by a loop ostomy bridge. **B**, Abdominal view of loop colostomy in transverse colon. (**A** courtesy Hollister Incorporated, Libertyville, Ill. Permission to use this copyrighted material has been granted by the owner, Hollister Incorporated. **B** from Hampton BG, Bryant RA: *Ostomies and continent diversions: nursing management*, St. Louis, 1992, Mosby.)

GI tract either removed or sewn closed (called Hartmann's pouch) and left in the abdominal cavity. End colostomies are a surgical treatment for colorectal cancer. In such cases, the rectum is sometimes removed. Patients with diverticulitis

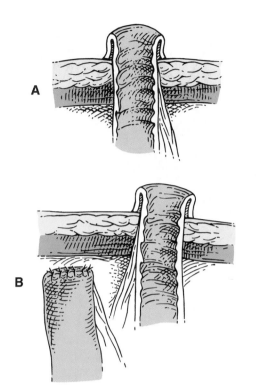

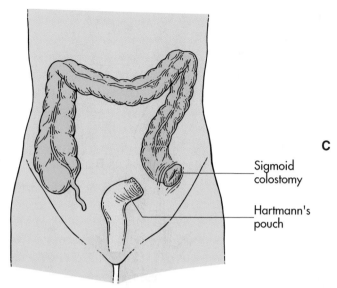

FIGURE **33-4** End colostomy. **A,** Cross-sectional view of end stoma. **B,** Cross-sectional view of end stoma with distal bowel oversewn and secured to anterior peritoneum at stoma site. **C,** Sigmoid colostomy. Distal bowel is oversewn and left in place to create Hartmann's pouch. (From Hampton BG, Bryant RA: *Ostomies and continent diversions: nursing management,* St. Louis, 1992, Mosby.)

often have a temporary end colostomy constructed with a Hartmann's pouch (Figure 33-4).

Unlike the loop colostomy, surgeons surgically sever the bowel in a double-barrel colostomy (Figure 33-5) and the two ends are brought out onto the abdomen. The double-barrel colostomy consists of two distinct stomas: the proximal functioning stoma and the distal nonfunctioning stoma (mucous fistula).

A stoma that produces frequent passage of liquid stool (e.g., an ileostomy) creates a management challenge. Skin protection is important because of the liquid and caustic nature of the output, which may cause contact dermatitis, fungal infections, or folliculitis (Wound, Ostomy, and Continence Nurses Society [WOCN], 2005). A pouch with a skin barrier surrounds the stoma, and the pouch is emptied several times a day. The pouching system is changed approximately every 3 to 5 days depending upon the type of system utilized.

A colostomy located in the descending or sigmoid portion of the colon discharges stool only once a day. Some patients choose to use removable pouches that are discarded rather than emptying a pouch. An option for the patient with a sigmoid stoma is to irrigate the stoma, training the bowel to empty stool at a specific time. A person who irrigates the stoma uses a small cap over the stoma for protection (Colwell and others, 2001).

**Alternative Procedures.** The ileoanal pouch anastomosis is a newer surgical procedure that is an option for some patients who need to undergo a colectomy, removal of the colon, for treatment of ulcerative colitis or familial polyposis. In this procedure the colon is removed, a pouch is created from the

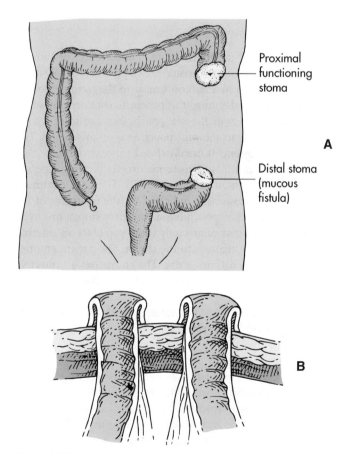

FIGURE **33-5** Double-barrel colostomy. **A,** Double-barrel colostomy in the descending colon. **B,** Cross-sectional view of double-barrel stoma. (From Hampton BG, Bryant RA: *Ostomies and continent diversions: nursing management,* St. Louis, 1992, Mosby.)

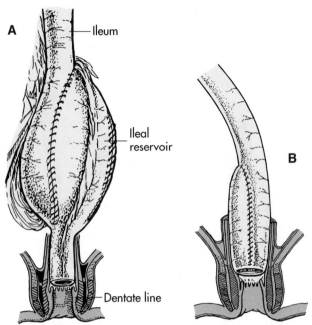

FIGURE **33-6** Ileoanal reservoirs (IARs). **A,** S-shaped configuration. **B,** J-shaped configuration. (From Hampton BG, Bryant RA: *Ostomies and continent diversions: nursing management,* St. Louis, 1992, Mosby.)

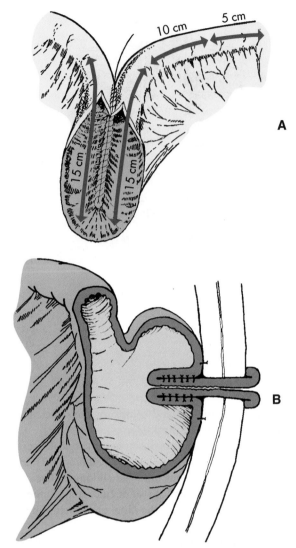

FIGURE **33-7** Construction of Kock continent ileostomy—Kock pouch. **A,** Two 15-cm limbs are used to create pouch, and one 15-cm limb is used to fashion a nipple valve and stoma. **B,** Distal limb is intussuscepted into reservoir to create a one-way valve and accomplish continence. Sutures or staples or both are placed to stabilize and maintain nipple. Anterior surface of reservoir is anchored to anterior peritoneal wall. (From Hampton BG, Bryant RA: *Ostomies and continent diversions: nursing management,* St. Louis, 1992, Mosby.)

end of the small intestine, and the pouch is attached to the anus (Figure 33-6). The ileoanal pouch provides for collection of waste material in a fashion similar to the rectum. Stool is evacuated from the anus; the patient is continent of stool. When surgeons create the ileal pouch, they also make a temporary ileostomy to allow the pouch anastomosis to heal. The temporary ileostomy is usually closed 3 months later.

The Kock continent ileostomy involves creating a pouch from the small intestine (Figure 33-7). The Kock continent ileostomy is occasionally indicated for the treatment of ulcerative colitis. The pouch has a continent stoma, or a type of nipple valve that drains only when you place an external catheter intermittently into the stoma. The patient empties the pouch several times a day. The stoma has a protective dressing or stoma cap (Colwell and others, 2001).

## Critical Thinking

### Synthesis

As you begin the problem-solving process of caring for a patient experiencing bowel elimination problems, it becomes important to reflect on the knowledge, experience, critical thinking attitudes, and standards of care that will improve patient outcomes. Assuming the proper attitudes of critical thinking will enable you to design an individualized approach to care.

**KNOWLEDGE.** Reflect on knowledge regarding normal anatomy and physiology of the GI tract, as well as knowledge regarding specific GI alterations. This information will help you more accurately focus your nursing assessment and identify alterations when they exist. Even insignificant alterations in bowel elimination produce significant health problems for the patient. For example, diarrhea leads to electrolyte imbalances, dehydration, and rectal soreness.

Abdominal pain is one of the most common complaints of patients who seek health care. Apply knowledge of the nature of pain (see Chapter 30) and pain assessment to accurately analyze elimination problems. This helps in determining if the pain causes the symptoms associated with altered bowel elimination or conversely if the bowel elimination problem results in pain or discomfort.

Functional bowel disorders make up the most frequently reported GI complaints. It is important that you have the knowledge from anatomy and physiology, as well as information from the psychosocial sciences, to understand and consider the psychological aspects associated with these diseases to provide appropriate care.

The intake of certain foods also reflects the patient's culture or beliefs. Foods in various cultures have different status relating to religion, availability, cost, and tradition. For example, some Hispanic Americans use certain hot foods (e.g., chocolate, cheese, and eggs) for conditions producing fever, and cold foods (e.g., fresh vegetables, dairy foods, and honey) are for disorders such as cancer or headaches (Giger and Davidhizar, 2004). Understand the patient's cultural heritage and the role diet plays in health promotion and maintenance (see Chapter 17).

When caring for patients from other cultures and ethnic groups, modifications of care are frequent. This is particularly of importance when you provide care related to your patients' elimination needs (Box 33-3).

A final area of knowledge is an understanding of those changes occurring as a result of the aging process. Far too often nurses discount an older adult's problems with intestinal elimination as an everyday complaint. Remember that what appears at the outset to be quite insignificant is sometimes a major problem to the patient physically and psychologically.

**EXPERIENCE.** Elimination alterations are common for many patients who seek health care. In the acute care environment numerous variables, including diet changes, medications, fluid restrictions, decreased activity, and diagnostic tests, cause major alterations to bowel function. You will provide better care to patients by reflecting on your previous experiences involving patients with similar alterations and similar lifestyle habits affecting elimination.

**ATTITUDES.** Apply all of the attitudes of critical thinking when caring for a patient with elimination problems. Creativity comes into play, especially when patients need adjustments in their diet and exercise planning or when caring for patients with a bowel diversion. Similarly, perseverance is important in selecting effective diet therapies and in finding the best appliances for ostomy patients. Confidence is an important factor in providing care to patients with bowel diversions or resections. Often these patients are very ill and in significant pain. Your confidence with moving and positioning the patient, handling stoma supplies, and managing pain will place the patient at ease and facilitate the recovery process.

**STANDARDS.** To establish regular bowel habits, patients require consistency in bowel care and training. It is possible to establish regular bowel habits by setting standards for appropriate nutritional and elimination support. For example, the Association for Parenteral and Enteral Nutrition (ASPEN) has specific guideline for nutritional support (see Chapter 31). The Wound, Ostomy, and Continence Nurses Society (WOCN,

---

**BOX 33-3   CULTURAL FOCUS**

As Vickie prepares to care for Mr. Gutierrez she learns that people from different cultures have different beliefs and practices. She knows that Mr. Gutierrez keeps many of his cultural practices and it is important that she understand early in his care how his culture and customs may impact her care plan. Elimination needs are very personal, and Vickie knows she needs to respect and be sensitive to her patient's elimination practices.

**Implications for Practice**

- Accommodate need for gender-congruent care among cultures emphasizing separate gender roles and female modesty such as African, Hispanic, Asian, Islamic, Arabic, Hindu, Jewish Orthodox, and Amish cultures.
- In any culture the presence and care of an ostomy presents unique challenges. New ostomies require monitoring and observation, and patients from other cultures may find this more invasive and embarrassing.
  - Most cultures consider bowel and urinary secretions as not fit for public display. However, exposure of the lower torso, which is needed for ostomy care, is generally avoided among Asians, Africans, Hispanics, Hindus, Muslims, Arabic, Orthodox Jewish, and Amish groups.
    - When caring for patients with ostomies from these cultures, it is helpful to assign gender-congruent caregivers if possible and to allow presence of a family member if requested by the patient.
- Provide for hygiene needs of patients.
  - Distinct hygienic practices are observed by certain cultures such as Hindus and Muslims that designate the left hand to perform unclean procedures such as bowel elimination.
  - Wash your hands before touching the patient, and use your right hand.
- Promote understanding of patients of the procedure to be done.
  - Use an interpreter if needed.
    - Repeat explanations because patient's anxiety about the loss of privacy can pose a distraction.

---

2004a, 2004b, 2005) has specific standards for ostomy care. Regardless of age or disease state, maintenance of bowel function and integrity is essential to well-being.

When assessing a patient's abdominal pain, make sure your findings are specific, clear, precise, and accurate. Although the intellectual standards for critical thinking apply to all symptoms, thorough pain assessment is critical. A multitude of problems are detectable on the basis of the nature of abdominal pain. Physicians or health care providers will collaborate with you on your assessment to identify the appropriate medical diagnosis.

Patients with alterations in bowel elimination, especially incontinence, are at risk for ridicule and shame on the part of some health care providers. This is especially true for providers with limited educational experience, to whom the task of patient hygiene is often delegated. It is your responsibility to make certain such individuals understand the needs of these patients and attend to their needs in a respectful way.

## Nursing Process

The needs and problems of patients experiencing alterations in bowel elimination are distinct and numerous. Incorporate assessment skills and use appropriate communication techniques throughout the care planning process.

### Assessment

Assessment of bowel elimination requires you to review any complaints the patient has affecting the GI system. Because the patient's chewing ability, recent intake of both solids and liquids, personal eating habits, and level of stress all influence bowel function, include this information in your assessment (Norton and Chelvanayagam, 2000).

**HEALTH HISTORY.** In determining the patient's bowel habits, remember "normal" is unique to each individual. Apply this knowledge in preparing questions for the patient interview to determine the presence and extent of GI alterations. Family members are usually helpful if the patient is unable to provide necessary information. You will organize much of the nursing history around factors that affect bowel elimination (Norton and Chelvanayagam, 2000):

1. Determine your patient's usual pattern of bowel elimination. Usual frequency and time of day are important, but you also determine if any changes in elimination patterns have occurred. Ask patient to make suggestions about the reason for any change.
2. Get the patient's description of usual characteristics of stool. Determine whether the stool is normally watery or formed, soft or hard, and the typical color. Ask the patient to describe a normal stool's shape and the number of stools per day.
3. Identify specific routines followed to promote normal elimination. Examples are drinking hot liquids, laxatives, eating specific foods, or taking time to defecate during a certain part of the day. If your patient uses a specific routine, be sure to ask about how the routine is followed.
4. Assess the use of artificial aids at home, for example, the use of enemas, laxatives, or special foods before having a bowel movement. Ask how often the patient uses them.
5. Determine the presence and status of artificial orifices. If the patient has an ostomy, assess the frequency of fecal drainage, character of feces, type of appliance used, and methods used to maintain the ostomy function.
6. Identify changes in appetite. Include changes in your patient's eating patterns and a change in weight, either loss or gain. If a change in weight is present, inquire if the patient planned the weight change, such as weight loss with a diet.
7. Ask about diet history, including the patient's dietary preferences. Is mealtime regular or irregular, and does the patient eat certain foods infrequently? This enables you to determine the intake of grains, fruits, meats, and vegetables.
8. Get a description of daily fluid intake. This includes the type and amount of fluid. Have the patient estimate the amount using common household measurements. You can ask the patient to give you a 24-hour diet recall during your assessment. You may also want to ask the patient to complete a 72-hour food intake diary for the next visit.
9. Get a history of surgery or illnesses affecting the GI tract. This information often helps to explain symptoms, the potential for maintaining or restoring a normal elimination pattern, and whether there is a family history of cancer involving the GI tract.
10. Ask about medication history. Determine whether the patient takes medications that alter defecation or fecal characteristics.
11. Assess the patient's emotional state. Observe patient's emotional state, including tone of voice and mannerisms, which will reveal significant behaviors indicating stress.
12. Get a history of exercise. Obtain a description of the type, frequency, and amount of daily exercise.
13. Get a history of pain or discomfort. Ask the patient whether there is a history of abdominal or anal pain. The location and nature of pain helps to locate the source of a problem (see Chapter 30).
14. Find out the patient's social history. If the patient is not independent in bowel management, determine methods and degree of assistance required.
15. Assess for mobility and dexterity. Determine your patient's ability to toilet independently or if the patient needs assistive devices or personnel.

**PHYSICAL ASSESSMENT.** Assess the status of GI function to detect factors that affect elimination, and gather data regarding the patient's elimination problems. Table 33-2 demonstrates how to focus your patient assessment to identify problems associated with bowel elimination. You will need to conduct an examination of the oral cavity, abdomen, and anus and rectal canal (see Chapter 13).

When a digital examination is necessary, inspect the fecal material on the glove for several characteristics (Table 33-3). If there are no feces on the glove, ask the patient to describe a typical stool, noting recent changes. The patient or primary caregiver is the most knowledgeable about changes. You also determine whether the patient passes an unusual amount of or little gas.

**LABORATORY AND DIAGNOSTIC EXAMINATIONS**
**Laboratory Tests.** Several laboratory tests are available to assist in diagnosing problems with the GI system, including the following blood tests:

Total bilirubin—a degraded product of hemoglobin excreted in the bile. Elevated in hepatobiliary diseases.
Alkaline phosphatase—an enzyme found in many tissues. Elevated in obstructive hepatobiliary diseases and carcinomas, bone tumors, and healing fractures.

## FOCUSED PATIENT ASSESSMENT                    TABLE 33-2

| Factors to Assess | Questions and Approaches | Physical Assessment Strategies |
|---|---|---|
| Chewing | Ask if patient has difficulty chewing. Ask if patient has dentures. | Inspect condition of teeth, tongue, gums, and mouth. Observe for fit of dentures, observing for sores or pressure areas from dentures. Observe patient eating meal, determine patient's ability to eat all types of foods. |
| Mobility | **In Ambulatory Patients** Ask patient about activity/exercise patterns. **For Patients With Restricted Mobility** Determine patient's frequency in using toileting facilities independently. Ask patient and family how much assistance patient needs for toileting. | Observe patient's gait. Observe patient's ability to assist with transfer, positioning, and activity. |
| Abdomen | Ask patient to relax and breathe normally. Ask if patient feels any gas or distention or if there is any pain or discomfort. If pain or discomfort is present, ask patient to point to the area of tenderness. | Observe all four abdominal quadrants, noting the presence of scars, masses, venous patterns, stomas, lesions, and peristaltic waves. Auscultate all four quadrants for the presence of bowel sounds; determine if these sounds are normal, hypoactive (less than 5 sounds per minute), hyperactive (greater than 35 sounds per minute), or absent (no auscultated bowel sounds). Gently palpate all four quadrants, noting areas of distention, masses, or pain. When pain is present, note the location. Percuss, or tap, all four quadrants. |
| Abdominal muscle contractility | Instruct patient to "bear down" while lightly palpating the abdominal wall. | Palpate lower abdomen for muscle contraction and distention. |
| Anal sphincter function | Ask if patient is able to sense bowel distention, because an inability to sense bowel distention impairs patient's ability to evacuate bowel. | Inspect anal sphincter at rest, and perform digital examination while asking patient to contract and relax sphincter. NOTE: A small amount of stool is normal; large amount or hard stool indicates impaired emptying of bowel. |

## TABLE 33-3   Fecal Characteristics

| Characteristic | Normal | Abnormal | Abnormal Cause |
|---|---|---|---|
| Color | Infant: yellow; adult: brown | White or clay | Absence of bile |
| | | Black or tarry (melena) | Iron ingestion or upper GI bleeding |
| | | Red | Lower GI bleeding, hemorrhoids, ingestion of beets |
| | | Pale with fat | Malabsorption of fat |
| | | Translucent mucus | Spastic constipation, colitis, excess straining |
| | | Bloody mucus | Blood in feces, inflammation, infection |
| Odor | Pungent; affected by food type | Noxious change | Blood in feces or infection |
| Consistency | Soft, formed | Liquid | Diarrhea, reduced absorption |
| | | Hard | Constipation |
| Frequency | Varies: infant 4 to 6 times daily (breast-fed) or 1 to 3 times daily (bottle fed); adult daily or 2 to 3 times a week | Infant more than 6 times daily or less than once every 1 to 2 days; adult more than 3 times a day or less than once a week | Hypomotility or hypermotility |
| Amount | 150 g per day (adult) | | |
| Shape | Resembles diameter of rectum | Narrow, pencil shaped | Obstruction, rapid peristalsis |
| Constituents | Undigested food, dead bacteria, fat, bile pigment, cells lining intestinal mucosa, water | Blood, pus, foreign bodies, mucus, worms | Internal bleeding, infection, swallowed objects, irritation, inflammation |
| | | Excess fat | Malabsorption syndrome, enteritis, pancreatic disease, surgical resection of intestine |

## SYNTHESIS IN PRACTICE

When Vickie prepared to conduct an assessment of Mr. Gutierrez, she reflected back on experiences with other patients in the home setting. She recalled one patient in particular who had elimination problems resulting from a diet consisting mainly of high-fat and high-carbohydrate foods. She thought that her involvement with that patient was likely help in the care of Mr. Gutierrez.

Vickie also reviewed her class notes on the anatomy and physiology of the GI system. Given Mr. Gutierrez's age, Vickie focused on reviewing the physiological changes that aging produces within the GI system. These changes include loss of teeth, taste bud atrophy, decreased secretion of gastric acid, and a slight decrease in small intestine motility.

Vickie will thoroughly assess Mr. Gutierrez's dietary intake by using a 24-hour diet recall. Being familiar with Mr. Gutierrez's

Hispanic heritage, Vickie anticipates certain food preferences and will need to assess these. Vickie knows Mr. Gutierrez does not like the food served at the long-term care center and frequently requests "home cooked" tortillas and green chili peppers from his niece.

The symptoms Mr. Gutierrez exhibits, no bowel movement in 2 days and a feeling of bloating, is associated with several different problems. Vickie plans a thorough and precise assessment, being sure to rule out any abdominal discomfort or other symptoms expected from elimination problems. Because problems with bowel elimination have been an ongoing concern for Mr. Gutierrez, Vickie will persevere as she begins to identify nursing diagnoses and outline goals of care. Vickie will need to avoid preconceived ideas regarding constipation in older adults. She will remain open to all the possibilities concerning changes in GI functioning.

---

| **BOX 33-4** | PROCEDURAL GUIDELINES FOR |

### Measuring Fecal Occult Blood

**Delegation Considerations:** You can delegate this skill to assistive personnel. However, it is your responsibility to assess the significance of the findings.

**Equipment:** Hemoccult test paper, Hemoccult developer, and wooden applicator (see illustration), disposable gloves.

1. Explain purpose of test and ways patient will assist. Some patients collect own specimen, if possible.
2. Perform hand hygiene.
3. Apply clean, disposable gloves.
4. Use tip of wooden applicator (see equipment illustration) to obtain a small portion of uncontaminated stool specimen. Be sure specimen is free of toilet paper.
5. Perform Hemoccult slide test:
   a. Open flap of slide, and, using a wooden applicator, thinly smear stool in first box of the guaiac paper. Apply a second fecal specimen from a different portion of the stool to slide's second box (see illustration).
   b. Close slide cover, and turn the packet over to reverse side (see illustration). Open cardboard flap, and apply two drops of developing solution on each box of guaiac paper. A blue color indicates a positive guaiac, or presence of fecal occult blood.

   c. Observe the color of the guaiac paper after 30 to 60 seconds.
   d. Dispose of test slide in proper receptacle.
6. Wrap wooden applicator in paper towel, remove gloves, and discard in proper receptacle.
7. Perform hand hygiene.
8. Record results of test; note any unusual fecal characteristics.

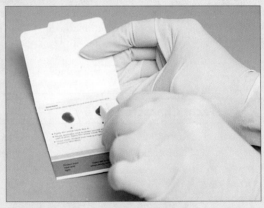

STEP **5a** Application of fecal specimen on guaiac paper.

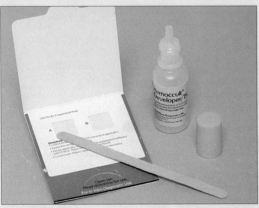

STEP **4** Equipment needed for fecal occult blood testing.

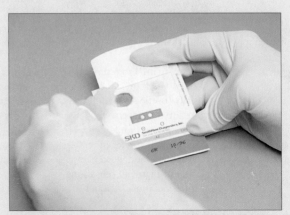

STEP **5b** Application of Hemoccult developing solution on the guaiac paper on the reverse side of test kit.

---

**BOX 33-5** **Screening for Colon Cancer**

**Risk Factors**

- Age: over 50 (more than 90% of cases diagnosed over age of 50)
- Personal or family history: colorectal cancer, polyps, inflammatory bowel disease
- Genetic predisposition
- Race: African Americans have highest colon cancer rates
- Diet: high intake of animal fats or red meat and low intake of fruits and vegetables
- Obesity and physical inactivity
- Smoking
- Alcohol consumption

**Warning Signs**

- Change in bowel habits (e.g., diarrhea, constipation, narrowing of stool lasting more than few days)

- Rectal bleeding or blood in stool
- A sensation of incomplete evacuation
- Cramping or gnawing stomach pain
- Decreased appetite
- Weakness and fatigue

*Beginning at age 50 both men and women should follow **one** of these five screening options.*

**Screening Tests**

- Yearly fecal occult blood test (FOBT) or fecal immunochemical test (FIT)*
- Flexible sigmoidoscopy every 5 years (FSIG)
- Yearly FOBT or FIT and flexible sigmoidoscopy every 5 years†
- A double contrast barium edema every 5 years
- A colonoscopy every 10 years

© 2004 American Cancer Society, Inc. www.cancer.org. Reprinted with permission.
*FOBT or FIT should be done at home following manufacturer's recommendations and not in the doctor's office.
†Combined testing is preferred over either annual FOBT or FIT, or FSIG every 5 years, alone.

---

Amylase—an enzyme secreted by the pancreas. Elevated in conditions of the pancreas, such as inflammation or tumors. Also elevated in cholecystitis, necrotic bowel, and diabetic ketoacidosis.

Carcinoembryonic antigen (CEA)—a protein. It is typically elevated in persons with cancers of the GI tract or hepatobiliary organs.

*Fecal Specimens.* Analysis of fecal contents will also detect alterations in GI functioning. A person who handles a specimen improperly will easily acquire bacteria. Follow standard precautions when coming in contact with the specimen (see Chapter 11). The patient is often capable of obtaining the specimen without assistance, if properly instructed. Make sure the patient understands not to mix feces with urine or water. The patient defecates into a clean, dry bedpan or special container placed under the toilet seat.

Laboratory tests for blood in the stool and stool cultures require only a small sample. Researchers believe that minimum abrasions of the intestinal mucosa cause blood loss of 1 to 3 ml daily in feces (Norton and Chelvanayagam, 2000). Blood loss of over 50 ml appears as **melena.** To detect quantities less than 50 ml of blood, you will need a laboratory analysis. Collect approximately an inch of formed stool or 15 to 30 ml of liquid diarrhea stool. Tests for measuring the output of fecal fat require the patient to collect stools for 3 to 5 days. All fecal material needs to be saved throughout the test period. Some tests require a chemical preservative.

After obtaining a specimen, tightly seal the container, complete laboratory requisition forms, and record all specimen collections in the patient's medical record. Avoid delays in sending specimens to the laboratory. Some tests require the stool to be warm. When stool specimens are allowed to stand at room temperature, bacteriological changes occur that alter test results.

A common test is the **fecal occult blood test (FOBT),** which measures microscopic amounts of blood in the feces (Box 33-4). It is a useful screening test for colon cancer (Box 33-5). One positive result does not confirm GI bleeding. The test is repeated at least 3 times while the patient refrains from ingesting foods and medications that cause a false-positive result. The FOBT is done in the patient's home or physician's or health care provider's office. FOBT is a screening tool, not a diagnostic tool (American Cancer Society [ACS], 2004). Current recommendations include the combination of yearly FOBT plus flexible sigmoidoscopy every 5 years. All positive tests should be followed up with colonoscopy (ACS, 2004).

When your patients are going to have an FBOT, it is important for you to instruct them in which foods to avoid, because some foods cause a false-positive test result. Examples of these foods and medications include red meat, poultry, fish, some raw vegetables, vitamin C, and aspirin (Ransohoff and Lang, 1997). Patients on anticoagulants are at risk for developing GI bleeding and are regularly screened with this test.

**Diagnostic Examinations.** For patients experiencing alterations in the GI system, there are a variety of radiological and diagnostic tests. The preparation and the test itself are often quite unpleasant for the patient. See Box 33-6 for an explanation of these tests.

**PATIENT EXPECTATIONS.** When you assess the patient's expectations of care, it is helpful to anticipate the patient's need for privacy and respect. Bowel elimination problems are embarrassing for some. Ask the patient what is important to ensure that you give care in a personal and professional way.

Because there is a direct link between nutrition and bowel elimination, consider the patient's cultural choices of foods and fluids. Sometimes the patient will have to make concessions on certain food selections. Methods of preparation are

---

**BOX 33-6** | **Radiological and Diagnostic Tests**

**Direct Visualization**

**Endoscopy**

Routine examination, such as a sigmoidoscopy or colonoscopy, uses a lighted fiber-optic tube to gain direct visualization of the upper GI tract (upper endoscopy) or large intestine (colonoscopy). The fiber-optic tubes contains a lens, forceps, and brushes for biopsy. If an endoscopy identifies a lesion, such as a polyp, a biopsy can be obtained. Normally the GI tract is free of polyps, tumors, inflammation, ulcerations, obstructions, or hernias.

**Indirect Visualization**

**Plain Film of Abdomen/Kidneys, Ureter, Bladder**

A simple x-ray film of the abdomen requiring no preparation.

**Barium Swallow/Enema**

An x-ray examination using an opaque contrast medium (barium, which is swallowed) to examine the structure and motility of the upper GI tract, including pharynx, esophagus, and stomach. The barium enema provides visualization of the structures of the lower GI tract.

**Ultrasound**

A technique that uses high-frequency sound waves to echo off body organs, creating a picture of the GI tract.

**Computed Tomography Scan**

An x-ray examination of the body from many angles utilizing a scanner analyzed by a computer.

**Magnetic Resonance Imaging**

A noninvasive examination that uses magnet and radio waves to produce a picture of the inside of the body.

---

also a concern, especially if tradition and cost are deciding factors.

When determining the patient's expectations, consider his or her normal bowel pattern. Some patients wish to have activities planned in order to maintain normal routines. If what is "normal" to the patient is unhealthy or promotes negative health practices, you first meet the patient's educational needs.

## Nursing Diagnosis

Gather data from the nursing assessment, validate the data, and analyze clusters of defining characteristics to identify relevant nursing diagnoses. Reflecting on each of your data sources is necessary in determining the correct diagnosis. Defining characteristics identified during your assessment sometimes apply to more than one diagnosis, so be clinically skillful in determining patterns that reveal the diagnosis that best fits the patient's situation. A concept map (Figure 33-8) shows how a nursing diagnosis of constipation is related to three other nursing diagnoses in the case of a patient who has had a hysterectomy. In this example the patient had surgery

and developed constipation as a result of reduced activity, decreased fluid and fiber intake, and pain medications.

In another example, a patient reports not having a bowel movement for several days. This defining characteristic applies to the diagnosis of *constipation* and *perceived constipation*. The difference is that on examination the patient with *constipation* has a dry, hard stool with abdominal or rectal fullness. In contrast, the patient with *perceived constipation* has expectation of having a stool daily, and in fact the stools are quite normal. There are a variety of nursing diagnoses that are relevant for patients with altered bowel elimination. Below is a listing of some examples (NANDA International, 2005):

- Activity intolerance
- Disturbed body image
- Bowel incontinence
- Constipation
- Risk for constipation
- Diarrhea
- Imbalanced nutrition
- Acute pain
- Chronic pain
- Toileting self care deficit
- Impaired skin integrity

It is important to establish the correct "related to" factor for a diagnosis. For example, with the diagnosis of *constipation* you distinguish between related factors of nutritional imbalance, exercise, medications, and emotional problems. Selection of the correct related factors for each diagnosis ensures that you will implement the appropriate nursing interventions. For example, the interventions for nutritional imbalance will be different than those for exercise or emotional problems.

## Planning

**GOALS AND OUTCOMES.** After you identify nursing diagnoses, you and the patient set goals and expected outcomes to direct interventions. When possible, these goals and outcomes incorporate the patient's elimination routines or habits as much as possible and reinforce those that promote health. In addition, consider the patient's preexisting health concerns. For example, one method of reducing the risk of constipation is to increase fluids to add bulk to the fecal material. However, if your patient is at risk for the development of congestive heart failure, you need to tailor the expected outcome of increasing fluid intake to the patient's cardiac function to safely handle an increase in the volume of fluid.

The goals and expected outcomes you establish need to be realistic. The outcomes provide measurable behaviors or physiological responses that indicate progress toward the goal of a normal bowel elimination pattern. Design nursing interventions to achieve the outcomes of care.

**SETTING PRIORITIES.** Defecation patterns vary among individuals. For this reason you and the patient work together to plan effective interventions to meet the patient's elimination needs and priorities (see care plan). A realistic

## CONCEPT MAP

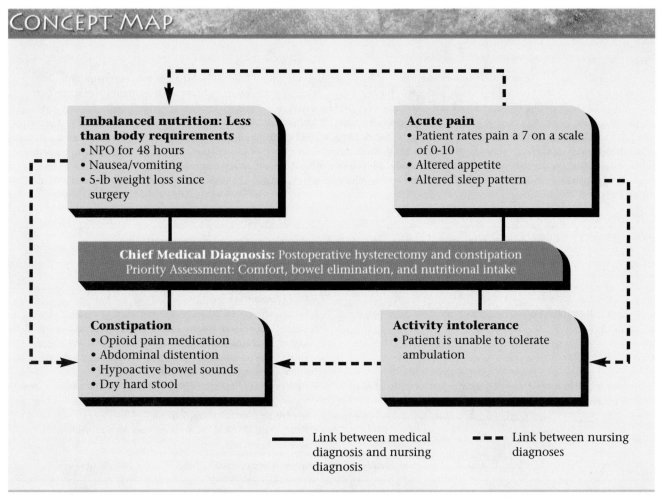

**Imbalanced nutrition: Less than body requirements**
- NPO for 48 hours
- Nausea/vomiting
- 5-lb weight loss since surgery

**Acute pain**
- Patient rates pain a 7 on a scale of 0-10
- Altered appetite
- Altered sleep pattern

**Chief Medical Diagnosis:** Postoperative hysterectomy and constipation
Priority Assessment: Comfort, bowel elimination, and nutritional intake

**Constipation**
- Opioid pain medication
- Abdominal distention
- Hypoactive bowel sounds
- Dry hard stool

**Activity intolerance**
- Patient is unable to tolerate ambulation

—— Link between medical diagnosis and nursing diagnosis

- - - Link between nursing diagnoses

FIGURE **33-8** Concept map for patient with postoperative hysterectomy and constipation.

time frame to establish a normal defecation pattern for one patient is sometimes very different for another. In addition, if the patient has a new ostomy resulting from cancer, the priority of coping with cancer and its treatment precedes the patient's need to independently manage care of the bowel diversion. In addition, when a bowel diversion is necessary, coping with changes in body image is a high priority for both the patient and family.

**CONTINUITY OF CARE.** Other health care team members are important resources for the patient and family. You will sometimes refer a patient with chronic constipation to a dietitian to plan a nutritionally balanced diet that incorporates the patient's food preferences and lifestyle.

Involvement of the family in the plan of care is important. When patients are disabled or debilitated, family members often become the primary caregivers. Patient and family education is important to promote understanding of ways to establish normal bowel function. If access to proper nutrition is a concern, community organizations that deliver meals to the home or that provide transportation for patients will be beneficial.

A clinical nurse specialist or wound, ostomy, and continence nurse specialist will provide guidance in the care and management of ostomy sites and problems involving incontinence or skin breakdown. In many institutions, members of the health care team work together in developing a critical pathway for patient care.

### ✿ Implementation

**HEALTH PROMOTION.** The factors that normally promote bowel elimination are appropriate interventions for helping patients develop normal bowel habits. It is important for you to teach your patient about the benefits and effects of a balanced diet, regular exercise, and stress management on bowel habits and their effects on developing a bowel routine. Teach your patients to try to develop a routine time for bowel evacuation. A good time is after a morning or evening meal when your patient does not feel rushed. Establishing a consistent time for bowel hygiene is just one evidence-based practice to avoid constipation (Box 33-7).

**Diet.** Depending on the patient's elimination problem, specific foods ensure proper nutrient intake and normal

## CARE PLAN  Constipation

### ASSESSMENT

From their first visit, Vickie and Mr. Gutierrez have been able to communicate without difficulty. Mr. Gutierrez complains of feeling **"full of gas"** but has not "passed any wind," perhaps in the last 2 days. Because of the feeling of fullness Mr. Gutierrez also states, "I really **haven't felt like eating today and have not eaten much for the last 4 days,** and I need to move my bowels. I took a laxative last night, and I think I need an enema." Vickie confirms that Mr. Gutierrez had his **last bowel movement 3 days ago.** The **stool was brown in color and hard.** On examination of the abdomen Vicki finds **hypoactive bowel sounds** in all four quadrants. His abdomen is soft but slightly distended. A medication history shows that Mr. Gutierrez frequently resorts to taking laxatives. An assessment of Mr. Gutierrez's diet reveals a high intake of corn tortillas and cheese and a low intake of fruits. His stove has not been working well, and he has been unable to prepare rice and beans. On the basis of the nursing history, Vickie estimates Mr. Gutierrez normally drinks about 1200 ml of fluid daily.

*Defining characteristics are shown in bold type.

---

### NURSING DIAGNOSIS  Constipation related to less than adequate fluid and dietary intake and chronic laxative use.

---

### PLANNING

| GOAL | EXPECTED OUTCOMES* |
|---|---|
| • Patient will establish and maintain a normal defecation pattern within 1 month. | **Bowel Elimination**<br>• Patient will have a bowel movement within 48 hours.<br>• Patient's abdomen will be soft, nondistended, and nontender within 24 hours.<br>• Patient will pass soft, formed stools at least every 3 days.<br>**Nutritional Status: Food and Fluid Intake** |
| • Patient will identify practices that reduce the risk for or prevent constipation within 2 weeks. | • Patient will increase the fiber content of his diet within 1 week.<br>• Patient will immediately discontinue laxative use and when needed will use fiber supplements.<br>• Patient will drink eight 8-ounce glasses of noncaffeine beverages within 3 days. |

*Outcomes classification label from Moorhead S, Johnson M, Maas M: *Nursing outcomes classification (NOC),* ed 3, St. Louis, 2004, Mosby.

---

### INTERVENTIONS†

**Constipation/Impaction Management**
• Instruct patient in a weekly menu plan, including foods high in fiber: brown rice, beans and rice, tomatoes, and wheat tortillas.

• Add bran flakes, bran, or fiber supplement to the diet.

• Consult with patient's niece and long-term care center to have patient's stove repaired.
• Educate patient about use of liquids to promote softening of stool and defecation; have patient drink noncaffeine beverage of choice.

• Encourage patient to try to establish a routine time for defecation, establishing a routine after breakfast or other meal.

### RATIONALE

High-fiber foods increase the bulk of the fecal contents, which in turn increases peristalsis and improves the movement of intestinal contents through the GI tract (Dosh, 2002; Doughty, 2000b).
Bran as flakes or fiber supplements add bulk to the feces and increase the number of soft-formed stools (Bliss and others, 2001). Dietary fiber, either through diet or supplement, reduces the need for laxatives (Doughty, 2000; Thompson and others, 2003).
Cooking facilities are necessary for preparation of selected food preferences.
Caffeine beverages cause the body to increase excretion of fluids and dehydrate the patient. Fluids help to keep fecal mass soft and increase stool bulk, causing increase in colon peristalsis (Ebersole, Hess, and Luggen, 2004).
With aging there are some normal changes in rectal sensation, and the body needs larger volumes to elicit the sensation to defecate. Using the normal gastrocolic reflex, which results in movement of colon contents approximately 1 hour after a meal, assists in establishing routine bowel habits (Ebersole and others, 2004).

†Intervention classification labels from Dochterman JM, Bulechek GM, editors: *Nursing interventions classification (NIC),* ed 4, St. Louis, 2004, Mosby.

---

### EVALUATION

• Ask patient to keep a diary of the types of foods and beverages ingested for 1 week, and review.
• Ask patient to describe the effect fluids and high-fiber foods have on elimination.

• Ask patient about frequency of laxative use.
• Ask patient to describe frequency and character of stool. Whenever possible, observe stool.
• Palpate abdomen for distention and tenderness.

## BOX 33-7 USING EVIDENCE IN PRACTICE

**Research Summary**

Multiple areas of research support the increasing evidence that low fat intake and increases in dietary fiber and bulk-forming foods reduce the patient's risk of colorectal cancers, digestive diseases, and other cancers (Anti and others, 1998; Bliss and others, 2001). Assisting patients and their families in different food selection and preparation practices helps to reduce the risks of GI disease. Give consideration to whether a patient is able to afford the foods recommended. In addition to solid foods, the patient needs to drink 2000 to 3000 ml of fluids daily, if not contraindicated by other medical conditions.

**Application to Nursing Practice**[*]

- Recommend fluid intake of at least 1.5 L per day. Preferred fluid is water because it is sodium-, caffeine-, and calorie-free. Patient will benefit from one to two glasses of fruit juice as well (Anti and others, 1998).
- Teach patients to avoid coffee, tea, and alcohol due to their diuretic properties.
- Suggest a high-fiber diet (25 to 30 g per day) to reduce constipation; as fiber passes though the colon, it acts as a sponge. As a result, bulkier and softer stools develop. In addition, the waste moves through the body more easily and results in more regular bowel movements. High-fiber diet is not for individuals who are immobile or who do not consume at least 1.5 L of fluid per day (Bliss and others, 2001).
- Teach patients to use a combination of insoluble and soluble fiber (e.g., bran, fruits, and vegetables) to prevent constipation.
- Assess the patient's ability to afford foods.
- Encourage physical activity in combination with adequate fluid intake and high-fiber diet to manage constipation. Walking once or twice a day for 15 to 20 minutes is sufficient.
- Suggest chair or bed exercises such as pelvic tilt, low trunk rotation, and single leg lifts for individuals who are unable to walk.
- Explain need to use laxatives with caution. A stepwise progression of laxatives is recommended: first bulk-forming laxatives, followed by stool softeners, osmotic, stimulants, suppositories, and enemas as a last resort.

*Modified from Hinrichs M, Huseboe J: *Evidenced-based protocol: management of constipation.* In Titler MG, series editor: Series on evidence based practice for older adults, Iowa City, 1998, The University of Iowa, Gerontological Nursing Interventions Research Center, Research Dissemination Core. For more information, http://www.nursing.uiowa.edu/center/gnirc/disseminatecore.htm.

defecation (see Boxes 33-1 and 33-7). When your patient has an ostomy, the location of the ostomy determines the type of diet needed for regular evacuation. Initially place patients on low-fiber diets to avoid stoma obstruction. Slowly add high-fiber foods one at a time over a period of several weeks. Maintain a high fluid intake. Teach your patient to avoid foods that cause blockage, such as organs, apples with tough skins, corn, and popcorn.

**Exercise.** An age-specific exercise program also assists patients in maintaining a healthy bowel pattern. Regular exercise, such as walking, biking, or swimming 30 minutes daily, promotes normal GI motility. Regular activity keeps the intestines working well (Dosh, 2002). Have a patient who experienced a period of immobilization from illness ambulate as soon as possible. Ambulation promotes peristalsis and a return to normal bowel function.

**Timing and Privacy.** One of the most important habits you will teach your patients regarding bowel habits is to take time for defecation. Ignoring the urge to defecate and not taking time to defecate completely are common causes of constipation. To establish regular bowel habits, a patient needs to respond to the urge to defecate. Prompt response will help the patient to reduce episodes of constipation.

Defecation is most likely to occur an hour after meals. If the patient attempts to defecate during the time when mass colonic peristalsis occurs, the chances of success are great. If a patient is restricted to bed or requires assistance in ambulating, you recommend use of a bedside commode or a bedpan or have a caregiver help the patient reach the bathroom. Patients will need prompt assistance before the urge disappears.

Some patients have previously established routines to assist them with defecation. When patients become hospitalized, health promotion habits become disrupted. Encourage patients to maintain as many of these regular practices as possible. Privacy is often a concern for patients. Health care providers often walk in and out of rooms without knocking, and many patients reside in semiprivate rooms or living areas. Remain acutely aware of the patient's need for modesty and privacy.

**Promotion of Normal Defecation.** To help patients evacuate contents normally and without discomfort, recommend interventions that stimulate the defecation reflex or increase peristalsis. One way to promote defecation is by having the patient assume a squatting position during defecation. Squatting increases pressure on the rectum and facilitates use of intraabdominal muscles. Patients who have difficulty in squatting because of muscular weakness or mobility limitations benefit from the use of elevated toilet seats. Regular toilets are too low for patients unable to lower themselves to a squatting position because of joint or muscle-wasting diseases or for those who have had abdominal surgery. With an elevated seat, the patient exerts less effort to sit or stand.

**ACUTE CARE.** When patients become acutely ill, this often affects the GI system first. Simple changes in activity levels, sleeping patterns, diet, and medications directly affect regular bowel habits. Surgical intervention creates additional elimination problems for the patient in acute care (e.g., discomfort from an abdominal incision, absent or decreased gastrointestinal peristalsis, or increased accumulation of intestinal gas following surgery). Sensitivity to the patient's need for the provision of as much self-care as possible will assist the patient in coping with the changes.

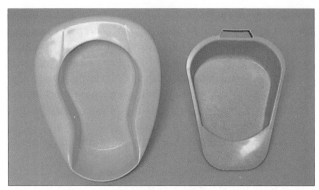

FIGURE **33-9** Types of bedpans. *From left:* Regular bedpan and fracture pan.

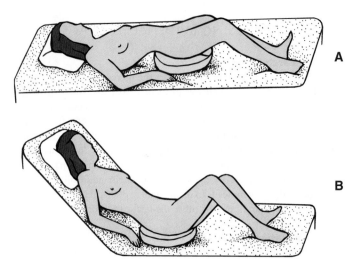

FIGURE **33-10** Positions on a bedpan. **A,** Improper positioning of a patient. **B,** Proper position reduces patient's back strain.

**Positioning on Bedpan.** A patient restricted to use of a bedpan for defecation will usually need assistance. Sitting on a bedpan is uncomfortable and awkward. Help position the patient comfortably. Two types of bedpans are available. The regular bedpan, made of metal or hard plastic, has a curved smooth upper end and a sharp-edged lower end and is about 5 cm (2 inches) deep. A fracture pan, designed for patients with body or leg casts or for whom the semi-Fowler's position is contraindicated, has a shallow upper end about 1.3 cm ($\frac{1}{2}$ inch) deep (Figure 33-9).

The upper end of either pan fits under the buttocks toward the sacrum, with the lower end just under the upper thighs. Make sure the pan is high enough so that feces enter it. The most important element for you to consider in positioning the patient is preventing muscle strain and discomfort. Never place a patient on a bedpan and then leave the bed flat unless activity restrictions demand it. This forces the patient to hyperextend the back to lift the hips onto the pan (Figure 33-10, *A*). It is often necessary to have the bed flat when placing the patient on a bedpan. In this case you then raise the head of the bed 30 to 45 degrees (Figure 33-10, *B*). Patients who have overhead trapeze frames are able to easily lift themselves by grasping the trapeze bar. Box 33-8 describes steps in assisting a patient with a bedpan.

For the more mobile patient, a bedside commode is a safe, effective alternative to a bedpan. Its use is less exhausting and allows the patient to assume a more "normal" or "familiar" position for defecation.

**Medications.** Some medications initiate and facilitate stool passage. **Cathartics** and **laxatives** have the short-term action of emptying the bowel. These agents are also used in bowel evacuation for patients undergoing GI tests and abdominal surgery. Although the terms *cathartic* and *laxative* are often used interchangeably, cathartics have a stronger and more rapid effect on the intestines.

Although patients usually take medications via the oral route, cathartics prepared as suppositories are more effective because of their stimulant effect on the rectal mucosa. Cathartic suppositories such as bisacodyl (Dulcolax) act

within 30 minutes. Give the suppository shortly before the patient's usual time to defecate or immediately after a meal. Teach patients about the potential harmful effects of repeated use of laxatives, such as permanent bowel damage, osteomalacia, and electrolyte imbalances (McKenry and Salerno, 2001). Make sure the patient understands that laxatives and cathartics are not for long-term maintenance of bowel function.

Cathartics are classified by the method by which the agent promotes defecation. Stimulant cathartics cause local irritation to the intestinal mucosa, increase intestinal motility, and inhibit reabsorption of water in the large intestine. The rapid movement of feces causes retention of water in the stool. The drugs cause formation of a soft to fluid stool in 6 to 8 hours.

Saline or osmotic agents contain a salt preparation that the intestines do not absorb. The cathartic draws water into the fecal mass. This osmotic action increases the bulk of the intestinal contents and enhances lubrication. Rapid bowel evacuation occurs in 1 to 3 hours.

Emollient or wetting agents are detergents and act as stool softeners to lower the surface tension of feces, allowing water and fat to penetrate the fecal material. These drugs also block absorption of water by the intestines. The fecal mass becomes large and soft, preventing the patient from straining during defecation. A bowel movement occurs within 12 to 24 hours.

Bulk-forming cathartics absorb water and increase solid intestinal bulk. The fecal bulk stretches the intestinal walls, stimulating peristalsis. Passage of stool will occur in 12 to 24 hours. Bulk-forming laxatives are the least irritating and safest of all cathartics. Encourage patients to take bulk cathartics with plenty of liquids.

Lubricants soften the fecal mass, thus easing the strain of defecation. Patients with painful hemorrhoids particularly benefit from a lubricant. The only lubricant laxative available is mineral oil. However, teach patients that the regular use of mineral oil interferes with absorption of the fat-soluble vita-

---

**BOX 33-8** PROCEDURAL GUIDELINES FOR

## Assisting Patient On and Off a Bedpan

**Delegation Considerations:** You can delegate the skill of assisting a patient onto a bedpan to assistive personnel. Be sure to inform and assist care provider in proper way to position patients who have mobility restrictions. Also instruct care provider about how to position patients who also have therapeutic equipment present, such as drains, intravenous catheters, or traction.

**Equipment:** Appropriate type of clean bedpan; bedpan cover; toilet tissue; specimen container (if necessary); plastic bag, clearly labeled with date, patient's name, and identification number; washbasin; washcloths; towels; soap; waterproof, absorbent pads; clean drawsheet (optional), disposable gloves

1. Assess the patient's level of mobility, strength, ability to help, and presence of any condition (e.g., orthopedic) that interferes with the use of a bedpan.
2. Explain the technique you will use in turning and positioning to the patient.
3. Offer the bedpan at a time that coincides with the duodeno-colic or mass peristaltic reflex.
4. Perform hand hygiene, and apply disposable gloves.
5. Close the room curtain for privacy.
6. If using a metal bedpan, hold it under warm running water for a couple of minutes, then dry.
7. Raise the bed to a comfortable working height, and be sure patient is positioned high in bed with head elevated 30 degrees (unless contraindicated). Raise the side rail opposite the side where you are standing.
8. Fold back top linen to patient's knees.
9. Assist with positioning: Instruct patient to bend knees and place weight on heels. Place your hand, palm up, under patient's sacrum, resting elbow on mattress. Then have patient lift hips while you slip bedpan into place with other hand.
10. Dependent patient: Lower head of bed flat, and have patient roll onto side opposite nurse. Apply powder lightly to lower back and buttocks (optional). Place bedpan firmly against buttocks and push down into mattress with open rim toward patient's feet. Keeping one hand against bedpan, place other hand around patient's fore hip (see illustration). Ask patient to roll onto pan, flat on bed. With patient positioned comfortably, raise head of bed 30 degrees.
11. Place rolled towel under lumbar curve of patient's back.
12. Place call light and toilet tissue within patient's reach, and keep side rails up as needed.
13. Remove bedpan as patient lifts hips up or as patient carefully rolls off pan and to side. Hold pan firmly as patient moves.
14. Assist in cleansing anal area. Wipe from pubic area toward anus. Replace top covers.
15. If you collect a specimen or intake and output, do not dispose of tissue in bedpan.
16. Have patient wash and dry hands.
17. Empty pan's contents, dispose of gloves, and perform hand hygiene.
18. Inspect stool for color, amount, consistency, odor, or presence of abnormal substances.

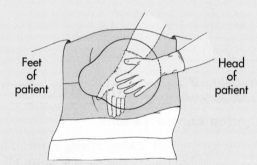

STEP **10** Place one hand against bedpan; place other hand around patient's fore hip.

---

mins A, D, E, and K. In addition, because this medication is an oil-based preparation, it causes a dangerous form of pneumonia when aspirated. Therefore warn patients with nausea and vomiting not to take the medication.

For patients with diarrhea, the most effective antidiarrheal agents are opiates. Antidiarrheal agents decrease intestinal muscle tone to slow the passage of feces. As a result, the body absorbs more water through the intestinal walls. Use antidiarrheal agents with caution because opiates are habit forming.

**Enemas.** An **enema** is an instillation of a preparation into the rectum and sigmoid colon. You will give an enema primarily to promote defecation by stimulating peristalsis. The volume of fluid instilled breaks up the fecal mass, stretches the rectal wall, and begins the defecation reflex. Enemas are also a vehicle for drugs that exert a local effect on rectal mucosa.

The most common use for an enema is temporary relief of constipation. Other indications include removing impacted feces; emptying the bowel before diagnostic tests, surgery, or childbirth; and beginning a program of bowel training. Discourage patients from relying on enemas to maintain bowel regularity. Enemas do not treat the cause of constipation. As with laxative abuse, frequent use will destroy normal defecation reflexes.

Cleansing enemas promote complete evacuation of feces from the colon. They act by stimulating peristalsis through the infusion of a large volume of solution or through local irritation of the colon's mucosa. Cleansing enemas include tap water, normal saline, low-volume hypertonic saline, and soapsuds solution. Each solution exerts a different osmotic effect, causing the movement of fluids between the colon and interstitial spaces beyond the intestinal wall. Infants and children will tolerate only normal saline because they are at risk for fluid imbalance (see Chapter 15).

Tap water is hypotonic and exerts a lower osmotic pressure than fluid in interstitial spaces. After infusion into the colon, tap water escapes from the bowel lumen into interstitial spaces. The net movement of water is low; the infused volume stimulates defecation before large amounts of water leave the bowel. Do not repeat tap water enemas, because water toxicity or circulatory overload will develop if the body absorbs large amounts of water.

Physiologically, normal saline is the safest solution to use because it exerts the same osmotic pressure as fluids in interstitial spaces around the bowel. The volume of infused saline stimulates peristalsis. Giving saline enemas does not create the danger of excess fluid absorption.

Hypertonic solutions infused into the bowel exert osmotic pressure that pulls fluids out of interstitial spaces. The colon fills with fluid, and the resultant distention promotes defecation. Patients unable to tolerate large volumes of fluid benefit most from this type of enema. A hypertonic solution of 120 to 180 ml (4 to 6 oz) is usually effective. The Fleet enema is the most common.

You add soap solution to tap water or saline to create the additional effect of intestinal irritation. Only pure castile soap is safe. Harsh soaps or detergents cause serious bowel inflammation.

A physician or health care provider will sometimes order a high or low cleansing enema. The terms *high* and *low* refer to the height and the pressure with which you deliver the fluid. You give high enemas to cleanse the entire colon. A low enema cleans only the rectum and sigmoid colon. After you infuse the enema, you ask the patient to turn from the left lateral to the dorsal recumbent, then over to the right lateral position. The position change helps fluid to reach the large intestine.

Oil-retention enemas lubricate the rectum and colon. The feces absorb the oil and become softer and easier to pass. To enhance action of the oil, the patient retains the enema for several hours if possible.

Certain enemas or enema administrations contain drugs. An example is sodium polystyrene sulfonate (Kayexalate), used to treat patients with dangerously high serum potassium levels. Skill 33-1 outlines the steps for enema administration.

*Text continued on p. 972*

## SKILL 33-1 | Administering a Cleansing Enema

### Delegation Considerations

You can delegate the skill of administering an enema to assistive personnel. Before delegating this skill, instruct the assistive personnel about:

- Proper ways to position patients who have mobility restrictions.
- Positioning of patients with therapeutic equipment present, such as drains, intravenous catheters, or traction.
- Signs and symptoms of patient not tolerating the procedure, and when to stop it. These signs and symptoms include abdominal pain more than a pressure sensation, abdominal cramping, abdominal distention, or rectal bleeding.
- The expected outcome of the enema and to immediately inform the nurse about the presence of blood in the stool or around the rectal area, any change in patient vital signs, or new symptoms so the nurse is able to further assess the patient.

### Equipment

- Disposable gloves
- Water-soluble lubricant

- Waterproof, absorbent pads
- Bath blanket
- Toilet tissue
- Bedpan, bedside commode, or access to toilet
- Wash basin, washcloths, towel, and soap
- Intravenous (IV) pole

*Enema Bag Administration*

- Enema container
- Tubing and clamp (if not already attached to container)
- Appropriate-size rectal tube:
  - Adult: 22 to 30 Fr
  - Child: 12 to 18 Fr
- Correct volume of warmed solution:
  - Adult: 750 to 1000 ml
  - Child:
    - 150 to 250 ml, infant
    - 250 to 350 ml, toddler
    - 300 to 500 ml, school-age child
    - 500 to 700 ml, adolescent

*Prepackaged Enema*

- Prepackaged enema container with rectal tip

| STEP | RATIONALE |
|---|---|

## ASSESSMENT

1. Assess status of patient: last bowel movement, normal versus most recent bowel pattern, bowel sounds, hemorrhoids, mobility, external sphincter control, presence of abdominal pain.

Determines factors indicating need for enema and influencing the type of enema used. Also establishes a baseline for bowel function.

2. Review medical record for presence of increased intracranial pressure, glaucoma, or recent rectal or prostate surgery.

These conditions contraindicate use of enemas.

3. Inspect abdomen for presence of distention.

Frequently a full colon or impacted bowel results in abdominal distention. Assessment of distention establishes a baseline for determining effectiveness of the enema.

4. Determine patient's level of understanding of purpose of enema.

Allows you to plan for appropriate teaching measures.

5. Check patient's medical record to clarify the rationale for the enema.

Determines purpose of enema administration: preparation for special procedure or relief of constipation.

6. Review physician's or health care provider's order for enema.

Enemas require a physician's or health care provider's order. Determines number and type of enema you will give.

- *Critical Decision Point:* "Enemas until clear" order means that you repeat enemas until patient passes fluid that is clear of fecal matter. Check agency policy, but usually patients receive only three consecutive enemas to avoid disruption of fluid and electrolyte balance.

## PLANNING

1. Collect appropriate equipment.
2. Correctly identify patient, and explain procedure.

Information promotes patient cooperation and reduces anxiety.

3. Assemble enema bag with appropriate solution and rectal tube.

## IMPLEMENTATION

1. Perform hand hygiene, and apply gloves.

Reduces transmission of microorganisms.

2. Provide privacy by closing curtains around bed or closing door.

Reduces embarrassment for patient.

3. Raise bed to appropriate working height for nurse: Stand on right side of bed, and raise side rail on opposite side.

Promotes good body mechanics and patient safety.

4. Assist patient into left side-lying (Sims') position with right knee flexed. Also place children in dorsal recumbent position.

Positioning allows enema solution to flow downward by gravity along natural curve of sigmoid colon and rectum, thus improving retention of solution.

- *Critical Decision Point:* If you suspect patient of having poor sphincter control, position on bedpan in a comfortable dorsal recumbent position. Patients with poor sphincter control are unable to retain all of the enema solution. Administering an enema with the patient sitting on the toilet is unsafe because the curved rectal tubing will scrape the rectal wall.

5. Place waterproof pad under hips and buttocks.

Prevents soiling of linen.

6. Cover patient with bath blanket, exposing only rectal area, clearly visualizing anus.

Provides warmth, reduces exposure of body parts, and allows patient to feel more relaxed and comfortable.

7. Separate buttocks, and examine perianal region for abnormalities including hemorrhoids, anal fissure, or rectal prolapse (Moppett, 1999).

Findings influence approach to the insertion of the enema tip. A prolapsed rectum is a contraindication for an enema (Moppett, 1999).

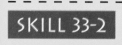

**SKILL 33-2** | **Inserting and Maintaining a Nasogastric Tube for Gastric Decompression**

## Delegation Considerations

The skill of inserting and maintaining an NG tube should not be delegated to assistive personnel. The nurse is responsible for the proper function and drainage of the nasogastric tube, all relevant assessments, and determining the patient's level of comfort. The nurse instead directs the assistive personnel to:

- Measure and record the drainage from an NG tube
- Provide oral and nasal hygiene measures
- Perform selected comfort measures, such as positioning, ice chips if allowed
- Anchor the tube to the patient's gown during routine care to prevent accidental displacement

## Equipment

- 14 or 16 Fr NG tube (smaller-lumen catheters are not used for decompression in adults because they must be able to remove thick secretions)

- Water-soluble lubricating jelly
- pH test strips (measure gastric aspirate acidity)
- Tongue blade
- Flashlight
- Emesis basin
- Asepto bulb or catheter-tipped syringe
- 1-inch (2.5-cm) wide hypoallergenic tape or commercial fixation device
- Safety pin and rubber band
- Clamp, drainage bag, or suction machine or pressure gauge if wall suction is to be used
- Towel
- Glass of water with straw
- Facial tissues
- Normal saline
- Tincture of benzoin (optional)
- Suction equipment
- Disposable gloves

| STEP | RATIONALE |
|---|---|

### ASSESSMENT

1. Inspect condition of patient's nasal and oral cavity.

2. Ask if patient has had history of nasal surgery, and note if deviated nasal septum is present.

3. Palpate patient's abdomen for distention, pain, and rigidity. Auscultate for bowel sounds.

4. Assess patient's level of consciousness and ability to follow instructions.

Baseline condition of nasal and oral cavity determines need for special nursing hygiene measures after tube placement.

Nurse should insert tube into ***uninvolved*** nasal passage. Procedure may be contraindicated if surgery is recent.

Baseline determination of level of abdominal distention and function later serves as comparison once tube is inserted. Decreased bowel sounds occur with peritonitis and paralytic ileus. In the presence of diminished or absent bowel sounds the abdomen should be auscultated for 5 minutes in all four quadrants to make sure that no sounds are missed and to localize specific sounds (Seidel and others, 2003).

Determines patient's ability to assist in procedure.

---

• ***Critical Decision Point:*** If patient is confused, disoriented, or unable to follow commands, obtain assistance from another staff member to insert the tube.

---

5. Determine if patient has had an NG tube insertion in the past and which nares was used.

6. Check medical record for physician's or health care provider's order, type of NG tube to be placed, and whether tube is to be attached to suction or drainage bag.

Procedure is uncomfortable and requires thorough explanation. Patient's previous experience will complement any explanations.

Procedure requires physician's or health care provider's order. Adequate decompression depends on NG suction.

---

### PLANNING

1. Prepare equipment at the bedside. Have a 4-inch (10-cm) piece of tape ready with one end split in half.

Ensures well-organized procedure. Tape will be used to initially hold tube in place after insertion.

| STEP | RATIONALE |
|---|---|
| 2. Identify patient, and explain procedure. Let patient know there will be a burning sensation in nasopharynx as tube is passed. | Identification prevents error of placing tube in wrong patient. Explanation gains patient's cooperation and ability to anticipate nurse's action. |
| 3. Position patient in high-Fowler's position with pillows behind head and shoulders. Raise bed to a horizontal level comfortable for the nurse. | Good body mechanics prevents injury to nurse or patient. |

## IMPLEMENTATION

| | |
|---|---|
| 1. Perform hand hygiene, and apply disposable gloves. | Reduces transmission of microorganisms. |
| 2. Place bath towel over patient's chest; give facial tissues to patient. Place emesis basin within reach. | Prevents soiling of patient's gown. Tube insertion through nasal passages may cause tearing and coughing with increased salivation. |
| 3. Pull curtain around the bed, or close room door. | Provides privacy. |
| 4. Stand on patient's right side if right-handed, left side if left-handed. | Allows easiest manipulation of tubing. |
| 5. Instruct patient to relax and breathe normally while occluding one nares. Then repeat this action for other nares. Select nostril with greater airflow. | Tube passes more easily through nares that is more patent. |
| 6. Measure distance to insert tube: | |
|    **a.** *Traditional method:* Measure distance from tip of nose to earlobe to xiphoid process (see illustration). | Tube should extend from nares to stomach; distance varies with each patient. |
|    **b.** *Hanson method:* First mark 50-cm point on tube, then do traditional measurement. Tube insertion should be to midway point between 50 cm (20 inches) and traditional mark. | |
| 7. Mark length of tube to be inserted with small piece of tape placed around tube so it can be easily removed. | Marks amount of tube to be inserted from nares to stomach. |
| 8. Curve 10 to 15 cm (4 to 6 inches) of end of tube tightly around index finger, then release. | Curving tube tip aids insertion and decreases stiffness of tube. |
| 9. Lubricate 7.5 to 10 cm (3 to 4 inches) of end of tube with water-soluble lubricating gel. | Minimizes friction against nasal mucosa and aids insertion of tube. |
| 10. Alert patient that procedure is to begin. | Decreases patient anxiety and increases patient cooperation. |
| 11. Initially instruct patient to extend neck back against pillow; insert tube slowly through nares with curved end pointing downward (see illustration). | Facilitates initial passage of tube through nares and maintains clear airway for open nares. |

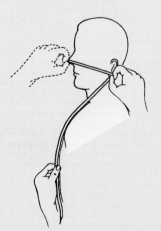

STEP **6a** Technique for measuring distance to insert NG tube.

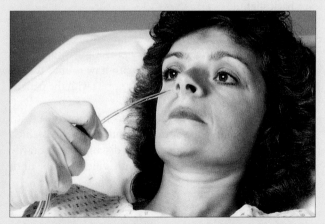

STEP **11** Insert NG tube with curved end pointing downward.

SKILL 33-2 | Inserting and Maintaining a Nasogastric Tube for Gastric Decompression—cont'd

| STEP | RATIONALE |
|---|---|
| 12. Continue to pass tube along floor of nasal passage, aiming down toward ear. When resistance is felt, apply gentle downward pressure to advance tube (do not force past resistance). | Minimizes discomfort of tube rubbing against upper nasal turbinates. Resistance is caused by posterior nasopharynx. Downward pressure helps tube curl around corner of nasopharynx. |
| 13. If resistance is met, try to rotate the tube and see if it advances. If still resistant, withdraw tube, allow patient to rest, relubricate tube, and insert into other nares. | Forcing against resistance can cause trauma to mucosa. Helps relieve patient's anxiety. |

• *Critical Decision Point:* If unable to insert tube in either nares, stop procedure and notify physician or health care provider.

| | |
|---|---|
| 14. Continue insertion of tube until just past nasopharynx by gently rotating tube toward opposite nares. | |
|    a. Once past nasopharynx, stop tube advancement, allow patient to relax, and provide tissues. | Relieves patient's anxiety; tearing is natural response to mucosal irritation, and excessive salivation may occur because of oral stimulation. |
|    b. Explain to patient that next step requires that patient swallow. Give patient glass of water unless contraindicated. | Sipping of water aids passage of NG tube into esophagus. |
| 15. With tube just above oropharynx, instruct patient to flex head forward, take a small sip of water, and swallow. Advance tube 2.5 to 5 cm (1 to 2 inches) with each swallow of water. If patient is not allowed fluids, instruct to dry swallow or suck air through straw. Advance tube with each swallow. | Flexed position closes off upper airway to trachea and opens esophagus. Swallowing closes epiglottis over trachea and helps move the tube into the esophagus. Swallowing water reduces gagging or choking. Water can be removed later from stomach by suction. |
| 16. If patient begins to cough, gag, or choke, withdraw slightly and stop tube advancement. Instruct patient to breathe easily and take sips of water. | Tubing may accidentally enter larynx and initiate cough reflex, and withdrawal of the tube reduces risk of laryngeal entry. Gagging is eased by swallowing water, which must be given cautiously to reduce the risk of aspiration. |

• *Critical Decision Point:* If vomiting occurs, assist patient in clearing airway; oral suctioning may be needed. Do not proceed until airway is cleared.

| | |
|---|---|
| 17. If patient continues to cough during insertion, pull tube back slightly. | Tube may enter larynx and obstruct airway. |
| 18. If patient continues to gag and cough or complains that the tube feels as though it is coiling in the back of the throat, check back of oropharynx using flashlight and tongue blade. If tube is coiled, withdraw it until the tip is back in the oropharynx. Then reinsert with the patient swallowing. | Tube may coil around itself in back of throat and stimulate gag reflex. |
| 19. After patient relaxes, continue to advance tube with swallowing until tape or mark on tube is reached, which signifies the tube is in the desired distance. Temporarily anchor tube to patient's cheek with a piece of tape until tube placement is verified. | Tip of tube should be within stomach to decompress properly. Anchoring of tube prevents accidental displacement while the tube placement is verified. |

| STEP | RATIONALE |
|---|---|
| **20.** Verify tube placement: Check agency policy for preferred methods for checking tube placement. | |
| **a.** Ask patient to talk. | Patient is unable to talk if NG tube has passed through vocal cords. |
| **b.** Inspect posterior pharynx for presence of coiled tube. | Tube is pliable and can coil up in back of pharynx instead of advancing into esophagus. |
| **c.** Aspirate gently back on syringe to obtain gastric contents, observing color (see illustration). | Gastric contents are usually cloudy and green, but may be off-white, tan, bloody, or brown in color. Aspiration of contents provides means to measure fluid pH and thus determine tube tip placement in gastrointestinal tract. |
| | Other common aspirate colors include the following: duodenal placement (yellow or bile stained), esophagus (may or may not have saliva-appearing aspirate). |
| **d.** Measure pH of aspirate with color-coded pH paper with range of whole numbers from 1 to 11 (see illustration). | Gastric aspirates have decidedly acidic pH values, preferably 4 or less, compared with intestinal aspirates, which are usually greater than 4, or respiratory secretions, which are usually greater than 6.0 (Metheny and others, 1993, 1994, 1998; Metheny and Titler, 2001). |

· *Critical Decision Point:* Be sure to use gastric (Gastroccult) pH test and not Hemoccult test.

| STEP | RATIONALE |
|---|---|
| **e.** Have ordered x-ray examination performed of chest/abdomen. | X-ray examination verifies initial placement of the tube (Metheny and Titler, 2001). |
| **f.** If tube is not in stomach, advance another 2.5 to 5 cm (1 to 2 inches) and repeat steps 20a-d to check tube position. | Tube must be in stomach to provide decompression. |
| **21.** Anchoring tube: | |
| **a.** After tube is properly inserted and positioned, either clamp end or connect it to drainage bag or suction machine. | Drainage bag is used for gravity drainage. Intermittent suction is most effective for decompression. Patient going to the operating room or for diagnostic tests often has tube clamped. |
| **b.** Tape tube to nose; avoid putting pressure on nares. Cut tape about 5 inches (12 cm), and split halfway. | Prevents tissue necrosis. Tape anchors tube securely. |
| (1) Before taping tube to nose, apply small amount of tincture of benzoin to lower end of nose and allow to dry (optional). Apply tape to nose, leaving the split end free. Be sure top end of tape over nose is secure. | Benzoin prevents loosening of tape if patient perspires. |

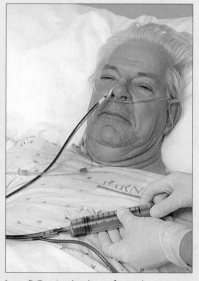

STEP **20c** Aspiration of gastric contents.

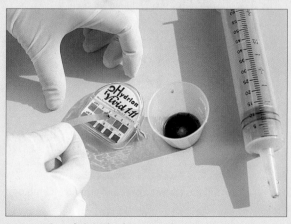

STEP **20d** Checking pH of gastric aspirate.

---
| SKILL 33-2 | Inserting and Maintaining a Nasogastric Tube for Gastric Decompression—cont'd |
---

| STEP | RATIONALE |
|---|---|
| (2) Carefully wrap two split ends of tape around tube (see illustration). | |
| (3) Alternative: Apply tube fixation device using shaped adhesive patch (see illustration). | |
| **c.** Fasten end of NG tube to patient's gown by looping rubber band around tube in slipknot. Pin rubber band to gown (provides slack for movement). Do not attach pin to NG tube itself. | Reduces pressure on nares if tube moves. |
| **d.** Unless physician or health care provider orders otherwise, head of bed should be elevated 30 degrees. | Helps prevent esophageal reflux and minimizes irritation of tube against posterior pharynx. |
| **e.** Explain to patient that sensation of tube should decrease somewhat with time. | Adaptation to continued sensory stimulus. |
| **f.** Remove gloves, and perform hand hygiene. | Reduces transmission of microorganisms. |
| **22.** Once placement is confirmed: | |
| **a.** Place a mark, either a red mark or tape, on the tube to indicate where the tube exits in the nose. | The mark or tube length is to be used as a guide to indicate whether displacement may have occurred. |
| **b.** Measure the tube length from nares to connector as an alternate method. | |
| **c.** Document the tube length in the patient record. | |
| **23.** Tube irrigation: | |
| **a.** Perform hand hygiene, and apply gloves. | Reduces transmission of microorganisms. |
| **b.** Check for tube placement in stomach (see step 20). Reconnect NG tube to connecting tube. | Prevents accidental entrance of irrigating solution into lungs. |
| **c.** Draw up 30 ml of normal saline into Asepto or catheter-tip syringe. | Use of saline minimizes loss of electrolytes from stomach fluids. |
| **d.** Clamp NG tube. Disconnect from connecting tubing, and lay end of connection tubing on towel. | Reduces soiling of patient's gown and bed linen. |
| **e.** Insert tip of irrigating syringe into end of NG tube. Remove clamp. Hold syringe with tip pointed at floor, and inject saline slowly and evenly. Do not force solution. | Position of syringe prevents introduction of air into vent tubing, which could cause gastric distention. Solution introduced under pressure can cause gastric trauma. |

---

• *Critical Decision Point:* Do not introduce saline through blue colored "pigtail" air vent of Salem sump tube.

---

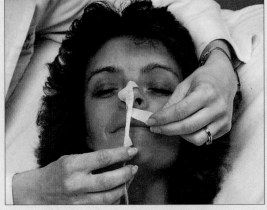

STEP **21b(2)** Tape is crossed over and around NG tube.

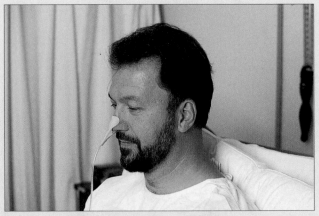

STEP **21b(3)** Patient with tube fixation device.

| STEP | RATIONALE |
|---|---|
| **f.** If resistance occurs, check for kinks in tubing. Turn patient onto left side. Repeated resistance should be reported to physician or health care provider. | Tip of tube may lie against stomach lining. Repositioning on left side may dislodge tube away from the stomach lining. Buildup of secretions will cause distention. |
| **g.** After instilling saline, immediately aspirate or pull back slowly on syringe to withdraw fluid. If amount aspirated is greater than amount instilled, record the difference as output. If amount aspirated is less than amount instilled, record the difference as intake. | Irrigation clears tubing, so stomach should remain empty. Fluid remaining in stomach is measured as intake. |
| **h.** Reconnect NG tube to drainage or suction. (If solution does not return, repeat irrigation.) | Reestablishes drainage collection; may repeat irrigation or repositioning of tube until NG tube drains properly. |
| **i.** Remove gloves, and perform hand hygiene. | Reduces transmission of microorganisms. |
| **24.** Discontinuation of NG tube: | |
| **a.** Verify order to discontinue NG tube. | Physician's or health care provider's order required for procedure. |
| **b.** Explain procedure to patient, and reassure that removal is less distressing than insertion. | Minimizes anxiety and increases cooperation. Tube passes out smoothly. |
| **c.** Perform hand hygiene, and apply disposable gloves. | Reduces transmission of microorganisms. |
| **d.** Turn off suction, and disconnect NG tube from drainage bag or suction. Remove tape or fixation device from bridge of nose, and unpin tube from gown. | Have tube free of connections before removal. |
| **e.** Stand on patient's right side if right-handed, left side if left-handed. | Allows easiest manipulation of tube. |
| **f.** Hand the patient facial tissue; place clean towel across chest. Instruct patient to take and hold a deep breath. | Patient may wish to blow nose after tube is removed. Towel may keep gown from getting soiled. Airway will be temporarily obstructed during tube removal. |
| **g.** Clamp or kink tubing securely, and then pull tube out steadily and smoothly into towel held in other hand while patient holds breath. | Clamping prevents tube contents from draining into oropharynx. Reduces trauma to mucosa and minimizes patient's discomfort. Towel covers tube, which can be an unpleasant sight. Holding breath helps to prevent aspiration. |
| **h.** Measure amount of drainage, and note character of content. Dispose of tube and drainage equipment into proper container. | Provides accurate measure of fluid output. Reduces transfer of microorganisms. |
| **i.** Clean nares, and provide mouth care. | Promotes comfort. |
| **j.** Position patient comfortably, and explain procedure for drinking fluids, if not contraindicated. | Depends on physician's or health care provider's order. Sometimes patients are allowed nothing by mouth (NPO) for up to 24 hours. When fluids are allowed, the order usually begins with a small amount of ice chips each hour and increases as patient is able to tolerate more. |
| **25.** Clean equipment and return to proper place. Place soiled linen in utility room or proper receptacle. | Proper disposal of equipment prevents spread of microorganisms and ensures proper exchange procedures. |
| **26.** Remove gloves, and perform hand hygiene. | Reduces transmission of microorganisms. |

## EVALUATION

| | |
|---|---|
| **1.** Observe amount and character of contents draining from NG tube. Ask if patient feels nauseated. | Determines if tube is decompressing stomach of contents. |
| **2.** Palpate patient's abdomen periodically, noting any distention, pain, and rigidity, and auscultate for the presence of bowel sounds. Turn off suction while auscultating. | Determines success of abdominal decompression and the return of peristalsis. The sound of the suction apparatus may be transmitted to abdomen and be misinterpreted as bowel sounds. |
| **3.** Inspect condition of nares and nose. | Evaluates onset of skin and tissue irritation. |
| **4.** Observe position of tubing. | Determines if tension is being applied to nasal structures. |
| **5.** Ask if patient feels sore throat or irritation in pharynx. | Evaluates level of patient's discomfort. |

---

SKILL 33-2 | Inserting and Maintaining a Nasogastric Tube for Gastric Decompression—cont'd

---

## RECORDING AND REPORTING

■ Record length, size, and type of gastric tube inserted and through which nostril it was inserted, patient's tolerance to procedure, confirmation of tube placement, character of gastric contents, pH value, whether the tube is clamped or connected to drainage or to suction, and the amount of suction supplied.

■ Record difference between amount of normal saline instilled and amount of gastric aspirate removed on intake and output (I&O) sheet. Record in nurses' notes or flow sheet amount and character of contents draining from NG tube every shift.

## UNEXPECTED OUTCOMES AND RELATED INTERVENTIONS

■ Patient's abdomen is distended or painful.
   • Assess patency of the tube.
   • Irrigate tube.
   • Verify that suction is on as ordered.

■ Patient complains of sore throat from dry, irritated mucous membranes.
   • Perform oral hygiene more frequently.
   • Ask physician or health care provider whether patient can suck on ice chips or throat lozenges.

■ Patient develops irritation or erosion of skin around nares.
   • Provide frequent skin care to area.
   • Retape tube to avoid pressure on naris.
   • Consider switching tube to other naris.

■ Patient develops signs and symptoms of pulmonary aspiration: fever, shortness of breath, or pulmonary congestion.
   • Perform complete respiratory assessment.
   • Notify physician or health care provider.
   • Obtain chest x-ray examination as ordered.
   • Clamp tubing and do not flush it or put any medications or feedings through it until tube placement is verified.

---

The stoma itself often has a series of small stitches around its perimeter. You will apply a pouch and skin barrier that do not constrict the stoma or traumatize healing tissues. Initially some patients will not need to empty the pouch over a postoperative colostomy frequently because drainage is diminished or lacking. Several days will pass before a patient's normal elimination pattern returns. In the case of an ileostomy, the patient will have frequent liquid stools when peristalsis returns (Erwin-Toth, 2001).

Many types of pouches and skin barriers are available (Schiff, 2000). Some pouches have skin barriers directly preattached and are called one-piece pouching systems. Some of these one-piece pouches already are precut to size by the manufacturer, whereas others you will custom cut to size for the patient's stoma measurement. Other systems are two separate pieces. You attach the pouch to the skin barrier by attaching it to the flange (a plastic ring) on the barrier. Often you will have to custom cut the skin barrier to the patient's specific stoma size. For two-piece systems you will use the skin barrier with flange with the corresponding-size pouch that fits that flange *from the same manufacturer* to use the system correctly without leakage. Understand how to use each of these different pouching systems (Figure 33-11). Modifications for preventing complications related to leakage of feces or urine are essential

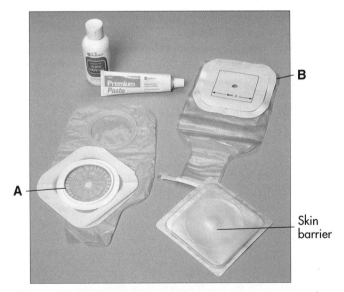

FIGURE **33-11** Examples of pouching systems. **A,** Two-piece detachable system. (NOTE: Skin barrier would need to be cut by the patient according to stoma size obtained by self-measurement.) The pouch opening is already precut by the manufacturer to fit the size of the flange on the skin barrier. **B,** One-piece pouch with skin barrier.

| BOX 33-10 | PATIENT TEACHING |

**Stoma Care (Conventional Incontinent Ileostomy)**

- Teach the patient that the drainage from the stoma site is very irritating to skin and to avoid contact if at all possible. If contact occurs, cleanse the area and determine that the pouch fits properly (WOCN, 2005).
- Instruct the patient to wash skin with plain water and dry the skin thoroughly (WOCN, 2004a).
- If soap is necessary, a mild soap should be used and the soap must be thoroughly rinsed off because the remaining residue will prevent the skin barrier from adhering to the skin (WOCN, 2004a).
- Instruct patient not to use moistened wipes, baby wipes, or towelettes that contain lanolin or other oils because they are skin irritants and interfere with adherence of the skin barrier (WOCN, 2004a).
- Tell the patient not to use creams or ointments on peristomal skin because they cause skin irritation and prevent the skin barrier from sticking to the skin.
- Teach the patient to routinely inspect the appearance of the stoma and surrounding skin. (Stomas are normally moist, shiny, and dark pink to red.) Bleeding around the stoma is minimal. Tell the patient to report excess bleeding, abnormal color, or edema to the nurse or physician or health care provider (WOCN, 2004a).
- Teach the patient how to select and apply a skin barrier and pouch. Include length of wear.
- Teach the patient how to empty and change the pouch. It needs emptying when one-third to one-half full.
- Teach the patient methods of reducing odor. Commercial deodorants are available.
- Tell the patient to carry ostomy supplies at all times.
- If yeast infections develop, instruct the patient to wash thoroughly but gently, pat dry, and apply medically prescribed antifungal powders to the irritated skin. The use of creams is not recommended because they interfere with adhering of the pouch (WOCN, 2004b).

(Erwin-Toth, 2001; Thompson, 2000). You need to perform meticulous skin care to prevent liquid stool from irritating skin around a stoma (Box 33-10).

You change the pouch when there is little drainage from the ostomy (e.g., before meals or at bedtime). Have the patient participate in the procedure as much as possible. The patient needs to learn to recognize the normal appearance of a stoma. Skill 33-3 describes the steps for pouching an ostomy.

A patient with an ostomy suffers a change in body image. The appearance of the stoma and accompanying body odors causes psychological stress. For the patient with a new ostomy, it is important for you to promote independence and acceptance of the ostomy. Early involvement in self-care promotes the patient's independence. Even simple tasks such as holding pieces of equipment during stoma pouching help the patient begin to adjust to bodily changes. Many patients benefit from the information and encouragement from ostomy support groups.

**Care of Hemorrhoids.** Many patients experience discomfort from alterations in elimination. The patient with hemorrhoids has pain when hemorrhoid tissues are directly irritated from passage of hard stool. The primary goal for the patient with hemorrhoids is soft-formed stools. Treatment includes proper diet, fluids, and regular exercise. Local heat provides temporary relief to swollen hemorrhoids. A sitz bath is the most effective means of heat application.

When hemorrhoids are present, it is important to prevent trauma to tissues. Use caution when inserting rectal thermometers, suppositories, or rectal tubes. A generous amount of lubricating jelly reduces friction. Often the patient is better able to insert an object safely into the rectum. You never attempt to force a thermometer or suppository into the rectum without full view of the anus.

**Maintenance of Skin Integrity.** The patient with diarrhea or fecal incontinence is at risk for skin breakdown when fecal contents remain on the skin (see Chapter 35). The same problem exists for the patient with an ostomy that drains liquid stool. Liquid stool is usually acidic and contains digestive enzymes. Irritation from repeated wiping with toilet tissue aggravates skin breakdown. Cleansing the skin after soiling helps but sometimes results in more irritation unless the skin is thoroughly dried (Colwell and others, 2001).

Instruct the patient about cleansing the anal area with mild soap and water after each passage of stool. When caring for a debilitated, incontinent patient who is unable to ask for assistance, check frequently for defecation. Protect the skin around anal areas with petrolatum jelly, zinc oxide, or other barrier ointments that hold moisture in the skin and protect the skin from irritation. Yeast infections of the skin develop easily. Do not use baby powder or cornstarch because they have no medicinal properties and they frequently cake on the skin and become difficult to remove.

## Evaluation

**PATIENT CARE.** You will evaluate the effectiveness of nursing interventions for the patient with alterations in bowel elimination by determining success in meeting the patient's expected outcomes and goals of care. Optimally the patient will be able to eliminate soft-formed stools regularly. In addition, the patient will gain the information necessary to establish a normal elimination pattern (Table 33-4).

Evaluate success of the plan by having the patient describe his or her elimination pattern following therapy. Focus on evaluating the character of the patient's stool. A return to a more normal, regular elimination pattern can take time. Periodically reevaluate the patient. A soft, nondistended abdomen is a desirable finding.

Evaluate an ostomy patient's success at self-care. Inspect the patient's peristomal skin, looking for impairment in skin

*Text continued on p. 989*

## SKILL 33-3 | Pouching an Ostomy

### Delegation Considerations

Do not delegate this skill to assistive personnel. The one exception in some agencies is care of an enterostomy (6 weeks or more postoperative). When delegating this skill, instruct the assistive personnel about:

- The expected amount, color, and consistency of drainage from the enterostomy
- The expected appearance of the stoma
- Special equipment needed to complete procedure
- When to report changes in the patient's stoma and surrounding skin integrity

### Equipment

- Pouch, clear drainable colostomy/ileostomy/urostomy in correct size for two-piece system (see Figure 33-11, *A*) or custom cut-to-fit, one-piece type with attached skin barrier (see Figure 33-11, *B*)
- Pouch closure device, such as a clamp or pouch valve
- Adhesive remover (optional)
- Clean disposable gloves
- Ostomy deodorant, if needed
- Gauze pads or washcloth
- Towel or disposable waterproof barrier
- Basin with warm tap water
- Scissors/pen
- Skin barrier such as sealant wipes or wafer
- Ostomy belt (optional)

| STEP | RATIONALE |
|---|---|

### ASSESSMENT

1. Perform hand hygiene, and put on clean gloves. Auscultate for bowel sounds.

   Reduces transmission of microorganisms. Documents presence of peristalsis. Absence of sounds may indicate a problem.

2. Observe skin barrier and pouch for leakage and length of time in place. Depending on type of pouching system used (such as opaque pouch), remove the pouch to fully observe the stoma. Clear pouches permit the viewing of the stoma without their removal.

   Determines likelihood of pouch loosening from stoma and failing to collect effluent. Routine observation allows for early detection of potential problems (Thompson, 2000). Leaking may indicate the need for a different pouch or sealant.

- *Critical Decision Point:* You do not need to change intact skin barriers that have no evidence of leakage daily. These are able to remain in place for 3 to 5 days (Ayello, 2000; Erwin-Toth, 2001).

3. Observe stoma for color, swelling, trauma, and healing; make sure stoma is moist and reddish pink. Assess type of stoma. Stomas are flush with the skin or are a budlike protrusion on the abdomen (see illustration).

   Stoma characteristics are one of the factors to consider when selecting an appropriate pouching system (WOCN, 2005).

- *Critical Decision Point:* When a new ostomy is present, it is important to measure the stoma with each pouching system change to determine correct size of equipment needed. The system may need modifications as the stoma size changes (WOCN, 2005). Follow each ostomy pouch manufacturer's directions and measuring guide to determine which size ostomy pouch to use based on patient's actual stoma measurement size (Erwin-Toth, 2000).

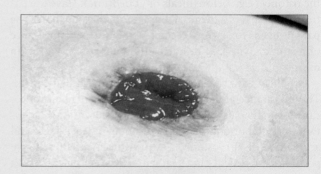

STEP **3** Normal bud stoma. (Courtesy Hollister, Incorporated, Libertyville, Ill. Permission to use this copyrighted material has been granted by the owner, Hollister International.)

| STEP | RATIONALE |
|------|-----------|
| 4. Observe abdominal contour and abdominal incision (if present). | Relationship of abdominal contour to stoma determines proper placement of pouch. The presence of pressure areas from the pouching system may necessitate the use of a new pouching system (WOCN, 2005). |
| 5. Observe effluent from stoma, and keep a record of intake and output. Ask patient about skin tenderness. | Plan on routine changing of skin barrier pouch at times of less effluent output. Generally avoid changing after meals, when gastrocolic reflux increases chance of fecal effluent output. |
| 6. When assessing skin for irritation, check that pouching system is not leaking. | Leaking indicates the need for a different type of pouch or sealant. |

• *Critical Decision Point:* Because of stoma and abdominal characteristics, some patients need their ostomy pouching system to curve outward to avoid leakage (see illustration for step 3) (Thompson, 2000).

| | |
|------|-----------|
| 7. To minimize skin irritation, avoid unnecessary changing of entire pouching system. You change a one-piece pouch with attached skin barriers or the skin barrier of a two-piece pouching system every 3 to 5 days, *not* daily. | Makes sure pouches are emptied when one-third to one-half full because weight of contents will dislodge skin seal, and ostomy drainage is irritating to the skin. Also, pouches collect flatus (gas), which will disrupt skin seal if it is not expelled. |
| 8. Assess abdomen for best type of pouching system to use. Consider:<br>a. Contour and peristomal plane | Determines pouching system selection and need for other equipment.<br>A firm/flat and round/hard abdomen usually needs a flexible or soft pouching system, whereas a flabby or soft abdomen usually needs a firmer system (see illustration for step 3). Stomas that are retracted or in skinfolds need convexity (curving outward), and different pouching systems are necessary to prevent leaking. |
| b. Presence of scars, incisions<br>c. Location and type of stoma | |

• *Critical Decision Point:* Pouching system options include the following:
  • One-piece pouch with skin barrier already attached; precut pouch and skin barrier; or two-piece pouch system, which consists of pouch that detaches from skin barrier and remains around patient's stoma for several days.
  • Two-piece pouches give patient choice of using either an open-ended or closed-ended pouch. This is because the patient is able to remove the pouch from the skin barrier to empty effluent. For some patients, accessory products, such as karaya paste or careful use of a pouch belt, will enhance the seal and prevent leakage (Erwin-Toth, 2001).
  • If excessive gas accumulation is present, determine the need for the patient to switch to a pouch with a vent or filter (WOCN, 2004a).

| | |
|------|-----------|
| 9. Assess the patient's self-care ability to determine the best type of pouching system to use. Assess the patient's vision, dexterity or mobility, and cognitive function. | Patients with poor vision will benefit by using yellow-tinted sunglasses to reduce glare and improve contrast and by using magnification mirrors (Jeffries and MacKay, 1997). Patients who also have mobility problems or spinal cord injuries will benefit by using equipment that has a longer pouch, which is easier to empty independently when sitting (Erwin-Toth, 2003; Thompson, 2000). Patients who have difficulty using their hands or who have limited vision will find a one-piece system or a precut pouch and skin barrier more desirable to use; others prefer being able to keep the skin barrier in place for several days and changing just the pouch For these patients the two-piece system is preferable. |

## SKILL 33-3 | Pouching an Ostomy—cont'd

| STEP | RATIONALE |
|------|-----------|
| 10. Remove existing pouch, if any, by gently pushing skin from adhesive barrier; properly dispose of soiled pouch (save clamp if attached to pouch). After skin barrier and pouch removal, assess skin around stoma, noting scars, folds, skin breakdown, and peristomal suture line, if present. | Prevents skin irritation and controls odor. Determines need for barrier paste to increase adherence of pouch to skin or to fill in irregularities. Many enterostomal pouch systems have a flexible adhesive, a pectin, karaya or synthetic wafer flange that assists in leak prevention. Karaya is a natural gum product that softens with body heat and conforms to the contours around the stoma. A deeper skin crease will need a paste to fill in the defect and prevent leakage (Erwin-Toth, 2000). |
| 11. Remove gloves, and perform hand hygiene. | Reduces transmission of microorganisms. |
| 12. Determine patient's emotional response and knowledge and understanding of an ostomy and its care. | Assists in determining how able the patient is to participate in care and also determines the need for teaching and information clarification (O'Shea, 2001; Secord and others, 2001). |

### PLANNING

| | |
|--|--|
| 1. Explain procedure to patient; encourage patient's interaction and questions. | Lessens anxiety and promotes patient's participation. |
| 2. Assemble equipment, and close room curtains or door. | Organization saves time, optimizes use of time, and conserves the patient's energy. Provides privacy. |

### IMPLEMENTATION

| | |
|--|--|
| 1. Position patient either standing or supine, and drape, leaving area around stoma exposed. If seated, position patient either on or in front of toilet. | When patient is supine, there are fewer skin wrinkles, which allows for ease of application of pouching system; maintains patient's dignity. |
| 2. Perform hand hygiene, and apply disposable gloves. | Reduces transmission of microorganisms. |
| 3. Place towel or disposable waterproof barrier under patient. | Protects bed linen. |

• *Critical Decision Point:* If portions of the skin barrier remain, use an adhesive remover to gently remove them. Improper removal of barrier will irritate patient's skin, cause skin tears, and result in poor adhering of the new pouch.

| | |
|--|--|
| 4. Cleanse peristomal skin gently with warm tap water using gauze pads or clean washcloth; do not scrub skin; dry completely by patting skin with gauze or towel. | Avoid use of soap because it leaves a residue on skin that interferes with pouch adhesion to skin. Skin needs to be dry as skin barrier; pouch does not adhere to wet skin, and moisture increases patient's risk for fungal infections. If blood appears on gauze pad, do not be alarmed. If rubbed, stomas ooze some blood as a result of cleaning process. Stoma's surface is highly vascular mucous membrane. Bleeding into pouch is abnormal (WOCN, 2004b). |

• *Critical Decision Point:* Adhesive removers should not be routinely used. However, adhesive removers may necessary when the patient's skin tears easily or there is a buildup of sticky residue over the peristomal skin. When adhesive removers are used, follow up with washing the skin with water and a mild soap to remove the oily coating on the skin from the adhesive remover (WOCN, 2004a).

| | |
|--|--|
| 5. Measure stoma for correct size of pouching system needed using the manufacturer's measuring guide (see illustration). | Ensures accuracy in determining correct pouch size needed. Stoma shrinks and does not reach usual size for 6 to 8 weeks (Thompson, 2000). |

| STEP | RATIONALE |
|---|---|
| **6.** Select appropriate pouch for patient based on patient assessment. With a custom cut-to-fit pouch, use an ostomy guide to cut opening on the pouch $\frac{1}{16}$ to $\frac{1}{8}$ inch larger than stoma before removing backing. Prepare pouch by removing backing from barrier and adhesive. With ileostomy, apply thin circle of barrier paste around opening in pouch; allow to dry (see illustrations A to C). | Size of pouch opening keeps drainage off skin and lessens risk of damage to stoma during peristalsis or activity. Change pouch and skin barrier whenever leaking. Change when patient is comfortable; before a meal is better because this avoids increased peristalsis and chance of evacuation during pouch change. Also, change pouch before or after tub bath or shower. Paste facilitates seal and protects skin. Stool is alkaline and contains enzymes, and this irritates skin; fecal bacteria colonize on skin and increase risk of infection. |

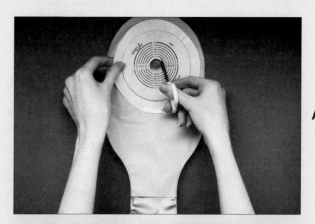

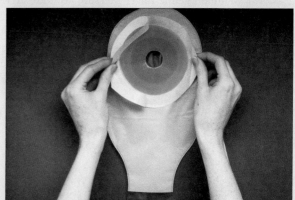

A

B

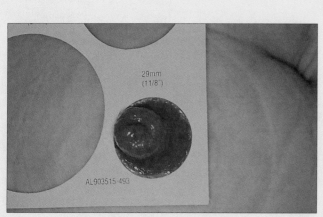

STEP **5** Measuring a stoma.

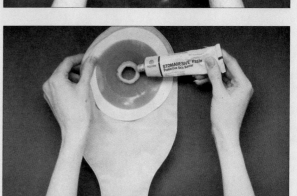

C

STEP **6** **A,** Cut-to-fit, one-piece drainable ostomy pouch. **B,** Removing the backing paper for the barrier of a one-piece pouch. **C,** Applying barrier paste to a one-piece ostomy pouch. (Courtesy ConvaTec, Princeton, NJ.)

Pouching an Ostomy—cont'd

| STEP | RATIONALE |
|---|---|

• *Critical Decision Point:* If patient has large amount of liquid stool from an ileostomy, consider using a "high-output" pouch that will contain this effluent and reduce frequency of pouch emptying.

| | |
|---|---|
| 7. Apply skin barrier and pouch. If creases next to stoma occur, use barrier paste to fill in; let dry 1 to 2 minutes. | Paste creates flat surface for pouch application. |

• *Critical Decision Point:* When applying skin barrier to stoma that is close to patient's abdominal incision, skin barrier may have to be trimmed to fit.

| | |
|---|---|
| **A. For One-Piece Pouching System** | |
| (1) Use skin sealant wipes on skin directly under adhesive skin barrier or pouch; allow to dry. Press adhesive backing of pouch and/or skin barrier smoothly against skin, starting from the bottom and working up and around sides. | Ensures smooth, wrinkle-free seal. Be aware of any irritated or open areas because the skin sealant wipes often contain alcohol (WOCN, 2004a). |
| (2) Hold pouch by barrier, center over stoma, and press down gently on barrier; bottom of pouch points toward patient's knees (see illustration). | A different positioning of the pouch is sometimes necessary to allow better gravity flow. For example, a patient confined to bed needs to have pouch positioned horizontally over the side of the abdomen (Thompson, 2000). |
| (3) Maintain gentle finger pressure around barrier for 1 to 2 minutes. | Gentle pressure and body heat assist in adhesion. |
| **B. If Using Two-Piece Pouching System** | |
| (1) Apply barrier-paste flange (barrier with adhesive) as in steps above for one-piece system. Then snap on pouch, and maintain finger pressure (see illustration). | Creates wrinkle-free, secure seal; decreases irritation from adhesive on skin. Some two-piece pouching systems have a snapping or clicking sound that occurs when attaching pouch to skin barrier. |
| **C.** For both pouching systems gently tug on pouch in a downward direction. | Determines that you have securely attached the pouch. |
| 8. Gently press on the pectin or karaya flange to facilitate adhesion. | A pectin, karaya, or synthetic skin barrier adds to security of keeping pouch system attached securely (Erwin-Toth, 2001). Some patients prefer a belt attached to the pouch for extra security. |

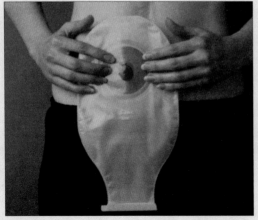

STEP **7A(2)** Applying a one-piece pouch. (Courtesy ConvaTec, Princeton, NJ.)

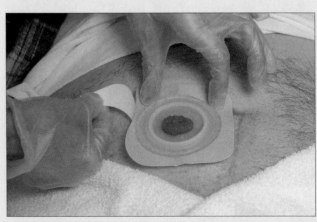

STEP **7B(1)** Application of a barrier-paste flange. (Courtesy ConvaTec, Princeton, NJ.)

| STEP | RATIONALE |
|------|-----------|

• *Critical Decision Point:* Make sure patient who chooses to wear an ostomy belt does not have the belt too tight. To check for appropriate tightness, make sure two fingers fit comfortably between the belt and the patient's skin.

| | |
|---|---|
| 9. Although many ostomy pouches are odorproof, explain to patient not to use "home remedies," which will harm the stoma, to control ostomy odor. Do not make a hole in pouch to release flatus. | Causes damage to pouch and defeats purpose of odorproof pouch. A hole for flatus will also allow effluent to leak. |

• *Critical Decision Point:* Never add aspirin to an ostomy pouch. It will cause stoma bleeding.

| | |
|---|---|
| 10. Fold bottom of drainable open-ended pouches up once, and close using a closure device such as a clamp (or follow manufacturer's instructions for closure). | Maintains secure seal to prevent leaking. |
| 11. Properly dispose of old pouch and soiled equipment. Some patients will also request you to spray the room with air freshener. | Lessens odors in room. |
| 12. Remove gloves, and perform hand hygiene. | Reduces transmission of microorganisms. |
| 13. Change one- or two-piece pouch every 3 to 7 days unless leaking. Pouch remains in place for tub bath or shower. After bath, pat adhesive dry. | Avoids unnecessary trauma to skin from too-frequent changes. If patient removes pouch for bathing, have the patient use a mild soap without oils or deodorants. Make sure patient rinses all soap residue off. Drying ensures adhesion of pouch and prevention of skin irritation under pouch (Erwin-Toth, 2001). |

## EVALUATION

| | |
|---|---|
| 1. Ask if patient feels discomfort around stoma. | Determines presence of skin irritation. |
| 2. Note appearance of stoma around skin and existing incision (if present) while removing pouch and cleansing skin. Reinspect condition of skin barrier and adhesive. Inspect edges of pouch for "tracking" of effluent under edges. This signals a potential leak due to skinfold or wrinkle. | Determines condition of tissues and progress of healing. Determines presence of leaks. |
| 3. Auscultate bowel sounds, and observe characteristics of stool. | Determines return of peristalsis and bowel elimination. |
| 4. Observe patient's nonverbal behaviors as you apply pouch. Ask if patient has any questions about pouching. | Indicates emotional response to stoma and readiness for teaching. Determines level of understanding of procedure (O'Shea, 2001). |

## RECORDING AND REPORTING

■ Chart type of pouch and skin barrier applied.
■ Record amount and appearance of stool or drainage in pouch, size of stoma, color of stool, texture, condition of peristomal skin, and sutures.
■ Document abdominal distention and excessive tenderness, nature and location of bowel sounds.
■ Record patient's level of participation and need for teaching.
■ Report any of the following to nurse in charge and/or physician or health care provider:
  • Abnormal appearance of stoma, suture line, peristomal skin, character of output, absence of bowel sounds
  • No flatus in 24 to 36 hours and no stool by third day

## UNEXPECTED OUTCOMES AND RELATED INTERVENTIONS

■ Skin around stoma is irritated; a rash with red papules or white pustules may be present. The patient may complain of burning or itching sensations.
  • Assess stoma for separation of mucosal layer of stoma from skin. Cleanse the area with normal saline, tap water, or noncytotoxic wound cleanser. Fill the separation to absorb drainage and provide healing (WOCN, 2005).
  • Determine if there is an undermining of pouch seal by fecal contents. Also indicates an allergic reaction, evident by erythema and blistering, usually confined to one area immediately under allergen (Erwin-Toth, 2000).

## SKILL 33-3 Pouching an Ostomy—cont'd

### UNEXPECTED OUTCOMES AND RELATED INTERVENTIONS—CONT'D

- Increase frequency of pouching system changes to provide wound care. Use a pouching system that allows access to the separation so the entire system does not need to be changed (WOCN, 2005).
- ■ Necrotic stoma is purple or black color, dry instead of moist texture, fails to bleed when washed gently, or has the presence of tissue sloughing.
  - Assess circulation to stoma.
  - Determine presence of excessive edema or excessive tension on bowel suture line.
  - Use transparent pouching system (WOCN, 2005).

- ■ Patient complains of irritation and burning around stoma.
  - Assess skin for breaks in integrity, skin inflammation, maceration, or infection.
  - Eliminate exposure of underlying skin to moisture or effluent.
  - If topical fungal infection is present, apply antifungal powder (WOCN, 2005).
  - If the patient has diabetes, assess serum glucose levels and determine the need for tighter controls to control risk for fungal infections (WOCN, 2005).
- ■ Patient refuses to view stoma or participate in care.
  - Obtain information about ostomy support groups in community.
  - Refer patient and family to other volunteer patients with an ostomy in community for individual support.

---

## OUTCOME EVALUATION

**TABLE 33-4**

| Nursing Action | Patient Response/Finding | Achievement of Outcome |
| --- | --- | --- |
| Review Mr. Gutierrez's diary of foods, and ask him about his intake as well. | Mr. Gutierrez described likes and dislikes, but admits to eating high-fat foods and little fruits and vegetables. | Mr. Gutierrez's intake of high-fiber foods is still limited. |
| Ask him about pattern of elimination over the last 2 weeks and laxative use. | Mr. Gutierrez says, "I still go about the same" but states that he thinks he now goes about every 2 days. Mr. Gutierrez has not used any laxatives. Bowel sounds are normal. Abdomen is soft and nontender with no distention. | He has bowel movements approximately every 2 days. His abdomen is less distended. |
| Ask Mr. Gutierrez about type and amount of fluid intake. | Mr. Gutierrez says he is drinking more water each day, "about six glasses." | Mr. Gutierrez's fluid intake is improving. |

---

## EVALUATION

Vickie returns to see Mr. Gutierrez 2 weeks later. Vickie is eager to determine if Mr. Gutierrez has made any changes in his diet and how his problems with bowel elimination have been progressing. Vickie is also anxious to learn if the niece has assisted in having Mr. Gutierrez's stove repaired.

Mr. Gutierrez tells Vickie that he has been eating bran cereal in the morning, has been eating rice and/or beans for dinner, and has added one fruit each day to his diet. He has been walking twice a day through the long-term care center. Although he does not have a bowel movement each day, his stools are much softer and easier to pass and he says he is less concerned. He has not taken a laxative for a stool since last talking with Vickie.

**Documentation Note**

"Problem with bowel elimination is improving. Abdomen is soft and nondistended; bowel sounds normal and audible in all quadrants. Because of the teaching plan, has altered eating habits to include more fiber, fruit, and fluids. Although concern over bowel habits has not ceased, does state he feels 'in better control' and has decreased laxative use. Niece assisted in having stove repaired."

integrity. Your evaluation will also include observing the patient change and empty an ostomy pouch or perform an irrigation. Evaluate the output or functioning of the ostomy or reservoir as well. In addition, consider the patient's self-esteem and evaluate it by the patient's response to and willingness to care for the ostomy.

**PATIENT EXPECTATIONS.** Using patient expectations identified during assessment, determine the patient's level of satisfaction with nursing care. Does the patient feel that you provided care respectfully, offering privacy and support

when necessary? Is the patient satisfied with the elimination pattern established? Are stools easier to manage?

Your goal for the patient with an ostomy is to achieve a realistic level of self-care and to maintain or reinforce a healthy body image. When discussing these issues with the patient, determine if the patient's participation in care helped the patient accept the ostomy. Were expectations of the patient unrealistic? Did the patient feel like a partner in care? Learning about the patient's level of satisfaction with care will go a long way toward helping future patients.

## KEY CONCEPTS

- Mechanical breakdown of food elements, GI motility, and selective absorption and secretion of substances by the large intestine influence the character of feces.
- Food high in fiber content and an increased fluid intake keep feces soft.
- The greatest danger from diarrhea is fluid and electrolyte imbalance.
- The location of an ostomy influences the consistency of stool.
- Assessment of an elimination pattern focuses on bowel habits, an analysis of factors that normally influence defecation, a review of recent changes in elimination, and a physical examination.
- A fecal occult blood test is for patients who are over 50 years of age, take anticoagulants, who have a bleeding disorder or GI disorder causing bleeding, or who are at risk for colon cancer.
- Consider frequency of defecation, fecal characteristics, and effect of foods on GI function when selecting a diet promoting normal elimination.
- Consider the patient's usual time of defecation in the administration of cathartics or laxatives.
- Proper administration of an enema requires the slow instillation of the proper volume of a warm solution.
- A continent ostomy provides control over when fecal material exits.
- Dangers during digital removal of stool include traumatizing the rectal mucosa and promoting vagal stimulation.
- Skin breakdown occurs after repeated exposure to liquid stool. This is especially true in patients with a stoma.

## CRITICAL THINKING IN PRACTICE

*While fulfilling your community service responsibility of taking blood pressure measurements at the senior citizens' center, one of the patients tells you that this morning after he had a bowel movement, he noticed bright red blood on the toilet tissue.*

1. What further data do you need to gather?
2. Mrs. Cavendish is a 40-year-old woman who has just had a colon resection for cancer 2 days ago, and she has a temporary colostomy ostomy.

a. Describe your assessment of the ostomy.
b. Describe your assessment of her abdomen and surgical wound.
3. Mrs. Cavendish has not looked at the ostomy. What effect will this have on her independence? What are some strategies that you will use to help her with this adjustment?

## NCLEX® REVIEW

1. Most nutrients and electrolytes are absorbed in the:
   1. Colon
   2. Stomach
   3. Esophagus
   4. Small intestine
2. During assessment your patient reveals that he has diarrhea and cramping every time he has ice cream. He attributes this to the cold nature of the food. However, you begin to suspect that these symptoms might be associated with:
   1. Food allergy
   2. Irritable bowel
   3. Lactose intolerance
   4. Increased peristalsis

3. You are assessing a 55-year-old patient who is in the clinic for a routine physical. You will only instruct the patient to obtain a fecal occult blood specimen:
   1. When there is a family history of polyps
   2. If patient reports rectal bleeding
   3. If a palpable mass is detected on digital examination
   4. As part of a routine examination, in accordance with American Cancer Society guidelines
4. Diarrhea that occurs with a fecal impaction is the result of:
   1. A clear liquid diet
   2. Irritation of the intestinal mucosa
   3. Seepage of stool around the impaction
   4. Inability of the patient to form a stool

5. You are caring for a patient with an established ostomy. The patient manages her colostomy on her own. However, she is now complaining of peristomal irritation. To determine the cause of this irritation, you must assess:
   1. Circulation to stoma and fit of pouch
   2. Quantity and consistency of fecal drainage in pouch
   3. Presence of signs of infection at the stoma or peristomal skin
   4. Circulation to stoma, quantity and consistency of fecal drainage, allergic response to ostomy products, fit of pouch, and presence of infection

6. A cleansing enema is ordered for a 55-year-old patient before intestinal surgery. The maximum amount given is:
   1. 150 to 200 ml
   2. 200 to 400 ml
   3. 400 to 750 ml
   4. 750 to 1000 ml

7. During the enema your patient begins to complain of pain. You note blood in the return fluid and rectal bleeding. Your actions are to:
   1. Stop the instillation
   2. Slow down the rate of instillation
   3. Stop the instillation and obtain vital signs
   4. Tell the patient to breathe slowly and relax

## REFERENCES

American Cancer Society: *Colon and rectal cancer: 2004*, Atlanta, 2004, The Society, www.cancer.org.

Annells M, Koch T: Older people seeking solutions to constipation: the laxative mire, *J Clin Nurs* 11(5):603, 2002.

Anti M and others: Water supplementation enhances the effect of high-fiber diet on stool frequency and laxative consumption in adult patients with functional constipation, *Hepatogastroenterology* 45(21):727, 1998.

Ayello EA: The ABCDs of stoma assessment and pouching, personal correspondence, 2000.

Bliss DZ and others: Fecal incontinence in hospitalized patients who are acutely ill, *Nurs Res* 49(2):101, 2000.

Bliss DZ and others: Supplementation with dietary fiber improves fecal incontinence, *Nurs Res* 50(4):203, 2001.

Colwell J and others: The state of the standard diversion, *J Wound Ostomy Continence Nurs* 28:6, 2001.

Dochterman JM, Bulechek GM, editors: *Nursing interventions classification (NIC)*, ed 4, St. Louis, 2004, Mosby.

Dosh SA: Evaluation and treatment of constipation, *J Fam Pract* 51(6):555, 2002.

Doughty D: A physiologic approach to bowel training, *J Wound Ostomy Continence Nurs* 23(1):46, 2000.

Doughty D: *Urinary and fecal incontinence nursing*, ed 2, St. Louis, 2006, Mosby.

Ebersole P, Hess P, Luggen AS: *Toward healthy aging: human needs and nursing response*, ed 6, St. Louis, 2004, Mosby.

Erwin-Toth P: Ostomies and fistulas: prevention and management of peristomal skin complications, *Adv Skin Wound Care* 13(4):175, 2000.

Erwin-Toth P: Caring for a stoma is more than skin deep, *Nursing* 31(5):36, 2001.

Erwin-Toth P: Ostomy pearls, *Adv Skin Wound Care* 16(3):146, 2003.

Giger JN, Davidhizar RE: *Transcultural nursing: assessment and intervention*, ed 4, St. Louis, 2004, Mosby.

Gong G: Relief of postoperative gas pain 'bed exercise': a new means of addressing an old problem, *Am J Nurs* 104(2):72A, 2004.

Hampton BG, Bryant RA: *Ostomies and continent diversions: nursing management*, St. Louis, 1992, Mosby.

Hinrichs M, Huseboe J: *Evidenced-based protocol: management of constipation*. In Titler MG, series editor: Series on evidence based practice for older adults, Iowa City, 1998, The University of Iowa, Gerontological Nursing Interventions Research Center, Research Dissemination Core. For more information, http://www.nursing.uiowa.edu/center/gnirc/disseminatecore.htm.

Jeffries C, MacKay AT: Improving stoma management in the low-vision patient, *J Wound Ostomy Continence Nurs* 24(6):302, 1997.

Lembo A, Camilleri M: Current concepts: chronic constipation, *N Engl J Med* 349(14):1360, 2003.

McCance KL, Huether SE: *Pathophysiology: the biologic basis for disease in adults and children*, ed 4, St Louis, 2002, Mosby.

McKenry LM, Salerno E: *Mosby's pharmacology in nursing*, ed 21, St. Louis, 2001, Mosby.

Metheny N and Titler M: Placement of feeding tubes, *Am J Nurs*, 101(5): 36, 2001.

Metheny N and others: Effectiveness of pH measurements in predicting feeding tube placement: an update, *Nurs Res* 42(6):324, 1993.

Metheny N and others: Visual characteristics from aspirates in feeding tubes as a method for predicting tube location, *Nurs Res* 43:282, 1994

Metheny N and others: pH, color, and feeding tubes, *RN* 61(1):277, 1998.

Moorhead S, Johnson M, Maas M: *Nursing Outcomes Classification (NOC)*, ed 3, St. Louis, 2004, Mosby.

Moppett S: Administration of an enema, *Nurs Times* 95:insert 2p, 1999.

NANDA International: *Nursing diagnoses: definitions and classifications 2005-2006*, Philadelphia, 2005, NANDA International.

Norton C, Chelvanayagam S: A nursing assessment tool of adults with fecal incontinence, *J Wound Ostomy Continence Nurs* 27:279, 2000.

O'Shea HS: Teaching the adult ostomy patient, *J Wound Ostomy Continence Nurs* 28(1):47, 2001.

Ransohoff DF, Lang CA: Screening for colorectal cancer with the fecal occult blood test: a background paper, *Ann Intern Med* 126:881, 1997.

Richmond J: Prevention of constipation through risk management, *Nurs Stand* 17(16):39, 2003.

Schiff L: Ostomy products, *RN* 63(11):71, 2000.

Secord C and others: Adjusting to life with an ostomy, *Can Nurse* 97(1):29, 2001.

Seidel HM and others: *Mosby's guide to physical examination*, ed 5, St. Louis, 2003, Mosby.

Thompson J: A practical ostomy guide, part I, *RN* 63(11):61, 2000.

Thompson MJ and others: Management of constipation, *Nurs Stand* 18(14-16):41, 2003.

Wound, Ostomy, and Continence Nurses Society: *Basic ostomy skin care: a guide for patients and healthcare providers*, Glenview, Ill, 2004a, The Society.

Wound, Ostomy, and Continence Nurses Society: *Peristomal skin complications: best practice for clinicians*, Glenview, Ill, 2004b, The Society.

Wound, Ostomy, and Continence Nurses Society: *Stoma complications: best practice for clinicians*, Glenview, Ill, 2005, The Society.

# CHAPTER 34

# Immobility

## MEDIA RESOURCES

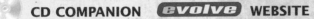

**CD COMPANION** *evolve* **WEBSITE**

http://evolve.elsevier.com/Potter/basic

- **NCLEX® Review**
- **Audio Glossary**
- **English/Spanish Audio Glossary**

## OBJECTIVES

- Describe mobility and immobility.
- Discuss the benefits and hazards of bed rest.
- Identify changes in metabolic rate associated with immobility.
- Describe physical changes associated with immobility.
- Describe physiological changes associated with immobility.
- Discuss factors that contribute to pressure ulcer formation.

- Describe psychosocial and developmental effects of immobilization.
- Complete a nursing assessment of an immobilized patient.
- Develop a nursing care plan for an immobilized patient.
- List appropriate nursing interventions for an immobilized patient.
- State evaluation criteria for the immobilized patient.

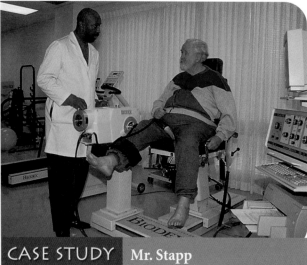

### CASE STUDY  Mr. Stapp

Bob Stapp is a 54-year-old man admitted to the rehabilitation center after a bilateral total knee replacement 3 days ago. Mr. Stapp expects to be at the center for 5 days, then he expects to go home and continue therapy on an outpatient basis. He says his health is good, except he has a "bit of sugar" and "can't seem to lose that 50 lb the doc wants me to." He plans to return to work in the steel mill, where he has worked for 28 years, as soon as he gets the physician's or health care provider's okay. His postoperative course has been as expected.

Mark Weber is a 48-year-old nursing student who is completing the second half of his first clinical experience in nursing. He is a retired fireman, divorced, and has a son who is also in nursing school at a nearby college. It is his first day at the center; he spent the first half of his clinical experience on an orthopedic unit in a community hospital.

### KEY TERMS

activities of daily living (ADLs), p. 992
anthropometric measurements, p. 996
bed rest, p. 993
bone resorption, p. 994
disuse osteoporosis, p. 994
diuresis, p. 993
footdrop, p. 994
hypercalcemia, p. 993
hypostatic pneumonia, p. 993
immobility, p. 993
instrumental activities of daily living (IADLs), p. 1011

ischemia, p. 995
isometric exercises, p. 1004
joint contracture, p. 994
mobility, p. 996
negative nitrogen balance, p. 993
orthostatic hypotension, p. 993
osteoporosis, p. 995
pathological fractures, p. 994
renal calculi, p. 995
thrombus, p. 994

## Scientific Knowledge Base

### Mobility

Mobility is the capacity to move around freely in the environment. It serves many purposes, including expressing emotion, self-defense, attaining basic needs, participating in recreational activities, and completing **activities of daily living (ADLs)** such as bathing, dressing, and eating. Mobility assists in maintaining the body's normal physiological activities and requires the functioning of the nervous and musculoskeletal systems.

A decline in a patient's mobility status sometimes results from many types of health problems. Patients with certain illnesses, injuries, or surgeries experience a period of immobilization. Factors that contribute to the extent of a patient's immobility (inability to move around freely), include length and severity of illness, emotional status, and physical condition. Immobilization is also used therapeutically to limit movement as in the application of a cast.

**BED REST.** **Bed rest** is an intervention in which a patient is restricted to bed for therapeutic reasons. Advantages of bed rest include decreasing the body's oxygen needs, reducing pain, and allowing the debilitated or ill patient to rest. The duration of bed rest depends on the type and nature of the illness or injury and the patient's prior state of health.

## Immobility

Immobility occurs when a patient is unable to move independently or is restricted for therapeutic reasons. Immobility results from pain, cognitive, or neurological changes and also from emotional changes such as depression.

No body system is immune to the hazardous effects of immobility (McCance and Huether, 2002; Puckree, Moonasur, and Govender, 2000). The greater the extent and longer the duration of immobility, the more pronounced the consequences.

**PHYSIOLOGICAL EFFECTS.** Each body system is at risk for impairment from immobility (Box 34-1). The severity of impairment depends on the patient's age, overall mental and physical health, and the extent of immobility. Despite a patient's age, impairment as a result of immobility affects the respiratory system, metabolism, fluid and electrolyte balance, gastrointestinal tract, cardiovascular system, musculoskeletal system, integument, and urinary elimination.

**RESPIRATORY CHANGES.** Decreased lung expansion, generalized respiratory muscle weakness, and stasis of secretions occur with immobility. These conditions often contribute to the development of atelectasis (collapse of alveoli) and **hypostatic pneumonia** (inflammation of the lung from stasis or pooling of secretions).

With decreased lung expansion and weakened respiratory muscles, secretions stagnate or pool in the dependent lung regions. In atelectasis, secretions block a bronchiole or a bronchus and the distal lung tissue (alveoli) collapses. Respiratory changes reduce the patient's ability to cough due to generalized muscle weakness. Mucus accumulates, particularly when the patient lies supine (flat position), providing an excellent medium for bacterial growth. Hypostatic pneumonia results.

**CHANGES IN METABOLISM.** Immobility disrupts normal metabolic functioning, decreasing the metabolic rate and altering the metabolism of carbohydrates, proteins, and fats. A patient's basal metabolic rate (BMR) decreases in response to reduced cellular energy and oxygen demands. However, in the presence of an infection, immobilized patients have an increased BMR as a result of fever or wound healing. Fever and wound repair increase cellular oxygen requirements (McCance and Huether, 2002).

Prolonged bed rest decreases the body's ability to produce insulin and metabolize glucose. When the body is unable to metabolize glucose, it begins to break down protein stores

---

| **BOX 34-1** | **Pathophysiology of Immobility** |
| --- | --- |

**Physiological Outcomes**

- ↓ Basal metabolic rate (BMR)
- ↓ Gastrointestinal motility
  - ↓ Nutrients/fluids
  - ↓ Appetite
- Shift in electrolyte balance
- ↓ O₂ availability/ischemia
  - ↓ O₂/CO₂ exchange
  - ↑ Respiratory muscle weakness
  - ↓ Lung expansion
  - ↑ Atelectasis/hypostatic pneumonia
- ↓ Cardiac output
  - ↑ Cardiac workload
  - ↑ Oxygen demand
  - ↑ Dependent edema
  - ↑ Clot formation (DVT)
- ↑ Muscle atrophy
  - ↓ Strength/flexibility/endurance
  - ↑ Joint contractures
- ↑ Disuse osteoporosis
- ↑ Bone resorption

**Psychological Outcomes**

- ↑ Stressors
- ↑ Depression
  - ↓ Self-identity
  - ↓ Self-esteem
- ↑ Behavioral changes
- ↑ Changes in sleep/wake cycles
- ↓ Coping successes
- ↑ Isolation
- ↑ Passive behaviors
- ↑ Sensory deprivation/overload

**Developmental Outcomes**

- ↑ Dependence
- ↑ Regression in development

---

for energy. Nitrogen is the end product of protein metabolism. Nitrogen balance provides a reliable indicator of protein use by the body. A **negative nitrogen balance** exists when the excretion of nitrogen from the breakdown of protein exceeds intake. A negative nitrogen balance predisposes your patient to problems with wound healing and normal tissue growth. Immobility causes a loss of lean body mass and an increased percentage of body fat.

**FLUID AND ELECTROLYTE BALANCES.** Major shifts in blood volume occur in immobile patients. **Diuresis** (increased urine excretion) occurs as a result of increased blood flow to the kidneys and expanded circulating blood volume. Diuresis causes the body to lose electrolytes, such as potassium and sodium. Diuresis also affects serum calcium levels. Immobility increases calcium resorption (loss) from bones, causing a release of excess calcium into circulation. This leads to **hypercalcemia** if the kidneys are unable to respond appropriately (Maher and others, 2002).

**GASTROINTESTINAL CHANGES.** Activity stimulates peristalsis. The immobile patient is at risk for constipation from lack of activity and from hypercalcemia, which depresses peristalsis. Constipation is sometimes so severe that fecal impaction occurs (see Chapter 33). Left untreated, a partial or complete bowel obstruction will occur.

**CARDIOVASCULAR CHANGES.** Orthostatic hypotension occurs in patients on bed rest and after prolonged sitting. **Orthostatic hypotension** is a drop of 20 mm Hg or more in systolic blood pressure or a decrease in diastolic blood pressure of more than 10 mm Hg when the patient rises from a lying or sitting position to a standing position (Ejaz and others, 2004). In the immobilized patient decreased circulating fluid volume, pooling of blood in the lower extremities, and decreased autonomic response occur. These factors result in decreased venous return, decreased central venous pressure and stroke volume, and a drop in systolic blood pressure when the patient stands (McCance and Huether, 2002).

Prolonged bed rest increases the heart's workload, producing a need for more oxygen. Bed rest also increases the resting heart rate 4 to 15 beats per minute. When the immobilized patient performs physical activity such as range-of-joint-motion (ROJM) exercises or ADLs, this increased rate is more pronounced.

Immobile patients are at risk for deep venous thrombosis (DVT). A **thrombus** is an accumulation of platelets, fibrin, clotting factors, and cellular elements of the blood attached to the interior wall of a vein or artery, sometimes occluding the lumen of the vessel. Three factors contribute to venous thrombus formation: (1) loss of integrity of the vessel wall (e.g., injury), (2) abnormalities of blood flow (e.g., slow blood flow in calf veins associated with bed rest), and (3) alterations in blood constituents (e.g., a change in clotting factors or increased platelet activity). These three factors are referred to as Virchow's triad (McCance and Huether, 2002). Two additional problems predispose the immobile patient to DVTs: (1) the weight of the legs on the bed compresses the blood vessels of the calves, causing stasis and injury to vessel linings; (2) the skeletal muscles in the legs lose their pumping action, leading to stasis and less blood returning to the heart.

Venous thrombi place the patient at risk for pulmonary emboli, a life-threatening complication. Pulmonary emboli are clots that move to the lung and block a portion of the pulmonary artery, which disrupts the blood flow to the lungs. Immobilized surgical and older adult patients are at high risk for developing pulmonary emboli (Byrne, 2001).

**MUSCULOSKELETAL CHANGES.** Immobility leads to loss of strength and endurance, decreased muscle mass, and decreased stability or balance. The body loses muscle strength when muscles are inactive. The rate of muscle decline will vary with the degree of immobility, but it is rapid while mobility and weight bearing are restricted. These effects are devastating to patients who are marginally functional with their ADLs.

Reduced endurance results when patients are immobile from changes in muscle strength and altered cardiovascular functioning. Muscle endurance decreases due to the inability of the cardiopulmonary system to meet the oxygen needs of the body. Reduced metabolism leads to a loss of muscle and body mass causing fatigue with prolonged activity.

As immobility progresses and muscles are not exercised, muscle mass continues to decrease. The muscle atrophies and the size of the muscle decreases. Immobility affects the leg muscles the most, which explains the difficulty older patients have in getting up out of a chair after periods of bed rest.

Immobility causes two skeletal changes. First, a **joint contracture** is an abnormal and possibly permanent condition

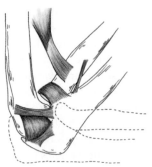

FIGURE **34-1** Flexion contracture of elbow resulting in permanent flexion of joint. Normally the elbow is able to extend to a 90-degree angle (*dotted line*) and to a 180-degree angle (*not shown*).

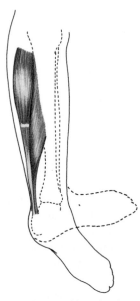

FIGURE **34-2** Footdrop. Ankle is fixed in plantar flexion.

characterized by fixation of the joint. Disuse, atrophy, and shortening of muscle fibers and surrounding joint tissues cause joint contracture. When a contracture occurs, the joint cannot maintain full ROJM (Figure 34-1). Contractures leave joints in nonfunctional positions, as seen in patients who are permanently curled in a fetal position.

One common and debilitating contracture is **footdrop** (Figure 34-2). When footdrop occurs, the foot is permanently in plantar flexion. Ambulation is difficult with the foot in this position because the patient cannot dorsiflex.

The second skeletal change is **disuse osteoporosis,** a disorder characterized by **bone resorption.** Immobilization increases the rate of bone resorption and bone tissue becomes less dense. Reduced bone density leads to disuse osteoporosis. Bone resorption also impairs calcium metabolism and causes calcium to be released in the blood, producing hypercalcemia. Patients with disuse osteoporosis are at risk for **pathological fractures,** a type of fracture that occurs as a result of bone weakness.

**Osteoporosis** is a major health concern in this country. This disease frequently affects women, whereas only 20% of men are diagnosed with the disease. The National Osteoporosis Foundation (NOF) (2002) reports that one out of two women will suffer the severe consequence of a pathological fracture as a result of primary osteoporosis. Although primary osteoporosis is different in origin from the osteoporosis that results from immobility, it is imperative for you to recognize that immobilized patients are at high risk for accelerated bone loss if they have primary osteoporosis.

**INTEGUMENT CHANGES.** The direct effect of pressure on the skin by immobility is compounded by the changes in metabolism. Older adult patients and patients with paralysis have a greater risk for developing pressure ulcers (see Chapter 35). Pressure affects cellular metabolism by decreasing or obliterating tissue circulation. When a patient lies in bed or sits in a chair, the weight of the body is on bony prominences. The longer the pressure is applied, the longer the period of **ischemia** (temporary decrease of blood flow to an organ or tissue) and therefore the greater the risk of skin breakdown (see Chapter 35). Any break in the skin's integrity is difficult to heal in the immobilized patient.

**URINARY ELIMINATION CHANGES.** Urine flows out of the renal pelvis and into the ureter and bladder because of gravitational forces when a patient is upright. When the patient is reclining or flat, the kidneys and ureters move toward a more level plane, and urine formed by the kidney enters the bladder against gravity. Because the peristaltic contractions of the ureters are not strong enough to overcome gravity, the renal pelvis fills before urine enters the ureters. This condition, called urinary stasis, increases the patient's risk of urinary tract infection and renal calculi. **Renal calculi** are calcium stones that lodge in the renal pelvis and pass through the ureters. Immobilized patients are at risk for calculi because of altered calcium metabolism and the resulting hypercalcemia.

## Nursing Knowledge Base

Monitoring or assisting patients with mobility is basic to nursing. Concepts that relate to mobility such as movement, exercise and rest, and posture are soundly grounded in many nursing theories. Immobilization leads to a variety of psychosocial responses. You will draw upon your assessment skills to fully understand the patient's initial condition and to monitor and evaluate care (see Chapter 13).

### Psychosocial Effects

Immobilization reduces a patient's independence and creates a sense of loss. As a result, emotional, intellectual, sensory, and sociocultural responses occur. The most common emotional changes are depression, sleep-wake disturbances, and impaired coping.

Some immobilized patients become depressed because of changes in self-concept (see Chapter 20). Depression is an affective disorder characterized by exaggerated feelings of sadness, melancholy, dejection, worthlessness, emptiness, and hopelessness. Depression can reduce a person's willingness to take part in activity, aggravating any immobile condition.

Immobilized patients require vigilant nursing care, such as repositioning every 2 hours, to avoid physical complications. You need to make sure to cluster nursing and medical interventions together as much as possible to ensure the patient receives sufficient sleep (see Chapter 29). Disruption of normal sleeping patterns will cause further behavioral changes.

Long-term immobility or bed rest affects usual coping patterns. Some immobilized patients withdraw and become passive. The passive patient demonstrates little interest in achieving independence or participating in care. Assess the patient's normal coping mechanisms, and develop a nursing care plan based on patient strengths.

### Developmental Effects

Developmental effects of immobility more commonly affect the very young and the older adult. The immobilized young or middle-age adult experiences few, if any, developmental changes.

When the infant, toddler, or preschooler is immobilized, it is usually because of trauma or the need to correct a congenital skeletal abnormality. Prolonged immobilization delays the child's motor skill and intellectual development. When caring for immobilized children, plan activities that provide physical and psychosocial stimuli (Hockenberry and others, 2003).

Immobilization of older adult patients increases their physical dependence on others and accelerates functional losses in physiological systems (Ebersole and others, 2004). Immobilization of older adults usually results from a degenerative disease, neurological trauma, or a chronic illness. For some patients immobilization occurs gradually and progressively, whereas for others—especially those who have had a cerebral vascular accident (CVA)—immobilization is sudden. Develop nursing care plans that encourage patient independence in as many self-care activities as possible.

## Critical Thinking

### Synthesis

As a nurse you gather information from a variety of sources when caring for patients. Integrating your knowledge and experience makes it possible to determine physical, psychosocial, and developmental needs of immobilized patients.

**KNOWLEDGE.** Understanding pathophysiology enables you to anticipate patients' limitations in mobility. These limitations are sometimes the direct result of musculoskeletal alteration, such as a broken ankle, or deconditioning from a chronic health problem, such as poor activity tolerance associated with cardiac problems. Nursing assessment enables you to determine the extent of any limitations. You need to assess the patient's developmental stage to determine current functional and mobility status and the health care needs of the patient. Knowledge gained from the study of human growth and development is essential to completing your assessment.

The use of proper body mechanics is important for you and your patient during positioning and transferring. The use of safe patient-handling equipment in conjunction with proper body mechanics significantly reduces work-related injuries in nurses (Nelson and Baptiste, 2004). Knowledge of the physiological changes associated with immobility enables you to identify complications and intervene appropriately. Patient teaching is essential to ensure rehabilitation following immobilization.

**EXPERIENCE.** You may have taken care of other patients who have had mobility restrictions. These experiences help you to anticipate the patient's need for comfort, pain control, positioning, and support of activities of daily living. Experiential learning will also occur during visits to a physical therapy unit in the hospital or in a community. Your experience with a variety of exercise strategies helps you develop health promotion activities or rehabilitation plans for your patients.

**ATTITUDE.** You need to be creative in designing solutions to improve the patient's mobility status. Speak with other health care providers to determine the best setting to provide care. Collaboration and creativity help you to establish an individualized rehabilitation program. Reflect on your own perceptions of the patient's mobility status. Self-reflection enables you to act as a patient advocate. It is your responsibility as a nurse to motivate the patient toward improved mobility and to identify ways in which the family may participate. The attitude of perseverance is essential for the nurse to coordinate patient care and work with patients experiencing psychological and developmental changes due to immobilization.

**STANDARDS.** It is important to promote your patient's independence while adhering to the prescribed rehabilitation plan and maintaining safety. Nursing policies and procedures offer standards for the safe use of transfer and positioning equipment. Be clear and specific when giving discharge instructions. Always use the ethical standard of autonomy in supporting patients to make decisions about their discharge needs. Also, use good evaluation standards in your care. Ask your patients to demonstrate required actions to ensure that you have communicated your directions accurately and that they have understood them completely.

Synthesis of knowledge, experience, attitudes, and standards is important in developing an individualized care plan for the immobilized patient. This plan of care will help to prevent complications, promote rehabilitation, and expedite discharge.

## Nursing Process

### Assessment

Mobility assessment focuses on patients' past and present mobility and the potential effects of immobility. Table 34-1 presents a focused patient assessment of immobility, pain associated with movement, and activity tolerance.

**MOBILITY.** Assessment of the patient's **mobility** focuses on range of motion, muscle strength, activity tolerance, gait, and posture. Table 34-2 describes the ROJM for all joints in the body. Observing the patient's posture while sitting and standing and assessing gait helps you to determine the type of assistance the patient requires for ambulation or transfer. Assess the patient for stiffness, swelling, pain, and unequal or limited movement. These data provide baseline information to evaluate the patient's overall level of mobility and coordination. Patient immobility leads to physical, psychosocial, and developmental changes.

**RESPIRATORY SYSTEM.** Perform a respiratory assessment at least every 2 hours for acutely ill patients with restricted activity. Monitor the patient's respiratory rate and oxygen saturation. Inspect chest wall movements, and auscultate the lungs to identify regions of diminished breath sounds. Focus auscultation for adventitious lung sounds on the dependent lung field because pulmonary secretions tend to accumulate in the lower lobes. If a patient has an atelectatic area, breath sounds will be asymmetrical. A complete respiratory assessment identifies the presence of secretions, and you will use this to determine nursing interventions necessary to maintain optimal respiratory function.

**METABOLIC SYSTEM.** When assessing the patient's metabolic functioning, use **anthropometric measurements** (body measures of height, weight, and skinfolds) to evaluate muscle atrophy. Intake and output records and laboratory data assist in evaluating fluid and electrolyte status. You assess a patient's nutritional status to determine the risk for nitrogen imbalance. A patient whose mobility is restricted often has a reduced appetite, altered gastrointestinal function, and a reduced capacity to self-feed.

Anorexia commonly occurs in immobilized patients. Assess food intake and the environment for unpleasant odors or noises that interfere with appetite. You can avoid nutritional imbalances if you learn the patient's previous dietary patterns and food preferences early in the immobilization (see Chapter 31).

Anthropometric measurements include height, weight, mid upper-arm circumference, and triceps skinfold measurements. Ideally, you perform this assessment early in the period of immobilization and repeat it at regular intervals. Chapter 13 discusses assessment of height and weight. A decrease in mid upper-arm circumference, measured in centimeters, or triceps skinfold, measured in millimeters, indicates a decline in muscle mass. After the initial assessment, take this measurement every 2 to 4 weeks, depending on the patient's age, previous physical condition, and the amount of immobility.

If an immobilized patient has a wound, the speed of healing indicates how well the body delivers nutrients to the tissues for use (see Chapter 35). The normal progression of wound healing indicates that the metabolic needs of the injured tissues are being met.

**CARDIOVASCULAR SYSTEM.** Cardiovascular assessment of the immobilized patient includes monitoring

## FOCUSED PATIENT ASSESSMENT

TABLE 34-1

| Factors to Assess | Questions and Approaches | Physical Assessment Strategies |
|---|---|---|
| Range of motion (ROJM) | Ask if patient has limited movement in joints.<br>Ask if patient has a history of connective tissue disorders, fractures, and/or damage to ligaments or tendons. | Observe patient's gait<br>Observe patient's ROJM for all joints.<br>Inspect joints for deformity.<br>Observe patient while performing self-care activities. |
| Pain | Ask if patient experiences pain or discomfort on movement.<br>Ask patient to rate pain on a 0-10 pain scale.<br>Ask patient to describe pain onset, duration, location, severity, precipitating factors, and relief measures.<br>Ask if patient needs pain medication before ambulating (with assistance), particularly after surgical procedure. | Observe for objective signs of pain such as grimacing, moaning, increasing respiratory rate, pulse, and blood pressure.<br>Inspect joints for redness or swelling, indicating potential inflammatory process. |
| Endurance and activity | Ask if patient feels fatigued.<br>Ask if patient is experiencing difficulty with ADLs because of muscle weakness.<br>Ask if patient is experiencing shortness of breath (SOB), dyspnea on exertion (DOE), palpitations, light-headedness, or dizziness. | Observe for signs of fatigue.<br>Observe patient's performance of ADLs.<br>Observe patient for pallor; obtain baseline vital signs.<br>Monitor oxygen saturation before and following activity. |

blood pressure, apical and peripheral pulses, and observing the venous system. Because of the risk for orthostatic hypotension, measure blood pressure when the patient moves from lying to a sitting or standing position. In this way, you are able to assess the patient's ability to tolerate postural changes.

Recumbency increases the cardiac workload and results in an increased pulse rate. In some patients, particularly the older adult, the heart is not able to tolerate the increased workload, and a form of cardiac failure develops. Document and report the absence of a peripheral pulse, particularly one that was previously present, after you make a complete circulatory assessment (see Chapter 13).

Edema indicates the heart's inability to handle the increased workload. Because fluid moves to dependent body regions, assessment of the immobilized patient includes the sacrum, legs, feet, and hips. If the heart is unable to tolerate the increased cardiac workload, the peripheral body regions such as the hands, feet, nose, and earlobes will be colder than the central body regions.

Assess the venous system for DVT. To assess for DVT, remove the patient's antiembolic stockings or sequential compression stockings once every 8 hours and observe the calves and thighs for unilateral leg swelling, redness, warmth, and tenderness. Ask the patient about calf pain. Assessing for Homans' sign, discomfort in the upper calf during forced dorsiflexion of the foot, is no longer an accurate predictor of DVT (Ramzi and Leeper, 2004; Riddle and Wells, 2004). Approximately half of all patients with DVTs are asymptomatic.

**MUSCULOSKELETAL SYSTEM.** The major musculoskeletal changes identified during assessment of an immo-

bilized patient include decreased muscle strength, loss of muscle tone and mass, and contractures. Patients with musculoskeletal injuries or chronic conditions require careful palpation of joints and extremities to reduce discomfort. Because immobilized patients are weakened, determine if difficulty in moving joints is the result of fatigue or decreased range of joint motion.

**SKIN INTEGRITY.** Continually assess the skin for signs of pressure ulcer formation. All immobilized patients are at high risk for developing pressure ulcers. Use of the Braden Scale (see Chapter 35) assesses a patient's risk for pressure ulcer formation. The type of risks then directs the interventions most appropriate to treat ulcers. The Braden Scale score then evaluates treatment outcomes.

**ELIMINATION SYSTEM.** Assess the patient's elimination status on each shift, and assess the total intake and output every 24 hours (see Chapter 15). Assessment of elimination also includes auscultation for bowel sounds, the frequency and consistency of bowel movements, and the patient's typical urine and bowel elimination patterns. Accurate assessment and documentation enable you to intervene before fecal impaction and urinary incontinence occur. You perform elimination assessment at the beginning and at the end of each shift or as necessary.

**PSYCHOSOCIAL CONDITION.** Changes in psychosocial status usually occur slowly. Observe for changes in emotional status (e.g., depression) and behavioral changes (e.g., cooperative patients who become argumentative or modest patients who begin to expose themselves repeatedly). Continual communication with family members is vital because they will identify and report changes in personality that you may not recognize.

| TABLE 34-2 | Range-of-Motion Exercises |

| Body Part | Type of Joint | Type of Movement | Range (Degrees) | Primary Muscles |
|---|---|---|---|---|
| Neck, cervical spine | Pivotal | *Flexion:* Bring chin to rest on chest | 45 | Sternocleidomastoid |
| | | *Extension:* Return head to erect position | 45 | Trapezius |
| | | *Hyperextension:* Bend head back as far as possible | 10 | Trapezius |
| | | *Lateral flexion:* Tilt head as far as possible toward each shoulder | 40-45 | Sternocleidomastoid |
| | | *Rotation:* Turn head as far as possible in circular movement | 180 | Sternocleidomastoid, trapezius |
| Shoulder | Ball and socket | *Flexion:* Raise arm from side position forward to position above head | 45-60 | Coracobrachialis, deltoid |
| | | *Extension:* Return arm to position at side of body | 180 | Latissimus dorsi, teres major, triceps brachii |
| | | *Hyperextension:* Move arm behind body, keeping elbow straight | 45-60 | Latissimus dorsi, teres major, deltoid |
| | | *Abduction:* Raise arm to side to position above head with palm away from head | 180 | Deltoid, supraspinatus |
| | | *Adduction:* Lower arm sideways and across body as far as possible | 320 | Pectoralis major |
| | | *Internal rotation:* With elbow flexed, rotate shoulder by moving arm until thumb is turned inward and toward back | 90 | Pectoralis major, latissimus dorsi, teres major, subscapularis |
| | | *External rotation:* With elbow in full circle, move arm until thumb is upward and lateral to head | 90 | Infraspinatus, teres major |
| | | *Circumduction:* Move arm in full circle (Circumduction is combination of all movements of ball-and-socket joint.) | 360 | Deltoid, coracobrachialis, latissimus dorsi, teres major |
| Elbow | Hinge | *Flexion:* Bend elbow so that lower arm moves toward its shoulder joint and hand is level with shoulder | 150 | Biceps brachii, brachialis, brachioradialis |
| | | *Extension:* Straighten elbow by lowering hand | 150 | Triceps brachii |
| Forearm | Pivotal | *Supination:* Turn lower arm and hand so that palm is up | 70-90 | Supinator, biceps brachii |
| | | *Pronation:* Turn lower arm so that palm is down | 70-90 | Pronator teres, pronator quadratus |
| Wrist | Condyloid | *Flexion:* Move palm toward inner aspect of forearm | 80-90 | Flexor carpi ulnaris, flexor carpi radialis |
| | | *Extension:* Move fingers and hand posterior to midline | 80-90 | Extensor carpi radialis brevis, extensor carpi radialis longus, extensor carpi ulnaris |
| | | *Hyperextension:* Bring dorsal surface of hand back as far as possible | 80-90 | Extensor carpi radialis brevis, extensor carpi radialis longus, extensor carpi ulnaris |
| | | *Abduction (radial deviation):* Bend wrist laterally toward fifth finger | up to 30 | Flexor carpi radialis, extensor carpi radialis brevis, extensor carpi radialis longus |
| | | *Adduction (ulnar deviation):* Bend wrist medially toward thumb | 30-50 | Flexor carpi ulnaris, extensor carpi ulnaris |
| Fingers | Condyloid hinge | *Flexion:* Make fist | 90 | Lumbricales, interosseus volaris, interosseus dorsalis |
| | | *Extension:* Straighten fingers | 90 | Extensor digiti quinti proprius, extensor digitorum communis, extensor indicis proprius |
| | | *Hyperextension:* Bend fingers back as far as possible | 30-60 | Extensor digitorum |
| | | *Abduction:* Spread fingers apart laterally | 30 | Interosseus dorsalis |
| | | *Adduction:* Bring fingers together laterally | 30 | Interosseus volaris |

| TABLE 34-2 | Range-of-Motion Exercises—cont'd | | | |
|---|---|---|---|---|
| **Body Part** | **Type of Joint** | **Type of Movement** | **Range (Degrees)** | **Primary Muscles** |
| Thumb | Saddle | *Flexion:* Move thumb across palmar surface of hand | 90 | Flexor pollicis brevis |
| | | *Extension:* Move thumb straight away from hand | 90 | Extensor pollicis longus, extensor pollicis brevis |
| | | *Abduction:* Extend thumb laterally (usually done when placing fingers in abduction and adduction) | 30 | Abductor pollicis brevis and longus |
| | | *Adduction:* Move thumb back toward hand | 30 | Adductor pollicis obliquus, adductor pollicis transversus |
| | | *Opposition:* Touch thumb to each finger of same hand | | Opponens pollicis, opponens digiti minimi |
| Hip | Ball and socket | *Flexion:* Move leg forward and up | 90-120 | Psoas major, iliacus, sartorius |
| | | *Extension:* Move leg behind body | 90-120 | Gluteus maximus, semitendinosus, semimembranosus |
| | | *Hyperextension:* Move leg behind body | 30-50 | Gluteus maximus, semitendinosus, semimembranosus |
| | | *Abduction:* Move leg laterally away from body | 30-50 | Gluteus medius, gluteus minimus |
| | | *Adduction:* Move leg back toward medial position and beyond if possible | 30-50 | Adductor longus, adductor brevis, adductor magnus |
| | | *Internal rotation:* Turn foot and leg toward other leg | 90 | Gluteus medius, gluteus minimus, tensor fasciae latae |
| | | *External rotation:* Turn foot and leg away from other leg | 90 | Obturatorius internus, obturatorius externus, quadratus femoris, piriformis, gemellus superior and inferior, gluteus maximus |
| | | *Circumduction:* Move leg in circle | 120-130 | Psoas major, gluteus maximus, gluteus medius, adductor magnus |
| Knee | Hinge | *Flexion:* Bring heel back toward back of thigh | 120-130 | Biceps femoris, semitendinosus, semimembranosus, sartorius |
| | | *Extension:* Return leg to floor | 120-130 | Rectus femoris, vastus lateralis, vastus medialis, vastus intermedius |
| Ankle | Hinge | *Dorsal flexion:* Move foot so that toes are pointed upward | 20-30 | Tibialis anterior |
| | | *Plantar flexion:* Move foot so that toes are pointed downward | 45-50 | Gastrocnemius, soleus |
| Foot | Gliding | *Inversion:* Turn sole of foot medially | 10 or less | Tibialis anterior, tibialis posterior |
| | | *Eversion:* Turn sole of foot laterally | 10 or less | Peroneus longus, peroneus brevis |
| Toes | Condyloid | *Flexion:* Curl toes downward | 30-60 | Flexor digitorum, lumbricalis pedis, flexor hallucis brevis |
| | | *Extension:* Straighten toes | 30-60 | Extensor digitorum longus, extensor digitorum brevis, extensor hallucis longus |
| | | *Abduction:* Spread toes apart | 15 or less | Abductor hallucis, interosseus dorsalis |
| | | *Adduction:* Bring toes together | 15 or less | Adductor hallucis, interosseus plantaris |

Evaluate your patients' readiness to improve their level of independence. Be prepared to adapt your teaching and motivational strategies to meet their expectations and needs.

You need to identify and correct any changes in the patient's sleep-wake cycle, such as difficulty falling asleep or frequent awakenings (see Chapter 29). Many sleep disruptions are preventable with an assessment of prior sleep habits and early intervention when you suspect problems. Observe for changes in the use of normal coping mechanisms to adapt to immobilization. Decreasing coping ability causes the patient to become disoriented, confused, or depressed.

**DEVELOPMENT.** Assessment of the immobilized patient includes developmental considerations. Assess a young child's developmental stage before immobilization. Developmental delays or regression occur with prolonged bed rest. Reassure parents that these developmental changes are usually temporary.

BOX 34-2 USING EVIDENCE IN PRACTICE

### Research Summary

It is widely known that decreased mobility contributes to physical and psychological impairment. Researchers know little, however, about the meaning of mobility to residents and nurses in long-term care facilities. It is important for nurses to understand the phenomena of mobility in order to develop strategies to maximize independence in long-term care residents.

The purpose of this study was to generate knowledge about the meaning of mobility from the perspective of both nurses and residents in long-term care. This knowledge is useful for developing strategies to support mobility in the institutionalized elder. The researchers interviewed 20 residents and 15 nurses in three long-term care facilities.

Both groups identified mobility as key to quality of life. The residents equated mobility with freedom, choice, and independence. Nurses valued mobility and associated it with freedom and autonomy. The nurses and the residents viewed having to "wait" for assistance as a barrier to mobility. Nurses identified further obstacles, such as heavy workload and lack of time. Residents focused on physical barriers such as steep ramps, crowded elevators, and negative attitudes of staff.

### Application to Nursing Practice

The results of this study help nurses provide quality nursing care. Mobility is central to residents' quality of life and well-being and nurses play an important role in assessing and assisting residents with their mobility needs. Nurses focus on minimizing obstacles to mobility and regularly coordinate with other health care professionals to meet residents' mobility needs. It is crucial that nurses use creative strategies to encourage mobility in elders because mobility is far more than merely the movement from one point to another.

Data from Bourret E and others: The meaning of mobility for residents and staff in long-term care facilities, *J Adv Nurs* 37(4):338, 2002.

### SYNTHESIS IN PRACTICE

As Mark prepares for an assessment on Mr. Stapp, he reviews the pathophysiology regarding the hazards of immobility. He gathers knowledge about knee replacement surgery and the expected postoperative physical therapy and rehabilitative measures. During a previous clinical experience, Mark cared for a patient who was recently diagnosed with diabetes mellitus. He knows that the presence of diabetes mellitus will affect Mr. Stapp's postoperative status in several ways. Wound healing is slower in patients with diabetes. In addition, because Mr. Stapp will be participating in a physical exercise program to increase knee mobility, his caloric requirements will need to change and Mark needs to monitor his blood glucose levels.

Mark knows that he needs to respect Mr. Stapp's need to be independent and desire to participate in rehabilitation. Although Mark and his patient are close in age, he knows that Mr. Stapp has his own life goals. He approaches this clinical experience with energy and creativity; he plans to implement individualized care to increase Mr. Stapp's mobility status and progression through rehabilitation.

Meeting the developmental needs of patients, especially older adults, with altered immobility is very important (Box 34-2). Developmental assessment of older adults enables you to determine the patient's ability to meet needs independently. A decline in developmental functioning prompts investigation to determine the reasons the change occurred and the interventions necessary to restore the patient to an optimal level of functioning (see Chapter 19).

### Nursing Diagnosis

Assessment reveals clusters of data that indicate whether a patient is at risk or if a mobility problem exists. Assessment also identifies pertinent defining characteristics that support the nursing diagnosis and probable cause of the nursing diagnosis. Locating the probable cause of the diagnosis, based on assessment data, is important to planning patient-centered goals and subsequent nursing interventions that will best help the patient.

An immobilized or partially immobilized patient will possibly have one or more nursing diagnoses:

- Activity intolerance
- Ineffective airway clearance
- Ineffective breathing pattern
- Risk for constipation
- Ineffective coping
- Risk for disuse syndrome
- Risk for falls
- Risk for deficient fluid volume
- Impaired gas exchange
- Risk for infection
- Risk for injury
- Risk for perioperative-positioning injury
- Impaired bed mobility
- Impaired physical mobility
- Impaired wheelchair mobility
- Risk for impaired skin integrity
- Disturbed sleep pattern
- Social isolation
- Ineffective tissue perfusion
- Impaired urinary elimination

The two diagnoses most directly related to mobility problems are *impaired physical mobility* and *risk for disuse syndrome*. *Impaired physical mobility* is for the patient who demonstrates functional limitations but is not completely immobile. For the patient who is immobile and at risk for multisystem complications, the more pertinent nursing diagnosis is *risk for disuse syndrome*. The list of potential nursing diagnoses related to immobility is more extensive when alterations in physical, psychosocial, or developmental functioning occur. Often these problems are interrelated, and it is imperative that nursing care focus on all dimensions.

## Planning

Active care planning focused on prevention of physical, psychosocial, and developmental complications is essential. Encouraging or providing for range of joint motion and patient repositioning is a first step in preventing serious complications such as pneumonia or pulmonary emboli. Routine monitoring of patients' skin condition using the Braden Scale helps avoid deterioration leading to infection or sepsis. Your attention to detail in care planning is critical.

**GOALS AND OUTCOMES.** Patients at risk for hazards of immobility require nursing care plans directed at meeting their actual and potential needs (see care plan). It is important to develop patient-centered goals aimed at preventing or reducing the hazards of immobility. You set realistic goals and outcomes mutually with the patient and family. A family who does too much or too little in an attempt to help the patient will seriously impede the patient's progress. Watching a family member walk slowly and using effort seems cruel, and some families excessively perform tasks that patients need to learn how to do for themselves. Patients often suffer immobility for a long time. Thus, setting sequential outcomes helps ensure progressive improvement over time.

**SETTING PRIORITIES.** Prioritize care by taking into consideration the patient's most immediate needs. Patients with impaired mobility have multiple diagnoses that affect mental and physical health (Figure 34-3). For example, you may need to relieve a patient's pain first before you can implement aggressive mobility activities. Because you are able to delegate many of the skills associated with care of the immobile patient, such as turning and applying antiembolic stockings, it is easy to overlook the potential complications of immobility until they occur. Therefore be vigilant in monitoring patients, reinforcing prevention techniques, and supervising assistive personnel in carrying out activities aimed at preventing complications of immobility.

**CONTINUITY OF CARE.** You will often need the help of another health team member, such as a physical or occupational therapist, when considering mobility needs. Collaboration of health care providers is important for patients in institutional and home settings. You begin discharge planning when a patient enters the health care system. Anticipating the patient's discharge from an institution, a referral is necessary to help the patient remain mobile or regain mobility at home.

## Implementation

Nursing interventions for the completely or partially immobilized patient focus on health promotion and prevention of complications. Specific interventions, in the acute care setting, focus on reducing complications by positioning and transferring patients correctly. In restorative and continuing care, you direct interventions at regaining and maximizing functional mobility and independence.

**HEALTH PROMOTION.** Structured exercise programs for immobile patients will improve their endurance, strength, overall health, and feelings of well-being. Exercise is recommended preoperatively for patients expected to have mobility restrictions after surgery.

Disuse and disease account for much of the functional decline in the older adult population. The older adult patient need not accept muscle deterioration as inevitable (Box 34-3). It is important that you be alert to prevent further disuse while the older adult is ill.

You will contribute to promoting health for many types of patients by encouraging or starting managed exercise programs (Box 34-4). Encourage hospitalized patients to do stretching, ROJM, and light walking, depending on their physical capabilities. Measure distances walked in feet and yards instead of "walked to the nurses' station and back to room." Adults also enjoy and benefit from exercise postoperatively. Activities other than traditional Western exercises, such as walking or swimming, are beneficial when patients return home (Box 34-5).

**Respiratory System.** Aim your interventions for the respiratory system at promoting expansion of the chest and lungs, preventing stasis of pulmonary secretions, and maintaining a patent airway.

***Promoting Expansion of the Chest and Lungs.*** Changing the position of the patient at least every 2 hours allows the dependent lung regions to reexpand. Reexpansion maintains the elastic recoil property of the lungs and clears the dependent lung regions of pulmonary secretions. Assess patients to determine if they need more frequent position changes (see Chapter 35). Expansion also is promoted through regular deep breathing exercises.

***Preventing Stasis of Pulmonary Secretions.*** Stagnant secretions accumulating in the bronchi and lungs of the immobilized patient lead to the growth of bacteria and the subsequent development of pneumonia. Changing the patient's position every 2 hours will reduce stagnation of secretions. This change rotates the dependent lung, mobilizing secretions.

Make sure the immobile patient has a fluid intake of at least 2000 ml per day, if not contraindicated, to help keep mucociliary clearance intact. In patients free from infection and with adequate hydration, pulmonary secretions will appear thin, watery, and clear. It is easy for the patient to remove these secretions with coughing. Without adequate hydration, secretions become thick, tenacious, and difficult to remove. One method for removing pulmonary secretions is chest physiotherapy (CPT). The use of this technique drains secretions from specific segments of the bronchi and lungs into the trachea and helps the patient expel the secretions by coughing (see Chapter 28).

**Metabolic System.** You design a dietary plan of carbohydrates, proteins, and fats to combat the effects of immobility. Carbohydrates are necessary to meet energy requirements. Proteins are necessary for tissue repair. Fats prevent further breakdown of nutritional stores. You determine the

## CARE PLAN  Impaired Physical Mobility

### ASSESSMENT

Mr. Bob Stapp, a 54-year-old patient, came to the rehabilitation hospital after bilateral **total knee replacement (TKR).** He has a history of smoking. He is **50 lb overweight.** He does not use his incentive spirometer. He is to **start physical therapy this afternoon.** He is reporting his **pain at a level 8** on the pain scale. He is experiencing difficulty **transferring himself independently to a chair from the bed. He can stand on his own with the aid of a walker.** He has **50-degree flexion of his knee.**

*Defining characteristics are shown in bold type.

### NURSING DIAGNOSIS Impaired physical mobility related to status postoperative total knee replacement as evidenced by activity restrictions and pain.

### PLANNING

#### GOAL

- Patient will rate his pain at a level of 3 or less on a 0 to 10 pain scale by discharge from the rehabilitation hospital.

- Patient will transfer independently to a chair from bed by day 3.

#### EXPECTED OUTCOMES*
##### Pain Control
- Patient will rate his pain no greater than a level 3 in the first 3 days.
- Patient will verbalize satisfaction with pain control measures.
##### Mobility
- Patient is able to assume sitting positin on side of bed.
- Patient is able to stand and bear weight during transfer to chair.

*Outcomes classification label from Moorhead S, Johnson M, Maas M: *Nursing outcomes classification (NOC),* ed 3, St. Louis, 2004, Mosby.

### INTERVENTIONS†
#### Pain Management
- Control environmental factors that influence Mr. Stapp's response to discomfort. Dim his room lights, and monitor noise level. Control his room temperature for comfort. Limit the number of Mr. Stapp's visitors.
- Teach use of nonpharmacological techniques for Mr. Stapp's pain reduction. Demonstrate use of massage for relaxation. Use distraction to reduce Mr. Stapp's awareness of pain and increase his pain tolerance.
- Monitor Mr. Stapp's satisfaction with pain management at specified intervals. Document his response to prescribed pain medication and nonpharmacological interventions.

#### Positioning
- Encourage Mr. Stapp to assume a comfortable position in bed or chair.

#### Medication Management
- Provide Mr. Stapp with optimal pain relief with prescribed analgesics. Administer prescribed pain medication on an around-the-clock schedule.
- Schedule ATC dosing to medicate Mr. Stapp before physical therapy to increase his participation, but evaluate the hazard of sedation. Medicate him 1 hour before.

#### Self-Care Assistance: Transfer
- Instruct patient on bed to chair transfer, using transfer belt and having two people assist with movement.
- Position bed and built-up chair to accommodate transfer within 50-degree flexion limit of the knees.

### RATIONALE

A darkened room, decreased noise level, and comfortable temperature (68° to 74° F) are best for rest and sleep.

Massage produces physical and mental relaxation and reduces pain. Useful forms of distraction include singing, praying, listening to music, and playing games (Austin, 2004).

Continuous evaluation and documentation of pain relief is necessary to determine if patient requires new or revised therapies (see Chapter 30).

Turning and repositioning reduce stimulation of pain and pressure receptors. Comfortable positioning will decrease patient's perception of pain.

Around-the-clock medication administration maintains a constant level of analgesia within therapeutic range (American Pain Society, 2003; Pasero, 2003).

Medicating patients before therapy or activity optimizes their level of comfort and maximizes their participation and benefit from treatment (American Pain Society, 2003).

Prevents injury during transfer.

Prevents strain on joints with limited range of joint motion.

†Intervention classification labels from Dochterman JM, and Bulechek GM, editors: *Nursing interventions classification (NIC),* ed 4, St. Louis, 2004, Mosby.

### EVALUATION
- Observe Mr. Stapp to determine if his environment is comfortable and restful.
- Ask Mr. Stapp how effective nonpharmacological relaxation techniques are.
- Request Mr. Stapp to report his pain level using the pain scale and if analgesic administration frequency is adequate.
- Observe Mr. Stapp for proper positioning to promote comfort.
- Discuss with Mr. Stapp his comfort level during physical therapy.

# CONCEPT MAP

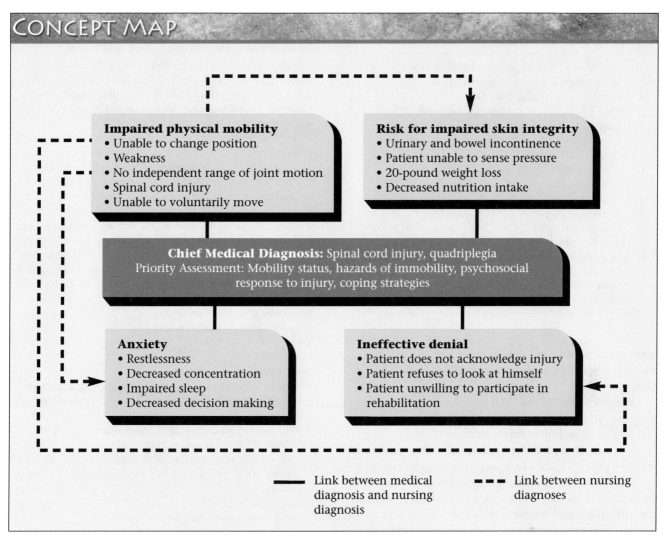

FIGURE **34-3** Concept map for patient with a spinal cord injury and quadriplegia.

---

| BOX 34-3 | CARE OF THE OLDER ADULT |
|---|---|

- Base program on individual assessment data (underlying conditions, medications, present activity level). Consult physician or health care provider for specific exercise restrictions before onset of exercise program.
- Use correct body mechanics, appropriate clothing, exercise-specific shoes, and sufficient hydration.
- Perform a gradual, extended exercise warm-up (e.g., 15 minutes) to maximize flexibility and decrease muscle injury.
- Begin at low level (40% to 50% of predicted maximal heart rate), and follow gentle exercise progression.

- Avoid sudden twisting movements, rapid movements, and rapid transitions from one movement to the next.
- Avoid exercises that tax vision and balance.
- Avoid sustained isometric contractions of greater than 10 seconds.
- Avoid exercise during acute viral infections.
- Stop exercising if cardiac dysrhythmias, angina, or excessive breathlessness occurs.
- Perform cool-down until heart rate returns to resting level to decrease postural hypotension and cardiac dysrhythmias.
- Modify exercise program based on individual's responses.

Modified from Ebersole P and others: *Toward healthy aging: human needs and nursing response*, ed 6, St. Louis, 2004, Mosby.

**Guidelines for Assisting Patients With Exercising**

1. Teach patients breathing skills to help reduce anxiety and to fully oxygenate tissues and expand lungs.
2. Always know patients' limitations.
3. Do not force a muscle or a joint during exercise.
4. Let each patient move at own pace.
5. Keep a record of the patient's progress, and provide feedback as patient exercises.
6. Maintain posture, body alignment, and good body mechanics during exercise.
7. Monitor vital signs before, during, and after exercise.
8. Stop exercising if patient has pain, shortness of breath, or a change in vital signs.
9. Make sure patients wear shoes and comfortable clothing.
10. Know what the patient's mobility skills were before hospitalization.
11. Be aware of any medical limitations (e.g., weight-bearing status, untreated fracture, cardiovascular disease).

**BOX 34-5** CULTURAL FOCUS

Culture influences our time orientation, health care practices, nutrition, religion, and family systems. Less attention has been given to the impact of culture on mobility and exercise. However, cultural influences have an important role in exercise and physical activity.

In many written materials, exercise is often described based on white, middle-class values. For example, not everyone has access to a tennis court or swimming pool at a local country club. Furthermore, many individuals do not feel comfortable in this environment. Certain cultures discourage involvement in organized recreational physical activities such as basketball, running, and aerobics (Johnson, 2000). Ethnic dancing is an effective activity that is more acceptable than the above organized sports activities in Western European countries (Jain, 2001). Other cultures emphasize exercise in terms of activities of daily living such as walking, gardening, and prayer/meditation. As an example, people from Bangladesh view prayer as a structured form of exercise. Muslims value participation in community activities and consider walking to the mosque a part of their weekly exercise regimen (Johnson, 2000).

**Implications for Practice**

- Evaluate patient's patterns of daily living and culturally prescribed activities before suggesting specific forms of exercise to patients.
- Help patients plan physical activities that are culturally acceptable (Melillo and others, 2001).
- Make exercise programs flexible and accommodate family and community responsibilities of the culture (Banks-Wallace, 2000).
- Encourage culturally specific interventions to help patients commit to exercise (Banks-Wallace, 2000).

specific caloric and diet prescription from the nutritional assessment in collaboration with a registered dietitian (see Chapter 31).

**Cardiovascular System.** You design nursing therapies to minimize or prevent orthostatic hypotension, increased cardiac workload, and thrombus formation.

*Reducing Orthostatic Hypotension.* After prolonged bed rest, patients usually have an increased pulse rate, a decrease in pulse pressure, and a drop in blood pressure with an increase in fainting when arising to a sitting or standing position (Black and Hawks, 2005). You need to attempt to get the patient moving as soon as the physical condition allows, even if this only involves dangling at the bedside or moving to a chair. This activity maintains muscle tone and increases venous return. **Isometric exercises,** those activities that involve muscle tension without muscle shortening, do not have any beneficial effect on preventing orthostatic hypotension but improve activity tolerance (see Chapter 25).

When transferring from a supine position into a chair, move the patient gradually. First obtain a baseline blood pressure and pulse with the patient in the supine position. Then raise the patient to a high-Fowler's position, and measure blood pressure and pulse again to detect decreases in blood pressure or elevations in pulse. Leave the patient in this position for 2 minutes to allow the body to adapt. Monitor the patient for dizziness or light-headedness. The patient is now ready to sit at the side of the bed with the feet on the floor. If there is no dizziness, assist the patient to a chair. When transferring an immobile patient for the first time, make sure you have the assistance of at least one other person (Lance and others, 2000).

*Preventing Thrombus Formation.* Proper positioning used with other therapies (e.g., anticoagulants and antiembolic stockings) helps reduce thrombus formation. When positioning patients, use caution to prevent pressure on the pos-

terior knee and deep veins in the lower extremities. Teach patients to avoid crossing the legs, sitting for prolonged periods of time, wearing tight clothing that constricts the legs or waist, putting pillows under the knees, and massaging the legs.

Range-of-joint-motion exercises reduce the risk of contractures and also aid in preventing thrombi (see Box 34-6). Activity causes contraction of the skeletal muscles, which exerts pressure on the veins to promote venous return. An increase in venous return reduces venous stasis. Specific exercises that help prevent thrombophlebitis are ankle pumps, foot circles, hip rotation, and knee flexion. Ankle pumps, sometimes called calf pumps, include alternating plantar flexion and dorsiflexion. Foot circles require the patient to rotate the ankle. While the patient is supine (lying on back) or sitting, he or she rotates the hip inward and outward. Knee flexion involves alternately extending and flexing the knee. These exercises aimed at preventing thrombus are sometimes called antiembolic exercises. Patients should do these exercises hourly while awake.

**Musculoskeletal System.** The immobilized patient needs to exercise to prevent excessive muscle atrophy, decreased endurance, and joint contractures. The amount of

| BOX 34-6 | **Incorporating Active Range-of-Joint-Motion Exercises Into Activities of Daily Living** |

Nodding head "yes" exercises *neck* (flexion).
Shaking head "no" exercises *neck* (rotation).
Moving right ear to right shoulder exercises *neck* (lateral flexion).
Moving left ear to left shoulder exercises *neck* (lateral flexion).
Reaching to turn on overhead light exercises *shoulder* (extension).
Reaching to bedside stand for book exercises *shoulder* (extension).
Scratching back exercises *shoulder* (hyperextension).
Rotating shoulders toward chest exercises *shoulder* (abduction).
Rotating shoulders toward back exercises *shoulder* (adduction).
Eating, bathing, shaving, and grooming exercise *elbow* (flexion and extension).
All activities requiring fine motor coordination, such as writing and eating, exercise *fingers* and *thumb* (flexion, extension, abduction, adduction, and opposition).
Walking exercises *hip* (flexion, extension, and hyperextension).
Moving to side-lying position exercises *hip* (flexion, extension, and abduction).
Moving from side-lying position exercises *hip* (extension and adduction).
Rolling feet inward exercises *hip* (internal rotation).
Rolling feet outward exercises *hip* (external rotation).
Walking exercises *knee* (flexion and extension).
Moving to and from a side-lying position exercises *knee* (flexion and extension).
Walking exercises *ankle* (dorsiflexion and plantar flexion).
Moving toe toward head of bed exercises *ankle* (dorsiflexion).
Moving toe toward foot of bed exercises *ankle* (plantar flexion).
Walking exercises *toes* (extension and hyperextension).
Wiggling toes exercises *toes* (abduction and adduction).

| BOX 34-7 | **PATIENT TEACHING** |

Mr. Stapp is interested in knowing what to expect when he returns home following his stay in the rehabilitation center. Mark Weber, his nursing student, develops the following discharge teaching plan.

**Outcome**
At the end of the teaching session Mr. Stapp will verbalize essential elements of his home care.

**Teaching Strategies**
• Assess Mr. Stapp's openness to learning.
• Determine appropriate teaching strategies based on Mr. Stapp's cognitive ability.
• Use common terminology to describe Mr. Stapp's home care plan.
• Address more complicated content early in the day.
• Assess Mr. Stapp's pain level before beginning the teaching session.
• Include instruction on activities such as use of assistive devices, application of antiembolic stockings, and use of analgesics.

**Evaluation Strategies**
• Use focused questions to evaluate Mr. Stapp's understanding of exercise regimen.
• Observe Mr. Stapp demonstrating use of assistive devices (cane, walker).
• Ask Mr. Stapp to describe the proper use of analgesics and anticoagulants.
• Evaluate Mr. Stapp's ability to correctly apply antiembolitic stockings.
• Have Mr. Stapp verbalize low-fat, high-protein foods that will promote weight loss and wound healing.
• Listen to Mr. Stapp describe signs and symptoms of wound infection.
• Ask Mr. Stapp to identify concerns about which he should contact his health care provider.

activity required to prevent physical disuse syndromes is only about 2 hours in a 24-hour period, and you schedule this regularly throughout the day based on individual patient needs. The best method to prevent complications from impaired mobility is to encourage ambulation (Jones, 2001).

If the patient is unable to move any part or all of the body, perform passive range-of-joint-motion exercises for all immobilized joints at least 3 or 4 times a day unless contraindicated. If one extremity is paralyzed, teach the patient to perform passive ROJM on the paralyzed limb and encourage the patient to engage in active ROJM with all other extremities. For patients on bed rest, incorporate active range-of-joint-motion exercises into their ADL schedule (Box 34-6).

The best nursing intervention is establishing an individualized progressive exercise program. A progressive exercise program gradually increases the patient's physical activity to reverse the deconditioning associated with immobility. Teaching is an important aspect for patients with limited mobility (Box 34-7). Depending on the setting and resources available, refer the patient for physical therapy to assist in setting up the exercise program.

**Skin Integrity.** The major risk to the skin from restricted mobility is the formation of pressure ulcers. Early identification of high-risk patients assists you in preventing pressure ulcers. Interventions aimed at prevention are positioning, skin care, and the use of pressure-relief devices. Change the immobilized patient's position according to the patient's activity level, perceptual ability, treatment protocols, and daily routines (see Chapter 35). Although turning every 1 to 2 hours is recommended for preventing ulcers, it is sometimes necessary to use devices for relieving pressure. Normally, the time a patient sits uninterrupted in a chair is 1 hour or less, but make sure to individualize this time interval. Reposition the patient frequently because uninterrupted pressure will cause skin breakdown. Teach patients who are able to move to shift their weight every 15 minutes. Make sure chair-bound patients have a pressure-reducing device for the chair (Agency for Healthcare Research and Quality [AHRQ], 2003).

**Elimination System.** Direct your interventions for maintaining optimal urinary functioning by keeping the patient well hydrated without causing bladder distention and the reflux of urine into the ureters and renal pelvis. Adequate hydration helps to prevent renal calculi and urinary tract infections. Timely toileting prevents bladder distention. Make sure the patient's urine is light yellow and comparable in amount to the fluid intake.

Monitor the frequency and amount of urinary output to further prevent bladder distention. A patient who continually dribbles urine and whose bladder is distended has reflex incontinence. If the immobilized patient does not have voluntary control of bladder elimination, bladder retraining is necessary. It will be necessary to insert a straight or indwelling Foley catheter (see Chapter 32) if the patient experiences bladder distention.

Record the frequency and consistency of bowel movements. A diet rich in fruits and vegetables helps to facilitate normal peristalsis. If a patient is unable to maintain normal bowel patterns, initiate a bowel training program and the physician or health care provider may order stool softeners, cathartics, or enemas (see Chapter 33).

**Psychosocial Problems.** Health promotion for the immobilized patient requires that you anticipate changes in psychosocial status and intervene with preventive measures. Provide routine and informal socialization for the patient. Plan activities to give the patient opportunities to interact with the staff. If possible, place the patient in a room with other mobile patients. If the patient remains in a private room, ask staff members to visit periodically throughout waking hours. Provide stimuli to maintain orientation and to entertain the patient.

Encourage patients to wear their glasses or dentures and to shave or apply makeup. These are normal activities to enhance body image. Encourage the patient to perform as much self-care as possible. Make sure hygiene and grooming articles are within easy reach so the patient can attend to personal needs.

**Developmental Changes.** Your care should stimulate the patient mentally, as well as physically, particularly with a young child. Incorporate play activities into the nursing care plan. Puzzles, for example, help patients develop fine motor skills. Place an immobilized child in a room with children of the same age who are mobile, unless a contagious disease is present (Hockenberry and others, 2003). Health promotion for older adults requires matching mobility needs with the patient's developmental limitations. Older adults benefit when exercise routines are mildly progressive. Walking, aquatic exercise, swimming, and gardening are good ways to promote range of joint motion and endurance.

**ACUTE CARE.** Patients in acute care settings demonstrate more rapid and pronounced complications of immobility because of the presence of multisystem involvement. In these patients you will design nursing interventions to reduce the impact of immobility on body systems and prepare the patient for restorative and continuing care. Interventions are used in combination with those outlined in the health promotion section to return the patient to an optimal level of function.

**Respiratory System.** Encourage the patient to cough and deep breathe every 1 to 2 hours while awake. This action expands all lobes of the lungs and prevents atelectasis. Coughing reduces the stasis of pulmonary secretions. Some immobile patients, particularly after surgery, will need to use an incentive spirometer to aid in deep breathing (see Chapter 28).

Postoperative patients who have undergone anesthesia need to cough and deep breathe to prevent atelectasis and stasis of secretions. Timely pain management for incisional discomfort is essential. Patients cough more effectively when their pain is under control. If a patient becomes drowsy from medication, actively reinforce coughing and deep breathing. Encouraging early ambulation helps prevent multiple pulmonary complications.

*Maintaining a Patent Airway.* Immobilized patients and those on bed rest are generally weakened. The cough reflex gradually becomes inefficient as the weakness progresses. If the patient is too weak or unable to cough up secretions, you maintain the patient's airway by using suctioning techniques (see Chapter 28). This usually involves oral or nasotracheal suctioning and suctioning of artificial airways. Suspect hypostatic bronchopneumonia if the patient develops a productive cough with greenish-yellow sputum, fever, and pain on breathing.

**Cardiovascular System.** Direct nursing interventions at reducing cardiac workload. When a patient moves up in bed or strains on defecation, a Valsalva maneuver occurs. The patient holds his or her breath and strains, increasing intrathoracic pressure, which decreases venous return and cardiac output. When the strain is released, venous return and cardiac output immediately increase, and systolic blood pressure and pulse pressure rise. These pressure changes produce a reflex bradycardia that is associated with sudden cardiac death, particularly in patients with heart disease. Teach the patient to breathe out while moving or being lifted up in bed to avoid straining. Interventions that reduce the risk of thrombus formation in the immobilized patient include leg exercises, encouraging fluids, and position changes. Instruct preoperative patients in exercise before surgery (see Chapter 37). Other interventions, such as antiembolic elastic stockings and sequential compression devices (SCDs), require a physician's or health care provider's order.

Elastic stockings aid in maintaining pressure on the muscles of the lower extremities to promote venous return. Make sure to apply the stockings properly (Box 34-8) and remove and reapply them at least every 8 hours. Improper application of stockings can lead to decreased circulation in the lower extremities. Always observe the status of circulation to the extremities (see Chapter 13) and check to be sure stockings are properly fitted.

SCDs consist of inflatable plastic sleeves wrapped around the legs. The sleeves are connected to an air pump that alternately inflates and deflates, providing rhythmic, external ex-

| **BOX 34-8** | PROCEDURAL GUIDELINES FOR |

## Applying Antiembolic Elastic Stockings

**Delegation Considerations:** You can delegate the skill of applying antiembolic elastic stockings to assistive personnel. Before delegation, instruct the assistive personnel to inform the patient:

- To avoid activities that promote venous stasis (e.g., crossing legs, wearing garters)
- To elevate legs while sitting and before applying stockings to improve venous return
- Not to massage legs
- To avoid wrinkles in the stockings
- To observe for allergic reactions, skin irritation, and thrombophlebitis

**Equipment:** tape measure, elastic support stockings

1. Assess patient for risk factors in Virchow's triad:
   a. *Hypercoagulability:* all patients with clotting disorders, fever, dehydration, pregnancy and first 6 weeks postpartum if the woman was confined to bed, and oral contraceptive use (especially if patient smokes)
   b. *Venous wall abnormalities:* local trauma, orthopedic surgeries, major abdominal surgery, varicose veins, atherosclerosis
   c. *Blood stasis:* immobility, obesity, pregnancy

2. Observe for signs, symptoms, and conditions that contraindicate use of antiembolitic elastic stockings. Signs and symptoms include:
   a. Dermatitis or open skin lesion
   b. Recent skin graft
   c. Decreased circulation in lower extremities as evidenced by cyanotic cool extremities, gangrenous conditions affecting the lower limb(s).

3. Assess and document the condition of the patient's skin and circulation to the legs (i.e., presence of pedal pulses, edema, discoloration of the skin, temperature, lesions, or abrasions).

4. Obtain physician's or health care provider's order.

5. Assess patient's or caregiver's understanding of application of antiembolic elastic stockings.

6. Assess the condition of the patient's skin and circulation to the leg and foot (e.g., presence of popliteal and pedal pulses, edema, discoloration of the skin, skin temperature, lesions, or cuts).

---

- *Critical Decision Point:* Clinical signs of thrombophlebitis vary according to the size and location of the thrombus. Signs and symptoms of superficial thrombosis include palpable veins and the surrounding area's being tender to the touch, reddened, and warm. Temperature elevation and edema may or may not be present. Signs and symptoms of DVT include swollen extremity; pain; warm, cyanotic skin; and temperature elevation. However, up to 80% of patients are asymptomatic. The Homans' sign (pain in calf on dorsiflexion of the foot) is no longer a reliable assessment. Fewer than 20% of patients have a positive Homans' sign (Phipps and others, 2003).

---

7. Use a tape measure to measure patient's legs to determine proper stocking size.

8. Explain procedure and reasons for applying stockings.

9. Perform hand hygiene. Provide hygiene to patient's lower extremities as needed.

10. Position patient in supine position.

11. Apply elastic stockings:
    a. Turn elastic stocking inside out up to the heel. Place one hand into stocking, holding heel. Pull top of stocking with the other hand inside out over foot of stocking.
    b. Place patient's toes into foot of elastic stocking, making sure that stocking is smooth (see illustration).
    c. Slide remaining portion of stocking over patient's foot, being sure that the toes are covered. Make sure the foot fits into the toe and heel position of the stocking (see illustration).
    d. Slide top of stocking up over patient's calf until stocking is completely extended. Be sure stocking is smooth and no ridges or wrinkles are present, particularly behind the knee (see illustration).
    e. Instruct patient not to roll stockings partially down.

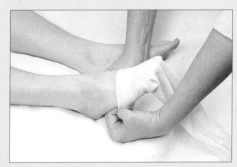

STEP **11b** Place toes into foot of stocking.

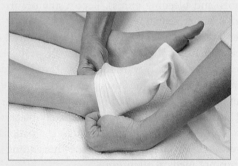

STEP **11c** Slide heel of stocking over foot.

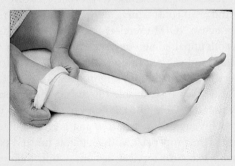

STEP **11d** Slide stocking up leg until completely extended.

*Continued*

---

**BOX 34-8** PROCEDURAL GUIDELINES FOR

**Applying Antiembolic Elastic Stockings, cont'd**

12. Reposition patient for comfort, and perform hand hygiene.
13. Remove stockings at least once per shift.
14. Inspect stockings for wrinkles or constriction.
15. Inspect elastic stockings to determine that there are no wrinkles, rolls, or binding.

16. Observe circulatory status of lower extremities. Observe color, temperature, and condition of skin. Palpate pedal pulses.
17. Observe the patient's response to wearing the antiembolitic elastic stockings.
18. Observe patient or caregiver applying stockings.

---

tremity compression (Box 34-9). Use of the SCDs on the legs decreases venous stasis by increasing venous return. In postoperative patients, keep these compression devices in place until the patient is ambulatory.

Immobilized patients are frequently on prophylactic (preventative) low-dose heparin therapy to minimize the risk of venous thromboembolism. Heparin is an anticoagulant that suppresses clot formation. This therapy requires a physician's or health care provider's order. Newer low-molecular-weight (LMW) heparins such as ardeparin and enoxaparin are being prescribed in place of older forms of unfractionated heparin. The LMW heparins have a more predicable anticoagulant effect (McHenry and Salerno, 2001). The drugs are given subcutaneously, usually every 12 hours until the risk of DVT declines. LMW heparin compared with unfractionated heparin reduces the occurrence of major hemorrhage as a side effect (van Dongen and others, 2005). Local irritation such as erythema, hematoma, and urticaria at injection sites is common. However, it is still wise to monitor the patient for signs of bleeding (e.g., increased bruising, guaiac-positive stools, and bleeding gums). Report any occurrence of hemorrhage immediately.

When you suspect DVT, do not massage the area. Report your assessment findings to the physician or health care provider immediately. Elevate the leg, with no pressure on the area of the leg with the suspected thrombus. If the patient complains of shortness of breath or severe chest pain, suspect a pulmonary embolus. Immediately place the patient in high-Fowler's position and check the patient's oxygen saturation. This complication is life-threatening and requires prompt medical attention.

**Musculoskeletal System.** The immobilized patient needs to receive some exercise to prevent excessive muscle atrophy and joint contractures. For patients on bed rest, incorporate active ROJM exercises into their daily schedules. Patients with impaired nervous, skeletal, or muscular system functioning and significant weakness often require help from the nurse to attain body alignment.

Several devices are available for maintaining proper patient positioning (Table 34-3). Pillows are commonly used to support body alignment. Before using a pillow, determine whether it is the proper size. A thick pillow under a patient's head causes excessive cervical flexion. A thin pillow under bony prominences is inadequate to protect skin and tissue from damage. When additional pillows are unavailable, use

folded sheets, blankets, or towels as positioning aids. The 30-degree semi-Fowler's position is for patients at risk for pressure ulcer development. Elevate the patient's calves on a pillow to avoid pressure on the heels. A trochanter roll prevents external rotation of the hips when the patient is in a supine position (Figure 34-4). Hand rolls maintain the hand, thumb, and fingers in a functional position. Hand-wrist splints are individually molded for the patient to maintain proper alignment of the thumb. A trapeze bar is a triangular device that hangs from a securely fastened overhead bar that is attached to the patient's bed frame (Figure 34-5). It is a useful device for helping to increase patient independence, maintain upper body strength, and reduce friction from movement in bed.

Some orthopedic and neurological conditions require more frequent passive ROJM exercises to restore the injured joint or extremity to maximal function. Patients with such conditions use automatic equipment for passive range-of-joint-motion exercises. The continuous passive motion (CPM) machine moves the extremity within a prescribed range for a specific period. This method is beneficial when the patient gradually increases ROJM of a particular joint. Studies over the last 5 years have yielded varying evidence about the effectiveness of CPM in patients with total knee replacements. Some studies noted short-term benefits, but long-term improvement in range of motion was questionable (Maher and others, 2002) (Figure 34-6).

**Psychosocial Problems.** Schedule nursing care between 10 PM and 7 AM to minimize sleep interruptions. Establish a balance between rest and the physiological effects of bed rest. Keep assessments to a minimum in a stable patient who is able to turn in bed unassisted. More seriously ill patients will need medications, assessments, and skin care during the night. Coordinate your nursing care to prevent as many interruptions as possible.

Finally, observe the patient for failure to cope with restricted mobility. If the nursing care plan is not improving the patient's coping patterns, outside assistance is necessary. Incorporate referrals to community resources into the care plan.

**Developmental Changes.** Immobilization or restricted mobility of an older adult requires complex care and innovative approaches. Inactive older adults are at risk for cognitive changes and depression as a result of immobilization, chronic illnesses, and medications. It is important to focus on activities to promote cognitive awareness of the patient's

| BOX 34-9 | PROCEDURAL GUIDELINES FOR |
|---|---|

## Applying Sequential Compression Devices

**Delegation Considerations:** You can delegate the skill of applying SCDs to assistive personnel. The nurse is responsible for assessing circulation in the extremities. Instruct the assistive personnel to:
- Notify nurse if patient complains of leg pain
- Notify nurse if discoloration develops in extremities

**Equipment:** sequential compression device (SCD) insufflator with air hoses attached, adjustable Velcro compression stockings/SCD sleeve, hygiene supplies

1. Assess patient for need for sequential compression stockings (see Box 34-8).
2. Obtain baseline assessment data about the status of circulation, pulse, and skin integrity on patient's lower extremities before initiating sequential compression stockings.
3. Perform hand hygiene. Provide hygiene to lower extremities, as needed.
4. Assemble and prepare equipment.
5. Arrange SCD sleeve under the patient's leg according to the leg position indicated on the inner lining of the sleeve (see illustration).
    a. Back of patient's ankle should line up with the ankle marking on inner lining of the sleeve.
    b. Position back of knee with the popliteal opening (see illustration).
6. Wrap SCD sleeve securely around patient's leg.
7. Verify fit of SCD sleeves by placing two fingers between patient's leg and sleeve (see illustration).
8. Attach SCD sleeve's connector to plug on mechanical unit. Arrows on compressor line up with arrows on plug from mechanical unit (see illustration).
9. Turn mechanical unit on. Green light indicates unit is functioning.
10. Observe functioning of unit for one complete cycle.
11. Reposition patient for comfort, and perform hand hygiene.
12. Remove compression stockings at least once per shift.
13. Monitor skin integrity and circulation to patient's lower extremities as ordered or as recommended by SCD manufacturer.

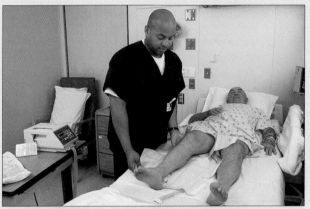

STEP **5** Correct leg position on inner lining.

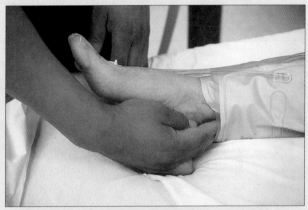

STEP **7** Check fit of SCD sleeve.

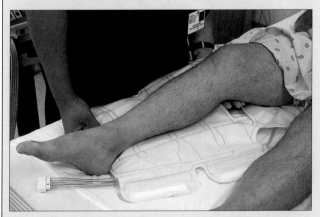

STEP **5b** Position back of patient's knee with the popliteal opening.

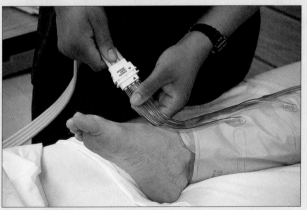

STEP **8** Align arrows when connecting to mechanical unit.

| TABLE 34-3 | Devices Used for Proper Positioning |
|---|---|
| **Devices** | **Uses and Descriptions** |
| Pillows | Pillows are readily available in most health care facilities, including the home. Make sure they are the appropriate size for the body part you will position. Pillows provide support, elevate body parts, and splint incisional areas, reducing postoperative pain during activity or coughing and deep breathing. |
| Foot boots | Foot boots maintain feet in dorsiflexion. Boots are made of rigid plastic or heavy foam and keep the foot flexed at the proper angle. Remove the foot boots at least every 4 hours to assess skin integrity and joint mobility. |
| Trochanter rolls | Trochanter rolls prevent external rotation of legs when patients are in the supine position. To form a trochanter roll, fold a cotton bath blanket or a sheet lengthwise to a width extending from the greater trochanter of the femur to the lower border of the popliteal space (see Figure 34-4). Place the blanket under the buttocks and then rolled away from the patient until the thigh is in the neutral position or an inward position with the patella facing upward. |
| Sandbags | Sandbags provide support and shape to body contours; they immobilize extremities and maintain specific body alignment. Sandbags are filled plastic tubes that you shape to body contours. They are used in place of, or in addition to, trochanter rolls. |
| Hand rolls | Hand rolls maintain the thumb slightly adducted and in opposition to the fingers; they maintain fingers in a slightly flexed position. The nurse evaluates the position of the hand roll to make certain the hand is indeed in a functional position. |
| Hand-wrist splints | Hand-wrist splints are individually molded for the patient to maintain proper alignment of the thumb in slight adduction and the wrist in slight dorsiflexion. Use these splints only for the patient for whom the splint was made. |
| Trapeze bar | The trapeze bar descends from a securely fastened overhead bar attached to the bed frame (see Figure 34-5). The trapeze allows the patient to use upper extremities to raise the trunk off the bed, to assist in transfer from bed to wheelchair, or to perform upper arm strengthening exercises. |
| Wedge pillow | A wedge or abductor pillow is a triangular-shaped pillow made of heavy foam. It is used to maintain the legs in abduction following total hip replacement surgery. |

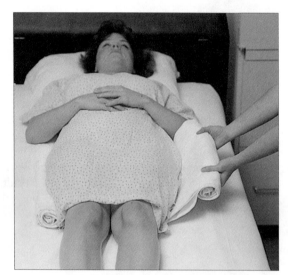

FIGURE **34-4** Trochanter roll.

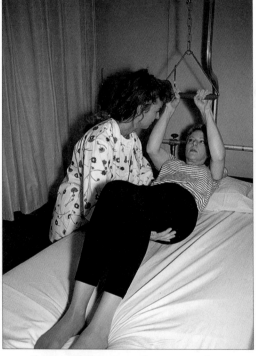

FIGURE **34-5** Patient using a trapeze bar.

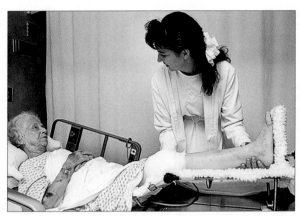

FIGURE **34-6** Continuous passive range-of-motion machine.

surroundings (see Chapter 36). Give explanations before starting care, and encourage the patient to make decisions about care. Plan nursing care to allow the older adult patient to perform as many ADLs as possible. Not only are older adults more susceptible to the hazards of immobility, but the consequences of immobility appear more quickly and become severe more rapidly.

**RESTORATIVE AND CONTINUING CARE.** The goal of restorative and continuing care for the immobilized patient is to maximize independence, increase endurance, and prevent injury. Restorative interventions focus on **instrumental activities of daily living (IADLs)** such as shopping, preparing meals, banking, and taking medications, in addition to ADLs.

You will use many of the same interventions as described in the health promotion and acute care sections, but the emphasis is on working collaboratively with patients, families, friends, and other health care professionals. Sometimes occupational or physical therapy is ordered. Your role is to work collaboratively with these professionals and reinforce exercises and teaching. Common items used to help the patient adapt to mobility limitations include walkers, canes, wheelchairs, and assistive devices such as toilet seat extenders, reaching sticks, special silverware, and clothing with Velcro closures.

### Evaluation

**PATIENT CARE.** You evaluate interventions for reducing the risks of immobility by comparing the patient's actual response to the expected outcomes for each goal (Table 34-4). If you do not achieve expected outcomes, you will need to revise the care plan. You base the success in meeting each outcome on the use of evaluative measures such as ROJM status, exercise tolerance, and fluid intake.

You will also evaluate outcomes designed to demonstrate normal function of specific systems and to prevent complications.

- Are the lungs clear?
- Is the patient's diet appropriate to promote tissue repair?
- Is the patient performing leg exercises regularly?

- Are bowel sounds present?
- Are there any areas of skin breakdown?
- Does the patient remain injury free?
- Is urinary output greater than 25 to 30 ml/hour?
- Is the patient experiencing depression or regression?

**PATIENT EXPECTATIONS.** People often take movement for granted. Patients who are immobile and dependent on others for some or all of their needs sometimes become overly dependent or try to do too much themselves too early. It is a difficult task finding the balance between independence and dependence. Patients will want control over their mobility that is personally satisfactory. For patients who are completely dependent on others for care, control over how and when things are done is very important. Do they feel they are treated with dignity? Do caregivers treat them as adults? Patients who are dependent on others for care sometimes see their demands as the only control they have over their lives.

For most patients with mobility problems, lack of control is often a major issue. Do they feel staff are considerate, and do staff protect their privacy? Are patients' preferences taken into consideration when planning care? Do caregivers talk to them or ignore them? It is helpful to remember that lack of movement is often associated with punishment in our society. We give children "time-outs," teens are "grounded," and people who do not receive promotions are seen as failures. It is therefore important to recognize that immobility possibly leads to fear, anger, grief, withdrawal, or hostility. If you are sensitive to these reactions and help the patient work through them, instead of responding negatively to the patient, you will make a big difference in the patient's outcome.

## OUTCOME EVALUATION

TABLE 34-4

| Nursing Action | Patient Response/Finding | Achievement of Outcome |
|---|---|---|
| Ask Mr. Stapp to rate his pain on a scale of 0 to 10. | Mr. Stapp's facial expressions show grimacing when he moves or uses the walker.<br>Rates his pain between 5 and 6 on the scale. | Outcome of pain control unmet. |
| Review Mr. Stapp's analgesic use over the last 48 hours. | A review of Mr. Stapp's medication administration record (MAR) shows that he is only getting analgesia when he requests, usually before physical therapy.<br>Mr. Stapp states that after he is medicated and before physical therapy his pain level is 2 or less. | Outcome of pain control partially met before physical therapy. |
| Ask Mr. Stapp about his perceptions of pain control. | Mr. Stapp doesn't want to get "hooked" on drugs and tries to "tough it out."<br>He thinks he should only take his medication before physical therapy. | Outcome of satisfaction with pain control measures unmet. |

## KEY CONCEPTS

- Normal physical mobility depends on intact and functioning nervous and musculoskeletal systems.
- The risk of disabilities related to immobilization depends on the extent and duration of the immobilization.
- Immobility results from illness or trauma or is prescribed for therapeutic reasons; it presents hazards in the physical, psychological, and developmental dimensions.
- Pressure ulcers, although often preventable, are one of the most common physical hazards of immobility.
- Effects of immobility include depression, behavioral changes, changes in the sleep-wake cycle, decreased coping abilities, and developmental delays.
- Assessment focuses on range of joint motion, musculoskeletal status, and complete physical examination for potential adverse effects in all body systems, as well as psychosocial and developmental effects.

- After identifying nursing diagnoses, plan and implement interventions to prevent or minimize the hazards and complications of immobilization.
- Adequate hydration measures reduce immobility-related complications in the respiratory and elimination systems.
- Elastic antiembolic stockings and sequential compression devices both improve venous return.
- The primary evaluation criterion for nursing care in the developmental dimension for immobilized patients is the prevention of any measurable decline in functioning or delay in development.
- Early mobilization helps to decrease the effects of bed rest.

## CRITICAL THINKING IN PRACTICE

*Mrs. Woods is an 80-year-old African-American woman admitted to your nursing floor following a left total hip arthroplasty. She has a history of hypertension (HTN) and coronary artery disease (CAD). Upon arrival to her room from the postanesthesia care unit (PACU) her vital signs are: temperature, 38.4° C; blood pressure, 174/92 mm Hg; pulse, 84 beats per minute; respirations, 22 breaths per minute. After you help to position her in semi-Fowler's position, she reports that her pain is at a level 6 on the 0 to 10 pain scale. In addition to morphine sulfate 2 to 4 mg intravenous push (IVP) for pain every 3 to 4 hours, Mrs. Woods has metoprolol 25 mg orally (PO) 2 times a day (bid), heparin 5,000 units sub-Q bid, and bisacodyl 10 mg PO daily ordered as scheduled medications.*

1. List three nursing interventions that you will initiate with Mrs. Woods to prevent respiratory complications due to immobility.
2. Administering bisacodyl will help to prevent what potentially life-threatening complication of constipation in an immobilized patient with heart disease?
3. How will you explain the purpose of heparin therapy to Mrs. Woods?
4. Identify five additional actions that will reduce the risk of clot formation in Mrs. Woods' condition.

## NCLEX® REVIEW

1. What is the most important objective of bed rest for a patient with bilateral pneumonia?
   1. Provide for uninterrupted sleep time
   2. Reduce the oxygen needs of the body
   3. Decrease the need for pain medication
   4. Prevent patient falls due to fatigue
2. Which patient is at greatest risk for developing the adverse effects of immobility?
   1. 3-year-old with a fractured femur
   2. 48-year-old following a thyroidectomy
   3. 78-year-old in traction for a broken hip
   4. 38-year-old following abdominal surgery
3. When assisting a patient with standing following a prolonged period of bed rest, what physical response should the nurse be most prepared to assess?
   1. Steadiness of gait
   2. Respiratory rate
   3. Orthostatic hypotension
   4. Dependent edema
4. What is the most important reason to encourage the use of antiembolic stockings? To facilitate:
   1. Early ambulation
   2. Venous return
   3. Arterial insufficiency
   4. Skin integrity
5. Which nursing intervention will best promote respiratory health in an immobile postoperative patient?
   1. Sequential compression device use
   2. Low-dose heparin therapy
   3. Incentive spirometry
   4. Isometric exercises
6. The nurse has six patient assignments on the day shift. After receiving report, which patient care responsibility would be the best to delegate to assistive personnel?
   1. Repositioning of an unstable cerebral vascular accident patient who is experiencing left-sided paralysis
   2. Teaching a postoperative hip arthroplasty patient how to use an incentive spirometer
   3. Application of antiembolic stockings on a patient admitted with dehydration and anemia
   4. Assessing a stage I sacral pressure ulcer on an older adult pneumonia patient to determine if it should have a DuoDerm dressing applied
7. What would be the highest priority nursing diagnosis for a patient first day postoperative knee replacement?
   1. Impaired skin integrity
   2. Impaired bed mobility
   3. Ineffective breathing pattern
   4. Acute pain
8. What population is most affected developmentally by prolonged bed rest?
   1. Infants
   2. Children
   3. Adults
   4. Older adults
9. What is the best nursing strategy to implement with an immobilized patient to avoid joint contractures?
   1. Ambulation
   2. Physical therapy
   3. Continuous passive motion (CPM)
   4. Range of joint motion (ROJM)

## REFERENCES

Agency for Healthcare Research and Quality (AHRQ): *Pressure ulcer prevention and treatment*, 2003, http://hstat.nlm.nih.gov/hq/Hquest/screen/TestBrowse/t/1049658066834/s/40521.

American Pain Society: *Analgesic use in the treatment of acute pain and cancer pain*, ed 6, Glenview, Ill, 2003, The Society.

Austin J: Mind-body therapies for the management of pain, *Clin J Pain* 20(1):27, 2004.

Banks-Wallace J: Staggering under the weight of responsibility: the impact of culture on physical activity among African American women, *J Multicult Nurs Health* 6(3):24, 2000.

Black J, Hawks J: *Medical-surgical nursing: clinical management for positive outcomes*, ed 7, Philadelphia, 2005, Elsevier.

Bourret E and others: The meaning of mobility for residents and staff in long-term care facilities, *J Adv Nurs* 37(4):338, 2002.

Byrne B: Deep vein thrombosis prophylaxis: the effectiveness and implications of using below-knee or thigh-length graduated compression stockings, *Heart Lung* 30(4):277, 2001.

Dochterman J, Bulechek GM, editors: *Nursing interventions classification (NIC)*, ed 4, St. Louis, 2004, Mosby.

Ebersole P and others: *Toward healthy aging: human needs and nursing response*, ed 6, St. Louis, 2004, Mosby.

Ejaz A and others: Characteristics of 100 consecutive patients presenting with orthostatic hypotension, *Mayo Clin Proc* 79(7):890, 2004.

Hockenberry M and others: *Wong's nursing care of infants and children*, ed 7, St. Louis, 2003, Mosby.

Jain S: Cultural dance: an opportunity to encourage physical activity and health in communities, *Am J Health Educ* 32(4):216, 2001.

Johnson M: Perceptions of barriers to healthy physical activity among Asian communities, *Sport Education & Society* 5(1):51, 2000.

Jones D: Successful aging: maintaining mobility in a geriatric patient population, *Long-Term Rehab* 14(9):46, 2001.

Lance R and others: Comparison of different methods of obtaining orthostatic vitals signs, *Clin Nurs Res* 9(4):479, 2000.

Maher A, Salmond S, Pellino T: *Orthopeadic nursing*, ed 3, Philadelphia, 2002, Saunders.

McCance K, Huether S: *Pathophysiology: the biologic basis for disease in adults and children*, ed 4, St. Louis, 2002, Mosby.

McKenry LM, Salerno E: *Mosby's pharmacology in nursing*, ed 21, St. Louis, 2001, Mosby.

Melillo K and others: Perceptions of older Latino adults regarding physical fitness, physical activity, and exercise, *J Gerontol Nurs* 27(9):38, 2001.

Moorhead S, Johnson M, Maas M: *Nursing outcomes classification (NOC)*, ed 3, 2004, Mosby.

National Osteoporosis Foundation: *American's bone health: the state of osteoporosis and low bone mass in our nations*, 2002, The Foundation.

Nelson A, Baptiste A: Evidence-based practices for safe patient handling and movement, *Online J Issues Nurs* 9(3):1, 2004, http://www.nursingworld.org/ojin/topic25/tpc25_3.htm.

Pasero C: *Intravenous patient-controlled analgesia for acute pain management*, self directed learning module, Pensacola, Fla, 2003, American Society for Pain Management Nursing.

Phipps W and others: *Medical-surgical nursing: health and illness perspectives*, ed 7, St. Louis, 2003, Mosby.

Piotrowski M and others: Massage as adjuvant therapy in the management of acute postoperative pain: a preliminary study, *J Am Coll Surg* 197(6):1037, 2003.

Puckree T, Moonasur R, Govender K: Bedrest alters respiratory muscle strength in patients immobilized due to fractured femurs, *S Afr Journal of Physiotherapy* 56(4):27, 2000.

Ramzi D, Leeper K: DVT and pulmonary embolism. I. Diagnosis, *Am Fam Physician* 69(12):2829, 2004.

Riddle D, Wells P: Diagnosis of lower-extremity deep vein thrombosis in outpatients, *Phys Ther* 84(8):729, 2004.

Van Dongen CJJ and others: Fixed dose subcutaneous low molecular weight heparins versus adjusted dose of unfractionated heparin for venous thromboembolism, The Cochrane Database of Systematic Reviews, Issue 4, 2005, http://www.cochrane.org/reviews/en/ab001100.html.

# CHAPTER 35

# Skin Integrity and Wound Care

## MEDIA RESOURCES

**CD COMPANION** *evolve* **WEBSITE**

http://evolve.elsevier.com/Potter/basic

- **NCLEX® Review**
- **Audio Glossary**
- **English/Spanish Audio Glossary**
- **Video Clips**

## OBJECTIVES

- Describe risk factors for pressure ulcer development.
- List the National Pressure Ulcer Advisory Panel (NPUAP) classification of pressure ulcer staging.
- Discuss the body's response during each phase of the wound healing process.
- Describe wound assessment criteria: anatomical location, size, type and percentage of wound tissue, volume and color of wound drainage, and condition of surrounding skin.
- Differentiate healing by primary and secondary intention.
- Discuss common complications of wound healing.

- Explain factors that impair or promote normal wound healing.
- Describe the purposes of and precautions taken with applying bandages and binders.
- Describe the mechanism of action of wound care dressings.
- Describe the differences in therapeutic effects of heat and cold.
- Complete an assessment for a patient with impaired skin integrity.
- List nursing diagnoses associated with impaired skin integrity.
- Develop a nursing care plan for a patient with impaired skin integrity.
- State evaluation criteria for a patient with impaired skin integrity.

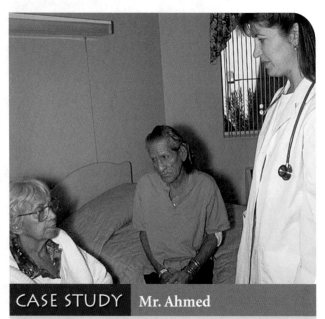

**CASE STUDY** Mr. Ahmed

Mr. Omar Ahmed, a 76-year-old accountant, has come to the hospital again, this time for treatment of pneumonia. Before admission he had been unable to eat and had lost more than 20 lb over the last 2 months. Three years ago he had coronary artery bypass surgery. As a precaution, he has been put on telemetry monitoring. He also has hypertension and type 2 diabetes mellitus. His mobility is limited because of his weakness, difficulty breathing, and acutely ill state. Mr. Ahmed is retired. He lives in a one-family home with his wife, Natalie. Their children and grandchildren live nearby and visit often. On admission his skin is intact. He complains that his "bottom hurts" from lying in bed.

Lynda Abraham is a junior nursing student who is completing her medical-surgical clinical experience on the medical nursing unit. This is her first hospital-based clinical practice.

**KEY TERMS**

abrasion, p. 1029
approximate, p. 1019
bandages, p. 1057
binders, p. 1057
blanchable hyperemia, p. 1017
cachexia, p. 1018
compress, p. 1060
debridement, p. 1036
dehiscence, p. 1022
drainage evacuators, p. 1057
ecchymosis, p. 1030
edema, p. 1018
eschar, p. 1019
evisceration, p. 1022
fistula, p. 1022
friction, p. 1017
granulation tissue, p. 1019

hematoma, p. 1022
hemostasis, p. 1022
induration, p. 1025
laceration, p. 1029
maceration, p. 1043
nonblanchable hyperemia, p. 1017
pressure ulcer, p. 1016
primary intention, p. 1019
secondary intention, p. 1019
shear, p. 1017
sitz bath, p. 1062
tissue ischemia, p. 1017
wound culture, p. 1030

## Scientific Knowledge Base

### Pressure Ulcers

**Pressure ulcer** (formerly called *pressure sore, decubitus ulcer,* or *bedsore*) is the term used to describe impaired skin integrity (Figure 35-1) resulting from pressure (Wound, Ostomy and Continence Nurses Society [WOCN], 2003). A patient experiencing decreased mobility, inadequate nutrition, decreased sensory perception, or decreased activity is at

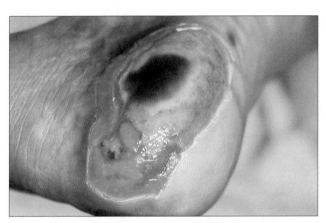

FIGURE **35-1** Pressure ulcer with tissue necrosis.

## BOX 35-1 USING EVIDENCE IN PRACTICE

### Research Summary

A pressure ulcer prevalence study was done to understand the scope of the problems for hospitalized patients with skin care issues. The study examined the number of patients who had pressure ulcers, the characteristics of those patients, and the stage and body location of the pressure ulcers. These hospital data were compared with prevalence rates at other comparable institutions.

All patients in the acute care hospital had head-to-toe skin assessments performed during an 8-hour period by a team of staff members. Included in the study were 513 adult and pediatric patients. For the adult patients the average age was 65 to 79 years, and for the pediatric patients it was less than 1 year.

### Results

The combined pressure ulcer prevalence (percentage of patients with skin breakdown in the hospital on that given day) was 26.3%; 29.2% of the adults and 13.1% of the children assessed had pressure ulcers. In the adults the group with the highest number of pressure ulcers were those ages 64 to 79, and the youngest group of children had the highest amount of pressure ulcers. It was found that there was an average of 2 ulcers per adult patient and 1.6 ulcers per child. The patient care units with the highest prevalence of pressure ulcers were the emergency department and the intensive care units. The most common body locations for pressure ulcers were the sacrum (22.1%), heels (14.8%), ears (12.9%), elbows (10.6%), and the buttocks (6.8%). Forty-eight percent of the ulcers were stage I, 36% stage II, 6% stage III-IV, and 10% unable to stage. This study concluded that patients at the extreme ends of the age spectrum had an increased risk of pressure ulcers. Stage I and II ulcers occurred the most frequently.

### Application to Nursing Practice

The results of this study help nurses to understand the patient population at risk for the development of pressure ulcers. This information can be compared with other similar health care settings and can serve as a benchmark for measuring clinical outcomes. Because the majority of ulcers were stage I and stage II ulcers, preventative measures should be put in place to help decrease the prevalence of pressure ulcers.

Data from Groeneveld A and others: The prevalence of pressure ulcers in a tertiary care pediatric and adult hospital, *J Wound Ostomy Continence Nurs* 31(3):108, 2004.

risk for pressure ulcer development. More than one million individuals develop pressure ulcers each year. Because pressure ulcers usually develop within the first 2 weeks of hospitalization, it is important to identify high-risk groups to target interventions (Box 35-1).

**Tissue ischemia** occurs when capillary blood flow is obstructed, as in the case of pressure. When pressure is relieved in a relatively short time, a phenomenon called reactive hyperemia occurs. Reactive hyperemia is a redness of the skin due to dilation of the superficial capillaries (WOCN, 2003). You can determine if reactive hyperemia is present by checking for blanching. The area, which appears red and warm, will blanche (turn lighter in color) following fingertip palpation (Figure 35-2). **Blanchable hyperemia** is harder to assess in patients with dark skin. The discoloration or redness appears as a deepening of normal ethnic color or a purple hue to the skin (Ayello and Lyder, 2001). This hyperemia usually resolves without tissue loss if pressure is reduced or relieved.

**Nonblanchable hyperemia** is redness that persists after palpation and indicates tissue damage (Figure 35-3). When you press a finger against the red or purple area, it does not turn lighter in color. Deep tissue damage is present and is commonly the first stage of pressure ulcer development. This stage of skin injury is also reversible if the pressure is relieved and the tissue protected.

**CONTRIBUTING FACTORS TO PRESSURE ULCER FORMATION.** In addition to pressure, other factors increase the patient's risk for developing pressure ulcers. The external factors include shear, friction, and moisture, and internal factors include nutrition, infection, and age.

**Shear.** **Shear** is the force exerted against the skin while the skin remains stationary and the bony structures move. For example, when the head of the bed is elevated, gravity causes the bony skeleton to pull towards the foot of the bed, while the skin remains against the sheets (Figure 35-4). The underlying tissue blood vessels are stretched and angulated, and blood flow is impeded to the deep tissue. Ulcers occur with large areas of undermined damage and less damage at the skin surface.

**Friction.** **Friction** is an injury to the skin that has the appearance of an abrasion. Friction results from two surfaces rubbing against one another. The body surfaces most at risk for friction are the elbows and heels because abrasion of these surfaces occurs when they are rubbed against the sheets during repositioning. A skin insult caused by friction looks like an abrasion or superficial laceration (Ayello and others, 2004).

**Moisture.** Moisture on the skin increases the risk of ulcer formation. Moisture reduces the skin's resistance to other physical factors such as pressure or shear. Moisture originates

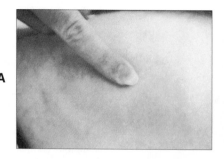
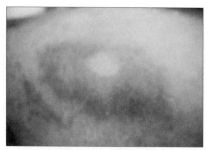

FIGURE **35-2 A,** Check for blanching by applying fingertip pressure. **B,** Area of blanchable hyperemia.

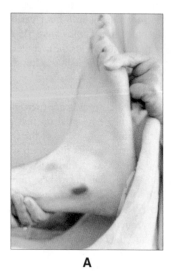
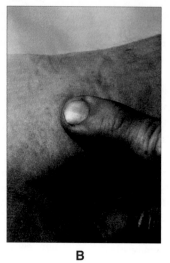
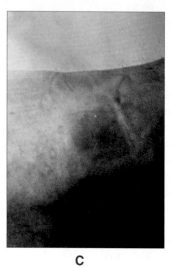

FIGURE **35-3 A,** Blanchable hyperemia. **B** and **C,** In nonblanchable hyperemia the area is darker than the surrounding skin and does not blanch with fingertip pressure.

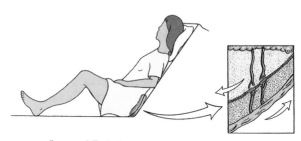

FIGURE **35-4** Shear exerted in the sacral area.

from wound drainage, perspiration, and/or fecal and urinary incontinence. Skin moisture and wetness from incontinence can cause skin breakdown (Fader, Bain, and Cottenden, 2004).

**Nutrition.** Poor nutrition, specifically severe protein deficiency, causes soft tissue to become susceptible to breakdown. Low protein levels cause edema or swelling, which contributes to problems with oxygen transport and the transport of nutrients (Mechanick, 2004).

Poor nutrition alters fluid and electrolyte balance. In patients with severe protein loss, hypoalbuminemia (serum albumin level below 3 g/100 ml) leads to a shift of fluid from the extracellular fluid volume to the tissues, resulting in

edema (Mathus-Vliegen, 2004). **Edema** increases the affected tissue's risk for pressure ulcer formation. The blood supply to the edematous tissue is decreased, and waste products remain because of the changing pressures in the capillary circulation and capillary bed.

**Cachexia** is generalized ill health and malnutrition, marked by weakness and emaciation, or extreme thinness. Basically the cachectic patient has lost the adipose tissue necessary to protect bony prominences from pressure.

**Infection.** Infection results from the presence of pathogens in the body. A patient with an infection usually has a fever. Infection and fever increase the metabolic needs of the body, making already hypoxic tissue more susceptible to ischemic injury. In addition, fever results in diaphoresis and increased skin moisture, which further predispose the patient to skin breakdown.

**Age.** Skin structure changes with age, causing a loss of dermal thickness and an increase in the risk of skin tears. Older adults are at highest risk for development of pressure ulcers; 60% to 90% of all pressure ulcers occur in patients over 65 years of age (Boynton and others, 1999). Neonates and young children (i.e., younger than 5 years old) are also at high risk for pressure ulcer occurrence (Quigley and Curley, 1996; WOCN, 2003).

## Origins of Pressure Ulcers

Pressure exerted against the skin surface causes pressure ulcers; usually a bone and the surface of the bed compress the skin. However, pressure ulcers also occur on any skin surface where pressure applied against the skin exceeds capillary closure pressure. Classic research identified that normal capillary pressure, the amount of pressure needed to keep the capillary open, is in the range of 12 to 32 mm Hg, depending on the location in the capillary (Landis, 1930). When the intensity of the pressure exerted to the capillary exceeds 12 to 32 mm Hg, this occludes the vessel, causing ischemic injury to the tissues it normally feeds. However, pressure to the tissue will not routinely result in pressure ulceration. Two other concepts, duration of the pressure and tissue tolerance, play a role.

High pressure over a short time and low pressure over a long time cause skin breakdown. Thus duration influences the effects of pressure; the longer the pressure is applied, the more likely tissue loss will occur. Tissue tolerance also plays an important role in pressure ulcer development. The integrity of the skin and the supporting structures influence the skin's ability to redistribute the pressure. The factors mentioned above—shear, friction, moisture, and the internal factors such as nutrition, infection, and age—alter the ability of the skin and supporting tissue to respond to the pressure (Ayello and others, 2004).

## Wound Classification

One method to classify pressure ulcers is to stage the ulcer according to tissue layer involvement. The National Pressure Ulcer Advisory Panel (NPUAP) (2005) supports the following staging system:

*Stage I:* An observable pressure ulcer–related alteration of intact skin whose indicators as compared to the adjacent or opposite area on the body include changes in one or more of the following: skin temperature (warmth or coolness), tissue consistency (firm or boggy feel), and/or sensation (pain, itching). The ulcer appears as a defined area of persistent redness in lightly pigmented skin, whereas in darker skin tones the ulcer appears with persistent red, blue, or purple hues (Figure 35-5, *A*).
*Stage II:* Partial-thickness skin loss involving epidermis, dermis, or both. The ulcer is superficial and presents as an abrasion, blister, or shallow crater (Figure 35-5, *B*).
*Stage III:* Full-thickness skin loss involving damage to, or necrosis of, subcutaneous tissue that extends down to, but not through, underlying fascia. The ulcer presents as a deep crater with or without undermining of surrounding tissue (Figure 35-5, *C*).
*Stage IV:* Full-thickness skin loss with extensive destruction, tissue necrosis, or damage to muscle, bone, or supporting structures (e.g., tendon or joint capsule). Undermining and sinus tracts are also associated with stage IV pressure ulcers (Figure 35-5, *D*).

There are limitations in staging: assessment of stage I pressure ulcers is difficult in patients with darkly pigmented skin. When **eschar** (dead, dry tissue) is present, accurate staging of the pressure ulcer is not possible until the eschar has sloughed or the wound has been debrided.

Wound assessment (regardless of cause) includes the following parameters: anatomical location, size (dimensions and depth of wound), type (viable or nonviable) and percentage of wound tissue (the proportion of tissue type), volume and color of wound drainage, and condition of surrounding skin (Baranoski and Ayello, 2004). These measures will assist in evaluating the progress of the wound, will drive decision making, and will provide assessment to evaluate wound healing.

## Wound Healing Process

The process of wound healing involves an orderly series of integrated physiological responses. Multiple factors promote or impede wound healing (Box 35-2). A wound with little or no tissue loss, such as a clean surgical incision, heals by **primary intention.** The skin edges **approximate,** or close together, and the risk of infection developing is slight. In contrast, a wound involving loss of tissue such as a severe laceration or a chronic wound such as a pressure ulcer heals by **secondary intention.** The skin edges cannot come together, and healing occurs gradually. A layer of granulation tissue covers the wound, wound contraction brings the wound edges together, and the wound closes with a scar. There are also instances in which a surgical wound is initially closed in the deep tissue layers; however, the subcutaneous fat and skin layers are left open. This method of wound closure is called *delayed primary closure.* The wound heals with a layer of **granulation tissue** at the edges and base, and several days after the initial wounding the wound edges are brought together with sutures or adhesive closures. The wound then heals by primary intention. An example of a wound closure by delayed primary closure occurs when a patient has a ruptured appendix. In some cases the surgeon is unsure if the appendix had microperforations and subsequent spilling of the intestinal contents into the abdomen and wound. Thus the surgeon will leave the incision open for up to 4 to 5 days following surgery. Then the surgeon assesses the wound, and, if after 4 to 5 days the surgeon does not note any clinical signs of infection, the wound is closed with either adhesive strips or sutures.

Wounds heal by one of two mechanisms: partial-thickness wound repair or full-thickness wound repair. Partial-thickness wound repair is necessary when there is loss of the epidermis and/or part of the dermis, such as wound healing by primary intention. Full-thickness wound repair is necessary when there is loss of the epidermis, dermis, and possible extension into subcutaneous layers, bone, and/or muscle.

**PARTIAL-THICKNESS WOUND REPAIR.** The body repairs wounds that heal by primary intention and shallow wounds that only involve loss of the epidermis and perhaps some of the dermis by resurfacing of the wound with new

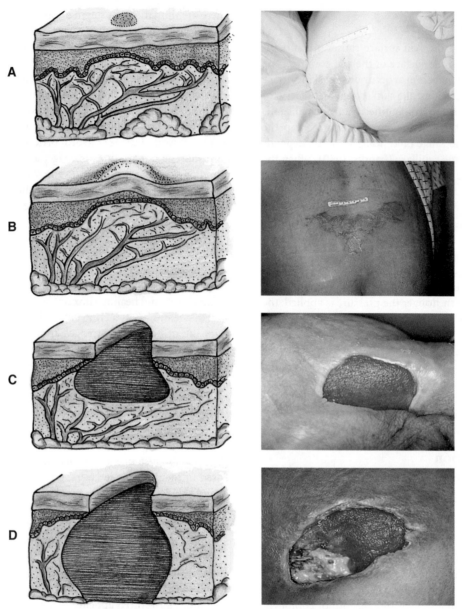

FIGURE **35-5 A,** Stage I pressure ulcer. **B,** Stage II pressure ulcer. **C,** Stage III pressure ulcer. **D,** Stage IV pressure ulcer. (Courtesy Laurel Wiersema-Bryant, RN, MSN, Clinical Nurse Specialist, Barnes Hospital, St. Louis.)

epidermal cells. The wounds go through several phases of wound healing.

**Inflammatory Response.** Erythema and edema are the first response, bringing white blood cells to the site. The wounded area appears red and swollen. If the exudate, or discharge, that brings the white blood cells to the area is allowed to dry, a scab will form. This response occurs for approximately 24 hours (Jones, Bale, and Harding, 2004).

**Epidermal Repair.** Epidermal cells begin migration across the wound, originating from the epidermal cells at the wound edges or the epidermal appendages. Peak epithelial proliferation occurs within 24 to 72 hours after injury. Wounds kept in a moist environment will heal in approximately 4 days (as opposed to 7 days when kept dry) because

new epithelial cells migrate across a moist surface. If a wound is dry, the cells have to find moisture below the skin surface (Waldrop and Doughty, 2000).

**Dermal Repair.** The epidermis thickens, anchors to adjacent cells, and resumes normal function. The new epidermis is pink, dry, and fragile. If dermal repair is necessary, dermal repair occurs concurrently with epidermal repair.

**FULL-THICKNESS WOUND REPAIR.** Full-thickness wounds involve tissue loss and are more common in chronic wounds such as pressure ulcers. Three phases are involved in healing a full-thickness wound.

**Inflammatory Phase.** The key events in the inflammatory phase are control of bleeding and the provision of a clean wound environment for wound healing. The first event

---

### BOX 35-2  Factors Influencing Wound Healing

**Age**

Blood circulation and oxygen delivery to the wound, clotting, inflammatory response, and phagocytosis are sometimes impaired in the very young and older adults. Risk of infection is greater.

Cell growth and differentiation in reconstruction are slower with advancing age.

Scar tissue never regains the tensile strength of noninjured skin, increasing the risk of altered body part function in older adults.

Age affects all phases of wound healing. A decline in the number of white blood cells places older adults at greater risk for a wound infection. A slowdown is common in the deposition of collagen in reepithelization.

**Nutrition**

Tissue repair and infection resistance depend on a balanced diet. Surgery, severe wounds, serious infections, and preoperative nutritional deficits increase nutritional requirements.

Nutrients provide raw materials needed for cellular activities that contribute to wound healing.

**Infection**

Wound infection prolongs the inflammatory phase, delays collagen synthesis, and prevents epithelialization.

**Obesity**

The less abundant supply of blood vessels in fatty tissue impairs delivery of nutrients and cellular elements needed for healing.

**Extent of Wound**

Wounds with extensive tissue loss heal by secondary intention and remain open for a prolonged period of time to heal.

**Tissue Perfusion**

Oxygen fuels the cellular function essential to the repair process. Chronic tissue hypoxia is associated with impaired collagen synthesis and reduced tissue resistance to infection.

**Smoking**

Functional hemoglobin levels decrease, impairing oxygen release to tissues.

**Immunosuppression**

Cortisone suppresses the inflammatory response, increasing the wound's vulnerability to infection.

Because steroids decrease the inflammatory response, detection of early signs of inflammation or infection is difficult.

Chemotherapeutic drugs and certain cancerous diseases interfere with leukocyte production and the immune response.

Immunosuppressive therapy impairs wound healing by preventing normal progression of the phases of wound healing.

**Diabetes Mellitus**

The patient with diabetes has small vessel disease that impairs tissue perfusion; thus oxygen delivery is poor.

An elevated blood glucose level impairs macrophage function. Risk of infection is increased because of poor wound healing.

Patients with diabetes demonstrate the following problems with wound healing: reduced collagen synthesis, decreased wound strength, and impaired white blood cell functioning. These adverse effects are at least in part due to poor glycemic control.

**Radiation**

Radiation therapy, which eventually results in fibrosis and vascular scarring, interferes with postoperative wound healing when surgery is delayed more than 4 to 6 weeks and irradiated tissues have become fragile and poorly perfused.

**Wound Stress**

Sustained stress (e.g., vomiting, abdominal distention, coughing) disrupts wound layers and tissue repair.

Modified from Waldrop J, Doughty D: Wound healing physiology in acute and chronic wounds. In Bryant RA, editor: *Acute and chronic wounds: nursing management,* ed 2, St. Louis, 2000, Mosby.

---

in this phase is hemostasis. Platelets cause coagulation and vasoconstriction. The platelets break down and release growth factors, which appear to initiate the entire wound-healing process (Jones and others, 2004). The inflammatory response brings white blood cells to the area, cleaning up the site and releasing additional growth factors. This phase lasts approximately 3 days in an acute clean wound, such as a surgical incision.

**Proliferative Phase.** The key events in the proliferative phase are production of new tissue, epithelialization, and contraction. New capillary networks form to provide oxygen and nutrients for new tissue and contribute to the synthesis of collagen. As collagen fibers and capillary networks continue to synthesize and increase in size, the wound begins to contract. The last component of this phase is epithelialization, in which the epithelial cells migrate and cover the defect. It is important to note that epithelialization occurs faster in a moist environment, supporting the role of moist wound dressings in wound care.

**Remodeling Phase.** The remodeling phase, which lasts up to 1 year, reorganizes the collagen to produce a more elastic, stronger collagen for the scar tissue. The tensile strength of the scar tissue is never more than 80% of the tensile strength in nonwounded tissue (Jones and others, 2004).

The phases of wound healing overlap, depending upon the patient's ability to heal and the type of wound. Acute wounds (most surgical wounds, for example) typically heal following the phases noted above; however, chronic wounds (some pressure ulcers, for example) appear to fail to negotiate one or more of the phases of wound healing.

## Complications of Wound Healing

Wound healing is not without complications. When caring for patients with wounds, you will observe the healing process while observing for complications.

**HEMORRHAGE.** Bleeding from an acute wound is normal during and immediately after initial trauma, but **hemostasis,** which is cessation of bleeding by vasoconstriction and coagulation, usually occurs within several minutes. Hemorrhage occurring later indicates a slipped surgical suture, a dislodged clot, infection, or the erosion of a blood vessel by a foreign object (e.g., a drain). Hemorrhage is external or internal. Symptoms of internal bleeding are hypovolemic shock and swelling of the affected body part. A **hematoma,** a collection of clotted blood, is a localized collection of blood underneath tissues, often appearing as a bluish swelling or mass. External hemorrhaging is usually more obvious because dressings covering the wound soon become saturated with blood. Surgical drains also drain blood. You will note a decrease in the patient's hemoglobin level and hematocrit.

**INFECTION.** Bacterial wound infection prevents healing by increasing tissue damage and altering the healing process. The chances of wound infection are greater when the wound contains dead or necrotic tissues, when foreign bodies are in or near the wound, and when the blood supply and local tissue defenses are lower than normal.

A contaminated or traumatic wound infection develops within 2 to 3 days; a surgical wound infection develops within 4 to 5 days. Locally, drainage is often yellow, green, or brown and odorous, depending on the causative organism. The wound edges will appear tense, swollen, and painful, with redness extending beyond the immediate wound edge. Systemic signs include fever, general malaise, and an elevated white blood cell count.

**DEHISCENCE.** When an acute wound fails to heal properly, the layers of skin and tissue separate. This most commonly occurs before collagen formation (3 to 11 days after injury). **Dehiscence** is the partial or total separation of layers of skin and tissue above the fascia in a wound that is not healing properly. Obese patients have a high risk for dehiscence because of constant strain on their wounds and the poor vascularity of fatty tissue. Dehiscence occurs most often in abdominal surgical wounds after a sudden strain such as coughing, vomiting, or sitting up in bed. Patients often report feeling as though something has given way. When serosanguineous drainage increases from a wound, be alert for dehiscence.

**EVISCERATION.** **Evisceration** occurs when wound layers separate below the fascial layer, and visceral organs protrude through the wound opening. It is a medical emergency requiring placement of sterile towels soaked in sterile saline over the extruding tissues to reduce chances of bacterial invasion and drying before surgical repair occurs.

**FISTULAS.** A **fistula** is an abnormal opening between two organs or between an organ and the skin. Fistulas result from wound-healing problems associated with trauma, infection, radiation exposure, or disease such as cancer. Fistulas increase the risks of infection, fluid and electrolyte imbalances, and skin breakdown from chronic drainage.

## Nursing Knowledge Base

A major aspect of nursing care is the maintenance of skin integrity and wound care. Nursing research has played an important role in developing guidelines for pressure ulcer care and prevention.

### Prediction and Prevention

In 1992 the Agency for Health Care Policy and Research (AHCPR) panel developed clinical guidelines for pressure ulcer prevention and treatment of pressure ulcers. These guidelines have assisted the health care providers in planning and implementing care for both prevention and treatment of the patient with a pressure ulcer. In 2003 the Wound, Ostomy and Continence Nurses Society (WOCN) developed the *Guideline for Prevention and Management of Pressure Ulcers.* Much like the process used to develop the AHCPR guidelines, a panel of experts performed extensive searches on available literature on pressure ulcers and established a level of evidence rating that provides the best evidence in the prevention and management of pressure ulcers available. This guideline has been accepted to the guideline resource component of the Agency for Healthcare Research and Quality, which has replaced the AHCPR. Predictive instruments for pressure ulcer development identify those patients at highest risk for pressure ulcers. Thus patients with little risk for pressure ulcer development will not have the unnecessary expense of preventive treatments and the risk of complications.

One reliable predictive tool is the Braden Scale. The Braden Scale is made of six subscales: sensory perception, moisture, activity, mobility, nutrition, and friction and shear (Table 35-1). A hospitalized adult with a score of 16 or below and an older adult at 18 or below are at risk for pressure ulcer development (Ayello and Braden, 2002; Bergstrom and others, 1998). This instrument is highly reliable in the identification of patients at greatest risk for pressure ulcers (Ayello and others, 2004; Bergstrom and others, 1987a, 1987b, 1998).

## Critical Thinking

### Synthesis

When you care for patients who have pressure ulcers or chronic wounds, competent nursing care that integrates information from all health-related sciences is needed. You are able to incorporate knowledge from courses, experiences, and appropriate standards of practice into the management of your patient's wound.

**KNOWLEDGE.** Performing a pressure ulcer risk assessment requires you to use a validated risk assessment tool. Knowing normal physiology and the impact of pressure on the skin enables you to practice preventive nursing mea-

2129254976

78033039376

## TABLE 35-1 Braden Scale for Predicting Pressure Sore Risk

| | | | | Score |
|---|---|---|---|---|
| **Sensory Perception**<br>Ability to respond meaningfully to pressure-related discomfort | **1. Completely limited:** Unresponsive (does not moan, flinch, or grasp) to painful stimuli due to diminished level of consciousness or sedation.<br><br>**or**<br><br>Limited ability to feel pain over most of body surface. | **2. Very limited:** Responds only to painful stimuli. Cannot communicate discomfort except by moaning or restlessness.<br><br>**or**<br><br>Has a sensory impairment that limits the ability to feel pain or discomfort over half of body. | **3. Slightly limited:** Responds to verbal commands but cannot always communicate discomfort or need to be turned.<br><br>**or**<br><br>Has some sensory impairment, which limits ability to feel pain or discomfort in 1 or 2 extremities. | **4. No impairment:** Responds to verbal commands. Has no sensory deficit that limits ability to feel or voice pain or discomfort. | |
| **Moisture**<br>Degree to which skin is exposed to moisture | **1. Constantly moist:** Perspiration, urine, etc. keeps skin moist almost constantly. Dampness is detected every time patient is moved or turned. | **2. Often Moist:** Skin is often, but not always, moist. Linen must be changed at least once a shift. | **3. Occasionally moist:** Skin is occasionally moist, requiring an extra linen change approximately once a day. | **4. Rarely moist:** Skin is usually dry; linen requires changing only at routine intervals. | |
| **Activity**<br>Degree of physical activity | **1. Bedfast:** Confined to bed. | **2. Confined to chair:** Ability to walk severely limited or nonexistent. Cannot bear own weight and/or must be assisted into chair or wheelchair. | **3. Walks occasionally:** Walks occasionally during day, but for very short distances, with or without assistance. Spends majority of each shift in bed or chair. | **4. Walks frequently:** Walks outside the room at least twice a day and inside the room at least once every 2 hours during waking hours. | |
| **Mobility**<br>Ability to change and control body position | **1. Completely immobile:** Does not make even slight changes in body or extremity position without assistance. | **2. Very limited:** Makes occasional slight changes in body or extremity position but unable to make frequent or significant changes independently. | **3. Slightly limited:** Makes frequent though slight changes in body or extremity position independently. | **4. No limitations:** Makes major and frequent changes in position without assistance. | |
| **Nutrition**<br>Usual food intake pattern | **1. Very poor:** Never eats a complete meal. Rarely eats more than one third of any food offered. Eats 2 servings or less of protein (meat or dairy products) per day. Takes fluids poorly. Does not take a liquid dietary supplement.<br><br>**or**<br><br>Is NPO and/or maintained on clear liquids or IVs for more than 5 days. | **2. Probably inadequate:** Rarely eats a complete meal and generally eats only about half of any food offered. Protein intake includes only 3 servings of meat or dairy products per day. Occasionally will take a dietary supplement.<br><br>**or**<br><br>Receives less than optimal amount of liquid diet or tube feeding. | **3. Adequate:** Eats over half of most meals. Eats a total of 4 servings of protein (meat, dairy products) each day. Occasionally will refuse a meal, but will usually take a supplement if offered.<br><br>**or**<br><br>Is on a tube-feeding or TPN regimen that probably meets most nutritional needs. | **4. Excellent:** Eats most of every meal. Never refuses a meal. Usually eats a total of 4 or more servings of meat and dairy products. Occasionally eats between meals. Does not require supplements. | |
| **Friction and shear** | **1. Problem:** Requires moderate to maximal assistance in moving. Complete lifting without sliding against sheets is impossible. Frequently slides down in bed or chair, requiring frequent repositioning with maximal assistance. Spasticity, contractions, or agitation leads to almost constant friction. | **2. Potential problem:** Moves feebly or requires minimal assistance. During a move skin probably slides to some extent against sheets, chair, restraints, or other devices. Maintains relatively good position in chair or bed most of the time but occasionally slides down. | **3. No apparent problem:** Moves in bed and in chair independently and has sufficient muscle strength to sit up completely during move. Maintains good position in bed or chair at all times. | | |

Instructions: Score patient in each of the six subscales. Maximum score is 23, indicating little or no risk. A score of = 16 indicates "at risk", ≤ 9 indicates high risk.

Copyright 1988. Used with permission of Barbara Braden, PhD, RN, Professor, Creighton University School of Nursing, Omaha, Nebraska and Nancy Bergstrom, Professor, University of Texas-Houston, School of Nursing, Houston, Texas.

sures. In addition, knowledge of normal healing patterns helps you to recognize alterations requiring intervention. In choosing interventions, consider the type of wound, the pain associated with it, conditions that affect healing, and the patient's psychological well-being.

**EXPERIENCE.** By observing the normal characteristics of a healing wound, you assess how your patient's wound is healing. This is especially important when your patient has some factors that impede wound healing, such as peripheral vascular disease, poor nutrition, or reduced mobility.

You are better able to assess a patient's wound by being able to draw from experience and recognize normal characteristics of wound healing. When caring for a patient who develops problems with wound healing, learn the clinical signs of complications. This is especially important when caring for a patient with darkly pigmented skin (Box 35-3). Reflecting on such experience prepares you to assess wounds more accurately.

**ATTITUDES.** Be observant when caring for an acutely ill patient; at times assessment for skin breakdown is overlooked because of other perceived priorities, such as respiratory or cardiac status. As a patient advocate, ensure that meticulous skin assessment and pressure ulcer prevention measures are incorporated in the plan of care. Skin assessment is important whenever a patient's health status changes (WOCN, 2003). Be aware that skin breakdown is sometimes unavoidable. However, the sooner you assess for and identify the risk factors for skin breakdown and plan interventions, the less severe the impaired skin integrity will be.

In the immediate postoperative period, some patients require well-thought-out modifications of wound care techniques. The dressing may not be changed, but you are responsible for ensuring that the dressing remains dry and intact. With knowledge about pressure ulcers, wounds, and normal wound healing, you will find creative measures to reduce the risks of impaired skin integrity and promote wound healing.

**STANDARDS.** The WOCN wrote the 2003 pressure ulcer guidelines to support clinical practice by providing consistent research-based clinical decisions. Box 35-4 has a summary of these guidelines. In addition, wound care protocols vary by agency policy. It is important that you know your agency's policy and practices regarding the use of skin care products, dressing materials, and frequency of dressing change.

## Nursing Process

### Assessment

Baseline and continual focused assessment data provide critical information about the patient's skin integrity and the increased risk for pressure ulcer development or impaired wound healing (Table 35-2). Although there are multiple factors that affect skin integrity, it is important that you identify and assess those factors relevant for your patient.

**PRESSURE ULCERS.** Perform assessment of the patient for risk of development of pressure ulcers using one

---

**BOX 35-3** CULTURAL FOCUS

**Skin Assessment for the Patient With Intact Darkly Pigmented Skin**

**Assess Localized Skin Color Changes**
Any of the following may appear:
- Skin color changes are different from usual skin tone.
- Appears darker than surrounding skin—purplish, bluish, eggplant.

**Importance of Lighting Source**
- Use natural or halogen light.
- Avoid fluorescent lamps.
- Avoid wearing tinted lenses when assessing skin color.

**Tissue Consistency**
- Skin is taut, shiny, or indurated; edema occurs with induration of more than 15 mm in diameter.
- Assess for edema/swelling.
- Assess for firm or boggy feel.

**Sensation**
- Assess for pain or changes in skin sensation, such as burning or itching.

**Assess Skin Temperature**
- Initially skin in the area of pressure may feel warmer than the surrounding skin.
- Subsequently skin may feel cooler than the surrounding skin.
- Feel areas of skin that are not involved in or around a pressure point to serve as a point of temperature reference.

Data from Bennett MA: Report of the Task Force on the implications for darkly pigmented intact skin in the prediction and prevention of pressure ulcers, *Adv Wound Care* 8(6):34, 1995; Henderson CT and others: Draft definition of stage I pressure ulcers: inclusion of persons with darkly pigmented skin, *Adv Wound Care* 10(5):16, 1997.

---

of the established predictive tools, such as the Braden Scale. Do this on admission to the agency, 24 to 48 hours after admission, at regular intervals, and when there is a significant change in the patient's condition. Ongoing assessment is important because the patient's condition may change; continual assessments will help identify changes that increase the patient's risk for pressure ulcer development. In addition to assessing the patient for potential risk factors, perform a skin assessment on a daily basis. The skin assessment provides for prompt problem identification and development of individualized interventions (Skill 35-1). Prompt identification of such patients enables nurses to individualize costly resources to appropriate patients and reduce their risk. When patients are identified as being at risk for pressure ulcers, specific prevention and ulcer treatment strategies are included in the plan of care (see Implementation section of this chapter).

**Skin.** Assessment for tissue pressure indicators includes visual and tactile inspection of the skin. Baseline assessment

---

**BOX 35-4** **Pressure Ulcer Prevention Points**

**Assessment**

1. Assess individual risk for developing pressure ulcers.
2. Perform a risk assessment (using a tool such as the Braden Scale) on entry to a health care setting, and repeat on a regularly scheduled basis or when there is a significant change in the patient's condition.
3. Assess for cognition, sensation, immobility, shear, friction, and incontinence.
4. Identify high-risk settings and groups to target prevention efforts to minimize risk.
5. Inspect skin and bony prominences at least daily.

**Skin Care and Early Treatment**

1. Continue preventative measures even when a patient has a pressure ulcer to prevent additional pressure areas from developing.
2. Clean and dry skin after each incontinent episode.
3. Use incontinence skin barriers such as creams, ointments, pastes, and film forming skin protectants as needed to protect and maintain intact skin.
4. Use turning or lift sheets or devices to turn or transfer patients.
5. Maintain head of bed at, or below 30 degrees or at the lowest level of elevation consistent with the patient's medical condition.
6. Avoid vigorous massage over bony prominences.

**Support Surfaces/Pressure Reduction**

1. Place at-risk individuals on a pressure reduction surface and on an ordinary hospital mattress.

2. Schedule regular and frequent turning and repositioning for bed- and chair-bound individuals. Turn at least every 2 to 4 hours on a pressure-reducing mattress or at least every 2 hours on a non–pressure-reducing mattress.
3. Reposition chair-bound individuals every hour if they are unable to perform pressure relief exercises every 15 minutes.

**Nutrition**

1. Maintain adequate nutrition that is compatible with the individuals' wishes or condition.
2. Consult a nutritionist in cases of suspected or identified nutritional deficiencies or when nutrition supplementation is necessary to prevent malnutrition.

**Patient/Caregiver Education**

1. Educate patient/caregiver about the causes and risk factors for pressure ulcer development and ways to minimize risk.
2. Include information on:
   a. Etiology of and risk factors for pressure ulcers
   b. Risk assessment tools and their application
   c. Skin assessment
   d. Selection/use of support surfaces
   e. Development with implementation of individualized programs of skin care
   f. Demonstration of positioning to decrease risk of tissue breakdown
   g. Accurate documentation of pertinent data

Data from Wound, Ostomy and Continence Nurses Society: *Guideline for prevention and management of pressure ulcers*, WOCN Clinical Practice Guidelines Series, Glenview, Ill, 2003, The Society.

---

determines the patient's normal skin characteristics and any actual or potential areas of breakdown. This is especially important with high-risk patients. The skin of an older adult patient is more fragile and has an increased risk for skin breakdown (Box 35-5). Pay particular attention to areas exposed to casts, traction, or splints. Perform systematic skin assessment at least once a day on those patients at greater risk for pressure ulcer development (WOCN, 2003).

Assess all areas of the skin, from head to toe, paying attention to any reddened areas or breaks in skin integrity. Document the assessment. When you notice hyperemia, document location, size, and color, and reassess the area after 1 hour. If you suspect nonblanchable hyperemia, outlining the affected area with a marker makes reassessment easier. Nonblanchable hyperemia is an early indicator of impaired skin integrity, but damage to the underlying tissue is sometimes more progressive. Palpate the tissues next to the observed area to acquire further data about **induration** and the damage to the skin and underlying tissues.

Assess patients with lightly pigmented skin for blanching with return to normal skin tones. Also note changes in color, temperature, and hardness of the surrounding skin and tissues. Use visual and tactile inspection over the body areas

most frequently at risk for pressure ulcer development (see Figure 35-6). When a patient lies in bed or sits in a chair, the body places weight heavily on certain bony prominences. Body surfaces subjected to the greatest weight or pressure are at greatest risk for pressure ulcer formation.

**Mobility.** Assessment includes documenting level of mobility, the potential effects of impaired mobility on skin integrity, and data regarding the quality of muscle tone and strength. For example, determine whether the patient is able to lift the weight off the ischial tuberosities and roll the body to a side-lying position. Some patients have adequate range of motion (ROM) to independently move into a more protective position. Finally, assess the patient's activity tolerance (see Chapter 25).

**Nutritional Status.** Malnutrition is associated with overall morbidity and mortality. Best practice involves monitoring the nutritional status as part of the total assessment (WOCN, 2003) (Box 35-6; see also Chapter 31). Inadequate caloric intake causes weight loss and a decrease in subcutaneous tissue, allowing bony prominences to compress and restrict circulation.

**WOUNDS.** The assessment of a patient's wound varies from one health care setting to another. It is important for

*Text continued on p. 1029*

## FOCUSED PATIENT ASSESSMENT

**TABLE 35-2**

| Factors to Assess | Questions and Approaches | Physical Assessment Strategies |
|---|---|---|
| Adequacy of the patient's sensory perception | Ask patient to respond to verbal commands; observe whether patient follows commands. Determine whether patient responds verbally, by moaning, or not at all. | Observe whether patient responds to verbal commands (no impairment). Apply painful stimuli to various body locations or reposition a bed-bound patient. If patient is unable to respond except by moaning, the patient has limited sensory perception. |
| Moisture | Observe patient's bed linens on a routine basis to assess for the presence of moisture. | Observe patient's skin, noting if it is dry (rarely moist) or seldom damp (occasionally moist) or if skin is often but not always wet (moist). Observe for wound drainage. |
| Activity | Determine patient's ability to use toileting facilities when needed. | Check whether the patient is incontinent of urine and stool; if almost constantly moist by fecal or urinary incontinence, this patient is constantly moist. |
| | Ask patient/family about the patient's level of physical activity. | Assess patient's ability to walk at least once every 2 hours while awake (walks frequently), or whether patient is only able to ambulate short distance (walks occasionally). Observe if patient is able to independently change positions in bed. |
| Nutrition | Ask patient and family about level of appetite and ability to eat a complete meal. | Observe patient eating: determine if patient takes most of the meal and if intake is balanced (excellent nutrition). Assess the amount of food the patient eats at meals for adequate nutrition, such as if patient finishes over half of meals, or whether patient is on tube feedings or TPN. Observe whether patient is eating less than one third of meal, taking fluids poorly, or NPO or on clear liquids for >3 days. Does the patient need assistance with feeding? |
| Friction and shear | Place patient in bed with head of bed in semi-Fowler's position; watch for sliding toward the foot of the bed. Ask patient if he or she needs assistance in moving up in bed or chair. | Assess if patient moves in bed and chair independently and if patient maintains a good position at all times (no apparent problem). Observe patient in bed and in a chair; if patient moves feebly or requires minimum assistance, this indicates a potential problem. Determine if patient requires moderate to maximum assistance in moving, and if the patient slides down in the bed and/or chair, which indicates a problem. |

*TPN,* Total parenteral nutrition; *NPO,* nothing by mouth.

---

**BOX 35-5**   CARE OF THE OLDER ADULT

- The older adult's skin is less tolerant to pressure, friction, and shear because of decreased elasticity from normal aging.
- The older adult's skin loses the ability to retain moisture within the dermis, resulting in less pliable tissue vulnerable to minor trauma.
- With aging the capacity for epidermal proliferation is decreased, so healing requires more time.
- The major change in aging skin is dryness, which affects as many as 59% to 85% of patients over the age of 64.

- The thinning of the dermis and flattening of the dermal-epidermal junction that occur in aging predispose the older adult's skin to tearing.
- Risk factors for skin tears include sensory loss, impaired nutritional status, impaired cognition, dependency on staff for activities of daily living, and the need for mechanical devices (e.g., lifts, wheelchairs).

Data from Bryant RA, Rolstad BS: Examining threats to skin integrity, *Ostomy Wound Management* 47(6):18, 2001.

| SKILL 35-1 | Assessment of Patient for Pressure Ulcer: Risk and Skin Assessment |

## Delegation Considerations

Assessment of adults for risk of pressure ulcers is the responsibility of the nurse. The nurse should instruct assistive personnel to report to the nurse:

- Any redness or break in the patient's skin
- Any abrasion from assistive devices
- Changes in patient's frequency of incontinence

## Equipment

- Risk assessment tool (e.g., Braden Scale)
- Skin assessment tool
- Documentation record
- Gloves

| STEP | RATIONALE |
|---|---|

## ASSESSMENT

1. Perform hand hygiene. Close door or bedside curatins.

2. Identify patient's risk for pressure ulcer formation using the Braden Scale; assign a score for each of the 6 subscales (see Table 35-1).

3. Obtain the risk score, and evaluate based upon patient's overall condition.

4. Conduct a systematic skin assessment of bony prominences. Wear examination gloves because you will be pressing on reddened areas and draining wound may be present. Look for areas of skin breakdown in the following locations (Figure 35-6):

   a. Inspect at-risk areas: back of head, shoulders, ribs, hips, sacral region, ischium, inner and outer knees, inner and outer ankles, heels, and feet.

Reduces transmission of microorganisms. Maintains patient privacy.

Identifies patients at risk for developing pressure ulcers, allowing you to initiate individualized preventive interventions (Ayello and Braden, 2002).

The score will predict the need for interventions to prevent skin breakdown (see Table 35-1).

Bony prominences are at high risk of skin breakdown because of high pressures exerted on these areas when patient is immobile. A finding of redness or impairment in skin integrity necessitates planning appropriate interventions.

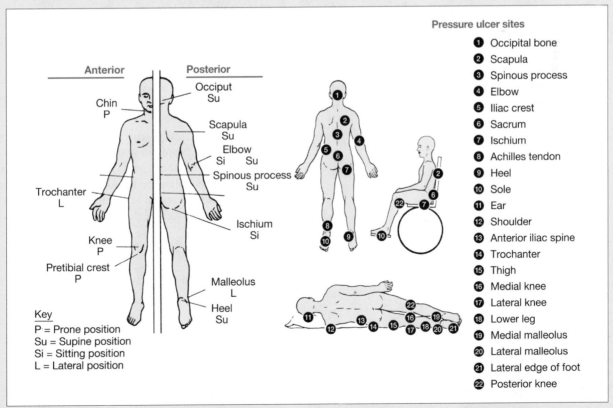

FIGURE 35-6 **A,** Bony prominences most frequently underlying pressure ulcers. **B,** Pressure ulcer sites. (From Trelease CC: Developing standards for wound care, *Ostomy Wound Manage* 20:46, 1988.)

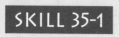

| SKILL 35-1 | Assessment of Patient for Pressure Ulcer: Risk and Skin Assessment—cont'd |
| --- | --- |

| STEP | RATIONALE |
| --- | --- |
| **5.** Assess the following potential areas of skin breakdown: | |
| a. Ears and nares | Cartilage that nasal cannulas or tubing compresses will develop pressure necrosis. |
| b. Lips | Oral airway and endotracheal tubes exert pressure if left in place for prolonged time periods. |
| c. Tube sites (e.g., gastrostomy or nasogastric tubes, Foley catheters, Jackson-Pratt drains) | Tubes exert pressure if taped snugly against skin or if there is stress at the insertion site. If moisture is present around tube insertion sites, leakage of bodily fluids will compromise skin integrity. |
| d. Orthopedic and positioning devices (e.g., casts, braces, cervical collar) | Improperly fitted or applied devices have the potential to cause pressure on adjacent skin and underlying tissue. |
| **6.** Assess all skin surfaces for the following: | |
| a. Absence of superficial skin layers | Damage of superficial skin layers is indicative of injury from friction or moisture. The area will be moist and sore to the touch. |
| b. Blisters | Suggests skin damage from friction and/or inappropriate tape removal. Blisters occur when the top layer of skin is pulled or rubbed, separating the epidermis from the dermis. |
| c. Any loss of epidermis and dermis | Indicates damage to skin. Determine the cause of this damage, and begin interventions to prevent further damage. |

## IMPLEMENTATION

| | |
| --- | --- |
| **1.** If any of the risk factors receive low scores on the risk assessment tool, consider one or more of the interventions listed in Box 35-4. | The identified risk factors can be eliminated or reduced by instituting appropriate interventions. |
| **2.** Assist patient when changing positions during the assessment. | Different positions (e.g., prone, supine, side-lying) are used when completing skin assessment. |
| **3.** When you note a reddened area, check for the following: | |
| a. Skin discoloration (e.g., redness in light-tone skin; purplish or bluish in darkly pigmented skin) (see Box 35-3) | May indicate that tissue was under pressure. |
| b. Blanchable erythema | Indicates pressure damage that will resolve. If the redness lightens under the application of pressure, make sure the vessels are intact and that there is no tissue damage present. |
| c. Nonblanchable erythema | Indicates potential damage to blood vessels and tissue damage. Once the blood vessels are damaged, the red area will not lighten in color because the tissue and blood vessels are inflamed. |
| d. Pallor or mottling | Persistent hypoxia in tissues alters circulation, and pallor or mottling may occur. |
| **4.** Remove gloves, perform hand hygiene, and reposition patient. | Reduces transmission of microorganisms. |

## EVALUATION

| | |
| --- | --- |
| **1.** Evaluate patient's skin regularly, especially those areas at high risk for breakdown. | Helps you determine success of prevention measures. |
| **2.** Compare current risk score with previous scores. | Allows you to provide individualized plan of care. |

## RECORDING AND REPORTING

- Record risk score and frequency of risk assessment.
- Record appearance of skin, especially pressure points.
- Describe positioning and turning schedule.
- Describe preventative skin interventions.
- Report changes in skin care protocol.
- Document consultation from skin/wound care specialists.

- Pressure areas become discolored or indurated or exhibit temperature changes.
  - Consult nurse specialist to revise skin care regimen for patient.
  - Consider supportive mattresses.

## UNEXPECTED OUTCOMES AND RELATED INTERVENTIONS

- Skin becomes mottled, reddened, or blistered.
  - Document and communicate interval for reevaluation of skin assessment.
  - Obtain physician's or health care provider's order for skin care or pressure reduction or relieving mattresses.

---

**BOX 35-6** **Nutritional Assessment and Management of Pressure Ulcers: WOCN 2003 Guideline Recommendations**

Perform nutritional assessment on entry to a new health care setting and whenever there is a change in an individual's condition that will increase the risk of malnutrition (see Chapter 31, Skill 31-1). Include the following parameters in the assessment:

a. Current and usual weight
b. History of involuntary weight loss or gain
c. Nutritional intake versus needs, incorporating protein, calorie, and fluid needs
d. Appetite
e. Dental health
f. Medical/surgical history or interventions that influence nutritional intake or absorption of nutrients.

g. Drug/nutrient interaction
  Assess laboratory parameters for nutritional status:
a. Standard measurements of protein status include albumin, transferrin, and prealbumin
b. Nutritional assessments, including protein markers, should be repeated to measure effectiveness of any interventions
c. Risk for malnutrition include:
  1. Age: <18 years or >64 years
  2. Weight: 5-10% loss in 1-6 months
  3. Albumin: <2.1 mg/dl (severe risk)
  4. Transferrin: <100 mg/dl (severe risk)
  5. Prealbumin: <7 mg/dl (severe risk)

---

you to be thorough in this assessment and accurately collect relevant data. Accurate and regular assessments of the patient's wounds drive treatment decisions and provide a baseline to evaluate the wounds' status (WOCN, 2003).

**Emergency Setting.** In an emergency the type of wound determines the criteria for inspection. After you stabilize a patient's cardiopulmonary status (see Chapter 28), inspect the wound for bleeding. An **abrasion,** or loss of the dermis, is usually superficial with little bleeding but some weeping (plasma leakage from damaged capillaries). A **laceration** is damage to the dermis and epidermis and is a torn, jagged wound. The depth and location of the laceration affect the extent of bleeding, with serious bleeding possible in lacerations greater than 5 cm (2 inches) long or 2.5 cm (1 inch) deep.

Puncture wounds bleed in relation to the depth and size of the wound; internal bleeding and infection are the primary dangers. Inspect the wound for contaminant material such as soil, broken glass, shreds of cloth, and foreign substances clinging to penetrating objects. Next, assess the size of the wound and the need for suturing or surface protection. When the injury is the result of trauma from a dirty penetrating object, determine if the patient has received a tetanus toxoid injection within the last year.

**Stable Setting.** Once an acute wound is stable after surgery or treatment, assess its progress toward healing. If a dressing covers the wound and there are written orders not to change it, inspect only the dressing and any external drains. If a dressing appears saturated with drainage, reinforce the secondary dressing pending a definitive response and orders from the physician or health care provider. Saturated dressings provide an excellent environment for bacterial growth, and you will need to inform the physician or health care provider of the color, odor, and estimate of drainage amount.

When you plan a dressing change, give the patient an analgesic at least 30 minutes before exposing a wound. Avoid accidentally removing or displacing underlying drains.

First, inspect the appearance of the wound, noting the anatomical location, size, approximation of wound edges, the presence of exudate, the condition of underlying tissue in an open wound, and signs of dehiscence, evisceration, or infection. Measure the length, diameter, or depth of wound using a centimeter measuring guide. Note any **ecchymosis,** skin discoloration or bruising caused by blood leakage into subcutaneous tissues after trauma to underlying vessels. The outer edges of a wound normally appear inflamed for the first 2 to 3 days, but this slowly disappears. When an infection develops, the wound edges are usually brightly inflamed, warm, tender, and swollen.

Next, assess the character of wound drainage by noting the amount, color, odor, and consistency. The amount of drainage depends on the location and extent of the wound. A simple method for estimating the volume of wound drainage is to report the number and type of dressings used and saturated over an interval of time. The color and consistency of drainage vary, depending on its components. Types of drainage include the following:

1. Serous: clear, watery plasma
2. Sanguineous: fresh bleeding
3. Serosanguineous: pale, more watery, a combination of plasma and red cells, may be blood-streaked
4. Purulent: thick, yellow, green, or brown, indicating the presence of dead or living organisms and white blood cells

If the drainage has a pungent or strong odor, an infection is likely. Objectively document the integrity of the wound and the character of drainage, describing the appearance by observable characteristics.

The presence of drains is another important assessment. A drain is used in a surgical wound if the health care provider expects a large amount of drainage and if keeping wound layers closed is especially important, because accumulated fluid under the tissues prevents closure. Drains lie under a dressing, extend through a dressing, or are connected to a drainage bag or suction apparatus. A pin or clip through a Penrose drain prevents it from slipping farther into a wound (Figure 35-7). As wound drainage decreases, the physician or health care provider slowly withdraws the drain or leaves orders for you to withdraw the drain a specified length over several days. First, observe the security of the drain and its location with respect to the wound. Next, note the character and amount of drainage if there is a collecting device. You need to pay particular attention to the flow of drainage through the tubing and notify the physician or health care provider of any sudden decrease that indicates a blocked drain or an increase indicating bleeding or infection.

In the case of a surgical wound, inspect the staples, sutures, or wound closures for irritation and note whether the closures are intact. You may choose to count sutures when the physician or health care provider has removed a portion of them. After the first few days when normal swelling

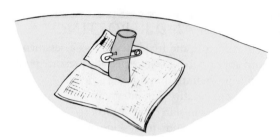

FIGURE **35-7** Penrose drain.

around closures usually has subsided, continued swelling sometimes indicates overly tight closures, which will cause wound separation or dehiscence. Early suture removal reduces formation of defects along the suture line and minimizes chances of unattractive scar formation.

When a wound exhibits swelling, separation of its edges, or redness in the periwound area, it is important to evaluate for the presence of cellulitis. Use light palpation to detect localized areas of tenderness or collection of drainage. Wearing sterile gloves, gently place your fingertips along the wound edges. If pressure causes fluid to be expressed from the wound, note the character of the drainage and collect a wound culture if needed. Sensitivity to such palpation is normal, but extreme tenderness indicates infection.

Pain assessment is an important component of wound assessment for detecting complications and planning for future wound care (see Chapter 30). Serious discomfort during inspection or palpation of the wound suggests underlying problems, whereas discomfort related to dressing removal or application calls for administration of analgesics before future dressing changes.

**Wound Cultures.** If you detect purulent (pus) or suspicious-looking drainage, this indicates a **wound culture.** Never collect a wound culture sample from old drainage, because resident colonies of bacteria grow in exudate. First clean the wound to remove skin flora. Aerobic organisms grow in superficial wounds exposed to the air, and anaerobic organisms tend to grow within body cavities. To collect an aerobic specimen, wipe a sterile swab from a culturette tube onto clean, healthy-looking tissue, return the swab to the culturette tube, cap the tube, and crush the inner ampule so that the medium for organism growth coats the swab tip (Stotts, 2000). Label the specimen appropriately, and send the labeled specimen to the laboratory immediately.

To collect an anaerobic specimen deep in a body cavity, use a sterile syringe tip to aspirate visible drainage from the inner wound, expel any air from the syringe, and inject contents into a special vacuum container with culture medium. In some institutions you place a cork over the needle to prevent entrance of air and send the syringe to the lab. Box 35-7 defines the procedure for a needle aspiration technique and the quantitative swab technique.

**PATIENT EXPECTATIONS.** When your patient has a pressure ulcer or a chronic wound, the course of treatment is usually costly and lengthy. Because your patient needs to be

## BOX 35-7 Recommendations for Standardized Techniques for Wound Cultures

### Needle Aspiration Procedure (Anaerobic Culture)

- Use a sterile 10-ml syringe with a 22-gauge needle.
- Aspirate 5 ml of air into the syringe.
- Clean intact skin with a disinfectant. Allow to dry.
- Insert needle into interior of the wound.
- Aspirate wound drainage, moving needle back and forth in two to four areas of the wound.
- Withdraw needle from wound; expel any remaining air from syringe.

### Quantitative Swab Procedure (Aerobic Culture)

- Obtain a sterile swab, sterile normal saline, and antiseptic solution.
- Clean wound surface with an antiseptic solution, and allow to dry.
- Moisten swab with normal saline.
- Swab wound in a $1 \times 1$ cm ($4$ cm$^2$) area of clean tissue.
- Apply pressure to express fluid from wound onto the sterile swab.

Modified from Stotts NS: Wound infection: diagnosis and management. In Bryant RA, editor: *Acute and chronic wounds: nursing management*, ed 2, St. Louis, 2000, Mosby.

## SYNTHESIS IN PRACTICE

When Lynda returns the next day, she finds that Mr. Ahmed has a stage II $1 \times 2$ inch ($2.5 \times 5$ cm) $\times \frac{1}{8}$ inch deep shallow wound on his sacrum. There is no necrotic tissue, and the wound bed has red moist tissue. When Lynda prepares to conduct a skin assessment on Mr. Ahmed, she recalls information about the pathogenesis of pressure ulcers and guidelines for skin assessment for patients with darkly pigmented skin. She will focus on determining changes in Mr. Ahmed's skin integrity.

Lynda observed care of a stage IV pressure ulcer during an experience in an extended care facility. From that experience she increased her knowledge about the debilitating effects of pressure ulcers. In addition, she was able to practice skin assessment techniques during her clinical experience in the extended care facility.

involved with the wound care management, it is important to know the patient's expectations. A patient who unrealistically expects rapid wound healing will be easily discouraged and not follow the treatment plan. Likewise, a patient who knows that the process is lengthy may unrealistically expect the area to heal without scarring. Knowing these expectations assists you in providing individualized care and helping the patient modify expectations when needed.

### 🔅 Nursing Diagnosis

A patient with actual or high risk for *impaired skin integrity* usually has one or more nursing diagnoses related to the condition. Assessment reveals clusters of data that indicate whether an actual or a risk for *impaired skin integrity* exists. After gathering appropriate assessment data, cluster defining characteristics to establish nursing diagnoses. For example, the destruction of the skin's surface clearly allows you to diagnose *impaired skin integrity*. The identification of nursing diagnoses related to wound healing helps you to anticipate the need for supportive or preventive care. There are many nursing diagnoses that are relevant to your patient who requires wound care:

- Risk for infection
- Impaired physical mobility
- Impaired bed mobility
- Imbalanced nutrition: less than body requirements
- Acute pain
- Chronic pain
- Situational low self-esteem

- Impaired skin integrity
- Risk for impaired skin integrity
- Ineffective tissue perfusion

Assess for related factors that contribute to each diagnostic statement. These related factors become the focus of your interventions. For example, the patient with *impaired skin integrity related to a surgical incision* requires a different set of interventions than the patient with *impaired skin integrity related to pressure and nutritional deficiency*. The patient whose surgical incision has increased drainage will require different and perhaps more frequent skin cleansing and dressings chosen to contain additional drainage.

### 🔅 Planning

Plan therapeutic interventions for your patients with actual or potential risks to skin integrity (see care plan). These therapies are designed according to severity of risks to the patient. Individualize the plan according to the patient's developmental stage and level of health.

**GOALS AND OUTCOMES.** You need to develop patient-centered goals aimed at preventing or reducing impaired skin integrity or promoting wound healing. Individualize care planning for the patient, taking into consideration the patient's most immediate needs. Assess all patients for risk of skin breakdown, and have skin and wound assessments performed on a routine basis. Integrate the information from the pressure ulcer risk and skin assessments into the plan of care, and write reasonable goals, such as "Patient will not develop further skin breakdown" and "Patient's wounds will demonstrate healing." Include the patient and the family in the assessment process so they will begin to see their contribution to reducing risk factors.

**SETTING PRIORITIES.** When planning care, establish priorities based on your comprehensive assessment, goals, and expected outcomes. Acute needs are immediate; however, also prioritize preventive interventions and institute them in a timely manner. Maintenance of skin integrity and promotion of wound healing prevent additional health care

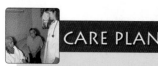

## CARE PLAN   Skin Integrity and Wound Care

### ASSESSMENT

Mr. Ahmed has **limited activity tolerance**. He **does not tolerate position changes or sitting out of bed**; he **wants to stay in a semi-Fowler's position** at all times. He complains of a **painful, burning sensation** in his sacral region. A 1 × 2 inch **open area** with a depth of ⅛ inch is present. The base of the **wound is red and moist**, and the **surrounding tissue is slightly reddened**. On palpation, **underlying skin is soft and indurated**.

*Defining characteristics are shown in bold type.

### NURSING DIAGNOSIS   Impaired skin integrity related to pressure over bony prominence in sacral region.

### PLANNING

| GOAL | EXPECTED OUTCOMES* |
|---|---|
| | *Tissue Integrity: Skin, Mucous Membranes* |
| • Pressure will be reduced to the sacral area, and the wound will show significant healing in 1 week. | • Wound will decrease in diameter in 7 days. |
| | • There will be no evidence of further wound formation in 3 days. |

*Outcomes classification label from Moorhead S, Johnson M, Maas M: *Nursing outcomes classification (NOC)*, ed 3, St. Louis, 2004, Mosby.

| INTERVENTIONS† | RATIONALE |
|---|---|
| **Pressure Management** | |
| • Post and implement a turning schedule. | Repositioning removes pressure. |
| • Obtain and place over the patient's mattress a static air overlay. | Reduces the amount of pressure on the bony prominences. |
| **Wound Care** | |
| • Cleanse wound and periwound skin; dry periwound skin. | Removes debris and old drainage from wound site, preventing further wound progression and/or skin breakdown (Ayello and others, 2004). |
| • Measure wound diameter and depth, assess the quality of the wound tissue, noting the condition of the periwound skin, and determine the presence of wound exudate at dressing change. | Cleansing of wounds is necessary at every wound dressing change. Wound assessment will provide a basis for determining effectiveness of wound treatment interventions (WOCN, 2003). |
| • Apply a hydrocolloid dressing to wound, as per order; extend the dressing 1½ inches beyond the wound edges. | The use of hydrocolloid dressing will support moist wound healing and protect the wound. |

†Intervention classification labels from Dochterman JM, Bulechek GM, editors: *Nursing interventions classification (NIC)*, ed 4, St. Louis, 2004, Mosby.

### EVALUATION

| | |
|---|---|
| • Compare wound assessment to determine progress (e.g., measure wound size; observe the appearance of the wound tissue at each dressing change). | • Observe all bony prominences when repositioning patient. |

---

issues. Skin and wound priorities include ongoing assessment of pressure ulcer risk and wound status, and providing interventions to control or eliminate contributing factors of pressure, shear, friction, moisture, and infection.

Consider other patient factors when setting priorities, including everyday activities and family factors. Sometimes you will need the help of another health care team member, such as a physical or occupational therapist, when considering mobility needs. These factors are important for patients in institutional and home settings.

**CONTINUITY OF CARE.** With the trend toward earlier discharge from health care settings, it is important to consider the patient's plan for discharge. Discharge planning begins when a patient enters the health care system. Anticipating the patient's discharge from an institution, a referral to a skilled nursing care facility or home care agency is necessary to help the patient remain mobile or regain mobility at home.

Patients and their families need to continue the objectives of wound management after discharge. Thus they will need to discuss the likelihood of the patient's returning home, returning home with the assistance of home nursing, or transferring to a skilled nursing facility for more care and observation.

### Implementation

**HEALTH PROMOTION.** Early identification of high-risk patients and their risk factors aids you in preventing pressure ulcers. Prevention minimizes the impact that risk factors or contributing factors will have on pressure ulcer development (see Box 35-4). Three major areas of nursing interventions for prevention of pressure ulcers are topical skin care, positioning and use of the 30-degree lateral position, and the use of support surfaces.

**Topical Skin Care.** Perform skin assessment daily, paying special attention to the bony prominences. Do not massage

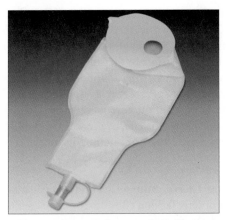

FIGURE **35-8** Hollister® Fecal Incontinence Collector. (Permission to use this copyrighted material has been granted by the owner, Hollister Incorporated.)

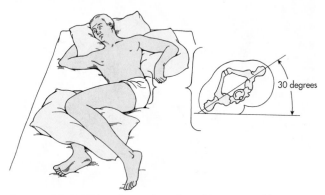

FIGURE **35-9** Thirty-degree lateral position to avoid pressure points. (From Pieper B: Mechanical forces: pressure, shear, friction. In Bryant RA, editor: *Acute and chronic wounds: nursing management,* ed 2, St. Louis, 2000, Mosby.)

reddened areas because reddened areas indicate tissue injury (Ayello and others, 2004). Massage to these areas further injures the tissue by causing breaks in the tissue capillaries. Examine skin for signs of dryness, cracking, edema, or excessive moisture. When you are cleansing the skin, use a mild cleansing agent. Soaps alter the skin's acid mantle, causing dryness and increasing the risk of skin infection. Skin lubrication will help keep the skin intact; consider using a moisturizer on a routine basis (WOCN, 2003). Keep the patient's skin clean and dry because this is an initial line of defense for preventing skin breakdown. The types of products available for skin care are numerous, and you need to match their uses to the specific needs of the patient.

For a patient who is incontinent of stool or urine, use a specialized incontinence cleanser. To protect the skin you apply a moisture-barrier product (generally petrolatum or dimethicone based) liberally to the exposed area. The moisture barrier will provide skin protection from the irritating effects of stool or urine and will allow you to clean the next incontinent episode easily. Apply the moisture barrier ointment after each cleansing. For skin that has become denuded or stripped from incontinence, use a barrier paste (zinc oxide based) that will stick to the irritated area and not be removed with each cleansing. You contain fecal incontinence using a fecal incontinence collector (Figure 35-8), an adhesive skin barrier attached to a drainable pouch applied around the anus to collect liquid stool. A fecal incontinence collector is used when the patient is experiencing frequent liquid bowel movements and has intact perirectal skin. Other external collection devices include male external catheters applied to the shaft of the penis to collect urine. Underpads and briefs are used to protect skin in patients incontinent of stool and urine. Most underpads and briefs have a plastic outer lining that holds moisture against skin. Diapers and underpads will irritate the skin if left under patients for prolonged periods of time. Select underpads, diapers, or briefs that are absorbent to wick incontinence moisture away from the skin versus trapping the moisture against the skin, which causes maceration (WOCN, 2003). When providing skin care to the incontinent patient, the health care team first assesses and treats the cause of the incontinence, then decides upon protection and/or collection interventions.

**Positioning.** Positioning interventions reduce pressure and shear to the skin. You change the immobilized patient's position according to activity level, perceptual ability, and daily routines (Bergstrom and others, 1987a, 1987b). Therefore a standard turning interval of 1 to 2 hours will not prevent pressure sore development in some patients. The WOCN (2003) recommends reducing shear by keeping the patient's head of bed below the 30-degree angle, using assistive devices when turning or transferring patients, using the bed gatch or footboard, and using the 30-degree lateral position (Figure 35-9).

When the patient is able to sit in the chair, reposition the patient every hour. In the sitting position, the pressure on the ischial tuberosities is greater than when in the supine position. In addition, assist or teach patients with the ability to shift weight every 15 minutes. Also, have the patient sit on gel or an air cushion to redistribute weight, decreasing the amount of weight on the ischial tuberosities.

The patient's heels are an area of concern because of the small surface area (Figure 35-10). Keep heels off the bed with a pillow under the lower leg or by the use of a heal protector (Ayello and others, 2004).

**Support Surfaces.** Support surfaces decrease the amount of pressure exerted over bony prominences by maximizing contact (allowing the body to touch the entire surface) and thereby redistributing weight over a large area. Support surfaces include mattresses, overlays, framed specialty beds, chair pads, table pads, and crib mattresses or pads (Table 35-3) In addition to reducing or relieving pressure, many of the support surfaces reduce shear and friction and decrease moisture.

Select an appropriate support surface based on your assessment findings (Box 35-8). A flow diagram (Figure 35-11)

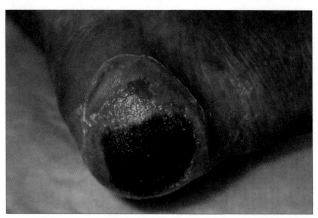

FIGURE **35-10** Formation of pressure ulcer on heel resulting from external pressure from mattress of bed. (Courtesy Janice Colwell, RN, MS, CWOCN, Clinical Nurse Specialist, University of Chicago Hospitals.)

will assist you in clinical decision making. When using a support surface, make sure there are minimal layers of bed linens between the patient and the surface. Position the patient as close as possible to the surface for it to be effective. Remember, even when using a support surface, you still need to reposition the patient. Once a support surface is in use, reevaluate the patient on a frequent basis to determine the continued need and the effectiveness of the product. Patient and caregiver education on the importance and use of the support product is essential (Box 35-9).

### ACUTE CARE

**Pressure Ulcers.** Address wound management principles in an orderly fashion (Box 35-10). Manage the etiology, pressure, shear, friction, and/or moisture as part of wound management (Skill 35-2).

| **TABLE 35-3** | **Support Surfaces** | | |
|---|---|---|---|
| Categories | Mechanism of Action | Indications | Examples of Manufacturers/ Product Names |
| **Low-Air-Loss System** | | | |
| Available in a full bed or as an overlay | Pressure relief device Bed: The entire surface is a powered, inflated surface with air loss Overlay: Powered surface, constant inflation and air loss at the surface; place over the bed mattress | Prevention of skin breakdown in patients who cannot be turned or have existing skin breakdown | Hill Rom/Flexicair Kinetic Concepts, Inc/First Step Select Crown Therapeutics/ Select Air Mattress |
| **Foam** | | | |
| Available as an overlay or in a full mattress | Reduces pressure and the cover (top) can reduce friction and shear Overlay: Placed on top of bed mattress Full mattress: Used in place of the usual mattress | Pressure reduction for high-risk patients | Bio Clinic/Bio Guard BG Industries/MaxiFloat |
| **Static Air-Filled Overlays** | | | |
| Available as an overlay | Interconnected air-filled cells, inflated to appropriate level Pressure relief or pressure reduction (depends on product) | High-risk patients | Crown Therapeutics/RoHo mattress Gaymar Industries/ Sof-Care |
| **Air-Fluidized Beds** | | | |
| Available as a bed | Bed frame with silicone-coated beads that become fluidized when air is pumped through the beads Pressure relief, anti-shear, anti-friction surface | For patients with burns or multiple stage III or stage IV pressure ulcers, protection of new grafts and flaps | Kinetic Concepts, Inc/FluidAir |
| **Kinetic Therapy** | | | |
| Available as a bed | Provides continuous passive motion, to promote mobilization of respiratory secretions; also provides low-air-loss therapy | Patients who are at risk for or have developed atelectasis and/or pneumonia | Hill Rom/Clinitron Hill Rom/Total Care Sport Kinetic Concepts, Inc/ TriaDyne |

| BOX 35-8 | **WOCN 2003 Pressure Reduction/Relief Recommendations** |
| --- | --- |

- Place at-risk individuals on a pressure reduction/relief surface and not on an ordinary hospital mattress.
- Pressure reducing or relief devices work by redistributing pressure over the bony prominences (see Table 35-3).
- Avoid using foam rings, donuts, and sheepskin for pressure reduction. Foam rings or donuts concentrate the pressure to the surrounding tissue.

- Use pressure relief devices in the operating room for individuals assessed to be at high risk for pressure ulcer development.
- Refer to professional health care specialists to select appropriate pressure reduction/relief devices for chairs, wheelchairs, and beds.

Data from Wound, Ostomy and Continence Nurses Society: *Guideline for prevention and management of pressure ulcers,* WOCN Clinical Practice Guidelines Series, Glenview, Ill, 2003, The Society.

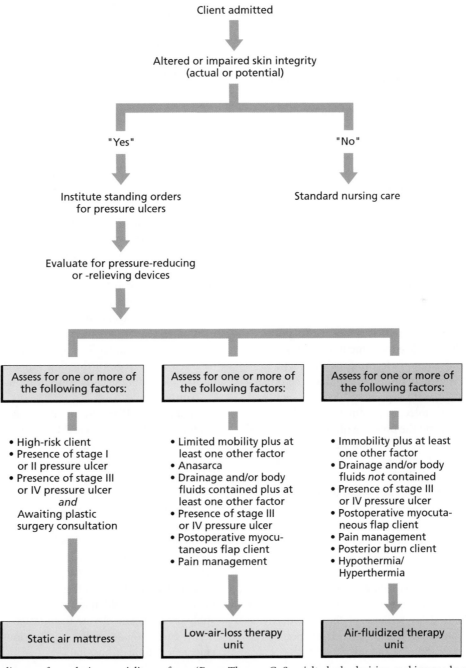

FIGURE **35-11** Flow diagram for ordering speciality surfaces. (From Thomas C: Specialty beds: decision making made easy, *Ostomy Wound Manage* 23:51, 1989.)

| BOX 35-9 | **Guidelines for Patient Education Regarding Therapeutic Surfaces** |
|---|---|

- Explain the rationale for utilization of support surfaces. Be sure the patient and family know that this will reduce pressure on the bony prominences by redistributing the pressure between the surface and the patient's skin.
- Teach patient and family the importance of minimal layers of linen or absorbent pads between patient and surface.
- Instruct in the importance of frequent position changes, demonstrating small shifts of weight.
- Demonstrate to patient and caregiver the procedure for lateral positioning at a 30-degree angle and the use of pillows to support various positions.

| BOX 35-10 | **Wound Healing Principles** |
|---|---|

1. Control or eliminate causative factors
   a. Pressure
   b. Shear
   c. Friction
   d. Moisture
2. Provide systemic support to reduce existing and potential cofactors
   a. Nutritional and fluid support
   b. Control of systemic conditions affecting wound healing
3. Maintain physiological wound environment
   a. Prevent and manage infection
   b. Cleanse wound
   c. Remove nonviable tissue (debridement)
   d. Manage exudates
   e. Eliminate dead space
   f. Control odor
   g. Protect wound
   h. Provide a moist environment

From Bryant RA and others: Pressure ulcer. In Bryant RA, editor: *Acute and chronic wounds: nursing management,* ed 2, St. Louis, 2000, Mosby.

The patient must receive systemic support to achieve wound healing. Concurrent cardiovascular or pulmonary disease decreases the amount of oxygen-rich hemoglobin available to be delivered to injured tissue. Oxygen is an essential element in angiogenesis, epithelialization, and resistance to infection. Interventions to maximize oxygen levels include use of pulmonary hygiene interventions, assessment and monitoring of tissue oxygen levels, and low-flow supplemental oxygen.

Wound healing depends on adequate nutrition. Protein intake is necessary to support new blood vessels and collagen synthesis. Carbohydrates, fats, and vitamins provide energy for cellular function. Interventions to support adequate nutritional intake are a nutritional referral, dietary supplements, and assessment of intake and output levels.

Certain medications (e.g., steroids) and medical conditions (e.g., diabetes) influence wound healing. Because hyperglycemia causes problems with wound healing, blood glucose control is essential.

A stable wound environment is necessary to promote healing. To maintain a stable environment it is important to control infection and promote cleansing, debridement, exudate management, control of dead space, and wound protection. Assess the patient with a pressure ulcer for signs and symptoms of a wound infection: redness, warmth of surrounding tissue, odor, and the presence of exudate. If any of these signs are present, consult with the health care team to determine if you should culture the wound and if systemic or topical antibiotics are indicated.

Cleanse pressure ulcers at each dressing change to promote removal of wound debris and bacteria from the wound surface (WOCN, 2003). Cleanse dirty wounds with irrigation; clean wounds require only gentle flushing with normal saline solution.

Necrotic tissue slows wound healing because it becomes a source for infection and a barrier for epithelialization (Schultz and others, 2003). If consistent with the patient's overall plan of care, plan a method for removal of the necrotic tissue (**debridement**). Types of debridement include mechanical, chemical, and autolytic (Singhal and others, 2001).

A moist wound environment supports wound healing; however, excessive wound moisture will macerate the wound edges and interfere with wound healing. Select a dressing that absorbs excessive moisture while providing the wound with the necessary hydration. Eliminate dead space by loosely filling all cavities with dressings. You need to fill wound cavities to support the growth of granulation tissue and to discourage infection.

It is important to involve the patient's family or other caregiver in management of pressure ulcers and their treatment. Frequently patients are discharged home and still require dressing changes. The patient's family or caregiver can be excellent sources for dressing support and identification of possible wound healing complications (Box 35-11).

**Wounds**

*First Aid for Wounds.* In an emergency setting use first aid measures for wound care. Under more stable conditions you are able to use a variety of interventions for wound healing. When a patient suffers a traumatic wound, first aid interventions include promoting hemostasis, cleansing the wound, and protecting the wound from further injury.

*HEMOSTASIS.* After assessing the type and extent of the wound, control bleeding from a laceration with application of direct pressure to the wound with a sterile or clean dressing. After bleeding subsides, an adhesive bandage strip or gauze dressing taped over the laceration allows skin edges to close and a blood clot to form. If a dressing becomes saturated with blood, add another layer of dressing, continue to apply pressure, and elevate the affected part. A physician or health care provider will suture serious lacerations in an emergency clinic or hospital.

*Text continued on p. 1041*

## SKILL 35-2 | Treating Pressure Ulcers

### Delegation Considerations

This skill is the responsibility of the nurse. Instruct the assistive personnel to:

- Report any wound drainage found on linens or intact skin that indicate the need to change the dressings or to use an alternative dressing.

### Equipment

- Disposable gloves (clean)
- Goggles and cover gown (*optional*)
- Plastic bag for dressing disposal
- Measuring device
- Cotton-tipped applicators
- Topical agent (as ordered)
- Cleansing agent (as ordered)
- Sterile solution container
- Washbasin, washcloths, towels
- Dressing of choice
- Hypoallergenic tape (if needed)
- Documentation records

| STEP | RATIONALE |
|---|---|

### ASSESSMENT

| STEP | RATIONALE |
|---|---|
| 1. Assess the patient's level of comfort and need for pain medication (Dallan, and others, 2004). Administer analgesic as needed. | The dressing change should not be a traumatic event for the patient; the majority of patients with pressure ulcers report pain at dressing change (Szor and Bourguignon, 1999). |
| 2. Determine if patient has allergies to topical agents. | Topical agents contain elements that may cause localized skin reactions. |
| 3. Review the order for topical agent or dressing. | Ensures that proper medication and treatment are administered to right patient. |

- *Critical Decision Point:* Determine if the order is consistent with established wound care guidelines and outcomes for the patient. If the order is not consistent with guidelines or varies from the identified outcome for the patient, review the order with the health care team.

| STEP | RATIONALE |
|---|---|
| 4. Assess each of the patient's pressure ulcer(s) and surrounding skin to determine ulcer characteristics, including the stage (see Figure 35-5). | Staging is a way of assessing a pressure ulcer, based on the depth of tissue destruction. |

- *Critical Decision Point:* To correctly stage a pressure ulcer, you need to be able to see the base of the wound. Therefore pressure ulcers that are covered with necrotic tissue cannot be staged until the eschar is debrided (NPUAP, 1989, 2000, 2003; WOCN, 2003). The nurse would document that the ulcer is unstagable.

| STEP | RATIONALE |
|---|---|
| 5. Assess the type of tissue in the wound bed. Color type indicates the type of tissue. Black tissue is necrotic tissue, yellow tissue is slough, and red tissue is granulation tissue. Chart the approximate amount of each tissue found in the wound bed. | The approximate percentage of each type of tissue in the wound provides critical information on the progress of wound healing and the choice of dressing. A wound with a high percentage of black tissue requires debridement, yellow tissue or slough tissue indicates the presence of an infection, and granulation tissue indicates a wound is beginning to heal. |
| 6. Assess need for revisions to therapy during each dressing change (WOCN, 2003). | Changes in the appearance of a wound can indicate that the topical therapy or type of dressing should be adjusted to continue to promote wound healing. |
| a. Note color, temperature, edema, moisture, and condition of skin around the ulcer. Modify the assessment technique based on the patient's individual skin color (see Box 35-3). | Skin condition at the ulcer edge may indicate progressive tissue damage. Maceration on the peri-wound skin may show the need to alter the choice of the wound dressing. |
| b. Measure the wound's length and width per agency protocol. | Consistency in how the wound is measured is important for determining wound progress. |

SKILL 35-2 | Treating Pressure Ulcers—cont'd

| STEP | RATIONALE |
|---|---|
| c. Measure the depth of the pressure ulcer using a sterile cotton-tipped applicator or other device that will allow measurement of wound depth. Place the applicator *gently* into the pressure ulcer until it touches the bottom. Mark the place on the applicator where it reaches the top of the wound, and then remove the applicator from the ulcer. Measure the distance from the tip of the applicator to the mark using a measuring tape or ruler to determine the depth of the pressure ulcer. | Depth measure is important for determining the amount of tissue loss. |
| d. Measure depth of undermining tissue. Use a cotton-tipped applicator, and gently probe under skin edges (see illustration). | Represents the loss of the underlying tissue and may indicate progressive tissue necrosis or ongoing injury from shearing. |
| 7. Remove gloves, discard appropriately, and perform hand hygiene. | Reduces transmission of microorganisms. Different wounds may be contaminated by different organisms. Failure to repeatedly perform hand hygiene can cause cross-wound contamination. |

## PLANNING

| | |
|---|---|
| 1. Explain procedure to patient and family. Individualize the teaching plan for older adult patients, taking into account the normal aging changes that affect learning. | Preparatory explanations relieve anxiety, correct any misconceptions about the ulcer and its treatment, and offer an opportunity for patient and family education. |
| 2. Prepare the following necessary equipment and supplies: | |
| a. Washbasin, warm water, soap, washcloth, and bath towel. | Used to bathe surrounding skin. |
| b. Normal saline or other wound-cleansing agent in sterile solution container. | Ulcer surface must be cleansed before the application of topical agents and a new dressing. |

• *Critical Decision Point:* Use only noncytotoxic agents to clean ulcers.

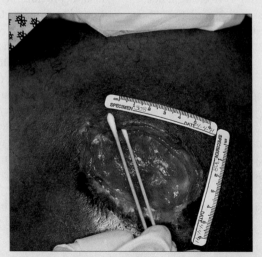

STEP **6b-d** Measuring length, width, and depth of pressure ulcer.

| STEP | RATIONALE |
|---|---|
| c. Prescribed topical agent (e.g., enzymatic agents, topical antibiotic). | Enzymes debride dead tissue to clean ulcer surface. Topical antibiotics are used to decrease the bioburden of the wound and should be considered for use if no healing is noted after 2 to 4 weeks of optimal care (AHCPR, 1994; WOCN, 2003). |

• *Critical Decision Point:* If using an enzymatic debriding agent, do not use wound-cleansing agents with metals.

| STEP | RATIONALE |
|---|---|
| d. Select an appropriate dressing and tape based on the pressure ulcer characteristics, purpose for which the dressing is intended, and patient care setting (see Table 35-5). | The dressing should maintain a moist environment for the wound while keeping the surrounding skin dry (AHCPR, 1994). |
| 3. Position patient to allow dressing removal, and position plastic bag for dressing disposal. | Area should be accessible for dressing change. Proper disposal of old dressing promotes proper handling of contaminated waste. |

## IMPLEMENTATION

| | |
|---|---|
| 1. Close room door or bedside curtains. Perform hand hygiene, and apply gloves. Open sterile packages and topical solution containers. (Goggles and moistureproof cover gown should be worn if potential for contamination from spray exists when cleansing the wound.) | Maintains patient privacy. Have supplies for easy application so that you can use supplies without contaminating them; reduces transmission of microorganisms. |
| 2. Remove bed linen and patient's gown to expose ulcer and surrounding skin. Keep remaining body parts draped. | Prevents unnecessary exposure of body parts. |
| 3. Gently wash skin surrounding ulcer with warm water and soap. | Cleansing of skin surface reduces bacteria. |
| 4. Rinse area thoroughly with water. | Soap can be irritating to skin. |
| 5. Gently dry skin thoroughly by patting lightly with towel. | Retained moisture causes maceration of skin layers. |
| 6. Perform hand hygiene, and change gloves. | Aseptic technique must be maintained during cleansing, measuring, and application of dressings. Refer to institutional policy regarding use of clean or sterile gloves. |
| 7. Cleanse ulcer thoroughly with normal saline or prescribed wound-cleansing agent. | Cleansing wound at each dressing change minimizes the trauma to the wound (WOCN, 2003). |
| 8. Use whirlpool treatments if needed to assist with wound debridement. Keep the wound directly away from the water jets. | Removes wound debris. Previously applied enzymes may require soaking for removal. Do not use whirlpool on clean granulating wounds. |
| 9. Apply topical agents, if prescribed. | |
| a. Enzymes: | Follow manufacturer's directions for frequency of application. Be aware of what solutions inactivate the enzymes, and avoid their use in wound cleaning. |
| (1) Using a wooden tongue blade, apply a small amount of enzyme debridement ointment directly to the necrotic areas on the base of pressure ulcer. Avoid getting the enzyme on the surrounding skin. The amount of enzyme should be the same as the amount of butter you would spread on bread. A thick layer of ointment is not necessary; a thin layer absorbs and acts more effectively. Do not apply enzyme to surrounding skin. | Proper distribution of ointment ensures effective action. Some enzymes can cause burning, paresthesia, and dermatitis to surrounding skin. |
| (2) Place gauze dressing directly over ulcer, and tape it in place. Follow specific manufacturer's recommendation for type of dressing material to use to cover a pressure ulcer when using enzymatic agent. | Protects wound and prevents removal of ointment during turning or repositioning. |

┌─────────────────────────────────────────────────
│ SKILL 35-2 ┆ Treating Pressure Ulcers—cont'd
└ ─ ─ ─ ─ ─ ─ ─ ─ ─ ─ ─ ─ ─ ─ ─ ─ ─ ─ ─ ─ ─ ─ ─

| STEP | RATIONALE |
|---|---|
| (3) If using an antibiotic solution, apply per order and cover with gauze pad. Generally, solution is applied every 12 hours. | |
| b. Hydrogel agents: | |
| (1) Cover surface of ulcer with hydrogel using applicator or gloved hand. | Provides a moist environment. |
| (2) Apply a secondary dressing, such as dry gauze, hydrocolloid, or transparent dressing over gel to completely cover ulcer. | Holds hydrogel against wound surface because hydrogel amphorous form (in tube) or sheet form does not adhere to the wound and requires a secondary dressing to hold it in place. |
| c. Calcium alginates: | Use in heavily draining wounds. |
| (1) Pack wound with alginate using applicator or gloved hand. | |
| (2) Apply a secondary dressing, such as dry gauze, foam, or hydrocolloid over alginate. | Holds alginate against wound surface. |
| 10. Reposition patient comfortably off pressure ulcer. | Avoids accidental removal of dressings. |
| 11. Remove gloves, and dispose of soiled supplies. Perform hand hygiene. | Reduces transmission of microorganisms. |

## EVALUATION

| | |
|---|---|
| 1. Observe skin surrounding ulcer for inflammation, edema, and tenderness. | A clean pressure ulcer should show evidence of healing within 2 to 4 weeks. |
| 2. Inspect dressings and exposed ulcers, observing for drainage, foul odor, and tissue necrosis. Monitor patient for signs and symptoms of infection, including fever and elevated white blood cell (WBC) count. | Ulcers can become infected. |
| 3. Compare subsequent ulcer measurements. | Allows comparison of serial measurements to assess wound healing. |
| 4. Use one of the scales designed to measure wound healing, such as the PUSH Scale (Thomas and others, 1997) or the PSST (Bates-Jensen, 1990). | Provides a standard method of data collection that will demonstrate wound progress, or lack thereof. |

## RECORDING AND REPORTING

- Record appearance of ulcer in patient's record.
- Describe type of topical agent used, dressing applied, and patient's response.
- Report any deterioration in ulcer appearance to nurse in charge or physician or heath care provider.

## UNEXPECTED OUTCOMES
## AND RELATED INTERVENTIONS

- Skin surrounding ulcer becomes macerated.
  - Reduce exposure of surrounding skin to topical agents and moisture.
  - Select a dressing that has increased moisture-absorbing capacity.

- Ulcer becomes deeper with increased drainage and/or development of necrotic tissue.
  - Review current wound care management.
  - Consult with multidisciplinary team regarding changes in wound care regimen.
  - Obtain wound cultures.
- Pressure ulcer extends beyond original margins.
  - Monitor for systemic signs and symptoms of poor wound healing, such as abnormal laboratory results (WBC, hemoglobin/hematocrit, serum albumin, serum prealbumin, total proteins), weight loss, and fluid imbalances.
  - Assess and revise current turning schedule.
  - Consider further pressure relieving devices (Table 35-4).

| TABLE 35-4 | Treatment Options by Ulcer Stage | | | | |
|---|---|---|---|---|---|
| Ulcer Stage | Ulcer Status | Dressing | Comments* | Expected Change | Adjuvants |
| I | Intact | None | Allows visual assessment. | Resolves slowly without epidermal loss over 7 to 14 days. | Turning schedule. Support hydration. Nutritional support. |
| | | Transparent dressing | Protects from shear. Do not use in the presence of excessive moisture. | | |
| | | Hydrocolloid | May not allow visual assessment. | | Pressure reduction mattress or chair cushion. |
| II | Clean | Composite film | Limits shear. | Heals through re-epithelialization. | See previous stage. Manage incontinence. |
| | | Hydrocolloid | Change when seal of dressing breaks, maximal wear time 7 days. | | |
| | | Hydrogel | Provides a moist environment. | | |
| III | Clean | Hydrocolloid | See stage II. | Heals through granulation and re-epithelialization. | See previous stages. Evaluate pressure relief needs. |
| | | Hydrogel Foam | Apply over wound to protect and absorb moisture. | | |
| | | Calcium alginate | Use when there is significant exudate. Cover with secondary dressing. | | |
| | | Gauze | Use with normal saline or other prescribed solution. Wring out excess solution, unfold to make contact with wound. | | |
| | | Growth factors | Use with gauze per manufacturer's instructions. | | |
| IV | Clean | Hydrogel | See stage III, clean. | Heals through granulation and re-epithelialization. | Surgical consult may be necessary for closure. See stages I, II, and III. |
| | | Calcium alginate | See stage III, clean. | | |
| | | Gauze | See stage III, clean. Fill all dead space with gauze. | | |
| | | Growth factors | Use with gauze. | | |
| | Eschar | Adherent film | Will facilitate softening of eschar. | Eschar will lift at the edges as healing progresses. | See previous stages. Surgical consult may be considered for debridement. |
| | | Hydrocolloid | Will facilitate softening of eschar. | | |
| | | Gauze plus ordered solution | Will deliver solution and wick wound drainage. | | May be considered for slow debridement. |
| | | Enzymes | | | |
| | | None | Rarely, if eschar is dry and intact, no dressing is used, allowing eschar to act as physiological cover. | | |

*As with *all* occlusive dressings, wounds should *not* be clinically infected.

Allow a puncture wound to bleed to remove dirt and other contaminants. If a penetrating object such as a knife blade is in a patient's body, do not remove the object. Removal will cause massive, uncontrolled bleeding. You apply pressure around the object but not on it or on surrounding tissues.

*CLEANSING.* Gentle cleansing of a wound removes contaminants that serve as sources of infection. However, vigorous cleaning causes bleeding or further injury. For abrasions, minor lacerations, and small puncture wounds, rinse the wound in running water, gently cleanse with mild soap and water, rinse, and apply an over-the-counter antiseptic. When

**PATIENT TEACHING**

Mrs. Ahmed is interested in learning how to change Mr. Ahmed's pressure ulcer dressing, so Lynda develops the following teaching plan:

**Outcome**
- At the end of the teaching session Mrs. Ahmed will perform an acceptable return demonstration of dressing application.

**Teaching Strategies**
- Plan a time Mrs. Ahmed is present and prepared to spend 30 minutes in two separate teaching sessions.
- Avoid using words that Mrs. Ahmed will not understand.
- Provide a brief description of what will be taught to both the patient and wife. Include the patient in all of the teaching even though he is unable to visualize the wound.
- Bring an extra dressing to the bedside to show Mrs. Ahmed what the dressing looks like and how to apply it.
- Use a pictorial guide of a pressure ulcer to help Mrs. Ahmed understand what the wound looks like and how it will progress if it shows signs of healing.
- Plan one session where Mrs. Ahmed will watch a demonstration of the wound being cleansed and the dressing applied. Plan a second session where she will do a return demonstration.
- At the end of each session ask Mrs. Ahmed how she felt doing the dressing and include Mr. Ahmed in this evaluation.

**Evaluation Strategies**
- Ask Mrs. Ahmed questions as she does the procedure to evaluate her understanding of each step.
- Ask Mrs. Ahmed what she will evaluate at each dressing change.
- Watch how Mrs. Ahmed handles the dressings and cleans the wound, and note any body language that indicates how she is feeling while doing the procedure.

a laceration is bleeding profusely, only brush away surface contaminants and concentrate on hemostasis until the patient reaches a clinic or hospital.

PROTECTION. Regardless of whether bleeding has stopped, protect the wound by applying a sterile or clean dressing, and immobilize the body part. A light dressing applied over minor wounds prevents entrance of microorganisms. In the case of small abrasions, it is acceptable to leave the wound open to air so that a scab will form.

The more extensive the wound, the larger the bandage required. In the home a clean towel or diaper is often the best dressing. A bulky dressing applied with pressure minimizes movement of underlying tissues and helps to immobilize the entire body part. A bandage or cloth wrapped around a penetrating object will immobilize it adequately.

**Dressings.** The use of dressings requires an understanding of wound healing and factors influencing healing. A variety of dressing materials are commercially available. Unless a dressing is suited to the characteristics of a wound, the dressing will stop wound repair.

The choice of dressing and the method of dressing a wound influence healing. The proper dressing does not allow a full-thickness wound to become dry with scab formation. When this occurs, the dermis dehydrates and crusts. As a result, a barrier forms against normal epidermal cell growth, slowing wound healing. Furthermore, dryness will increase discomfort. Ideally a dressing provides a moist environment to promote normal epidermal cell migration. The proper dressing will also absorb drainage to prevent pooling of exudate that promotes bacterial growth and prevents wound drainage from coming into contact with intact skin.

For surgical wounds that heal by primary intention, dressings are commonly removed as soon as drainage stops. Frequently the physician or health care provider removes the dressing 24 to 48 hours postoperatively. This coincides with initial epithelialization, so when the physician or health care provider removes the primary dressing, it reduces the risk of infection.

*Purposes.* A dressing serves several purposes. It discourages wound exposure to microorganisms. However, if a wound has minimal drainage, the natural formation of a fibrin seal eliminates the need for a dressing. A pressure dressing promotes hemostasis by exerting localized, downward pressure over an actual or potential bleeding site and fosters normal healing by eliminating dead space in underlying tissues. Assess skin color, pulses in distal extremities, patient comfort, and any changes in sensation to ensure pressure dressings do not interfere with circulation.

A dry dressing promotes healing by allowing the wound to heal by primary intention and absorbing minimal oozing of wound drainage. When a wound is healing by secondary intention, you use a dressing to provide a moist environment. You moisten the gauze with a solution, usually normal saline, wring it out, unfold it, and lightly pack it into the wound. The purpose of a moist gauze dressing is to act as a sponge, absorbing excessive wound drainage, while providing a moist environment. You change the dressing when it is saturated or if it begins to dry out. You always cover a moist dressing with a dry, secondary dressing.

A firmly taped or wrapped dressing supports or immobilizes a body part, minimizing movement of the underlying incision and traumatized tissues. Finally, a dressing promotes thermal insulation to the wound surface and protects it from the dehydrating effects of air.

*Types.* Dressings vary by type of material and mode of application (dry or moist). They are easy to apply, comfortable, and made of materials that promote wound healing.

Gauze is the most common dressing type. Gauze does not interact with wound tissues and thus causes little wound irritation. Gauze is available in different textures and in squares, rectangles, and rolls of various lengths and widths. Gauze dressings are best for wounds with moderate drainage, deep wounds, undermining, and tunnels. You apply gauze either moist or dry. Wet-to-dry (also called moist-to-dry) dressings are useful in debriding wounds. You moisten the primary gauze layer that touches the wound surface. This dressing should not be so moist that it will never dry out. The moistened gauze increases the absorptive ability of the dressing to collect exudate. You then cover the moist gauze with a secondary layer of dry gauze. Be sure the moist gauze does not cover the normal skin to prevent **maceration.**

Transparent film dressings are clear sheets coated on one side with an adhesive. The adhesive side will not stick to the wound because of the moisture and will trap moisture over the wound bed, providing a moist environment. The film is impermeable to fluid but semipermeable to oxygen. This type of dressing is used as a primary dressing in wounds with minimal tissue loss that have very little wound drainage. You change the dressing when the seal is broken.

Hydrocolloid dressings are made of gelling agents and have an adhesive wound surface. They come in a variety of sizes and shapes and are used to cover wounds, extending the hydrocolloid dressing at least $1\frac{1}{2}$ inches beyond the wound margin. Hydrocolloids form a gel as they interact with the wound surface. Because hydrocolloids are occlusive, they protect the wound from surface contaminants and you can leave them over a wound for several days. When removed, you will note a gel over the wound base; the gel maintains a moist environment to support healing and washes away during wound cleansing.

Hydrogel dressings are available in sheets or in a gel in a tube (amorphous). They contain a high percentage of water and are indicated for wounds that require moisture, either a wound with granulation (maintaining the moist wound environment needed for healing) or a wound that has a high percentage of necrotic tissue (the hydrogel facilitates debridement by softening the dead tissue). Hydrogels maintain moisture in some wounds for 1 to 3 days.

A new treatment for chronic wounds is the wound Vacuum Assisted Closure (known as The Wound V.A.C.® System). Wound closure applies negative pressure to the wound to promote and accelerate healing. You place an open foam sponge in the wound bed and a drainage/suction tube in the interior of the foam dressing. Then you seal the foam and the tube with a transparent dressing, and connect the tube to a prescribed amount of negative pressure, which creates a suction. All air is pulled out of the wound by the suction, making an airtight seal. This therapy provides removal of excess wound fluid to stimulate granulation tissue and to decrease wound bacteria (see Skill 35-4, p. 1049). This therapy has reduced healing time in chronic wounds and has resulted in early grafting of wounds (Broussard and others, 2000).

***Changing Dressings.*** To prepare for changing a dressing, you need to know the type of dressing, any underlying drains used, and the type of supplies needed for wound care. You can adjust the type and amount of dressings if the amount of drainage changes or if a wound becomes deeper. Notifying the physician or health care provider of any change is essential.

The order for changing a dressing usually indicates the dressing type, frequency of changing, and solutions or ointments you will apply. An order to "reinforce dressing prn" (add dressings without removing existing ones as needed) is common immediately after surgery, when the physician or health care provider does not want accidental disruption of the suture line or loss of hemostasis. A patient's medical or operating room record usually reveals whether drains are present. After the initial dressing change, communicate on the care plan the type of dressing materials and solutions to use and the type and location of drains.

Use aseptic technique during dressing change procedures (see Chapter 11). It is also essential for the patient to understand the steps of the procedure beforehand so he or she experiences less anxiety. Describe normal signs of the healing process, and offer to answer questions about the procedure or wound.

If a patient needs to care for a wound at home, you will demonstrate dressing changes to the patient and family and then provide an opportunity for practice. In the home, wound healing stabilizes so that sterile technique is usually unnecessary. However, patients need to learn clean technique. Make sure the patient is able to change a dressing independently or with assistance from a family member before discharge unless home care will be provided. Skill 35-3 outlines the steps for applying moist saline dressings.

***Securing Dressings.*** Use tape, ties, or bandages and cloth binders to secure a dressing over a wound site. The choice of anchoring depends on the wound size, location, drainage, frequency of dressing changes, and the patient's level of activity. You most often use tape strips to secure dressings if the patient does not react to tape. Hypoallergenic paper, plastic, and woven fabric tapes minimize skin reactions. Adhesive tape, the most likely anchor to cause skin irritation, adheres well to the skin's surface, whereas elastic adhesive tape compresses closely around pressure bandages and permits more movement of a body part (O'Brien and Reilly, 1995).

Tape is available in various widths; choose a size that sufficiently secures the dressing. Make sure the tape crosses the dressing and adheres to several inches of skin on each side. When securing the dressing, press the tape gently, exerting pressure away from the wound. Never apply tape over irritated skin. Apply a skin barrier to the skin around the wound so that the tape is secured to the skin barrier rather than to sensitive skin. To remove tape safely, loosen the tape ends and gently release the tape from the patient's skin by pressing the skin away from the tape.

To avoid repeated removal of tape from sensitive skin, secure dressings with reusable Montgomery ties (see Skill 35-3, step 16). Each tie consists of a long strip; half contains an adhesive backing to apply to the skin, and the other half folds back and contains a cloth tie that you tie across a dressing and untie at dressing changes. A large, bulky dressing requires two or more sets of Montgomery ties. To provide even support to a wound and immobilize a body part, apply elastic gauze or cloth bandages and binders over a dressing.

***Comfort Measures.*** Any wound can be painful, depending on the extent of tissue injury. You will use several tech-

*Text continued on p. 1053*

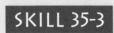

**SKILL 35-3** | **Applying Dressings: Dry or Wet-to-Dry and Transparent**

## Delegation Considerations

The care of acute new wounds and those that require sterile technique or a wet-to-dry dressing may not be delegated to assistive personnel. In some states, you can delegate certain aspects of wound care. This sometimes includes the changing of a dry dressing or changing the top dressing. The *assessment* of the wound must be completed by the nurse. Before you delegate any aspect of care:

- Discuss any unique modifications of the skill, such as the need for special tape or methods to secure the dressing.
- Instruct about signs of infection or poor wound healing that must be immediately reported.

## Equipment

- Clean disposable gloves
- Sterile gloves
- Sterile dressing set (scissors, forceps) *(may be optional, check institution policy)*

- Sterile drape *(optional)*
- Dressings: fine mesh gauze, sterile dressings, abdominal (ABD) pads, transparent
- Sterile basin *(optional)*
- Antiseptic ointment (as prescribed)
- Cleansing solution as prescribed
- Sterile normal saline or prescribed solution
- Tape, ties, or bandage as needed (include nonallergic tape if necessary)
- Protective waterproof underpad
- Waterproof bag
- Adhesive remover *(optional)*
- Measurement device *(optional)*: tape measure, camera (optional)
- Protective gown, mask, goggles used when spray from wound is a risk
- Additional lighting if needed (e.g., flashlight, treatment light)

| STEP | RATIONALE |
|---|---|

### ASSESSMENT

1. Assess size of wound to be dressed (see Skill 35-2).

Assists in planning for proper type and amount of supplies needed.

2. Assess location of wound.

Determines dressing type needed and if assistance is needed to hold dressings in place.

3. Ask patient to rate pain using a scale of 0 to 10.

Removal of dressing can be painful; patient may require pain medication before dressing change to allow drug's peak effect during procedure.

4. Assess patient's knowledge of purpose of dressing change.

Determines level of support and explanation required by patient.

5. Assess need and readiness for patient or family member to participate in dressing wound.

Prepares patient or family member if dressing must be changed at home.

6. Review medical orders for dressing change procedure.

Indicates type of dressing or applications to use.

7. Identify patients with risk factors for wound-healing problems (e.g., aging, prematurity, obesity, diabetes, compromised circulation, poor nutritional status, immunosuppressive drugs, irradiation in area of wound, high levels of stress, steroids)

Risk factors have the potential to affect wound healing and resistance to pathogens (Myer, 2000; Wysocki, 2002).

### PLANNING

1. Explain procedure to patient.

Decreases patient's anxiety.

2. Position patient to allow access to area to be dressed.

Facilitate application of dressing.

3. Plan dressing change to occur 30 minutes following administration of analgesic.

Dressing change is better tolerated by patient if pain medication has been administered at least 30 minutes before dressing change.

| STEP | RATIONALE |
|---|---|

## IMPLEMENTATION

1. Close room or cubicle curtains. Perform hand hygiene. Apply gown, goggles, and mask if risk of spray exists.

   Provides for privacy and reduces transmission of microorganisms.

2. Position patient comfortably, and drape to expose only wound site. Instruct patient not to touch wound or sterile supplies.

   Draping provides access to the wound yet minimizes unnecessary exposure.

3. Place disposable bag within reach of work area. Fold top of bag to make cuff. Put on clean disposable gloves.

   Ensures easy disposal of soiled dressings. Prevents contamination of bag's outer surface. Prevents transmission of infectious organisms.

4. Remove tape: pull parallel to skin, toward dressing, and hold down uninjured skin. If over hairy areas, remove in the direction of hair growth. Remove remaining adhesive from skin.

   Pulling tape toward dressing reduces stress on suture line or wound edges and reduces irritation and discomfort (Nelson and Dilloway, 2002).

5. With clean-gloved hand or forceps remove dressings. Carefully remove outer secondary dressing first, and then remove inner primary dressing that is in contact with the wound bed. If drains are present, slowly and carefully remove dressings one layer at a time. Keep soiled undersurface from patient's sight.

   The purpose of the primary dressing is to remove necrotic tissue and exudate. Appearance of drainage may be upsetting to patient. Avoids accidental removal of drain.

---

• *Critical Decision Point:* In wet-to-dry dressing, the inner primary dressing if applied properly will have dried and will adhere to underlying tissues; do not moisten it. It is incorrect technique and a common error by some clinicians to moisten the dried gauze before removing it so it does not stick to the wound. This defeats the purpose of using this type of dressing and reduces the amount of debris the dressing will remove (Ramundo and Wells, 2000).

---

6. Inspect wound for color, edema, drains, exudate, and integrity (see illustration). Observe appearance of drainage on dressing. Assess for odor. Gently palpate the wound edges for drainage, bogginess, or patient report of increased pain. Measure wound size (length, width, and depth [if indicated]) (see Skill 35-2).

   Provides assessment of drainage and of wound's condition. Indicates status of healing. Presence of bleeding during this type of dressing change is an indication that healthy tissue is being injured (Capasso and Munro, 2003).

---

• *Critical Decision Point:* Dressings that are heavily saturated with exudate indicate a need to add more absorbent gauze dressing to the wound. Assess the wound for any changes in color, drainage, odor, or edema.

---

7. Describe the appearance of the wound and any indicators of wound healing to the patient.

   Wounds may appear unsettling and frightening to patients; it is helpful for the patient to know that the wound appearance is as expected and that healing is taking place.

8. Dispose of soiled dressings in disposable bag. Remove gloves by pulling them inside out. Dispose of gloves in bag. Perform hand hygiene.

   Reduces transmission of microorganisms to other persons.

9. Open sterile dressing tray or individually wrapped sterile supplies. Place on bedside table (see illustration).

   Sterile dressings remain sterile while on or within sterile surface. Preparation of all supplies prevents break in technique during dressing change.

10. Open prescribed cleansing solution, and pour over sterile gauze.

    Keeps supplies sterile. Solution may be packaged to spray/pour directly on wound. Microorganisms move from nonsterile environment through dressing package to dressing itself by capillary action.

---

• *Critical Decision Point:* If sterile drape or gauze packages become wet from solution, repeat preparation of supplies.

---

## SKILL 35-3 ¦ Applying Dressings: Dry or Wet-to-Dry and Transparent—cont'd

| STEP | RATIONALE |
|---|---|

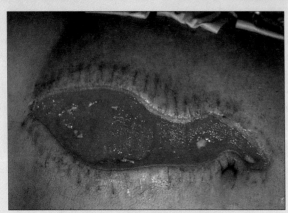

STEP **6** Abdominal wound, with beefy red granulation tissue present and attached wound edges. (From Bryant RA: *Acute and chronic wounds: nursing management,* ed 2, St. Louis, 2000, Mosby.)

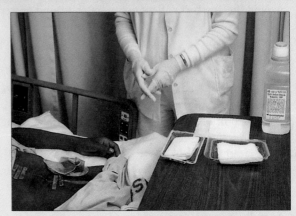

STEP **9** Sterile supplies on bedside table.

11. Put on gloves, clean or sterile depending on institution policy.

Sterile gloves allow handling of sterile supplies without contamination. Follow the guidelines of the health care institution related to clean versus sterile gloves. There is insufficient research to support either sterile or clean gloves as being more effective in decreasing infection and improving wound healing (Gray and Doughty, 2001).

12. Cleanse wound:
    a. Use separate swab for each cleansing stroke, or spray wound surface.

    Prevents contaminating previously cleaned area.

    b. Clean from least contaminated area to most contaminated.

    Cleansing in this direction prevents introduction of organisms into wound.

    c. Cleanse around the drain (if present), using circular stroke starting near drain and moving outward and away from the insertion site.

    Correct aseptic technique in cleansing prevents contamination of wound.

13. Use dry gauze to blot in same manner as in step 12 to dry wound. Dry thoroughly.

Drying reduces excess moisture, which could eventually harbor microorganisms. Transparent dressings do not adhere to damp surfaces.

14. Apply antiseptic ointment if ordered, using same technique as for cleansing.

Helps reduce growth of microorganisms.

15. Apply dressings to incision or wound site:

A dressing protects wound, prevents infection, and provides comfort.

   a. **Dry Dressing**
     (1) Apply loose woven gauze as contact layer.

Promotes proper absorption of drainage.

     (2) Cut 4 × 4 gauze flat to fit around drain if present or use precut split drain flat.

Secures drain and promotes drainage absorption at site.

     (3) Apply additional layers of gauze as needed.

Layering ensures proper coverage and optimal absorption.

     (4) Apply thicker woven pad (e.g., Surgipad, abdominal dressing).

This type of dressing is often used for postoperative wounds. Soft dressings over wounds protect the wound from irritation and provide support (West and Gimbel, 2000).

   b. **Wet-to-Dry Dressing (Moist-to-Dry)**
     (1) Place fine mesh gauze in container of sterile solution.

| STEP | RATIONALE |
|------|-----------|

• *Critical Decision Point:* Open or "fluff" the woven gauze that will be placed directly against the wound bed. Sometimes "packing strip" may be used to pack the wound (see illustration A for step 15b(2). When using packing strip, with a sterile scissor cut the amount of dressing that is anticipated to be used to pack the wound. Do not let the packing strip touch the side of the bottle. Pour prescribed solution over the packing gauze or strip to moisten it. Contact layer must be totally moistened to increase dressing's absorptive abilities (Ramundo and Wells, 2000).

| | |
|---|---|
| (2) Wring out excess fluid, and apply moist fluffed woven-mesh gauze or packing strip directly onto wound surface without having the gauze touch the surrounding skin (see illustration *A*). | Moist gauze absorbs drainage and adheres to debris (Hess, 2000). The inner gauze should be moist but not dripping wet. The moist gauze must be able to dry in the wound. Having the inner gauze too wet so it does not dry is a common error in technique for this type of dressing. |

• *Critical Decision Point:* If wound is deep, gently lay moistened woven gauze over wound surface with forceps until all surfaces are in contact with moist gauze and the wound is loosely filled. Fill the wound, but avoid packing the wound too tightly or having the gauze extend beyond the top of the wound (see illustration B).

| | |
|---|---|
| (3) Make sure any dead space from sinus tracts, undermining, or tunneling is loosely packed with gauze. | Do not overpack the wound too tightly; it can cause wound trauma when the dressing is removed (Ramundo and Wells, 2000). |
| (4) Apply dry sterile gauze over wet gauze. | Dry layer pulls moisture from wound. |
| (5) Cover the packed wound with a secondary dressing such as an ABD pad, Surgipad, or gauze | Protects wound from entrance of microorganisms. |
| c. **Transparent Dressing** | |
| (1) Apply dressing according to manufacturer's direction. Do not stretch film during application. Avoid wrinkles in film. | Wrinkles provide a tunnel for exudate to accumulate. |
| 16. Secure dressing with roll gauze (for circumferential dressings) (see illustrations), tape, Montgomery ties or straps (which are applied perpendicular to the wound) (see illustration), or binder. | Supports wound and ensures placement and stability of dressing. |

• *Critical Decision Point:* If areas of redness appear from tape, paper tape or alternatives such as elastic bandage, Kerlix, or a binder may be used to secure dressing. Sometimes strips of a hydrocolloid dressing are placed on the skin under the Montgomery ties to further protect the skin.

| | |
|---|---|
| 17. Remove gloves, gown if worn, and dispose of them in bag. Dispose of all supplies. Remove goggles if worn. | Reduces transmission of microorganisms. Clean environment enhances patient comfort. |
| 18. Assist patient to comfortable position. | Promotes patient's sense of well-being. |
| 19. Perform hand hygiene. | Reduces transmission of microorganisms. |

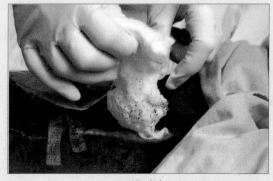

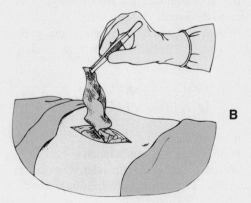

STEP **15b(2) A**, Packing wound. **B**, Wound packed loosely, until wound is filled.

| SKILL 35-3 | Applying Dressings: Dry or Wet-to-Dry and Transparent—cont'd |
|---|---|

| STEP | RATIONALE |
|---|---|

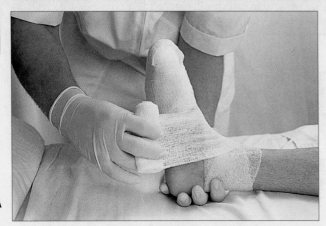 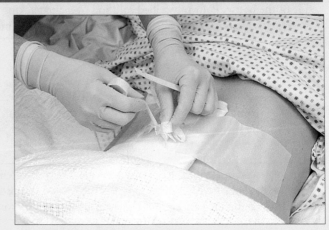

A                                                                            B

STEP **16 A,** Application of roll gauze. **B,** Securing Montgomery ties.

## EVALUATION

1. Inspect condition of wound and presence of any drainage.

   Determines rate of healing.

2. Ask if patient has pain during procedure.

   Pain may be early indication of wound complication or result of dressing pulling tissue.

3. Inspect condition of dressing at least every shift.

   Determines status of wound drainage.

4. Ask patient to describe steps and techniques of dressing change.

   Evaluates patient's learning.

## RECORDING AND REPORTING

■ Chart in the nurses' notes appearance of wound, color, presence and characteristics of exudate, change in wound characteristics, especially drainage amount, type and amount of dressings applied, and tolerance of patient to dressing change.

■ Report unexpected appearance of wound drainage or accidental removal of drain, bright red bleeding, or evidence of wound dehiscence or evisceration.

■ Write your initials, date, and time of dressing change on a piece of tape in ink (not marker), and place on dressing.

## UNEXPECTED OUTCOMES AND RELATED INTERVENTIONS

■ Wound drainage increases.
  • Increase frequency of dressing changes.
  • Notify physician or health care provider, who may consider drain placement or alternate dressing method.

■ Wound bleeds during dressing change.
  • Assess patient medication history and history of bleeding disorder.
  • If excessive, may need to apply pressure.
  • Observe color and amount of drainage.
  • Notify physician or health care provider.

■ Patient reports sensation that "something has given way under the dressing."
  • Remove dressing, and inspect wound for dehiscence or evisceration.
  • Protect wound. Cover with sterile moist dressing.
  • Instruct patient to lie still.
  • Remain with patient to monitor vital signs.
  • Notify physician or health care provider.

■ Skin around wound margins becomes red, macerated, or excoriated.
  • The outer layer of the wet-to-dry dressing is too moist.
  • Securing method for dressing is causing irritation. Change to paper tape.

| SKILL 35-4 | Wound Vacuum Assisted Closure |

## Delegation Considerations

The skill of wound Vacuum Assisted Closure should not be delegated to assistive personnel. Instruct assistive personnel to:

- Report to the nurse any change in the patient's temperature or level of comfort
- Change in the pressure of the V.A.C. unit
- Any change in the integrity of the Wound V.A.C. dressing

## Equipment

- The V.A.C.® System (requires physician's or health care provider's order) (Figure 35-12)
- V.A.C.® foam dressing
- Tubing for connection between V.A.C.® unit and V.A.C.® dressing
- Gloves, clean and sterile
- Scissors, sterile
- Waterproof bag for disposal
- Skin preparation/skin barrier
- Moist washcloth
- Linen bag
- Protective gown, mask, goggles (used when spray from wound is a risk)

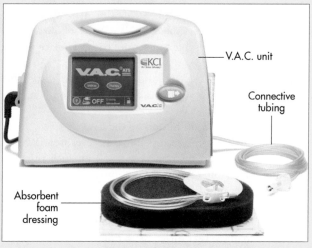

FIGURE **35-12** The V.A.C.® System. *Top to bottom:* V.A.C. System itself, connective tubing to go between V.A.C. system and dressing, absorbent foam dressing. (Courtesy Kinetic Concepts, Inc [KCI], San Antonio, Tex.)

| STEP | RATIONALE |
| --- | --- |

## ASSESSMENT

1. Assess location, appearance, and size of wound to be dressed (see Skill 35-2).

Allows you to gather information regarding status of wound healing, presence of complications, and type of supplies and assistance needed to apply V.A.C.® dressing.

2. Review physician's or health care provider's orders for frequency of dressing change, type of foam to use, and amount of negative pressure to be used.

Physician or health care provider orders frequency of dressing changes and special instructions.

3. Assess patient's level of comfort using a scale of 0 to 10.

Patient who is comfortable during procedure is less likely to move suddenly, causing wound or supply contamination.

4. Assess patient's and family member's knowledge of purpose of dressing.

Identifies patient's learning needs. Prepares patient and family if dressing will need to be changed at home.

## PLANNING

1. Collect equipment and arrange at bedside.

Organizes procedure.

2. Explain procedure to patient.

Relieves anxiety and promotes understanding of healing process.

3. Position patient to allow access to wound site.

Facilitates application of dressing.

## IMPLEMENTATION

1. Close room door or cubicle curtains.

Provides for patient privacy and reduces transmission of organisms.

2. Position patient, expose wound site, and cover patient.

Draping provides access to wound while minimizing exposure. Positioning ensures patient comfort during procedure.

## SKILL 35-4 | Wound Vacuum Assisted Closure—cont'd

| STEP | RATIONALE |
|---|---|
| 3. Cuff top of disposable waterproof bag, and place within reach of work area. | Cuff prevents accidental contamination of top of outer bag. |
| 4. Perform hand hygiene, and put on clean disposable gloves. If risk of spray exists, apply protective gown, goggles, and mask. | Reduces transmission of infectious organisms from soiled dressings to nurse's hands. |
| 5. Push therapy on/off button on the V.A.C.® | Deactivates therapy. |
| 6. Raise the tubing connectors above the level of the Wound V.A.C. unit, and disconnect tubes from each other to drain fluids into canister. Before lowering, tighten clamp on canister tube. | Allows for proper drainage of fluid in drainage tubing (KCI, 2003). The V.A.C.® canister unit should be changed when full or at least once a week to control odor (KCI, 2003). |
| 7. With dressing tube unclamped, introduce 10 to 30 ml of normal saline, if ordered, into tubing to soak underneath foam. Let set for 15 to 30 minutes. | Facilitates loosening of foam when tissue adheres to foam (KCI, 2003; Krasner, 2002). |
| 8. Gently stretch transparent film horizontally, and slowly pull up from the skin. | Reduces stress on suture line or wound edges and reduces irritation and discomfort. |
| 9. Remove the old V.A.C.® dressing, observing appearance and drainage on dressing. Use caution to remove dressing around drains. Dispose of soiled dressings in waterproof bag. Remove gloves by pulling them inside out, and dispose of them in waterproof bag. Avoid having patient see old dressing because the sight of wound drainage may be upsetting to the patient. Perform hand hygiene. | Determines dressings needed for replacement. Avoids accidental removal of drains. Reduces transmission of microorganisms. |
| 10. Apply sterile or clean gloves. Irrigate the wound with normal saline or other solution ordered by the physician or health care provider. Gently blot to dry (see Skill 35-5). | Irrigation removes wound debris and cleanses wound bed. |
| 11. Measure wound as ordered: at baseline, first dressing change, weekly, and discharge from therapy. Remove and discard gloves. Perform hand hygiene. | Provides objective measure of wound healing progress in response to negative pressure therapy (KCI, 2003). |

- *Critical Decision Point:* Wound cultures may be ordered on a routine basis. Obtain cultures during the dressing change when drainage looks purulent, there is change in amount or color, or drainage has a foul odor (Chua and others, 2000).

| STEP | RATIONALE |
|---|---|
| 12. Depending on the type of wound, apply sterile or new clean gloves. | Fresh sterile wounds require sterile gloves. Chronic wounds may require clean technique. Do not use the same gloves worn to remove old dressing because cross contamination may occur. |
| 13. Select appropriate foam dressing depending on wound type and stage of healing. Use sterile scissors to cut foam to exact wound size, making sure to fit the size and shape of the wound, including tunnels and undermined areas. | Black polyurethane (PU) foam has larger pores and is most effective in stimulating granulation tissue and wound contraction. White polyvinyl alcohol (PVA) soft foam is denser with smaller pores and is used when the growth of granulation tissue needs to be restricted (KCI, 2003; Mendez-Eastman, 1998). |

- *Critical Decision Point:* Use of black foam may cause patients to experience more pain because of excessive wound contraction. Patients may need to be switched to the PVA soft foam.

| STEP | RATIONALE |
|---|---|
| 14. Gently place foam in wound, being sure that the foam is in contact with entire wound base, margins, and tunneled and undermined areas (see illustration). | Maintains negative pressure to entire wound. Edges of the foam dressing must be in direct contact with the patient's skin (Mendez-Eastman, 1998). |
| 15. Insert tubing to foam in the wound (see illustration). | Tubing will connect to negative pressure from the V.A.C.® System to the wound foam. |

- *Critical Decision Point:* For deep wounds regularly reposition tubing to minimize pressure on wound edges. Patients with restricted mobility or sensation must be repositioned frequently so that they do not lie on the tubing and cause skin damage (KCI, 2003).

| STEP | RATIONALE |
|------|-----------|

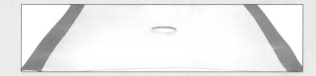

STEP **14** Dressing application. Properly sized foam to cover wound.

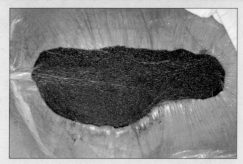

STEP **17 B,** Foam dressing, transparent dressing, and V.A.C.® System tubing secured over existing wound. (Courtesy Kinetic Concepts, Inc [KCI], San Antonio, Tex.)

 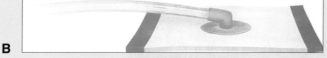

STEPS **15 A,** Wrinkle-free transparent dressing applied over foam. **B,** Secure tubing to the foam and transparent dressing unit (see step 17). (Courtesy Kinetic Concepts, Inc [KCI], San Antonio, Tex.)

16. Apply skin protectant, such as skin preparation or Stomahesive wafer, to skin around the wound.

Protects periwound skin from injury that may result from the occlusive dressing and will help decrease pain associated with wound margins (Krasner, 2002).

17. Apply the V.A.C.® transparent dressing, covering the V.A.C.® foam and 3 to 5 cm of surrounding healthy tissue (see illustration *A*). Make sure transparent dressing is wrinkle-free. Secure tubing to transparent film, aligning drainage hole to ensure an occlusive seal (see illustration *B*). Make sure not to apply tension to drape and tubing.

Ensure that the wound is properly covered and a negative pressure seal can be achieved. Excessive tension may compress foam dressing, impede wound healing, and produce a shear force on periwound area (KCI, 2003).

• ***Critical Decision Point:*** The wound must stay sealed to avoid wound desiccation. Wounds around joints and near the sacrum are problem areas to seal. An airtight seal can be assisted by shaving hair around wound, cutting transparent film to extend 3 to 5 cm beyond wound parameter, avoiding wrinkles in transparent film, patching leaks with transparent film, and using multiple small strips of transparent film to hold dressing in place before covering dressing with large piece of transparent film (Chua and others, 2000).

18. Secure tubing several centimeters away from the dressing.

Prevents pull on the primary dressing, which can cause leaks in the negative pressure system (Chua and others, 2000; KCI, 2003).

19. After the wound is completely covered, connect the tubing from the dressing to the tubing from the canister and the V.A.C.® System.

Intermittent or continuous negative pressure can be administered at 50 mm Hg to 175 mm Hg, according to physician's or or health care provider's orders and patient comfort. The average is 125 mm Hg (Chua and others, 2000; KCI, 2003).

   a. Remove canister from sterile packaging, and push into the V.A.C.® System until a click is heard. **An alarm will sound if the canister is not properly engaged.**

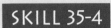

## SKILL 35-4 ┆ Wound Vacuum Assisted Closure—cont'd

| STEP | RATIONALE |
|---|---|
| b. Connect the dressing tubing to the canister tubing. Make sure both clamps are open. | |
| c. Place the V.A.C.® System on a level surface, or hang from the foot of the bed. **The V.A.C.® System will alarm and deactivate therapy if the unit is tilted beyond 45 degrees.** | |
| d. Press in green-lit power button, and set pressure as ordered. | |
| 20. Discard soiled dressing change materials properly. Perform hand hygiene. | Reduces transmission of microorganisms. |
| 21. Inspect the V.A.C.® System to verify that negative pressure is achieved. | Negative pressure is achieved when an airtight seal is achieved. |
| a. Verify that display screen reads THERAPY ON. | |
| b. Be sure clamps are open and tubing is patent. | |
| c. Identify air leaks by listening with stethoscope or by moving hand around edges of wound while applying light pressure. | |
| d. If a leak is present, use strips of transparent film to patch areas around the edges of the wound. | |
| 22. Assist patient to a comfortable position. | Enhances patient comfort and relaxation. |

## EVALUATION

| | |
|---|---|
| 1. Inspect condition of wound on ongoing basis; note drainage and odor. | Determines status of wound healing. |
| 2. Ask patient to rate pain using a scale of 0 to 10. | Determines patient's level of comfort following the procedure. |
| 3. Verify airtight dressing seal, and correct negative pressure setting. | Determines effective negative pressure being applied. |
| 4. Observe patient's or family member's ability to perform dressing change. | Indicates patient and family learning has occurred. |

## RECORDING AND REPORTING

■ Record wound appearance, color and characteristics of any drainage, presence of wound healing, and patient tolerance to procedure. Record date and time of new dressing on the dressing as per agency policy.

■ Report any brisk, bright red bleeding, evidence of poor wound healing, evisceration or dehiscence, and possible wound infection.

## UNEXPECTED OUTCOMES AND RELATED INTERVENTIONS

■ Wound appears inflamed and tender, drainage has increased, and an odor is present.
- Notify physician or health care provider.
- Obtain wound culture.

■ Patient reports increase in pain.
- If using black foam, switch to PVA foam.

■ Patient needs more analgesic support when V.A.C. is initiated.
- Reduce negative pressure.

■ Negative pressure seal has broken.
- Take preventive measures; before applying the transparent dressing; clip hair around wound, avoid wrinkles in transparent dressing, and avoid use of adhesive remover because it will leave a residue that interferes with adherence.
- Reinforce with transparent dressing strips.

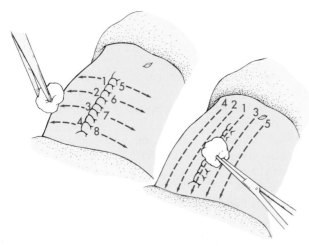

FIGURE **35-13** Methods for cleansing wound site.

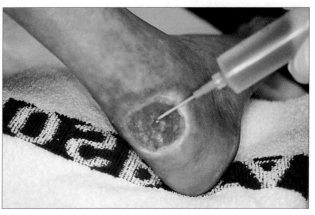

FIGURE **35-15** Wound irrigation using 35-ml syringe and 10-gauge catheter to facilitate removal of necrotic slough tissue.

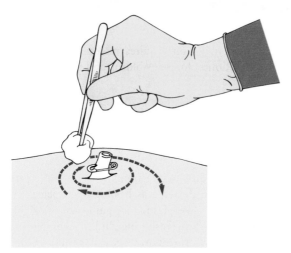

FIGURE **35-14** Cleansing of drain site.

niques to minimize discomfort. Careful removal of tape, gentle cleansing of wound edges, and gentle manipulation of dressings and drains minimize stress on sensitive tissues. Proper turning and positioning of the patient also reduce strain on the wound. Administration of analgesic medications 30 to 60 minutes before dressing changes (depending on a drug's time of peak action) also reduces discomfort (Rook, 1996) (see Chapter 30).

**Wound Cleansing.** Wound cleansing removes surface bacteria, preventing the invasion of healthy tissue. Normal saline effectively cleanses when delivered to the wound site with adequate force to agitate and wash away bacteria (Rolstad and others, 2000). Do not use povidone-iodine (e.g., Betadine), hydrogen peroxide, and acetic acid to irrigate a clean, granular wound. These solutions are toxic to fibroblasts, a key component in wound healing. Apply the following concepts when cleaning wounds:

1. Cleanse in a direction from the least contaminated area to the most contaminated, such as from the wound or inci-

sion to the surrounding skin (Figure 35-13) or from an isolated drain site to the surrounding skin (Figure 35-14).
2. Use light friction when applying antiseptics locally to the skin.
3. When irrigating, allow the solution to flow from the least contaminated to the most contaminated area.

**Wound Irrigation.** Irrigation is a way of cleansing wounds of exudate and debris. You use an irrigating syringe to flush the area with a constant flow of solution. Irrigations are useful for cleaning open deep wounds or sensitive or inaccessible body parts. Administer the prescribed solution (usually normal saline) at body temperature to enhance comfort and provide local cleansing application.

When irrigating clean wounds, use sterile technique and an irrigation system with a safe pressure (4 to 15 psi) to prevent trauma to the newly formed granulation tissue (WOCN, 2003). An example of a safe wound cleansing and irrigation system is a 35-ml syringe and a 19-gauge needle, which has a psi of 8. This method provides an ideal solution pressure for cleansing wounds while minimizing tissue trauma (Figure 35-15). Make sure the syringe tip is over but not sticking into the wound. Skill 35-5 lists steps for wound irrigation.

**Suture Care.** A surgeon closes a wound by bringing the edges as close together as possible to reduce the formation of scar tissue while minimizing trauma and tension and controlling bleeding. Sutures are threads or wires made of silk, steel, cotton, nylon, and polyester (Dacron) and are used to sew body tissues together. Dacron sutures minimize scar formation. Surgeons frequently use steel staples, a type of outer skin closure, because they result in less tissue trauma while providing extra strength (Figure 35-16). It is also common to see wounds closed with Steri-Strips, a sterile tape applied along both sides of a wound to keep the edges closed (Figure 35-17, p. 1057).

Policies vary at institutions as to who removes sutures. If you remove sutures, a physician's or health care provider's order is necessary. Be familiar with the types of suture methods (Figure 35-18, p. 1058).

*Text continued on p. 1057*

## SKILL 35-5 | Performing Wound Irrigation

### Delegation Considerations

The skill of wound irrigation should not be delegated to assistive personnel. In some settings you can delegate the cleansing of chronic wounds using *clean* technique to assistive personnel. It is your responsibility to assess the wound and evaluate wound care interventions. Before any delegation, instruct assistive personnel to:

- Report any changes in the patient's comfort level, wound drainage, or increase in temperature
- Report any bright red drainage

### Equipment

- Irrigant/cleansing solution (volume 1 to 2 times the estimated wound volume)
- Irrigation delivery system depending on amount of pressure desired:
  - Sterile irrigation 35-ml syringe with sterile soft angio-cath or 19-gauge needle (WOCN, 2003)
- Clean gloves
- Sterile gloves
- Waterproof underpad, if needed
- Dressing supplies
- Disposable waterproof bag
- Gown, goggles, mask for risk of spray

| STEP | RATIONALE |
|---|---|

### ASSESSMENT

1. Review physician's or health care provider's order for irrigation of open wound and type of solution to be used.

Open wound irrigation requires medical order including type of solution(s) to use (Waldrop and Doughty, 2000).

2. Assess recent recording of signs and symptoms related to patient's open wound:
   a. Extent of impairment of skin integrity, including size of wound (measure length, width, and depth). Wounds should be measured in centimeters and in the following order: length, width, and depth.

This assesses volume of irrigation solution needed. Data also used as baseline to indicate change in condition of wound.

   b. Elevation of body temperature.

May indicate response to infection.

   c. Drainage from wound (amount and color). Amount can be measured by part of dressing saturated or in terms of quantity (e.g., scant, moderate, copious).

Expect amount to decrease as healing takes place. Serous drainage is clear like plasma; sanguineous or bright red drainage indicates fresh bleeding; serosanguineous drainage is pink; purulent drainage is thick and yellow, pale green, or white.

   d. Odor. Must state whether or not there is odor. More frequent cleansing is needed if wound has a foul odor (AHCPR, 1994).

Strong odor indicates infectious process.

   e. Wound color.

Color represents a balance between necrotic tissue and new scar tissue. Proper selection of wound products, based on the color of the wound, facilitates removal of necrotic tissue and promotes new tissue growth (Rolstad and others, 2000).

   f. Consistency of drainage.

Type and color of drainage is dependent on moisture of the wound and type of organisms present.

   g. Culture reports.

Chronic wounds heal by secondary intention, and they are often colonized with bacteria.

   h. Stage of healing of the patient's wound.

Patient's wound characteristics determine type and amount of pressure to use during irrigation.

   i. Dressing: dry and clean; evidence of bleeding, profuse drainage.

Provides an initial assessment of present wound drainage.

3. Assess comfort level or pain on a scale of 0 to 10, and identify symptoms of anxiety.

Discomfort may be related directly to wound or indirectly to muscle tension or immobility. Anxiety results from multiple factors (e.g., surgery, diagnosis, awaiting pathology reports) and anticipation of unknown nursing interventions (e.g., first wound irrigation).

4. Assess patient for history of allergies to antiseptics, tapes, or dressing material.

Known allergies suggest application of a sample of prescribed antiseptic as skin test before flushing wound with large volume of solution or selection of different tape or dressing material.

| STEP | RATIONALE |
|---|---|

## PLANNING

1. Explain procedure of wound irrigation and cleansing.

   Information will reduce patient's anxiety.

2. Administer prescribed analgesic 30 to 45 minutes before starting wound irrigation procedure.

   Promotes pain control and permits patient to move more easily and be positioned to facilitate wound irrigation (Dochterman and Bulechek, 2004).

3. Position patient.
   a. Position comfortably to permit gravitational flow of irrigating solution through wound and into collection receptacle (see illustration).

   Directing solution from top to bottom of wound and from clean to contaminated area prevents further infection. Position patient during planning stage keeping in mind the bed surfaces needed for later preparation of equipment.

   b. Position patient so that wound is vertical to collection basin. Place container of irrigant/cleaning solution in basin of hot water to warm solution to body temperature.

   Warmed solution increases comfort and reduces vascular constriction response in tissues.

   c. Place padding or extra towel in the bed.

   Protects bedding.

   d. Expose wound only.

   Prevents chilling of patient.

## IMPLEMENTATION

1. Perform hand hygiene.

   Reduces transmission of microorganisms.

2. Form cuff on waterproof biohazard bag, and place it near bed.

   Cuffing helps to maintain large opening, thereby permitting placement of contaminated dressing without touching refuse bag itself.

3. Close room door or bed curtains.

   Maintains privacy.

4. Apply gown and goggles.

   Protects nurse from splashes or sprays of blood and body fluids.

5. Apply clean gloves, and remove soiled dressing and discard in waterproof bag. Discard gloves.

   Reduces transmission of microorganisms.

6. Prepare equipment; open sterile supplies.

7. Apply sterile gloves.

   Prevents transfer of microorganisms to wound surface.

8. To irrigate wound with wide opening:
   a. Fill 35-ml syringe with irrigation solution.

   Flushing wound helps remove debris and facilitates healing by secondary intention.

   b. Attach 19-gauge angiocatheter.

   Provides ideal pressure for cleansing and removal of debris (Ramundo and Wells, 2000).

   c. Hold syringe tip 2.5 cm (1 inch) above upper end of wound and over area being cleansed.

   Prevents syringe contamination. Careful placement of the syringe prevents unsafe pressure of the flowing solution.

   d. Using continuous pressure, flush wound; repeat steps 8a, b, and c until solution draining into basin is clear.

   Clear solution indicates all debris has been removed.

9. To irrigate deep wound with very small opening:
   a. Attach soft angiocatheter to filled irrigating syringe.

   Catheter permits direct flow of irrigant into wound. Expect wound to take longer to empty when opening is small.

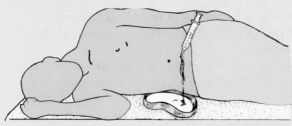

STEP **3a** Position of patient for abdominal wound irrigation.

┌─────────────────────────────────────────────┐
│ SKILL 35-5 │ Performing Wound Irrigation—cont'd
└─────────────────────────────────────────────┘

| STEP | RATIONALE |
|------|-----------|
| b. Lubricate tip of catheter with irrigating solution; then gently insert tip of catheter, and pull out about 1 cm (½ inch). | Removes tip from fragile inner wall of wound. |

• *Critical Decision Point:* Do not force catheter into the wound because this could cause tissue damage.

| | |
|------|-----------|
| c. Using slow, continuous pressure, flush wound. | Use of slow mechanical force of a stream of solution loosens particulate matter on the wound surface and promotes healing (Ramundo and Wells, 2000). |

• *Critical Decision Point:* CAUTION: Splashing may occur during this step.

| | |
|------|-----------|
| d. Pinch off catheter just below syringe while keeping catheter in place. | Prevents aspiration of solution into syringe and contamination of sterile solution. |
| e. Remove and refill syringe. Reconnect to catheter, and repeat until solution draining into basin is clear. | |

• *Critical Decision Point:* Pulsatile high-pressure lavage may be the irrigation of choice for necrotic wounds. The amount of irrigant is wound-size dependent. Pressure settings on the device should remain between 8 and 15 psi. Do not use pulsatile high-pressure lavage on exposed blood vessels, muscle, tendon, and bone. This type of irrigation should not be used with graft sites and should be used with caution in patients receiving anticoagulant therapy (Ramundo and Wells, 2000).

| | |
|------|-----------|
| 10. When indicated, obtain cultures after cleansing with nonbacteriostatic saline. | Routine culturing of open wounds is not recommended by AHCPR (1994). AHCPR (1994) recommends using quantitative bacterial cultures (tissue biopsy or wound fluid by needle aspiration) rather than swab cultures, which often detect only surface bacterial contaminants. |

• *Critical Decision Point:* Consider culturing a wound if it has a foul, purulent odor; inflammation surrounds the wound; a nondraining wound begins to drain; or patient is febrile.

| | |
|------|-----------|
| 11. Dry wound edges with gauze; dry patient if shower or whirlpool is used. | Prevents maceration of surrounding tissue from excess moisture. |
| 12. Apply appropriate dressing (see Skill 35-3). | Maintains protective barrier and healing environment for wound. |
| 13. Remove gloves, mask, goggles, and gown. | Prevents transfer of microorganisms. |
| 14. Assist patient to comfortable position. | |
| 15. Dispose of equipment and soiled supplies, and perform hand hygiene. | Reduces transmission of microorganisms. |

## EVALUATION

| | |
|------|-----------|
| 1. Assess type of tissue in wound bed. | Identifies wound healing progress and determines type of wound cleansing and dressing needed. |
| 2. Inspect dressing periodically. | Determines patient's response to wound irrigation and need to modify plan of care. |
| 3. Evaluate skin integrity. | Determines if extension of wound has occurred. |
| 4. Observe patient for signs of discomfort. | Patient's pain should not increase as a result of wound irrigation. |
| 5. Observe for presence of retained irrigant. | Retained irrigant is a medium for bacterial growth and subsequent infection. |

## RECORDING AND REPORTING

■ Record wound irrigation and patient response in progress notes.

■ Immediately report any evidence of fresh bleeding, sharp increase in pain, retention of irrigant, or signs of shock to attending physician or health care provider.

## UNEXPECTED OUTCOMES AND RELATED INTERVENTIONS

■ Bleeding or serosanguineous drainage appears.
  • Flush wound during next irrigation using less pressure.
  • Notify physician or health care provider of bleeding.

■ Opening in suture line extends.
  • Notify physician or health care provider.
  • Reevaluate amount of pressure to use for next wound irrigation.

■ Retained fluid and debris appear.
  • Increase amount of fluid used during irrigation.
  • Increase amount of pressure when flushing wound.
  • Make sure wound is clear of retained fluid and debris before applying dressing.

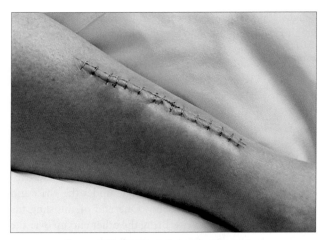

FIGURE **35-16** Wound closed with staples.

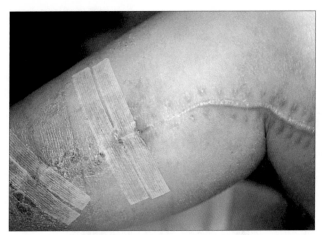

FIGURE **35-17** Steri-Strips placed over incision for closure.

***Drainage Evacuation.*** When drainage interferes with healing, you achieve drainage evacuation by using a drain or a drainage tube with continuous suction. **Drainage evacuators** are convenient, portable units that connect to tubular drains within a wound bed and exert a safe, constant, low-pressure vacuum to remove and collect drainage (Figure 35-19, p. 1058). Ensure that suction is exerted and that all connection points between the evacuator and tubing are intact. The evacuator collects drainage that is assessed for volume and character. When the evacuator fills, measure output by emptying the contents into a graduated cylinder, and immediately reset the evacuator to apply suction. You apply special skin barriers, similar to those used with ostomies (see Chapter 33) around drain sites. Skin barriers placed around a leaking drain protect the skin from the effluent.

**Bandages and Binders.** A simple gauze dressing is often not enough to immobilize or provide support to a wound. **Bandages** and **binders** applied over or around dressings will provide extra protection and therapeutic benefits by creating pressure over a body part, immobilizing a body part, supporting a wound, reducing or preventing edema, securing a splint, or securing dressings.

Bandages are available in rolls of various widths and materials, including gauze, elasticized knit, elastic webbing, flannel, and muslin. Gauze bandages are lightweight and inexpensive, mold easily around contours of the body, and permit air circulation to underlying skin to prevent maceration. Elastic bandages conform well to body parts but are also used to exert pressure over a body part.

Binders are bandages made of large pieces of material to fit a specific body part. An arm sling and a breast binder are two examples of binders. A binder reduces stress on a wound.

***Principles for Application of Bandages and Binders.*** Correctly applied bandages and binders do not cause injury to underlying or nearby body parts or create discomfort for the patient. Before applying a bandage or binder, perform the following steps:

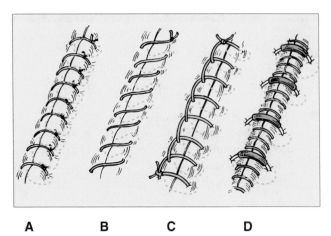

**A**  **B**  **C**  **D**

FIGURE **35-18** Examples of suturing methods. **A,** Intermittent. **B,** Continuous. **C,** Blanket continuous. **D,** Retention.

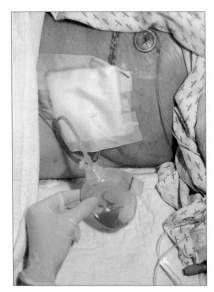

FIGURE **35-19** Jackson-Pratt drain and reservoir.

1. Inspect the skin for abrasions, edema, discoloration, or exposed wound edges.
2. Cover exposed wounds or open abrasions with a sterile dressing.
3. Assess the condition of underlying dressings, and change if they are soiled.
4. Assess the skin of underlying body parts and parts that will be distal to the bandage for signs of circulatory impairment (coolness, pallor or cyanosis, diminished or absent pulses, swelling, numbness, and tingling) to provide a means for comparing changes in circulation after bandage application.

Table 35-5 outlines the principles of bandage and binder application. After you apply a bandage, assess, document, and immediately report any changes in circulation, comfort level, body function such as ventilation, and skin integrity.

After you apply a bandage, you loosen or readjust it as necessary, but seek an order before loosening or removing a bandage applied by the physician or health care provider. Explain to the patient that any bandage or binder will feel relatively firm or tight; assesses the bandage carefully to be sure it is applied properly and is providing therapeutic benefit, and replace bandages when they become soiled.

***Binder Application.*** Binders are especially designed for the body part to be supported. The most common types of binders are the breast binder, abdominal binder, and sling (Box 35-12).

*BREAST BINDER.* A breast binder looks like a tight-fitting sleeveless vest. It conforms to the shape of the chest wall and is available in different sizes. Breast binders provide support after breast surgery or exert pressure to reduce lactation after childbirth. They do not impair chest expansion. However, if a patient develops pulmonary secretions, encourage active pulmonary hygiene exercises.

*ABDOMINAL BINDER.* An abdominal binder supports large incisions that are vulnerable to stress when the patient moves or coughs. It is a rectangular piece of cotton or elasticized material with many tails attached to the two longer sides or long extensions on each side to surround the abdomen (Figure 35-20).

*SLINGS.* Slings support arms with muscular sprains or fractures. A commercially made sling consists of a long sleeve that extends to the elbow and a strap that fits around the neck. In the home, patients can use a large triangular piece of cloth as a sling. The patient sits or lies supine for a sling application (Figure 35-21). Instruct the patient to bend the affected arm, bringing the forearm straight across the chest. The open sling fits under the patient's arm and over the chest, with the base of the triangle under the wrist and the triangle's point at the elbow. One end of the sling fits around the back of the neck. Bring the other end up over the affected arm while supporting the extremity. Tie the two ends at the side of the neck so that the knot does not press against the cervical spine. You can fold the loose fold at the elbow evenly around the elbow and pin it. To prevent the formation of dependent edema, make sure the lower arm is always supported at a level above the elbow.

***Bandage Application.*** Rolls of bandage secure or support dressings over irregularly shaped body parts. Each roll has a free outer end and a terminal end at the center. The rolled portion of the bandage is its body, and you place its outer surface against the patient's skin or dressing. Box 35-13 describes essential points when applying an elastic bandage.

**Heat and Cold Therapy.** The local application of heat and cold to an injured body part provides therapeutic benefits. Before using these therapies, however, understand normal body responses to local temperature variations, assess the integrity of the body part, determine the patient's ability to sense temperature variations, and ensure proper operation of equipment. You are legally responsible for the safe administration of all heat and cold applications.

***Body Responses to Heat and Cold.*** Exposure to heat and cold will cause systemic and local responses. Systemic responses occur through heat loss mechanisms (sweating or

| TABLE 35-5 | Principles for Bandage and Binder Application |
|---|---|
| **Principle** | **Rationale** |
| Position body part you will bandage in comfortable position of normal anatomical alignment. | Bandages cause restriction in movement. Immobilization in normal functioning position reduces risks of deformity or injury. |
| Prevent friction between and against skin surfaces by applying gauze or cotton padding. | Skin surfaces in contact with each other (e.g., between toes, under breasts) rub against each other to cause abrasion or chafing. Bandages over bony prominences rub against skin to cause breakdown. |
| Apply bandages securely to prevent slippage during movement. | Friction between bandage and skin causes skin breakdown. |
| When bandaging extremities, apply bandage first at distal end and progress toward trunk. | Gradual application of pressure from distal toward proximal portion of extremity promotes venous return and minimizes risk of edema or circulatory impairment. |
| Apply bandages firmly, with equal tension exerted over each turn or layer. Avoid excess overlapping of bandage layers. | Equal tension prevents unequal pressure distribution over bandaged body part. Localized pressure causes circulatory impairment. |
| Position pins, knots, or ties away from wound or sensitive skin areas. | Pins and ties used to secure bandages and binders exert localized pressure and irritation. |

vasodilation) or mechanisms promoting heat conservation (vasoconstriction or piloerection) and heat production (shivering) (see Chapter 12). Local responses to heat and cold occur through stimulation of temperature-sensitive nerve endings within the skin.

The body's adaptive ability creates the major problem in protecting patients from injury resulting from temperature extremes. A person initially feels an extreme change in temperature but within a short time hardly notices the temperature variation. This phenomenon is dangerous because a person insensitive to heat and cold extremes is at risk for serious tissue injury. Recognize patients most at risk for injuries from heat and cold applications (Table 35-6).

*Local Effects of Heat and Cold.* Heat and cold stimuli create different physiological responses. The choice of heat or cold therapy depends on the local responses desired for wound healing (Table 35-7).

Heat generally is therapeutic. If heat is applied for 1 hour or more, however, a reflex vasoconstriction reduces blood flow as the body attempts to control heat loss from the area. The periodic removal and reapplication of local heat will restore vasodilation. Continuous exposure to heat damages epithelial cells, causing redness, localized tenderness, and even blistering of the skin.

Prolonged exposure of the skin to cold results in a reflex vasodilation. The cell's inability to receive adequate blood flow and nutrients results in tissue ischemia. The skin initially takes on a reddened appearance, followed by a bluish-purple mottling with numbness and a burning type of pain. Tissues will actually freeze from exposure to extreme cold.

*Factors Influencing Heat and Cold Tolerance.* The body's response to heat and cold therapies depends on the following factors:

1. *Duration of application.* A person is better able to tolerate short exposures to any temperature extremes.

2. *Body part.* The neck, inner aspect of the wrist and forearm, and perineal regions are more sensitive to temperature variations. The foot and the palm of the hand are less sensitive.

3. *Damage to body surface.* Exposed skin layers are more sensitive to temperature variations.

4. *Prior skin temperature.* The body responds best to minor temperature adjustments.

5. *Body surface area.* A person is less tolerant of temperature changes over a large area of the body.

6. *Age and physical condition.* The very young and old are most sensitive to heat and cold. If a patient's physical condition reduces the reception or perception of sensory stimuli, the tolerance to temperature extremes is high, but the risk of injury is also high.

*Assessment for Temperature Tolerance.* Before applying heat or cold therapies, first observe the area you will treat so that you are able to later evaluate therapy-related skin changes. Alterations in skin integrity, such as abrasions, open wounds, edema, bruising, bleeding, or localized areas of inflammation, increase the risk of thermal injury. Identify conditions that contraindicate heat or cold therapy. *Do not* apply heat over an active area of bleeding (risk of continued bleeding) or an acute localized inflammation such as appendicitis (risk of rupture). If the patient has cardiovascular problems, it is unwise to apply heat to large portions of the body because massive vasodilation will disrupt blood supply to vital organs. Cold is contraindicated if the site of injury is edematous or the patient has impaired circulation or is shivering (may intensify shivering and reduce blood flow).

Also assess the patient's sensory function and ability to recognize when heat or cold becomes excessive. If a patient has peripheral vascular disease, observe circulation to the extremities. If a patient is confused or unresponsive, observe skin temperature, circulation, and integrity frequently after

---

**BOX 35-12** PROCEDURAL GUIDELINES FOR

## Applying Abdominal or Breast Binders

**Delegation Considerations:** You can delegate the application of an abdominal or breast binder to others. It is the responsibility of a professional nurse to assess the area where the binder will be applied and to assess the patient's comfort level after application.

**Equipment:** abdominal binder/breast binder; clean disposable gloves; pins, metal fasteners as indicated by type of binder used

1. Observe patient with need for support of thorax or abdomen. Observe ability to breathe deeply and cough effectively.
2. Review medical record if medical prescription for particular binder is necessary and reasons for application.
3. Inspect skin for actual or potential alterations in integrity. Observe for irritation, abrasion, skin surfaces that rub against each other, or allergic response to adhesive tape used to secure dressing.
4. Inspect any surgical dressing.
5. Assess patient's comfort level, using analog scale of 0 to 10 (see Chapter 30) and noting any objective signs and symptoms.
6. Gather necessary data regarding size of patient and appropriate binder.
7. Explain procedure to patient.
8. Perform hand hygiene, and apply gloves (if likely to contact wound drainage).
9. Close curtains or room door.
10. Apply binder.

   **a. Abdominal binder:**
   (1) Position patient in supine position with head slightly elevated and knees slightly flexed.
   (2) Fanfold far side of binder toward midline of binder.
   (3) Instruct and assist patient in rolling away from you toward raised side rail while firmly supporting abdominal incision and dressing with hands.
   (4) Place fanfolded ends of binder under patient.
   (5) Instruct or assist patient in rolling over folded ends toward you.

   (6) Unfold and stretch ends out smoothly on far side of bed.
   (7) Instruct patient to roll back into supine position.
   (8) Adjust binder so that supine patient is centered over binder using symphysis pubis and costal margins as lower and upper landmarks.
   (9) Close binder. Pull one end of binder over center of patient's abdomen. While maintaining tension on that end of binder, pull opposite end of binder over center and secure with Velcro closure tabs, metal fasteners, or horizontally placed safety pins (see Figure 35-21).
   (10) Assess patient's comfort level.
   (11) Adjust binder as necessary.

   **b. Breast binder:**
   (1) Assist patient in placing arms through binder's armholes.
   (2) Assist patient to supine position in bed.
   (3) Pad area under breasts if necessary.
   (4) Using Velcro closure tabs or horizontally placed safety pins, secure binder at nipple level first. Continue closure process above and then below nipple line until entire binder is closed.
   (5) Make appropriate adjustments, including individualizing fit of shoulder straps and pinning waistline darts to reduce binder size.
   (6) Instruct and observe skill development in self-care related to reapplying breast binder.

11. Remove gloves, and perform hand hygiene.
12. Observe site for skin integrity, circulation, and characteristics of the wound. (Periodically remove binder and surgical dressing to assess wound characteristics.)
13. Evaluate comfort level of patient, using analog scale of 0 to 10 and noting any objective signs and symptoms.
14. Evaluate patient's ability to ventilate properly, including deep breathing and coughing.

---

therapy begins. Finally, assess the condition of all equipment used, checking for cracked cords, frayed wires, damaged insulation, exposed heating components, leaks, and evenness of temperature distribution.

*Patient Education and Safety.* Before application of heat or cold therapy, make sure the patient understands its purpose, the symptoms of temperature exposure, and the precautions taken to prevent injury. Box 35-14 provides hints for safely applying heat and cold therapy.

*Applying Heat and Cold.* A prerequisite to using heat or cold application is a physician's or health care provider's order, which includes the body site to be treated and the type, frequency, and duration of application. The correct temperature to use for heat and cold applications varies according to agency policy.

*Choice of Moist or Dry.* You administer heat and cold applications in dry or moist forms. Consider the type of wound

or injury, location of the body part, and presence of drainage or inflammation when selecting dry or moist applications.

*Warm Moist Compresses.* A warm, moist compress improves circulation, relieves edema, and promotes concentration of pus and drainage. A **compress** is a piece of gauze dressing moistened in a prescribed warmed solution. A pack is a larger cloth or dressing applied to a larger body area.

Heat from warm compresses evaporates quickly. To maintain a constant temperature, change the compress frequently or apply a warm aquathermic pad or waterproof heating pad over the compress. Because moisture conducts heat, make sure any device's temperature setting is lower for a moist compress than for a dry application. A layer of plastic wrap or a dry towel will insulate the compress and retain heat. Moist heat promotes vasodilation and evaporation of heat from the skin's surface. For this reason a patient feels chilly. Control drafts, and keep the patient covered with a blanket or robe.

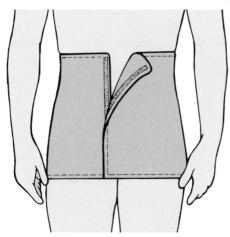

FIGURE **35-20** Abdominal binder secured with Velcro.

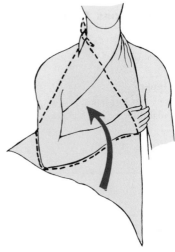

FIGURE **35-21** Application of a sling.

---

**BOX 35-13**  PROCEDURAL GUIDELINES FOR

## Applying Elastic Bandages

**Delegation Considerations:** Do not delegate the application of elastic bandages to assistive personnel. It is the nurse's responsibility to assess the area, apply the wrap, and then again assess the area for signs of circulatory occlusion (coolness of area wrapped, pain in the area, change in color of tissue in area).

**Equipment:** correct width and number of elastic bandages; clips, adhesive tape, or mesh dressing to secure elastic bandage; gloves if wound drainage is present

1. Review patient's medical record and order for application of elastic bandage.
2. Inspect areas to be bandaged for
    a. Intact skin
    b. Abrasions
    c. Draining wounds
    d. Skin discoloration
3. Note circulation to the area requiring an elastic bandage.
    a. Palpate skin, noting temperature, color.
    b. Palpate pulse, noting pulse quality.
    c. Observe extremity for edema or dehydration.
4. Determine level of function of affected extremity.
5. Assess level of pain severity to area (scale 0 to 10).
6. Explain procedure to patient.
7. Perform hand hygiene, and apply gloves, if indicated.
8. Close curtains or room door.

9. Hold roll of elastic bandage in dominant hand, and use other hand to tightly hold the beginning of bandage at distal body part.
10. Apply bandage from distal point toward proximal boundary, stretching the bandage slightly, using a variety of bandage turns to cover various body shapes. Prevent uneven bandage tension or circulatory impairment by overlapping turns by one-half to two-thirds width of bandage roll. NOTE: Be sure bandage is smooth (without creases).
11. Secure each roll with clip or tape before applying additional roll(s).
12. When finished with application, secure last elastic roll with clip, adhesive tape, or mesh to prevent wrap from becoming dislodged and thus decreasing extremity support.
13. Remove gloves, and perform hand hygiene.
14. Evaluate circulation to bandaged area every 4 hours.
    a. Palpate distal pulse.
    b. Palpate skin, noting temperature every 4 hours.
    c. Observe skin color.
15. Determine patient's level of comfort, using analog scale of 0 to 10 and noting any objective signs and symptoms.
16. Observe for changes from baseline assessment in level of extremity function.

---

***Warm Soaks.*** Immersion of a body part in a warmed solution promotes circulation, lessens edema, increases muscle relaxation, and allows application of medicated solution. You also accomplish a soak by wrapping the body part in dressings and saturating them with the warmed solution.

Position the patient comfortably, place waterproof pads under the area you will treat, and heat the solution to the patient's tolerance. Check the temperature by placing a small amount of solution on the inside of the forearm. After immersing the body part, cover the container and extremity with a towel to reduce heat loss. It is usually necessary to remove the cooled solution and the body part and add heated solution after about 10 minutes. The problem is to keep the solution at a constant temperature. Never add a hotter solution while the body part remains immersed. After any soak, dry the body part thoroughly to prevent maceration.

***Sitz Bath.*** The patient who has had rectal surgery or an episiotomy during childbirth or who has painful hemorrhoids

| TABLE 35-6 | Conditions That Increase Risk of Injury From Heat and Cold Application |
|---|---|
| **Condition** | **Risk Factors** |
| Very young; older adults | Thinner skin layers in children and older adults increase risk of burns; older adults have reduced sensitivity to pain. |
| Open wounds, broken skin | Subcutaneous tissue is more sensitive to temperature variations. |
| Areas of edema or scar formation | There is reduced sensation to temperature stimuli because of scar formation. |
| Peripheral vascular disease (e.g., diabetes, arteriosclerosis) | Body's extremities are less sensitive to temperature and pain stimuli because of circulatory impairment and local tissue injury; cold application further compromises blood flow. |
| Confusion or unconsciousness | There is reduced perception of sensory or painful stimuli. |
| Spinal cord injury | Alterations in nerve pathways prevent reception of sensory or painful stimuli. |

| TABLE 35-7 | Therapeutic Effects of Heat and Cold Applications | |
|---|---|---|
| **Physiological Response** | **Therapeutic Benefit** | **Examples of Conditions Treated** |
| **Heat Therapy** | | |
| Vasodilation | Improves blood flow to injured body part | Arthritis or degenerative joint disease |
| Reduced blood viscosity | Promotes delivery of nutrients and removal of wastes | Localized joint pain or muscle strains |
| Reduced muscle tension | | Low back pain |
| Increased tissue metabolism | Improves delivery of leukocytes and antibiotics to wound site | Menstrual cramping |
| Increased capillary permeability | Promotes muscle relaxation | Hemorrhoidal, perianal, and vaginal inflammation |
| | Reduces pain from spasm or stiffness | Local abscesses |
| | Increases blood flow | |
| | Provides local warmth | |
| | Promotes movement of waste products and nutrients | |
| **Cold Therapy** | | |
| Vasoconstriction | Reduces blood flow to injured site, preventing edema formation | Immediately after direct trauma (e.g., sprains, strains, fractures, muscle spasms) |
| Local anesthesia | Reduces inflammation | Superficial laceration or puncture wound |
| Reduced cell metabolism | Reduces localized pain | Minor burn |
| Increased blood viscosity | Reduces oxygen needs of tissues | After injections |
| Decreased muscle tension | Promotes blood coagulation at injury site | Arthritis or joint trauma |
| | Relieves pain | |

or vaginal inflammation will benefit from a **sitz bath,** a bath in which only the pelvic area is immersed in warm fluid. The patient sits in a special tub or chair or in a basin that fits on the toilet so that the legs and feet remain out of the water. Immersing the entire body causes widespread vasodilation and negates the effect of local heat to the pelvic area.

The desired temperature for a sitz bath depends on whether the purpose is to promote relaxation or to clean a wound. It is often necessary to carefully add warm water during the procedure, which usually lasts 20 minutes. A disposable basin contains an attachment that resembles an enema bag and allows the gradual introduction of warmer water.

Prevent overexposure by draping bath blankets around the patient's shoulders and thighs and controlling drafts. Make sure the patient is able to sit in the basin or tub with feet flat on the floor and without pressure on the sacrum or thighs. Because exposure of a large portion of the body to heat causes extensive vasodilation, assess the patient's pulse

and facial color and ask whether the patient feels light-headed or nauseated.

*Aquathermia (Water-Flow) Pads.* The aquathermia pad is useful for treating muscle sprains and areas of mild inflammation or edema (Figure 35-22). The unit consists of a waterproof plastic or rubber pad connected by two hoses to an electrical control unit that has a heating element and motor. Distilled water circulates through hollowed channels within the pad to the control unit where water is heated or cooled (depending on temperature setting). Although the units are safer than the conventional heating pad, you still check for equipment malfunctions. You fix the temperature setting by inserting a plastic key into the temperature regulator. If the water in the unit runs low, simply add distilled water to the reservoir at the top of the control unit.

To avoid burning the patient's skin, fold a thin cloth or pillowcase over the heating pad; use tape, ties, or a gauze roll to hold the pad in place. Never use pins. Observe the skin

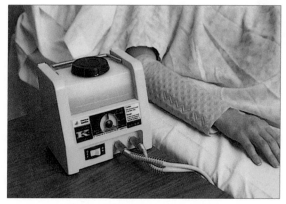

FIGURE **35-22** Aquathermia pad.

frequently for signs of burning. An application lasts only 20 to 30 minutes, and the patient does not lie on the pad.

*Commercial Hot Packs.* Commercially prepared, disposable hot packs apply warm, dry heat to an injured area. Striking, kneading, or squeezing the pack mixes chemicals that release heat. Package directions recommend the time for heat application.

*Hot-Water Bottles.* The hot-water bottle is an economical means of applying heat to an injured body part. Many patients use them in the home. Give patients and family members the following instructions about the safe use of water bottles:

1. Ensure that there are no leaks. Fill the bottle with warm tap water, secure the cap, and turn the bottle upside down.
2. Fill the bag only two-thirds full, expel air at the top, and secure the cap. The bag is then easier to mold over a body part.
3. Wipe off moisture on the outside of the bag.
4. Never apply a water bottle directly to the skin surface. Cover it with a towel or pillowcase.
5. Keep the bottle in place for 20 to 30 minutes.

*Electric Heating Pads.* Another conventional form of heat therapy is the heating pad, an electric coil enclosed within a waterproof pad covered with cotton or flannel cloth. The pad is connected to an electric cord that has a temperature-regulating unit for a high, medium, or low setting. Advise patients to avoid using the high setting and to never lie on the pad. Another precaution to note is that a safety pin inserted through a pad will result in an electrical shock.

*Cold Moist Compresses.* The procedure for applying cold moist compresses is the same as that for warm compresses. Apply cold compresses for 20 minutes at a temperature of 15° C (59° F) to relieve inflammation and swelling. Compresses are clean or sterile. Observe for adverse reac-

tions such as burning or numbness, mottling of the skin, redness, extreme paleness, or a bluish skin discoloration.

*Cold Soaks.* The procedure for preparing cold soaks and immersing a body part is the same as for warm soaks. The desired temperature for a 20-minute soak is 15° C (59° F). Take precautions to protect the patient from chilling.

*Ice Bag or Collar.* For a patient who has a muscle sprain, localized hemorrhage, or hematoma or has undergone dental surgery, an ice bag is ideal to prevent edema formation, control bleeding, and anesthetize the body part. Proper use of the bag requires the following:

1. Fill the bag with water, secure the cap, invert to check for leaks, and pour out the water.
2. Fill the bag two-thirds full with crushed ice so that the bag molds easily over a body part.
3. Release air from the bag by squeezing its sides before securing the cap (because excess air interferes with conduction of cold).
4. Wipe off excess moisture.
5. Cover the bag with a flannel cover, towel, or pillowcase.
6. Apply the bag to the injury site for 30 minutes; you reapply the bag in an hour.

*Commercial Cold Packs.* Commercially prepared single-use ice packs come in various sizes and shapes. When you squeeze or knead the pack, an alcohol-based solution is released inside to create the cold temperature. The soft outer coverings are usually safe to apply directly to the skin surface.

**RESTORATIVE AND CONTINUING CARE.** Some chronic wounds are the result of underlying pathological conditions that continue long after wound healing occurs. Healing for a pressure ulcer or a chronic wound is lengthy and requires continuity of care from the acute care setting to the restorative care setting. In this setting, you use many of the principles and interventions detailed in the acute care section. Continue diligent assessment to identify those patients at risk for impaired skin integrity, and institute preventive measures as needed.

Despite efforts with wound care, wound healing will not occur if the patient is malnourished. Tissue repair requires more protein, carbohydrates, fats, vitamins, minerals, water,

## OUTCOME EVALUATION

TABLE 35-8

| Nursing Action | Patient Response/Finding | Achievement of Outcome |
|---|---|---|
| Measure wound size. | Ulcer is 2 × 2.5 cm. | Wound diameter is decreasing. |
| Observe wound and any drainage, noting color, amount, and type of drainage. | Serous drainage present. Wound color remains beefy red. | Ulcer remains, but signs of healing are present. |
| Palpate underlying skin around wound. | Underlying skin around wound remains intact with no palpable tissue change. | No evidence of advancing pressure ulcer or tissue damage. |
| Ask Mr. Ahmed about any discomfort or new sensations of burning or tingling at wound site. | Mr. Ahmed does not notice any decrease in level of comfort or any new "pain or burning." | No evidence of new tissue damage. |
| Ask Mr. Ahmed about his food intake. | Mr. Ahmed reports that his appetite is increasing, and he eats most of his meals. Review of caloric count for the last week documents that Mr. Ahmed's nutritional intake has increased. | He is improving nutritional intake. |

## EVALUATION

Lynda Abraham has completed her clinical experience with Mr. Ahmed. His pressure ulcer is still present, but it is reduced in size and is healing. No other sites of nonblanchable erythema were noted, and the rest of his skin remains intact. He is going to be discharged to his home in 2 days. Lynda has taught Mr. Ahmed's wife how to do the dressing changes and how to assess her husband's skin for signs of increased risk for or actual further skin breakdown. On her last day of this clinical experience, Lynda has prepared to refer her patient to a home care agency. Lynda, with the help of her instructor, has devised a plan of care for the home; Lynda and her instructor are meeting with the home care nurse today when she visits Mr. and Mrs. Ahmed in the hospital.

**Documentation Note**

"Small amount of serous drainage from stage II pressure ulcer on his sacrum. Wound is 2.5 × 2.5 cm × ⅛ inch deep, with beefy red tissue. Mrs. Ahmed cleansed the wound with normal saline and applied a hydrocolloid dressing. Maintained aseptic technique and correctly assessed skin. She reminds her husband to change his position every 1½ to 2 hours. Awaiting visit from home care nurse."

and oxygen than normal tissue metabolism (see Chapter 31). In addition, the delivery of nutritional substances to tissues depends on a healthy circulatory system. Malnutrition causes an insufficient supply of the necessary nutritional elements and alterations in blood vessel integrity. Therefore work closely with dietitians to provide a well-balanced diet, and educate the patient about the importance of good dietary habits. For patients weakened or debilitated by illness, supportive nutritional therapies will become necessary. The surgical patient who is well nourished and has no complications requires at least 0.8 g of protein per kilogram daily for nutritional maintenance. Supplemental tube feedings (enteral feedings) introduce nutrients directly into the gastrointestinal tract. If a patient is unable to tolerate enteral feedings, the physician or health care provider will often order parenteral (intravenously administered) nutrition.

The patient with a wound that restricts mobility or has the potential to compromise the function of a joint sometimes requires additional physical and/or occupational therapy. Work closely with the physical therapist in monitoring the patient's activity and tolerance for exercise. It is important to optimize activity within the patient's physical limitations and return function as rapidly as possible.

### ✸ Evaluation

**PATIENT CARE.** You evaluate nursing interventions for reducing and treating pressure ulcers determining the patient's response to nursing therapies and determining whether you achieved each goal (Table 35-8). The primary goals are to prevent injury to the skin and tissues, to reduce injury to the skin and underlying tissues, and to restore skin integrity. Also evaluate specific interventions designed to promote skin integrity and to teach the patient and family to reduce future threats to skin integrity. In addition, evaluate the patient's and family's need for additional support services, and initiate the referral process.

**PATIENT EXPECTATIONS.** The patient and caregiver need to understand how to prevent or treat pressure ulcers. Some patients enter into the wound-healing phase with unrealistic expectations regarding duration of care. Collect evaluation data about the patient's perception of wound care management. Patients with chronic wounds are often cared for in their home settings and have certain expectations about their level of comfort, lifestyle, independence, and privacy. Therefore you determine from the patient whether you respected and met his or her expectations.

## KEY CONCEPTS

- Wounds with partial-thickness tissue loss heal by epidermal repair, and full-thickness wounds heal by forming scar tissue.
- A clean surgical incision with little tissue loss heals by primary intention.
- Wounds healing by secondary intention proceed through three overlapping phases: inflammation, proliferation, and remodeling.
- When there is extensive tissue loss, a wound heals by secondary intention.
- The chances of wound infection are greater when the wound contains dead or necrotic tissue, when foreign bodies lie on or near the wound, and when blood supply and tissue defenses are reduced.
- Physical stress from vomiting, coughing, or sudden muscular contraction causes separation of wound edges, dehiscence.
- Wound assessment includes anatomical location, size (dimensions and depth of wound), type and percentage of wound tissue, volume and color of wound drainage, and condition of surrounding skin.

- Wound drains remove secretions within tissue layers to promote wound closure.
- Never collect a wound culture from old drainage.
- Principles of wound management include controlling or eliminating the cause, providing systemic support to reduce existing and potential cofactors, and maintaining a physiological local wound environment.
- A moist environment supports wound healing.
- When cleaning wounds or drain sites, clean from the least to most contaminated area.
- Apply a bandage or binder in a manner that does not impair circulation or irritate the skin.
- The safe use of heat or cold therapy requires an assessment of the patient's sensory function, identification of risk factors, and understanding of the physiological effects of heat and cold.
- An acute sprain, fracture, or bruise responds best to cold applications.
- Warm applications are effective for improving circulation to wound sites and promoting muscle relaxation.

## CRITICAL THINKING IN PRACTICE

1. A patient has two Jackson-Pratt drainage collectors on the right side of the abdomen. What nursing assessments do you make to ensure proper functioning of this system? Can you delegate any aspects of care for this type of drainage collector? Explain the rationale for your answer.
2. Your 85-year-old African-American male patient is admitted to the hospital with a diagnosis of left cerebral vascular accident. He has right-sided weakness, and he cannot turn or walk without assistance. He also has difficulty swallowing, and he is incontinent of urine and stool. What risk factors, if any, for pressure ulcers does this pa-

tient have? What characteristics do you assess this patient for to monitor for a stage I pressure ulcer? How do you accomplish this?
3. Upon assessing a patient for risk development of a pressure ulcer using the Braden Scale, you note that she scores very low on the moisture subscale. You determine that the patient is incontinent of liquid stool at least 4 times in 24 hours. What are some of the possible interventions that you will plan for this patient to protect her skin from fecal incontinence?

## NCLEX® REVIEW

1. When repositioning an immobile patient, you notice redness over a bony prominence. When the area is assessed, the red spot blanches with fingertip pressure, indicating:
   1. A local skin infection requiring antibiotics
   2. This patient has sensitive skin and requires special bed linen
   3. A stage III pressure ulcer, needing the appropriate dressing
   4. Blanchable hyperemia
2. Pressure injury to the skin results from:
   1. Blood vessel damage from repeated injections
   2. Continual exposure of the skin to fecal or urinary incontinence
   3. Compression of the skin by two surfaces for a prolonged period of time
   4. Excessive dryness of the epidermis, allowing damage to the dermis

3. The topical management of a clean, granular wound healing by secondary intention requires:
   1. A moist wound dressing
   2. An antibiotic cream applied twice a day
   3. Whirlpool treatments to stimulate granulation tissue
   4. A treatment plan that allows the wound to be exposed to air for 15 minutes twice a day
4. When obtaining a wound culture to determine the presence of a wound infection, the specimen should be taken from:
   1. The necrotic tissue
   2. The wound drainage
   3. The drainage on the dressing
   4. Clean, healthy-looking tissue
5. Postoperatively the patient with a closed abdominal wound reports a sudden "pop" after coughing. When you examine the surgical wound site, the sutures are

open and pieces of small bowel are noted at the bottom of the now opened wound. The correct intervention would be:

1. To allow the area to be exposed to air until all drainage has stopped
2. To place several cold packs over the area, protecting the skin around the wound
3. To cover the area with sterile saline-soaked towels and immediately notify the surgical team
4. To cover the area with sterile gauze, place a tight binder over the area, and ask the patient to remain in bed for 30 minutes

6. Serous drainage from a wound is defined as:
   1. Fresh bleeding
   2. Thick and yellow
   3. Clear, watery plasma
   4. Beige to brown and foul smelling

7. Interventions to manage a patient who is experiencing fecal and urinary incontinence include:
   1. Use of a large absorbent diaper, changing when saturated
   2. Keeping the buttocks exposed to air at all times
   3. Utilization of an incontinence cleanser, followed by application of a moisture-barrier ointment
   4. Frequent cleansing, application of an ointment, and covering the area with a thick absorbent towel

8. The best description of a hydrocolloid dressing is:
   1. A seaweed derivative that is highly absorptive
   2. Premoistened gauze, placed over a granulating wound
   3. A debriding enzyme that is used to remove necrotic tissue
   4. A dressing that forms a gel that interacts with the wound surface

9. A binder placed around a surgical patient with a new abdominal wound is indicated for:
   1. Collection of wound drainage
   2. Reduction of abdominal swelling
   3. Reduction of stress on the abdominal incision
   4. Stimulation of peristalsis (return of bowel function) from direct pressure

10. Application of a warm compress is indicated:
    1. To relieve edema
    2. For a patient who is shivering
    3. To promote healing by stimulating blood flow
    4. To protect bony prominences from pressure ulcers

11. Vacuum Assisted Closure is defined as:
    1. Wound protection from bacteria or other contaminants, preventing overgrowth of bacteria in the wound base
    2. A system that provides continuous irrigant in the wound bed, stimulating granulation tissue
    3. A wound management system that uses negative pressure to the wound to promote and accelerate healing
    4. A method to clean the wound bed of necrotic tissue without the use of toxic solutions

## REFERENCES

Agency for Health Care Policy and Research, Panel for Prediction and Prevention of Pressure Ulcers in Adults: *Pressure ulcers in adults: prediction and prevention,* Clinical Practice Guideline No. 3, AHCPR Pub No. 92-0047, Rockville, Md, 1992, Agency for Health Care Policy and Research, Public Health Service, U.S. Department of Health and Human Services.

Agency for Health Care Policy and Research, Panel for the Treatment of Pressure Ulcers in Adults: *Treatment of pressure ulcers,* Clinical Practice Guideline No.15, Pub No. 95-0653, Rockville, Md, 1994, Agency for Health Care Policy and Research, Public Health Service, U.S. Department of Health and Human Services.

Ayello EA, Braden B: How and why do pressure ulcer risk assessment, *Adv Skin Wound Care* 15(3):125, 2002.

Ayello EA, Lyder CH: Pressure ulcers in person of color: race and ethnicity. In Cuddigan J, editor: Pressure ulcers in America: prevalence, incidence, and implications for the future, Reston, Va, 2001, National Pressure Ulcer Advisory Panel.

Ayello EA and others: Pressure ulcers. In Baranoski S, Ayello EA. *Wound care essentials: practice principles,* Philadelphia, 2004, Lippincott Williams & Wilkins.

Baranoski S, Ayello EA: Wound assessment. In Baranoski S, Ayello EA. *Wound care essentials: practice principles,* Philadelphia, 2004, Lippincott Williams & Wilkins.

Bates-Jensen B: New pressure ulcer status tool, *Decubitus* 3(3):14, 1990.

Bennett MA: Report of the Task Force on the implications for darkly pigmented intact skin in the prediction and prevention of pressure ulcers, *Adv Wound Care* 8(6):34, 1995.

Bergstrom N and others: A clinical trial of the Braden Scale for predicting pressure sore risk, *Nurs Clin North Am* 22(2):417, 1987a.

Bergstrom N and others: The Braden Scale for predicting pressure sore risk, *Nur Res* 36:205, 1987b.

Bergstrom NL and others: Predicting pressure ulcer risk: a multisite study of the predictive validity of the Braden Scale, *Nurs Res* 47(5):261, 1998.

Boynton PR and others: Meeting the challenges of healing chronic wounds in older adults, *Nurs Clin North Am* 34(4):921, 1999.

Broussard CL and others: Adjuvant wound therapies. In Bryant RA, editor: *Acute and chronic wounds: nursing management,* ed 2, St. Louis, 2000, Mosby.

Bryant RA, editor: *Acute and chronic wounds: nursing management,* ed 2, St. Louis, 2000, Mosby.

Bryant RA, Rolstad BS: Examining threats to skin integrity, *Ostomy Wound Manage* 47(6):18, 2001.

Bryant RA and others: Pressure ulcer. In Bryant RA, editor: *Acute and chronic wounds: nursing management,* ed 2, St. Louis, 2000, Mosby.

Capasso V, Munro BH: The cost and efficiency of two wound treatments, *AORN J* 77(5):984, 2003.

Chua PC and others: Vacuum Assisted Closure, *Am J Nurs* 100(12):45, 2000.

Dallan LE and others: Pain management and wounds. In Baranoski S, Ayello EA. *Wound care essentials: practice principles*, Philadelphia, 2004, Lippincott Williams & Wilkins.

Dochterman JM, Bulechek GM, editors: *Nursing interventions classification (NIC)*, ed 4, St. Louis, 2004, Mosby.

Fader M, Bain D, Cottenden A: Effects of absorbent incontinence pads on pressure management mattresses, *J Adv Nurs* 48(6):569, 2004.

Gray M, Doughty DB: Clean versus sterile technique when changing wound dressings, *J Wound Ostomy Continence Nurs* 28(3):125, 2001.

Groeneveld A and others: The prevalence of pressure ulcers in a tertiary care pediatric and adult hospital, *J Wound Ostomy Continence Nurs* 31(3):108, 2004.

Henderson CT and others: Draft definition of stage I pressure ulcers: inclusion of persons with darkly pigmented skin, *Adv Wound Care* 10(5):16, 1997.

Hess CT: How to use gauze dressings, *Nursing* 30(9):88, 2000.

Jones V, Bale S, Harding K: Acute and chronic wound healing. In Baranoski S, Ayello EA: *Wound care essentials: practice principles*, Philadelphia, 2004, Lippincott Williams & Wilkins.

KCI USA: *The V.A.C.: Vacuum Assisted Closure—guidelines for use, physician and caregiver reference manual*, Product information, San Antonio, Tex, 2003.

Krasner DL: Managing wound pain in patients with vacuum assisted closure devices, *Ostomy Wound Manage* 48(5):38, 2002.

Landis EM: Micro-injection studies of capillary blood pressure in human skin, *Heart* 15:209, 1930.

Mathus-Vliegen EMH: Old age, malnutrition and pressure sores: an ill fated alliance, *J Gerontol A Biol Sci Med Sci* 59(4):355, 2004.

Mechanick JI: Practical aspects of nutritional support of wound-healing patients, *Am J Surg* 188 (suppl to July 2004):52S, 2004.

Mendez-Eastman S: When wounds won't heal, *RN* 61(10):20, 1998.

Moorhead S, Johnson M, Maas M: *Nursing outcomes classification (NOC)*, ed 3, St. Louis, 2004, Mosby.

Myer AH: The effects of aging on wound healing, *Top Geriatr Rehabil* 19(2):1, 2000.

National Pressure Ulcer Advisory Panel: Pressure ulcer prevalence, cost and risk assessment: consensus development conference statement, *Decubitus* 2(2):24, 1989.

National Pressure Ulcer Advisory Panel: *Facts about reverse staging*, NPUAP position paper, 2000, http://www.npuap.org.

National Pressure Ulcer Advisory Panel: *PNUAP staging report*, 2003, http://www.npuap.org.

National Pressure Ulcer Advisory Panel: *Pressure ulcer staging*, 2005, http://www.npuap.org.postin4.html.

Nelson DB, Dilloway MA: Principles, products, and practical aspects of wound care, *Crit Care Nurs Q* 25(1):33, 2002.

O'Brien JM, Reilly NJ: Comparison of tape products on skin integrity, *Adv Wound Care* 8(6):26, 1995.

Pieper B: Mechanical forces: pressure, shear, friction. In Bryant RA, editor: *Acute and chronic wounds: nursing management*, ed 2, St. Louis, 2000, Mosby.

Quigley SM, Curley MAQ: Skin integrity in the pediatric population: preventing and managing pressure ulcers, *J Soc Pediatr Nurs* 1(1):7, 1996.

Ramundo J, Wells J: Wound debridement. In Bryant RA: *Acute and chronic wounds: nursing management*, St. Louis, 2000, Mosby.

Rolstad BS and others: Principles of wound management. In Bryant RA, editor: *Acute and chronic wounds: nursing management*, ed 2, St. Louis, 2000, Mosby.

Rook JL: Wound care pain management, *Adv Wound Care* 9(6):24, 1996.

Schultz GS and others: Wound bed preparation: a systematic approach to wound management, *Wound Repair Regen* 11(suppl 1): S1, 2003.

Singhal A and others: Options for nonsurgical debridement of necrotic wounds, *Adv Skin Wound Care* 14:96, 2001.

Stotts NA: Wound infection: diagnosis and management. In Bryant RA, editor: *Acute and chronic wounds: nursing management*, ed 2, St. Louis, 2000, Mosby.

Szor JK, Bourguignon C: Description of pressure ulcer pain at rest and dressing change, *J Wound Ostomy Continence Nurs* 26(3):115, 1999.

Thomas C: Specialty beds: decision-making made easy, *Ostomy Wound Manage* 23:51, 1989.

Thomas DR and others: Pressure ulcer scale for healing: derivation and validation of the PUSH Tool, *Adv Wound Care* 10(5):96, 1997.

Trelease CC: Developing standards for wound care, *Ostomy Wound Manage* 20:46, 1988.

Waldrop J, Doughty D: Wound healing physiology in acute and chronic wounds. In Bryant RA, editor: *Acute and chronic wounds: nursing management*, ed 2, St. Louis, 2000, Mosby.

West JM, Gimbel M: Acute surgical and traumatic wound healing. In Bryant RA: *Acute and chronic wounds: nursing management*, ed 2, St. Louis, 2000, Mosby.

Wound, Ostomy and Continence Nurses Society: *Guideline for prevention and management of pressure ulcers*, WOCN Clinical Practice Guidelines Series, Glenview, Ill, 2003, The Society.

Wysocki AB: Evaluating and managing open skin wounds: colonization versus infection, *AACN Clin Issues* 13(3):382, 2002.

# CHAPTER 36

# Sensory Alterations

## MEDIA RESOURCES

CD COMPANION    *evolve*  WEBSITE

http://evolve.elsevier.com/Potter/basic

- **NCLEX® Review**
- **Audio Glossary**
- **English/Spanish Audio Glossary**

## OBJECTIVES

- Differentiate among the processes of reception, perception, and reaction to sensory stimuli.
- Discuss common causes and effects of sensory alterations.
- Discuss common sensory changes that occur with aging.
- Identify factors to assess in determining a patient's sensory status.
- Describe behaviors indicating sensory alterations.

- Develop a care plan for patients with visual, auditory, tactile, gustatory, and olfactory alterations.
- Describe nursing interventions that promote effective communication with patients who have sensory alterations.
- Describe conditions in the health care agency or patient's home that you will adjust to promote meaningful sensory stimulation.
- Discuss ways to maintain a safe environment for patients with sensory alterations.

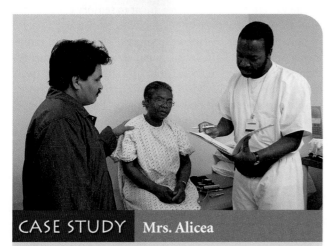

## CASE STUDY  Mrs. Alicea

Mrs. Alicea is a 73-year-old woman who is at the senior health center for her routine 6-month checkup. She has been visiting the senior center on a regular basis for the past 8 years. Mrs. Alicea has lived alone since her husband died 1 year ago. She lives in a single-story, four-room home a few miles away from the health center. Her son, Rico, lives 5 minutes away. Rico drives Mrs. Alicea to her health care visits. Six months ago Mrs. Alicea reported a progressive hearing loss. Today when she enters the clinic she reports "having trouble seeing."

Peter Morris, a 33-year-old junior nursing student assigned to the senior health center, is learning to conduct assessments and to develop health promotion plans for visiting patients. For the past month, Peter has been attending his clinical rotation at the center and participating in teaching health promotion activities. He is enjoying this rotation because he is learning more about geriatric patients and is finding that they are very independent and capable of productive lifestyles.

## KEY TERMS

accommodation, p. 1071
age-related macular degeneration, p. 1070
auditory, p. 1069
cataracts, p. 1070
diabetic retinopathy, p. 1070
glaucoma, p. 1070
gustatory, p. 1069
Meniere's disease, p. 1072
olfactory, p. 1069
ototoxic, p. 1071
presbycusis, p. 1071

presbyopia, p. 1072
proprioception, p. 1069
refractive errors, p. 1078
sensory deficits, p. 1070
sensory deprivation, p. 1070
sensory overload, p. 1070
tactile, p. 1069
tinnitus, p. 1071
visual, p. 1069

People are unique because they are able to sense a variety of stimuli from changes in their environment. To maintain coordination, the body assimilates sensory input from vestibular, visual, and proprioceptive systems (Sandhaus, 2002). The sense organs of sight (**visual**), hearing (**auditory**), touch (**tactile**), smell (**olfactory**), taste (**gustatory**), balance, and the body's ability to sense its position and movement in space (**proprioception**) produce special senses and initiate reflexes important for homeostasis. People learn about the environment from healthy sensory organs. When sensory function is altered, the patient's ability to relate to and function within the environment changes. As a nurse, you must understand and help to meet the needs of patients with sensory alterations and recognize when patients are at risk for developing sensory problems. Your nursing care helps patients learn to alter their environment for improved safety.

## Scientific Knowledge Base

### Normal Sensation

When a person's nervous system is intact, he or she feels and reacts to sensations. Perception or awareness of sensations depends on a region of the cerebral cortex where specialized brain cells interpret the quality and nature of each sensory stimulus. Sensory experiences include reception, perception, and reaction. People react to stimuli that are most meaningful to them. When a person attempts to react to every stimulus within his or her environment or when stimuli are lacking, sensory alterations occur.

### Types of Sensory Alterations

Many factors influence the capacity to receive or perceive sensations (Box 36-1). In your nursing experience you will care for patients with **sensory deficits, sensory deprivation,** and **sensory overload.** When patients suffer from more than one sensory alteration, their ability to function and relate within the environment becomes impaired.

**SENSORY DEFICITS.** Four major diseases cause impaired vision in Americans age 40 and over. They are **age-related macular degeneration, glaucoma, cataracts,** and **diabetic retinopathy** (National Eye Institute, 2004a). The National Eye Institute predicts that age-related macular degeneration will affect 2.9 million people; glaucoma, 3.3 million people; cataracts, 30.1 million people; and diabetic retinopathy, 7.2 million people by 2020.

A sensory deficit occurs when problems with sensory reception or perception exist (Box 36-2). Patients are not able to receive certain stimuli (e.g., light and sound), or stimuli are distorted (e.g., blurred vision from cataracts and abnormal taste sensation from xerostomia). A sudden sensory loss caused by injury or as a side effect to medications (Box 36-3) causes fear, anger, and feelings of helplessness. Some patients withdraw socially to cope with the loss (Moore and Miller, 2003). In addition, the patient's safety is threatened because the person is unable to respond normally to stimuli. When a deficit is chronic or develops gradually, the patient learns to rely on unaffected senses. Some senses even become more acute to compensate for an alteration. For example, a blind patient often develops an acute sense of hearing. Changes in sensory deficits cause patients to change their behaviors in adaptive or maladaptive ways.

**SENSORY DEPRIVATION.** Sensory deprivation occurs when inadequate quality or quantity of stimuli impairs perception. Reduced sensory input (hearing loss), confusion, and a restricted environment (bed rest) are three types of sensory deprivation. These effects sometimes produce cognitive changes such as the inability to solve problems, poor task performance, and disorientation. Second, affective changes, which include boredom, restlessness, increased anxiety, or emotional liability, occur. Lastly, perceptual changes such as reduced attention span, disorganized visual and motor coordination, and confusion of sleeping and waking states also occur.

Children often demonstrate behaviors related to sensory deprivation by a higher-than-normal level of anxiety that causes restlessness, difficulty with problem solving, and depression (Hockenberry and others, 2003). In adults the symptoms of sensory deprivation are similar to psychological illness, confusion, symptoms of severe electrolyte imbalance, or the influence of psychotropic drugs. Accurate diagnosis of a problem is crucial.

**SENSORY OVERLOAD.** When a person receives multiple sensory stimuli, the brain has difficulty distinguishing the stimuli that causes a sensory overload to occur. The person no longer perceives the environment in a way that makes sense. Overload prevents a meaningful response to a stimulus by the brain. As a result, thoughts race, attention moves in many directions, and restlessness occurs. The patient demonstrates panic, confusion, and aggressiveness. Sleep loss is common. Sensory overload causes a state similar to sensory deprivation.

Acutely ill patients easily develop sensory overload because of noise in the health care environment. The constant monitoring of patients, noise from equipment, and the nursing activities of turning, repositioning, and administering treatments bombard patients with stimuli. Some patients are more sensitive to sensory overload than others. Behavioral changes are easily confused with mood swings or disorientation.

## Nursing Knowledge Base

Thirty-four million Americans are hearing impaired (Sommer and Sommer, 2002). Eighty million Americans have eye diseases that will lead to blindness, while 14 million will have low vision (American Federation for the Blind, 2004b). By 2020, 5.5 million Americans over the age of 40 will have a diagnosis of blindness or low vision (National Eye Institute, 2004a). The population of the United States is growing older. The American Association of Retired Persons (AARP) (2004) estimated that 71.5 million people will reach 65 years of age by 2030. As a nurse, stay informed of new health care and nursing knowledge as it pertains to the older adult population and the effects of diverse sensory changes.

There is a relationship between hearing loss, self-esteem, and communication (Slaven, 2003). Hearing impairments cause a person to experience loss and fear. A patient feels a loss of control, independence, or self-esteem. Feelings of grief, anger, isolation, depression, and loneliness are also common. Knowledge regarding the effects of sensory loss is important for you to assess how a sensory impairment influences a patient's self-concept and ability to communicate and function in the everyday world.

Older adults who experience sensory deficits often withdraw from social activities. The risk of social isolation, depression, fear, and low self-esteem interferes with their ability to care for themselves and interact with others. According to research, older adult patients who have a good support system, understand their vision loss, and have a higher income and education level have a better attitude toward their sensory loss

## BOX 36-1  Factors That Influence Sensory Function

### Age

**Infants**

Binocular vision begins at 6 weeks and is well established by 4 months. During the second year of life, infants discriminate shapes, objects, and colors.

Neonates respond to loud noises. Within a year infants visually locate the source of noises.

Newborns react to strong odors such as alcohol and vinegar by turning their heads. Newborns discriminate their own mother's milk.

**Children**

Refractive errors are the most common types of visual disorders in children and are treated with corrective lenses. Serious visual impairment affects a child's ability to play and socialize. All senses develop and become coordinated with each other. A toddler will visually inspect an object, turn it over, taste it, smell it, and touch it several times while investigating it (Hockenberry and others, 2003).

**Adults**

Visual changes include presbyopia and the need for glasses for reading (ages 40 to 50). Also, the cornea, which assists with light refraction to the retina, becomes flatter and thicker. These aging changes lead to astigmatism. Pigment loss from the iris and collagen fibers build up in the anterior chamber, which increases the risk of glaucoma by decreasing the reabsorption of intraocular fluid (Ebersole and others, 2004).

**Older Adults**

Hearing changes associated with aging include decreased hearing acuity, speech intelligibility, and pitch discrimination, which is referred to as **presbycusis.** Low-pitched sounds are easiest to hear, but it is difficult to hear conversation over background noise. It is also difficult to discriminate consonants (*f, z, s, th, ch, p, k, t,* and *g*). Vowels that have a low pitch are easier to hear. Speech sounds are distorted, and there is a delayed reception and reaction to speech. A decrease in active sebaceous glands causes the cerumen to become dry and completely obstruct the external auditory canal (Ebersole and others, 2004).

Visual changes include reduced visual fields, increased glare sensitivity, impaired night vision, reduced **accommodation,** reduced depth perception, and reduced color discrimination. Many of these symptoms occur because the pupils in the older adult take longer to dilate and constrict secondary to weaker iris muscles. Color vision decreases because the retina is duller and the lens yellows. Older adults require 3 times as much light to see objects as they did when they were in their 20s (Ebersole and others, 2004).

Olfactory and taste changes begin around age 50 and include a loss of cells in the olfactory bulb of the brain and a decrease in the number of sensory cells in the nasal lining. Reduced sensitivity to odors is common. Aging causes taste buds to atrophy, to lose efficiency in relaying flavor, and to reduce in number. Reduced taste discrimination is common. Sweet taste is the last sense to go (Ebersole and others, 2004).

Proprioceptive changes include an increased difficulty with balance and coordination. Older adults cannot avoid obstacles as quickly, nor are they able to prevent an accident from happening to themselves when fast action is necessary. The automatic response to protect and brace oneself when falling is slower (Ebersole and others, 2004).

Older adults experience tactile changes, including declining sensitivity to pain, pressure, and temperature secondary to peripheral vascular disease and neuropathies (Ebersole and others, 2004).

### Medications

**Ototoxic** medications (see Box 36-3), such as analgesics, antibiotics, or diuretics, affect hearing acuity, balance, or both, with the most common symptom being **tinnitus** (ringing in the ears). Ototoxicity causes a progressive or continuing hearing loss that in many patients goes unnoticed (McKenry and Salerno, 2003). Hearing loss is not always permanent depending upon the extent of damage and the length of time that the drug is given. Patients with renal failure have an increased sensitivity to ototoxic drugs (McKenry and Salerno, 2003).

### Environment

Excessive environmental stimuli result in sensory overload, marked by confusion, disorientation, and inability to make decisions. Restricted environmental stimulation leads to sensory deprivation. Poor quality of environment worsens sensory impairment.

### Preexisting Illnesses

Peripheral vascular disease causes reduced sensation in the extremities and impaired cognition. Chronic diabetes causes reduced vision or blindness or peripheral neuropathy. Some neurological disorders, such as stroke, impair sensory reception (Phipps and others, 2003).

### Smoking

Chronic tobacco use atrophies the taste buds and affects olfactory function.

### Noise Levels

Constant exposure to high noise levels causes hearing loss.

---

(Houde and Huff, 2003). Education by the nurse about disease process, available social services, assistive devices, and the need for annual physical examinations helps provide the older patient with better coping abilities and health maintenance.

Managing patients with sensory alterations challenges you to apply nursing research and information from your practice to assist patients with participating in their environment, remaining socially interactive, and continuing to be productive. In addition, your application of critical thinking principles helps you to promote patients' sensory function and to protect them from possible injury (Box 36-4).

| BOX 36-2 | Common Sensory Deficits |
|---|---|

### Visual

**Presbyopia**—Gradual decline in ability of the lens to accommodate or to focus on close objects. Reduces ability to see near objects clearly.

**Cataract**—Cloudy or opaque areas in part of the lens or the entire lens. Interferes with passage of light through the lens, causing problems with glare and blurred vision. Cataracts usually develop gradually, without pain, redness, or tearing in the eye (Houde and Huff, 2003).

**Dry eyes**—Result when tear glands produce too few tears, resulting in itching, burning, or even reduced vision.

**Glaucoma**—A slowly progressive increase in intraocular pressure that causes progressive pressure against the optic nerve, resulting in peripheral visual loss, decreased visual acuity with difficulty adapting to darkness, and a halo effect around lights, if untreated (Houde and Huff, 2003).

**Diabetic retinopathy**—Pathological changes secondary to increased pressure in the blood vessels of the retina result in decreased vision or vision loss due to hemorrhage and macular edema (Walker and Rodgers, 2002).

**Age-related macular degeneration**—The macula (specialized portion of the retina responsible for central vision) degenerates as a result of aging and loses its ability to function efficiently. First signs include blurring of reading matter, distortion or loss of central vision, sensitivity to glare, and distortion of objects (Houde and Huff, 2003).

### Hearing

**Presbycusis**—A common progressive hearing disorder in older adults.

**Cerumen accumulation**—Buildup and hardening of earwax in the external auditory canal causes conduction deafness.

### Balance

**Dizziness and disequilibrium**—Common condition in older adulthood, usually resulting from vestibular dysfunction and precipitated by change in position of the head to the rest of the body.

**Meniere's disease**—Cause is unknown but diagnosis is based on clinical symptoms of intermittent hearing loss, vertigo, tinnitus, and pressure sensation in ears (Ervin, 2004; Meniere's Disease Information Center, 2004).

### Taste

**Xerostomia**—Decrease in salivary production that leads to thicker mucus and a dry mouth. Interferes with the ability to eat and leads to appetite and nutritional problems.

### Neurological

**Peripheral neuropathy**—Commonly associated with diabetes, alcoholism, and peripheral vascular disease (Ebersole and others, 2004). Symptoms include numbness and tingling of the affected area and stumbling gait.

**Hemiplegia**—Caused by a thrombus, hemorrhage, or embolus affecting a blood vessel leading to or within the brain. Creates altered proprioception with marked incoordination and imbalance. Loss of sensation and motor function in extremities controlled by the affected area of the brain also occurs.

| BOX 36-3 | Examples of Medications Reported to Cause Ototoxicity |
|---|---|

**Antibiotics**

Aminoglycosides
Clarithromycin
Vancomycin
Polymyxin B
Polymyxin C
Erythromycin

**Analgesics/NSAIDs**

Aspirin
Ibuprofen

**Diuretics**

Ethacrynic acid
Furosemide
Bumetanide

**Antineoplastic Agents**

Bleomycin
Cisplatin

From McKenry L, Salerno E: *Pharmacology in nursing*, ed 21, St. Louis, 2003, Mosby.
*NSAID,* Nonsteroidal antiinflammatory drug.

## Critical Thinking

### Synthesis

As you apply the nursing process for patients with sensory alterations, you need to analyze and integrate information from a variety of sources. Learn to anticipate the kind of information necessary to form good clinical judgments. A combination of past patient care experiences and the application of scientific and nursing knowledge assists you in selecting an individualized plan of care for the patient.

**KNOWLEDGE.** A number of factors cause sensory alterations. Knowledge of those factors, the normal components of a sensory experience, and anatomy and physiology help you to understand how a particular alteration affects a patient's function. Knowing the pathophysiological changes of sensory organ disorders will also help you to anticipate how sensory changes affect a patient. When you are able to identify characteristics of sensory alterations and the interventions to minimize them, you implement a comprehensive plan of care.

Depending on the patient's problem, use your knowledge of communication principles (see Chapter 9) to select the best method to communicate with the patient. Patients with

USING EVIDENCE IN PRACTICE

**Research Summary**

A study of older men with impaired vision secondary to age-related macular degeneration interviewed the men at home and asked them to describe the effect of their vision changes on everyday life. The men cherished their present level of independence, and they became creative in developing strategies to overcome their problems. In addition, they confronted their fear of the unknown with hope and optimism.

**Application to Nursing Practice**

This information assists in understanding the patient's continued need for independence. As you develop a plan of care for visually impaired patients, encourage the patients to discuss what they think is important in their care and what goals are important to them. Also, because these patients want to remain independent, some will not ask for assistance when they need it. Work with patients and families to determine how to make the environment safe while promoting the patients' independence and meeting their individualized health care needs (American Federation for the Blind, 2004a). Use large print, and post telephone numbers of friends or social service agencies next to the patient's phone for easy access. When patients are losing their eyesight, provide factual information about the disease and answer their questions truthfully.

Data from American Federation for the Blind: *Creating a comfortable environment for older individuals who are visually impaired,* 2004a, http://www.afb.org; Moore L, Miller M: Older men's experiences of living with severe visual impairment, *J Adv Nurs* 43(1):10, 2003.

hearing impairment require different communication approaches to obtain a complete and accurate nursing assessment and to deliver interventions effectively. You also need to have a good knowledge of pharmacology because a variety of medications affect sensory function. Being able to anticipate the side effects of medications allows you to prepare patients for possible sensory changes.

**EXPERIENCE.** Many of us have experienced altered sensory function or encountered this experience while interacting with family, friends, or patients. Previous personal or clinical experiences with sensory changes help you to anticipate the patient's care needs. How do individuals adapt to hearing aids and glasses? What adjustments do they make to function safely in their homes? What communication techniques are necessary when speaking to individuals with hearing impairment? Such experiences will help you to choose successful nursing interventions when caring for patients in a variety of health care settings.

**ATTITUDES.** Critical thinking attitudes assist you in becoming a more disciplined thinker. Creativity is often necessary to find the right solutions for your patient's problems. For example, living in a nonstimulating home environment may be a cause of your patient's sensory deprivation. Working with the patient, you suggest changes to the environment that improve the quality of stimulation and reduce

the patient's risk for injury. Curiosity applies when a patient shows unexplained behavioral changes. Asking why and being curious help you to assess a less obvious sensory problem.

**STANDARDS.** An important ethical standard to follow when assisting patients with sensory alterations is preservation of autonomy (see Chapter 5). For the patient to regain independence, do not override autonomy with the principle of beneficence. You need to remember that although professionals believe they know what is best, patients have to live with the sensory alteration and adapt to the consequences of their own choices. The Americans with Disabilities Act (ADA) requires health care institutions to provide for interpreters when a patient with disabilities needs to consent for surgery or other invasive procedures in order to establish understanding and to maintain confidentiality (Sommer and Sommer, 2002).

## Nursing Process

### Assessment

When assessing your patients, consider age and other factors that influence sensory function. Collect a complete nursing history by examining how a sensory deficit affects a patient's lifestyle, self-care ability, psychosocial adjustment, health promotion habits, and safety. Focus the assessment on the quality and quantity of stimuli within the patient's environment.

**PATIENTS AT RISK.** Learn to conduct a sensory assessment for any patient at risk for sensory alteration. The older adult is obviously in a high-risk group because of normal physiological changes associated with aging. Older patients often do not report certain sensory changes, assuming the change is a part of aging (Halle, 2002; Moore and Miller, 2003). Patients who are immobilized by bed rest, physical impediments (e.g., casts or traction), or chronic disability are unable to experience all the normal sensations of free movement. Such conditions lead to sensory deprivation. Always remain alert for any behavioral changes common to sensory deprivation. Patients isolated in a health care setting or at home due to conditions such as active tuberculosis are often restricted to a private room and unable to enjoy normal interactions with visitors.

A hospital environment is full of sensory stimuli. When ill or hospitalized, a patient is often confined to an unfamiliar and unresponsive environment. This does not mean that all hospitalized patients experience sensory overload. Assess carefully those patients subjected to high stress levels (e.g., intensive care unit [ICU] environment, long-term hospitalization, and multiple therapies).

**SENSORY STATUS.** The nursing history is a tool for assessing the nature and characteristics of sensory alterations. Assessment categories include the type and extent of sensory impairment, the onset and duration of symptoms, and whether there are factors that aggravate or relieve symptoms. Often you will observe such characteristics by watching the patient perform routine activities of daily living (ADLs) in

## FOCUSED PATIENT ASSESSMENT

**TABLE 36-1**

| Factors to Assess | Questions and Approaches | Physical Assessment Strategies |
|---|---|---|
| Sensory status | Ask if patient has difficulty seeing, hearing, sensing touch, or maintaining balance.<br>Ask when the difficulty started. | Assess patient's vision, hearing, balance, and sense of touch.<br>Observe patient behaviors during conversation and while watching the patient perform IADLs and ADLs.<br>Observe home for factors that obstruct or support vision changes. |
| Self-care management in home and community care settings | Ask if the patient with a visual alteration is able to prepare a meal or write a check.<br>Ask if the patient with decreased tactile sensation is able to dress or bathe safely using hot water. | Observe patient in the home, in the kitchen while preparing a meal.<br>Observe patient during dressing and bathing. |
| Health promotion practices | Ask the patient to explain how he or she practices ear/eye hygiene.<br>Ask if the patient has difficulty with routine care of glasses, hearing aids, contact lenses.<br>Ask patient about activity/work where eye injuries are possible. Is he or she wearing safety glasses/eye shields? Ear noise protective gear? | Find out when the patient last had an eye or ear screening.<br>Observe ear/eye routine care.<br><br>Check for appropriate eye protection with eye shields and safety glasses or face shields (Occupational Safety and Health Administration, 2004). |

the home or health care setting. Table 36-1 provides examples of factors to assess, relevant questions to address with your patient, and appropriate physical assessment strategies.

**PATIENT'S LIFESTYLE.** Learn about a patient's perception of a sensory loss to find out how the patient's quality of life has been influenced. Ask patients to describe any problems the sensory alteration creates for their normal daily routines and lifestyle. Does a sensory alteration change a patient's ability to retain social relationships, continue performing at work or school, or function within the home?

**SOCIALIZATION.** The amount and quality of contact with family members or friends determines whether a patient with sensory alterations becomes isolated. Assess if a patient lives alone and whether family, friends, or neighbors frequently visit. The absence of visitors at home or to a health care setting creates a sense of monotony that contributes to social isolation. Also assess the patient's social skills and level of satisfaction in the support given by family and friends.

**SELF-CARE MANAGEMENT.** A patient's functional ability incorporates ADLs (e.g., grooming, bathing, dressing, and toileting) and instrumental activities of daily living (IADLs) (e.g., grocery shopping, writing a check, and using a phone). If a sensory alteration impairs a patient's functional ability, planning for discharge from a health care setting and providing resources within the home become necessary. You need to consider the activities patients normally do for themselves and how the sensory alteration impairs their functioning (see Table 36-1).

**PSYCHOSOCIAL ADJUSTMENT.** Because sensory changes alter a patient's behavior, family and friends are often the best resources for this information. Some patients are unaware of or unwilling to discuss such changes. Assess if the patient has shown any recent mood swings (e.g., outbursts of anger, depression or fear). Sensory alterations also cause changes in the patient's orientation and ability to concentrate.

**HEALTH PROMOTION PRACTICES.** Assess the daily routines patients follow in maintaining sensory function. The information will determine the patient's need for education or referral to appropriate resources (see Table 36-1).

**HAZARDS.** Make sure the home environment is healthy, comfortable, and safe. A thorough home assessment will help you provide options for ways to make the home safe. First assess the home setting for any hazards that increase the risk for injury (e.g., poorly lit stairs). A home safety checklist is usually available in most home care agencies. The type of sensory alteration makes certain home features more hazardous than others. Patients with visual problems will require more light. Patients with hearing deficits sometimes require safety alarms with visual signals. Those with severe hearing impairments need to have a telecommunication device for the deaf (TDD). The TDD has a keyboard and displays numbers and letters that provide messages to the hearing impaired from another TDD (Sommer and Sommer, 2002).

In a health care setting, assess for any factors that will be dangerous to the patient. Assess a patient's hospital room for clutter, unnecessary equipment, and obstacles in the path leading to the bathroom. Also ask the patient about barriers or obstacles the patient perceives as potentially dangerous.

**MEANINGFUL STIMULI.** Meaningful stimuli reduce the incidence of sensory deprivation. In the home, check for the use of bright colors, comfortable furnishings, adequate lighting, good ventilation, and clean surroundings. Also ob-

## SYNTHESIS IN PRACTICE

While Peter prepares to assess Mrs. Alicea, he recalls what he has learned about the pathophysiology of eye disorders. Peter will focus on the "warning signs" of eye problems, determining which, if any, of the signs Mrs. Alicea has experienced. Because Mrs. Alicea reportedly has hearing and visual losses, Peter will consider the communication approaches best suited for conducting a successful assessment. It will be helpful for Peter to position himself so that Mrs. Alicea is able to see his face clearly. Peter also needs to speak slowly and enunciate words clearly, giving time for Mrs. Alicea to respond to questions. Avoidance of questions answered by "yes" or "no" will require Mrs. Alicea to provide more detailed answers, ensuring that she has heard the questions correctly.

Peter respects Mrs. Alicea's cultural background and explores the role Rico plays in supporting his mother. The Hispanic culture shows respect for elders and authority figures by not maintaining direct eye contact. They also engage in "small talk" before discussing the serious aspects of the interview, because being direct is considered rude (Tate, 2003). Providing time for small talk will help Peter to gather a complete assessment. Self-disclosure is for those whom the individual knows well. It will thus be important for Peter to express caring and respect for Mrs. Alicea to be successful with the assessment. Hispanic patients value health practitioners who are informal and friendly and who include family members in the interactions. Taking time to listen is also important. Family interdependence takes precedence over independence (Galanti, 2003). Rico will play a key role in Mrs. Alicea's ability to maintain self-care. Is Rico the primary individual who offers assistance with IADLs or other activities?

Peter's own grandmother has bilateral cataracts. Peter has witnessed how his grandmother has adjusted in order to continue activities she enjoys. Peter has learned in class that you can make a variety of adaptations to maximize the sensory functions a patient still has. Peter will plan to discover if Mrs. Alicea has made any adaptations in her home environment. Creativity will be an important attitude to exercise.

serve for presence of pets, family pictures, television, a clock, or calendar. In a health care setting, note if patients have roommates, visitors, or any personal items such as pictures. A patient will become disoriented in a barren environment that gives few signals for normal sensory perception. Meaningful stimuli influence the patient's alertness and the ability to participate in self-care.

**ENVIRONMENT.** Excessive environmental stimuli causes sensory overload. In an acute care setting the frequency of observations, tests, and procedures is often stressful to the patient. The location of a patient's room near repetitive or loud noises (e.g., nurses' station or supply room) contribute to sensory overload. In addition, explore a loud television or roommate or a bright room light as possible contributing factors. Patients who are in pain, traction, or restricted by a cast are also at risk for excessive stimulation. Your responsibility as a nurse is to reduce or eliminate excessive stimuli.

**COMMUNICATION METHODS.** To understand the quality of patients' communication, assess whether they have trouble speaking, understanding, reading, or writing. Next, ask the patient what communication method they prefer (Sommer and Sommer, 2002). Patients with existing sensory deficits often develop alternative ways of communicating. Some hearing-impaired patients read lips, use sign language, wear a hearing aid, or read and write notes. The visually impaired learn to detect voice tones and inflections to identify the emotional tone of a conversation. To assess communication methods, sit facing the patient, speaking in a normal tone. Disorganized speech, long periods of silence, or a patient who continually asks you to repeat your sentence indicates a sensory deficit in the patient. Some patients also exhibit signs and symptoms of confusion or respond in an inappropriate manner secondary to their hearing impairment.

**PHYSICAL EXAMINATION.** Patients with known or suspected sensory deficits resulting from visual and hearing losses, spinal cord injury, or peripheral neuropathies will require complete and detailed sensory examinations (see Chapter 13). Table 36-2 summarizes behaviors of sensory deficits. If you suspect the patient has a sensory deprivation, observation during history taking, physical examination, or care will provide information about the person's condition. Also observe the patient's physical appearance and behavior, measure cognitive ability, and assess emotional stability. At this time, also remember that factors other than sensory deprivation or overload cause impaired perception (e.g., medications, pain, or electrolyte imbalances).

**PATIENT EXPECTATIONS.** When conducting an assessment, review the patient's expectations. Some patients enter the health care system willingly, whereas others experience confusion or unfamiliarity in that environment. Many patients have a definite plan as to how they want their care delivered. Some patients expect you to either perform care or provide equipment for them so they will properly care for their sensory aids (glasses or hearing aids). Asking patients what they expect helps you to know if you need special communication methods. Some patients request that family members or friends help with their care. Begin by asking, "What do you expect from the nursing staff to feel you are being well cared for?" "Now that I better understand what affects your ability to see/hear, what do you expect in the care we will be providing you?"

### Nursing Diagnosis

After assessment, review all available data and look for patterns of defining characteristics that represent nursing diagnoses relating to sensory alterations. For example, asking others to repeat spoken words, inappropriate response to questions, head tilting, social avoidance, irritability, ear pain, and withdrawal are defining characteristics for the nursing diagnosis *disturbed sensory perception: auditory*. Validate your findings by collaborating with a colleague or asking the patient to self-rate his or her hearing on a scale of 1 to 10, 1 representing perfect hearing and 10 representing deafness.

| TABLE 36-2 | Behaviors Indicating Sensory Deficits |
|---|---|
| **Behavior Indicating Deficit (Children)** | **Behavior Indicating Deficit (Adults)** |
| **Vision** | |
| Self-stimulation, including eye rubbing, body rocking, sniffing, arm twirling; hitching (using legs to propel while in sitting position) instead of crawling | Poor coordination, squinting, underreaching or overreaching for objects, persistent repositioning of objects, impaired night vision, accidental falls |
| **Hearing** | |
| Frightened when unfamiliar people approach, no reflex or purposeful response to sounds, failure to be awakened by loud noise, slow or absent development of speech, greater response to movement than to sound, avoidance of social interaction with others | Blank looks, decreased attention span, lack of reaction to loud noises, increased volume of speech, positioning of head toward sound, smiling and nodding of head in approval when someone speaks, use of other means of communication such as lip reading or writing, complaints of ringing in ears |
| **Touch** | |
| Inability to perform developmental tasks related to grasping objects or drawing, repeated injury from handling of harmful objects (e.g., hot stove, sharp knife) | Clumsiness, overreaction or underreaction to painful stimulus, failure to respond when touched, avoidance of touch, sensation of pins and needles, numbness |
| **Smell** | |
| Difficult to assess until child is 6 or 7 years old, difficulty discriminating unpleasant odors | Failure to react to noxious or strong odors, increased body odor, decreased sensitivity to odors |
| **Taste** | |
| Inability to tell whether food is salty or sweet, possible ingestion of strange-tasting things | Change in appetite, excessive use of seasoning and sugar, complaints about taste of food, weight change |
| **Position Sense** | |
| Clumsiness, extraneous movement, excessive arm swinging in those with hyperactivity or learning difficulty | Poor balance and spatial orientation, shuffling gait, reduced response to brace self when falling, more precise and deliberate movements |

The following are examples of nursing diagnoses that may be used for patients with sensory alterations.

- Anxiety
- Disturbed body image
- Fear
- Hopelessness
- Risk for injury
- Deficient knowledge
- Risk for loneliness
- Powerlessness
- Bathing/hygiene self-care deficit
- Dressing/grooming self-care deficit
- Risk for situational low self-esteem
- Disturbed sensory perception
- Impaired social interaction
- Social isolation

Next, determine the likely related factor for the nursing diagnosis to ensure that you select appropriate interventions. For example, impacted cerumen is the cause of a patient's hearing alteration. In this case, regular ear canal irrigation will improve auditory perception (Phipps and others, 2003).

If the patient's auditory alteration is related to altered sensory reception from nerve deafness, nursing interventions of alternative communication methods will be more successful in minimizing the patient's hearing impairment.

## Planning

The patient's plan of care depends on your assessment of the patient's perception and acceptance of the sensory alteration and how well the patient has adjusted to the loss (see care plan).

**GOALS AND OUTCOMES.** The patient will be able to work with you in adapting to the environment and remaining safe and productive if the plan includes clear goals and attainable outcomes. Make sure goals not only meet the immediate needs of the patient, but also strive towards rehabilitation. Some sensory alterations are short term, requiring only temporary interventions. Permanent sensory alterations require long-term goals, with a series of outcomes that the patient reaches over time. For example, if a patient suffers an injury causing blindness, the long-term goal of "managing self-care within the home" will require numerous short-term outcomes and outcomes that require progressive advancement. Examples of outcomes include

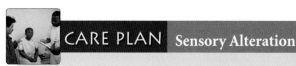

## CARE PLAN  Sensory Alteration

### ASSESSMENT

Mrs. Alicea comes to the clinic reporting **"having trouble seeing,"** especially with **"having a hard time judging distances between objects, which seems worse at night."** Peter spends 20 minutes speaking with Mrs. Alicea and finds the patient needs to have questions repeated several times. Mrs. Alicea **cannot judge steps clearly** and has also noticed a sensitivity to glare. In addition, when the patient tries to read or sew, **her vision is blurred even with glasses.** On physical examination, Mrs. Alicea's corneas appear opaque and there is a **reduction in accommodation.** Her external auditory canals are free from cerumen. Motor function and peripheral sensation appear intact. Mrs. Alicea reports that it has been about 2 years since she has been to an eye doctor. Peter also speaks with Rico, Mrs. Alicea's son. Peter recalls the importance of inspecting the home of a patient with a sensory alteration for safety hazards. Rico has made a safety environmental check but asks Peter for any tips he has, considering Mrs. Alicea's condition.

*Defining characteristics are shown in bold type.

### NURSING DIAGNOSIS Risk for injury related to visual alterations from cataracts.

### PLANNING

| GOAL | EXPECTED OUTCOMES* |
|---|---|
| | RISK CONTROL: VISUAL IMPAIRMENT |
| • Patient's home environment is safe and free of hazards within 4 weeks. | • Patient will report an increased sense of home safety and independence within 4 weeks. |
| | • Patient and son will make recommended changes to home environment within 4 weeks. |

*Outcomes classification label from Moorhead S, Johnson M, Maas M: *Nursing outcomes classification (NOC),* ed 3, St. Louis, 2004, Mosby.

| INTERVENTIONS† | RATIONALE |
|---|---|
| **Environmental Management: Safety** | |
| • Recommend son install a nonglare work surface in the kitchen area. | Sensitivity to glare increases markedly because of the clouding of lens and vitreous that result in scattering of light that passes through the lens (American Federation for the Blind, 2004a). |
| • Teach son methods to improve environmental safety such as installation of handrails along stairs, securing carpeting, removal of throw rugs, and painting of stairs. | A decrease in visual acuity and depth perception places the patient at risk for falls in the presence of environmental hazards (Ebersole and others, 2004). |
| • Recommend son install incandescent lights in the home. | The intensity of lighting needs to be 3 times as powerful for older adults to produce the same results (Ebersole and others, 2004). |
| • Have patient make appointment with ophthalmologist within the next 4 weeks. | Older adults need routine eye examination at least annually. Patient is presenting symptoms of cataracts (National Eye Institute, 2004b). |
| **Communication Enhancement: Visual Deficit** | |
| • Explain use of a pocket magnifier, and offer list of locations where to purchase one. | Magnifier enlarges visual images when reading or doing close work (Ebersole and others, 2004). |

†Intervention classification labels from Dochterman JM, Bulechek GM, editors: *Nursing interventions classification (NIC),* ed 4, St. Louis, 2004, Mosby.

### EVALUATION

- Ask Mrs. Alicea to describe changes in her perception of safety and independence.
- Have Mrs. Alicea describe her perception of risk for accidents in the home.
- Ask Mrs. Alicea and her son to discuss changes made in the home to reduce environmental hazards.
- During a home visit observe for removal of hazards in the home.

---

"Patient will learn to ambulate within the home in 2 weeks" and "Patient will perform ADLs within 4 weeks."

**SETTING PRIORITIES.** After selecting nursing diagnoses and mutually agreed-upon goals and outcomes, work with the patient in setting priorities. Generally you will rank diagnoses in order of importance based on the patient's safety, personal desires, and needs. When setting priorities, safety is a top priority. However, some patients prefer to learn about ways to communicate more effectively or about adaptive methods that will enable participation in favorite activities (e.g., a hobby). Sometimes the patient needs to change the way self-care activities, communication, and socialization are performed.

**CONTINUITY OF CARE.** Review all resources available to patients when you develop a plan of care. The family plays a key role in providing meaningful stimulation and learning ways to help a patient adjust to any limitations once the patient returns home. Teach hospitalized patients and their families how to adapt interventions to their lifestyles. Encourage patients to participate in family and social activities. Referral to resources such as occupational therapists, social service, and speech therapists ensures a multidisciplinary approach. Community resources, such as the American Foundation for the Blind, American National Red Cross, Lions Club, provide information to assist patients and families with discharge planning and home needs.

## Implementation

Nursing interventions involve the patient and family in order to maintain a safe, pleasant, and stimulating sensory environment. Effective interventions help the patient with sensory alterations to function safely with existing deficits and to continue a normal lifestyle.

**HEALTH PROMOTION.** Good sensory function begins with prevention. When a patient seeks health care, provide interventions that reduce risk for sensory losses. Educate older adult patients about having eye and ear examinations annually.

**Screening and Prevention.** Children need appropriate visual screenings to prevent visual impairment (Hockenberry and others, 2003). Three common interventions include screening women considering pregnancy for rubella and syphilis; advocating adequate prenatal care to prevent premature birth, which results in infants' being exposed to excessive oxygen during care; and periodic screening of all children for congenital blindness and visual impairment caused by **refractive errors** and strabismus. Vision problems occur in approximately 20% to 30% of school-age children (Halle, 2002). Children also need to receive immunizations for rubella (see Chapter 11).

Nearsightedness is common during childhood. School nurses usually conduct routine vision testing of school-age and adolescent children. Your role as a nurse is one of detection, education, and referral. Parents need to know the signs of visual impairment (e.g., failure to react to light and reduced eye contact from the infant). Parents need to report any signs to their health care provider.

Trauma is a common cause of blindness in children. Examples include injury from flying objects or penetrating wounds. Parents and children need education on ways to avoid eye trauma (e.g., wearing safety devices and buying only "safe" toys). Safety equipment is in sport and department stores.

Adults need routine visual screenings. If left undetected and untreated, glaucoma leads to permanent visual loss. The American Academy of Ophthalmology (2004) recommends regular medical eye examinations every 2 to 4 years for those over 40 years old. Patients 65 years and older need examinations every 1 to 2 years, especially those who are of African descent because of their increased risk of diabetes, have a family history of glaucoma, have a serious eye injury, or are taking steroid medications.

Adults are at risk for eye injury when playing sports and working in jobs involving exposure to chemicals or flying objects. The Occupational Safety and Health Administration (OSHA) (2004) has guidelines for workplace safety. Employers must have employees wear eye goggles and/or use equipment that reduces risk of injury. You will play a role in reinforcing eye safety at work as well as when participating in activities that places the adult at risk for eye injury.

In the United States hearing impairment is common. At-risk children include those with a family history of childhood hearing impairment, perinatal infection (rubella, herpes, or cytomegalovirus), low birth weight, chronic ear infection, and Down syndrome. Advise pregnant women to seek early prenatal care, avoid ototoxic drugs, and undergo testing for syphilis and rubella.

Chronic middle ear infections are a common cause of hearing impairment in children. These children need periodic auditory testing. Exposure to loud or high-intensity noise is a risk factor for hearing loss. Advise both children and parents to take precautions and use earplugs or earphones to block high-decibel sound.

In adults, guidelines for hearing screening are variable. If a patient works or lives in a high noise level environment, an annual screening is recommended. The most important concept for adults to understand is hearing loss is not a natural part of aging. Once a patient reports a hearing loss, regular testing becomes necessary.

**Use of Assistive Aids.** Patients with sensory deficits often require use of assistive aids. Patients who wear corrective lenses, eyeglasses, or hearing aids need to keep them accessible, functional, and clean (see Chapter 27). A family member or friend also needs to know how to clean these aids. Contact lens wearers are subject to serious eye infections, caused by infrequent lens disinfection, contamination of lens storage cases or contact lens solutions, and use of homemade saline. Reinforce proper lens care in any health maintenance discussions.

A wide variety of cosmetically acceptable hearing aids that enhance a person's hearing ability are currently available (Box 36-5). A person who sees the need for good hearing will likely be influenced to wear hearing aids (Sommer and Sommer, 2002). Offer patients information on the benefits of hearing aid use. Family members or friends who support the use of the aid will influence the patient to use the aid as instructed.

**Promoting Meaningful Stimulation.** You will help patients make their environments more stimulating by considering the normal physiological changes that accompany sensory deficits (Box 36-6). When the patient ages, the pupil loses the ability to adjust to light. You reduce this sensitivity to glare by reducing the amount of bright light in the person's living environment. Cerumen impaction is a reversible cause of conductive hearing loss in older adults. Irrigation of the canal with tepid water in a 60-ml syringe will remove cerumen (Phipps and others, 2003). Cold water irrigation will cause the patient to become dizzy and vomit.

---

**BOX 36-5  Care of Hearing Aids**

- Protect hearing aids from water, alcohol, hairspray, perspiration, and cologne.
- Store hearing aids and batteries with a desiccant or in an electric dryer.
- Regularly remove cerumen from aid by using wax loop or device supplied with aid.
- Encourage patients to visit audiologist at least annually.

---

**BOX 36-6  Promoting Sensory Stimulation**

- Reduce glare by eliminating waxed floors and shiny surfaces exposed to bright sunlight, installing tinted glass or sheer curtains over large windows, and using soft and diffused lighting.
- Teach use of assistive devices to improve visual acuity (e.g., pocket magnifiers, telescopic lens eyeglasses, large-print books, clocks, watches).
- Recommend introducing brighter colors (e.g., red, orange, yellow) into the home environment so that patients are able to differentiate between surfaces and room objects.
- Explain how to maximize hearing reception or minimize effects of hearing loss by increasing amplification on TVs or radios and using recorded music in low-frequency sound.
- Promote sense of taste through good oral hygiene, serving well-seasoned and differently textured foods, avoiding blending or mixing foods, and chewing food thoroughly.
- Enhance the sense of smell by removing unpleasant odors from the environment and introducing pleasant smells such as mild room deodorizers or fragrant flowers.

---

Some patients experience reduced tactile sensations in a limited portion of their body. Touch therapy helps to stimulate existing function. If the patient is willing, your brushing and combing the patient's hair, giving a back rub, and touching of the arms or shoulders increase tactile contact. Turning and positioning also improve the quality of tactile sensation.

**Creating a Safe Environment.** Patients become less secure within their home and workplace when they have a sensory alteration. An actual or potential sensory loss determines the type of safety precautions necessary. Security is necessary for a person to feel independent. Make recommendations for improving safety within a patient's living environment without restricting the patient's independence. Be sure the patient helps to choose any changes made in the home.

*Visual Adaptations.* When a patient experiences a decrease in visual acuity, peripheral vision, adaptation to the dark, or depth perception, safety is a concern. With reduced peripheral vision a patient cannot see panoramically. With reduced depth perception, a person is unable to judge how far away objects are located. The home safety assessment helps you identify hazards in the patient's living environment. Remove clutter such as footstools or electrical cords.

Arrange furniture so that a patient is able to move about easily without fear of tripping or running into objects. Make sure all flooring is in good repair, and remove all throw rugs. Stairwells need to be well lighted and have securely fastened handrails extending the full length of the stairs.

Front and back entrances to the home and work areas need good lighting. Light fixtures need high-wattage bulbs with wider illumination. A light switch located at the top and bottom of stairwells adds an additional safety element. Replace fluorescent lighting with incandescent lights.

Driving is sometimes a safety hazard for older adults. A sensitivity to glare creates a problem for driving at night with headlights. Reduced peripheral vision prevents a driver from seeing cars in the next lane. Reduced vision, complicated by a decrease in reaction time, reduced hearing, and decreased strength in the legs and arms, seriously limit an older adult's driving skills. To minimize patients' risk, encourage them to drive only in familiar areas and not during rush hour. Urge patients to drive defensively and to avoid driving at night or at dusk. Older adults need to drive slowly but not so slowly that they create a safety problem for other drivers.

Some patients have problems seeing dials or controls on electrical appliances and equipment when they are unable to contrast colors. Use color contrasts (e.g., tape, paint, or nail enamel) to highlight dials. Tour the patient's home to find opportunities for color coding.

*Hearing Adaptations.* Individuals need to hear environmental sounds such as fire alarms, alarm clocks, phones, or doorbells. Change or amplify the sound of these devices to a more low-pitched, buzzerlike quality. Signaling devices, such as a flashing light on a phone, allow the hearing impaired greater independence. Sound lamps that respond with light to the sounds of babies crying, smoke detectors, and burglar alarms are also available. Advise family and friends who call the patient regularly to let the phone ring for a longer period.

*Smell and Tactile Adaptations.* The patient with a reduced sensitivity to odors is often unable to smell leaking gas, a smoldering cigarette, fire, or tainted food. Make sure the patient uses smoke detectors and takes precautions such as checking ashtrays or placing cigarette butts in water. Also advise the patient to check food package dates and inspect the appearance of food. Patients with reduced tactile sensation need to use water bottles or heating pads cautiously and never use the high setting. Make sure the temperature on the home water heater is no higher than 120° F.

**Communication.** Individuals need to interact with people around them. The type of sensory loss influences the methods and styles of communication you use during interactions with patients. Some patients with a hearing impairment are able to speak normally. To more clearly hear what a person communicates, family and friends need to learn to move away from background noise, rephrase rather than repeat sentences, be positive, and have patience. On the other hand, some deaf patients have serious speech alterations. Deaf patients use sign language, use lip reading, write with

---

**BOX 36-7** PATIENT TEACHING

Rico tells Peter that he is concerned about communicating well with his mother now that she is having some hearing deficits. Peter develops the following teaching plan for Rico:

**Outcome**
- At the end of the teaching session, Rico will be able to verbalize understanding of four strategies he will take to improve communication with his mother.

**Teaching Strategies**
- Approach a person with hearing difficulties from the front, and gently touch his or her arm so you will not startle him or her (McConnell, 2002).
- Face the person, and stand or sit on the same level. Be sure your face and lips are illuminated to promote lip reading. Do not stand in front of the light. Avoid glare and shadows. Do not speak with something in your mouth. Keep your hands away from your mouth (Sommer and Sommer, 2002).
- Speak slowly, and articulate clearly. Use a normal tone of voice and inflections of speech. Avoid slang or jokes (Sommer and Sommer, 2002).

- Avoid eating, chewing, or smoking while speaking (McConnell, 2002).
- When you are not understood, rephrase rather than repeat the conversation (Sommer and Sommer, 2002).
- Use visible expressions. Speak with your hands, your face, and your eyes.
- Do not shout. Loud sounds are usually higher pitched and prevent hearing by accentuating vowel sounds and concealing consonants. If speaking loudly is necessary, speak in lower tones (Sommer and Sommer, 2002).
- Talk toward the person's best or normal ear.
- Avoid speaking from another room or while walking away. Reduce or eliminate background noise.
- Use written information to enhance the spoken word (McConnell, 2002).

**Evaluation Strategies**
- Ask Rico to verbalize at least four communication approaches.
- Ask Rico to role-play with you and use some of the communication strategies that you discussed.

---

pad and pencil, or learn to use a computer for communication (Box 36-7).

**ACUTE CARE.** Some hospitalized patients are treated for sensory deficits (e.g., acute eye infection) and some have preexisting sensory problems. You need to know the patient's health history to appropriately support self-care activities while promoting a safe environment.

**Orientation to the Environment.** Be sure to completely orient patients with sensory impairments to a care setting. Always keep your name tag visible, address the patient by name, explain the patient's location, and frequently include the time and date in conversations. Repeating explanations in short and simple terms reduces confusion. Encourage family and friends not to argue with or contradict a confused patient but to explain calmly their location, identity, and time of day.

Patients with serious visual impairments need to feel comfortable in knowing the boundaries of their environment. The patient needs to walk through a room and feel the walls to establish a sense of direction. Remember to approach the blind patient from the front. Explain the location of objects within the room, such as chairs or equipment. It is important to keep all objects in the same place and position. Moving an object, even a short distance creates a safety hazard. You will need to reorient the patient frequently by describing the location of key items. Place necessary objects such as the call light, patient-controlled analgesia (PCA) button, glasses, water, or facial tissue in front of patients to prevent falls caused by reaching. A night-light in the bathroom will help reduce falls by decreasing the time required for the eyes to adapt to the dark. Also, ask the patient how to

arrange objects so ambulation is easier. Remove clutter and unnecessary equipment. Always keep the path to the bathroom clear. Make sure doors are completely closed or open to prevent injury from a partially opened door (Houde and Huff, 2003).

**Safety Measures.** Assist patients with acute visual impairments with walking. Stand at the patient's nondominant side, approximately one step in front, as you describe the course of movement (Figure 36-1). The patient uses the nondominant hand to grasp your elbow or upper arm. You then walk one-half step ahead and slightly to the patient's side. The patient's shoulder is directly behind your shoulder. Relax, and walk at a comfortable pace. Warn the patient when approaching doorways, and tell the patient whether the door opens in or out. Do not leave a patient with visual impairment alone in an unfamiliar area.

A patient with a hearing impairment will have difficulty hearing typical hospital sounds such as an intravenous pump alarm, nurse intercom system, or nurse instructions (Slaven, 2003). Always visit the patient's bedside more frequently. Never restrict both arms of deaf or hearing-impaired patients with intravenous lines or restraints. Always alert the entire multidisciplinary team when a patient has a sensory alteration.

**Controlling Sensory Stimuli.** You reduce sensory overload by organizing the patient's care to control for excessive stimuli. Combining activities such as dressing changes, bathing, and vital sign assessment in one visit prevents the patient from becoming overly fatigued. Coordination with other departments will reduce the time needed for tests and

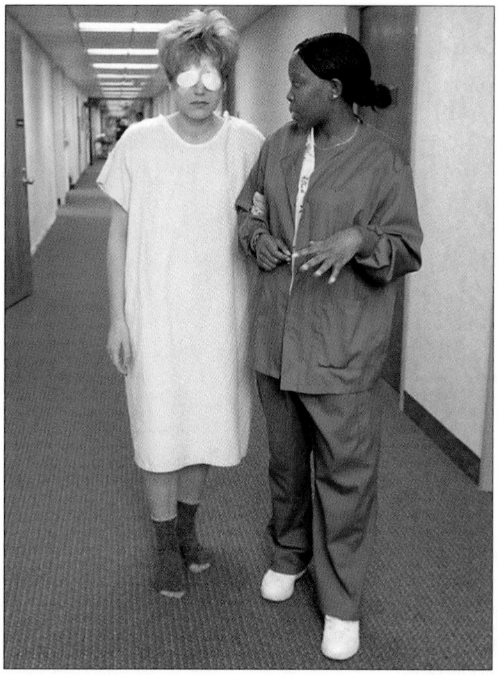

FIGURE **36-1** Nurse assists visually impaired patient with ambulation.

BOX 36-8 **Introducing Stimuli Into the Care Setting**

**Visual**

Open the drapes to the patient's room.
Raise the head of the bed, and draw back dividing curtains or partitions.
Provide attractive decorations on tables or cabinets, such as fresh flowers, plants, a picture, or greeting cards.
Provide talking books and large-print reading material.

**Auditory**

Sit down and speak with the patient. Make the conversation meaningful.
Turn on a radio with the type of music the patient enjoys.
A favorite radio or television program is stimulating.

**Taste and Smell**

Provide attractive, taste-appealing meals. Be sure tableware and glasses are clean. Make sure warm foods are served warm and cold foods are served cold.
Provide a variety of textures, aromas, and flavors to enhance the patient's appetite.

examinations. The patient needs time for rest and quiet. Perform routine nursing procedures as quietly as possible. Encourage a family member to sit quietly with a patient or involve the patient in an undemanding repetitive activity such as combing hair.

Try to control extraneous noise in and around a patient's room, such as television volume and visitors. Turn off bedside equipment not in use. Close the patient's room door if necessary. Hospital staff needs to control loud laughter or conversation at the nurses' station. In addition to controlling excess stimuli, try to introduce meaningful stimulation (Box 36-8) that makes the environment pleasing and comfortable.

**RESTORATIVE AND CONTINUING CARE.** After patients have experienced a sensory loss, they need to adjust to continue a normal lifestyle. Many of the interventions previously discussed under health promotion are adaptable for the home setting. The home environment needs to be healthy, comfortable, and safe. Suggest changes in a person's home environment after you assess the home setting for any hazards that increase the risk for injury.

**Promoting Self-Care.** Patients who have had surgery related to a sensory deficit need a plan of care that allows them to return safely to their home environment. Most patients have same-day surgical procedures (see Chapter 37). Family members or friends need to understand how the patient's sensory impairment will affect the ability to perform normal ADLs and IADLs and the factors that lessen or worsen sensory problems. Community resources discussed in the planning section will be useful.

Patients with sensory impairments are able to continue independent self-care activities. In the case of eating meals, you arrange food on the plate and condiments, salad, or drinks around the plate according to numbers on the face of a clock (Figure 36-2). The patient will become oriented to the items after the family member explains each item's location. Patients will need assistance in arranging self-care items, such as clothing, hygiene, food supplies, and utensils in a consistent location to continue managing daily care activities.

The visually impaired patient will also need assistance in reaching the bathroom safely. Safety bars need to be installed near the toilet. A bar that is a different color from the wall is easier to see. Never place towels on safety bars because this interferes with a person's grasp.

If tactile sense is decreased, the patient will dress more easily with zippers or Velcro strips, pullover sweaters or blouses, and elasticized waists. If the patient has a partial paralysis, you dress the affected side first. Some patients also need assistance with basic grooming such as brushing, combing, shaving, and shampooing hair.

**Socialization.** Interacting with others is difficult for many patients. A patient with a hearing loss will become embarrassed and exhausted after asking people to continuously repeat what they say. Patients often lose the motivation to engage in social activities and withdraw from interaction. Introduce therapies to reduce loneliness, particularly for older adult patients (Box 36-9). Family members need to learn to focus on a person's ability rather than his or her disability. Never assume that a hearing impaired person does not wish to speak.

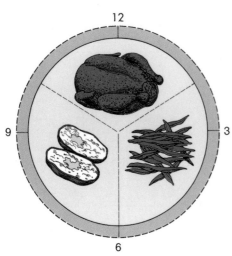

12

9

3

6

FIGURE **36-2** Arrange food on a plate and orient patient to placement based on numbers on a clock face.

## Evaluation

**PATIENT CARE.** It is important to evaluate whether care measures maintain or improve a patient's ability to interact and function within the environment. Adapt evaluation measures to determine whether actual outcomes are the same as expected outcomes (Table 36-3). Be sure a patient with a hearing deficit hears your questions about responses to treatment. When expected outcomes have not been achieved, there is a need to change interventions or add new ones.

If nursing care has been directed at improving or maintaining sensory acuity, evaluate the integrity of the sensory organs and the patient's ability to perceive stimuli. This often involves a simple vision or hearing assessment by asking the patient to perform a self-care skill. When you teach patients in order to improve their sensory function, you need to know if the patient is following recommended therapies and meeting mutually set goals. Asking the patient to explain or demonstrate a newly learned self-care skill is an effective evaluative measure.

**PATIENT EXPECTATIONS.** It is important to learn if patients think they are receiving appropriate care. A sensory deficit is potentially embarrassing and threatens a person's self-image. Does the patient feel comfortable relating to you? Was the patient able to maintain the plan of care for assistive devices? Did the patient think you were exhibiting a caring, professional approach? Asking patients if nursing care successfully met their expectations will provide valuable knowledge when you care for other patients with similar sensory problems.

- Recommend alterations in living arrangements if physical isolation is a factor.
- Give older adults extra time to communicate.
- Assist patients in keeping contact with people important to them.
- Encourage and facilitate socialization (Houde and Huff, 2003).
- Help patients acquire information about support groups.
- Arrange for security escort services as needed.
- Link patients with religious organizations attuned to the social needs of older adults.
- Bring a pet into the home (for hearing impaired only).

## EVALUATION

One month has passed since Mrs. Alicea's last visit to the senior health care center. Today Peter sits down and talks with both the patient and Rico. He learns that Mrs. Alicea is no longer having difficulty with glare because Rico changed the lights in the house to incandescent bulbs. Rico also reports that he plans to install some sheer curtains Mrs. Alicea chose last week, to hang over the large window in the living room. Mrs. Alicea also tells Peter that Rico has made a "few changes around the house," including rearranging furniture, securing the rugs, and removing extension cords. After purchasing a magnifier at a local drug store, Mrs. Alicea is able to read the newspaper and medication labels more easily.

On examination, Mrs. Alicea's visual acuity continues to reveal blurring when she tried to read an informational pamphlet. Her pupils continue to respond slowly to accommodation. Peter inquires as to whether Mrs. Alicea has made an appointment with her ophthalmologist. She confirms that the appointment is within the next 2 weeks.

Overall, Mrs. Alicea confides, "I think I have been helped with the ideas we talked about last time. I feel a little better about getting around the house and doing the things I like to do." When asked if he has noticed any changes in his mother's actions, Rico states, "She seems less fearful of possibly falling."

**Documentation Note**

"Patient visited clinic this morning as scheduled. Has implemented measures at home to improve her visual acuity and sensitivity to glare. Son supportive in making necessary home environment changes. Plans to make additional ones. Patient has set an appointment with ophthalmologist within next 2 weeks."

## OUTCOME EVALUATION

TABLE 36-3

| Nursing Action | Patient Response/Finding | Achievement of Outcome |
|---|---|---|
| Ask Mrs. Alicea if she visited ophthalmologist. | She visited ophthalmologist; new eyeglass prescription was written. | Outcome met. Encourage annual eye examinations in the future. |
| Observe Mrs. Alicea walk through home and down stairs. | She is able to walk with steady, purposeful gait. | Outcome met. |
| Conduct a home visit, and reassess the home environment. | Son has changed all lightbulbs in the halls and stairways. He removed all throw rugs. He also painted edges of stairs. | Home environment has improved. Recommend that son change the work surface in the kitchen to decrease glare. |

## KEY CONCEPTS

- Sensory perception depends on a region in the cerebral cortex where specialized brain cells interpret the quality and nature of sensory stimuli.
- Because a patient learns to rely on unaffected senses after a sensory loss, you design interventions to preserve function of these senses.
- Aging results in a gradual decline of acuity in all senses.
- Environmental stimuli in a hospital, such as an intensive care unit, place a patient at risk for sensory overload.
- The extent of support from family members and significant others influences the quality of sensory experiences.
- Assessment of sensory function includes a physical examination and measurement of functional abilities.
- The presence of cerumen in the external auditory canal is a common cause of hearing loss in older adults.
- A patient's self-rating of hearing is an important defining characteristic for disturbed sensory perception (auditory).
- Sensory losses create loneliness and impair the ability to socialize.

- An assessment of environment includes identifying hazards, sources of meaningful stimulation, and the amount of stimuli.
- Prenatal screening and childhood immunizations prevent sensory alterations in the newborn and child.
- The care plan for patients with sensory alterations includes participation by family members.
- Patients with visual impairments need to learn boundaries within the environment to ambulate safely.
- Patients with existing hearing deficits are able to learn alternative ways to communicate.
- Nursing care for patients with sensory alterations includes using stronger sensory stimuli, compensating with other senses, and modifying the environment to maximize remaining sensory function.
- To prevent sensory overload, control stimuli, orient the patient to the environment, and promote rest by minimizing interruptions.
- Safety is a top concern when setting priorities for patients who experience sensory deprivation.

## CRITICAL THINKING IN PRACTICE

*Mr. Gale is a 70-year-old man who lives alone in a high-rise for older adults. His apartment is on the seventh floor and consists of a bedroom, bathroom, kitchen, and living area. Mr. Gale is visually impaired due to a diagnosis of glaucoma 3 years ago. He also has prebycusis. The community health nurse is coming to Mr. Gale's apartment to complete an initial assessment of his health and safety needs.*

- - - - - - - - - - - - - - - -

1. The nurse starts her visit by introducing herself outside the apartment door and showing Mr. Gale her identification badge. The nurse shows her badge because:
   a. Patients with glaucoma have impaired central vision
   b. She wanted the patient to know her name
   c. Mr. Gale must identify anyone asking to come into his apartment
   d. Mr. Gale is unable to read with his vision impairment
2. When speaking to Mr. Gale, the nurse knows that it is easier for the patient to understand a spoken conversation when you:

   a. Approach a patient quietly from behind
   b. Use a louder than normal tone of voice
   c. Select a public area to have a spoken conversation
   d. Use your hands and eyes as visual aids while speaking
3. Because Mr. Gale has a hearing and vision impairment, the assessment data that best indicate signs of sensory deprivation include:
   a. Diminished anxiety
   b. Altered ability to concentrate
   c. Improved completion of tasks
   d. Decreased need for physical stimulation
4. During the home visit you notice that Mr. Gale's environment is poorly illuminated. A priority intervention you will include is:
   a. Using fluorescent lightening
   b. Recommending muted colors
   c. Doubling the amount of light fixtures throughout the house
   d. Placing incandescent, higher wattage lightbulbs into light fixtures

## NCLEX® REVIEW

1. Normal physiological changes in sensory input of the older adult patient may include:
   1. Decreased sensitivity to glare
   2. Increased number of taste buds
   3. Increased peripheral neuropathy
   4. Difficulty discriminating vowel sounds

2. When assessing a patient whose regimen includes use of nonsteroidal antiinflammatory drugs (NSAIDs), you should be aware that a common side effect includes:
   1. Ototoxicity
   2. Loss of taste
   3. Optic irritation
   4. Alteration in perception

3. A hospitalized older adult patient is often disoriented to his or her environment. An intervention to properly introduce stimuli would be to:
   1. Keep the room darkened
   2. Introduce an all-talk radio program
   3. Speak with the patient in muted tones
   4. Draw back dividing curtains or partitions

4. When you are performing a home assessment, the observation that would be most significant for the safety of a patient with peripheral neuropathy includes:
   1. Cluttered walkways
   2. Absence of smoke detectors
   3. Lack of bathroom safety bars
   4. Improper water heater setting

5. Because hearing impairment is one of the most common disabilities among children, an intervention you teach parents is to:
   1. Avoid activities in which crowds and loud noises occur
   2. Delay childhood immunizations until hearing can be verified
   3. Take precautions when involved in activities associated with high-intensity noises
   4. Prophylactically administer antibiotics to reduce the incidence of infections

6. A patient has an acute attack of Meniere's disease. The nurse should anticipate which of these clinical manifestations?
   1. Anxiety, insomnia, paranoia
   2. Ear pain, imbalance, photophobia
   3. Blurred vision, headache, and diaphoresis
   4. Vertigo, hearing impairment, tinnitus

## REFERENCES

American Academy of Ophthalmology: *Comprehensive adult medical eye evaluation,* San Francisco, 2004, The Academy.

American Association of Retired Persons: *A profile of older adults,* 2004, http://research.aarp.org.

American Federation for the Blind: *Creating a comfortable environment for older individuals who are visually impaired,* 2004a, http://www.afb.org.

American Federation for the Blind: *Quick facts and figures on blindness and low vision,* 2004b, http://www.afb.org.

Dochterman JM, Bulecheck GM, editors: *Nursing interventions classification (NIC),* ed 4, St. Louis, 2004, Mosby.

Ebersole P and others: *Toward healthy aging,* ed 6, St. Louis, 2004, Mosby.

Ervin S: Meniere's disease: identifying classic symptoms and current treatments, *Nurs Stand* 18(12):156, 2004.

Galanti G: The Hispanic family and male-female relationships: an overview, *J Transcult Nurs* 14(3):180, 2003.

Halle C: Achieve new vision screening objectives, *Nurse Pract* 27(3):15, 2002.

Hockenberry MC and others: *Wong's nursing care of infants and children,* ed 7, St. Louis, 2003, Mosby.

Houde S, Huff M: Age-related vision loss in older adults: a challenge for gerontological nurses, *J Gerontol Nurs* 29(4):25, 2003.

McConnell E: How to converse with a hearing impaired patient, *RN* 32(8):20, 2002.

McKenry L, Salerno E: *Mosby's pharmacology in nursing,* ed 21, St. Louis, 2003, Mosby.

Meniere's Disease Information Center: *What is Meniere's disease,* 2004, http://www.menieresinfo.org.

Moore L, Miller M: Older men's experiences of living with severe visual impairment, *J Adv Nurs* 43(1):10, 2003.

Moorhead S, Johnson M, Maas M: *Nursing outcomes classification (NOC),* ed 3, St. Louis, 2004, Mosby.

National Eye Institute: *Vision loss from eye diseases will increase as Americans age,* 2004a, http://www.nei.nih.gov.

National Eye Institute: *Vision: national eye health education program (NEHEP),* 2004b, http://www.nei.nih.gov.

Occupational Safety and Health Administration: *Eye protection for the workplace,* 2004, U.S. Department of Labor, http://www.osha.gov.

Phipps W and others: *Medical-surgical nursing: health and illness perspectives,* ed 7, St. Louis, 2003, Mosby.

Sandhaus S: Stop the spinning: diagnosing and managing vertigo, *Nurse Pract* 27(8):11, 2002.

Slaven A: Communication and the hearing impaired patient, *Nurs Stand* 18(12):39, 2003.

Sommer S, Sommer N: When your patient is hearing impaired, *RN* 65(12):28, 2002.

Tate D: Cultural awareness: bridging the gap between caregivers and Hispanic patients, *J Contin Educ Nurs* 34(5):213, 2003.

Walker R, Rodgers J: Diabetic retinopathy, *Nurs Stand* 16(45):46, 2002.

# CHAPTER 37

# Surgical Patient

## MEDIA RESOURCES

**CD COMPANION** **evolve** **WEBSITE**

http://evolve.elsevier.com/Potter/basic

- **NCLEX® Review**
- **Audio Glossary**
- **English/Spanish Audio Glossary**
- **Video Clip**

## OBJECTIVES

- Explain the concept of perioperative nursing care.
- Differentiate among classifications of surgery and types of anesthesia.
- List factors to include in the preoperative assessment of a surgical patient.
- Design a preoperative teaching plan.
- Prepare a patient for surgery.

- Explain the differences in caring for the patient undergoing outpatient surgery versus the patient undergoing inpatient surgery.
- Describe intraoperative factors that affect a patient's postoperative course.
- Identify factors to assess in a patient in postoperative recovery.
- Describe the rationale for nursing interventions designed to prevent postoperative complications.

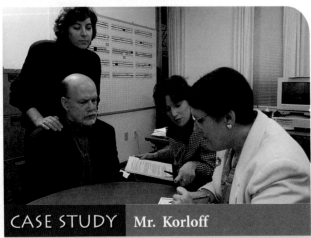

### CASE STUDY    Mr. Korloff

Mr. Korloff is a 53-year-old man who has been experiencing abdominal pain for 2 months. Following a series of diagnostic tests, he is now scheduled for an elective laparoscopic cholecystectomy. Mr. Korloff is originally from Russia and has lived in the United States for 20 years. He speaks English quite well but still has a Russian accent. He is a vice president for an international business firm. He is widowed and has two adult daughters, both born in Russia before coming to the United States. The daughters are married and live in the same neighborhood as Mr. Korloff.

Sue Collins is a nursing student assigned to the preadmission center at the local hospital where she has been working for 2 weeks. She is completing her last clinical rotation and will graduate in 1 month. Sue is 30 years old, is married, and has no children. She plans to seek employment in a hospital on a general surgery floor after graduation. Sue's father recently had surgery for prostate cancer.

### KEY TERMS

antiembolism stockings, p. 1110
atelectasis, p. 1087
bronchospasm, p. 1092
circulating nurse, p. 1112
conscious sedation, p. 1114
convalescence, p. 1115
dehiscence, p. 1089
embolism, p. 1089
evisceration, p. 1123
general anesthesia, p. 1114
laryngospasm, p. 1092
malignant hyperthermia, p. 1091
moderate sedation/ analgesia, p. 1114
nasogastric (NG) tube, p. 1110
operating bed, p. 1089
operating room, p. 1111

outpatient, p. 1086
paralytic ileus, p. 1119
perioperative nursing, p. 1086
postanesthesia care unit (PACU), p. 1115
preanesthesia care unit, p. 1112
preoperative teaching, p. 1090
presurgical care unit (PSCU), p. 1112
pulmonary hygiene, p. 1092
recovery, p. 1115
regional anesthesia, p. 1114
scrub nurse, p. 1112
sequential compression stockings, p. 1110

This chapter synthesizes many concepts and skills previously presented in this text. You will recognize these previously learned areas and apply this information to the surgical patient in the preoperative and postoperative phases.

**Perioperative nursing** care includes nursing care given before (preoperative), during (intraoperative), and after (postoperative) surgery. Today surgery takes place in a variety of settings, including hospitals, ambulatory surgery centers, clinics, physicians' or health care provider's offices, and even mobile units. Minor surgeries are performed on an **outpatient** basis, with the patient entering the setting, undergoing surgery, and being discharged the same day. Many patients undergoing surgery enter the setting as outpatients

| TABLE 37-1 | **Classification for Surgical Procedures** | |
|---|---|---|
| Type | Description | Example |
| **Seriousness** | | |
| Major | Involves extensive reconstruction or alteration in body parts; poses great risks to well-being | Coronary artery bypass, colon resection, removal of larynx, resection of lung lobe |
| Minor | Involves minimal alteration in body parts; often designed to correct deformities; involves minimal risks compared with major procedures | Cataract extraction, facial plastic surgery, tooth extraction |
| **Urgency** | | |
| Elective | Performed on basis of patient's choice; not essential and is not always necessary for health | Bunionectomy, facial plastic surgery, hernia repair, breast reconstruction |
| Urgent | Necessary for patient's health, will possibly prevent additional problems from developing (e.g., tissue destruction, impaired organ function); not necessarily an emergency | Excision of cancerous tumor, removal of gallbladder for stones, vascular repair for obstructed artery (e.g., coronary artery bypass) |
| Emergency | Must be done immediately to save life or preserve function of body part | Repair of perforated appendix, repair of traumatic amputation, control of internal hemorrhaging |
| **Purpose** | | |
| Diagnostic | Surgical exploration that allows physician or health care provider to confirm diagnosis; sometimes involves removal of tissue for further diagnostic testing | Exploratory laparotomy (incision into peritoneal cavity to inspect abdominal organs), breast mass biopsy |
| Ablative | Amputation or removal of diseased body part | Amputation, removal of appendix, cholecystectomy |
| Palliative | Relieves or reduces intensity of disease symptoms; will not produce cure | Colostomy, removal of necrotic tissue, resection of nerve roots |
| Reconstructive/ restorative | Restores function or appearance to traumatized or malfunctioning tissues | Internal fixation of fractures, scar revision |
| Procurement for transplant | Removal of organs and/or tissues from a person pronounced brain dead for transplantation into another person | Kidney, cornea, or liver transplant |
| Constructive | Restores function lost or reduced as result of congenital anomalies | Repair of cleft palate, closure of atrial septal defect in heart |
| Cosmetic | Performed to improve personal appearance | Blepharoplasty to correct eyelid deformities; rhinoplasty to reshape nose |

for preoperative screening and testing and are admitted to the hospital after surgery. Oftentimes patients requiring extensive preoperative care are admitted to the hospital before surgery. The principles of caring for perioperative patients are the same regardless of the setting.

## Scientific Knowledge Base

### Classification of Surgery

Surgical procedures are classified according to the seriousness, urgency, and purpose of surgery (Table 37-1). For example, a breast biopsy, done for diagnostic purposes, is classified as urgent and done on an outpatient basis. Knowing the classification will help you to plan appropriate preoperative and postoperative care for each patient.

### Surgical Risk Factors

Knowledge regarding the physiology of stress (see Chapter 22) and risk factors that affect how a patient responds to the stress of surgery is necessary to anticipate patient needs for preoperative preparation, teaching, and postoperative care. Smoking has a significant association with postoperative pulmonary complications, specifically pneumonia and **atelectasis.** Smoking also increases the risk of circulatory and infectious complications (Moller and others, 2002). Patients who are 70 years or older, have a productive cough, and diabetes mellitus are more likely to develop cardiac and pulmonary complications (Hulzebos and others, 2003; Scales and Master, 2003).

**AGE.** Very young and older patients are at greater surgical risk as a result of an immature or a declining physiological status. Maintaining the patient's normal body temperature is a concern during surgery. When compared with an adult, an infant has a proportionately greater surface area and less subcutaneous fat, placing these patients at risk for wide temperature variations. In addition, general anesthetics inhibit shivering, a protective reflex to maintain body temperature, and cause vasodilation, which results in heat loss. During surgery an infant also has difficulty in maintaining a normal circulatory blood volume. The total blood volume of infants is considerably less than that of older children and

| TABLE 37-2 | Physiological Factors That Place the Older Adult at Risk During Surgery | |
|---|---|---|
| **Alterations** | **Risks** | **Nursing Implications** |
| **Cardiovascular System** | | |
| Degeneration of myocardium and valves | Reduces cardiac reserve. | Assess baseline vital signs and patient's fluid volume status. |
| Rigid arteries and reduction in sympathetic and parasympathetic innervation to heart | Predisposes patient to postoperative hemorrhage and hypertension. | Instruct patient in techniques for performing leg exercises and proper turning. |
| Increase in calcium and cholesterol deposits within small arteries; thickened arterial walls | Increases risk for clot formation in lower extremities. | Apply elastic stockings, sequential compression devices (SCDs). |
| **Integumentary System** | | |
| Decreased subcutaneous tissue and increased fragility of skin | Patient is prone to pressure ulcers and skin tears. | Assess skin every 2 hours or more often; pad all bony prominences during surgery. Turn or reposition every 2 hours if possible. |
| **Pulmonary System** | | |
| Rib cage stiffened and reduced in size | Reduces vital capacity. | Instruct patient in proper technique for coughing, deep breathing, splinting incision, and use of inspirometers. |
| Reduced range of movement in diaphragm | Greater residual capacity or volume of air left in lung after normal breath, reducing amount of new air brought into lungs with each inspiration. | When possible, have patient ambulate and sit in chair frequently. |
| Stiffened lung tissue and enlarged air spaces | Reduces blood oxygenation levels. | Provide supplemental oxygen when ordered. |
| Decreased ability to cough and clear upper airway | Increases the risk of postoperative pulmonary infection. | Have patient cough, deep breathe, and use inspirometer every 2 hours. |
| **Renal System** | | |
| Reduced blood flow to kidneys | Increases risk for damage to renal tissues. | For patients hospitalized before surgery, determine baseline urinary output for 24 hours. |
| Reduced glomerular filtration rate and excretory times | Limits ability to eliminate drugs or toxic substances. | Maintain adequate hydration. |
| Reduced bladder capacity | Voiding frequency increases, and larger amount of urine stays in bladder after voiding. | Instruct patient to notify nurse immediately when sensation of bladder fullness develops. |
| | Sensation of need to void sometimes does not occur until bladder is full. | Keep call light and bedpan within easy reach. |
| **Neurological System** | | |
| Sensory losses, including reduced tactile sense and increased pain tolerance | Patient is less able to respond to early warning signs of surgical complications. | Orient patient to surrounding environment. Observe for nonverbal signs of pain. |
| Decreased reaction time | Patient becomes easily confused after anesthesia. | Reorient frequently. Keep side rails up and room free from clutter. |
| **Metabolic System** | | |
| Reduced number of red blood cells and hemoglobin levels | Reduces ability to carry adequate oxygen to tissues. | Administer necessary blood products. Monitor blood test results. |
| Change in total amounts of body potassium and water volume | Increases risk for fluid or electrolyte imbalance. | Monitor fluid and electrolyte levels. |

adults, creating a risk for both dehydration and overhydration. With advancing age a patient's physical capacity to adapt to the stress of surgery lessens because of deterioration of certain body functions. Table 37-2 summarizes physiological factors that place older adult patients at risk during surgery.

**NUTRITION.** Normal tissue repair and resistance to infection depend on adequate nutrition. Surgery increases the need for nutrients. Postoperatively a patient requires at least 1500 kilocalories per day to maintain energy reserves. Additional protein, carbohydrates, zinc, and vitamins A, B, C, and K are necessary for proper wound healing (see Chapters 31 and 36). A malnourished patient is prone to poor tolerance of anesthesia, negative nitrogen balance, delayed postoperative recovery, infection, and delayed wound healing (Black and Hawks, 2005).

**OBESITY.** An obese patient usually has reduced ventilatory capacity because of the upward pressure against the diaphragm caused by an enlarged abdomen. There is also an increased risk of aspiration during the administration of anesthesia (Scales and Master, 2003). The recumbent and supine positions required on the **operating bed** (table) for surgery further limit the obese patient's ventilation. The increased workload of the heart and atherosclerotic blood vessels often results in compromised cardiovascular function. Because of these physiological changes, obese patients often have difficulty in resuming normal physical activity after surgery. Hypertension, coronary artery disease, type 2 diabetes mellitus, and congestive heart failure are common in this population. Obese patients are more susceptible to developing **embolism,** atelectasis, and pneumonia postoperatively than nonobese patients (Black and Hawks, 2005).

In addition, excess weight placed on skin over bony prominences restricts blood flow and results in impaired skin integrity. The obese patient is susceptible to poor wound healing and wound infection because fatty tissue contains a poor blood supply and slows the delivery of essential nutrients and antibodies needed for healing. It is often difficult to close the surgical wound of an obese patient because of the thick adipose layer. The risk for **dehiscence** and **evisceration** is increased because of these factors (see Chapter 35).

**IMMUNOCOMPETENCE.** Radiation and chemotherapeutic drugs used for cancer therapy, immunosuppressive agents used to prevent rejection after organ transplantation, steroids such as prednisone used to treat a variety of inflammatory conditions, and disorders affecting the immune system such as acquired immunodeficiency syndrome (AIDS) all render the body vulnerable to infection because they suppress the body's immune system. Patients with immunosuppression have an increased risk of infection following surgery. For example, the patient with cancer often has radiotherapy before surgery to reduce the size of the cancerous tumor in order to remove it surgically. Radiation causes fibrosis and vascular scarring in the radiated area. This causes tissues to become fragile and poorly oxygenated, increasing the risk of wound infection. Ideally surgery takes place 4 to 6 weeks after the completion of radiation treatments to avoid wound-healing problems.

**FLUID AND ELECTROLYTE BALANCE.** The body responds to surgery as a form of trauma. As a result of the adrenocortical stress response, hormonal reactions cause sodium and water retention and potassium loss within the first 2 to 5 days after surgery. Severe protein breakdown creates a negative nitrogen balance. The severity of the stress response influences the degree of fluid and electrolyte imbalance. The more extensive the surgery is, the more severe the physiological stress. Patients with preexisting renal, fluid and electrolyte, gastrointestinal, respiratory, or cardiovascular problems are at greatest risk for operative complications. For example, a patient who is dehydrated from vomiting preoperatively is at greater risk for hypovolemic shock (see Chapter 15).

**PREGNANCY.** When dealing with a pregnant patient, be prepared to consider the needs of both the pregnant woman and her unborn fetus. For this reason surgery is only for urgent or emergent reasons, such as appendicitis or trauma. The enlarged uterus displaces abdominal organs and distorts landmarks, making surgery more complex.

Anesthetics and medication cause fetal abnormalities during the first trimester. During pregnancy the following maternal physiological changes occur that make monitoring this surgical patient very difficult (Rothrock, 2003):

1. Cardiac output and respiratory tidal volume increase to keep up with the increase in metabolic rate and blood pressure decreases, making interpretation of vital signs and recognition of hypovolemic shock more difficult.
2. The high level of progesterone relaxes the lower esophageal sphincter (LES) and decreases gastrointestinal motility, which slows gastric emptying, resulting in an increased risk for aspiration of stomach contents.
3. Normal laboratory values change during pregnancy and include a decrease in hemoglobin and hematocrit, blood urea nitrogen (BUN), and albumin because of hemodilution from an increase in plasma volume at the beginning of the third trimester. Blood loss will exceed 1000 ml for signs and symptoms of hypovolemia to be manifested.
4. Near term there is an increase in white blood cells beyond the normal range for that of nonpregnant women who have no infection.
5. Fibrinogen levels are increased and clotting time is decreased, increasing the risk of deep vein thrombosis.

In addition, the pregnant patient and her family experience increased psychological stress because of fear of fetal loss or deformity. The perioperative team has to address these concerns.

## Nursing Knowledge Base

The concept of perioperative nursing stresses the importance of providing continuity of care for the surgical patient using the nursing process. In some hospitals, perioperative nurses assess a patient's health status preoperatively, identify specific patient needs, teach and counsel, attend to the patient's needs in the operating room (OR), and then follow the patient's recovery. However, in other institutions, different nurses care for the surgical patient during each phase of the surgical experience. Therefore adequate verbal and written information from each perioperative nurse is essential to ensure continuity of care. Your major responsibility as a perioperative nurse is safe, consistent, and effective nursing care during each phase of the perioperative experience.

## Critical Thinking

### Synthesis

It is important that you synthesize knowledge, experience, attitudes, and standards when planning and providing care for a patient having surgery. Doing so will help you prevent complications, promote rehabilitation, and promote a timely discharge of patients to their home.

**KNOWLEDGE.** It is essential that you have a strong knowledge base in anatomy and physiology, principles of aseptic technique (see Chapter 11), pharmacology (see Chapter 14), and teaching-learning principles (see Chapter 10). In addition, you need to understand the effect surgical procedures and medications will have on different body systems. You also need to understand the normal stress response in order to anticipate potential complications during the perioperative experience. Your role as the perioperative nurse in infection control is based on knowledge of microbiology, the immune system, and aseptic technique. Effective **preoperative teaching** starts when you first assess the patient's and family's readiness and ability to learn and requires a knowledge base of teaching and communication principles and the planned surgical procedure.

**EXPERIENCE.** Any personal experience with surgery helps you to understand the anxiety of the patient and family, as well as to explain some of the physical sensations that the patient will experience. Previous experiences with surgical patients enable you to anticipate questions that the patient and family will ask and help focus preoperative teaching. In addition, past experiences will help you recognize physiological changes in patients more quickly so that you are able to initiate preventive and/or corrective measures early.

**ATTITUDES.** Key attitudes for a perioperative nurse are responsibility and authority. The nurse is a patient advocate. When a patient consents to surgery and receives an anesthetic agent that alters the level of consciousness, health care providers have the responsibility for protecting the patient. You are accountable to the patient for maintaining the rights of the patient when the patient cannot speak on his or her own behalf.

Perioperative nurses also need to be creative in developing plans of care that incorporate the patients' individual differences. For example, you position pregnant patients on the operating bed in a way that promotes venous return. Placing a wedge under the right hip to displace the uterus to the left corrects the problem. Assess each patient, and use the most appropriate padding and positioning techniques possible to prevent injury.

Your attitude about the discipline of nursing is also important when caring for surgical patients. The surgical patient will experience numerous routines necessary both for preparation for surgery and for an efficient and optimal re-

covery. You will systematically follow the current standards of practice to ensure high-quality care for each patient.

**STANDARDS.** The application of critical thinking intellectual standards is important for the surgical patient, particularly if the patient has preexisting physical or psychological factors that will influence the outcomes of surgery. Be very precise, accurate, and complete in gathering assessment data, and use a logical, relevant, and well-thought-out approach in making clinical decisions because the patient's condition can change quickly.

The Association of periOperative Registered Nurses (AORN) has established standards of practice for nurses in perioperative clinical practice. The standards cover practices that ensure safety of the patient, appropriate monitoring and evaluation, infection-control practices, and timely and effective nursing interventions. As the perioperative nurse, you are responsible for following these standards (AORN, 2006). The Joint Commission on Accreditation of Healthcare Organizations (JCAHO) (2006) has developed a Patient Safety Goal to eliminate wrong-patient, wrong-procedure surgery.

## Preoperative Surgical Phase

Surgical patients enter the health care setting in different stages of health. Some patients enter the facility feeling relatively healthy while awaiting elective surgery. Other patients enter in great distress when facing emergency surgery. Many tests and procedures are often necessary to ensure that surgery is indicated and that the patient is in optimum condition for surgery. During these tests and procedures the patient meets many health care personnel who play a role in the patient's care and recovery. Family members or friends also play an important role by providing support through their presence, but they also face many of the same stressors as the patient.

Some patients have preoperative preparation several days before the day of surgery. Preadmission testing is often done in the hospital, physician's or health care provider's office, or outpatient laboratory. With this testing completed, the patient usually enters the hospital the day surgery is performed. Many hospitals have special outpatient or "ambulatory" surgery units for elective surgery, where patients come to the hospital, have surgery, and return home on the same day. Outpatient surgery is also performed in freestanding clinics and ambulatory surgery centers. The more traditional preoperative routine involves the patient entering the hospital the day before surgery. Be able to properly prepare the patient for surgery regardless of where the patient enters the health care setting.

## Nursing Process

### Assessment

Your assessment of the surgical patient establishes a normal baseline for the patient and alerts you to special needs and potential intraoperative and postoperative complications.

You will need good communication skills to gather information and screen patients for potential risk factors for surgery (Scales and Master, 2003).

**NURSING HISTORY.** The preoperative history includes key elements that pertain to the surgical patient's risks and needs. In the ambulatory surgical setting the history is sometimes less detailed than when the patient is hospitalized the evening before surgery; however, the basic information outlined below is necessary for competent care in each setting. If a patient is unable to relate all the necessary information, interview family members or significant others. As with any admission to a health care facility, you include information concerning advance directives. Ask if the patient has a durable power of attorney for health care and a living will (see Chapter 4), and include a copy in the chart. The law requires this for patients of all ages and for all surgical procedures.

**Medical History.** A review of the patient's medical history includes past illnesses and the primary reason for seeking medical care. Candidates for surgery are screened for major medical conditions that will increase the risk for complications (Table 37-3). If a patient is at increased risk, surgery as an outpatient is not advisable. Ask women of childbearing age about the date of their last menstrual period (LMP), if their last period was "typical" for them, and if they have had unprotected sex in the last month. Because many women do not know that they are pregnant early in the first trimester, many institutions require a pregnancy test when a patient of childbearing age is scheduled for surgery and has not had surgical sterilization.

**Previous Surgeries.** Past experience with surgery reveals potential physical and psychological responses to a procedure and alerts you to special needs and risk factors. Complications such as anaphylaxis or **malignant hyperthermia** during previous surgery alert you to the need for preventive measures and availability of emergency equipment. A history of postoperative complications, such as persistent vomiting or excessive pain, also alerts you to the possible need for different medications. Reports of severe anxiety before a previous surgery identify the need for additional emotional support, medications, and preoperative teaching.

| TABLE 37-3 | Medical Conditions That Increase the Risks of Surgery |
|---|---|
| **Type of Condition** | **Reason for Risk** |
| Bleeding disorders (thrombocytopenia, hemophilia) | Disorders increase risk of hemorrhaging during and after surgery. |
| Diabetes mellitus | Diabetes increases susceptibility to infection and impairs wound healing from altered glucose metabolism and associated circulatory impairment. Fluctuating blood glucose levels cause central nervous system (CNS) alterations during anesthesia. Stress of surgery causes increases in blood glucose levels. |
| Heart disease (recent myocardial infarction, dysrhythmias, congestive heart failure) and peripheral vascular disease | Stress of surgery causes increased demands on myocardium to maintain cardiac output. General anesthetic agents depress cardiac function. |
| Hypertension | Hypertension increases the risk of cardiovascular complications during anesthesia (e.g., stroke, tissue oxygenation). |
| Upper respiratory infection | Infection increases risk of respiratory complications during anesthesia (e.g., pneumonia, spasm of laryngeal muscles). |
| Renal disease | Renal disease alters the excretion of anesthetic drugs and their metabolites. Acid-base balance is altered, increasing risk of surgical complications. |
| Liver disease | Liver disease alters metabolism and elimination of drugs administered during surgery and impairs wound healing and clotting time because of alterations in protein metabolism. |
| Fever | Fever predisposes patient to fluid and electrolyte imbalances and often indicates underlying infection. |
| Chronic respiratory disease (emphysema, bronchitis, asthma) | Respiratory disease reduces patient's means to compensate for acid-base alterations. Anesthetic agents reduce respiratory function, increasing risk for severe hypoventilation. |
| Immunological disorders (leukemia, acquired immunodeficiency syndrome [AIDS], bone marrow depression, organ transplantation and use of chemotherapeutic drugs) | Immunological disorders increase risk of infection and delay wound healing after surgery. |
| Abuse of alcohol and street drugs | Patients who abuse drugs sometimes have underlying disease (human immunodeficiency virus [HIV], hepatitis) and altered wellness, which affect healing. Alcohol addiction causes unpredictable reactions to anesthesia. Persons develop withdrawal symptoms during and after surgery. |
| Chronic pain | Regular use of pain medications often results in higher tolerance. Increased doses of narcotics or analgesics are frequently necessary to achieve postoperative pain control. |

**Medication History.** Review whether the patient is taking any medications that predispose him or her to surgical complications (Table 37-4). Many medications interact unpredictably with anesthetic agents during surgery (McKenry and Salerno, 2003). If a patient regularly uses prescription or over-the-counter (OTC) medications, or herbal supplements, some physicians or health care providers will decide to temporarily discontinue the drugs before surgery or adjust the dosages. Instruct patients to ask the physician or health care provider whether they should take their usual medications the morning of surgery. If the patient is having inpatient surgery, all prescription drugs taken before surgery are automatically discontinued after surgery unless reordered. Be vigilant in reviewing the surgeon's preoperative orders so that you do not forget any medication the patient needs to take before the operation. It is very important that as the patient moves through the different areas during the surgical procedure that a complete list of the patient's medications is accurately communicated from nurse to nurse (JCAHO, 2004).

**Allergies.** Allergies to medications, topical agents used to prepare the skin for surgery, and latex create significant risks for the surgical patient. An allergic response to any agent is potentially fatal, depending on its severity. Latex allergies are on the rise (see Chapter 11). A latex allergy manifests as contact dermatitis with redness, inflammation, and blisters; as contact urticaria with pruritus, redness, and swelling; or as hay fever–like symptoms and anaphylaxis.

All health care workers need to know about their patient's allergies. In most health care agencies, if allergies exist, the patient receives an allergy identification band to wear during the surgery and until the patient is discharged. Allergies are also often listed on the front of the patient's chart, on the medical order sheet, and on the patient's medication administration record. You need to verify your patient's allergies before, during, and after surgery.

**Smoking Habits.** The patient who smokes is at a greater risk for postoperative pulmonary complications than a nonsmoker. Smoking decreases ciliary movement of mucus from the lower airways upward, increases mucus production, and causes bronchial constriction, thus increasing airway obstruction. After surgery this patient will have greater difficulty clearing the airways of mucous secretions and is at increased risk for **bronchospasm** and **laryngospasm.** Use this information to plan aggressive postoperative **pulmonary hygiene,** including more frequent turning, deep breathing, coughing, use of incentive spirometry, and chest physical therapy (PT) if ordered. Smoking causes hypercoagulability of the blood and increased risk of clot formation (Black and Hawks, 2005). You also need to add measures to decease risk of clot formation such as pulsatile stockings, deep breathing, leg exercises, and early ambulation to the plan of care.

**Alcohol and Controlled Substance Use and Abuse.** The surgical team needs to be aware of the use of alcohol and controlled substances by patients to prepare for adverse reactions, such as withdrawal, that may occur during surgery. Increased tolerance to opioids occurs with opioid use, resulting in an increased need for anesthesia and postoperative analgesics (Black and Hawks, 2005).

**Family Support.** Determine the extent of the patient's support from family members or friends. Surgery often re-

---

| TABLE 37-4 | Drugs With Special Implications for the Surgical Patient |
|---|---|
| **Drug Class** | **Effects During Surgery** |
| Antibiotics | Antibiotics potentiate action of anesthetic agents. If taken within 2 weeks before surgery, aminoglycosides (gentamicin, tobramycin, neomycin) will cause mild respiratory depression from depressed neuromuscular transmission. |
| Antidysrhythmics | Antidysrhythmics reduce cardiac contractility and heart rate and impair cardiac conduction during anesthesia. |
| Anticoagulants | Anticoagulants alter normal clotting factors and thus increase risk of hemorrhaging during and after surgery. Discontinue them at least 48 hours before surgery. Aspirin is a common medication that alters clotting mechanisms. |
| Anticonvulsants | Long-term use of certain anticonvulsants (e.g., phenytoin [Dilantin], phenobarbital) alters metabolism of anesthetic agents. |
| Antihypertensives | Antihypertensives interact with anesthetic agents and cause bradycardia, hypotension, and impaired circulation. They inhibit synthesis and storage of norepinephrine in sympathetic nerve endings. |
| Corticosteroids | With prolonged use, corticosteroids cause adrenal atrophy, which reduces the body's ability to withstand stress and results in hypotension during surgery. Before and during surgery, dosages are sometimes temporarily increased. |
| Insulin | Patients with diabetes often need less insulin after surgery because their nutritional intake is decreased. However, stress response and intravenous (IV) administration of glucose solutions increase insulin dosage requirements after surgery. |
| Diuretics | Diuretics potentiate electrolyte imbalances (particularly potassium), increasing the risk of dysrhythmias during and after surgery. |
| Nonsteroidal antiinflammatory drugs (NSAIDs) | NSAIDs inhibit platelet aggregation and prolong bleeding time, increasing susceptibility to bleeding during and after surgery. |

sults in temporary disability that often requires direct care and assistance from significant others during recovery. The patient does not always immediately assume the same level of physical activity and often returns home with dressings to change or exercises to perform. You ask questions to determine the condition of the patient's home environment and factors that will interfere with postoperative restrictions or care activities. For example, the patient receives discharge instructions that state no stair climbing due to limited mobility. When you talk to the patient and family you discover that the bathroom in the home is on the second floor. In this case, you will need to make sure that the patient has a commode to use on the lower level of the home.

**Occupation.** Surgery often results in physical alterations that hinder or prevent a person from returning to work. Assess the patient's occupational history to anticipate the effect surgery will have on convalescence and eventual work performance. This prepares you to explain any restrictions the patient will have when returning to work.

**Feelings.** Surgery causes anxiety and a feeling of loss of control for most patients. Many families are concerned about the ability of the patient to return to a productive life and the impact recovery will have on the family. You will need to detect the patient's feelings about having surgery from both verbal and nonverbal cues. A patient who is fearful will ask many questions or be very quiet, will seem uneasy when strangers enter the room, or will actively seek the company of friends and relatives.

It is often difficult to assess feelings thoroughly when ambulatory surgery is scheduled because of the limited time you will spend with the patient. As the nurse in an outpatient surgical program, telephone the patient at home before surgery or interview the patient during a preadmission testing visit. For hospital inpatients, choose a time for discussion after preliminary admitting or diagnostic tests are complete. The patient's ability to share feelings depends in part on your willingness to ask questions, listen, be supportive, and clarify misconceptions.

**Cultural and Spiritual Factors.** Cultural differences in the use of both verbal and nonverbal communication require you to validate interpretation of cues with the patient and family. This is especially important after you conduct the initial preoperative assessment and then look for changes in the patient's status after surgery. For example, patients from Asian cultures often remain silent out of respect, not fear. Individuals from Central America usually prefer to have many family members and friends surrounding them and helping to express their needs. In some cultures women follow what the significant male member of their family dictates; therefore it is very important to explain everything to your female patient's husband, father, or brother in order for her to participate in the plan of care (Giger and Davidhizar, 2004). When doing this, make sure to have permission from the patient to share personal health information. Many cultural and religious taboos exist concerning the body, who cares for the physical needs of others, and treatments appropriate for healing, so it is important to explore these issues with the patient and/or family. Although it is important to recognize and plan for differences based on culture, remember that not all members of one family always hold the beliefs of a particular religion or culture. Asking relevant questions of each patient concerning cultural and spiritual beliefs and expectations will further individualize your nursing care (see Chapters 17 and 18). The spiritual beliefs of the patient help the patient cope with fears and anxieties related to the upcoming surgery. Make sure to help the patient get the spiritual help that is requested before surgery. For example, contact the hospital chaplain that the patient has asked to speak to before going to surgery (Box 37-1).

**Coping Resources.** Assessment of a patient's feelings and self-concept helps to reveal whether the patient has the ability to cope with the stress of surgery. It is also valuable to ask the patient about stress management. If the patient has had previous surgery, discuss with the patient the behaviors that helped to resolve past tension or nervousness. You will often

---

| **BOX 37-1** | CULTURAL FOCUS |
| --- | --- |

In preparing her preoperative teaching Sue discovers that Russian-Americans, such as Mr. Korloff, expect the nurse to be warm and caring. Nurses are expected to help patients cope with their health problems. Russian-Americans expect the nurse to be friendly, using open inviting nonverbal postures, and a friendly smile. They freely share health problems with nurses conveying this friendly, caring behavior. Russian-Americans are also willing to follow teaching provided by nurses who they feel are sincere, competent, and trustworthy. They value receiving immediate information and answers from health care workers and follow up on health care instructions when they fully understand them. Russian-Americans typically have strong family ties and values. The father usually plays a primary role in the function of the family. Using the knowledge of Russian-Americans Sue gained from her reading and past experience, she developed a culturally competent plan of care for Mr. Korloff.

**Implications for Practice**
- Sue assesses Mr. Korloff's opinions about surgery first and then works to include the family.
- Sue assesses the level of involvement of Mr. Korloff's daughters in his surgical preparation and care.
- Sue provides Mr. Korloff's preoperative teaching in a warm, caring, open manner using frequent smiles and hand gestures.
- Sue speaks slowly and clearly in a low, calm voice using simple words.
- Sue provides an explanation of the importance of preoperative exercises so Mr. Korloff will understand why the exercises are important and will be more willing to do them after surgery.
- Sue determines that Mr. Korloff's daughters are close to their father and includes them in the teaching session.

From Giger JN, Davidhizar RE: *Transcultural nursing: assessment and intervention*, ed 4, St. Louis, 2004, Mosby.

need to instruct the patient on relaxation exercises (see Chapter 30), which help control anxiety.

**Body Image.** Surgical removal of a diseased tissue or organ often leaves permanent disfigurement or alteration in body function. Concern over mutilation, change in sexuality, or loss of a body part compounds a patient's fears. Individuals react differently, depending on age, culture, occupation, self-image, and degree of self-esteem. Encourage patients to express these concerns. The patient facing even temporary disability or sexual dysfunction requires understanding and support (see Chapter 20).

**Patient Expectations.** It is important to identify the patient's and family's perceptions and expectations regarding surgery, recovery, and health care providers. This information provides you with information to plan interventions for teaching and emotional preparation and provides the basis for evaluation of care. For example, some patients have expectations regarding pain control and the use of pain medications that are unrealistic. Patients who are prepared to experience pain and taught the proper use of pharmacological and non-pharmacological pain-relief measures tend to require less medication (LaMontagne and others, 2003; Rothrock, 2003).

Patients and family members often have misconceptions about surgery. It is important to discuss with them their understanding of the purpose of the tests, the possible outcomes, and the persons responsible for informing them of results and providing follow-up care. When a patient is well prepared and knows what to expect, reinforce the patient's knowledge.

You will face an ethical dilemma when a patient is unaware of the real reason for surgery. In such a case, speak with the physician or health care provider before revealing specific information related to the medical diagnosis to prevent confusion and to alert the physician or health care provider that clarification is necessary.

**PHYSICAL EXAMINATION.** You will conduct a partial or complete physical examination (see Chapter 13), depending on the setting and nature of the surgery. The assessment focuses on findings related to the patient's medical history and on body systems that surgery or anesthesia will affect (Table 37-5).

**General Survey.** Gestures and body movements reflect decreased energy or weakness caused by illness. Height and body weight are important indicators of nutritional status and are used to calculate medication dosages. Preoperative vital signs provide a baseline with which to compare alterations that occur during and after surgery. Anesthetic agents and medications produce vital sign changes. Preoperative assessment of vital signs is also important in ruling out fluid and electrolyte abnormalities (see Chapter 15).

An elevated temperature is cause for concern. If the patient has an underlying infection, surgery will often be postponed until the infection is treated or resolved. An elevated body temperature also alters drug metabolism and increases the risk of fluid and electrolyte imbalances.

**Head and Neck.** Assessment of oral mucous membranes reveals the level of hydration. Dehydration increases the risk for the development of serious fluid and electrolyte imbal-

ances during surgery. During the oral examination, identify loose or capped teeth because they often become dislodged during endotracheal intubation. You need to note any dentures your patient has to protect them from loss or damage.

Inspection of the soft palate and nasal sinuses sometimes reveals sinus drainage indicative of respiratory or sinus infection. To rule out the possibility of local or systemic infection, palpate for cervical lymph node enlargement. Also inspect the jugular veins for distention. Excess fluid within the circulatory system or failure of the heart to contract efficiently frequently leads to jugular vein distention. A patient with heart disease or fluid overload is at risk for cardiovascular complications during surgery.

**Skin.** Conduct a thorough inspection of the patient's skin overlying all body parts, especially bony prominences. During surgery a patient lies in a fixed position, often for several hours. Avoid positioning a patient over an area where the skin shows signs of pressure over bony prominences. A patient is susceptible to skin breakdown if the skin is thin or dry or has poor turgor (see Chapter 35).

**Thorax and Lungs.** A decline in ventilatory function, assessed through breathing pattern and chest excursion, indicates a patient's risk for respiratory complications. Serious pulmonary congestion often causes postponement of surgery. For example, narrowing of the airways, as occurs with chronic lung disease (CLD, formerly known as chronic obstructive pulmonary disease [COPD]) increases the risk of airway obstruction because of bronchospasm related to endotracheal intubation and anesthesia.

**Heart and Vascular System.** If the patient has heart disease, assess the apical pulse. After surgery compare the rate and rhythm of the patient's pulse with preoperative baseline values.

Assessment of peripheral pulses, color, and temperature of extremities is particularly important for the patient undergoing vascular surgery, the patient undergoing surgery on an extremity using a tourniquet, or when applying constricting bandages or casts to an extremity after surgery. Postoperative color changes, change in sensation, or development of a weak or absent pulse in a patient who had adequate circulation before surgery indicates impaired circulation.

**Abdomen.** Alterations in gastrointestinal function after surgery often result in decreased or absent bowel sounds and distention. You need to recognize whether the patient is simply obese or the abdomen has become distended. Assessment of preoperative bowel sounds and normal elimination pattern is useful as a baseline. If surgery requires manipulation of portions of the gastrointestinal tract or if a general anesthetic is used, normal peristalsis sometimes does not return and bowel sounds are absent or diminished for up to several days.

**Neurological Status.** A patient's level of consciousness will change as a result of general anesthesia. However, after the effects of anesthesia disappear, the patient will return to the preoperative level of responsiveness.

Spinal or epidural anesthesia causes temporary paralysis of the lower extremities. Be aware of preexisting weakness or impaired mobility of the lower extremities to avoid becom-

## FOCUSED PATIENT ASSESSMENT

TABLE 37-5

| Factors to Assess | Questions and Approaches | Physical Assessment Strategies |
|---|---|---|
| Significant medical history and previous surgeries | Ask patient about condition requiring surgery and expectations derived from having surgery.<br>Ask if patient experiences conditions that increase risk of surgery (see Table 37-3) and how each is being treated.<br>Ask patient for list of past surgeries with approximate dates.<br>Ask patient about family history of cardiac, renal, liver, and endocrine diseases. | Monitor vital signs, and note any abnormalities.<br>Inspect neck for jugular vein distention (cardiac disease, fluid overload).<br>Inspect skin for turgor, dryness, surgical scars, rashes, skin breakdown.<br>Auscultate heart, lungs, vascular system, and abdomen for abnormal sounds (murmurs, congestion, bruits, absence of bowel sounds).<br>Palpate heart, vascular system, abdomen for abnormalities (thrill, masses).<br>Assess extremities for decreased sensation, hair loss, clubbed fingers, deformed nails, sluggish capillary reflex, color. |
| Medication history and allergies | Ask patient for detailed list of all prescription, OTC, and herbal medications.<br>Ask patient about instructions from surgeon concerning taking or omitting any medications preoperatively.<br>Ask patient and/or family about any personal and/or family history of allergic responses to medications (including anesthetics) or environmental factors (e.g., latex, foods).<br>Ask patient about manifestations of allergic reactions. | Inspect any medication containers brought in by patient or family.<br>Monitor laboratory values for any evidence of side effects of medications or drug levels, if ordered.<br><br>Observe skin and mucous membranes for any evidence of allergic response. |
| Diet history | Ask patient about any medical, cultural, religious, or personal dietary restrictions. | Assess for evidence of nutritional alterations (rash, dry skin, hair loss, decreased muscle mass, obesity). |

## SYNTHESIS IN PRACTICE

As Sue prepares to conduct the preadmission assessment of Mr. Korloff, she will recall what she has learned regarding risk factors for patients undergoing surgery. Mr. Korloff has had a history of heart disease in the past, according to the referral note. Five years ago he was treated for a cardiac dysrhythmia but has had no further problems. Sue will plan to question Mr. Korloff thoroughly about any potential cardiac symptoms.

Sue's knowledge of laparoscopic surgery will help her anticipate the types of postoperative problems Mr. Korloff is likely to develop, such as food intolerance and abdominal or referred pain from the carbon dioxide gas used during laparoscopy. Sue's expe-

rience with her own father after surgery will help her to explain some of the sensations that Mr. Korloff will experience, such as a sore throat from the endotracheal tube used for administering anesthesia. She will also need to draw on her experiences with patients she cared for after laparoscopic cholecystectomies during her previous rotation on a general surgery floor. She will inform Mr. Korloff and his daughters that he will have intravenous (IV) fluids infusing until he tolerates oral fluids and that he will likely experience only mild discomfort. Mr. Korloff will be able to get out of bed the evening of surgery, and if all goes well he will likely be discharged the next day.

ing alarmed when full motor function does not return immediately after the procedure.

**RISK FACTORS.** Knowledge of preoperative risk factors discussed earlier will enable you to take necessary precautions in planning care.

**DIAGNOSTIC SCREENING.** Before a patient has surgery, diagnostic tests screen for preexisting abnormalities. Patients scheduled for elective surgery take these tests as an outpatient on or before the morning of surgery. If tests reveal severe problems, the surgeon or anesthesiologist will cancel surgery until the condition stabilizes. As the preoper-

ative nurse, you are responsible for coordinating the completion of tests and for verifying that the patient is prepared properly. You also review diagnostic results as they become available, alerting the surgeon and/or anesthesiologist of findings and planning appropriate therapy.

Screening tests depend on the condition of the patient and the nature of the surgery. Table 37-6 summarizes routine screening tests. In addition, the patient will need a blood type and screen if transfusions are necessary. Additional preoperative tests include a urinalysis screen for urinary tract infections, renal disease, or diabetes mellitus; and a 12-lead

| TABLE 37-6 | Common Laboratory Blood Tests |

| | | Significance | |
|---|---|---|---|
| Test | Normal Values* | Low | High |
| **Complete Blood Count (CBC)** | | | |
| Hemoglobin (Hgb) | Female: 12-15 g/dl; male: 13.6-17.2 g/dl | Anemia | Polycythemia |
| Hematocrit (Hct) | Female: 35%-47%; male: 42%-52% | Fluid overload | Dehydration |
| Platelet count | 150,000-400,000/mm³ | Decreased clotting | Increased thrombosis |
| White blood cell count | 4500-11,000/mm³ | Immunosuppression | Infection |
| **Blood Chemistry (SMA 7 or CHEM 7)** | | | |
| Sodium (Na) | 137-145 mEq/L | Hyponatremia/fluid overload | Hypernatremia/dehydration |
| Potassium (K) | 3.5-5.0 mEq/L | Cardiac dysrhythmias | Renal disease |
| Chloride (Cl) | 97-107 mEq/L | Follows shifts in sodium blood levels | |
| Carbon dioxide (CO₂) | 22-30 mEq/L | Indirect measurement of bicarbonate (HC₃⁻) | |
| Blood urea nitrogen (BUN) | 5-20 mg/dl | Liver disease/fluid overload | Renal disease/ dehydration |
| Glucose | 70-105 mg/dl fasting | Hypoglycemia/insulin reaction | Hyperglycemia/diabetes mellitus |
| Creatinine | Female: 0.5-1.1 mg/dl; male: 0.6-1.2 mg/dl | Malnutrition | Renal disease |
| **Coagulation Studies** | | | |
| Prothrombin time (PT) | 10-15 sec | Risk of thrombosis | Risk of hemorrhage Coumadin response |
| Partial thromboplastin time (PTT) | <35 sec | Risk of thrombosis | Risk of hemorrhage |
| Activated PTT (APTT) | 30-40 sec | Activators added to PTT reagent to shorten time | Heparin response |

From Chernecky CC, Berger BJ: *Laboratory tests and diagnostic procedures*, ed 4, Philadelphia, 2004, Saunders.
*Normal ranges vary slightly among laboratories.

electrocardiogram to determine the normality of the heart rate and rhythm. A chest x-ray study to assess the size and shape of the heart, presence of lung lesions and chest wall abnormalities, and position of the diaphragm and the aorta is also a common preoperative test.

## Nursing Diagnosis

Cluster defining characteristics gathered during assessment to identify appropriate nursing diagnoses and related factors. The nature and type of surgery, as well as the patient's age and health status, suggest defining characteristics for many nursing diagnoses. The diagnoses establish direction for care during one or all of the surgical phases. For example, a patient's restlessness, poor eye contact, and expressed concern about the results of surgery point to the diagnosis of *anxiety*. However, you need to validate the assessment to avoid misdiagnosis. In the assessment above, restlessness also indicates pain. Therefore you need to ensure that you identify the nursing diagnosis that best fits your patient's problem. Nursing diagnoses for the preoperative patient may include:

- Anxiety
- Decisional conflict
- Compromised family coping
- Ineffective coping
- Fear
- Risk for imbalanced fluid volume
- Hopelessness
- Deficient knowledge
- Imbalanced nutrition: less than body requirements
- Imbalanced nutrition: more than body requirements
- Powerlessness
- Ineffective role performance
- Risk for impaired skin integrity
- Disturbed sleep pattern
- Risk for spiritual distress

A diagnosis and its related factors offer direction to the most effective nursing interventions. Make sure the related factors are accurate to avoid inappropriate interventions. For example, *anxiety related to deficient knowledge of perioperative rou-*

*tines* will require you to offer thorough instruction preoperatively and immediately postoperatively. However, *anxiety related to threat of ineffective role performance* will require counseling and coaching during the postoperative recovery. If the threat is real, it is necessary to notify social services.

Preoperatively, nursing diagnoses focus on the intraoperative and postoperative risks a patient face. Preventive care is essential to manage the surgical patient effectively.

## ❀ Planning

It is essential to include the patient, family, and primary caregiver in any discussions before surgery. Involving the patient early minimizes surgical risks and postoperative complications. Structured preoperative teaching reduces the amount of anesthesia and postoperative pain medication needed, decreases the occurrence of postoperative urinary retention, promotes an earlier return to normal oral intake, and decreases length of hospital stay (Rothrock, 2003). Patients informed about the surgical experience are less likely to be fearful and are able to prepare for expected outcomes.

**GOALS AND OUTCOMES.** The plan of care begins in the preoperative phase, and you modify it during the intraoperative and postoperative phases (see care plan). The goals of care for the surgical patient include the following:

Understanding the physiological and psychological responses to surgery
Understanding intraoperative and postoperative events
Achieving emotional and physiological comfort and rest
Achieving return of normal physiological function after surgery (e.g., return of normal vital signs, fluid and electrolyte balance, muscle function)
Remaining free of surgical wound infection
Remaining safe from harm during the perioperative period

Outcomes established for each goal of care provide measurable behavioral evidence to determine the patient's progress toward meeting stated goals.

**SETTING PRIORITIES.** You establish individualized care by prioritizing nursing diagnoses and interventions based on the assessed needs of each patient. Setting priorities requires clinical judgment. For example, if a patient has *anxiety* and *deficient knowledge,* the patient's priority is deficient knowledge. In this case you will need to instruct the patient in order to relieve the anxiety. Your approach to each patient needs to be thorough and reflect your understanding of the implications of the patient's age, physical and psychological health, educational level, cultural and religious practices, and stated and/or written wishes concerning advance medical directives.

**CONTINUITY OF CARE.** For the ambulatory surgical patient the preoperative planning phase usually occurs in the outpatient surgery setting before or on the morning of surgery. Ideally, it begins in the surgeon's office and continues in the home. This gives the patient time to think about the surgical experience, make necessary physical preparations, and ask questions about postoperative procedures. Well-planned preoperative care ensures that the patient is well informed and ac-

tively participates during recovery. The family or significant others also play an active supportive role for the patient.

Planning also requires referral to other members of the health care team. Patients who will require aggressive pulmonary rehabilitation, such as those having thoracic surgery, are referred to a respiratory therapist. Many patients and their families benefit from referral to pastoral care, especially if the procedure is an emergency or is life threatening.

## ❀ Implementation

Preoperative nursing interventions provide the patient with an understanding of the physical and psychological aspects of surgical intervention.

**INFORMED CONSENT.** A surgeon cannot legally perform surgery nor can an anesthesia care provider administer an anesthetic until a patient understands the need for the procedure and the steps involved, as well as the risks, expected results, and alternative treatments. Chapter 4 summarizes issues and guidelines for informed consent. All consent forms need to be signed before you administer any preoperative medications that alter the patient's consciousness. The primary responsibility for informing the patient rests with the surgeon and anesthesia care personnel (Fogg, 2003). However, if the patient is confused or uncertain about the procedure, you have an ethical obligation to contact the surgeon and/or anesthesia care provider so that further discussion and clarification are provided to meet the patient's information and emotional needs. The patient always has the right to refuse surgery or treatment even after giving written consent (Iocono, 2000).

**HEALTH PROMOTION.** Health promotion activities during the preoperative phase focus on prevention of complications, health maintenance, and support of possible rehabilitation needs postoperatively.

**Preoperative Teaching.** Patient education relieves anxiety, increases patient satisfaction, speeds up the recovery process, decreases the amount of perceived pain, and facilitates a more rapid return to work or normal functioning (Lewis and others, 2002). Preoperative teaching provided in a systematic, structured, and interactive format has a positive influence on patients' recovery (Lewis and others, 2002). Structured teaching often influences the following postoperative factors:

1. *Ventilatory function:* Teaching improves the ability and willingness to deep breathe and cough effectively.
2. *Physical functional capacity:* Teaching increases understanding and willingness to ambulate and resume activities of daily living.
3. *Sense of well-being:* Patients who are prepared for surgery experience less anxiety and report a greater sense of psychological well-being (Shuldham, 1999).
4. *Length of hospital stay:* Teaching frequently reduces the patient's length of hospital stay by preventing or minimizing postoperative complications.
5. *Anxiety about pain and amount of pain medication needed for comfort:* Patients who learn about pain and ways to relieve it are less anxious about the pain, ask for what they need, and actually require less pain medication.

thing that contradicts the surgeon's explanation. One way to avoid contradictions is to first ask what the surgeon has told the patient. If the patient has little or no understanding about the surgery, you refer the patient back to the surgeon for additional information.

PREOPERATIVE ROUTINES. You will need to explain certain preoperative routines. For example, your patient needs to have a chest x-ray examination. You explain the test and why it is necessary. Knowing what tests are planned and why will increase the patient's sense of control.

The anesthesiologist will visit with the patient to complete a preanesthesia assessment either during the preoperative admission process or when the patient is in the presurgical care unit. The patient and family need to know about this visit, so they can ask any questions they have or provide necessary information.

The patient and family need to understand that the patient can have no oral intake (either food or liquids) for approximately 2 hours (clear liquids) before surgery. The patient also cannot have any meat or fried foods 8 hours before surgery, unless explicitly specified by the anesthesiologist or surgeon (American Society of Anesthesiologists Task Force on Perioperative Fast, 1999). During the use of general anesthesia, the muscles relax and gastric contents can reflux into the esophagus. The anesthetic eliminates the patient's ability to gag. Therefore the patient is at risk for aspiration of food or fluids from the stomach into the lungs. The physician's or health care provider's orders provide additional guidance for routines you explain to the patient (e.g., IV therapy, preoperative medications, or insertion of a urinary catheter or a nasogastric tube).

INTRAOPERATIVE ROUTINES. The scheduled operative time is only an anticipated time. Unanticipated delays occur for many reasons that have nothing to do with your patient. Emphasize that the scheduled time is a rough estimate and the actual time will possibly be sooner or later than the scheduled time. Tell family members where to wait, and inform them that the surgeon will speak to them when the surgery is completed. Communicate excessive delays to the family if they occur.

POSTOPERATIVE ROUTINES. The patient and family want to know about postoperative events. If they understand routine postoperative vital sign monitoring, they are less likely to worry when nurses perform these assessments. You also explain if the patient is to have IV lines, dressings, or drainage tubes. It is important to neither overprepare nor underprepare the patient and family. You cannot predict all the patient's requirements, and a patient may be misinformed about a therapy that may not be initiated. Contradictions between your explanations and reality cause anxiety.

SENSORY PREPARATION. Provide the patient with information about sensations typically experienced before, during, and after surgery. Preparatory information helps patients anticipate the steps of a procedure and form a realistic image of the surgical experience. When sensations occur as predicted, the patient is better at coping with the experiences. For example, the operating room is very bright and cool.

Explain that you will apply a cuff for a noninvasive blood pressure monitor to the patient's arm. This monitor makes a hum and a beep, and the cuff tightens around the patient's arm. Informing the patient about these and other sensations in the operating room will reduce anxiety before the patient is anesthetized, which will help decrease the amount of anesthetic needed for induction. Other postoperative sensations to describe include blurred vision from ophthalmic ointment, dryness of the mouth or the sensation of a sore throat resulting from an endotracheal tube, pain at the incision site, tightness of the dressings, and feeling cold.

PAIN RELIEF. One of the surgical patient's greatest fears is pain. The family is also concerned about the patient's comfort. Preoperative preparation regarding pain and pain control helps the patient to cope with the pain. Patient-controlled analgesia (PCA) is common and provides the patient with control over pain. Explain to the patient how to operate the pump and the importance of administering medication as soon as pain becomes persistent (see Chapter 30). Analgesics will not provide adequate pain relief if the patient waits until the pain becomes excruciating before using or requesting an analgesic. Encourage the patient to use analgesics as needed and not be fearful of any dependence on pain medications following surgery.

If epidural, intramuscular, or oral analgesics will be used, the patient needs to know the schedule for these drugs. Encourage the patient to inform nurses as soon as pain becomes a persistent discomfort. The patient needs to also know it takes time for a drug to act and that the drug will rarely eliminate all the discomfort. In addition, inform the patient and family of other therapies available for pain relief, such as focused breathing and relaxation, distraction, and the use of a K-pad or an ice pack.

**Postoperative Exercises.** Every preoperative teaching program includes explanation and demonstration of the five postoperative exercises: diaphragmatic breathing, incentive spirometry, controlled coughing, turning, and leg exercises (Skill 37-1).

Diaphragmatic breathing improves lung expansion and oxygen delivery without using excess energy. The patient learns to use the diaphragm during deep breathing to take slow, deep, and relaxed breaths. Eventually the patient's lung volume improves. Deep breathing also helps to clear any anesthetic gases from the airways.

To facilitate deep breathing the physician or health care provider often orders an incentive spirometer for the patient (see Chapter 28). Incentive spirometry encourages forced inspiration. The therapy is effective in preventing atelectasis postoperatively.

Coughing assists in removing retained mucus in the airways. A deep, productive cough is more beneficial than merely clearing the throat. The patient needs to anticipate postoperative discomfort and understand the importance of coughing, even when it is difficult. Teach the patient to splint an abdominal incision to minimize pain during coughing and to ask for pain medications as needed.

*Text continued on p. 1108*

# SKILL 37-1 | Teaching Postoperative Exercises

## Delegation Considerations

Postoperative exercise teaching cannot be delegated. Assistive personnel reinforce and assist patients in performing postoperative exercises.

## Equipment

- Pillow (optional; used to splint surgical incision when coughing)
- Incentive spirometer
- Elastic stockings or sequential compression stockings

| STEP | RATIONALE |
|---|---|

## ASSESSMENT

1. Assess patient's risk for postoperative respiratory complications: review medical history to identify presence of chronic pulmonary condition (e.g., emphysema, asthma), any condition that affects chest wall movement, history of smoking, and presence of reduced hemoglobin (low red blood cell [RBC] count).

   General anesthesia predisposes patient to respiratory problems because lungs do not fully inflate during surgery, cough reflex is suppressed, and mucus collects within airway passages. After surgery patient will have reduced lung volume and require greater efforts to deep breathe and cough; inadequate lung expansion leads to atelectasis and pneumonia. Patient is at greater risk for developing respiratory complications if chronic lung conditions are present. Smoking damages ciliary clearance and increases mucus secretion. A reduced hemoglobin level leads to inadequate oxygenation.

2. Auscultate lungs.

   Establish as baseline for postoperative comparison.

3. Assess patient's ability to cough and deep breathe by having patient take a deep breath and observing movement of shoulders, chest wall, and abdomen. Observe chest excursion during a deep breath. Ask patient to cough after taking a deep breath.

   Reveals maximum potential for chest expansion and ability to cough forcefully; serves as baseline to measure patient's ability to perform exercises postoperatively. Diaphragmatic breathing allows for greater lung expansion, improved ventilation, and increased blood oxygenation. Coughing loosens and removes secretions from the pulmonary alveoli.

4. Assess patient's risk for postoperative thrombus formation (older patients, immobilized patients, patients with personal or family history of clots, women over 35 years who smoke and are taking oral contraceptives). Observe the calves for redness, warmth, and tenderness. Palpate pedal pulses. Observe for a Homan's sign, calf pain, or dorsiflexion of the foot. Compare legs for bilateral equality.

   Thrombus forms when venous stasis, hypercoagulability, and vein trauma exist simultaneously (Lewis and others, 2004). Following general anesthesia circulation slows, resulting in a greater tendency for clot formation. Immobilization results in decreased muscular contraction in lower extremities, which promotes venous stasis. The physical stress of surgery creates a hypercoagulable state in most individuals. Manipulation and positioning during surgery sometimes cause trauma to leg veins.

---

• *Critical Decision Point:* A Homan's sign is not always present when a deep vein thrombosis exists (Day, 2003, Urbano, 2001). Checking for Homan's sign may be contraindicated in a suspected DVT; some researchers think that vigorous dorsiflexion may dislodge a thrombus. If a thrombus is suspected, notify physician and refrain from manipulating extremity any further. Surgery will usually be postponed. Antiembolism stockings or sequential compression stockings may be ordered for patients at risk for thrombus formation.

---

5. Assess patient's ability to move independently while in bed.

   Patients confined to bed rest, even for limited periods, will need to turn regularly. Determines existence of any mobility restrictions.

6. Assess patient's willingness and capability to learn exercises; note attention span, anxiety, level of consciousness, and language level.

   Ability to learn depends on readiness, ability, and learning environment.

7. Assess family members' or significant other's willingness to learn and to support patient postoperatively.

   Encourage family member or significant other to coach patient on exercise performance.

8. Assess patient's medical orders preoperatively and postoperatively.

   Some patients will require adaptations in way to perform exercises.

| SKILL 37-1 | Teaching Postoperative Exercises—cont'd |

| STEP | RATIONALE |
|---|---|
| (6) Instruct patient to breathe normally for short period. | Prevents hyperventilation and fatigue. |
| (7) Have patient repeat maneuver until goals are achieved. | Ensures correct use of spirometer. |
| (8) Perform hand hygiene. | Reduces transmission of microorganisms. |
| **C. Positive Expiratory Pressure Therapy and "Huff" Coughing** | |
| (1) Perform hand hygiene. | Reduces transmission of microorganisms. |
| (2) Set positive expiratory pressure (PEP) device for setting ordered. | Higher settings require more effort. |
| (3) Instruct patient to assume semi-Fowler's or high-Fowler's position, and place nose clip on patient's nose (see illustration). | Promotes optimum lung expansion and expectoration of mucus. |
| (4) Have patient place lips around mouthpiece. Instruct patient to take a full breath and then exhale 2 or 3 times longer than inhalation. Repeat pattern for 10 to 20 breaths. | Ensures that patient does all breathing through mouth. Ensures that patient uses the device properly. |
| (5) Remove device from mouth, and have patient take a slow, deep breath and hold for 3 seconds. | Promotes lung expansion before coughing. |
| (6) Instruct patient to exhale in quick, short, forced "huffs." | "Huff" coughing, or forced expiratory technique, promotes bronchial hygiene by increasing expectoration of secretions. |
| **D. Controlled Coughing** | |
| (1) Explain importance of maintaining an upright position. | Position facilitates diaphragm excursion and enhances thorax expansion. |

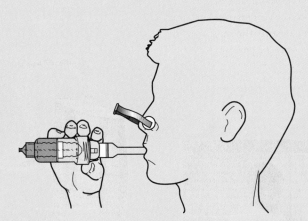

STEP **1C(3)** Diagram of use of positive expiratory pressure device.

| STEP | RATIONALE |
|---|---|
| (2) If surgical incision will be either abdominal or thoracic, teach patient to place pillow or bath blanket over incisional area and place hands over pillow to splint incision. During breathing and coughing exercises, press gently against incisional area for splinting or support. You do this with the hands (see illustrations). | Surgical incision cuts through muscles, tissues, and nerve endings. Deep breathing and coughing exercises place additional stress on suture line and cause discomfort. Splinting incision with hands or pillow provides firm support and reduces incisional pulling. |
| (3) Demonstrate coughing. Take two slow, deep breaths, inhaling through nose and exhaling through mouth. | Deep breaths expand lungs fully so that air moves behind mucus and facilitates effects of coughing. |
| (4) Inhale deeply a third time, and hold breath to count of three. Cough fully for two or three consecutive coughs without inhaling between coughs. (Tell patient to push all air out of lungs.) | Consecutive coughs help remove mucus more effectively and completely than one forceful cough. |

---

• *Critical Decision Point:* Coughing is often contraindicated after brain, spinal, head, neck, or eye surgery due to a potential increase in intracranial pressure.

---

| STEP | RATIONALE |
|---|---|
| (5) Caution patient against just clearing throat instead of coughing. Explain that coughing will not cause injury to incision (see illustrations). | Clearing throat does not remove mucus from deeper airways. Postoperative incisional pain makes it harder to cough effectively. |
| (6) Have patient continues to practice coughing exercises, splinting imaginary incision. Instruct the patient to cough 2 or 3 times every hour while awake. | Stresses value of deep coughing with splinting to effectively expectorate mucus with minimal discomfort. |
| (7) Instruct patient to examine sputum for consistency, odor, amount, and color changes. | Sputum consistency, odor, amount, and color changes indicate the presence of a pulmonary complication, such as pneumonia. |
| **E. Turning** | |
| (1) Instruct patient to assume supine position and move toward left side of bed by bending knees and pressing heels against the mattress to raise and move buttocks (see illustration). | Positioning begins on left side of bed so that turning to right side will not cause patient to roll toward bed's edge. Buttocks lift prevents shearing force from body movement against sheets. |

---

• *Critical Decision Point:* If patient has decreased strength or mobility on the right side, have patient assume position on the left side of the bed. Also, use pull sheet to turn patient.

---

| STEP | RATIONALE |
|---|---|
| (2) Instruct patient to place the right hand over incisional area to splint it. | Splinting incision supports and minimizes pulling on suture line during turning. |
| (3) Instruct patient to keep right leg straight and flex left knee up (see illustration). | Straight leg stabilizes the patient's position. Flexed left leg shifts weight for easier turning. |

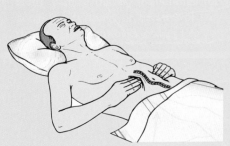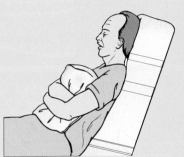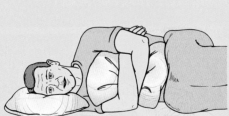

STEP **1D(2)** Techniques for splinting incision. (From Lewis S and others: *Medical-surgical nursing: assessment and management of clinical problems,* ed 6, St. Louis, 2004, Mosby.)

Leg exercises and turning improve blood flow to the extremities and thus reduce venous stasis, reducing the risk for clot formation and subsequent pulmonary emboli. Contractions of lower leg muscles promote venous return, making it difficult for clots to form. Turning also helps to mobilize pulmonary secretions and increases ventilation and perfusion of the lungs. After explaining each exercise, demonstrate it. Then, while acting as a coach, ask the patient to demonstrate each exercise.

**Activity Resumption.** The type of surgery a patient has affects how quickly the patient is able to resume normal physical activity and regular eating habits. Explain that it is normal for the patient to progress gradually in activity and eating. If the patient tolerates activity and diet well, activity levels will progress more quickly. For example, if the patient is not nauseated following cholecystectomy, encourage ambulation the night of surgery.

**Promotion of Nutrition.** The surgical patient is vulnerable to fluid and electrolyte imbalances as a result of inadequate preoperative intake, excessive fluid loss during surgery, and the stress response. A patient usually takes nothing by mouth after midnight before the morning of surgery to reduce risks of vomiting and aspirating emesis during surgery. Instruct the patient to eat and drink sufficient amounts before fasting to ensure adequate fluid and nutrition intake. Make sure the patient's diet includes foods high in protein, with sufficient amounts of carbohydrates, fat, and vitamins. Instruct the patient and family members regarding preoperative fasting requirements and oral medication use. Notify the surgeon and anesthesiologist as soon as possible if the patient eats or drinks during the fasting period.

For hospitalized patients, remove all fluids and solid foods from the bedside and post a sign over the bed to alert hospital personnel and family members about fasting restrictions. Instruct the patient to rinse the mouth with water or mouthwash and brush the teeth, but instruct the patient not to swallow anything, even clear liquids. Patients may take oral medications with sips of water if ordered by the physician or health care provider. Notify the dietary department to cancel meals. A patient who is at home the evening before surgery needs to understand the importance of not taking food or fluids and be willing to follow restrictions.

**Promotion of Rest.** Rest is essential for normal healing. Anxiety about surgery interferes with the ability to relax or sleep. The underlying conditions necessitating surgery are often painful, further impairing rest. Frequent visits by staff members, diagnostic testing, and physical preparation for surgery consume a large amount of time, and the patient has few opportunities to reflect on events. Make sure that the patient's individual needs are met. The patient and family need time to express feelings about surgery, either together or separately. The patient's level of anxiety influences the frequency of discussions, and you will need to encourage expression of these concerns.

Attempt to make the patient's environment quiet and comfortable. The surgeon often orders a sedative-hypnotic or an-

tianxiety agent for the night before surgery. Sedative-hypnotics affect and promote sleep. Antianxiety agents act on the cerebral cortex and limbic system to relieve anxiety. An advantage to ambulatory surgery or same-day surgical admissions is that the patient is able to sleep at home the night before surgery.

**ACUTE CARE.** The degree of preoperative physical preparation depends on the patient's health status, the surgery, and the surgeon's preferences. A seriously ill patient will receive more supportive care than the patient facing a less serious elective procedure.

**Minimize Risk of Surgical Wound Infection.** The risk of developing a surgical wound infection depends on the amount and type of microorganisms contaminating a wound, the susceptibility of the host, and the condition of the wound at the end of the operation. All three factors interact, determining the risk for infection (see Chapter 11).

The skin is a favorite site for microorganisms to grow and multiply. Without proper skin preparation, the risk of postoperative wound infection is high. Many surgeons have patients bathe or shower with an antimicrobial soap the evening before surgery. Some physicians or health care providers order patients to bathe or shower more than once, whereas others have patients give special attention to cleansing the proposed operative site. If the surgical procedure involves the head, neck, or upper chest area, the patient also is required to shampoo the hair. Surgeons generally order hair removal only if the hair has the potential to interfere with exposure, closure, or dressing of the surgical site. This is done as close to the time of surgery as possible (AORN, 2006).

**Prevention of Bowel Incontinence and Contamination.** The patient will often receive a bowel preparation (e.g., a cathartic or an enema) if surgery involves the lower gastrointestinal system. Manipulation of portions of the gastrointestinal tract during surgery results in absence of peristalsis for 24 hours and sometimes longer. Enemas and cathartics, such as GoLYTELY, cleanse the gastrointestinal tract to prevent problems with incontinence or constipation. An empty bowel reduces risk of injury to the intestines and minimizes contamination of the operative wound in case a portion of the bowel is incised or opened. Chapter 33 summarizes enema administration.

**Interventions on Day of Surgery.** On the morning of surgery, complete the routine procedures discussed in the following sections before releasing the patient for surgery.

*Documentation.* Before the patient goes to the operating room, check the medical record to be sure all relevant laboratory and test results are present. Check all consent forms for completeness and accuracy of information. A preoperative checklist (Figure 37-1) provides guidelines for ensuring completion of all nursing interventions. Also check the nurses' notes to be sure documentation is current. This is especially important if the patient experienced unpredicted problems the night before surgery.

*Assessment of Vital Signs.* Make a final assessment of vital signs, and document them on the preoperative checklist and in the nurses' notes. If the preoperative vital signs are abnormal, notify the surgeon because surgery needs to be postponed.

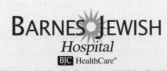

## SURGICAL/PROCEDURE CHECKLIST

### Complete this side for inpatients and outpatients
### having any invasive procedure

Please check (✔) the appropriate box (☐) and fill in the blank(s) as needed.

ADDRESSOGRAPH

Date of Procedure: _____    Type of Procedure: _____

Off Floor Reports printed and placed in chart: ☐ Yes  ☐ No  ☐ N/A: _____

| ITEM | Yes/Initials | NA | COMMENT | Date |
|---|---|---|---|---|
| Face sheet in chart | | | | |
| Consent to Surgery or Other Procedure signed | | | ☐ To be signed in treatment area. | |
| **SPECIALTY**  Consent signed | | | ☐ To be signed in treatment area.<br>   (Specify) | |
| Transfusion consent signed | | | | |
| ID Band on | | | | |
| Allergies Noted: ☐ Armband<br>   ☐ Medication Record<br>   ☐ Allergies/Sensitivities<br>   Record/Override Order Form | | | | |
| Height & Weight documented | | | | |
| Dentures, eyeglasses, contact lenses, nail polish, hairpins, prosthesis, jewelry removed | | | | |
| Surgical/Procedural skin prep done | | | | |
| Patient in hospital gown/pajamas | | | | |
| Patient has been NPO since: _____ | | | | |
| Voided or catheterized | | | | |
| Vital Signs taken and documented | | | | |
| Patient is on isolation | | | (Specify) | |
| History & physical in chart | | | | |
| Lab work in chart (Printed Off Floor reports) | | | | |
| Urinalysis in chart | | | | |
| EKG in chart | | | | |
| Chest X-ray (done if ordered) | | | | |
| Change in condition/VS reported to: | | | | |
| Valuables/Inventory checklist done | | | | |
| Pre-Operative meds given: | | | | |
| Addressograph plate in chart | | | | |
| Patient transferred to Surgical/Procedure area in HIS | | | | |
| Mode of travel: ☐ Amb ☐ W/C ☐ Stretcher ☐ Bed | | | | |
| Operative Site Marked | | | ☐ Site to be marked in holding area | |
| Case Cancelled | | | | |

Family contact during surgery:

Name: _____    Location: _____    Phone: _____

| INITIALS | SIGNATURES | INITIALS | SIGNATURES |
|---|---|---|---|
| | | | |
| | | | |

BJ 2-3343-465 (10/12/05) Page 1 of 2  TAB: TREATMENT     **DO NOT WRITE BELOW THIS LINE**

BJ 2-3343-465

FIGURE **37-1** Surgical/Procedure Checklist. (Courtesy Barnes-Jewish Hospital, St. Louis, Missouri.)

***Hygiene.*** Basic hygiene measures remove skin contamination and increase the patient's comfort. If the patient is unwilling or unable to take a complete bath, a partial bath is refreshing and removes irritating secretions or drainage from the skin. Because the patient cannot wear personal nightwear to the operating room, provide a clean hospital gown and instruct the patient to remove all other articles of clothing, including undergarments. After having nothing by mouth throughout the night, the patient usually has a very dry mouth. Offer mouthwash and toothpaste, again cautioning the patient not to swallow anything.

***Preparation of Hair and Removal of Cosmetics.*** During surgery the anesthesiologist positions the patient's head to put an endotracheal tube into the airway (see Chapter 28). This involves manipulation of the hair and scalp. To avoid injury, ask the patient to remove hairpins or clips. Also, have patients remove hairpieces or wigs. Patients can braid long hair. The patient will wear a disposable hat to contain hair before entering the operating room.

During and after surgery the anesthesia care provider and nurses assess skin and mucous membranes to determine the patient's level of oxygenation, circulation, and fluid balance. You will usually apply a pulse oximeter to a finger to monitor oxygen saturation of the blood. For these reasons, have patients remove all makeup (lipstick, powder, blush, nail polish) and artificial fingernails to expose normal skin and nail coloring. Anything in or around the eye will irritate or injure the eye during surgery. Therefore have patients remove contact lenses, false eyelashes, and eye makeup. Eyeglasses usually remain in the room, or you can give them to the family immediately before the patient enters the operating room.

***Removal of Prostheses.*** It is easy for any type of prosthetic device to become lost or damaged during surgery. The patient removes all removable prosthetics for safekeeping. If the patient has a brace or splint, check with the surgeon to determine whether it should remain with the patient, to be reapplied after surgery.

Although patients need to remove hearing aids, eyeglasses, and contact lenses, do not have them do this until just before the surgery. Allowing the patient to wear these aids facilitates communication and increases the patient's sense of control. Refer to the institution's policies for clarification.

Having dentures in place provides a better seal for ventilation during intubation in the operating room. Therefore in some settings dentures are in place until after the first stages of anesthesia. The dentures are then removed. For many patients, removing dentures is embarrassing. If the patient removes the dentures before surgery, provide privacy. Place dentures in special containers, and label with the patient's name for safekeeping to prevent breakage. Assess the patient for loose teeth. A broken tooth can become dislodged during insertion of an endotracheal tube and obstruct the airway.

You will need to inventory and secure all prosthetic devices, give prosthetics to family members or significant others, or keep the devices at the patient's bedside. Follow agency policy, and document where these devices are located.

***Preparation of Bowel and Bladder.*** Some patients receive an enema or cathartic the morning of surgery. If so, give it at least 1 hour before the patient leaves, allowing time for the patient to defecate without rushing.

You do not prepare the bladder until the morning of surgery. Instruct the patient to void just before leaving for the operating room. If the patient is unable to void, enter a notation on the preoperative checklist. An empty bladder minimizes incontinence and injury to the bladder during surgery. An empty bladder also makes abdominal organs more accessible during surgery. The surgeon will order an indwelling catheter if the surgery is long or the incision is in the lower abdomen (see Chapter 32).

***Application of Antiembolism Devices.*** Many physicians or health care providers order **antiembolism stockings** to be worn during surgery. They maintain compression of small veins and capillaries of the lower extremities. The constant compression forces blood into larger vessels, thus promoting venous return and preventing venous stasis (Chapter 34). When correctly sized and properly applied, antiembolism stockings reduce the risk of thrombi (see Chapter 34). **Sequential compression stockings** are also for promoting venous return. These stockings are attached to an air pump that inflates and deflates the stockings, applying intermittent pressure sequentially from the ankle to the knee.

***Promotion of Patient's Dignity.*** During preoperative preparations, care will become depersonalized unless you maintain the patient's privacy and reduce sources of anxiety. Ambulatory and same-day surgical admission patients often sit in a waiting room before surgery. To protect patients' modesty, allow patients to wear underclothes when possible and provide cover robes. Ensure hospitalized patients their privacy by closing room curtains or doors during preoperative preparation. Allow family to stay until the patient goes to the operating room.

***Performing Special Procedures.*** Sometimes a patient's condition requires special interventions before surgery. The surgeon's orders state the need to start IV infusions, to insert a Foley catheter or **nasogastric (NG) tube** for greater decompression (see Chapter 33), or to administer medications.

***Safeguarding Valuables.*** If a patient has valuables, turn them over to family members or secure them for safekeeping in a designated location. Many facilities require patients to sign a release to free the institution of responsibility for lost valuables. Prepare a list with a description of items, place a copy with the patient's chart, and give a copy to a designated family member. Patients are often reluctant to remove wedding rings or religious medals. Tape a wedding band in place; however, do not create a tourniquet with the tape. If there is a risk that the patient will experience swelling of the hand or fingers, remove the band. Many hospitals allow patients to pin religious medals to their gowns, although the risk of loss increases (Phillips, 2004).

## EVALUATION

It is the morning of Mr. Korloff's surgery, and Sue admits him to the hospital with the help of one of his daughters. She checks that the informed consent has been signed and witnessed. She completes his physical assessment, which focuses on assessing breath sounds, condition of his skin, and vital signs. Sue also completes the preoperative checklist. She asks Mr. Korloff if he has any questions about the nature or purpose of the surgery. Sue also reviews with Mr. Korloff and his daughter the events that will occur in the holding area and the postanesthesia care unit (PACU). She asks if they are frightened or anxious about any aspect of the procedure or routine, and she addresses their concerns. Sue then reviews with Mr. Korloff the exercises that were in the booklet he received in the mail. Sue has Mr. Korloff demonstrate coughing and deep breathing, while reinforcing its importance once surgery is over. She then gives Mr. Korloff a hospital gown and cover-up and shows him to the changing area. After he has removed his clothes and put on the hospital gown, Sue accompanies Mr. Korloff and his daughter to the holding area.

**Documentation Note**

"Patient admitted for scheduled laparoscopic cholecystectomy. BP 142/84, P 88, R 18, T 98.9° F. Lungs are clear to auscultation bilaterally with normal excursion. Skin warm and dry; no evidence of lesions. Patient remained NPO during the night. Reviewed instructions on postoperative exercises, and patient is able to demonstrate coughing and deep breathing. Daughters will be in waiting area during procedure."

*Administering Preoperative Medications.* Typically, the physician or health care provider orders preoperative drugs for you to give before the patient leaves for the operating room. You provide all nursing care measures before giving the preoperative medication. Although some preoperative drugs administered, such as benzodiazepines, opioids, antiemetics, and anticholinergics, usually do not induce sleep, they do cause dry mouth and dizziness. If the drug causes drowsiness or dizziness, keep the side rails in the up position, the bed in the low position, and the call bell within easy reach for the patient. Instruct the patient to remain in bed until the surgical nursing assistant or transporter arrives to take the patient to the operating room and to call for assistance if there is a need to get out of bed.

### Evaluation

Evaluation of the preoperative goals and outcomes of the plan of care begins before surgery and extends into the postoperative period, providing direction for future interventions. For some patients, surgery is an emergency. Others will require procedures up until surgery. This leaves little time for evaluation. For some measures, such as those to prevent infection, you perform evaluation postoperatively when you are able to determine the outcome.

**PATIENT CARE.** Determine if the patient and family have adequate preoperative preparation by asking the patient to describe the surgical procedure, its purpose, and the postoperative care. By having the patient and family describe the reasons for postoperative exercises and spirometry you evaluate the patient's understanding of the physiological and psychological responses to surgery. Evaluate adequacy of preoperative teaching by asking the patient to demonstrate exercises. Evaluate anxiety by monitoring pulse and blood pressure, facial expressions, and verbal interactions. In addition, ask the patient if he or she remains anxious or fearful of any aspect of the surgery.

**PATIENT EXPECTATIONS.** Determine if the patient's and family's expectations have been met up to this point. Spend time talking with the patient and family to learn if they are satisfied with their preparation and the approach used by the nursing staff. Knowing this information assists you in helping the patient to redefine realistic expectations. In emergency situations this becomes more difficult to evaluate. The family often becomes the focus of the evaluation if the patient is unable to respond or is in a condition that prevents a meaningful discussion.

### Transport to the Operating Room

Personnel in the **operating room** notify the nursing unit or preoperative surgery holding area when it is time for surgery. In many hospitals a nursing assistant or a transporter brings a wheelchair or stretcher for transporting the patient. The transporter checks the patient's identification bracelet against the patient's medical record to be sure the correct person is going to surgery. When using a stretcher to transport a patient, the nurses and transporter assist the patient with safely transferring from bed to stretcher. The ambulatory surgery patient, if able and not medicated, often walks to the operating room, providing more control over the event.

Provide the family with an opportunity to visit before the patient goes to the operating room. Then direct the family to the appropriate waiting area. If the patient has been hospitalized before surgery and will be returning to the same nursing unit, prepare the bed and room for the patient's return. You will be better prepared for postoperative care if the room is ready before the patient's return.

Include the following in a postoperative bedside unit:

1. Sphygmomanometer, stethoscope, and thermometer
2. Emesis basin
3. Clean gown
4. Washcloth, towel, and facial tissues
5. IV pole and pump
6. Suction equipment (if needed)
7. Oxygen equipment (if ordered)
8. Extra pillows for positioning the patient comfortably
9. Bed pads to protect bed linen from drainage
10. PCA pump and tubing if ordered
11. Bed raised to stretcher height with bed linen turned back and furniture moved to accommodate the stretcher

## Intraoperative Surgical Phase

Care of the patient during surgery requires careful preparation and knowledge of the events that will occur during the surgical procedure.

### Nurse's Role During Surgery

A nurse usually assumes one of two roles in the operating room: **circulating nurse** or **scrub nurse** (Figure 37-2). The circulating nurse, who is a licensed registered nurse (RN), cares for the patient while in the operating room by completing a preoperative assessment, establishing and implementing the intraoperative plan of care, evaluating the care, and providing for the continuity of care postoperatively. The circulating nurse assists the anesthesiologist or nurse anesthetist with endotracheal intubation, calculating blood loss and urinary output, and administering blood. This nurse monitors sterile technique and a safe operating room environment, assists the surgeon and scrub nurse by operating nonsterile equipment and providing additional instruments and supplies, and maintains accurate and complete documentation.

The scrub nurse, who is an RN, a licensed practical nurse (LPN), or a surgical technician, is responsible for maintaining a sterile field during the surgical procedure and adhering to strict surgical asepsis. This nurse assists with applying surgical drapes and hands the surgeon instruments, sponges, sutures, and other supplies.

**PREANESTHESIA CARE UNIT.** In most hospitals the patient enters a **preanesthesia care unit (PACU)** or **presurgical care unit (PSCU)** (sometimes called a holding area) outside the operating room, where preoperative preparations are completed. Nurses in the PSCU are usually part of the operating room staff and wear surgical scrub suits.

In the PSCU a nurse, nurse anesthetist, or anesthesiologist will insert an IV catheter into the patient's vein to establish a route for fluid replacement, IV drugs, and blood or blood products if needed. They will also administer preoperative medications and/or conscious sedation at this time.

If a patient needs to have hair removed around the surgical site, this is done in a private area near the operating room immediately before surgery. AORN-recommended practices include the use of electric or battery-operated clippers for preoperative hair removal when needed. Clippers minimize the risk of irritation and small cuts, which predispose the patient to infection. Make sure to follow the manufacturer's guidelines if you use a depilatory to remove hair (AORN, 2006). Consult the physician's or health care provider's order sheet and the institution's policy and procedure manual regarding hair removal.

### Admission to the Operating Room

The circulating nurse transfers the patient to the operating room. The patient is usually still awake and will notice nurses and physicians or health care providers wearing sur-

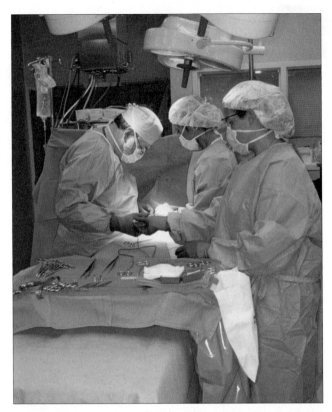

FIGURE **37-2** Nurses in the operating room. (Courtesy OFS Healthcare.)

gical masks, protective eye wear, and gowns. You, along with other staff members, carefully transfer the patient to the operating bed, being sure the stretcher and bed are locked in place. After being transferred to the operating bed, the patient is secured to the bed with safety straps. Just before starting the surgical procedure, the surgical team takes a "time out" for a final verification of the right patient, right procedure, and right site. This final "time out" is part of JCAHO Universal Protocol for Eliminating Wrong-Site, Wrong-Patient, Wrong-Procedure Surgery (JCAHO, 2006).

## Nursing Process

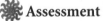 **Assessment**

As a nurse in the PSCU, you will conduct a special preoperative assessment to verify the patient is ready for surgery and to plan intraoperative care. Ask the patient his or her name, and compare the response with the identification band and chart. Then review consent forms, allergies, medical history, physical assessment findings, and test results. Verify with the patient the type of surgery and the surgical site (Table 37-7). Pay special attention to the psychological comfort of the patient. Also perform a brief assessment of key body systems (see Table 37-5).

## FOCUSED PATIENT ASSESSMENT

TABLE 37-7

| Factors to Assess | Questions and Approaches | Physical Assessment Strategies |
|---|---|---|
| The right patient | Ask patient to state full name. | Inspect patient identification band for patient name and date of birth. |
| The right surgical procedure on the right body part | Ask patient to state in his or her own words what has to be done in surgery and where, and compare with operative permit. | Inspect and palpate body part to add any physical evidence of need for surgery (redness, edema, pain). Sometimes there is none, depending on the nature of the surgery. |
| The right set of data in chart | Verify and clarify with patient any medical, surgical, medication, and allergy history found in preoperative assessment. | Inspect skin for stated surgical scars. |
| | | Observe for the presence and patency of ordered tubes and lines (NG, Foley, IV). |
| | Review findings from laboratory reports, diagnostic tests, x-ray films, and electrocardiogram (ECG) ordered. | |
| The right frame of mind of patient | Discuss with patient expected outcomes of surgery. | Observe for signs of fear and anxiety. |
| | Ask patient how he or she feels about surgery. | Monitor vital signs for indications of excessive anxiety. |
| | If patient changes mind about surgery, notify surgeon. Surgery will be canceled or postponed. | Compare vital signs to baseline. |

## Nursing Diagnosis

Review preoperative nursing diagnoses, and modify them to individualize the care plan in the operating room. You add additional diagnoses and related factors based on the patient's condition, specific surgical intervention, and method and type of anesthesia. Nursing diagnoses for the intraoperative patient may include:

- Risk for latex allergy response
- Risk for aspiration
- Decreased cardiac output
- Risk for deficient fluid volume
- Impaired gas exchange
- Risk for infection
- Risk for perioperative-positioning injury
- Powerlessness
- Impaired skin integrity
- Ineffective thermoregulation
- Ineffective tissue perfusion
- Impaired urinary elimination

Nursing care in the operating room also includes monitoring for *latex allergy response* and prevention of *perioperative-positioning injury*. These diagnoses provide direction for both intraoperative and postoperative care for this patient.

## Planning

**GOALS AND OUTCOMES.** Some patient-centered outcomes of preoperative care extend into the intraoperative phase. These include remaining free of infection and achieving psychological and physical comfort. Additional goals include maintaining skin integrity, therapeutic body tempera-

ture, and fluid and electrolyte balance. You measure goal achievement through outcome criteria, such as the presence of intact skin, without redness or irritation; body temperature within the patient's normal range; stable vital signs and adequate urinary output.

Priority setting and continuity of care come from the plan of care and any additional information from oral and written reports of the preadmission area and/or the presurgical care unit.

## Implementation

A major focus of intraoperative care is to prevent injury and complications related to anesthesia, surgery, positioning, and equipment used. As the perioperative nurse you act as an advocate for the patient during surgery. Protect the patient's dignity and rights at all times.

**ACUTE CARE**

**Physical Preparation.** After securing the patient safely, first apply small plastic electrodes on the chest and extremities for continuous electrocardiographic monitoring during surgery. A monitor displays the heart's electrical activity. Next, apply a blood pressure cuff around the patient's arm for the anesthesiologist to measure the blood pressure. Attach a pulse oximeter probe to the patient's finger or earlobe, which allows measurement of the oxygen saturation of the blood and an evaluation of ventilation.

**Psychological Support.** Entering the operating room is stressful for most patients. Reassure the patient, and remain at the patient's side until after anesthesia is induced. Offering a hand to hold is often helpful. If the patient is awake during surgery, give this support throughout the surgical procedure.

**Introduction of Anesthesia.** The nature and extent of a patient's surgery and the patient's current physical status in-

| TABLE 37-8 | Examples of Complications of Anesthesia |
| --- | --- |
| **Type** | **Complications** |
| General anesthesia | Aspiration of vomitus |
| | Cardiac irregularities |
| | Decreased cardiac output |
| | Hypotension |
| | Hypothermia |
| | Hypoxia |
| | Laryngospasm |
| | Malignant hyperthermia |
| | Nephrotoxicity |
| | Respiratory depression |
| Regional anesthesia | Hypotension |
| Epidural | Hypothermia |
| Spinal | Injury to spinal cord |
| | Injury to numb legs |
| | Respiratory paralysis |
| | Spinal headache |
| Local anesthesia | Anaphylactic shock |
| | Hives |
| | Rash |
| Conscious sedation | Aspiration |
| | Decreased level of consciousness |
| | Hypoxemia |
| | Respiratory depression |

fluence the type of anesthesia administered in surgery. It is especially important postoperatively that you know the complications to watch for after a patient has had anesthesia (Table 37-8).

*General Anesthesia.* Under **general anesthesia** the patient loses all sensations, consciousness, and reflexes, including gag and blink reflexes. The patient's muscles relax, and he or she experiences amnesia. General anesthesia is for major procedures requiring extensive tissue manipulation or anytime analgesia, muscle relaxation, immobility, and control of autonomic nervous system are required. This includes minor procedures, especially with children (Burden, 2000).

*Regional Anesthesia.* **Regional anesthesia** results in loss of sensation in an area of the body by anesthetizing sensory pathways. This type of anesthesia is accomplished by injecting a local anesthetic along the pathway of a nerve from the spinal cord (Rothrock, 2003). Administration techniques include peripheral nerve blocks and spinal, epidural, and caudal blocks. There are risks involved with regional anesthetics, particularly in the case of spinal and epidural anesthesia. The patient requires careful monitoring during and immediately after regional anesthesia.

*Local Anesthesia.* Local anesthesia involves loss of sensation at the desired site by inhibiting peripheral nerve conduction. Local anesthesia is usually for minor procedures performed in ambulatory surgery. Local anesthetics are also for patients receiving general or regional anesthesia. Long-acting

local anesthetics are sometimes injected into the incision at the end of the patient's surgery for postoperative pain relief.

*Moderate Sedation/Analgesia (Conscious Sedation).* IV **moderate sedation/analgesia** or **conscious sedation** is routinely used for diagnostic or therapeutic procedures that do not require complete anesthesia but simply a decreased level of consciousness. The patient needs to maintain respirations and respond appropriately to physical and verbal stimuli. Advantages to IV conscious sedation include adequate sedation, diminished anxiety, amnesia, pain relief, mood alteration, enhanced patient cooperation, stable vital signs, and the rapid recovery with minimal risk (American Society of Anesthesiologists, 2004).

As the nurse assisting with the administration of conscious sedation, you must be certified in the care of these patients. You also need to be able to assess, diagnose, and intervene if a complication arises. Skill in airway management, oxygen delivery, and use of resuscitation equipment is essential (AORN, 2006). Document vital signs, oxygen saturation, auscultation of breath sounds and heart rhythm, and level of consciousness every 15 minutes during the procedure and the immediate recovery period (American Society of Anesthesiologists, 2002; AORN, 2006).

Support any patient who remains awake by explaining procedures, encouraging questions, and warning the patient when unpleasant sensations will be experienced. In some settings music is provided to mask unpleasant sounds and to promote relaxation.

**Positioning.** You position the patient during surgery to provide good access to and exposure of the operative site and to promote adequate circulatory and respiratory function. Make sure the positioning does not impair neuromuscular structures or skin integrity. When using general anesthesia, the nursing personnel and surgeon usually do not position the patient until the anesthesia care provider notifies them that the patient is intubated and has entered the stage of complete relaxation.

You need to consider the patient's comfort and safety. It is sometimes difficult to understand why patients feel a wide range of discomfort after surgery. The alert person maintains normal range of motion by pain and pressure receptors. If a joint is extended too far, pain stimuli warn that muscle and joint strain is too great. In an anesthetized patient, normal defense mechanisms do not guard against joint damage and muscle stretch and strain. The patient's muscles are so relaxed that it is relatively easy to place the patient in a position he or she normally does not assume while awake. The patient often remains in a given position for several hours. Once the patient awakens, musculoskeletal pain is significant.

Intraoperative nursing care also includes interventions to prevent infection and injury to the patient, to maintain fluid and electrolyte balance, and to control the patient's temperature (Table 37-9).

**Documentation of Intraoperative Care.** During the intraoperative phase, the nursing staff continues the estab-

| TABLE 37-9 | Intraoperative Nursing Care | |
|---|---|

| Outcomes | Interventions |
|---|---|
| Patient will be free of infection. | Maintain standard precautions. |
| | Monitor surgical asepsis. |
| | Perform surgical skin scrub. |
| Patient will be free of injury. | Apply sterile surgical drapes. |
| | Perform accurate sponge, needle, and instrument counts. |
| | Provide grounding for electrosurgical cautery. |
| | Provide eye protection when using a laser. |
| Patient will maintain body temperature. | Warm room. |
| | Monitor body temperature. |
| | Warm irrigating solutions. |
| | Apply warming blanket immediately after surgery. |
| Patient will maintain fluid and electrolyte balance. | Monitor blood loss, NG drainage, and urinary output. |
| | Provide blood products as ordered. |
| | Monitor type and flow rate of IV fluids. |

## EVALUATION

Mr. Korloff's surgery is complete, and he is transferred to the PACU. Sue has requested that she accompany Mr. Korloff into the PACU. He received general anesthesia, and the procedure was uneventful. Mr. Korloff did not receive any blood or blood products. He did receive Ringer's lactate solution intravenously via a catheter in the left lower forearm. Small gauze dressings were applied to the four small abdominal puncture wounds. At this time the priorities are to maintain Mr. Korloff's vital signs and airway, which is established with an oral airway, and to protect him from injury during transport to the PACU.

lished plan of care and modifies it as needed. Throughout the surgical procedure keep an accurate record of patient care activities and procedures performed by operating room personnel. This record provides useful data for the nurse who cares for the patient postoperatively.

## Evaluation

You evaluate many interventions implemented during the intraoperative phase postoperatively, because complications (e.g., infection) often arise days after surgery.

**PATIENT CARE.** After surgery, perform a postoperative evaluation of the patient. Inspect the skin under the grounding pad and areas of the skin where equipment or positioning has exerted pressure. Monitor body temperature during the procedure and immediately postoperatively to assess thermoregulation. Obtain vital signs and auscultate lung sounds to assess pulmonary and fluid and electrolyte status.

**PATIENT EXPECTATIONS.** Question a patient who is not receiving general anesthesia frequently during the procedure regarding pain, numbness, and perceived room temperature. This determines if the analgesia is adequate and if the patient is comfortable in regard to position and temperature.

When the patient is having major surgery, it is very important to keep the family informed. Typically, family members want to know if surgery is progressing without problems. Many hospitals provide phones within waiting areas that allow nursing staff to reach families and to explain the progress of the surgery. Also, if you are on the surgical nursing unit, you can walk by the waiting area to give the families additional information and support.

## Postoperative Surgical Phase

Following surgery, a patient's postoperative course involves two phases: the immediate **recovery** period and **convalescence.** For an ambulatory surgical patient the immediate recovery period normally lasts only 1 to 2 hours, and convalescence will occur at home. For a hospitalized patient the immediate postoperative period often lasts a few hours, with convalescence taking 1 or more days, depending on the extent of surgery and the patient's response.

### Recovery

During recovery it is important for you to be very conscientious in monitoring the surgical patient and making the clinical judgments necessary to determine if the patient is progressing as expected. This is a time when the patient's condition will change very quickly. Immediately after surgery the patient goes to the **postanesthesia care unit (PACU)** for close monitoring (Figure 37-3). Before the patient arrives, you, as the PACU nurse, will receive a report from the surgical team in the operating room to determine the patient's most current status, nursing care priorities, and the need for special equipment. The report will include information about anesthetic agents given during surgery, IV fluids and blood products administered, status of the wound including the presence of drainage devices, and whether the patient has had any surgical complications, such as excessive

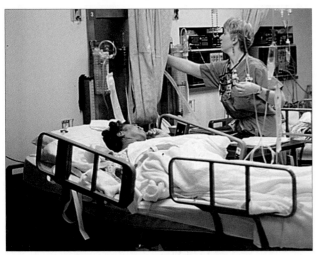

FIGURE **37-3** Nurse in postanesthesia care unit (PACU).

blood loss. The information from the report will allow you to monitor the patient, assess for change, and take appropriate preventive action. While the patient is in the PACU, conduct ongoing assessments every 15 minutes or more often.

**POSTANESTHESIA CARE IN AMBULATORY SURGERY.** The postanesthesia care of ambulatory surgery patients occurs in two phases. Phase 1 is essentially the same as described for hospitalized patients in the PACU. Phase 2, however, prepares the patient for discharge and self-care. The patient receiving only local anesthesia is usually admitted directly to the phase 2 area. In phase 2, encourage the patient to gradually sit up on the stretcher or recliner and begin to take ice chips or sips of water or other clear liquids after regaining full alertness.

Phase 2 postanesthesia care occurs in a room equipped with medical recliner chairs, side tables, and footrests. Kitchen facilities for preparing light snacks and beverages are in the area, along with bathrooms. The phase 2 environment promotes the patient's and family's comfort and well-being until discharge. Continue to monitor the patient but not at the same intensity as in phase 1. In phase 2, initiate postoperative teaching with the patient and family members (Box 37-4). After the patient's condition becomes stable, he or she is discharged.

### Convalescence

Once it has been determined a patient is stable, usually within 2 to 3 hours, the anesthesia provider or surgeon transfers the hospitalized patient to a postoperative nursing unit, whereas the ambulatory surgical patient will return home. Unstable patients remain in the PACU or go to an intensive care unit for more intense monitoring and care. During convalescence you will consider the goals of care established during the preoperative and intraoperative phases, because your aim is to support the patient in returning to normal physiological function. In addition, you direct your nursing care toward facilitating a patient's smooth transition

home. This is a time to encourage family participation in the patient's plan of care. The family provides coaching during postoperative exercises and important psychosocial support to the patient.

## Nursing Process

### Assessment

The parameters that you assess for a surgical patient are basically the same during recovery and convalescence. When the patient enters the PACU, perform a rapid assessment of the respiratory and circulatory status of the patient and attach electronic monitors. Make assessments while considering the patient's surgical risks and the type of surgery performed. For example, if a patient has a history of smoking and underwent abdominal surgery involving a high abdominal incision, you will be concerned about the status of respirations. The patient's pain could potentially reduce ventilation, which leads to the development of atelectasis.

Once a patient reaches a postoperative nursing unit, you perform the vital sign measurements and assessments less often, usually every 15 to 30 minutes initially, then hourly, and then less often per physician's or health care provider's orders. Check the institution's policy on vital signs following surgery. Table 37-10 summarizes a focused postoperative assessment.

**RESPIRATION.** Assess the quality of the patient's respirations and the patency of the airway. A patient receiving a general anesthetic often has an artificial airway still in place when arriving in the PACU. Certain anesthetic agents and opioids often continue to cause respiratory depression. Thus be especially alert for slow, shallow breathing. Assess respiratory rate, rhythm, and depth and quality of ventilatory movement. Auscultate lung sounds to identify any abnormalities such as rales, which are caused by retained secretions, or wheezing, resulting from laryngospasm. If breathing is unusually shallow, place your hand over the patient's face or mouth to feel exhaled air. Pulse oximetry reflecting 92% to 100% saturation is within normal limits unless the physician or health care provider orders other limits (see Chapter 12).

# FOCUSED PATIENT ASSESSMENT

**TABLE 37-10**

| Factors to Assess | Questions and Approaches | Physical Assessment Strategies |
|---|---|---|
| Respirations | Review baseline vital signs for current comparison. | Monitor respiratory rate, rhythm, and depth every 15 min × 4 or until stable, then every 30 min × 2, and then every hour × 4. |
| | Review history for medical conditions involving respiratory system, medications taken, and any allergies. | Observe for symmetry of chest wall movements, color of skin and mucous membranes. |
| | Review report of type of anesthesia and agents used. | Auscultate breath sounds for rales, wheezing, decreased or absent sounds. |
| | Review report of any medications given during surgery or after that affect respiratory function (analgesics, antianxiety agents). | Apply pulse oximeter to detect $O_2$ saturation. |
| | Ask patient to breathe deeply and cough when awake. | |
| Circulation | Review baseline vital signs for current comparison. | Monitor pulse rate and rhythm as well as blood pressure every 15 min × 4 or until stable, then every 30 min × 2, and then every hour × 4 or more often as patient's condition warrants. |
| | Review report of amount of blood loss and any replacement blood or blood products. | Assess level of consciousness and symptoms of restlessness or altered mental status. |
| | Review intake of IV fluids as to type and amount to date. | Observe skin, nail beds, and mucous membranes for color and hydration. Auscultate lungs for signs of congestion. |
| | Review current IV orders as to type of fluid and infusion rate. | Palpate peripheral pulses distal to surgical site, tight dressing, tourniquet, or cast if present. |
| | Ask if patient experiences dizziness and/or visual disturbances when changing positions. | Inspect for amount of bleeding on dressing, in drainage systems (NG suction, Hemovac, Jackson-Pratt drain, Foley catheter) and underneath patient. |
| | | Monitor ECG if ordered. |
| Infection control | Review patient history for risk factors for infection (contaminated surgical site, history of diabetes mellitus, human immunodeficiency virus [HIV], or use of immunosuppressing drugs [Prednisone]). | Monitor patient temperature and white blood cell count as indicated. |
| | Review patient history for risk factors of poor wound healing. | Observe surgical wound for redness, edema, warmth, purulent drainage, and dehiscence. |
| | Ask patient about symptoms of urinary tract or respiratory tract infections. | Inspect any output (urine, wound drainage) for color, consistency, and odor. |
| Gastrointestinal function | Review report for history of problems with gastrointestinal function. | Inspect for abdominal distention caused by gas or bleeding. |
| | Ask patient about symptoms of nausea, cramping, anorexia. | Auscultate for bowel sounds in all four quadrants at least every shift until discharge. |
| | Ask patient about symptoms of return of bowel function (passing flatus, having bowel movement). | Palpate abdomen for firmness caused by gas, fluid, or mass. |
| | | Monitor NG tube for patency and NG tube output for color and amount of drainage if present. |
| | | Observe patient's ability and willingness to tolerate fluids and food. |
| | | Advance diet only with return of active bowel sounds. |
| Comfort | Review symptoms of pain before surgery, type of anesthesia, location of surgery, and expected level of pain associated with this type of surgery (large incision or laparoscopic procedure). | Observe for signs and symptoms of discomfort (restlessness; elevated pulse, respirations, blood pressure; grimaces; guarding. |
| | Review history of pain medication use before surgery and since. | Observe patient for individualized manner of dealing with pain and discomfort. |
| | Review any history of alcohol or illicit drug use. | Assess for any side effects of pain medication (altered mental status, depressed respirations, bradycardia, orthostatic hypotension, nausea or vomiting, urinary retention, constipation). |
| | Ask patient to rate pain on a 0-10 scale before and after each administration of pain medication. | |
| | Assess previous pain management techniques. | |

Once a patient is on a surgical nursing unit, respirations have usually stabilized. Frequent auscultation of lung sounds is still important because the patient is still at risk for developing pneumonia unless he or she follows postoperative exercises routinely. Remember that pain control will be important during convalescence so that the patient coughs and deep breathes with relative ease.

**CIRCULATION.** The patient is at risk for cardiovascular complications from actual or potential blood loss at the surgical site, side effects of anesthesia, electrolyte imbalances, and depression of normal circulatory regulating mechanisms. Continuous electrocardiographic (ECG) monitoring is routine in the PACU to detect rhythm and rate disturbances. Assessment of heart rate and rhythm and blood pressure reveals the patient's cardiovascular status. Compare preoperative vital signs with postoperative values to determine the patient's status.

Assess circulatory perfusion, especially for patients who have had procedures that impair circulation, such as vascular surgery, use of a tourniquet, or application of casts or tight dressings. Always be alert to the amount of bleeding that occurs after surgery and the possibility of hemorrhage. The risk for hemorrhage continues for several days postoperatively. Blood loss occurs externally through a drain or incision or internally within the surgical wound. Either type of hemorrhage is indicated by a fall in blood pressure; elevated heart and respiratory rates; thready pulse; cool, clammy, pale skin; and restlessness.

**TEMPERATURE CONTROL.** The operating room environment is cool, and the patient's depressed level of body function results in a lowering of metabolism and fall in body temperature. When patients begin to awaken in the PACU, they often complain of feeling cold and uncomfortable. Shivering is not always a sign of hypothermia, but rather a side effect of certain anesthetic agents. Measure body temperature to direct for interventions. On a surgical unit, monitoring of body temperature is important for detecting early occurrence of wound infection. If a patient develops a fever, report it to the surgeon immediately.

**NEUROLOGICAL FUNCTION.** In the PACU the patient is usually drowsy but reacts to verbal commands. However, drugs, electrolyte and metabolic changes, pain, oxygen saturation, and emotional factors influence level of consciousness. Normally as anesthetic agents are metabolized, the patient's reflexes return, he or she regains muscle strength, and a normal level of orientation returns. Check for pupillary and gag reflexes, hand grasp, and movements of the extremities (see Chapter 13). If a patient has had surgery involving a portion of the neurological system, conduct a more thorough neurological assessment.

Once a patient returns to a surgical nursing unit, a sudden change in consciousness is not normal. However, routine detailed neurological assessment is unnecessary unless a patient is slow to awaken fully or has had surgery involving the neurological system.

**FLUID AND ELECTROLYTE BALANCE.** Because of the surgical patient's risk for fluid and electrolyte abnormal-

ities, assess hydration status and monitor cardiac and neurological function for signs of electrolyte alterations (see Chapter 15). Routinely inspect the IV catheter and insertion site to be sure it is patent, no signs of infiltration are present, and the IV fluids are infusing properly. It is important that a good venous access is available in case the patient requires fluid and/or blood replacement. IV fluids will continue on the surgical nursing unit, sometimes for several days. If the IV catheter is in place for over 24 hours, routinely assess for the presence of phlebitis. An IV catheter will remain in place depending on the type of surgery, the medications the patient receives, and how well the patient tolerates continuation of oral fluids and food.

Monitoring and accurate recording of intake and output help to assess fluid balance, as well as renal and cardiac function. Measure all sources of input (e.g., IV fluids and oral intake) and output (e.g., NG tubes, drains, and urine), and consult with the physician or health care provider if appropriate.

**SKIN INTEGRITY AND CONDITION OF THE WOUND.** Thoroughly assess the condition of the patient's skin. A rash often indicates a drug sensitivity or allergy. Abrasions or petechiae result from inadequate padding during positioning or restraining on the operating bed. If a patient has burns or serious injury to the skin, communicate this information by completing an incident report (see Chapter 4).

The surgical wound sometimes has no dressing, or it is covered with gauze or transparent dressing that protects the wound site. For open wounds or during the changing of a dressing, observe the appearance of the suture line and note the color, odor, and consistency of any drainage (see Chapter 35). Estimate the amount of drainage by noting the extent and area of the dressing covered (example: lower half of dressing saturated with sanguineous drainage). If a patient has a wound drainage system, monitor the output routinely and note the character of drainage. Keep the drainage tubes patent. A sudden increase in drainage indicates possible hemorrhage.

A critical time for wound healing is 24 to 72 hours after surgery (see Chapter 35). A patient exerts physical stress on a wound from coughing, vomiting, or movement. Inadequate nutrition, impaired circulation, and metabolic alterations further impair healing. Observe the incision for signs of dehiscence and evisceration. Notify the surgeon of any area of dehiscence. Evisceration is a medical emergency. In the event of evisceration, cover any exposed abdominal contents with gauze soaked with sterile normal saline. Prepare an IV infusion set for rapid infusion of IV fluids.

If a wound becomes infected, it usually occurs 3 to 6 days after surgery, when the patient is at home. Ongoing observation of the wound includes inspection for redness, increased warmth, edema, and purulent drainage. Instruct the patient to assess the wound and immediately report any signs and symptoms of wound infection to the surgeon.

**GENITOURINARY FUNCTION.** Spinal anesthesia often prevents the patient from feeling bladder fullness or distention and causes urinary retention for up to 6 to 8 hours. Palpate the lower abdomen just above the symphysis pubis

## SYNTHESIS IN PRACTICE

### Postoperative Assessment and Planning

Mr. Korloff's stay in the PACU is uneventful except for pain in the right shoulder. Air is put into the abdominal cavity during a laparoscopy. The air causes referred pain. In the PACU Mr. Korloff's pain was a 7 on a 10-point scale.

It is the evening of the day of Mr. Korloff's surgery. Mr. Korloff is in the nursing division for an overnight stay because of his previous cardiac history. He performs deep breathing and coughing exercises and uses the incentive spirometer as ordered. Because he is ambulating frequently in the hall, with the assistance of his daughters, he is not performing postoperative leg exercises. The IV fluids were discontinued just before he left the PACU. Mr. Korloff was able to tolerate a clear liquid diet and had adequate bowel sounds. He rates his pain as 5 on a 10-point scale, continuing to note some discomfort in the shoulder area. His pain has been controlled with an oral pain medication, acetaminophen with codeine, which he receives every 3 to 4 hours ATC. His vital signs are within normal limits compared to preoperative values, and his lungs are clear on auscultation. The four small abdominal puncture wounds are without drainage or redness.

for bladder distention. A full bladder is painful and is often the cause of a patient's restlessness, agitation, or high blood pressure. If the patient has a Foley catheter (see Chapter 32), make sure there is a continuous flow of urine of at least 30 ml/hour in adults or 1 to 2 ml/kg/hour in infants and children. Observe the color and odor of urine. Surgery involving portions of the urinary tract normally causes bloody urine for at least 12 to 24 hours.

**GASTROINTESTINAL FUNCTION.** Anesthetic agents slow gastrointestinal motility and cause nausea. In addition, manipulation of the intestines during abdominal surgery further impairs peristalsis. You will normally hear faint or absent bowel sounds in all four quadrants during the immediate recovery phase. Normal bowel sounds usually return in about 24 hours, unless major abdominal surgery was performed. **Paralytic ileus,** loss of function of the intestine which causes abdominal distention, is always a possibility after abdominal surgery. On the surgical nursing unit ask whether the patient is passing flatus, an important sign indicating return of normal bowel function. Inspect the abdomen for distention caused by gas. Distention also develops if internal bleeding occurs in a patient who has had abdominal surgery. If an NG tube is in place, assess the patency of the tube (see Chapter 31) and the color and amount of any drainage.

**COMFORT.** As a patient awakens from general anesthesia, the sensation of discomfort often becomes prominent. Some patients perceive pain before regaining full consciousness. Acute incisional pain causes the patient to become restless and frequently causes changes in vital signs. Pain management is perhaps one of the most important priorities in postoperative care. If a patient has a PCA de-

vice, have the patient begin using it as soon as possible. It is difficult for patients to begin deep breathing and coughing exercises and to eventually begin turning and ambulation when they have pain, particularly if there is an abdominal or chest incision.

The patient who had regional or local anesthesia usually does not experience pain initially, because the incisional area is still anesthetized. You need to be skilled at assessing levels of pain and be alert to the patient's need for pain medication. Pain scales are an effective method of assessing pain, evaluating the response to analgesics, and objectively documenting the severity of a patient's pain (see Chapter 30).

### Nursing Diagnosis

Based on your assessment and information gathered from the reports of members of the surgical team, you will identify nursing diagnoses that apply to your patient. Nursing diagnoses that give direction to the continuing care of the patient in the PACU and on the surgical nursing unit include:

- Activity intolerance
- Ineffective airway clearance
- Anxiety
- Disturbed body image
- Ineffective breathing pattern
- Impaired verbal communication
- Risk for constipation
- Risk for deficient fluid volume
- Risk for infection
- Impaired physical mobility
- Nausea
- Imbalanced nutrition: less than body requirements
- Acute pain
- Disturbed sleep pattern
- Delayed surgical recovery
- Ineffective therapeutic regimen management
- Ineffective tissue perfusion
- Impaired urinary elimination
- Impaired spontaneous ventilation

Be sure to analyze and validate assessment data and cluster findings to identify correct nursing diagnoses. For example, a finding of *anxiety* manifested by restlessness could be related to *acute pain, urinary retention,* or *ineffective tissue perfusion.* Further assessment and clustering of findings will lead to the correct diagnosis.

### Planning

Because of the critical nature of the immediate postoperative period, the plan of care in the PACU always involves close monitoring of the patient and frequent assessments to ensure stable physiological function. On the surgical nursing unit, your care will become more focused on facilitating the patient's recovery. Nursing care will be based on your nursing assessment and the surgeon's postoperative orders. Typical postoperative orders include the following:

1. Frequency of vital signs monitoring and special assessments
2. Types of IV fluids and rate of infusion
3. Postoperative medications (especially those for pain and nausea)
4. Oxygen therapy or incentive spirometry
5. Fluids and food allowed by mouth
6. Level of activity the patient is allowed to resume
7. Position that patient is to maintain while in bed
8. Intake and output measures
9. Laboratory tests and x-ray studies

**GOALS AND OUTCOMES.** During recovery in the PACU, goals of care include returning the patient to normal physiological functioning without complications and maintaining physical and psychological comfort. Examples of outcomes include stable vital signs within the patient's normal range, patent airway, palpable peripheral pulses, oxygen saturation over 95%, an intact incision with minimal wound drainage, and balanced intake and output. Another outcome is for the patient to be awake and oriented to the PACU environment with the ability to move all extremities and to verbalize pain relief and decreased anxiety.

Once the patient is on the surgical nursing unit, goals are more long term. Maintenance of pain control with improvement in physiological function is still a priority. Adequate wound healing without the presence of infection, restoration of nutrition, the patient's return to a functional state of health, and maintenance of self-concept and body image are additional goals. Examples of measurable outcomes include the following: patient states level of pain relief is acceptable, appetite and nutritional intake return to previous or improved state, and patient states willingness to participate in discharge instruction.

**SETTING PRIORITIES.** While in the PACU, a patient's priorities usually center on physiological needs. As you review preoperative and intraoperative data, as well as your ongoing assessments in the PACU, you will determine how a patient is progressing and set priorities on developing needs. For example, if a patient begins to awaken without complications but urinary output is less than normal, you consult with the physician or health care provider to determine if IV fluids need to be increased to prevent dehydration. Data indicating any immediate postoperative complications such as hemorrhage will require you to alter your plan of care and to take necessary emergency measures.

The patient's physical status often changes on the surgical nursing unit, so it remains important to be alert for developing complications. Focus priorities on returning the patient to preoperative functioning or better. Patients will generally have many nursing diagnoses (Figure 37-4). However, management of acute pain will often be the priority of postoperative nursing care. If a surgical patient's pain is properly managed, ambulation will begin earlier, deep breathing and coughing will be less difficult, and the patient will have a better sense of well-being. In addition, you will begin to prepare the patient for discharge by providing the patient and family necessary instruction and ensuring that adequate resources are available in the home. Monitoring the patient for any psychosocial problems such as body image disturbance or altered coping will also be important during convalescence.

**CONTINUITY OF CARE.** Continuity of nursing care between the OR, the PACU, and the surgical nursing unit depends on good communication among all members of the nursing and surgical team. Nursing staff within each area must be able to convey clear and accurate information about the patient's status and medications to the next nurse who assumes care for the patient. For example, you need to thoroughly describe the condition of a wound so that each nurse knows what to anticipate during wound assessment and care. In that way you will be able to detect any signs of poor wound healing early.

The ambulatory surgical patient will likely be discharged home with family members or friends. It is essential that the patient and family understand continuing care needs of the patient. Usually the ambulatory surgery nursing staff has discharge instruction sheets available. When you care for patients on surgical nursing units, be sure to consider the patient's continuing care needs in the home. Referral to home care services or a clinical nurse specialist in wound care or ostomy care, for example, will provide valuable assistance.

### Implementation

Critical thinking is important in the postoperative care of the surgical patient because you need to consider the interrelationship of all body system, and the effect of the therapies. The patient remains at risk for a variety of postoperative complications (Table 37-11) unless you provide aggressive care and unless the patient becomes actively involved in recovery and convalescence. Review the patient's perioperative teaching, and reinforce as needed (Box 37-5). If the patient is an older adult, the gerontological nursing practice guidelines in Box 37-6 will be helpful.

**RESPIRATION.** Following general anesthesia, a patient in the PACU often has an oral or nasal airway inserted to maintain a patent airway until regular breathing at a normal rate resumes. This airway is not taped in place. As respiratory function returns, ask the patient to expel the airway. The patient's ability to do so signifies a return of a normal gag reflex.

One of your greatest concerns following surgery is airway obstruction resulting from weakness of pharyngeal or laryngeal muscle tone (from the effects of anesthetics), aspiration of emesis, accumulation of secretions in the pharynx or trachea or bronchial tree, or laryngeal or subglottic edema. Often the tongue causes airway obstructions. The following measures maintain airway patency:

1. *Position the patient on one side with the face downward and the neck slightly extended* (Figure 37-5, p. 1124). A small, folded towel supports the head. Neck extension prevents occlusion of the airway at the pharynx. When the face is turned downward, the tongue moves forward

## CONCEPT MAP

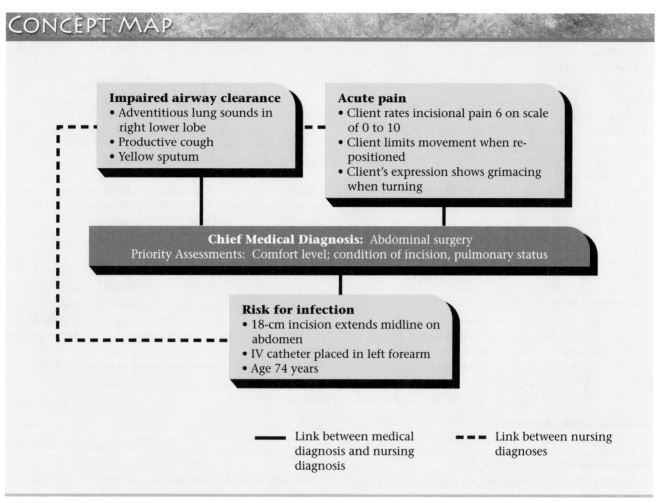

**Impaired airway clearance**
- Adventitious lung sounds in right lower lobe
- Productive cough
- Yellow sputum

**Acute pain**
- Client rates incisional pain 6 on scale of 0 to 10
- Client limits movement when re-positioned
- Client's expression shows grimacing when turning

**Chief Medical Diagnosis:** Abdominal surgery
Priority Assessments: Comfort level; condition of incision, pulmonary status

**Risk for infection**
- 18-cm incision extends midline on abdomen
- IV catheter placed in left forearm
- Age 74 years

—— Link between medical diagnosis and nursing diagnosis

- - - Link between nursing diagnoses

FIGURE **37-4** Concept map for surgical patient with abdominal surgery.

and mucous secretions flow out of the mouth instead of accumulating in the pharynx. If the nature of the surgery prevents turning the patient on one side, the head of the bed is slightly elevated and the patient's neck slightly extended, with the head turned to the side. Never position the patient with arms over or across the chest, because this reduces maximum chest expansion.

2. *Suction the artificial airway and oral cavity for mucous secretions as necessary* (see Chapter 28). Avoid continually eliciting the gag reflex, which will cause vomiting. Before removing an airway, suction the back of the airway to remove any mucous plugs or secretions.

3. *Begin deep breathing and coughing exercises* as soon as the patient responds to instructions.

4. *Administer oxygen as ordered,* and monitor oxygen saturation with a pulse oximeter.

Once a patient reaches a surgical nursing unit, begin aggressive pulmonary hygiene. The patient will participate actively if your preoperative instruction was effective. Remember, have the family help coach patients in completing their exercises. Encourage diaphragmatic breathing exercises every

hour while the patient is awake. Follow diaphragmatic breathing by having the patient use the incentive spirometer. Have the patient try to reach the inspiratory volume achieved preoperatively on the spirometer. Proper use of the spirometer will ensure a maximum inspiration. Encourage regular turning and early ambulation. Walking causes the patient to assume a position that does not restrict chest wall expansion, stimulates an increased respiratory rate, and improves circulation. Assist patients who are restricted to bed to turn side-to-side every 1 to 2 hours while awake and to sit when possible. If a patient develops pulmonary secretions, encourage coughing exercises followed by deep breathing at least once an hour. Be sure to maintain pain control so that the patient achieves a full, productive cough. Provide frequent oral hygiene to help the patient expectorate mucus easily. If the patient is not allowed to have anything by mouth (NPO) or is on a limited fluid intake, the mouth easily becomes dry. Finally, initiate postural drainage and suctioning if the patient is too weak or unable to cough secretions (see Chapter 28).

**CIRCULATION.** In the PACU it is important to monitor for changes in blood pressure or heart rate. The surgeon

| TABLE 37-11 | **Common Postoperative Complications** |
|---|---|

| Complication | Cause |
|---|---|
| **Respiratory System** | |
| *Atelectasis*   Collapse of alveoli with retained mucous secretions. Signs and symptoms: elevated respiratory rate, dyspnea, fever, crackles over involved lobes of lungs, productive cough. | Caused by inadequate lung expansion. Greater risk in patients with upper abdominal surgery who have pain during inspiration and repress deep breathing. |
| *Pneumonia*   Inflammation of alveoli caused by infectious process. Usually develops in lower dependent lobes of lung if patient is immobilized. Signs and symptoms: fever, chills, productive cough, chest pain, purulent mucus, dyspnea. | Caused by poor lung expansion with retained secretions. *Diplococcus pneumoniae*, a resident bacterium in the respiratory tract, causes most cases of pneumonia. |
| *Hypoxia*   Inadequate concentration of oxygen in arterial blood. Signs and symptoms: restlessness, dyspnea, hypertension, tachycardia, diaphoresis, cyanosis. | Respirations depressed by anesthetics or analgesics. Increased retention of mucus with impaired ventilation occurs from pain, poor positioning, or poor coughing and deep breathing. |
| *Pulmonary embolism*   Clot blocking pulmonary artery and disrupting blood flow to one or more lobes of lung. Signs and symptoms: dyspnea, sudden chest pain, cyanosis, tachycardia, hypotension. | Immobilized surgical patient with preexisting circulatory or coagulation disorders is at high risk. |
| **Circulatory System** | |
| *Hemorrhage*   Loss of large amount of blood externally or internally in short period of time. Signs and symptoms: same as for hypovolemic shock. | Slipping of suture or dislodged clot at incisional site. Patients with coagulation disorders are at greater risk. |
| *Hypovolemic shock*   Reduced perfusion of tissues and cells from loss of circulatory fluid volume. Signs and symptoms: hypotension, weak and rapid pulse, cool and clammy skin, rapid breathing, restlessness, reduced urine output. | In surgical patient, hemorrhage usually causes hypovolemic shock. |
| *Thrombophlebitis*   Inflammation of vein (usually in leg), often accompanied by clot formation. Signs and symptoms: swelling and inflammation of involved site, aching or cramping pain. Vein feels hard, cordlike, and sensitive to touch. | Venous stasis is aggravated by prolonged sitting or immobilization, trauma to vessel wall, and hypercoagulability of blood increase risk of vessel inflammation. |
| *Thrombus*   Formation of clot attached to interior wall of vein or artery, which occludes vessel lumen. Symptoms include localized tenderness along vein, swollen calf or thigh in affected leg. Decreased pulse below thrombus (if arterial). | Venous stasis and vessel trauma. Venous Injury is usually common after surgery of legs, abdomen, pelvis, and major vessels. Patients with major surgery or trauma to these areas are at risk for thrombus formation. |
| *Embolus*   Piece of thrombus that has dislodged and circulates in bloodstream until it lodges in another vessel, commonly lungs, heart, or brain. | Thrombi also form from increased coagulability of blood. |
| **Gastrointestinal System** | |
| *Paralytic ileus*   Nonmechanical obstruction of the bowel caused by physiological, neurogenic, or chemical imbalance may be associated with decreased peristalsis. Common in initial hours following surgery. | Handling of intestines during surgery can lead to loss of peristalsis for a few hours to several days. |
| *Abdominal distention*   Retention of air within intestines. Signs and symptoms: increased abdominal girth, complaint of fullness and "gas pains." | Caused by slowed peristalsis from anesthesia, bowel manipulation, or immobilization. |
| *Nausea and vomiting*   Symptoms of improper gastric emptying or chemical stimulation of vomiting center. Patient complains of gagging or feeling full or sick to stomach. | Caused by severe pain, abdominal distention, fear, medications, eating or drinking before peristalsis returns, and initiation of gag reflex. |
| **Genitourinary System** | |
| *Urinary retention*   Involuntary accumulation of urine in bladder as result of loss of muscle tone. Signs and symptoms: inability to void, restlessness, and bladder distention occurring 6-8 hours postoperatively. | Caused by effects of anesthesia, narcotic analgesics, local manipulation of tissues surrounding bladder, and poor positioning of patient, which impairs voiding reflex. |
| Urinary tract infection caused by bacteria or yeast contamination. Possible symptoms: pain, itching, burning, urgency, and frequency. | Frequently results after bladder catheterization. |

| TABLE 37-11 | Common Postoperative Complications—cont'd | |
|---|---|---|

| Complication | Cause |
|---|---|
| **Integumentary System** | |
| *Wound infection*   An invasion of deep or superficial wound tissues by pathogenic microorganisms. Signs and symptoms: warm, red, and tender skin around incision, fever and chills, purulent drainage. It usually appears 3-6 days postoperatively. | Caused by poor aseptic technique and/or contaminated wound before surgical exploration. Chronically ill, obese, or immunosuppressed patient are at high risk. |
| *Wound dehiscence*   Separation of wound edges at suture line. Signs and symptoms: increased drainage and appearance of underlying tissues occurring 6-8 days after surgery. | Caused by malnutrition, obesity, preoperative radiation to surgical site, old age, poor circulation to tissues, and unusual strain on suture line from coughing. |
| *Wound evisceration*   Protrusion of internal organs and tissues through incision. It usually occurs 6-8 days after surgery. | See Wound dehiscence. Patient with dehiscence is at risk for developing evisceration. |
| **Nervous system** | |
| *Intractable pain*   Pain that is not amenable to analgesia or pain relief measures. | Related to wound, dressing, anxiety, or patient positioning. |

| BOX 37-5 | PATIENT TEACHING |
|---|---|

Mr. Korloff tells Sue that the plan is for discharge tomorrow. In their conversation he says to Sue that he hopes he will remember all of the care she taught him before surgery. Sue develops the following teaching plan for Mr. Korloff:

**Outcome**
- At the end of the teaching session, Mr. Korloff is able to verbalize understanding of his discharge teaching.

**Teaching Strategies**
- Explain the rationale for postoperative exercises so Mr. Korloff will know how the exercises will benefit him.
- Demonstrate coughing, deep breathing, and leg exercises to Mr. Korloff.
- Encourage Mr. Korloff to practice postoperative exercises every 1 to 2 hours.
- Reinforce the need for the patient to ask for pain medication before pain becomes severe.
- Encourage patient to avoid smoking because nicotine accelerates the metabolism of pain medication, resulting in shorter duration of effect.

- Teach nonpharmacological means of pain control, such as slow deep breathing, progressive relaxation, and use of tactile stimulation, such as back rubs (see Chapter 30).
- Teach the names, purpose, and timing of medications that patient will continue at home.
- Teach signs and symptoms of hemorrhage, wound infection, and dehiscence.
- Instruct in proper hand hygiene.
- Demonstrate wound care techniques that are necessary after discharge (see Chapter 35).
- Review high-protein foods needed for wound healing.

**Evaluation Strategies**
- Use open-ended questions.
- Have Mr. Korloff provide return demonstration of the coughing, deep breathing, and leg exercises, hand hygiene, and wound care techniques.
- Ask Mr. Korloff to identify food to include in his diet.
- Have Mr. Korloff verbalize wound care and abnormal signs and symptoms of wound healing to report to the physician or health care provider.

usually writes an order indicating which changes to report. However, use critical thinking and notify the surgeon when there is a significant change or a continuous negative trend in vital signs. If hemorrhage is external, observe for increased bloody drainage on dressings or through drains. If a dressing becomes saturated, the blood will ooze down the patient's sides and collect in a pool under bedclothes. Always check under the patient for drainage whether or not the dressing is saturated. When hemorrhage is internal, the operative site becomes swollen and tight, and a hematoma develops. Report the first signs of suspected hemorrhaging to

the surgeon immediately. Maintain the IV infusion, monitor vital signs continuously, continue oxygen, and raise the patient's legs in a modified Trendelenburg's position to promote venous return until the patient's condition stabilizes.

Early measures directed at preventing venous stasis will prevent deep vein thrombosis during convalescence. On the surgical nursing unit, begin the following interventions as soon as possible:

1. *Encourage a patient to perform leg exercises at least every hour while awake unless contraindicated by surgery.*

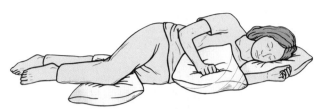

FIGURE **37-5** Position of patient during recovery from general anesthesia. (From Lewis S and others: *Medical-surgical nursing: assessment and management of clinical problems,* ed 6, St. Louis, 2004, Mosby.)

---

**BOX 37-6** CARE OF THE OLDER ADULT

- If the patient will be on bed rest for more than 24 hours, an order for subcutaneous heparin or enoxaparin is necessary to prevent deep vein thrombosis.
- Intake and output is maintained longer postoperatively because perfusion of kidneys is compromised and the older adult frequently decreases oral intake of fluids to minimize voiding frequency.
- Any fluid, electrolyte, or acid-base imbalance will quickly alter mental status. Older adults often need to be closer to the nurses' station and be monitored more frequently for confusion, disorientation, or decreased level of consciousness. Fall precautions are necessary.
- Patients with increased pain tolerance need to be appropriately medicated when they indicate they have pain. Ask patients often to rate their pain, and give them treatment options. Offer pain medications before painful procedures (e.g., dressing changes, walking in the hallway, getting up in a chair).
- Pain medication is more likely to cause altered mental status in older adults, increasing the need to monitor for confusion and disorientation.
- Metabolism of drugs is slowed in older patients, so the effects of medication persist for a longer period of time.
- Nutritional deficits are common, and diets high in protein, calcium, and vitamins B and C are necessary for wound healing and positive nitrogen balance. Carbohydrate intake is essential for energy and to spare protein use for wound healing. Increase iron intake if the patient is anemic.
- Older adults have more difficulty with constipation because of decreased peristalsis, decreased activity and abdominal muscles, and decreased neurological stimulation. Orders for a stool softener and/or extra fiber are accompanied by increased fluid intake despite the resulting increased need to void.

---

2. *Apply elastic antiembolism stockings or pneumatic compression stockings as ordered by the physician or health care provider* (see Chapter 34). Often these devices are on the patient in the operating room. The stockings need to be removed every 8 hours and left off for 1 hour. Do a thorough assessment of the skin of the legs at this time.
3. *Encourage early ambulation.* Most patients are ordered to ambulate the evening of surgery, depending on the severity of surgery and the patient's condition. The degree of

activity allowed progresses as the patient's condition improves. Before ambulation, assess vital signs.

Abnormalities often contraindicate ambulation. If vital signs are normal, first assist the patient with sitting on the side of the bed. Dizziness is a sign of postural hypotension (see Chapter 12). Check the patient's blood pressure again and ensure that the patient is not dizzy to determine if ambulation is safe. Assist with ambulation by standing at the patient's side and helping to either hold or move equipment. During the first few times out of bed, the patient often walks only a few feet. Tolerance improves each time. Evaluate the patient's tolerance to activity by periodically assessing pulse rate.

4. *Avoid positioning the patient in a manner that interrupts blood flow to the extremities.* While the patient is in bed, do not place pillows or rolled blankets directly under the knees. Compression of the popliteal vessels causes a thrombus to form. When sitting in a chair, have the patient elevate the legs on a footstool, avoiding hyperextension of the knee. Never allow the patient to sit with one leg crossed over the other.
5. *Administer anticoagulant drugs if ordered.* Small doses of anticoagulants, such as heparin given subcutaneously, reduce risk for thrombus formation. Orthopedic patients often receive low doses of aspirin for anticoagulation.
6. *Promote adequate fluid intake orally or intravenously.* Adequate hydration prevents the concentration of platelets and red blood cells and thus prevents formation of small clots within blood vessels. Adequate hydration also promotes tissue healing and liquefies respiratory secretions.

**TEMPERATURE CONTROL.** Due to the cool temperature in the operating room, the patient is usually cool when arriving in the PACU. Provide specially warmed blankets or other warming devices (e.g., warming mattress). Increasing body warmth causes the patient's metabolism to rise and circulatory and respiratory functions to improve. Patients often still feel cold when reaching a surgical nursing unit. Offer extra blankets or apply a loose-fitting pair of socks to the feet.

**NEUROLOGICAL FUNCTION.** Deep breathing and coughing help to expel retained anesthetic gases and increase the patient's level of consciousness. Try to arouse the patient by calling his or her name in a moderate tone of voice, noting whether the patient responds appropriately. If the patient remains asleep or is unresponsive, waken them through touch or by gently moving a body part. If you need a painful stimulus to wake the patient, then notify the anesthesia care provider. Orientation to the environment is important in maintaining alertness. Explain that surgery is complete, and describe all procedures and nursing measures performed.

**FLUID AND ELECTROLYTE BALANCE.** The patient's only source of fluid intake immediately after surgery is intravenously; therefore it is important to maintain patency of the IV catheter (see Chapter 15). Once an ambulatory surgical patient awakens and is able to tolerate water without gastrointestinal upset, the IV line is usually removed. A more seriously ill patient will require an IV line to receive blood products, depending on the amount of blood lost during surgery. The physician or health care provider orders a prescribed solution and rate for each IV infusion. Most often IV solutions are infused through a pump to ensure correct volume delivery.

**GENITOURINARY FUNCTION.** A full bladder is painful and causes a patient awakening from surgery to become restless or agitated. Patients who have abdominal surgery or surgery of the urinary system frequently have indwelling catheters inserted until voluntary control of urination returns. If a catheter is in place and urinary output is less than 30 ml/hour in an adult patient and 1 to 2 ml/kg/hour in infants and children, check for catheter occlusion or kinking and notify the surgeon if measured output does not improve.

During convalescence the following measures promote normal urinary elimination (see Chapter 32):

1. Assist the patient in assuming normal positions for voiding.
2. Check the patient frequently for the need to void when a catheter is not in place. The feeling of bladder fullness and urgency to void is often sudden, and you need to respond promptly when the patient calls for assistance.
3. Assess for bladder distention. The patient's physician or health care provider usually orders a straight urinary catheter to be inserted if a patient does not void within 8 hours of surgery or sooner if the bladder is distended. Even if the patient has been NPO for hours, IV fluids give the renal system sufficient fluid to excrete urine. Continued difficulty in voiding requires an indwelling catheter, although the risk for urinary tract infection increases.
4. Monitor intake and output. If the patient's urine is dark and concentrated, notify the surgeon. A patient easily becomes dehydrated. Remember, if the output is less than 30 ml/hour in adults or 1 to 2 ml/kg/hour in infants and children, the patient is experiencing acute renal insufficiency or failure, and you need to notify the surgeon immediately.

**GASTROINTESTINAL FUNCTION.** Minimize a patient's nausea during recovery in the PACU by avoiding sudden movement of the patient. If the patient has an NG tube, maintain tube patency with normal saline irrigations as ordered (see Chapter 31). Occlusion of an NG tube causes the accumulation of gastric contents in the stomach. Because stomach emptying slows under anesthesia, the accumulated contents cannot escape, and nausea and vomiting develop. Normally a patient does not receive fluids to drink in the PACU because of the risk of vomiting and altered mental status from general anesthesia. Use a moist cloth or swab to relieve dryness of the patient's lips and mouth. If the patient is nauseated, give prescribed medication to prevent vomiting and aspiration.

Interventions for preventing gastrointestinal complications during convalescence promote the return of normal elimination and faster resumption of normal nutritional intake. It takes several days for a patient who has had surgery on gastrointestinal structures to resume a normal dietary intake. Normal peristalsis does not usually return for 24 to 48 hours.

In contrast, the patient whose gastrointestinal tract is unaffected directly by surgery simply endures the effects of anesthesia before resuming dietary intake. Follow these guidelines:

1. *Maintain a gradual progression in dietary intake.* Immediately after surgery, a patient receives only IV fluids. Once the surgeon orders a resumption of oral intake, you will first provide clear liquids, such as water, apple juice, gelatin, or decaffeinated tea or coffee, after nausea subsides. Overloading with large amounts of fluids leads to distention and vomiting. If the patient tolerates liquids without nausea, advance the diet to full liquids, followed by a light diet of solid foods, and finally a regular diet, stressing the importance of foods that are high in protein and vitamin C. Patients who have had abdominal surgery are usually NPO the first 24 hours or until the return of bowel sounds.
2. *Promote ambulation and exercise.* Physical activity stimulates a return of peristalsis. The patient who suffers abdominal distention and "gas pain" will often obtain relief while walking.
3. *Maintain an adequate fluid intake.* Fluids keep fecal material soft for easy passage.
4. *Administer fiber supplements, stool softeners, enemas, and rectal suppositories as ordered.* Constipation or distention often develops postoperatively related to side effects of anesthetic agents and pain medication.
5. *Stimulate the patient's appetite* by removing sources of noxious odors and providing small servings of nonspicy foods.
6. *Assist the patient to sit* (if possible) during mealtime to minimize pressure on the abdomen.
7. *Provide frequent oral hygiene.*
8. *Provide meals when the patient is rested and free from pain.* A patient will often lose interest in eating if he or she is exhausted by activities such as ambulation before mealtime.

**COMFORT.** The anesthesiologist or nurse anesthetist orders medications for pain management in the PACU. IV opioid analgesics, such as morphine sulfate, are the drugs of choice for the immediate postoperative period. Administer morphine intravenously, titrating it as ordered until pain relief is achieved. Morphine depresses vital signs and level of consciousness, but at appropriate doses this is rare. However, acute pain often causes low blood pressure. In such a situation an analgesic improves vital sign values. Be skilled at determining the proper dose of an analgesic and knowing possible side effects. Once a patient is awake, a PCA pump may be ordered. If the patient has an epidural catheter, caution is needed if additional analgesics are ordered (see Chapter 30).

A patient's pain increases as the effects of anesthesia wear off once the patient reaches the surgical nursing unit. The patient becomes more aware of surroundings and more perceptive of discomfort. The incisional area is only one source of pain. Irritation from drainage tubes, tight dressings, or casts and the muscular strains caused from positioning on the operating bed also cause discomfort.

Pain significantly slows recovery. The patient in pain becomes reluctant to perform necessary postoperative exercises. Assess the patient's pain thoroughly. Do not assume that the pain is incisional in origin. When the patient requests pain medication, determine the nature and character of the pain. Patients have the most surgical pain during the first 24 to 48 hours after surgery. Provide analgesics as often as allowed. IV or epidural PCA systems allow the patient to administer analgesics from specially prepared pumps (see Chapter 30). A PCA device is attached to the IV line, or the analgesic is given via an epidural catheter, as with fentanyl or morphine. The patient controls the amount of analgesia received within set doses and times ordered by the surgeon or anesthesia care provider. You program the doses and frequencies of pain medication into the pump. PCA medication is delivered at a preprogrammed basal rate, a bolus dose at specified intervals as needed, or both. When a patient is receiving pain medications through a PCA pump, make sure to document respirations and level of consciousness. Documentation of frequent objective pain assessment using a pain scale, appropriate nursing interventions, and evaluation of the patient's response must be in every patient's medical record as of January 2001 according to the JCAHO 2000 standards (Sandlin, 2000).

**PROMOTING WOUND HEALING.** Leave surgical dressings in place the first 24 hours after surgery to reduce the risk of infection. During this time you simply add an extra layer of gauze on top of the original dressing if drainage develops. Mark or draw around the drainage on the dressing. Date and time the marking on the dressing. This will provide you with a means to monitor increasing amounts of drainage. Notify the physician or health care provider if bleeding is excessive. In certain types of surgery the surgeon will choose to use no dressing at all.

During convalescence continue close observation of the surgical wound. If a wound becomes infected, it usually occurs 3 to 6 days after surgery. Always use aseptic technique during dressing changes and wound care. Surgical drains need to remain patent so that accumulated secretions are removed from the incision site. Observation of the wound identifies early signs and symptoms of infection (see Chapter 35).

To ensure continuity of care be sure that all staff are aware of the proper materials to use in a dressing change. It is not uncommon for patients to feel discomfort during an extensive dressing change, so offer a pain medication 5 to 30 minutes before the procedure. Time the procedure to begin when the pain medication begins to work. For example, oral pain medications take about 30 minutes to begin working; therefore give oral pain medication 30 minutes before the procedure. Pain medications given IV push usually only take 5 to 10 minutes to work. In this case give the IV pain medication about 5 to 10 minutes before the dressing change.

If you anticipate that the patient will need to continue dressing changes in the home, plan instruction at a time when the patient is alert and comfortable, and family caregivers are present. Be sure at the time of discharge that a patient knows how to obtain the materials needed for the dressing change.

**MAINTAINING SELF-CONCEPT.** During a patient's convalescence, the appearance of wounds, bulky dressings, and extruding drains and tubes threatens a patient's self-concept. The nature of the surgery often also creates a permanent change in body image. If surgery leads to impairment in body function, the patient's role within the family and community often changes significantly. Observe the patient for alterations in self-concept (see Chapter 20). Some patients show revulsion toward their appearance by refusing to look at an incision or carefully covering dressings with bedclothes. The fear of not being able to return to a functional role in the family or at a previously held job even causes the patient to avoid participating in the care plan.

The family or significant other frequently plays an important role in efforts to improve the patient's self-concept. Help the family to accept the patient's needs and still encourage independence. The following measures maintain the patient's self-concept:

1. *Provide privacy* during dressing changes or wound inspection by closing room curtains and draping the patient so that only the dressing and incisional area are exposed.
2. *Maintain the patient's hygiene.* A complete bath the first day after surgery usually makes the patient feel renewed. Offer a clean gown and washcloth if the gown becomes soiled. Keep the patient's hair neatly combed, and offer frequent oral hygiene, especially for the patient who is NPO.
3. *Prevent drains from overflowing.* You typically measure the drainage sets every 8 hours for output recording, but sometimes you will need to empty and measure them more often if drainage is excessive.
4. *Maintain a pleasant environment.* Store or remove all unused supplies, and keep the bedside orderly and clean.
5. *Offer opportunities for the patient to discuss feelings about appearance.* Patients worry about permanent scarring. When the patient chooses to look at an incision for the first time, make sure the area is clean. Eventually the patient will care for the incision site by applying simple dressings or bathing.
6. *Give the family opportunities to discuss ways to promote the patient's self-concept.* Encouraging independence is difficult for a family member who has a strong desire to assist the patient in any way. By knowing about the appearance of a wound or incision, family members will be supportive during dressing changes.

**RESTORATIVE AND CONTINUING CARE.** There are other postoperative care activities promote a patient's return to a functional state of health. Throughout the postoperative convalescent period promote the patient's independence and active participation in care. When a patient is in pain or suffers from postoperative complications, there is little motivation for self-care. The goals you set for a patient's involvement need to be realistic. It is unrealistic to involve the patient if movement is highly restricted or if participation increases the patient's discomfort.

## OUTCOME EVALUATION

TABLE 37-12

| Nursing Action | Patient Response/Finding | Achievement of Outcome |
|---|---|---|
| Observe Mr. Korloff's willingness and ability to turn, deep breathe with incentive spirometer, and cough every 1 to 2 hours while awake. | He is able and willing to turn, deep breathe, and cough every 2 hours without assistance. He is able to use incentive spirometer to 1500 ml. | Breath sounds clear in all lobes and equal bilaterally. |
| Observe Mr. Korloff performing leg exercises every 1 to 2 hours while awake until he is ambulating. | He is able to perform ankle circles and calf pumping every 2 hours without difficulty. He refused to do quadriceps setting and leg lift exercises. | Lower extremities warm and pink with brisk capillary refill. |
| Ambulate Mr. Korloff progressively starting first morning postoperatively as ordered. | He is able to ambulate in room and in hall by postoperative day 1 without assistance. | No redness, edema, excessive warmth, or pain in either calf noted. |
| Monitor intake and output every shift. | Intake: IV 1000 ml Output: Foley 950 ml<br>    PO <u>400 ml</u>         Void <u>300 ml</u><br>Total    1400 ml    Total 1250 ml | Intake and output within normal limits. |
| Monitor infusion of IV solutions via pump as ordered. | IV solution of D₅NS infusing via pump at 125 ml/hour without signs of redness or edema. | |
| Ask Mr. Korloff if he has nausea. | He denies nausea and is taking clear fluids PO. | |
| Encourage early voiding postoperatively or after catheter removal. | He is able to void 300 ml in bathroom without difficulty within 2 hours after surgery or Foley catheter removed. | Mr. Korloff is able to resume oral fluid intake and normal urinary elimination without difficulty. |
| Monitor for bladder distention and urinary retention with overflow. | No bladder distention noted. | |

Keep the patient and family informed of progress made toward recovery. Many patients become depressed if they think recovery is slow. Explain the length of time expected to reach a level of maximal recovery. For some patients, surgery also causes permanent physical limitations that require time to accept.

You plan care daily, keeping in mind the ultimate goals for recovery. From the moment the patient enters the hospital, anticipate and plan for the patient's return home.

Involvement of family members in the care plan facilitates early discharge and adequate care at home. Instruct family members in care activities. If family members are unable to assist the patient, work with the surgeon, social worker, and/or discharge planner for referrals to home care agencies to provide services at home.

## 🌀 Evaluation

**PATIENT CARE.** As a PACU nurse you continuously evaluate the effectiveness of interventions and the patient's response. The patient's condition can change quickly. Your evaluation of the patient's status involves ongoing measurement of vital signs, pulse oximetry, wound drainage, intake and output, and other physical assessments. The Glasgow Coma Scale (see Chapter 13) evaluates the patient's level of consciousness and return of motor function. You may need to increase frequency of assessments based on the patient's response to anesthesia. If evaluation reveals the patient is recovering from anesthesia, the surgeon will discharge the patient from the PACU.

On the surgical nursing unit evaluate the effectiveness of care on the basis of expected outcomes resulting from nursing interventions (Table 37-12). Your evaluation will occur over several days. It is important to evaluate the patient's clinical progress by observing the patient's participation in postoperative exercises, self-care activities, and ambulation. Evaluate the ambulatory surgical patient's outcomes by making a postoperative telephone call to the patient's home. The call, usually placed 24 hours after surgery, reassures the patient that you are concerned and allows you to evaluate the progress of recovery and to answer any questions the patient or family has.

**PATIENT EXPECTATIONS.** In the PACU some patients are not able to voice expectations. However, evaluation of pain is critical. Because pain is subjective, you validate it by frequently ask the patient how he or she feels. If possible, use a pain assessment scale. Note the patient's movement and positioning, because nonverbal behaviors indicate if a patient is comfortable. If pain is not adequately relieved, you need to change the dosage or type of medication. Also evaluate the patient's level of anxiety by assessing presence of any concerns or fears. Further explanation of postoperative progress and procedures reduces anxiety.

As the patient progresses through convalescence, physical and psychological comfort continues to be typical expectations of patients and families. Also evaluate if the patient feels prepared for discharge from the acute care facility. Is the patient able to explain the required care to continue following discharge? Have the patient demonstrate any procedures such as wound care or medication administration. Give the patient and family numerous opportunities to ask questions about what to anticipate once the patient returns home.

## EVALUATION

Mr. Korloff progressed well and is ready for discharge the day after surgery. He expresses relief that everything went well and that he will be able to return to work, hopefully by next week. Sue continues to care for him on the surgical patient care unit. Sue explains how to remove the gauze on the puncture sites and tells Mr. Korloff to bathe and shower tomorrow. Symptoms the patient and family need to watch for are redness, swelling, bile-colored drainage or pus from the abdominal wounds, severe abdominal pain, nausea, vomiting, and fever greater than 100° F or chills. Any of these symptoms need to be reported to Mr. Korloff's physician or health care provider immediately. His daughters observed the puncture sites and are able to identify symptoms of complications.

Mr. Korloff is ready for discharge and plans to stay with one of his daughters over the weekend. Sue makes a follow-up surgical appointment for Mr. Korloff and gives him the surgeon's phone number in case he has any questions or concerns once he returns home.

**Documentation Note**

"Abdominal puncture sites dry and intact, without redness. Discharge teaching provided to patient and daughters. Repeated signs and symptoms of complications; wound care instructions; activity restrictions; and follow-up appointment time, date, and place. Patient and daughter verbalize understanding of all discharge teaching."

## KEY CONCEPTS

- Perioperative nursing includes professional nursing care given to the surgical patient before, during, and after surgery.
- Previous illnesses and past surgeries affect the patient's ability to tolerate surgery.
- Older adult patients are at greater surgical risk because of their declining physiological status.
- All medications taken before surgery are automatically discontinued after surgery unless a physician or health care provider reorders the drugs.
- Family members and significant others are important in assisting patients with physical limitations and in providing emotional support postoperatively.
- Preoperative assessment of vital signs and physical findings provides an important baseline with which to compare postoperative assessment data.
- Primary responsibility for informed consent rests with the surgeon.
- Structured preoperative teaching positively influences postoperative recovery.

- If hair around the incision needs to be removed, clip it as close as possible to the time of surgery to minimize the risk of infection.
- In ambulatory surgery, nurses use the limited time available to assess, prepare, and educate patients for surgery.
- Nurses within the operating room focus on protecting the patient from potential harm.
- Postoperative assessment centers on the body systems most likely to be affected by surgery.
- Because a surgical patient's condition may change rapidly during recovery, you monitor the patient's status at least every 15 minutes until stable.
- Postoperative nursing interventions focus on prevention of complications.
- The risk of postoperative complications increases when the patient does not become actively involved in recovery.
- From the time of admission the nurse plans for the surgical patient's discharge.

## CRITICAL THINKING IN PRACTICE

*Mr. Watson is a 72-year-old patient admitted for a right total hip replacement. He has a history of emphysema. Because of this, he takes daily doses of theophylline and prednisone to improve his breathing. Mr. Watson also has atrial fibrillation and takes warfarin sodium (Coumadin) 2 mg daily.*

- - - - - - - - - - - - - - - - - - -

1. Based on Mr. Watson's history you recognize that he is at most risk for what complications related to surgery? (Mark all that apply.) Explain your answers.
   a. Atelectasis
   b. Bleeding
   c. Paralytic ileus
   d. Infection
   e. Urinary retention
   f. Hypothermia
2. You assess Mr. Watson's preoperative laboratory values. Which value needs to be called to the physician or health care provider?

   a. Prothrombin time (PT) 12 seconds
   b. White blood cell (WBC) count 9500/mm$^3$
   c. Platelet count 75,000/mm$^3$
   d. Serum potassium 4.2 mEq/L

*Mr. Watson's surgery is completed. He returns to the orthopedic surgery unit after an uneventful stay in PACU.*

- - - - - - - - - - - - - - - - - - -

3. Six hours after he has returned from surgery, you notice that Mr. Watson's dressing has a 5-cm area of serosanguineous drainage on it. What nursing interventions should you take at this time? (Mark all that apply.)
   a. Hold pressure over the incision for 5 minutes.
   b. Notify the physician or health care provider of the bleeding.
   c. Assess Mr. Watson's vital signs.
   d. Reinforce the dressing with gauze pads.
   e. Remove the dressing, and assess for bleeding.

4. You are caring for Mr. Watson the first postoperative day and assess rales when auscultating his lungs. Which nursing diagnosis best addresses this problem?
   a. Impaired gas exchange
   b. Risk for aspiration
   c. Excess fluid volume
   d. Ineffective airway clearance
5. Mr. Watson is to get up to the chair today for the first time. What is a priority nursing intervention to carry out related to his activity?

a. Administer oral pain medication 30 minutes before getting him up.
b. Use a Hoyer lift to transfer him from the bed to the chair.
c. Have Mr. Watson pivot on his right foot when moving.
d. Instruct him to rest 30 minutes before getting up.
6. It is the third postoperative day for Mr. Watson. During your morning assessment you find that his abdomen is distended. What might this indicate? What additional assessment data should be gathered?

## NCLEX® REVIEW

1. A priority nursing intervention to prevent respiratory complications after surgery in older adults is:
   1. Ambulate the patient every 2 hours
   2. Monitor intake and output every shift
   3. Increase fluid intake during first 24 hours
   4. Encourage the patient to turn, deep breathe, and cough frequently
2. You must ask each patient preoperatively for the name and dose of all prescription and over-the-counter medications taken before surgery because they:
   1. May cause allergies to develop
   2. May interact with anesthetic agents
   3. Will need to be reordered after surgery
   4. Should be taken the morning of surgery with sips of water
3. A patient with a prothrombin time (PT) or an activated partial thromboplastin time (APTT) greater than normal needs to be monitored closely for:
   1. Anemia
   2. Bleeding
   3. Infection
   4. Cardiac dysrhythmias
4. You review the laboratory results of the patient you are preparing for surgery. Which laboratory value interacts with anesthesia to increase the risk of cardiac dysrhythmias?
   1. Hematocrit 44%
   2. Potassium 3.1 mEq/L
   3. Creatinine 0.9 mg/dl
   4. Platelet count 184,000/mm³
5. You are checking your patient 2 hours after he returns from surgery. Which assessment finding requires immediate attention?

1. Nasogastric tube drained 50 ml of tea-colored liquid.
2. Skin is pale, cool, and dry.
3. Foley catheter drained 30 ml of urine for past 2 hours.
4. Patient very drowsy but responds promptly to voice.
6. Which factor contributes to the risk of poor wound healing in obese patients?
   1. Resumption of activity is delayed.
   2. Ventilatory capacity is decreased.
   3. Intestinal peristalsis is delayed.
   4. Fatty tissue has a poor blood supply.
7. Which statement made by the patient having hernia surgery indicates a need for further teaching?
   1. I'll use a clean disposable razor to shave the hair on my lower abdomen before surgery.
   2. I will not eat or drink anything after midnight.
   3. I'll splint my incision with a pillow before I cough.
   4. I'll have my wife bring me to the hospital 2 hours before my surgery.
8. In the PACU you note that the patient is having difficulty breathing because of an airway obstruction. You would first:
   1. Suction the pharynx and bronchial tree
   2. Give oxygen through a mask at 10 L/min
   3. Position the patient so that the tongue falls forward
   4. Ask the patient to use an incentive spirometer
9. Which nursing intervention is most effective to prevent the postoperative complication of deep vein thrombosis?
   1. Frequent coughing exercises
   2. Early ambulation
   3. Use of inspirometer
   4. Turning every 2 hours

## REFERENCES

American Society of Anesthesiologists: Practice guidelines for sedation and analgesia by nonanesthesiologists, *Anesthesiology* 96:1004, 2002.

American Society of Anesthesiologists: *Distinguished monitored anesthesia care from moderate sedation/analgesia (conscious sedation)*, 2004, http://www.asahq.org/publicationsAndservices/standards/35.htm.

American Society of Anesthesiologists Task Force on Perioperative Fast: Practice guidelines for preoperative fasting and the use of pharmacologic agents to reduce the risk of pulmonary aspiration: application to healthy patients undergoing elective procedures, *Anesthesiology* 90(3):896, 1999.

Association of periOperative Registered Nurses: *Standards, recommended practices, and guidelines,* Denver, 2006, The Association.

Bernier MR and others: Preoperative teaching received and valued in a day surgery setting, *AORN J* 77(3):563, 2003.

Black JM, Hawks JH: *Medical-surgical nursing: clinical management for positive outcomes,* ed 7, St. Louis, 2005, Saunders.

Burden N: *Ambulatory surgical nursing,* ed 2, London, 2000, Saunders.

Chernecky CC, Berger BJ: *Laboratory tests and diagnostic procedures,* ed 4, Philadelphia, 2004, Saunders.

Day MW: Recognizing and management: DVT—deep vein thrombosis, *Nursing* 33(5):36, 2003.

Dochterman JM, Bulechek GJ: *Nursing interventions classification (NIC),* ed 4, St. Louis, 2004, Mosby.

Fogg D: Expiration dates; alcohol disinfection; OR consents, local anesthesia, marking surgical site, moderate sedation, *AORN J* 78(2):295, 2003.

Giger JN, Davidhizar RE: *Transcultural nursing: assessment and intervention,* ed 4, St. Louis, 2004, Mosby.

Hulzebos EHJ and others: Reduction of postoperative pulmonary complications on the basis of preoperative risk factors in patients who had undergone coronary artery bypass surgery, *Phys Ther* 83(1):8, 2003.

Iocono M: Informed consent, *J Perianesth Nurs* 15(3):180, 2000.

Joint Commission on Accreditation of Healthcare Organizations: 2006 National Patient Safety Goals: Goal 4: eliminate wrong-site, wrong-patient, wrong-procedure surgery, 2006, http://www.Jcipatientsafety.org.

Joint Commission on Accreditation of Healthcare Organizations: *2005 Ambulatory care national patient safety goals,* 2004, http://www/jcaho.org.

LaMontagne L and others: Effects of coping instruction in reducing young adolescents' pain after major spinal surgery, *Orthop Nurs* 22(6):398, 2003.

Lewis C and others: Patient knowledge, behavior and satisfaction with the use of a preoperative DVD, *Orthop Nurs* 21(6):41, 2002.

Lewis S and others: *Medical-surgical nursing: assessment and management of clinical problems,* ed 6, St. Louis, 2004, Mosby.

Lowdermilk D, Perry SE: *Maternity nursing,* ed 6, St. Louis, 2003, Mosby.

McKenry LM, Salerno E: *Mosby's pharmacology in nursing,* ed 21, St. Louis, 2003, Mosby.

Moller M and others: Effect of preoperative smoking intervention on postoperative complications: a randomized clinical trial, *Lancet* 359:114, 2002.

Moorhead S, Johnson J, Maas M: *Nursing outcomes classification (NOC),* ed 3, St. Louis, 2004, Mosby.

Mordiffi SZ and others: Information provided to surgical patients versus information needed, *AORN J* 77(3):546, 2003.

*Mosby's medical, nursing, and allied health dictionary,* ed 6, St. Louis, 2002, Mosby.

Phillips N: *Berry and Kohn's operating room technique,* ed 10, St. Louis, 2004, Mosby.

Rothrock J: *Alexander's care of the patient in surgery,* ed 12, St. Louis, 2003, Mosby.

Sandlin D: The new Joint Commission on Accreditation of Healthcare Organization's requirements for pain assessment and treatment: a pain in the assessment? *J Perianesth Nurs* 15(3):182, 2000.

Scales BA, Master R: Screening high-risk patients for the ambulatory setting, *J Perianesth Nurs* 18(5):307, 2003.

Shuldham C: A review of the impact of pre-operative education on the recovery from surgery, *Int J Nurs Stud* 37:171, 1999.

Urbano EL: Homan's sign in the diagnosis of deep vein thrombosis, *Hosp Physician* 37(3)22, 2001.

# Glossary

**abduction** (Chapter 25) Movement of a limb away from the body.

**abrasion** (Chapter 35) Scraping or rubbing away of epidermis; may result in localized bleeding and later weeping of serous fluid.

**absorption** (Chapters 14, 31) Passage of drug molecules into the blood. Factors influencing drug absorption include route of administration, ability of the drug to dissolve, and conditions at the site of absorption.

**acceptance** (Chapter 23) Fifth stage of Kübler-Ross's stages of dying. An individual comes to terms with a loss rather than submitting to resignation and hopelessness.

**accessory muscles** (Chapter 28) Muscles in the thoracic cage that assist with respiration.

**accommodation** (Chapter 36) Process of responding to the environment through new activity and thinking and changing the existing schema or developing a new schema to deal with the new information. For example, a toddler whose parent consistently corrected him when he called a horse a "doggie" accommodates and forms a new schema for horses.

**accountability** (Chapters 5, 24) State of being answerable for one's actions— a nurse answers to himself or herself, the patient, the profession, the employing institution such as a hospital, and society for the effectiveness of nursing care performed.

**accreditation** (Chapter 8) Process whereby a professional association or nongovernmental agency grants recognition to a school or institution for demonstrated ability to meet predetermined criteria.

**acculturation** (Chapter 17) The process of adapting to and adopting a new culture.

**acne** (Chapter 27) Inflammatory, papulopustular skin eruption, usually occurring on the face, neck, shoulders, and upper back.

**acromegaly** (Chapter 13) Chronic metabolic condition caused by overproduction of growth hormone and characterized by gradual, marked enlargement and elongation of bones of the face, jaw, and extremities.

**active listening** (Chapter 9) Listening attentively with the whole person—mind, body, and spirit. It includes listening for main and supportive ideas, acknowledging and responding, giving appropriate feedback, and paying attention to the other person's total communication, including the content, the intent, and the feelings expressed.

**active range-of-motion (ROM) exercise** (Chapter 25) Completion of exercise to the joint by the patient while doing activities of daily living or during joint assessment.

**active strategies of health promotion** (Chapter 1) Activities that depend on the patient's being motivated to adopt a specific health program.

**active transport** (Chapter 15) Movement of materials across the cell membrane by means of chemical activity that allows the cell to admit larger molecules than would otherwise be possible.

**activities of daily living (ADLs)** (Chapter 34) Activities usually performed in the course of a normal day in the patient's life, such as eating, dressing, bathing, brushing the teeth, or grooming.

**activity tolerance** (Chapter 25) Kind or amount of exercise or work a person is able to perform.

**actual loss** (Chapter 23) Loss of an object, person, body part or function, or emotion that is overt and easily identifiable.

**actual nursing diagnosis** (Chapter 7) A judgment that is clinically validated by the presence of major defining characteristics.

**acuity recording** (Chapter 8) Mechanism by which entries describing patient care activities are made over a 24-hour period. The activities are then translated into a rating score, or acuity score, that allows for a comparison of patients who vary by severity of illness.

**acute care** (Chapter 2) Pattern of health care in which a patient is treated for an acute episode of illness, for the sequelae of an accident or other trauma, or during recovery from surgery.

**acute illness** (Chapter 1) Illness characterized by symptoms that are of relatively short duration, are usually severe, and affect the functioning of the patient in all dimensions.

**adduction** (Chapter 25) Movement of a limb toward the body.

**adolescence** (Chapter 19) The period in development between the onset of puberty and adulthood. It usually begins between 11 and 13 years of age.

**adult day care centers** (Chapter 2) Facility for the supervised care of older adults, providing activities such as meals and socialization during specified day hours.

**advanced sleep phase syndrome** (Chapter 29) Common in older adults, a disturbance in sleep manifested as early waking in the morning with an inability to get back to sleep. It is believed that this syndrome is caused by advancing of the body's circadian rhthym.

**adventitious sounds** (Chapters 13, 29) Abnormal lung sounds heard with auscultation.

**adverse effect** (Chapter 14) Harmful or unintended effect of a medication, diagnostic test, or therapeutic intervention.

**adverse reaction** (Chapter 7) Any harmful, unintended effect of a medication, diagnostic test, or therapeutic intervention.

**advocacy** (Chapter 5) Process whereby a nurse objectively provides patients with the information they need to make decisions and supports the patients in whatever decisions they make.

**afebrile** (Chapter 12) Without fever.

**affective learning** (Chapter 10) Acquisition of behaviors involved in expressing feelings in attitudes, appreciation, and values.

**afterload** (Chapter 28) Resistance to left ventricular ejection; the work the heart must overcome to fully eject blood from the left ventricle.

**age-related macular degeneration** (Chapter 36) Progressive disorder in which the macula (the specialized portion of the retina responsible for central vision) degenerates as a result of aging and loses its ability to function efficiently. First signs include blurring of reading matter, distortion or loss of central vision, sensitivity to glare, and distortion of objects.

**agnostic** (Chapter 18) Individual who believes that any ultimate reality is unknown or unknowable.

**airborne precautions** (Chapter 11) Safeguards designed to reduce the risk of transmission of infectious agents through the air a person breathes.

**alarm reaction** (Chapter 22) Mobilization of the defense mechanisms of the body and mind to cope with a stressor. The initial stage of the general adaptation syndrome.

**aldosterone** (Chapter 15) Mineralocorticoid steroid hormone produced by the adrenal cortex with action in the renal tubule to regulate sodium and potassium balance in the blood.

**allergic reactions** (Chapter 14) Unfavorable physiological response to an allergen to which a person has previously been exposed and to which the person has developed antibodies.

**alopecia** (Chapter 13) Partial or complete loss of hair; baldness.

**Alzheimer's disease** (Chapter 19) Disease of the brain parenchyma that causes a gradual and progressive decline in cognitive functioning.

**AMBULARM** (Chapter 26) Device used for the patient who climbs out of bed unassisted and is in danger of falling. This device is worn on the leg and signals when the leg is in a dependent position such as over the side rail or on the floor.

**amino acid** (Chapter 31) Organic compound of one or more basic groups and one or more carboxyl groups. Amino acids are the building blocks that construct proteins and the end products of protein digestion.

**anabolism** (Chapter 31) Constructive metabolism characterized by conversion of simple substances into more complex compounds of living matter.

**analgesic** (Chapter 30) Relieving pain; drug that relieves pain.

**analogies** (Chapter 10) Resemblances made between things otherwise unlike.

**anaphylactic reactions** (Chapter 14) Hypersensitive condition induced by contact with certain antigens.

**aneurysm** (Chapter 13) Localized dilations of the wall of a blood vessel, usually caused by atherosclerosis, hypertension, or a congenital weakness in a vessel wall.

**anger** (Chapter 23) Second stage of Kübler-Ross's stages of dying. During this stage an individual resists loss by expressing extreme displeasure, indignation, or hostility.

**angiotensin** (Chapter 15) Polypeptide occurring in the blood, causing vasoconstriction, increased blood pressure, and the release of aldosterone from the adrenal cortex.

**anion gap** (Chapter 15) Difference between the concentrations of serum cations and anions, determined by measuring the concentrations of sodium cations and chloride and bicarbonate anions.

**anions** (Chapter 15) Negatively charged electrolytes.

**anthropometric measurements** (Chapter 34) Body measures of height, weight, and skinfolds to evaluate muscle atrophy.

**anthropometry** (Chapter 31) Measurement of various body parts to determine nutritional and caloric status, muscular development, brain growth, and other parameters.

**antibodies** (Chapter 11) Immunoglobulins, essential to the immune system, that are produced by lymphoid tissue in response to bacteria, viruses, or other antigens.

**anticipatory grief** (Chapter 23) Grief response in which the person begins the grieving process before an actual loss.

**antidiuretic hormone (ADH)** (Chapter 15) Hormone that decreases the production of urine by increasing the reabsorption of water by the renal tubules. ADH is secreted by cells of the hypothalamus and stored in the posterior lobe of the pituitary gland.

**antiembolic stockings** (Chapter 37) Elasticized stockings that prevent formation of emboli and thrombi, especially after surgery or during bed rest.

**antigen** (Chapter 11) Substance, usually a protein, that causes the formation of an antibody and reacts specifically with that antibody.

**antipyretic** (Chapter 12) Substance or procedure that reduces fever.

**anxiolytics** (Chapter 23) Drugs used primarily to treat episodes of anxiety.

**aphasia** (Chapter 13) Abnormal neurological condition in which language function is defective or absent; related to injury to speech center in cerebral cortex, causing receptive or expressive aphasia.

**apical pulse** (Chapter 12) Heartbeat as listened to with the bell or diaphragm of a stethoscope placed on the apex of the heart.

**apnea** (Chapter 12) Cessation of airflow through the nose and mouth.

**apothecary system** (Chapter 14) System of measurement. The basic unit of weight is a grain. Weights derived from the grain are the gram, ounce, and pound. The basic measure for fluid is the minim. The fluidram, fluid ounce, pint, quart, and gallon are measures derived from the minim.

**approximate** (Chapter 35) To come close together, as in the edges of a wound.

**arcus senilis** (Chapter 13) Opaque ring, gray to white in color, that surrounds the periphery of the cornea. The condition is caused by deposits of fat granules in the cornea. Occurs primarily in older adults.

**asepsis** (Chapter 11) Absence of germs or microorganisms.

**aseptic technique** (Chapter 11) Any health care procedure in which added precautions are used to prevent contamination of a person, object, or area by microorganisms.

**assault** (Chapter 4) Unlawful threat to bring about harmful or offensive contact with another.

**assertive communication** (Chapter 9) Type of communication based on a philosophy of protecting individual rights and responsibilities. It includes the ability to be self-directive in acting to accomplish goals and advocate for others.

**assessment** (Chapter 7) First step of the nursing process; activities required in the first step are data collection, data validation, data sorting, and data documentation. The purpose is to gather information for health problem identification.

**assimilation** (Chapter 17) To become absorbed into another culture and to adopt its characteristics.

**assisted living** (Chapter 2) Residential living facilities in which each resident has his or her own room and shares dining and social activity areas.

**associative play** (Chapter 19) Form of play in which a group of children participates in similar or identical activities without formal organization, direction, interaction, or goals.

**atelectasis** (Chapters 28, 34, 37) Collapse of alveoli, preventing the normal respiratory exchange of oxygen and carbon dioxide.

**atheist** (Chapter 18) Individual who does not believe in the existence of God.

**atherosclerosis** (Chapter 13) Common arterial disorder characterized by yellowish plaques of cholesterol, lipids, and cellular debris in the inner layers of the walls of the large- and medium-size arteries.

**atrioventricular (AV) node** (Chapter 28) A portion of the cardiac conduction system located on the floor of the right atrium; it receives electrical impulses from the atrium and transmits them to the bundle of His.

**atrophied** (Chapter 13) Wasted or reduced size or physiological activity of a part of the body caused by disease or other influences.

**attachment** (Chapter 19) Initial psychosocial relationship that develops between parents and the neonate.

**attentional set** (Chapter 10) Internal state of the learner that allows focusing and comprehension.

**auditory** (Chapter 36) Related to, or experienced through, hearing.

**auscultation** (Chapter 13) Method of physical examination; listening to the sounds produced by the body, usually with a stethoscope.

**auscultatory gap** (Chapter 12) Disappearance of sound when obtaining a blood pressure; typically occurs between the first and second Korotkoff sounds.

**authority** (Chapter 24) The right to act in areas in which an individual has been given and accepts responsibility.

**autologous transfusion** (Chapter 15) Procedure in which blood is removed from a donor and stored for a variable period before it is returned to the donor's own circulation.

**autonomy** (Chapter 5) Ability or tendency to function independently.

**back-channeling** (Chapter 7) Active listening technique that prompts a respondent to continue telling a story or describing a situation. Involves use of phrases such as "Go on," "Uh huh," and "Tell me more."

**bacteriuria** (Chapter 32) Presence of bacteria in the urine.

**balance** (Chapter 25) Position when the person's center of gravity is correctly positioned so that falling does not occur.

**bandages** (Chapter 35) Available in rolls of various widths and materials including gauze, elasticized knit, elastic webbing, flannel, and muslin. Gauze bandages are lightweight and inexpensive, mold easily around contours of the body, and permit air circulation to underlying skin to prevent maceration. Elastic bandages conform well to body parts but can also be used to exert pressure over a body part.

**bargaining** (Chapter 23) Third stage of Kübler-Ross's stages of dying. A person postpones the reality of a loss by attempting to make deals in a subtle or overt manner with others or with a higher being.

*baridi* (Chapter 17) A condition among the Bena people of Tanzania, this illness is attributed to disrespectful behavior within the family or transgression of cultural taboos. The person experiences physical and psychological symptoms and is usually treated by a traditional healer, who has the person make a public admission or an apology or who treats the person with herbal remedies.

**basal cell carcinoma** (Chapter 13) Malignant epithelial cell tumor that begins as a papule and enlarges peripherally, developing a central crater that erodes, crusts, and bleeds. Metastasis is rare.

**basal metabolic rate (BMR)** (Chapter 12) Amount of energy used in a unit of time by a fasting, resting subject to maintain vital functions.

**battery** (Chapter 4) Legal term for touching of another's body without consent.

**bed boards** (Chapter 25) Boards placed under the mattress of a bed that provide extra support to the mattress surface.

**bed rest** (Chapter 34) Placement of the patient in bed for therapeutic reasons for a prescribed period.

**benchmarking** (Chapter 24) Identifying best practices and comparing them to the organization's current practices for the purpose of improving performance. This process helps to support the institution's claims of quality care delivery.

**beneficence** (Chapter 5) Doing good or active promotion of doing good. One of the four principles of the ethical theory of deontology.

**benign breast disease (fibrocystic)** (Chapter 13) A benign condition characterized by lumpy, painful breasts and sometimes nipple discharge. Symptoms are more apparent before the menstrual period. Known to be a risk factor for breast cancer.

**bereavement** (Chapter 23) Response to loss through death; a subjective experience that a person suffers after losing a person with whom there has been a significant relationship.

**biases and prejudices** (Chapter 17) Beliefs and attitudes associating negative permanent characteristics to people who are perceived as different from oneself.

**bilineally** (Chapter 17) Kinship that extends to both the mother's and father's sides of the family.

**binders** (Chapter 35) Bandages made of large pieces of material to fit specific body parts.

**bioethics** (Chapter 5) Branch of ethics within the field of health care.

**biological clock** (Chapter 29) Cyclical nature of body functions; functions controlled from within the body are synchronized with environmental factors; same meaning as biorhythm.

**biotransformation** (Chapter 14) The chemical changes that a substance undergoes in the body, such as by the action of enzymes.

**blanchable hyperemia** (Chapter 35) Redness of the skin due to dilation of the superficial capillaries. When pressure is applied to the skin, the area blanches, or turns a lighter color.

**body image** (Chapter 20) Persons' subjective concept of their physical appearance.

**body mechanics** (Chapter 25) Coordinated efforts of the musculoskeletal and nervous systems to maintain proper balance, posture, and body alignment.

**bone resorption** (Chapter 34) Destruction of bone cells and release of calcium into the blood.

**borborygmi** (Chapter 13) Audible abdominal sounds produced by hyperactive intestinal peristalsis.

**botanica** (Chapter 17) Place that sells religious and herbal remedies.

**bradycardia** (Chapter 12) Slower-than-normal heart rate; heart contracts fewer than 60 times per minute.

**bradypnea** (Chapter 12) Abnormally slow rate of breathing.

**bronchospasm** (Chapter 37) An excessive and prolonged contraction of the smooth muscle of the bronchi and bronchioles resulting in an acute narrowing and obstruction of the respiratory airway.

**bruit** (Chapter 13) Abnormal sound or murmur heard while auscultating an organ, gland, or artery.

**buccal** (Chapter 14) Of or pertaining to the inside of the cheek or the gum next to the cheek.

**buccal cavity** (Chapter 27) Consists of the lips surrounding the opening of the mouth, the cheeks running along the side walls of the cavity, the tongue and its muscles, and the hard and soft palate.

**buffer** (Chapter 15) Substance or group of substances that can absorb or release hydrogen ions to correct an acid-base imbalance.

**bundle of His** (Chapter 28) A portion of the cardiac conduction system that arises from the distal portion of the atrioventricular (AV) node and extends across the AV groove to the top of the intraventricular septum, where it divides into right and left bundle branches.

**cachexia** (Chapter 35) Malnutrition marked by weakness and emaciation, usually associated with severe illness.

**capitation** (Chapter 2) Payment mechanism in which a provider (e.g., health care network) receives a fixed amount of payment per enrollee.

**carbohydrates** (Chapter 31) Dietary classification of foods comprising sugars, starches, cellulose, and gum.

**carbon monoxide** (Chapter 26) Colorless, odorless, poisonous gas produced by the combustion of carbon or organic fuels.

**cardiac index** (Chapter 28) The adequacy of the cardiac output for an individual. It takes into account the body surface area (BSA) of the patient.

**cardiac output (CO)** (Chapters 12, 28) Volume of blood expelled by the ventricles of the heart, equal to the amount of blood ejected at each beat, multiplied by the number of beats in the period of time used for computation (usually 1 minute).

**cardiopulmonary rehabilitation** (Chapter 28) Actively assisting the patient with achieving and maintaining an optimal level of health through controlled physical exercise, nutrition counseling, relaxation and stress management techniques, prescribed medications and oxygen, and compliance.

**cardiopulmonary resuscitation (CPR)** (Chapter 28) Basic emergency procedures for life support consisting of artificial respiration and manual external cardiac massage.

**care** (Chapter 5) To feel concern or interest in one who has sorrow or difficulties.

**caring** (Chapter 16) Universal phenomenon that influences the way we think, feel, and behave in relation to one another.

**carriers** (Chapter 11) Persons or animals who harbor and spread an organism that causes disease in others but do not become ill.

**case management** (Chapter 2) Organized system for delivering health care to an individual patient or group of patients across an episode of illness and/or a continuum of care; includes assessment and development of a plan of care, coordination of all services, referral, and follow-up; usually assigned to one professional.

**case management plan** (Chapter 8) A multidisciplinary model for documenting patient care that usually includes plans for problems, key interventions, and expected outcomes for patients with a specific disease or condition.

**catabolism** (Chapter 31) Breakdown of body tissue into simpler substances.

**cataplexy** (Chapter 29) Condition characterized by sudden muscular weakness and loss of muscle tone.

**cataracts** (Chapter 36) An abnormal progressive condition of the lens of the eye characterized by loss of transparency.

**cathartics** (Chapter 33) Drugs that act to promote bowel evacuation.

**catheterization** (Chapter 32) Introduction of a catheter into a body cavity or organ to inject or remove fluid.

**cations** (Chapter 15) Positively charged electrolytes.

**center of gravity** (Chapter 25) Midpoint or center of the weight of a body or object.

**centigrade** (Chapter 12) Denotes temperature scale in which 0° is the freezing point of water and 100° is the boiling point of water at sea level; also called Celsius.

**cerumen** (Chapter 13) Yellowish or brownish waxy secretion produced by sweat glands in the external ear.

**chancres** (Chapter 13) Skin lesions or venereal sores (usually primary syphilis) that begin at the site of infection as papules and develop into red, bloodless, painless ulcers with a scooped-out appearance.

**change-of-shift report** (Chapter 8) Report that occurs between two scheduled nursing work shifts. Nurses communicate information about their assigned patients to nurses working on the next shift of duty.

**channel** (Chapter 9) Method used in the teaching-learning process to present content: visual, auditory, taste, smell. In the communication process, a method used to transmit a message: visual, auditory, touch.

**charting by exception (CBE)** (Chapter 8) Charting methodology in which data are entered only when there is an exception from what is normal or expected. Reduces time spent documenting in charting. It is a shorthand method for documenting normal findings and routine care.

**chest percussion** (Chapter 28) Striking of the chest wall with a cupped hand to promote mobilization and drainage of pulmonary secretions.

**chest physiotherapy (CPT)** (Chapters 28, 34) Group of therapies used to mobilize pulmonary secretions for expectoration.

**chest tube** (Chapter 28) A catheter inserted through the thorax into the chest cavity for removing air or fluid, used after chest or heart surgery or pneumothorax.

**chronic illness** (Chapter 1) Illness that persists over a long time and affects physical, emotional, intellectual, social, and spiritual functioning.

**circadian rhythm** (Chapter 29) Repetition of certain physiological phenomena within a 24-hour cycle.

**circulating nurse** (Chapter 37) Assistant to the scrub nurse and surgeon whose role is to provide necessary supplies, dispose of soiled instruments and supplies, and keep an accurate count of instruments, needles, and sponges used.

**civil law** (Chapter 4) Statutes concerned with protecting a person's rights.

**climacteric** (Chapter 19) Physiological, developmental change that occurs in the male reproductive system between the ages of 45 and 60.

**clinical criteria** (Chapter 7) Objective or subjective signs and symptoms, clusters of signs and symptoms, or risk factors.

**clinical decision making** (Chapter 26) A problem-solving approach that nurses use to define patient problems and select appropriate treatment.

**closed-ended question** (Chapter 7) A form of question that limits a respondent's answer to one or two words.

**clubbing** (Chapter 13) Bulging of the tissues at the nail base that is caused by insufficient oxygenation at the periphery, resulting from conditions such as chronic emphysema and congenital heart disease.

**code of ethics** (Chapters 5, 24) Formal statement that delineates a profession's guidelines for ethical behavior; a code of ethics sets standards or expectations for the professional to achieve.

**cognitive learning** (Chapter 10) Acquisition of intellectual skills that encompass behaviors such as thinking, understanding, and evaluating.

**collaborative interventions** (Chapter 7) Therapies that require the knowledge, skill, and expertise of multiple health care professionals.

**collaborative problem** (Chapter 7) Physiological complication that require the nurse to use nursing-prescribed and physician-prescribed interventions to maximize patient outcomes.

**colloid osmotic pressure** (Chapter 15) Abnormal condition of the kidney caused by the pressure of concentrations of large particles, such as protein molecules, that will pass through a membrane.

**colon** (Chapter 33) Portion of the large intestine from the cecum to the rectum.

**colonization** (Chapter 11) The presence and multiplication of microorganisms without tissue invasion or damage.

**comforting** (Chapter 16) Acts toward another individual that display both an emotional and physical calm. The use of touch, establishing presence, the therapeutic use of silence, and the skillful and gentle performance of a procedure are examples of comforting nursing measures.

**common law** (Chapter 4) One source for law that is created by judicial decisions as opposed to those created by legislative bodies (statutory law).

**communicable disease** (Chapter 11) Any disease that can be transmitted from one person or animal to another by direct or indirect contact or by vectors.

**communication** (Chapter 9) Ongoing, dynamic series of events that involves the transmission of meaning from sender to receiver.

**community health nursing** (Chapter 3) A nursing approach that combines knowledge from the public health sciences with professional nursing theories to safeguard and improve the health of populations in the community.

**community-based nursing** (Chapter 3) The acute and chronic care of individuals and families to strengthen their capacity for self-care and promote independence in decision making.

**competence** (Chapter 5) Specific range of skills necessary to perform a task.

**complete bed bath** (Chapter 27) Bath in which the entire body of a patient is washed in bed.

**compress** (Chapter 35) Soft pad of gauze or cloth used to apply heat, cold, or medications to the surface of a body part.

**computer-based patient record (CBCR)** (Chapter 8) Comprehensive computerized system used by all health care practitioners to permanently store information pertaining to a patient's health status, clinical problems, and functional abilities.

**concentration** (Chapter 14) Relative content of a component within a substance or solution.

**concentration gradient** (Chapter 15) Gradient that exists across a membrane separating a high concentration of a particular ion from a low concentration of the same ion.

**concept map** (Chapter 7) A care-planning tool that assists in critical thinking and forming associations between a patient's nursing diagnoses and interventions.

*confianza* (Chapter 17) Trust.

**confidentiality** (Chapter 5) The act of keeping information private or secret; in health care, the nurse only shares information about a patient with other nurses or health care providers who need to know private information about a patient in order to provide care for the patient; information can only be shared with the patient's consent.

**conjunctivitis** (Chapter 13) Highly contagious eye infection. The crusty drainage that collects on eyelid margins can easily spread from one eye to the other.

**connectedness** (Chapter 18) Having close spiritual relationships with oneself, others, and God or another spiritual being.

**connotative meaning** (Chapter 9) The shade or interpretation of a word's meaning influenced by the thoughts, feelings, or ideas people have about the word.

**conscious sedation** (Chapter 37) Administration of central nervous system depressant drugs and/or analgesics to provide analgesia, relieve anxiety, and/or provide amnesia during surgical, diagnostic, or interventional procedures.

**constipation** (Chapter 33) Condition characterized by difficulty in passing stool or an infrequent passage of hard stool.

**consultation** (Chapter 7) Process in which the help of a specialist is sought to identify ways to handle problems in patient management or in the planning and implementing of programs.

**contact precautions** (Chapter 11) Safeguards designed to reduce the risk of transmission of epidemiologically important microorganisms by direct or indirect contact.

**continent urinary diversion (CUR)** (Chapter 32) Surgical diversion of the drainage of urine from a diseased or dysfunctional bladder. Patient uses a catheter to drain the pouch.

**convalescence** (Chapter 37) Period of recovery after an illness, injury, or surgery.

**coping** (Chapter 22) Making an effort to manage psychological stress.

**core temperature** (Chapter 12) Temperature of deep structures of the body.

**cough** (Chapter 28) Sudden, audible expulsion of air from the lungs. The person breathes in, the glottis is partially closed, and the accessory muscles of expiration contract to expel the air forcibly.

**counseling** (Chapter 7) A problem-solving method used to help patients recognize and manage stress and to enhance interpersonal relationships; it helps patients examine alternatives and decide which choices are most helpful and appropriate.

**crackles** (Chapter 13) Fine bubbling sounds heard on auscultation of the lung; produced by air entering distal airways and alveoli, which contain serous secretions.

**crime** (Chapter 4) Act that violates a law and that may include criminal intent.

**criminal law** (Chapter 4) Concerned with acts that threaten society but may involve only an individual.

**crisis** (Chapter 22) Transition for better or worse in the course of a disease, usually indicated by a marked change in the intensity of signs and symptoms.

**crisis intervention** (Chapter 22) Use of therapeutic techniques directed toward helping a patient resolve a particular and immediate problem.

**critical pathways** (Chapters 7, 8) Tools used in managed care that incorporate the treatment interventions of caregivers from all disciplines who normally care for a patient. Designed for a specific care type, a pathway is used to manage the care of a patient throughout a projected length of stay.

**critical period of development** (Chapter 19) A specific phase or period when the presence of a function or reasoning has its greatest effect on a specific aspect of development.

**critical thinking** (Chapter 6) The active, purposeful, organized, cognitive process used to carefully examine one's thinking and the thinking of other individuals.

**crutch gait** (Chapter 25) A gait achieved by a person using crutches.

**cue** (Chapter 7) Information that a nurse acquires through hearing, visual observations, touch, and smell.

**cultural and linguistic competence** (Chapter 17) A set of congruent behaviors, attitudes, and policies that come together in a system, agency, or among professionals that enables effective work in cross-cultural situations.

**cultural assessment** (Chapter 17) A systematic and comprehensive examination of the cultural care values, beliefs, and practices of individuals, families, and communities.

**cultural awareness** (Chapter 17) Gaining in-depth awareness of one's own background, stereotypes, biases, prejudices, and assumptions about other people.

**cultural care accommodation or negotiation** (Chapter 17) Adapting or negotiating with the patient/families to achieve beneficial or satisfying health outcomes.

**cultural care preservation or maintenance** (Chapter 17) Retaining and/or preserving relevant care values so that patients are able to maintain their well-being, recover from illness, or face handicaps and/or death.

**cultural care repatterning or restructuring** (Chapter 17) Reordering, changing, or greatly modifying a patient's/family's customs for new, different, and beneficial health care pattern.

**cultural competence** (Chapter 17) Process in which the health care professional continually strives to achieve the ability and availability to work effectively with individuals, families, and communities.

**cultural encounters** (Chapter 17) Engaging in cross-cultural interactions; refining intercultural communication skills; gaining in-depth understanding of others and avoiding stereotypes; and cultural conflict management.

**cultural imposition** (Chapter 17) Using one's own values and customs as an absolute guide in interpreting behaviors.

**cultural knowledge** (Chapter 17) Obtaining knowledge of other cultures; gaining sensitivity to, respect for, and appreciation of differences.

**cultural pain** (Chapter 17) The feeling a patient has after a health care worker disregards the patient's valued way of life.

**cultural skills** (Chapter 17) Communication, cultural assessment, and culturally competent care.

**culturally congruent care** (Chapter 17) Care that fits the people's valued life patterns and sets of meanings generated from the people themselves. Sometimes this differs from the professionals' perspective on care.

**culturally ignorant or blind** (Chapter 17) Uneducated about other cultures.

**culture** (Chapter 17) Integrated patterns of human behavior that include the language, thoughts, communications, actions, customs, beliefs, values, and institutions of racial, ethnic, religious, or social groups.

**culture-bound syndromes** (Chapter 17) Illnesses restricted to a particular culture or group because of its psychosocial characteristics.

**culture care theory** (Chapter 17) Leininger's theory that emphasizes culturally congruent care.

**culturological nursing assessment** (Chapter 17) A systematic and comprehensive examination of the cultural care values, beliefs, and practices of individuals, families, and communities.

**cutaneous stimulation** (Chapter 30) Stimulation of a person's skin to prevent or reduce pain perception. A massage, warm bath, hot and cold therapies, and transcutaneous electrical nerve stimulation are some ways to reduce pain perception.

**cyanosis** (Chapters 13, 28) Bluish discoloration of the skin and mucous membranes caused by an excess of deoxygenated hemoglobin in the blood or a structural defect in the hemoglobin molecule.

**DAR (data, action, patient response)** (Chapter 8) The format used in focus charting for recording patient information.

**data analysis** (Chapter 7) Logical examination of and professional judgment about patient assessment data; used in the diagnostic process to derive a nursing diagnosis.

**data cluster** (Chapter 7) A set of signs or symptoms that are grouped together in logical order.

**database** (Chapter 7) Store or bank of information, especially in a form that can be processed by computer.

**debridement** (Chapter 35) Removal of dead tissue from a wound.

**decentralized management** (Chapter 24) An organizational philosophy that brings decisions down to the level of the staff. Individuals best informed about a problem or issue participate in the decision-making process.

**decision making** (Chapter 6) Process involving critical appraisal of information that results from recognition of a problem and ends with the generation, testing, and evaluation of a conclusion. Comes at the end of critical thinking.

**defecation** (Chapter 33) Passage of feces from the digestive tract through the rectum.

**defendant** (Chapter 4) Individual or organization against whom legal charges are brought in a court of law.

**defining characteristics** (Chapter 7) Related signs and symptoms or clusters of data that support the nursing diagnosis.

**dehiscence** (Chapters 35, 37) Separation of a wound's edges, revealing underlying tissues.

**dehydration** (Chapter 15) Excessive loss of water from the body tissues, accompanied by a disturbance of body electrolytes.

**delegation** (Chapter 24) Process of assigning another member of the health care team to be responsible for aspects of patient care; for example, assigning nurse assistants to bathe a patient.

**delirium** (Chapter 19) An acute confusional state, which is potentially reversible and is often due to a physical cause.

**dementia** (Chapter 19) A generalized impairment of intellectual functioning that interferes with social and occupational functioning.

**denial** (Chapter 23) Unconscious refusal to admit an unacceptable idea.

**denotative meaning** (Chapter 9) Meaning of a word shared by individuals who use a common language. The word "baseball" has the same meaning for all individuals who speak English, but the word "code" denotes cardiac arrest primarily to health care providers.

**dental caries** (Chapter 27) Abnormal destructive condition in a tooth caused by a complex interaction of food, especially starches and sugars, with bacteria that form dental plaque.

**deontology** (Chapter 5) Traditional theory of ethics that proposes to define actions as right or wrong based on the characteristics of fidelity to promises, truthfulness, and justice. The conventional use of ethical terms such as *justice, autonomy, beneficence,* and *nonmaleficence* constitutes the practice of deontology.

**depression** (1) (Chapter 19) A reduction in happiness and well-being that contributes to physical and social limitations and complicates the treatment of concomitant medical conditions. It is usually reversible with treatment. (2) (Chapter 23) Fourth stage of Kübler-Ross's stages of dying. In this stage the person realizes the full impact and significance of the loss.

**dermis** (Chapter 27) Sensitive vascular layer of the skin directly below the epidermis composed of collagenous and elastic fibrous connective tissues that give the dermis strength and elasticity.

**determinants of health** (Chapter 1) The many variables that influence the health status of individuals or communities.

**detoxify** (Chapter 14) To remove the toxic quality of a substance; the liver acts to detoxify chemicals in drug compounds.

**development** (Chapter 19) Qualitative or observable aspects of the progressive changes one makes in adapting to the environment.

**developmental crises** (Chapter 22) Crises associated with normal and expected phases of growth and development, for example, the response to menopause; same as maturational crises.

**diabetic retinopathy** (Chapter 36) A disorder of retinal blood vessels. Pathological changes secondary to increased pressure in the blood vessels of the retina result in decreased vision or vision loss due to hemorrhage and macular edema.

**diagnosis-related group** (DRG) (Chapters 2, 8) Group of patients classified to establish a mechanism for health care reimbursement based on length of stay; classification is based on the following variables: primary and secondary diagnosis, comorbidities, primary and secondary procedures, and age.

**diagnostic process** (Chapter 7) Mental steps (data clustering and analysis, problem identification) that follow assessment and lead directly to the formulation of a diagnosis.

**diagnostic reasoning** (Chapter 6) Process that enables an observer to assign meaning and to classify phenomena in clinical situations by integrating observations and critical thinking.

**diaphoresis** (Chapter 12) Secretion of sweat, especially profuse secretion associated with an elevated body temperature, physical exertion, or emotional stress.

**diaphragmatic breathing** (Chapter 28) Respiration in which the abdomen moves out while the diaphragm descends on inspiration.

**diarrhea** (Chapter 33) Increase in the number of stools and the passage of liquid, unformed feces.

**diastolic** (Chapter 12) Pertaining to diastole, or the blood pressure at the instant of maximum cardiac relaxation.

**dietary reference intake** (DRI) (Chapter 31) Information on each vitamin or mineral to reflect a range of minimum to maximum amounts that avert deficiency or toxicity.

**diffusion** (Chapters 12, 15, 28) Movement of molecules from an area of high concentration to an area of lower concentration.

**digestion** (Chapter 31) Breakdown of nutrients by chewing, churning, mixing with fluid, and chemical reactions.

**direct care interventions** (Chapter 7) Treatments performed through interaction with the patient. For example, a patient may require medication administration, insertion of an intravenous infusion, or counseling during a time of grief.

**discharge planning** (Chapter 2) Activities directed toward identifying future proposed therapy and the need for additional resources before and after returning home.

**discrimination** (Chapter 17) Prejudicial outlook, action, or treatment.

**disease** (Chapter 17) Malfunctioning or maladaptation of biological or psychological processes.

**disinfection** (Chapter 11) Process of destroying all pathogenic organisms, except spores.

**disorganization and despair** (Chapter 23) One of Bowlby's four phases of mourning where an individual endlessly examines how and why the loss occurred.

**distress** (Chapter 22) Damaging stress; one of the two types of stress identified by Selye.

**disuse osteoporosis** (Chapter 34) Reductions in skeletal mass routinely accompanying immobility or paralysis.

**diuresis** (Chapter 34) Increased rate of formation and excretion of urine.

**documentation** (Chapter 8) Written entry into the patient's medical record of all pertinent information about the patient. These entries validate the patient's problems and care and exist as a legal record.

**dominant culture** (Chapter 17) The customs, values, beliefs, traditions, and social and religious views held by a group of people that prevail over another secondary culture.

**dorsiflexion** (Chapter 25) Flexion toward the back.

**drainage evacuators** (Chapter 35) Convenient portable units that connect to tubular drains lying within a wound bed and exert a safe, constant, low-pressure vacuum to remove and collect drainage.

**droplet precautions** (Chapter 11) Safeguards designed to reduce the risk of droplet transmission of infectious agents.

**dysmenorrhea** (Chapter 13) Painful menstruation.

**dysphagia** (Chapter 31) Difficulty in swallowing, commonly associated with obstructive or motor disorders of the esophagus.

**dyspnea** (Chapters 13, 28) Sensation of shortness of breath.

**dysrhythmia** (Chapters 12, 13, 28) Deviation from the normal pattern of the heartbeat.

**dysuria** (Chapter 32) Painful urination resulting from bacterial infection of the bladder and obstructive conditions of the urethra.

**ecchymosis** (Chapter 35) Discoloration of the skin or bruise caused by leakage of blood into subcutaneous tissues as a result of trauma to underlying tissues.

**ectropion** (Chapter 13) Eversion of the eyelid, exposing the conjunctival membrane and part of the eyeball.

**edema** (Chapters 13, 25, 35) Abnormal accumulation of fluid in interstitial spaces of tissues.

**egocentric** (Chapter 19) Developmental characteristic wherein a toddler is only able to assume the view of his or her own activities and needs.

**electrocardiogram (ECG)** (Chapter 28) Graphic record of the electrical activity of the myocardium.

**electrolyte** (Chapter 15) Element or compound that, when melted or dissolved in water or other solvent, dissociates into ions and can carry an electrical current.

**electronic infusion device** (Chapter 15) A piece of medical equipment that delivers intravenous fluids at a prescribed rate through an intravenous catheter.

**embolism** (Chapter 37) Abnormal condition in which a blood clot (embolus) travels through the bloodstream and becomes lodged in a blood vessel.

**emic worldview** (Chapter 17) An insider or native perspective.

**empathy** (Chapter 9) Understanding and acceptance of a person's feelings and the ability to sense the person's private world.

**endogenous infections** (Chapter 11) Infections produced within a cell or organism.

**endorphins** (Chapters 22, 30) Hormones that act on the mind like morphine and opiates, producing a sense of well-being and reducing pain.

**enema** (Chapter 33) Procedure involving introduction of a solution into the rectum for cleansing or therapeutic purposes.

**enteral nutrition (EN)** (Chapter 31) Provision of nutrients through the gastrointestinal tract when the patient cannot ingest, chew, or swallow food but can digest and absorb nutrients.

**entropion** (Chapter 13) Condition in which the eyelid turns inward toward the eye.

**environment** (Chapter 9) All of the many factors, such as physical and psychological, that influence or affect the life and survival of a person.

**epidermis** (Chapter 27) Outer layer of the skin that has several thin layers of skin in different stages of maturation; shields and protects the underlying tissues from water loss, mechanical or chemical injury, and penetration by disease-causing microorganisms.

**epidural infusion** (Chapter 30) Type of nerve block anesthesia in which an anesthetic is intermittently or continuously injected into the lumbosacral region of the spinal cord.

**erythema** (Chapter 13) Redness or inflammation of the skin or mucous membranes that is a result of dilation and congestion of superficial capillaries; sunburn is an example.

**eschar** (Chapter 35) A thick layer of dead, dry tissue that covers a pressure ulcer or thermal burn; it may be allowed to be sloughed off naturally or it may need to be surgically removed.

**ethical dilemma** (Chapter 5) Dilemma existing when the right thing to do is not clear. Resolution requires the negotiation of differing values among those involved in the dilemma.

**ethical principles** (Chapter 5) Set of guidelines for a profession's expectations and standards of behavior for its members.

**ethics** (Chapter 5) Principles or standards that govern proper conduct.

**ethics of care** (Chapter 5) Delivery of health care based on ethical principles and standards of care.

**ethnicity** (Chapter 17) A shared identity related to social and cultural heritage such as values, language, geographical space, and racial characteristics.

**ethnocentrism** (Chapter 17) A tendency to hold one's own way of life as superior to others.

**ethnohistory** (Chapter 17) Significant historical experiences of a particular group.

**etic worldview** (Chapter 17) An outsider's perspective.

**etiology** (Chapter 7) Study of all factors that may be involved in the development of a disease.

**eupnea** (Chapter 12) Normal respirations that are quiet, effortless, and rhythmical.

**eustress** (Chapter 22) Stress that protects health; one of the two types of stress identified by Selye.

**evaluation** (Chapter 7) Determination of the extent to which established patient goals have been achieved.

**evidence-based knowledge** (Chapter 6) Knowledge that is derived from the integration of best research, clinical expertise, and patient values.

**evidence-based practice** (Chapter 2) The use of current best evidence from nursing research, clinical expertise, practice trends, and patient preferences to guide nursing decisions about care provided to patients.

**evisceration** (Chapters 35, 37) Protrusion of visceral organs through a surgical wound.

**exacerbations** (Chapter 30) Increases in the seriousness of a disease or disorder as marked by greater intensity in signs or symptoms.

**excessive daytime sleepiness** (Chapter 29) Extreme fatigue felt during the day. Signs of this include falling asleep at inappropriate times, such as while eating, talking, or driving. May indicate a sleep disorder.

**excoriation** (Chapter 13) Injury to the skin's surface caused by abrasion.

**exhaustion stage** (Chapter 22) Phase that occurs when the body can no longer resist the stress; when the energy necessary to maintain adaptation is depleted.

**exogenous infection** (Chapter 11) Infection originating outside an organ or part.

**exostosis** (Chapter 13) An abnormal benign growth on the surface of a bone.

**expected outcomes** (Chapter 7) Expected conditions of a patient at the end of therapy or of a disease process, including the degree of wellness and the need for continuing care, medications, support, counseling, or education.

**extended care facility** (Chapter 2) An institution devoted to providing medical, nursing, or custodial care for an individual over a prolonged period, such as during the course of a chronic disease or during the rehabilitation phase after an acute illness.

**extension** (Chapter 25) Movement by certain joints that increases the angle between two adjoining bones.

**extracellular fluid (ECF)** (Chapter 15) Portion of body fluids composed of the interstitial fluid and blood plasma.

**exudate** (Chapter 11) Fluid, cells, or other substances that have been slowly discharged from cells or blood vessels through small pores or breaks in cell membranes.

**face-saving** (Chapter 17) A way of speaking or acting that preserves dignity.

**Fahrenheit** (Chapter 12) Denotes temperature scale in which 32° is the freezing point of water and 212° is the boiling point of water at sea level.

**faith** (Chapter 18) Set of beliefs and a way of relating to self, others, and a supreme being.

*fajita* (Chapter 17) Cotton binder used on a newborn's abdomen among Hispanics and Filipinos to prevent gas and umbilical hernia.

**family** (Chapter 21) Group of interacting individuals composing a basic unit of society.

**family as context** (Chapter 21) Nursing perspective in which the family is viewed as a unit of interacting members having attributes, functions, and goals separate from those of the individual family members.

**family diversity** (Chapter 21) The unique needs and characteristics of each member in a family.

**family durability** (Chapter 21) A system of support for a family that includes immediate and extended family members.

**family forms** (Chapter 21) Patterns of people considered by family members to be included in the family.

**family functioning** (Chapter 21) Processes families use to achieve their goals.

**family hardiness** (Chapter 21) Internal strengths and durability of the family unit; characterized by a sense of control over the outcome of life events and hardships, a view of change as beneficial and growth-producing, and an active rather than passive orientation in responding to stressful life events.

**family health** (Chapter 21) Determined by the effectiveness of the family's structure, the processes that the family uses to meet its goals, and internal and external forces.

**family as patient** (Chapter 21) A nursing approach that takes into consideration the effect of one intervention on all members of a family.

**family resiliency** (Chapter 21) A family's ability to cope with expected and unexpected stressors.

**family structure** (Chapter 21) Based on organization (i.e., ongoing membership) of the family and the pattern of relationships.

*farmacia* (Chapter 17) Place to obtain prescribed medications.

**febrile** (Chapter 12) Pertaining to or characterized by an elevated body temperature.

**fecal impaction** (Chapter 33) Accumulation of hardened fecal material in the rectum or sigmoid colon.

**fecal incontinence** (Chapter 33) Inability to control passage of feces and gas from the anus.

**fecal occult blood test (FOBT)** (Chapter 33) Measures microscopic amounts of blood in the feces.

**feces** (Chapter 33) Waste or excrement from the gastrointestinal tract.

**feedback** (Chapter 9) Process in which the output of a given system is returned to the system.

**felony** (Chapter 4) Crime of a serious nature that carries a penalty of imprisonment or death.

**feminist ethics** (Chapter 5) Ethical approach that focuses on relationships of those involved in an ethical dilemma rather than traditional abstract principles of deontology.

**fever** (Chapter 12) Elevation in the hypothalamic set point, so that body temperature is regulated at a higher level.

**fictive** (Chapter 17) Nonblood kin; considered family in some collective cultures.

**fidelity** (Chapter 5) The agreement to keep a promise.

**fight or flight response** (Chapter 22) The total physiological response to stress that occurs during the alarm reaction stage of the general adaptation syndrome. Massive changes in all body systems prepare a human being to choose to flee or to remain and fight the stressor.

**filtration** (Chapter 15) The straining of fluid through a membrane.

**fistula** (Chapter 35) Abnormal passage from an internal organ to the body surface or between two internal organs.

**flashback** (Chapter 22) A recollection so strong that the individual thinks he or she is actually experiencing the trauma again or seeing it unfold before his or her eyes.

**flatus** (Chapter 33) Intestinal gas.

**flora** (Chapter 11) Microorganisms that live on or within a body to compete with disease-producing microorganisms and provide a natural immunity against certain infections.

**flow sheets** (Chapter 8) Documents on which frequent observations or specific measurements are recorded.

**fluid volume deficit (FVD)** (Chapter 15) A fluid and electrolyte disorder caused by failure of the body's homeostatic mechanisms to regulate the retention and excretion of body fluids. The condition is characterized by decreased output of urine, high specific gravity of urine, output of urine that is greater than the intake of fluid in the body, hemoconcentration, and increased serum levels of sodium.

**fluid volume excess (FVE)** (Chapter 15) A fluid and electrolyte disorder characterized by an increase in fluid retention and edema, resulting from failure of the body's homeostatic mechanisms to regulate the retention and excretion of body fluids.

**focus charting** (Chapter 8) A charting methodology for structuring progress notes according to the focus of the note, for example, symptoms and nursing diagnosis. Each note includes data, actions, and patient response.

**focused cultural assessment** (Chapter 17) Method of evaluating a patient's ethnohistory, biocultural history, social organization, and religious and spiritual beliefs to find issues that are most relevant to the problem at hand.

**food poisoning** (Chapter 26) Toxic processes resulting from the ingestion of a food contaminated by toxic substances or by bacteria-containing toxins.

**foot boots** (Chapter 25) Soft, foot-shaped devices designed to reduce the risk of footdrop by maintaining the foot in dorsiflexion.

**footdrop** (Chapters 25, 34) An abnormal neuromuscular condition of the lower leg and foot, characterized by an inability to dorsiflex, or evert, the foot.

**friction** (Chapters 25, 35) Effects of rubbing or the resistance that a moving body meets from the surface on which it moves; a force that occurs in a direction to oppose movement.

**functional health illiteracy** (Chapter 10) The inability of an individual to obtain, interpret, and understand basic information about health.

**functional health patterns** (Chapter 7) Method for organizing assessment data based on the level of patient function in specific areas, for example, mobility.

**functional nursing** (Chapter 24) Method of patient care delivery in which each staff member is assigned a task that is completed for all patients on the unit.

**future orientation** (Chapter 17) Time dimension emphasized by dominant American culture. It is characterized by direct communication and is focused on task achievement, whereas past orientation communication is circular and indirect and is focused on group harmony.

**gait** (Chapter 25) Manner or style of walking, including rhythm, cadence, and speed.

**gastrostomy feeding tube** (Chapter 31) The insertion of a feeding tube, through a stoma, into the stomach for the purpose of providing enteral nutrition.

**general adaptation syndrome (GAS)** (Chapter 22) Generalized defense response of the body to stress, consisting of three stages: alarm, resistance, and exhaustion.

**general anesthesia** (Chapter 37) Intravenous or inhaled medications that cause the patient to lose all sensation and consciousness.

**geriatrics** (Chapter 19) Branch of health care dealing with the physiology and psychology of aging and with the diagnosis and treatment of diseases affecting older adults.

**gerontology** (Chapter 19) The study of all aspects of the aging process and its consequences.

**gingivae** (Chapter 13) Gums of the mouth; a mucous membrane with supporting fibrous tissue that overlies the crowns of unerupted teeth and encircles the necks of those teeth that have erupted.

**glaucoma** (Chapter 36) An abnormal condition of elevated pressure within an eye caused by obstruction of the outflow of aqueous humor. Often results in peripheral visual loss, decreased visual acuity with difficulty adapting to darkness, and a halo effect around lights, if untreated.

**globalization** (Chapter 2) Worldwide scope or application.

**glomerulus** (Chapter 32) Cluster or collection of capillary vessels within the kidney involved in the initial formation of urine.

**gluconeogenesis** (Chapter 31) Formation of glucose or glycogen from substances that are not carbohydrates, such as protein or lipid.

**glucose** (Chapter 31) The primary fuel for the body, needed to carry out major physiological functions.

**glycogen** (Chapter 31) Polysaccharide that is the major carbohydrate stored in animal cells.

**glycogenesis** (Chapter 31) The process for storage of glucose in the form of glycogen in the liver.

**goals** (Chapter 7) Desired results of nursing actions, set realistically by the nurse and patient as part of the planning stage of the nursing process.

**Good Samaritan laws** (Chapter 4) Legislation enacted in some states to protect health care professionals from liability in rendering emergency aid, unless there is proven willful wrong or gross negligence.

**graduated measuring container** (Chapter 32) Receptacle for volume measurement.

**granny midwives** (Chapter 17) Amateur health practitioners that assist in labor and delivery.

**granulation tissue** (Chapter 35) Soft, pink, fleshy projections of tissue that form during the healing process in a wound not healing by primary intention.

**graphic record** (Chapter 8) Charting mechanism that allows for the recording of vital signs and weight in such a manner that caregivers can quickly note changes in the patient's status.

**grief** (Chapter 23) Form of sorrow involving the person's thoughts, feelings, and behaviors, occurring as a response to an actual or perceived loss.

**grieving process** (Chapter 23) Sequence of affective, cognitive, and physiological states through which the person responds to and finally accepts an irretrievable loss.

**grounded** (Chapter 26) Connection between the electric circuit and the ground, which becomes part of the circuit.

**growth** (Chapter 19) Measurable or quantitative aspect of an individual's increase in physical dimensions as a result of an increase in number of cells. Indicators of growth include changes in height, weight, and sexual characteristics.

**guided imagery** (Chapter 30) Method of pain control in which the patient creates a mental image, concentrates on that image, and gradually becomes less aware of pain.

**gustatory** (Chapter 36) Pertaining to the sense of taste.

*halal* (Chapter 17) Foods permissible for Muslims to eat.

**hand rolls** (Chapter 25) Rolls of cloth that keep the thumb slightly adducted and in opposition to the fingers.

**hand-wrist splints** (Chapter 25) Splints individually molded for the patient to maintain proper alignment of the thumb, slight adduction of the wrist, and slight dorsiflexion.

*haram* (Chapter 17) Foods prohibited by Muslim religious standards.

**health** (Chapter 1) Dynamic state in which individuals adapt to their internal and external environments so that there is a state of physical, emotional, intellectual, social, and spiritual well-being.

**health belief model** (Chapter 1) Conceptual framework that describes a person's health behavior as an expression of the person's health beliefs.

**health beliefs** (Chapters 1, 10) Patient's personal beliefs about levels of wellness, which can motivate or impede participation in changing risk factors, participating in care, and selecting care options.

**health care–associated infection** (Chapter 11) An infection that was not present or incubating at the time of admission to a health care setting.

**health care problems** (Chapter 7) Any conditions or dysfunctions that the patient experiences as a result of illness or treatment of an illness.

**health promotion** (Chapter 1) Activities such as routine exercise and good nutrition that help patients maintain or enhance their present levels of health and reduce their risk of developing certain diseases.

**health promotion model** (Chapter 1) Defines health as a positive, dynamic state, not merely the absence of disease. The health promotion model emphasizes well-being, personal fulfillment, and self-actualization rather than reacting to the threat of illness.

**health status** (Chapter 1) Description of health of an individual or community.

**heat exhaustion** (Chapter 26) Abnormal condition caused by depletion of body fluid and electrolytes resulting from exposure to intense heat or the inability to acclimatize to heat.

**heat stroke** (Chapter 12) Continued exposure to extreme heat raising the core body temperature to 40.5° C (105° F) or higher.

**hematemesis** (Chapter 13) Vomiting of blood, indicating upper gastrointestinal bleeding.

**hematoma** (Chapter 35) Collection of blood trapped in the tissues of the skin or an organ.

**hematuria** (Chapter 32) Abnormal presence of blood in the urine.

**hemolysis** (Chapter 15) Breakdown of red blood cells and release of hemoglobin that may occur after administration of hypotonic intravenous solutions, causing swelling and rupture of erythrocytes.

**hemoptysis** (Chapter 28) Coughing up blood from the respiratory tract.

**hemorrhoids** (Chapter 13, 33) Permanent dilation and engorgement of veins within the lining of the rectum.

**hemostasis** (Chapter 35) Termination of bleeding by mechanical or chemical means or by the coagulation process of the body.

**hemothorax** (Chapter 28) Accumulation of blood and fluid in the pleural cavity between the parietal and visceral pleurae.

**hernia** (Chapter 13) Protrusion of an organ through an abnormal opening in the muscle wall of the cavity that surrounds it.

*hilots* (Chapter 17) Amateur health practitioners that assist in labor and delivery among Filipinos.

**holistic** (Chapter 18) Of or pertaining to the whole; considering all factors.

**holistic health** (Chapter 1) Comprehensive view of the person as a biopsychosocial and spiritual being.

**home care** (Chapter 2) Health service provided in the patient's place of residence for the purpose of promoting, maintaining, or restoring health or minimizing the effects of illness and disability.

**homeostasis** (Chapter 15) State of relative constancy in the internal environment of the body, maintained naturally by physiological adaptive mechanisms.

**hope** (Chapters 18, 23) Confident, yet uncertain, expectation of achieving a future goal.

**hospice** (Chapters 2, 23) System of family-centered care designed to help terminally ill persons be comfortable and maintain a satisfactory lifestyle throughout the terminal phase of their illness.

**Hoyer lift** (Chapter 25) A mechanical device that uses a canvas sling to easily lift dependent patients for transfer.

**humidification** (Chapter 28) Process of adding water to gas.

**humor** (Chapter 9) Coping strategy based on an individual's cognitive appraisal of a stimulus that results in behavior such as smiling, laughing, or feelings of amusement that lessen emotional distress.

**hydrocephalus** (Chapter 13) Abnormal accumulation of cerebrospinal fluid in the ventricles of the brain.

**hydrostatic pressure** (Chapter 15) Pressure caused by a liquid.

**hypercalcemia** (Chapter 34) Greater-than-normal amount of calcium in the blood.

**hypercapnia** (Chapter 28) Greater-than-normal amounts of carbon dioxide in the blood; also called hypercarbia.

**hyperextension** (Chapter 25) Position of maximal extension of a joint.

**hyperglycemia** (Chapter 31) Elevated serum glucose levels.

**hypertension** (Chapter 12) Disorder characterized by an elevated blood pressure persistently exceeding 120/80 mm Hg.

**hyperthermia** (Chapter 12) Situation in which body temperature exceeds the set point.

**hypertonic** (Chapter 15) Situation in which one solution has a greater concentration of solute than another solution; therefore the first solution exerts greater osmotic pressure.

**hypertonicity** (Chapter 13) Excessive tension of the arterial walls or muscles.

**hyperventilation** (Chapter 28) Respiratory rate in excess of that required to maintain normal carbon dioxide levels in the body tissues.

**hypnotics** (Chapter 29) Class of drug that causes insensibility to pain and induces sleep.

**hypostatic pneumonia** (Chapter 34) Pneumonia that results from fluid accumulation as a result of inactivity.

**hypotension** (Chapter 12) Abnormal lowering of blood pressure that is inadequate for normal perfusion and oxygenation of tissues.

**hypothermia** (Chapter 26) Abnormal lowering of body temperature below 35° C, or 95° F, usually caused by prolonged exposure to cold.

**hypotonic** (Chapter 15) Situation in which one solution has a smaller concentration of solute than another solution; therefore the first solution exerts less osmotic pressure.

**hypotonicity** (Chapter 13) Reduced tension of the arterial walls or muscles.

**hypoventilation** (Chapter 28) Respiratory rate insufficient to prevent carbon dioxide retention.

**hypovolemia** (Chapters 15, 28) Abnormally low circulating blood volume.

**hypoxemia** (Chapter 28) Arterial blood oxygen level less than 60 mm Hg; low oxygen level in the blood.

**hypoxia** (Chapter 28) Inadequate cellular oxygenation that may result from a deficiency in the delivery or use of oxygen at the cellular level.

**identity** (Chapter 20) Component of self-concept characterized by one's persisting consciousness of being oneself, separate and distinct from others.

**idiosyncratic reaction** (Chapter 14) Individual sensitivity to effects of a drug caused by inherited or other bodily constitution factors.

**illness** (1) (Chapter 1) Abnormal process in which any aspect of a person's functioning is diminished or impaired compared with that person's previous condition. (2) (Chapter 17) The personal, interpersonal, and cultural reaction to disease.

**illness behavior** (Chapter 1) Ways in which people monitor their bodies, define and interpret their symptoms, take remedial actions, and use the health care system.

**illness prevention** (Chapter 1) Health education programs or activities directed toward protecting patients from threats or potential threats to health and toward minimizing risk factors.

**imam** (Chapter 17) Muslim priest.

**immobility** (Chapter 34) Inability to move about freely, caused by any condition in which movement is impaired or therapeutically restricted.

**immunity** (Chapter 11) The quality of being insusceptible to or unaffected by a particular disease or condition.

**immunization** (Chapter 26) A process by which resistance to an infectious disease is induced or augmented.

**implementation** (Chapter 7) Initiation and completion of the nursing actions necessary to help the patient achieve health care goals.

**impression management** (Chapter 17) The ability to interpret the others' behavior within their own context of meanings and behave in a culturally congruent way to achieve desired outcomes of communication.

**incentive spirometry** (Chapter 28) Method of encouraging voluntary deep breathing by providing visual feedback to patients of the inspiratory volume they have achieved.

**incident rates** (Chapter 3) The rate of new cases of a disease in a specified population over a defined period of time.

**incident report** (Chapter 8) Confidential document that describes any patient accident while the person is on the premises of a health care agency (occurrance report).

**independent practice association (IPA)** (Chapter 2) Managed care organization that contracts with physicians or health care providers who usually are members of groups and whose practices include fee-for-service and capitated patients.

**indirect care interventions** (Chapter 7) Treatments performed away from the patient but on behalf of the patient or group of patients.

**induration** (Chapters 13, 35) Hardening of a tissue, particularly the skin, because of edema or inflammation.

**infection** (Chapter 11) The invasion of the body by pathogenic microorganisms that reproduce and multiply.

**inference** (1) (Chapter 7) A judgment or interpretation of informational cues. (2) (Chapter 6) Taking one proposition as a given and guessing that another proposition follows.

**infiltration** (Chapter 15) Dislodging an intravenous catheter or needle from a vein into the subcutaneous space.

**inflammation** (Chapter 11) Protective response of body tissues to irritation or injury.

**informed consent** (Chapter 4) Process of obtaining permission from a patient to perform a specific test or procedure, after describing all risks, side effects, and benefits.

**infusion pump** (Chapter 15) Device that delivers a measured amount of fluid over a period of time.

**infusions** (Chapter 14) Introduction of fluid into the vein, giving intravenous fluid over time.

**inhalation** (Chapter 14) Method of medication delivery through the patient's respiratory tract. The respiratory tract provides a large surface area for drug absorption. Inhalation can be through the nasal or oral route.

**injections** (Chapter 14) Parenteral administration of medication; four major sites of injection: subcutaneous, intramuscular, intravenous, and intradermal.

**insensible water loss** (Chapter 15) Water loss that is continuous and is not perceived by the person.

**insomnia** (Chapter 29) Condition characterized by chronic inability to sleep or remain asleep through the night.

**inspection** (Chapter 13) Method of physical examination by which the patient is visually systematically examined for appearance, structure, function, and behavior.

**instillation** (Chapter 14) To cause to enter drop by drop, or very slowly.

**institutional ethics committee** (Chapter 5) An interdisciplinary committee that discusses and processes ethical dilemmas that arise within a health care institution.

**instrumental activities of daily living (IADLs)** (Chapter 34) Activities that are necessary to be independent in society beyond eating, grooming, transferring, and toileting and include such skills as shopping, preparing meals, banking, and taking medications.

**integrated delivery network (IDN)** (Chapter 2) Set of providers and services organized to deliver a coordinated continuum of care to the population of patients served at a capitated cost.

**interpersonal communication** (Chapter 9) Exchange of information between two persons or among persons in a small group.

**interstitial fluid** (Chapter 15) Fluid that fills the spaces between most of the cells of the body and provides a substantial portion of the liquid environment of the body.

**interview** (Chapter 7) Organized, systematic conversation with the patient designed to obtain pertinent health-related subjective information.

**intracellular fluid** (Chapter 15) Liquid within the cell membrane.

**intradermal (ID)** (Chapter 14) Injection given between layers of the skin, into the dermis. Injections are given at a 5- to 15-degree angle.

**intramuscular (IM)** (Chapter 14) Injections given into muscle tissue. The intramuscular route provides a fast rate of absorption that is related to the muscle's greater vascularity. Injections are given at a 90-degree angle.

**intraocular** (Chapter 14) Method of medication delivery that involves inserting a medication disk, similar to a contact lens, into the patient's eye.

**intrapersonal communication** (Chapter 9) Communication that occurs within an individual; that is, persons "talk with themselves" silently or form an idea in their own mind.

**intravascular fluid** (Chapter 15) Fluid circulating within blood vessels of the body.

**intravenous** (Chapter 14) Injection directly into the bloodstream. Action of the drug begins immediately when given intravenously.

**intubation** (Chapter 28) Insertion of a breathing tube through the mouth or nose into the trachea to ensure a patent airway.

**intuition** (Chapter 6) The inner sensing that something is so.

**irrigation** (Chapter 14) Process of washing out a body cavity or wounded area with a stream of fluid.

**ischemia** (Chapter 34) Decreased blood supply to a body part, such as skin tissue, or to an organ, such as the heart.

**isolation** (Chapter 11) Separation of a seriously ill patient from others to prevent the spread of an infection or to protect the patient from irritating environmental factors.

**isometric exercises** (Chapter 34) Activities that involve muscle tension without muscle shortening, do not have any beneficial effect on preventing orthostatic hypotension, but may improve activity tolerance.

**isotonic** (Chapter 15) Situation in which two solutions have the same concentration of solute; therefore both solutions exert the same osmotic pressure.

**jaundice** (Chapter 13) Yellow discoloration of the skin, mucous membranes, and sclera caused by greater-than-normal amounts of bilirubin in the blood.

**jejunostomy tube** (Chapter 31) Hollow tube inserted into the jejunum through the abdominal wall for administration of liquefied foods to patients who have a high risk of aspiration.

**joint contracture** (Chapter 34) Abnormality that may result in permanent condition of a joint, is characterized by flexion and fixation, and is caused by disuse, atrophy, and shortening of muscle fibers and surrounding joint tissues.

**joints** (Chapter 25) Connections between bones; classified according to structure and degree of mobility.

**judgment** (Chapter 5) Ability to form an opinion or draw sound conclusions.

**justice** (Chapter 5) The ethical standard of fairness.

**Kardex** (Chapter 8) Trade name for card-filing system that allows quick reference to the particular need of the patient for certain aspects of nursing care.

**karma** (Chapter 17) Asian Indian belief that attributes mental illness to past deeds in one's previous life.

**Korotkoff sound** (Chapter 12) Sound heard during the taking of blood pressure using a sphygmomanometer and stethoscope.

**kyphosis** (Chapter 13) Exaggeration of the posterior curvature of the thoracic spine.

*la cuarantena* (Chapter 17) Period of rest and restricted physical activity after childbirth that usually lasts 40 days.

*la dieta* (Chapter 17) Diet.

**laceration** (Chapter 35) Torn, jagged wound.

**language** (Chapter 9) Code that conveys specific meaning as words are combined.

**laryngospasm** (Chapters 28, 37) Sudden uncontrolled contraction of the laryngeal muscles, which in turn decreases airway size.

**law** (Chapter 5) Rule, standard, or principle that states a fact or a relationship between factors.

**laxatives** (Chapter 33) Drugs that act to promote bowel evacuation.

**learning** (Chapter 10) Acquisition of new knowledge and skills as a result of reinforcement, practice, and experience.

**learning objective** (Chapter 10) Written statement that describes the behavior a teacher expects from an individual after a learning activity.

**left-sided heart failure** (Chapter 28) Abnormal condition characterized by impaired functioning of the left ventricle due to elevated pressures and pulmonary congestion.

**leukoplakia** (Chapter 13) Thick, white patches observed on oral mucous membranes.

**licensed practical nurse (LPN)** (Chapter 24) Also known as the licensed vocational nurse (LVN), or in Canada, registered nurse's assistant (RNA); trained in basic nursing skills and the provision of direct patient care.

**licensed vocational nurse (LVN)** (Chapter 24) The LVN is the same as a licensed practical nurse (LPN), an individual trained in the United States in basic nursing techniques and direct patient care who practices under the supervision of a registered nurse. The LVN is licensed by a board after completing what is usually a 12-month educational program and passing a licensure examination. In Canada an LVN is called a certified nursing assistant.

**lipids** (Chapter 31) Compounds that are insoluble in water but soluble in organic solvents.

**lipogenesis** (Chapter 31) Process during which fatty acids are synthesized.

**living wills** (Chapter 4) Instruments by which a dying person makes wishes known.

**local anesthesia** (Chapter 30) Loss of sensation at the desired site of action.

**logroll** (Chapter 25) Maneuver used to turn a reclining patient from one side to the other or completely over without moving the spinal column out of alignment.

**lordosis** (Chapter 13) Increased lumbar curvature.

**maceration** (Chapters 27, 35) Softening and breaking down of skin from prolonged exposure to moisture.

*mal de ojo* (Chapter 17) Evil eye.

**malignant hyperthermia** (Chapters 12, 37) Autosomal dominant trait characterized by often fatal hyperthermia in affected people exposed to certain anesthetic agents.

**malpractice** (Chapter 4) Injurious or unprofessional actions that harm another.

**malpractice insurance** (Chapter 4) Type of insurance to protect the health care professional. In case of a malpractice claim, the insurance pays the award to the plaintiff.

**managed care** (Chapter 2) Health care system in which there is administrative control over primary health care services. Redundant facilities and services are eliminated, and costs are reduced. Preventive care and health education are emphasized.

**Maslow's hierarchy of needs** (Chapter 1) A model, developed by Abram Maslow, used to explain human motivation.

**matrilineal** (Chapter 17) Kinship that is limited to only the mother's side.

**maturation** (Chapter 19) The genetically determined biological plan for growth and development. Physical growth and motor development are a function of maturation.

**maturational loss** (Chapter 23) Loss, usually of an aspect of self, resulting from the normal changes of growth and development.

**Medicaid** (Chapter 2) State medical assistance to people with low incomes, based on Title XIX of the Social Security Act. States receive matching federal funds to provide medical care and services to people meeting categorical and income requirements.

**medical asepsis** (Chapter 11) Procedures used to reduce the number of microorganisms and prevent their spread.

**medical diagnosis** (Chapter 7) Formal statement of the disease entity or illness made by the physician or health care provider.

**medical record** (Chapter 7) Patient's chart; a legal document.

**Medicare** (Chapter 2) Federally funded national health insurance program in the United States for people over 65 years of age. The program is administered in two parts. Part A provides basic protection against costs of medical, surgical, and psychiatric hospital care. Part B is a voluntary medical insurance program financed in part from federal funds and in part from premiums contributed by people enrolled in the program.

**medication abuse** (Chapter 14) Maladaptive pattern of recurrent medication use.

**medication allergy** (Chapter 14) Adverse reaction to a medication such as rash, chills, or gastrointestinal disturbances. Once a drug allergy occurs, the patient can no longer receive that particular medication.

**medication dependence** (Chapter 14) Maladaptive pattern of medication use in the following patterns: using excessive amounts of the medication, increased activities directed toward obtaining the medication, withdrawal from professional or recreational activities, and so on.

**medication error** (Chapter 14) Any event that could cause or lead to a patient's receiving inappropriate drug therapy or failing to receive appropriate drug therapy.

**medication interaction** (Chapter 14) The response when one drug modifies the action of another drug. The interaction can potentiate or diminish the actions of another drug, or it may alter the way a drug is metabolized, absorbed, or excreted.

**melanoma** (Chapter 13) Group of malignant neoplasms, primarily of the skin, that are composed of melanocytes. Common in fair-skinned people having light-colored eyes and in persons who have had a sunburn.

**melena** (Chapters 13, 33) Abnormal black, sticky stool containing digested blood, indicative of gastrointestinal bleeding.

**menarche** (Chapter 19) Onset of a girl's first menstruation.

**Meniere's disease** (Chapter 36) A chronic disease of the inner ear characterized by recurrent episodes of vertigo, progressive sensorineural hearing loss, which may be bilateral, and tinnitus.

**menopause** (Chapter 19) Physiological cessation of ovulation and menstruation that typically occurs during middle adulthood in women.

**message** (Chapter 9) Information sent or expressed by sender in the communication process.

**metabolic acidosis** (Chapter 15) Abnormal condition of high hydrogen ion concentration in the extracellular fluid caused by either a primary increase in hydrogen ions or a decrease in bicarbonate.

**metabolic alkalosis** (Chapter 15) Abnormal condition characterized by the significant loss of acid from the body or by increased levels of bicarbonate.

**metabolism** (Chapter 31) Aggregate of all chemical processes that take place in living organisms, resulting in growth, generation of energy, elimination of wastes, and other functions concerned with the distribution of nutrients in the blood after digestion.

**metacommunication** (Chapter 9) Dependent not only on what is said but also on the relationship to the other person involved in the interaction. It is a message that conveys the sender's attitude toward the self and the message and the attitudes, feelings, and intentions toward the listener.

**metastasize** (Chapter 13) Spread of tumor cells to distant parts of the body from a primary site, for example, lung, breast, or bowel.

**metered-dose inhaler (MDI)** (Chapter 14) Device designed to deliver a measured dose of an inhalation drug.

**metric system** (Chapter 14) Logically organized decimal system of measurement; metric units can easily be converted and computed through simple multiplication and division. Each basic unit of measurement is organized into units of 10.

**microorganisms** (Chapter 11) Microscopic entities, such as bacteria, viruses, and fungi, capable of carrying on living processes.

**micturition** (Chapter 32) Urination; act of passing or expelling urine voluntarily through the urethra.

**milliequivalent per liter (mEq/L)** (Chapter 15) Number of grams of a specific electrolyte dissolved in 1 L of plasma.

**mind mapping** (Chapter 7) A graphic approach to represent the connections between concepts and ideas (e.g., nursing diagnoses) that are related to a central subject (e.g. the patient's health problems).

**minerals** (Chapter 31) Inorganic elements essential to the body because of their role as catalysts in biochemical reactions.

**minimum data set (MDS)** (Chapter 2) Required by the Omnibus Budget Reconciliation Act of 1987, the MDS is a uniform data set established by the Department of Health and Human Services. The MDS serves as the framework for any state-specified assessment instruments used to develop a written and comprehensive plan of care for newly admitted residents of nursing facilities.

**misdemeanor** (Chapter 4) Lesser crime than a felony; the penalty is usually a fine or imprisonment for less than 1 year.

**mobility** (Chapter 34) Person's ability to move about freely.

**moderate sedation/analgesia/conscious sedation** (Chapter 37) Administration of central nervous system depressant drugs and/or analgesics to provide analgesia, relieve anxiety, and/or provide amnesia during surgical, diagnostic, or interventional procedures. Routinely used for diagnostic or therapeutic procedures that do not require complete anesthesia but simply a decreased level of consciousness.

**monosaturated fatty acid** (Chapter 31) A fatty acid in which some of the carbon atoms in the hydrocarbon chain are joined by double or triple bonds. Monounsaturated fatty acids have only one double or triple bond per molecule and are found as components of fats in such foods as fowls, almonds, pecans, cashew nuts, peanuts, and olive oil.

**morals** (Chapter 5) Personal conviction that something is absolutely right or wrong in all situations.

**motivation** (Chapter 10) Internal impulse that causes a person to take action.

**mourning** (Chapter 23) The process of grieving.

**murmurs** (Chapter 13) Blowing or whooshing sounds created by changes in blood flow through the heart or by abnormalities in valve closure.

**muscle tone** (Chapter 25) Normal state of balanced muscle tension.

**myocardial contractility** (Chapter 28) Measure of stretch of the cardiac muscle fiber. It can also affect stroke volume and cardiac output. Poor contraction decreases the amount of blood ejected by the ventricles during each contraction.

**myocardial infarction** (Chapter 28) Necrosis of a portion of cardiac muscle caused by obstruction in a coronary artery.

**myocardial ischemia** (Chapter 28) Condition that results when the supply of blood to the myocardium from the coronary arteries is insufficient to meet the oxygen demands of the organ.

**NANDA International** (Chapter 7) North American Nursing Diagnosis Association, organized in 1973, which formally identifies, develops, and classifies nursing diagnoses.

**narcolepsy** (Chapter 29) Syndrome involving sudden sleep attacks that a person cannot inhibit; uncontrollable desire to sleep may occur several times during a day.

**nasogastric (NG) tube** (Chapter 37) Tube passed into the stomach through the nose for the purpose of emptying the stomach of its contents or for delivering medication and/or nourishment.

**nebulization** (Chapter 28) Process of adding moisture to inspired air by the addition of water droplets.

**necessary losses** (Chapter 23) Losses that every person experiences.

**necrotic** (Chapter 11) Of or pertaining to the death of tissue in response to disease or injury.

**negative health behaviors** (Chapter 1) Practices actually or potentially harmful to health, such as smoking, drug or alcohol abuse, poor diet, and refusal to take necessary medications.

**negative nitrogen balance** (Chapter 34) Condition occurring when the body excretes more nitrogen than it takes in.

**negligence** (Chapter 4) Careless act of omission or commission that results in injury to another.

**neonate** (Chapter 19) Stage of life from birth to 1 month of age.

**nephrons** (Chapter 32) Structural and functional units of the kidney containing renal glomeruli and tubules.

**neurotransmitter** (Chapter 30) Chemical that transfers the electrical impulse from the nerve fiber to the muscle fiber.

**nociceptors** (Chapter 30) Somatic and visceral free nerve endings of thinly myelinated and unmyelinated fibers. They usually react to tissue injury but may also be excited by endogenous chemical substances.

**nocturia** (Chapter 29) Urination at night; can be a symptom of renal disease or may occur in persons who drink excessive amounts of fluids before bedtime.

**nonblanchable hyperemia** (Chapter 35) Redness of the skin due to dilation of the superficial capillaries. The redness persists when pressure is applied to the area, indicating tissue damage.

**nonmaleficence** (Chapter 5) The fundamental ethical agreement to do no harm. Closely related to the ethical standard of beneficence.

**nonrapid eye movement (NREM) sleep** (Chapter 29) Sleep that occurs during the first four stages of normal sleep.

**nonshivering thermogenesis** (Chapter 12) Occurs primarily in neonates. Because neonates cannot shiver, a limited amount of vascular brown adipose tissue present at birth can be metabolized for heat production.

**nonverbal communication** (Chapter 9) Communication using expressions, gestures, body posture, and positioning rather than words.

**normal sinus rhythm (NSR)** (Chapter 28) The wave pattern on an electrocardiogram that indicates normal conduction of an electrical impulse through the myocardium.

**nosocomial** (Chapter 32) Infection acquired during hospitalization or stay in a health care facility.

**numbing** (Chapter 23) One of Bowlby's four phases of mourning. It is characterized by the lack of feeling or feeling stunned by the loss. May last a few days or many weeks.

**Nurse Practice Acts** (Chapter 4) Statutes enacted by the legislature of any of the states or by the appropriate officers of the districts or possessions that describe and define the scope of nursing practice.

**nurse-initiated interventions** (Chapter 7) The response of the nurse to the patient's health care needs and nursing diagnoses. This type of intervention is an autonomous action based on scientific rationale that is executed to benefit the patient in a predicted way related to the nursing diagnosis and patient-centered goals.

**nursing diagnosis** (Chapter 7) Formal statement of an actual or potential health problem that nurses can legally and independently treat. The second step of the nursing process, during which the patient's actual and potential unhealthy responses to an illness or condition are identified.

**nursing health history** (Chapter 7) Data collected about a patient's present level of wellness, changes in life patterns, sociocultural role, and mental and emotional reactions to illness.

**nursing intervention** (Chapter 7) Any treatment, based upon clinical judgment and knowledge, that a nurse performs to enhance patient outcomes.

**nursing process** (Chapters 6, 7) Systematic problem-solving method by which nurses individualize care for each patient. The five steps of the nursing process are assessment, diagnosis, planning, implementation, and evaluation.

**nursing-sensitive outcomes** (Chapter 19) Outcomes that are within the scope of nursing practice; consequences or effects of nursing interventions that result in changes in the patient's symptoms, functional status, safety, psychological distress, or costs.

**nurturant** (Chapter 16) Behavior that involves caring for or fostering the well-being of another individual.

**nutrients** (Chapter 31) Foods that contain elements necessary for body function, including water, carbohydrates, proteins, fats, vitamins, and minerals.

**obesity** (Chapter 31) Abnormal increase in the proportion of fat cells, mainly in the viscera and subcutaneous tissues of the body.

**objective data** (Chapter 7) Information that can be observed by others; free of feelings, perceptions, prejudices.

**occurrence report** (Chapter 4) Confidential document that describes any patient accident while the person is on the premise of a health care agency. (See incident report.)

**olfactory** (Chapter 36) Pertaining to the sense of smell.

**oncotic pressure** (Chapter 15) The total influence of the protein on the osmotic activity of plasma fluid.

**open-ended question** (Chapter 7) A form of question that prompts a respondent to answer in more than one or two words.

**operating bed** (Chapter 37) Table for surgery.

**operating room** (Chapter 37) (1) Room in a health care facility in which surgical procedures requiring anesthesia are performed. (2) Informal: a suite of rooms or an area in a health care facility in which patients are prepared for surgery, undergo surgical procedures, and recover from the anesthetic procedures required for the surgery.

**ophthalmic** (Chapter 14) Drugs given into the eye, in the form of either eye drops or ointments.

**ophthalmoscope** (Chapter 13) Instrument used to illuminate the structures of the eye in order to examine the fundus, which includes the retina, choroid, optic nerve disc, macula, fovea centralis, and retinal vessels.

**opioid** (Chapters 14, 30) Drug substance, derived from opium or produced synthetically, that alters perception of pain and that with repeated use may result in physical and psychological dependence (narcotic).

**oral hygiene** (Chapter 27) Condition or practice of maintaining the tissues and structures of the mouth.

**orthopnea** (Chapters 13, 28) Abnormal condition in which a person must sit or stand up to breathe comfortably.

**orthostatic hypotension** (Chapters 12, 25, 34) Abnormally low blood pressure occurring when a person stands up.

**osmolality** (Chapter 15) Concentration or osmotic pressure of a solution expressed in osmoles or milliosmoles per kilogram of water.

**osmolarity** (Chapter 15) Osmotic pressure of a solution expressed in osmoles or milliosmoles per kilogram of the solution.

**osmoreceptors** (Chapter 15) Neurons in the hypothalamus that are sensitive to the fluid concentration in the blood plasma and regulate the secretion of antidiuretic hormone.

**osmosis** (Chapter 15) Movement of a pure solvent through a semipermeable membrane from a solution with a lower solute concentration to one with a higher solute concentration.

**osmotic pressure** (Chapter 15) Drawing power for water, which depends on the number of molecules in the solution.

**osteoporosis** (Chapters 13, 34) Disorder characterized by abnormal rarefaction of bone, occurring most frequently in postmenopausal women, in sedentary or immobilized individuals, and in patients on long-term steroid therapy.

**ostomy** (Chapter 33) Surgical procedure in which an opening is made into the abdominal wall to allow the passage of intestinal contents from the bowel (colostomy) or urine from the bladder (urostomy).

**otoscope** (Chapter 13) Instrument, with a special ear speculum, used to examine the deeper structures of the external and middle ear.

**ototoxic** (Chapters 13, 36) Having a harmful effect on the eighth cranial (auditory) nerve or the organs of hearing and balance.

**outcome** (Chapter 24) Condition of a patient at the end of treatment, including the degree of wellness and the need for continuing care, medication, support, counseling, or education.

**outliers** (Chapter 2) Patients with extended lengths of stay beyond allowable inpatient days or costs.

**outpatient** (Chapter 37) Patient who has not been admitted to a hospital but receives treatments in a clinic or facility associated with the hospital.

**oxygen saturation** (Chapter 12) The amount of hemoglobin fully saturated with oxygen, given as a percent value.

**oxygen therapy** (Chapter 28) Procedure in which oxygen is administered to a patient to relieve or prevent hypoxia.

**pain** (Chapter 30) Subjective, unpleasant sensation caused by noxious stimulation of sensory nerve endings.

**palliative care** (Chapter 23) A level of care that is designed to relieve or reduce intensity of uncomfortable symptoms but not to produce a cure. Palliative care relies on comfort measures and use of alternative therapies to help individuals become more at peace during end of life.

**pallor** (Chapter 13) Unnatural paleness or absence of color in the skin.

**palpation** (Chapter 13) Method of physical examination whereby the fingers or hands of the examiner are applied to the patient's body for the purpose of feeling body parts underlying the skin.

**palpitations** (Chapter 13) Bounding or racing of the heart associated with normal emotions or a heart disorder.

**Papanicolaou (Pap) smear** (Chapter 13) Painless screening test for cervical cancer. Specimens are taken of squamous and columnar cells of the cervix.

**parallel play** (Chapter 19) Form of play among a group of children, primarily toddlers, in which each one engages in an independent activity that is similar but not influenced by or shared with the others.

**paralytic ileus** (Chapters 13, 37) Usually temporary paralysis of intestinal wall that may occur after abdominal surgery or peritoneal injury and that causes cessation of peristalsis. Leads to abdominal distention and symptoms of obstruction.

**parenteral administration** (Chapter 14) Giving medication by a route other than the gastrointestinal tract.

**parenteral nutrition (PN)** (Chapters 15, 31) The administration of a nutritional solution into the vascular system.

**parteras** (Chapter 17) Lay midwives.

**partial bed bath** (Chapter 27) Bath in which body parts that might cause the patient discomfort if left unbathed (i.e., face, hands, axillary areas, back, and perineum) are washed in bed.

**passive range-of-motion (PROM) exercises** (Chapter 25) Range of movement through which a joint is moved with assistance.

**passive strategies of health promotion** (Chapter 1) Activities that involve the patient as the recipient of actions by health care professionals.

**pathogenicity** (Chapter 11) Ability of a pathogenic agent to produce a disease.

**pathogens** (Chapters 11, 26) Microorganisms capable of producing disease.

**pathological fractures** (Chapter 34) Fractures resulting from weakened bone tissue; frequently caused by osteoporosis or neoplasms.

**patient-centered care** (Chapter 2) Concept to improve work efficiency by changing the way patient care is delivered.

**patient-controlled analgesia (PCA)** (Chapter 30) Drug delivery system that allows patients to self-administer analgesic medications when they want.

**patrilineal, patrilineally** (Chapter 17) Kinship that is limited to only the father's side.

**perceived loss** (Chapter 23) Loss that is less obvious to the individual experiencing it. Although easily overlooked or misunderstood, a perceived loss results in the same grief process as an actual loss.

**perception** (Chapter 30) Persons' mental image or concept of elements in their environment, including information gained through the senses.

**percussion** (Chapter 13) Method of physical examination whereby the location, size, and density of a body part is determined by the tone obtained from the striking of short, sharp taps of the fingers.

**perfusion** (Chapter 12) (1) Passage of a fluid through a specific organ or an area of the body. (2) Therapeutic measure whereby a drug intended for an isolated part of the body is introduced via the bloodstream.

**perineal care** (Chapter 27) Procedure prescribed for cleaning the genital and anal areas as part of the daily bath or after various obstetrical and gynecological procedures.

**perioperative nursing** (Chapter 37) Refers to the role of the operating room nurse during the preoperative, intraoperative, and postoperative phases of surgery.

**peripherally inserted central catheter (PICC)** (Chapter 15) Alternative intravenous access when the patient requires intermediate-length venous access greater than 7 days to 3 months. Intravenous access is achieved by inserting a catheter into a central vein by way of a peripheral vein.

**peristalsis** (Chapters 13, 33) Rhythmical contractions of the intestine that propel gastric contents through the length of the gastrointestinal tract.

**peritonitis** (Chapter 13) Inflammation of the peritoneum produced by bacteria or irritating substances introduced into the abdominal cavity by a penetrating wound or perforation of an organ in the gastrointestinal tract or the reproductive tract.

**PERRLA** (Chapter 13) Acronym for "pupils equal, round, reactive to light, accommodative"; the acronym is recorded in the physical examination if eye and pupil assessments are normal.

*personalismo* (Chapter 17) Personalistic.

**petechiae** (Chapter 13) Tiny purple or red spots that appear on skin as minute hemorrhages within dermal layers.

**pharmacokinetics** (Chapter 14) Study of how drugs enter the body, reach their site of action, are metabolized, and exit from the body.

**phlebitis** (Chapters 13, 15) Inflammation of a vein.

**physician-initiated interventions** (Chapter 7) Based on the physician's response to a medical diagnosis, the nurse responds to the physician's written orders.

**PIE note** (Chapter 8) Problem-oriented medical record; the four interdisciplinary sections are the database, problem list, care plan, and progress notes.

**placebos** (Chapter 30) Dosage form that contains no pharmacologically active ingredients but may relieve pain through psychological effects.

**plaintiff** (Chapter 4) Individual who files formal charges against an individual or organization for a legal offense.

**planning** (Chapter 7) Process of designing interventions to achieve the goals and outcomes of health care delivery.

**plantar flexion** (Chapter 25) Toe-down motion of the foot at the ankle.

**pleural friction rub** (Chapter 13) Adventitious lung sound caused by inflamed parietal and visceral pleura rubbing together on inspiration.

**pneumothorax** (Chapter 28) Collection of air or gas in the pleural space.

**point of maximal impulse (PMI)** (Chapter 13) Point where the heartbeat can most easily be palpated through the chest wall. This is usually the fourth intercostal space at the midclavicular line.

**point of view** (Chapter 5) A way of looking at issues that reflects an individual's culture and societal influences.

**poison** (Chapter 26) Any substance that impairs health or destroys life when ingested, inhaled, or absorbed by the body in relatively small amounts.

**poison control center** (Chapter 26) One of a network of facilities that provides information regarding all aspects of poisoning or intoxication, maintains records of their occurrence, and refers patients to treatment centers.

**polypharmacy** (Chapters 14, 19) Use of a number of different drugs by a patient who may have one or several health problems.

**polyunsaturated fatty acid** (Chapter 31) Fatty acid that has two or more carbon double bonds.

**population** (Chapter 3) A collection of individuals who have in common one or more personal or environmental characteristics.

**positive health behaviors** (Chapter 1) Activities related to maintaining, attaining, or regaining good health and preventing illness. Common positive health behaviors include immunizations, proper sleep patterns, adequate exercise, and nutrition.

**postanesthesia care unit (PACU)** (Chapter 37) Area adjoining the operating room to which surgical patients are taken while still under anesthesia.

**postmortem care** (Chapter 23) Care of a patient's body after death.

**postural drainage** (Chapter 28) Use of positioning along with percussion and vibration to drain secretions from specific segments of the lungs and bronchi into the trachea.

**postural hypotension** (Chapter 12) Abnormally low blood pressure occurring when an individual assumes the standing posture; also called orthostatic hypotension.

**posture** (Chapter 25) Position of the body in relation to the surrounding space.

**power of attorney for health care** (Chapter 4) A person designated by the patient to make health care decisions for the patient if the patient becomes unable to make his or her own decisions.

**preadolescence** (Chapter 19) Transitional developmental stage that occurs between childhood and adolescence.

**preanesthesia care unit** (Chapter 37) Area outside the operating room where preoperative preparations are completed.

**preload** (Chapter 28) Volume of blood in the ventricles at the end of diastole, immediately before ventricular contraction.

**preoperative teaching** (Chapter 37) Instruction regarding a patient's anticipated surgery and recovery given before surgery. Instruction includes, but is not limited to, dietary and activity restrictions, anticipated assessment activities, postoperative procedures and pain relief measures.

**presbycusis** (Chapter 36) Hearing loss associated with aging. It usually involves both a loss of hearing sensitivity and a reduction in the clarity of speech.

**presbyopia** (Chapter 36) Gradual decline in ability of the lens to accommodate or to focus on close objects. Reduces ability to see near objects clearly. This condition commonly develops with advancing age.

**prescriptions** (Chapter 14) Written directions for a therapeutic agent (e.g., medication, drugs).

**presence** (Chapter 16) The deep physical, psychological, and spiritual connection or engagement between a nurse and patient.

**present time orientation** (Chapter 17) Time dimension that focuses on what is happening here and now. Communication patterns are circular, and this time orientation is in conflict with the dominant organizational norm in health care that emphasizes punctuality and adherence to appointments.

**pressure ulcer** (Chapter 35) Inflammation, sore, or ulcer in the skin over a bony prominence.

**presurgical care unit (PSCU)** (Chapter 37) Area outside the operating room where preoperative preparations are completed.

**preventive nursing actions** (Chapter 7) Nursing actions directed toward preventing illness and promoting health to avoid the need for primary, secondary, or tertiary health care.

**primary appraisal** (Chapter 22) Evaluating an event for its personal meaning related to stress.

**primary care** (Chapter 2) First contact in a given episode of illness that leads to a decision regarding a course of action to resolve the health problem.

**primary intention** (Chapter 35) Primary union of the edges of a wound, progressing to complete scar formation without granulation.

**primary nursing** (Chapter 24) Method of nursing practice in which the patient's care is managed, for the duration, by one nurse, who directs and coordinates other nurses and health care personnel. When on duty, the primary nurse cares for the patient directly.

**primary prevention** (Chapter 1) First contact in a given episode of illness that leads to a decision regarding a course of action to prevent worsening of the health problem.

**turgor** (Chapter 13) Normal resiliency of the skin caused by the outward pressure of the cells and interstitial fluid.

**unsaturated fatty acid** (Chapter 31) Fatty acid in which an unequal number of hydrogen atoms are attached and the carbon atoms attach to each other with a double bond.

**ureterostomy** (Chapter 32) Diversion of urine away from a diseased or defective bladder through an artificial opening in the skin.

**urinal** (Chapter 32) Receptacle for collecting urine.

**urinary diversion** (Chapter 32) Surgical diversion of the drainage of urine, such as a ureterostomy.

**urinary incontinence** (Chapter 32) Inability to control urination.

**urinary reflux** (Chapter 32) Abnormal, backward flow of urine.

**urinary retention** (Chapter 32) Retention of urine in the bladder; condition frequently caused by a temporary loss of muscle function.

**urine hat** (Chapter 32) Receptacle for collecting urine that fits toilet.

**urometer** (Chapter 32) Device for measuring frequent and small amounts of urine from an indwelling urinary catheter system.

**urosepsis** (Chapter 32) Organisms in the bloodstream.

**utilitarianism** (Chapter 5) Ethic that proposes that the value of something is determined by its usefulness. The greatest good for the greatest number of people constitutes the guiding principle for action in a utilitarian model of ethics.

**utilization review (UR) committees** (Chapter 2) Physician-supervised committees to review admissions, diagnostic testing, and treatments provided by physicians or health care providers to patients.

**validation** (Chapter 7) Act of confirming, verifying, or corroborating the accuracy of assessment data or the appropriateness of the care plan.

**Valsalva maneuver** (Chapter 33) Any forced expiratory effort against a closed airway, such as when an individual holds the breath and tightens the muscles in a concerted, strenuous effort to move a heavy object or to change positions in bed.

**value** (Chapter 5) Personal belief about the worth of a given idea or behavior.

**valvular heart disease** (Chapter 28) Acquired or congenital disorder of a cardiac valve characterized by stenosis and obstructed blood flow or valvular degeneration and regurgitation of blood.

**variances** (Chapter 8) The unexpected event that occurs during patient care and that is different from what is predicted on a CareMap. Variances or exceptions are interventions or outcomes that are not achieved as anticipated. Variance may be positive or negative.

**variant** (Chapter 17) Differing from a set standard.

**vascular access devices** (Chapter 15) Catheters, cannulas, or infusion ports designed for long-term, repeated access to the vascular system.

**vasoconstriction** (Chapter 12) Narrowing of the lumen of any blood vessel, especially the arterioles and the veins in the blood reservoirs of the skin and abdominal viscera.

**vasodilation** (Chapter 12) Increase in the diameter of a blood vessel caused by inhibition of its vasoconstrictor nerves or stimulation of dilator nerves.

**venipuncture** (Chapter 15) Technique in which a vein is punctured transcutaneously by a sharp rigid stylet (e.g., a butterfly needle), a cannula (e.g., an angiocatheter that contains a flexible plastic catheter), or a needle attached to a syringe.

**ventilation** (Chapters 12, 28) Respiratory process by which gases are moved into and out of the lungs.

**verbal communication** (Chapter 9) The sending of messages from one individual to another or to a group of individuals through the spoken word.

**vertigo** (Chapter 13) Sensation of dizziness or spinning.

**vibration** (Chapter 28) Fine, shaking pressure applied by hands to the chest wall only during exhalation.

**virulence** (Chapter 11) The ability of an organism to rapidly produce disease.

**visual** (Chapter 36) Related to, or experienced through, vision.

**vital signs** (Chapter 12) Temperature, pulse, respirations, and blood pressure.

**vitamins** (Chapter 31) Organic compounds essential in small quantities for normal physiological and metabolic functioning of the body. With few exceptions, vitamins cannot be synthesized by the body and must be obtained from the diet or dietary supplements.

**voiding** (Chapter 32) The process of urinating.

**vulnerable populations** (Chapters 2, 3) A collection of individuals who are more likely to develop health problems as a result of excess risks, limits in access to health care services, or being dependent on others for care.

**wellness** (Chapter 1) Dynamic state of health in which an individual progresses toward a higher level of functioning, achieving an optimum balance between internal and external environments.

**wellness education** (Chapter 1) Activities that teach people how to care for themselves in a healthy manner.

**wellness nursing diagnosis** (Chapter 7) Clinical judgment about an individual, group, or community in transition from a specific level of wellness to a higher level of wellness.

**wheezes, wheezing** (Chapters 13, 28) Adventitious lung sound caused by a severely narrowed bronchus.

**work redesign** (Chapter 2) Formal process used to analyze the work of a certain work group and to change the actual structure of the jobs performed.

**worldview** (Chapter 17) A cognitive stance or perspective about phenomena characteristic of a particular cultural group.

**wound culture** (Chapter 35) Specimen collected from a wound to determine the specific organism that is causing an infectious process.

**yearning and searching** (Chapter 23) The second phase of Bowlby's phases of mourning. It is characterized by emotional outbursts of tearful sobbing and acute distress.

**Z-track injection** (Chapter 14) Technique for injecting irritating preparations into muscle without tracking residual medication through sensitive tissues.

# Appendix A

# Common Abbreviations

*NOTE: Abbreviations in common use can vary widely from place to place. Each institution's list of acceptable abbreviations is the best authority for its records.*

| | | | | | | | |
|---|---|---|---|---|---|---|---|
| °C | degrees centigrade | cg | centigram | ESRD | end-stage renal disease | IEP | immunoelectrophoresis |
| °F | degrees Fahrenheit | CHF | congestive heart fail- | EST | electroshock therapy | Ig | immunoglobulin |
| μm | micrometer | | ure | ʒ | fluid ounce | IgA, etc. | immunoglobulin A, |
| ʒ | dram | CHO | carbohydrate | FANA | fluorescent antinuclear | | etc. |
| aa | of each | Cl | chlorine | | antibody test | IM | intramuscular |
| ABG | arterial blood gas | cm | centimeter | FBS | fasting blood sugar | IOP | intraocular pressure |
| ac | before meals | cm³ | cubic centimeter | Fe | iron | IPPB | intermittent positive |
| ad lib | freely as desired | CNS | central nervous system | FEV | forced expiratory vol- | | pressure breathing |
| ADLs | activities of daily | c/o | complains of | | ume | IV | intravenous |
| | living | CO | carbon monoxide | FHR | fetal heart rate | IVP | intravenous push; in- |
| Ag | silver, antigen | CO₂ | carbon dioxide | FRC | functional residual | | travenous pyelogram |
| AIDS | acquired immuno | COPD | chronic obstructive pul- | | capacity | IVU | intravenous urogram |
| | deficiency syndrome | | monary disease | FSH | follicle-stimulating | JRA | juvenile rheumatoid |
| ALS | amyotrophic lateral | CPK | creatine | | hormone | | arthritis |
| | sclerosis | | phosphokinase | FUO | fever of unknown | K | potassium |
| AM | morning | CPR | cardiopulmonary re- | | origin | kg | kilogram |
| ama | against medical advice | | suscitation | Fx, fx | fracture, fractional | KUB | kidney, ureters, and |
| AMI | acute myocardial | CSF | cerebrospinal fluid | | urine test | | bladder (radiograph) |
| | infarction | CT | computed tomography | g, gm, | gram | KVO | keep vein open |
| amp | ampule | CVA | cerebrovascular acci- | Gm | | L | liter |
| ARC | AIDS-related complex | | dent, costovertebral | Gc, GC | gonococcus | L&A | light and |
| ARDS | adult respiratory dis- | | angle | GI | gastrointestinal | | accommodation |
| | tress syndrome | CVP | central venous | gr | grain | LBBB | left bundle branch |
| AS | aortic stenosis | | pressure | grav I, II, | pregnancy one, two, | | block |
| ASD | atrial septal defect | D&C | dilation and curettage | III, etc. | three, etc. | LE | lupus erythematosus |
| Ba | barium | D₅W | 5% dextrose in water | gt, gtt | drop, drops | LGV | lymphogranuloma |
| BE | barium enema | db, dB | decibel | GTT | glucose tolerance test | | venereum |
| bid | two times a day | dc | discontinue | GU | genitourinary | LLL | left lower lobe |
| BM, bm | bowel movement | DIC | disseminated | GYN, | gynecological | LLQ | left lower quadrant |
| BMR | basal metabolic rate | | intravascular | Gyn | | LMP | last menstrual period |
| BP | blood pressure | | coagulation | h, hr | hour | LNMP | last normal menstrual |
| BPH | benign prostatic | diff | differential blood | H⁺ | hydrogen ion | | period |
| | hypertrophy | | count | H&P | history and physical | LP | lumbar puncture |
| BRP | bathroom privileges | dil | dilute | | examination | LUL | left upper lobe |
| BSA | body surface area | DJD | degenerative joint dis- | HAV | hepatitis A virus | LUQ | left upper quadrant |
| BUN | blood urea nitrogen | | ease | Hb | hemoglobin | LVH | left ventricular hyper- |
| c̄ | with | dl | deciliter | HBAg | hepatitis B antigen | | trophy |
| Ca | calcium, cancer, | DNR | do not resuscitate | HBV | hepatitis B virus | m | meter |
| | carcinoma | DOE | dyspnea on exertion | Hct, HCT | hematocrit | m, min, | minum |
| CAD | coronary artery | dx, Dx | diagnosis | HDL | high-density | MAP | mean arterial pressure |
| | disease | EBV | Epstein-Barr virus | | lipoprotein | mcg | microgram |
| cap | capsule | ECF | extracellular fluid | Hg | mercury | MCH | mean corpuscular |
| CAT | computed axial | ECG | electrocardiogram | Hgb | hemoglobin | | hemoglobin |
| | tomography | ECHO | echocardiography | HIV | human immunodefi- | MCHC | mean corpuscular he- |
| cath | catheter, catheterize | ECT | electroconvulsive | | ciency (AIDS) virus | | moglobin |
| CBC | complete blood count | | therapy | HLA | human lymphocyte | | concentration |
| CBR | complete bed rest | EDC | estimated date of | | antigen | MCV | mean cell volume; |
| CC | chief complaint | | confinement | h/o | history of | | mean corpuscular |
| CCU | coronary care unit, | EDD | estimated date of | H₂O | water | | volume |
| | critical care unit | | delivery | HSV2 | herpes simplex virus, | mg | milligram |
| CDC | Centers for Disease | EEG | electroencephalogram | | type 2 | Mg | magnesium |
| | Control and | EKG | electrocardiogram | I&O | intake and output | MG | myasthenia gravis |
| | Prevention | elix | elixir | IC | inspiratory capacity | MI | myocardial infarction |
| CEA | carcinoembryonic | EMG | electromyogram | ICP | intracranial pressure | MICU | medical intensive care |
| | antigen | ENG | electronystagmography | ICU | intensive care unit | | unit |
| CFT | complement-fixation | ER | emergency room | IDDM | insulin-dependent dia- | ml | milliliter |
| | test | ERG | electroretinogram | | betes mellitus | mm | millimeter |

mm³ — cubic millimeter
mm Hg — millimeters of mercury
MRI — magnetic resonance imaging
MS — multiple sclerosis
MW — molecular weight
N — nitrogen
Na — sodium
NICU — neonatal intensive care unit
NIH — National Institutes of Health
nm — nanometer
NMR — nuclear magnetic resonance
NPO — nothing by mouth
NS — normal saline
O₂ — oxygen
OD — right eye; optical density; overdose
OL — left eye
OOB — out of bed
ORIF — open reduction and internal fixation
OS — left eye
OT — occupational therapy
OTC — over-the-counter
ou — both eyes
oz, ℥ — ounce
P&A — percussion and auscultation
PaCO₂ — partial pressure of carbon dioxide (arterial blood)
PaO₂ — partial pressure of oxygen (arterial blood)
para I, II, etc. — unipara, bipara, etc.
PAT — paroxysmal atrial tachycardia
pc — after meals
PCG — phonocardiogram
PCO₂ — partial pressure of carbon dioxide
PCP — pulmonary capillary pressure, phencyclidine
PCV — packed cell volume
PCWP — pulmonary capillary wedge pressure
PD — interpupillary distance; postural drainage

PE — pulmonary embolism, physical examination
PEEP — positive end-expiratory pressure
PEG — pneumoencephalography
per — through, by way of
PERRLA — pupils equal, round, and reactive to light and accommodation
PET — positron emission tomography
PG — prostaglandin
pH — hydrogen ion concentration (acidity and alkalinity)
PID — pelvic inflammatory disease
PKU — phenylketonuria
PM — postmortem
pm — evening
PMS — premenstrual syndrome
PND — paroxysmal nocturnal dyspnea, postnasal drip
PO, po — orally
PO₂ — partial pressure of oxygen
PPD — purified protein derivative
ppm — parts per million
prn — when required, as often as necessary
PT — physical therapy; prothrombin time
PTT — partial thromboplastin time
PUO — pyrexia of unknown origin
PVC — premature ventricular contraction
q — every
q2h — every 2 hours
q3h — every 3 hours
q4h — every 4 hours
qh — every hour
qid — four times a day
qn — every night
qns — quantity not sufficient
RBBB — right bundle branch block
RBC — red blood cell
RDS — respiratory distress syndrome

Rh+ — positive Rh factor
Rh− — negative Rh factor
RHD — rheumatic heart disease
RLL — right lower lobe
RLQ — right lower quadrant
RML — right middle lobe
R/O — rule out
ROM — range of motion
ROS — review of systems
RS — Reiter's syndrome
RSV — Rous sarcoma virus
RUL — right upper lobe
RUQ — right upper quadrant
Rx — take; treatment
s̄ — without
SB — sternal border
sib — sibling
SICU — surgical intensive care unit
SIDS — sudden infant death syndrome
Sig — write on label
SLE — systemic lupus erythematosus
sol — solution, dissolved
sos — if necessary
sp gr, SG, sg — specific gravity
SR — sedimentation rate
ss — half
SSS — sick sinus syndrome; specific soluble substance; short-stay surgery
stat — immediately
STD — sexually transmitted disease
STS — serologic test for syphilis
Sub-Q — subcutaneous
susp — suspension
SV — stroke volume
T₃ — triiodothyronine
T₄ — tetraiodothyronine
T&A — tonsillectomy and adenoidectomy
TAB — typhoid and paratyphoid A and B
TAH — total abdominal hysterectomy
TAT — tetanus antitoxin; thematic apperception test

TB, TBC — tuberculosis
TBG — thyroxin-binding globulin
TG — triglyceride
TIA — transient ischemic attack
TIBC — total iron-binding capacity
tid — three times a day
TKO — to keep open
TLC — total lung capacity; thin-layer chromatography
TPN — total parenteral nutrition
TPR — temperature, pulse, and respirations
tr, tinct — tincture
TSH — thyroid-stimulating hormone
TST — triple sugar iron test
UA — urinalysis
UGI series — upper gastrointestinal series
UIBC — unsaturated iron-binding capacity
URI — upper respiratory infection
US — ultrasound
UTI — urinary tract infection
V&T — volume and tension
VC — vital capacity
VD — venereal disease
VDA — visual discriminatory acuity
VDH — valvular disease of the heart
VDRL — Venereal Disease Research Laboratories
VLDL — very-low-density lipoprotein
VS — vital signs
VSD — ventricular septal defect
V_T — tidal volume
W/V — weight/volume
WBC — white blood cell, white blood count
WNL — within normal limits
WR — Wassermann reaction

$T_3$ — triiodothyronine
$T_4$ — tetraiodothyronine
$V_T$ — tidal volume

# Appendix B

# Overview of CDC Hand Hygiene Guidelines

The Centers for Disease Control and Prevention released recommendations for hand hygiene in health care settings in 2002. Hand hygiene is a general term that applies to hand washing, antiseptic hand wash, antiseptic hand rub, or surgical hand antisepsis. Hand washing refers to washing hands thoroughly with plain soap and water. An antiseptic hand wash is defined as washing hands with water and soap containing an antiseptic agent. Antimicrobials effectively reduce bacterial counts on the hands and often have residual antimicrobial effects for several hours. An antiseptic hand rub means to apply an antiseptic alcohol-based waterless product to all surfaces of the hands to reduce the number of microorganisms present. Surgical hand antisepsis is an antiseptic hand wash or antiseptic hand rub performed preoperatively by surgical personnel.

Evidence suggests that hand antisepsis, the cleansing of hands with an antiseptic hand rub, is more effective in reducing nosocomial infections than plain hand washing.

## Follow These Guidelines in the Care of *All Patients*

Wash hands when hands are visibly dirty or contaminated with proteinaceous material or are visibly soiled with blood or other body fluids; wash hands preferably with an antimicrobial soap and water or a nonantimicrobial soap and water. The recommended duration for lathering hands is *at least 15 seconds* and preferably 30 seconds.

- Wash hands with soap and water before eating.
- Wash hands with soap and water and after using the restroom.
- Wash hands if exposed to spore-forming organisms such as *Clostridium difficile* or *Bacillus anthracis*. The physical action of washing and rinsing hands is recommended because alcohols, chlorhexidine, iodophors, and other antiseptic agents have poor activity against spores.

If hands are not visibly soiled, use an alcohol-based hand rub for routinely decontaminating the hands in all of the following clinical situations:

- Before having direct contact with clients
- Before donning sterile gloves
- Before inserting indwelling urinary catheters, peripheral vascular catheters, or other invasive devices that do not require a surgical procedure
- After contact with a client's intact skin (e.g., after taking a pulse or blood pressure, lifting a client)
- After contact with body fluids or excretions, mucous membranes, nonintact skin, and wound dressings *if hands are not visibly soiled*
- When moving from a contaminated body site to a clean body site during client care

- After contact with inanimate objects (e.g., medical equipment) in the immediate vicinity of the client
- After removing gloves

Note that an antiseptic hand wash may be performed in all situations when an alcohol-based hand rub is indicated. Antimicrobial-impregnated wipes (i.e., towelettes) are not a substitute for using an alcohol-based hand rub or antimicrobial soap.

## Method for Decontaminating Hands

*When using an alcohol-based hand rub, apply product to palm of one hand and rub hands together, covering all surfaces of hands and fingers, until hands are dry. Follow the manufacturer's recommendations regarding the volume of product to use.*

## Follow These Guidelines for Surgical Hand Antisepsis

Surgical hand antisepsis reduces the resident microbial count on the hands to a minimum. See Skill 37-1, p. 1102, for the surgical hand scrub procedure.

The CDC recommends using an antimicrobial soap and scrubbing hands and forearms for the length of time recommended by the manufacturer, usually 2 to 6 minutes. Refer to agency policy for time required.

When using an alcohol-based surgical hand-scrub product with persistent activity, follow the manufacturer's instructions. Before applying the alcohol solution, prewash hands and forearms with a nonantimicrobial soap and dry hands and forearms completely. After application of the alcohol-based product as recommended, allow hands and forearms to dry thoroughly before donning sterile gloves.

## General Recommendations for Hand Hygiene

Use hand lotions or creams to minimize the occurrence of irritant contact dermatitis associated with hand antisepsis or hand washing.

Do not wear artificial fingernails or extenders when having direct contact with clients at high risk (e.g., those in intensive care units or operating rooms).

Keep natural nail tips less than $\frac{1}{4}$ inch long.

Wear gloves when contact with blood or other potentially infectious materials, mucous membranes, and nonintact skin could occur.

Remove gloves after caring for a client. Do not wear the same pair of gloves for the care of more than one client.

Change gloves during client care if moving from a contaminated body site to a clean body site. This includes when working under isolation precautions.

Data from Centers for Disease Control and Prevention, Hospital Infection Control Practice Advisory Committee, HICPAC/SHEA/ APIC/IDSA Hand Hygiene Task Force: Guideline for hand hygiene in health-care settings, *MMWR Recommend Rep* 51(RR-16):1, 2002. Available at www.cdc.gov/handhygiene.

# Answers for NCLEX® Review Questions

**Chapter 1**
1. 4
2. 4
3. 3
4. 4
5. 3
6. 1
7. 4
8. 3
9. 4
10. 3
11. 4
12. 4
13. 4
14. 1

**Chapter 2**
1. 4
2. 1
3. 2
4. 1
5. 2
6. 3
7. 2
8. 4

**Chapter 3**
1. 2
2. 3
3. 1
4. 1
5. 4

**Chapter 4**
1. 3
2. 3
3. 2
4. 4
5. 4
6. 4
7. 2
8. 2

**Chapter 5**
1. 4
2. 4
3. 2
4. 3
5. 1
6. 1
7. 3
8. 3

**Chapter 6**
1. 4
2. 2
3. 3
4. 1
5. 3
6. 3

**Chapter 7**
1. 3
2. 4
3. 1

4. 1
5. 4

**Chapter 8**
1. 4
2. 2
3. 3
4. 3
5. 2
6. 3
7. 4
8. 1
9. 3

**Chapter 9**
1. 4
2. 3
3. 3
4. 4
5. 4
6. 4
7. 2
8. 3

**Chapter 10**
1. 3
2. 2, 3, 5
3. 3
4. 3
5. 1
6. 4
7. 2

**Chapter 11**
1. 1
2. 3
3. 3
4. 2
5. 4
6. 4

**Chapter 12**
1. 1
2. 1
3. 4
4. 2
5. 3
6. 3
7. 1
8. 2
9. 1
10. 4

**Chapter 13**
1. 2
2. 3
3. 2
4. 3
5. 4
6. 4
7. 3
8. 2
9. 3
10. 4
11. 4

12. 1
13. 1
14. 3
15. 1
16. 3
17. 2

**Chapter 14**
1. 1
2. 1
3. 2
4. 4
5. 4
6. 2
7. 4
8. 2
9. 2
10. 3

**Chapter 15**
1. 4
2. 3
3. 2
4. 2
5. 3
6. 2
7. 2
8. 3

**Chapter 16**
1. 2
2. 4
3. 4
4. 4
5. 3
6. 3
7. 4
8. 1

**Chapter 17**
1. 2
2. 1
3. 1
4. 1
5. 2
6. 2
7. 4
8. 1
9. 1
10. 1

**Chapter 18**
1. 2
2. 2
3. 3
4. 3
5. 4
6. 2, 3, 5
7. 4
8. 1

**Chapter 19**
1. 3
2. 4
3. 2

4. 2
5. 1
6. 4
7. 2

**Chapter 20**
1. 1
2. 3
3. 1
4. 4
5. 2
6. 2
7. 2

**Chapter 21**
1. 1
2. 3
3. 4
4. 4
5. 4
6. 3

**Chapter 22**
1. 4
2. 4
3. 4
4. 3
5. 4
6. 3
7. 4

**Chapter 23**
1. 2
2. 4
3. 3
4. 2
5. 3
6. 2

**Chapter 24**
1. 3
2. 2
3. 4
4. 3
5. 3
6. 4
7. 1
8. 1

**Chapter 25**
1. 2
2. 2
3. 1
4. 2
5. 1
6. 2
7. 1
8. 1

**Chapter 26**
1. 2
2. 1
3. 1
4. 4
5. 3, 5, 6

6. 1
7. 2
8. 3
9. 1
10. 4

**Chapter 27**
1. 3
2. 2
3. 4
4. 3
5. 2
6. 4

**Chapter 28**
1. 3
2. 3
3. 3
4. 3
5. 3
6. 2
7. 4

**Chapter 29**
1. 4
2. 3
3. 1
4. 4
5. 2
6. 3
7. 1
8. 2
9. 4
10. 2

**Chapter 30**
1. 6
2. Neuropathic
3. 2
4. 3
5. 3
6. 1
7. 1
8. 2

**Chapter 31**
1. 4
2. 2
3. 2
4. 3
5. 4
6. 4
7. 1

**Chapter 32**
1. 3
2. 3
3. Penile
4. 3
5. 1
6. 3
7. 1
8. 1
9. 2

**Chapter 33**
1. 4
2. 3
3. 4
4. 3
5. 4
6. 4
7. 3

**Chapter 34**
1. 2
2. 3
3. 3
4. 2
5. 3
6. 3
7. 3
8. 2
9. 4

**Chapter 35**
1. 4
2. 3
3. 1
4. 4
5. 3
6. 3
7. 3
8. 4
9. 3
10. 3
11. 3

**Chapter 36**
1. 4
2. 1
3. 4
4. 4
5. 3
6. 4

**Chapter 37**
1. 4
2. 2
3. 2
4. 2
5. 3
6. 4
7. 1
8. 3
9. 2

# Index

# Patient Teaching

# Care of the Older Adult

# Nursing Care Plans

# Cultural Focus